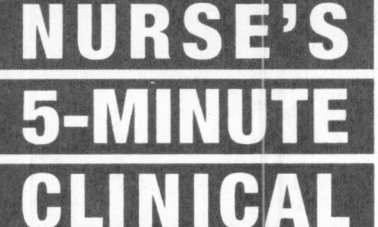

Diseases

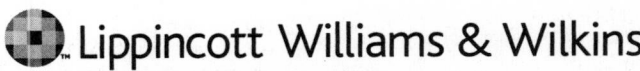

Lippincott Williams & Wilkins
a Wolters Kluwer business
Philadelphia · Baltimore · New York · London
Buenos Aires · Hong Kong · Sydney · Tokyo

STAFF

Executive Publisher
Judith A. Schilling McCann, RN, MSN

Editorial Director
H. Nancy Holmes

Clinical Director
Joan M. Robinson, RN, MSN

Senior Art Director
Arlene Putterman

Editorial Project Manager
Ann E. Houska

Clinical Project Manager
Beverly Ann Tscheschlog, RN, BS

Editors
Julie M. Catagnus, Amy Moshier

Clinical Editor
Kathryn Henry, RN, BSN, CCRC

Copy Editors
Kimberly Bilotta (supervisor), Scotti Cohn,
Heather Ditch, Jen Fielding, Dona Perkins,
Irene Pontarelli, Lisa Stockslager,
Dorothy P. Terry, Pamela Wingrod

Designers
Matie Anne Patterson (project manager),
Joseph John Clark, BJ Crim

Digital Composition Services
Diane Paluba (manager), Joyce Rossi Biletz,
Donna S. Morris

Manufacturing
Beth J. Welsh

Editorial Assistants
Megan L. Aldinger, Karen J. Kirk,
Linda K. Ruhf

Design Assistant
Georg W. Purvis IV

Indexer
Barbara Hodgson

The clinical treatments described and recommended in this publication are based on research and consultation with nursing, medical, and legal authorities. To the best of our knowledge, these procedures reflect currently accepted practice. Nevertheless, they can't be considered absolute and universal recommendations. For individual applications, all recommendations must be considered in light of the patient's clinical condition and, before administration of new or infrequently used drugs, in light of the latest package-insert information. The authors and publisher disclaim any responsibility for any adverse effects resulting from the suggested procedures, from any undetected errors, or from the reader's misunderstanding of the text.

5MCCD010906

Library of Congress
Cataloging-in-Publication Data

Nurse's 5-minute clinical consult diseases.
    p. ; cm.
  Includes bibliographical references and index.
  1. Nursing—Handbooks, manuals, etc. I.
Lippincott Williams & Wilkins. II. Title: Nurse's
five-minute clinical consult diseases.
  [DNLM: 1. Nursing Care—methods—Handbooks.
2. Clinical Medicine—Handbooks. 3. Nursing
Assessment—methods—Handbooks. 4. Patient
Education—Handbooks. WY 49 N97295 2007]
RT51.N87 2007
610.73—dc22
ISBN 1-58255-511-7 (alk. paper)   2006017007

Contents

Contributors and consultants

Katrina D. Allen, RN, MSN, CCRN
ADN Faculty
Faulkner State Community College
Bay Minette, Ala.

Sharron Elaine Ballard, APRN,BC, MSN, FNP
Associate Clinical Professor
Texas Women's University College of Nursing
Dallas

Lynn Cherry, RN, MSN
Education Specialist
Henry Ford Health System
Detroit

Marsha L. Conroy, RN, BA, MSN, APN
Nurse Educator
Cuyahoga Community College
Cleveland

Kim Cooper, RN, MSN
Nursing Department Program Chair
Ivy Tech Community College
Terre Haute, Ind.

Lillian Craig, RN, MSN, FNP-C
Family Nurse Practitioner
Internal Medicine Private Practice
Borger, Tex.

Eileen Croke, RN, MSN, EdD, ANP, GNP, LNC-C
Associate Professor Nursing
California State University
Long Beach

Anne D'Antuono, RN, PhD, APRN,BC, NPP
Faculty
St. Vincent Catholic Medical Centers
School of Nursing
Fresh Meadows, N.Y.

Shelba Durston, RN, MSN, CCRN
Nursing Instructor
San Joaquin Delta College
Stockton, Calif.
Staff Nurse
San Joaquin General Hospital
French Camp, Calif.

Merita Konstantacos, RN, MSN
Consultant
Clinton, Ohio

Cynthia A. Prows, RN, MSN
Clinical Nurse Specialist, Genetics
Children's Hospital Medical Center
Cincinnati

Kimberly Such-Smith, RN, BSN, LNC
Legal Nurse Consultant/Case Manager/Healthcare Advocate
Nursing Analysis & Review, LLC
Byron, Minn.

Allison J. Terry, RN, MSN, PhD
Nurse Consultant
Alabama Board of Nursing
Montgomery

NURSE'S 5-MINUTE CLINICAL CONSULT

Diseases

Abortion

OVERVIEW

- Expelled products of conception from the uterus before fetal viability
- May be spontaneous (miscarriage) (see *Types of spontaneous abortion*)
- May be therapeutic (elective) to preserve the mother's mental or physical health in cases of rape, unplanned pregnancy, or such medical conditions as maternal cardiac dysfunction or fetal abnormality

PATHOPHYSIOLOGY

- May result from fetal, placental, or maternal factors

Fetal factors

- Defective embryologic development
- Faulty implantation of fertilized ovum
- Failure of the endometrium to accept the fertilized ovum
- Usually cause abortion to occur between 9 and 12 weeks' gestation

Placental factors

- Premature separation of a normally implanted placenta
- Abnormal placental implantation
- Abnormal platelet function
- Usually cause abortion to occur around 14 weeks' gestation when the placenta takes over the hormone production necessary to maintain pregnancy

Maternal factors

- Maternal age
- Severe maternal illness that causes pyrexia or severe fetal hypoxia (such as pneumonia or rubella)
- Usually cause abortion to occur between 11 and 19 weeks' gestation

CAUSES

Spontaneous abortion

- Abnormalities of the reproductive organs
- Blood group incompatibility and Rh isoimmunization
- Diabetes mellitus
- Environmental toxins
- Fetal factors
- Incompetent cervix
- Lowered estriol secretion
- Maternal infection
- Placental factors
- Recreational drug use
- Severe malnutrition
- Surgery that necessitates manipulation of the pelvic organs
- Thyroid gland dysfunction
- Trauma

INCIDENCE

- Up to 15% of all pregnancies end in miscarriage.
- About 30% of first pregnancies end in miscarriage.
- At least 75% of miscarriages occur during the first trimester.
- Frequency of legally induced abortions is increasing in the United States.

COMPLICATIONS

- Anemia
- Coagulation defects
- Disseminated intravascular coagulation
- Hemorrhage
- Infection
- Psychological issues of loss and failure

ASSESSMENT

HISTORY

- Pink discharge for several days or scant brown discharge for several weeks before onset of cramps and increased vaginal bleeding
- Cramps that appear for a few hours, intensify, and then occur more frequently
- Continued cramps and bleeding if any uterine contents remain (cramps and bleeding may subside if entire contents expelled)

PHYSICAL FINDINGS

- Vaginal bleeding
- Cervical dilation
- Passage of nonviable products of conception

DIAGNOSTIC TEST RESULTS

LABORATORY

- Serum human chorionic gonadotropin levels are decreased, suggesting spontaneous abortion.
- Cytologic analysis shows evidence of products of conception.
- Serum hemoglobin levels and hematocrit are decreased from blood loss.

IMAGING

- Ultrasonography reveals presence or absence of fetal heart tones or of empty amniotic sac.

TREATMENT

GENERAL

- Accurate evaluation of uterine contents needed before treatment
- The progression of spontaneous abortion can't be prevented, except in those cases involving an incompetent cervix
- Hospitalization to control severe hemorrhage

ACTIVITY

- Bed rest

MEDICATIONS

- Transfusion with packed red blood cells or whole blood (severe bleeding)
- I.V. oxytocin (stimulates uterine contractions)
- $Rh_o(D)$ immune globulin for an Rh-negative woman with a negative indirect Coombs' test

Therapeutic abortion

- Administration of mifepristone followed by administration of misoprostol on day 3 if spontaneous abortion hasn't occurred
- Injection of hypertonic saline solution into the amniotic sac
- Injection of prostaglandin into the amniotic sac
- Insertion of a prostaglandin vaginal suppository

SURGERY

- Dilatation and curettage (D&C) if remnants remain in the uterus
- D&C if first-trimester induced abortion
- Surgical reinforcement of the incompetent cervix (cerclage) to prevent abortion

NURSING CONSIDERATIONS

NURSING DIAGNOSES

- Anxiety
- Compromised family coping
- Dysfunctional grieving
- Ineffective coping
- Risk for infection

EXPECTED OUTCOMES

The patient will:

- express feelings of comfort and decreased anxiety
- seek support systems and exhibit adequate coping behaviors
- communicate feelings about the situation
- demonstrate effective coping mechanisms
- remain free from all signs and symptoms of infection.

NURSING INTERVENTIONS

- Don't allow bathroom privileges because the patient may expel uterine contents without knowing it.
- Inspect bedpan contents carefully for intrauterine material.
- Save all sanitary pads for evaluation.
- Give prescribed drugs.
- Provide perineal care.
- Provide emotional support and counseling.
- Encourage expression of feelings.
- Help the patient develop effective coping strategies.

MONITORING

- Amount, color, and odor of vaginal bleeding
- Vital signs
- Intake and output
- Pain

PATIENT TEACHING

GENERAL

Be sure to cover:

- the disorder, diagnosis, and treatment
- vaginal bleeding or spotting
- bleeding that lasts longer than 8 to 10 days or excessive bleeding
- importance of reporting signs of bright red blood immediately
- signs of infection, such as fever and foul-smelling vaginal discharge
- gradual increase in daily activities
- schedule for returning to work (normally within 1 to 4 weeks)
- abstinence from intercourse until examined by practitioner
- prevention of spontaneous abortion
- contraceptive information
- avoidance of tampons until examined by practitioner
- follow-up examination.

DISCHARGE PLANNING

- Refer the patient for professional counseling if indicated.

RESOURCES

Organizations

American College of Obstetricians and Gynecologists: *www.acog.org*
American Society for Reproductive Medicine: *www.asrm.org*
National Abortion Federation: *www.prochoice.org*
National Abortion Rights Action League: *www.naral.org*

Selected references

Taylor, D., et al. "Care for Women Choosing Medication Abortion," *Nurse Practitioner* 29(10):65-70, October 2004.

Types of spontaneous abortion

Depending on clinical findings, a spontaneous abortion (miscarriage) may be threatened or inevitable; incomplete or complete; or missed, habitual, or septic. Here's how the seven types compare.

THREATENED ABORTION

Bloody vaginal discharge occurs during the first half of pregnancy. About 20% of pregnant women have vaginal spotting or actual bleeding early in pregnancy; of these, about 50% abort.

INEVITABLE ABORTION

The membranes rupture and the cervix dilates. As labor continues, the uterus expels the products of conception.

INCOMPLETE ABORTION

The uterus retains part or all of the placenta. Before 10 weeks' gestation, the fetus and placenta usually are expelled together; after the 10th week, they're expelled separately. Because part of the placenta may adhere to the uterine wall, bleeding continues. Hemorrhage is possible because the uterus doesn't contract and seal the large vessels that fed the placenta.

COMPLETE ABORTION

The uterus passes all the products of conception. Minimal bleeding usually accompanies complete abortion because the uterus contracts and compresses the maternal blood vessels that fed the placenta.

MISSED ABORTION

The uterus retains the products of conception after the death of the fetus. Uterine growth ceases; uterine size may even seem to decrease. Prolonged retention of the dead products of conception may cause coagulation defects such as disseminated intravascular coagulation.

HABITUAL ABORTION (RECURRENT PREGNANCY LOSS)

Spontaneous loss of three or more consecutive pregnancies constitutes habitual abortion.

SEPTIC ABORTION

Infection accompanies abortion. This may occur with spontaneous abortion but usually results from an illegal abortion or from the presence of an intrauterine device.

Abruptio placentae

OVERVIEW

- Premature separation of the placenta from the uterine wall
- Usually occurs after 20 weeks' gestation, most commonly during the third trimester
- Common cause of bleeding during the second half of pregnancy
- Fetal prognosis depends on gestational age and amount of blood loss
- Good maternal prognosis if hemorrhage can be controlled
- Classified according to degree of placental separation and severity of maternal and fetal symptoms (see *Degrees of placental separation in abruptio placentae*)
- Also called *placental abruption*

PATHOPHYSIOLOGY

- Spontaneous rupture of blood vessels at the placental bed possibly due to lack of resiliency or to abnormal changes in uterine vasculature
- Condition possibly complicated by hypertension or by an enlarged uterus that can't contract sufficiently to seal off the torn vessels
- Bleeding that continues unchecked, possibly shearing off the placenta partially or completely

CAUSES

- Exact cause unknown
- Advanced maternal age
- Amniocentesis
- Chronic or gestational hypertension
- Cocaine use
- Diabetes mellitus
- Dietary deficiency
- Fibroid tumors
- Multiparity
- Pressure on the vena cava from an enlarged uterus
- Short umbilical cord
- Smoking
- Traumatic injury

INCIDENCE

- Abruptio placentae is most common in multigravida women older than age 35, women with gestational hypertension, and women who use cocaine.

COMPLICATIONS

- Hemorrhage
- Shock
- Renal failure
- Disseminated intravascular coagulation (DIC)
- Maternal death
- Fetal death

ASSESSMENT

HISTORY
Marginal separation
- Mild to moderate vaginal bleeding
- Vague lower abdominal discomfort
- Mild to moderate abdominal tenderness

Central placental separation (about 50% placental separation)
- Continuous abdominal pain
- Moderate dark red vaginal bleeding
- Severe or abrupt onset of symptoms

Complete abruptio placentae (70% placental separation)
- Abrupt onset of agonizing, unremitting uterine pain
- Moderate vaginal bleeding

PHYSICAL FINDINGS
Marginal separation
- Fetal monitoring possibly indicating uterine irritability
- Strong and regular fetal heart tones

Central abruptio placentae
- Vital signs possibly indicating impending shock
- Tender uterus remaining firm between contractions
- Barely audible or irregular and bradycardic fetal heart tones
- Labor that usually starts within 2 hours and proceeds rapidly

Complete abruptio placentae
- Vital signs that indicate rapidly progressive shock
- Absence of fetal heart sounds
- Tender uterus with boardlike rigidity
- Possible increased uterine size in severe concealed abruptions

---

Degrees of placental separation in abruptio placentae

MARGINAL SEPARATION
Internal bleeding between the placenta and uterine wall characterize mild separation. The separation is at the outer edges of the placenta.

CENTRAL PLACENTAL SEPARATION
In central placental separation, the placenta separates in the center, and there may be concealed bleeding.

COMPLETE SEPARATION
External hemorrhage is also characteristic of complete separation.

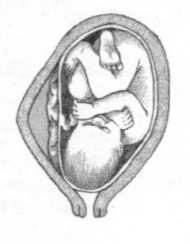
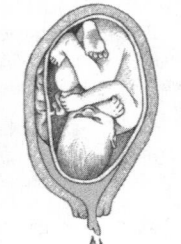
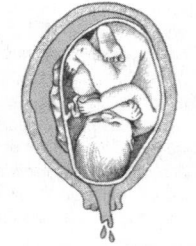

LABORATORY
- Serum hemoglobin (Hb) level and platelet count are decreased.
- Fibrin split products show progression of abruptio placentae and detection of DIC.

IMAGING
- Ultrasonography may rule out placenta previa.

OTHER
- Pelvic examination is performed under double setup conditions to prepare for an emergency cesarean delivery.

TREATMENT

GENERAL
- Assess, control, and restore amount of blood loss.
- Deliver the neonate.
- Prevent coagulation disorders.
- Vaginal delivery is needed if placental separation is severe with no signs of fetal life, unless contraindicated by uncontrolled hemorrhage or other complications.

⚡ **WARNING** *Because of possible fetal blood loss through the placenta, a pediatric team should be ready at delivery to assess and treat the neonate for shock, blood loss, and hypoxia.*

⚡ **WARNING** *Complications of abruptio placentae require prompt appropriate treatment. With a complication such as DIC, the patient needs immediate intervention with platelets and whole blood, as ordered, to prevent exsanguination.*

DIET
- Nothing to eat or drink until delivery of the fetus

ACTIVITY
- Bed rest until delivery of the fetus

MEDICATIONS
- I.V. fluid infusion (by large-bore catheter) as ordered

SURGERY
- Cesarean delivery if the fetus is in distress

NURSING CONSIDERATIONS

NURSING DIAGNOSES
- Acute pain
- Anxiety
- Compromised family coping
- Deficient fluid volume
- Dysfunctional grieving
- Fear
- Ineffective coping
- Ineffective tissue perfusion: Cardiopulmonary

EXPECTED OUTCOMES
The patient will:
- express feelings of comfort and decreased pain
- express feelings of decreased anxiety
- seek support systems and exhibit adequate coping behaviors
- maintain balanced fluid volume
- communicate feelings about the situation
- express feelings of decreased fear
- demonstrate effective coping mechanisms
- maintain hemodynamic stability.

NURSING INTERVENTIONS
- Insert an indwelling urinary catheter.
- Obtain blood specimens for Hb level and hematocrit, coagulation studies, and type and crossmatching.
- Give emotional support during labor.
- Provide information regarding progress and condition of fetus during labor.
- Encourage verbalization of feelings.
- Help the patient develop effective coping strategies.
- Give I.V. fluids and blood products.

MONITORING
- Maternal vital signs
- Central venous pressure
- Intake and output

- Vaginal bleeding
- Fetal heart rate (electronically)
- Progression of labor

PATIENT TEACHING

GENERAL
Be sure to cover:
- the disorder, diagnosis, and treatment
- signs of placental abruption
- possibility of an emergency cesarean delivery
- possibility of the delivery of a premature neonate
- changes to expect in the postpartum period
- possibility of neonatal death
- factors affecting survival of neonate
- importance of frequent monitoring and prompt management to reduce risk of death.

DISCHARGE PLANNING
- Refer the patient for professional counseling if indicated.

RESOURCES
Organizations
American College of Obstetricians and Gynecologists: *www.acog.org*
American Society for Reproductive Medicine: *www.asrm.org*

Selected references
Grossman, N.B. "Blunt Trauma in Pregnancy," *American Family Physician* 70(7):1303-10, October 2004.
Korby, J. "Abruptio Placentae," *Nursing* 32(4):96, February 2004.

Acceleration-deceleration injuries

- Injury resulting from sharp hyperextension and flexion of the neck that damage muscles, ligaments, disks, and nerve tissue
- Excellent prognosis; symptoms usually subside with symptomatic treatment
- Also called *whiplash*

PATHOPHYSIOLOGY
- Unexpected force causes the head to jerk back and then forward.
- The neck bones snap out of position, causing injury.
- Irritated nerves can interfere with blood flow and transmission of nerve impulses.
- Pinched nerves can affect certain body part functions.

CAUSES
- Fall
- Motor vehicle accident
- Sports accident

RISK FACTORS
- Absence of head restraint in automobile
- Osteoporosis
- Driving under the influence of alcohol or drugs

INCIDENCE
- One million cases occur each year in the United States.
- The average age of these patients is the late 40s.

COMPLICATIONS
- Temporomandibular disorder

HISTORY
- Mechanism of injury
- Pain initially minimal but increases 12 to 72 hours after the accident
- Dizziness
- Headache
- Back pain
- Shoulder pain
- Vision disturbances
- Tinnitus

PHYSICAL FINDINGS
- Neck muscle asymmetry
- Reduced neck mobility
- Gait disturbances
- Rigidity or numbness in the arms
- Tenderness at the exact location of the injury
- Decreased active and passive range of motion

IMAGING
- Full cervical spine X-rays rule out cervical fracture.

TREATMENT

GENERAL
- Soft cervical collar (see *Applying a cervical collar*)
- Ice packs

ACTIVITY
- Physical therapy
- Limited activity during the first 72 hours after the injury
- Limited neck movement
- Limited strenuous activities, such as lifting and contact sports, until full recovery has been established (which may take more than 2 years)

MEDICATIONS
- Oral analgesics (acetaminophen, nonsteroidal anti-inflammatory drugs, opioids)
- Muscle relaxants
- Corticosteroids

SURGERY
- Surgical stabilization may be necessary in severe cervical acceleration-deceleration injuries

NURSING CONSIDERATIONS

NURSING DIAGNOSES
- Acute pain
- Anxiety
- Impaired physical mobility
- Risk for posttrauma syndrome

EXPECTED OUTCOMES
The patient will:
- express feelings of increased comfort and decreased pain
- express feelings of decreased anxiety
- attain the highest degree of mobility possible
- state feelings and fears about the injury.

NURSING INTERVENTIONS
- Protect the patient's spine during all care.
- Give prescribed drugs.
- Apply a soft cervical collar.

MONITORING
- Pain control
- Response to medications
- Complications
- Neurologic status

PATIENT TEACHING

GENERAL
Be sure to cover:
- activity restrictions
- proper application of soft cervical collar
- medication administration, dosage, and possible adverse effects
- instructions about driving and the use of alcohol while taking an opioid.

DISCHARGE PLANNING
- Refer the patient to a neurologist, as indicated.

RESOURCES
Organizations
American Academy of Neurology: *www.aan.com*
American Academy of Orthopaedic Surgeons: *www.aaos.org*

Selected references
Atlas of Pathophysiology, 2nd ed. Philadelphia: Lippincott Williams & Wilkins, 2005.
Bemis, P.A. *Emergency Nursing Bible*, 2nd ed. Rockledge, Fla.: National Nurses in Business Association, Inc., 2004.
O'Shea, R.A. *Principles and Practice of Trauma Nursing*. Philadelphia: Elsevier, 2006.

Applying a cervical collar

Cervical collars are used to support an injured or weakened cervical spine and to maintain alignment during healing. The soft cervical collar, made of spongy foam, provides gentler support and reminds the patient to avoid cervical spine motion.

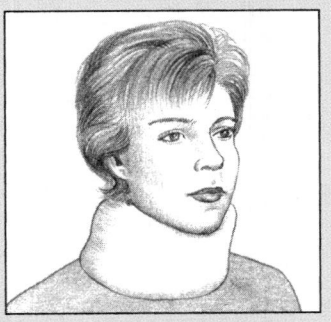

Acne vulgaris

- Inflammatory disorder of the sebaceous gland contiguous with a hair follicle (pilosebaceous follicle)
- Possibly developing in distinctive pilosebaceous units (sebaceous follicles)
- Acne lesions: Inflammatory (pustules, papules, and nodules) and noninflammatory (closed and open comedones) lesions
- Good prognosis with treatment

PATHOPHYSIOLOGY

- Begins with sebum accumulation that obstructs the pilosebaceous unit
- Keratinous and sebaceous material and bacteria accumulation in the pilosebaceous follicle
- Rupture, then inflammation from keratinous and sebaceous material becoming exposed to the dermis
- *Propionibacterium acnes:* produces substances that promote inflammation
- In noninflammatory acne, open comedones (blackheads), or closed comedones (whiteheads); accumulated material causing distention of the follicle and thinning of follicular canal walls
- Inflammatory acne developing in closed comedones when the follicular wall ruptures, expelling sebum into the surrounding dermis and initiating inflammation
- Pustule formation when the inflammation is close to the surface; papule and cystic nodule formation when the inflammation is deeper, causing mild to severe scarring

CAUSES

- Exact cause unknown
- Excessive sebum production
- Follicular hyperkeratinization
- Hormonal dysfunction
- Proliferation of *P. acnes*

Causes of acne flare-ups

- Menstrual cycle
- Stress
- Trauma
- Tropical climates

- Rubbing from tight clothing
- Environmental exposure to coal tar derivatives, certain chemicals, cosmetics, or hair pomades
- Hormonal contraceptives containing norethindrone and norgestrel; testosterone
- Anabolic agents
- Corticotropin, gonadotropins, corticosteroids (prolonged use)
- Iodine- or bromine-containing drugs
- Trimethadione
- Phenytoin
- Isoniazid
- Lithium
- Halothane

INCIDENCE

- Acne vulgaris affects nearly 75% of adolescents, although lesions can appear as young as age 8.
- The disorder affects males more often and more severely than females.
- Acne vulgaris occurs in females at an earlier age than males and tends to affect them for a longer time, sometimes into adulthood.
- The disorder tends to be familial.

COMPLICATIONS

- Deep cystic process
- Gross inflammation
- Abscess formation
- Secondary bacterial infection
- Acne scars

HISTORY

- Presence of one or more predisposing factors
- Seasonal or monthly eruption patterns
- Pain and tenderness around area of infected follicle

PHYSICAL FINDINGS

- Acne lesions, commonly located on the face, neck, shoulders, chest, and upper back
- Red and swollen area around the infected follicle
- Acne plugs that appear as closed or open comedones
- Oily and thickened skin
- Visible scars

LABORATORY

- Culture and sensitivity of pustules or abscesses show organism causing secondary bacterial infection.
- Skin lesion cultures rule out gram-negative folliculitis.

OTHER

- History and physical examination findings include visualization of acne pustules.

TREATMENT

GENERAL
◆ Treatment for causative factors

DIET
◆ Well-balanced

ACTIVITY
◆ Regular exercise

MEDICATIONS
◆ Antibacterials
◆ Anticomedonals
◆ Keratinolytics
◆ Anti-inflammatories
◆ Antiandrogens
◆ Antisebaceous agents
◆ Tretinoin
◆ Isotretinoin

SURGERY
◆ Comedo extraction
◆ Intralesional steroids
◆ Cryosurgery
◆ Dermabrasion
◆ Glycolic or salicylate acid peels

> **AGE FACTOR** *Tetracycline is con-traindicated during pregnancy and childhood because it may cause permanent discoloration of teeth (in children younger than age 8), enamel defects, and bone growth retardation. Erythromycin is an alternative for these patients.*

> **WARNING** *Because isotretinoin (Accutane) is known to cause birth defects, the manufacturer, with Food and Drug Administration approval, recommends pregnancy testing before dispensing, dispensing only a 30-day supply, repeat pregnancy testing throughout the treatment period, effective contraception during treatment, and informed consent of the patient or parents regarding the danger of the drug.*

NURSING CONSIDERATIONS

NURSING DIAGNOSES
◆ Disturbed body image
◆ Impaired skin integrity
◆ Risk for infection
◆ Situational low self-esteem

EXPECTED OUTCOMES
The patient will:
◆ verbalize feelings about body image
◆ exhibit improved or healed wounds or lesions
◆ remain free from all signs and symptoms of infection
◆ express positive feelings about self.

NURSING INTERVENTIONS
◆ Give prescribed drugs.
◆ Help the patient identify and eliminate predisposing factors.
◆ Encourage good personal hygiene and the use of oil-free skin care products.
◆ Discourage picking or squeezing of the lesions.
◆ Encourage the patient to verbalize his feelings.
◆ Encourage the patient to develop interests that support a positive self-image and de-emphasize appearance.

MONITORING
◆ Liver function studies, CBC counts, and serum triglyceride levels with isotretinoin use
◆ Complications
◆ Sensitivity reactions
◆ GI disturbances
◆ Mood changes (with isotretinoin)
◆ Serial pregnancy testing (with isotretinoin)
◆ Liver dysfunction
◆ Response to treatment
◆ Skin and mucous membranes

PATIENT TEACHING

GENERAL
Be sure to cover:
◆ the disorder and treatment
◆ medications and potential adverse reactions
◆ when to notify the practitioner
◆ signs and symptoms of infection
◆ causative factors associated with acne flare-up
◆ well-balanced diet
◆ adequate rest
◆ stress management.

RESOURCES
Organizations
American Academy of Dermatology: *www.aad.org*
Dermatology Foundation: *www.dermatologyfoundation.org*

Selected references
Ceilley, R.I. "Advances in the Topical Treatment of Acne and Rosacea," *Journal of Drugs in Dermatology* 3(5 suppl):S12-22, September-October 2004.
Fernandez, C., et al. "A Randomized Double-Blind Study to Assess the Effects of Salicylic Acid Compared to Placebo in Patients with Mild to Moderate Acne," *Journal of Dermatological Treatment* 16(5-6):287-94, 2005.

Acquired immunodeficiency syndrome and human

OVERVIEW

- Human immunodeficiency virus (HIV) type I — retrovirus causing acquired immunodeficiency syndrome (AIDS)
- Renders patients susceptible to opportunistic infections, unusual cancers, and other abnormalities
- Marked by progressive failure of the immune system
- Transmitted by contact with infected blood or body fluids and associated with identifiable high-risk behaviors

PATHOPHYSIOLOGY

- HIV strikes helper T cells bearing the CD4 antigen.
- The antigen serves as a receptor for the retrovirus, letting it enter the cell.
- After invading a cell, HIV replicates (leading to cell death) or becomes latent.
- HIV infection leads to profound pathology, either directly, through destruction of CD4+ T cells, other immune cells, and neuroglial cells, or indirectly, through the secondary effects of CD4+ T-cell dysfunction and resultant immunosuppression.

CAUSES

- Infection with HIV, a retrovirus

RISK FACTORS

- Sharing of I.V. drug needles or syringes
- Unprotected sexual intercourse
- Placental transmission
- History of sexually transmitted disease
- Homosexual lifestyle
- Contact with infected blood

INCIDENCE

- The average time between exposure to the virus and diagnosis of AIDS is 8 to 10 years, but shorter and longer incubation times have been recorded.

COMPLICATIONS

- Repeated opportunistic infections
- Neoplasms
- Premalignant diseases
- Organ-specific syndrome

ASSESSMENT

HISTORY

- A mononucleosis-like syndrome after a high-risk exposure and inoculation; may then remain asymptomatic for years
- In the latent stage, laboratory evidence of seroconversion the only sign of HIV infection

PHYSICAL FINDINGS

- Persistent generalized adenopathy
- Nonspecific symptoms (weight loss, fatigue, night sweats, fevers)
- Neurologic symptoms resulting from HIV encephalopathy
- Opportunistic infection or cancer (Kaposi's sarcoma)

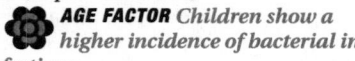 **AGE FACTOR** *Children show a higher incidence of bacterial infections.*

DIAGNOSTIC TEST RESULTS

LABORATORY

- CD4+ T-cell count of 200 cells/ml or more confirms HIV infection.
- Screening test (enzyme-linked immunosorbent assay) and confirmatory test (Western blot) detect the presence of HIV antibodies, which indicate HIV infection.

TREATMENT

GENERAL

- Variety of therapeutic options for opportunistic infections (the leading cause of morbidity and mortality in patients infected with HIV)
- Disease-specific therapy for a variety of neoplastic and premalignant diseases and organ-specific syndromes
- Symptom management (fatigue and anemia)

DIET

- Well-balanced

ACTIVITY

- Regular exercise as tolerated, with adequate rest periods

MEDICATIONS

- Immunomodulatory agents
- Anti-infective agents
- Antineoplastic agents
- Highly active antiretroviral therapy

Primary therapy

- Protease inhibitors
- Nucleoside reverse transcriptase inhibitors
- Nonnucleoside reverse transcriptase inhibitors

immunodeficiency virus

NURSING DIAGNOSES
◆ Activity intolerance
◆ Compromised family coping
◆ Disturbed body image
◆ Fatigue
◆ Hopelessness
◆ Imbalanced nutrition: Less than body requirements
◆ Impaired skin integrity
◆ Ineffective coping
◆ Ineffective sexuality patterns
◆ Powerlessness
◆ Risk for deficient fluid volume
◆ Risk for infection
◆ Social isolation

EXPECTED OUTCOMES
The patient will:
◆ perform activities of daily living without fatigue
◆ seek support systems and exhibit adequate coping behaviors
◆ verbalize feelings about changed body image
◆ develop adequate coping mechanisms and support systems
◆ express feelings of energy and decreased fatigue
◆ express feelings and concerns
◆ consume required caloric intake
◆ exhibit improved or healed wounds or lesions
◆ demonstrate effective coping skills
◆ voice feelings about changes in sexual identity and social response to disease, and follow safer sex practices
◆ express feelings of having greater control over the current situation
◆ have balanced intake and output
◆ remain free from signs and symptoms of infection
◆ maintain social interaction to the extent possible.

NURSING INTERVENTIONS
◆ Help the patient to cope with an altered body image, the emotional burden of serious illness, and the threat of death.
◆ Avoid glycerin swabs for mucous membranes. Use normal saline or bicarbonate mouthwash for daily oral rinsing.

◆ Ensure adequate fluid intake during episodes of diarrhea.
◆ Provide meticulous skin care, especially in the debilitated patient.
◆ Encourage the patient to maintain as much physical activity as he can tolerate. Make sure his schedule includes time for exercise and rest.

MONITORING
◆ Fever, noting any pattern
◆ Skin integrity
◆ Signs of illness, such as cough, sore throat, or diarrhea
◆ Swollen, tender lymph nodes
◆ Laboratory values
◆ Calorie intake
◆ Progression of lesions in Kaposi's sarcoma
◆ Opportunistic infections or signs of disease progression
◆ Compliance with medication regimen

GENERAL
Be sure to cover:
◆ medication regimens
◆ importance of informing potential sexual partners, caregivers, and health care workers of HIV infection (see *Preventing HIV transmission*)
◆ signs of impending infection and the importance of seeking immediate medical attention
◆ symptoms of AIDS dementia and its stages and progression.

DISCHARGE PLANNING
◆ Refer the patient to a local support group.
◆ Refer the patient to hospice care as indicated.

RESOURCES
Organizations
Center for AIDS Prevention Studies: *www.caps.ucsf.edu*
Centers for Disease Control and Prevention: *www.cdc.gov*

Selected references
Kasper, D.L., et al., eds. *Harrison's Principles of Internal Medicine*, 16th ed. New York: McGraw-Hill Book Co., 2005
Oyeyemi, A., et al. "Caring for Patients Living with AIDS: Knowledge, Attitude and Global Level of Comfort," *Journal of Advanced Nursing* 53(2):196-204, January 2006.

Preventing HIV transmission

◆ Use precautions in all situations that risk exposure to blood, body fluids, and secretions. Diligently practicing standard precautions can prevent the inadvertent transmission of human immunodeficiency virus (HIV), hepatitis B, and other infectious diseases that are transmitted by similar routes.
◆ Teach the patient and his family, sexual partners, and friends about the prevention of disease transmission to others.
◆ Tell the patient not to donate blood, blood products, organs, tissue, or sperm.
◆ If the patient uses I.V. drugs, caution him not to share needles.

◆ Inform the patient that high-risk sexual practices for HIV transmission are those that exchange body fluids, such as vaginal or anal intercourse without a condom.
◆ Discuss safer sex practices, such as hugging, petting, mutual masturbation, and protected sexual intercourse. Emphasize that abstinence is the most effective way to prevent transmission.
◆ Advise women of childbearing age to avoid pregnancy. Explain that an infant may become infected before birth, during delivery, or during breast-feeding.

Acute poststreptococcal glomerulonephritis

- Renal disease in which the glomeruli become inflamed
- Usually associated with a postinfectious state, commonly a streptococcal infection of the respiratory tract or, less commonly, a skin infection such as impetigo
- Up to 95% of children and 70% of adults recover fully
- In elderly patients it may progress to chronic renal failure within months
- Relatively common
- Also called *acute glomerulonephritis*

PATHOPHYSIOLOGY
- Antigen-antibody complexes are produced in response to group A beta-hemolytic streptococcus infection.
- Antigen-antibody complexes are trapped in the glomerular capillary membranes.
- Inflammatory damage results, impeding glomerular function.
- Immune complement may further damage the glomerular membrane.
- Damaged and inflamed glomeruli lose the ability to be selectively permeable
- Red blood cells (RBCs) and proteins then filter through as the glomerular filtration rate decreases.
- Uremic poisoning may result.

CAUSES
- Untreated group A beta-hemolytic streptococcus infection, especially of the respiratory tract

RISK FACTORS
- Impetigo

INCIDENCE
- Acute poststreptococcal glomerulonephritis occurs most commonly in boys ages 3 to 7; can occur at any age

COMPLICATIONS
- Progressive deterioration of renal function

HISTORY
- Untreated respiratory streptococcal infection within the last 1 to 3 weeks
- Decreased urination
- Smoky or coffee-colored urine
- Fatigue
- Dyspnea and orthopnea

PHYSICAL FINDINGS
- Oliguria
- Mild to moderate periorbital edema
- Mild to severe hypertension
- Bibasilar crackles (with heart failure)

LABORATORY
- Electrolyte levels are imbalanced.
- Blood urea nitrogen (BUN) and creatinine levels are elevated.
- Serum protein levels are decreased.
- The presence of RBCs, white blood cells, mixed cell casts, and protein in the urine indicate renal failure.
- Levels of fibrin degradation products and C3 protein are increased.

   AGE FACTOR *Proteinuria in an elderly patient usually isn't as pronounced as it is in a younger patient.*

- Elevated antistreptolysin-O titers (in 80% of patients), elevated streptozyme and anti-DNase B titers, and low serum complement levels verify recent streptococcal infection.
- Group A beta-hemolytic streptococci are revealed by throat culture.

IMAGING
- Kidney-ureter-bladder radiography reveals bilateral kidney enlargement.

DIAGNOSTIC PROCEDURES
- Renal biopsy or assessment of renal tissue confirms diagnosis.

TREATMENT

GENERAL
◆ Correction of electrolyte imbalances (possible dialysis)

DIET
◆ Sodium and fluid restriction
◆ High-calorie, low-protein, low-sodium, low-potassium

ACTIVITY
◆ Bed rest

MEDICATIONS
◆ Antibiotics for 7 to 10 days if streptococcal infection
◆ Loop diuretics, such as metolazone or furosemide

NURSING CONSIDERATIONS

NURSING DIAGNOSES
◆ Acute pain
◆ Decreased cardiac output
◆ Excess fluid volume
◆ Fatigue
◆ Imbalanced nutrition: Less than body requirements
◆ Impaired gas exchange
◆ Impaired physical mobility
◆ Risk for infection
◆ Risk for injury

EXPECTED OUTCOMES
The patient will:
◆ express feeling of comfort and relief from pain
◆ maintain adequate cardiac output
◆ maintain fluid balance
◆ express feelings of energy and decreased fatigue
◆ consume required caloric intake
◆ maintain adequate ventilation
◆ perform activities of daily living within the confines of the disorder
◆ remain free from all signs and symptoms of infection
◆ remain free from injury.

NURSING INTERVENTIONS
◆ Give prescribed drugs.
◆ Encourage the patient to verbalize feelings about his diagnosis.
◆ Provide support.

MONITORING
◆ Vital signs
◆ Electrolyte values and serum creatinine and BUN levels
◆ Urine creatinine clearance test results
◆ Intake and output
◆ Daily weight

PATIENT TEACHING

GENERAL
Be sure to cover:
◆ the disorder, diagnosis, treatment, prognosis, and possible complications
◆ importance of follow-up examinations to monitor renal function
◆ medication administration, dosage, and possible adverse effects.

DISCHARGE PLANNING
◆ Refer the patient to appropriate resources for information and support.

RESOURCES
Organizations
American Association of Kidney Patients: *www.aakp.org*
National Institute of Diabetes & Digestive & Kidney Diseases: *www.niddk.nih.gov*

Selected references
Diseases, 4th ed. Philadelphia: Lippincott Williams & Wilkins, 2006.
Hahn, R.G., et al. "Evaluation of Poststreptococcal Illness," *American Family Physician* 71(10):1949-54, May 2005.

Acute pyelonephritis

OVERVIEW

- Bacterial infection of the renal parenchyma
- Affecting one or both kidneys
- Good prognosis; extensive permanent damage rare
- Also called *acute infective tubulointerstitial nephritis*

PATHOPHYSIOLOGY

- Infection spreads from the bladder to the ureters to the kidneys, commonly through vesicoureteral reflux.
- Vesicoureteral reflux may result from congenital weakness at the junction of the ureter and bladder.
- Bacteria refluxed to intrarenal tissues may create colonies of infection within 24 to 48 hours.
- Female anatomy allows for higher incidence of infection.

CAUSES

- Bacterial infection of the kidneys
- *Escherichia coli* the most common colonized organism
- Microorganisms the same as those that cause lower urinary tract infection (UTI)

RISK FACTORS

- Renal procedures that involve instrumentation such as cystoscopy
- Hematogenic infection such as septicemia
- Sexual activity in women
- Pregnancy
- Neurogenic bladder
- Obstructive disease
- Renal diseases
- Structural abnormalities
- Lower UTI

INCIDENCE

- Acute pyelonephritis is more common in women than in men.
- Community-acquired cases occur in 15 per 100,000 annually.
- Hospital-acquired cases occur in 7 per 10,000 annually.

COMPLICATIONS

- Renal calculi
- Renal failure
- Renal abscess
- Multisystem infection
- Septic shock
- Chronic pyelonephritis

ASSESSMENT

HISTORY

- Pain over one or both kidneys, occasionally suprapubic
- Urinary urgency and frequency
- Burning during urination
- Dysuria, nocturia, hematuria
- Anorexia, vomiting, diarrhea
- Fatigue, malaise, weakness
- Symptoms that develop rapidly over a few hours or a few days
- Chills, rigors

PHYSICAL FINDINGS

- Mild to moderate suprapubic pain
- Pain on flank palpation (costovertebral angle tenderness)
- Cloudy urine
- Ammonia-like or fishy odor to urine
- May or may not be febrile
- If present, fever of 102° F (38.9° C) or higher
- Shaking chills
- Negative pelvic examination findings

DIAGNOSTIC TEST RESULTS

LABORATORY

- Urinalysis and culture and sensitivity testing reveal pyuria, significant bacteriuria, low specific gravity and osmolality, and slightly alkaline urine pH, or proteinuria, glycosuria, and ketonuria (less frequent).
- White blood cell count, neutrophil count, and erythrocyte sedimentation rate are increased.

IMAGING

- Kidney-ureter-bladder radiography reveals calculi, tumors, or cysts in the kidneys or urinary tract.
- Excretory urography shows asymmetrical kidneys, possibly indicating a high frequency of infection.

GENERAL

- Identification and correction of predisposing factors for infection, such as obstruction or calculi
- Short courses of therapy for uncomplicated infections
- Rest

DIET

- Increased fluid intake

MEDICATIONS

- 14-day course of antibiotics (I.V. or oral fluoroquinolone is drug of choice)
- Urinary analgesics such as phenazopyridine (Azo-Standard)
- Antipyretics as needed

NURSING DIAGNOSES

- Acute pain
- Excess fluid volume
- Fatigue
- Impaired physical mobility
- Impaired urinary elimination
- Ineffective tissue perfusion: Renal
- Risk for infection

EXPECTED OUTCOMES

The patient will:

- report increased comfort
- maintain fluid balance
- express feelings of energy and decreased fatigue
- perform activities of daily living within the confines of the disorder
- maintain urine specific gravity within the designated limits
- identify risk factors that exacerbate decreased tissue perfusion and modify lifestyle appropriately
- develop no signs or symptoms of infection.

NURSING INTERVENTIONS

- Give prescribed drugs.

MONITORING

- Vital signs
- Intake and output
- Characteristics of urine
- Pattern of urination
- Daily weight
- Renal function studies

GENERAL

Be sure to cover:

- the disorder, diagnosis, and treatment
- avoidance of bacterial contamination by following hygienic toileting practices (wiping the perineum from front to back after bowel movements for women)
- proper technique for collecting a clean-catch urine specimen
- drug administration, dosage, and possible adverse effects
- routine checkup for patients with a history of UTI
- signs and symptoms of recurrent infection.

RESOURCES

Organizations

American Association of Kidney Patients: *www.aakp.org*
National Institute of Diabetes & Digestive & Kidney Diseases: *www.niddk.nih.gov*

Selected references

Diseases, 4th ed. Philadelphia: Lippincott Williams & Wilkins, 2006.
Ramakrishnan, K., and Scheid, D.C. "Diagnosis and Management of Acute Pyelonephritis in Adults," *American Family Physician* 71(5):933-42, March 2005.

Acute respiratory distress syndrome LIFE-THREATENING DISORDER

OVERVIEW

- Severe form of alveolar injury or acute lung injury
- A form of noncardiogenic pulmonary edema; may be difficult to recognize
- Hallmark sign is hypoxemia despite increased supplemental oxygen
- A four-stage syndrome; can rapidly progress to intractable and fatal hypoxemia
- Little or no permanent lung damage occurring in patients who recover
- May coexist with disseminated intravascular coagulation (DIC)
- Also known as *adult respiratory distress syndrome* and *shock lung, stiff lung, white lung, wet lung,* or *Da Nang lung*

PATHOPHYSIOLOGY

- Increased permeability of the alveolocapillary membranes allows fluid to accumulate in the lung interstitium, alveolar spaces, and small airways, causing the lung to stiffen.
- Ventilation is impaired, reducing oxygenation of pulmonary capillary blood.
- Elevated capillary pressure increases interstitial and alveolar edema.
- Alveolar closing pressure then exceeds pulmonary pressures leading to closure and collapse of the alveoli.

CAUSES

- Acute miliary tuberculosis
- Anaphylaxis
- Aspiration of gastric contents
- Diffuse pneumonia (especially viral)
- Drug overdose
- Gestational hypertension
- Hemodialysis
- Idiosyncratic drug reaction
- Indirect or direct lung trauma (most common)
- Inhalation of noxious gases
- Leukemia
- Massive blood transfusion
- Near drowning
- Oxygen toxicity
- Pancreatitis
- Prolonged coronary artery bypass grafting

- Thrombotic thrombocytopenic purpura
- Uremia
- Venous air embolism

INCIDENCE

- Patients with three concurrent causes have an 85% probability of developing acute respiratory distress syndrome.

COMPLICATIONS

- Metabolic acidosis
- Respiratory acidosis
- Cardiac arrest
- Multiple organ dysfunction syndrome

ASSESSMENT

HISTORY

- Causative factor (one or more)
- Dyspnea, especially on exertion

PHYSICAL FINDINGS

Stage I
- Shortness of breath, especially on exertion
- Normal to increased respiratory and pulse rates
- Diminished breath sounds

Stage II
- Respiratory distress
- Use of accessory muscles for respiration
- Pallor, anxiety, and restlessness
- Dry cough with thick, frothy sputum
- Bloody, sticky secretions
- Cool, clammy skin
- Tachycardia and tachypnea
- Elevated blood pressure
- Basilar crackles

Stage III
- Respiratory rate more than 30 breaths/minute
- Tachycardia with arrhythmias
- Labile blood pressure
- Productive cough
- Pale, cyanotic skin
- Crackles and rhonchi possible

Stage IV
- Acute respiratory failure with severe hypoxia
- Deteriorating mental status (may become comatose)
- Pale, cyanotic skin
- Lack of spontaneous respirations
- Bradycardia with arrhythmias
- Hypotension
- Metabolic and respiratory acidosis

DIAGNOSTIC TEST RESULTS

LABORATORY

- Arterial blood gas (ABG) analysis initially shows a partial pressure of arterial oxygen (Pao_2) less than 60 mm Hg and a partial pressure of arterial carbon dioxide ($Paco_2$) less than 35 mm Hg.
- ABG analysis later shows increased $Paco_2$ (more than 45 mm Hg), decreased bicarbonate levels (less than 22 mEq/L), and decreased Pao_2 despite oxygen therapy.
- Gram stain and sputum culture and sensitivity show infectious organisms.
- Blood cultures reveal infectious organisms.
- Toxicology tests show drug ingestion in overdose.
- Serum amylase level is increased in pancreatitis.

IMAGING

- Chest X-rays show early bilateral infiltrates; in later stages, chest X-rays show a ground-glass appearance and, eventually, "whiteouts" of both lung fields.

DIAGNOSTIC PROCEDURES

- Pulmonary artery catheterization shows a pulmonary artery wedge pressure between 12 and 18 mm Hg.

TREATMENT

GENERAL

- Treatment of the underlying cause
- Correction of electrolyte and acid-base imbalances

For mechanical ventilation
- Target low tidal volumes; use of increased respiratory rates
- Target plateau pressures less than or equal to 40 cm H_2O
- Positive end-expiratory pressure (PEEP) as necessary

DIET
- Fluid restriction
- Tube feedings or parenteral nutrition

ACTIVITY
- Bed rest

MEDICATIONS
- Humidified oxygen
- Bronchodilators
- Diuretics

For mechanical ventilation
- Sedatives
- Opioids
- Neuromuscular blocking agents
- Short course of high-dose corticosteroids if fatty emboli or chemical injury is present
- Sodium bicarbonate if severe metabolic acidosis is identified
- Fluids and vasopressors if hypotensive
- Antimicrobials if nonviral infection is identified
- Prone positioning to help with perfusion to the lungs

SURGERY
- Possible tracheostomy

NURSING CONSIDERATIONS

NURSING DIAGNOSES
- Anxiety
- Decreased cardiac output
- Fatigue
- Fear
- Imbalanced nutrition: Less than body requirements
- Impaired gas exchange
- Impaired physical mobility
- Ineffective tissue perfusion: cardiopulmonary
- Risk for impaired skin integrity
- Risk for infection

EXPECTED OUTCOMES
The patient will:
- express feelings of comfort and decreased anxiety
- maintain adequate cardiac output
- express feelings of energy and decreased fatigue
- verbalize feelings of anxiety and fear
- consume required caloric intake
- maintain a patent airway
- maintain joint mobility and range of motion (ROM)
- maintain hemodynamic stability
- maintain skin integrity
- develop no signs or symptoms of infection.

NURSING INTERVENTIONS
- Give prescribed drugs.
- Maintain a patent airway.
- Perform tracheal suctioning as necessary.
- Ensure adequate humidification.
- Reposition the patient often.
- Consider prone positioning for alveolar recruitment.
- Administer tube feedings or parenteral nutrition as ordered.
- Allow periods of uninterrupted sleep.
- Perform passive ROM exercises.
- Provide meticulous skin care.
- Reposition the endotracheal tube (ET) per facility policy.
- Provide emotional support.
- Provide alternative communication means.

MONITORING
- Vital signs and pulse oximetry
- Hemodynamics
- Intake and output
- Respiratory status (breath sounds, ABG results)
- Mechanical ventilator settings
- Sputum characteristics
- Level of consciousness
- Daily weight
- Laboratory studies
- Response to treatment
- Complications, such as cardiac arrhythmias, DIC, GI bleeding, infection, malnutrition, and pneumothorax
- Nutritional status

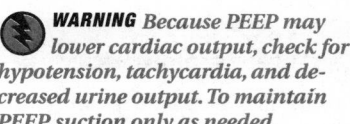 **WARNING** *Because PEEP may lower cardiac output, check for hypotension, tachycardia, and decreased urine output. To maintain PEEP, suction only as needed.*

For mechanical ventilation
- Ventilator settings
- Cuff pressure
- Complications of mechanical ventilation
- ET position and patency
- Signs and symptoms of stress ulcer

PATIENT TEACHING

GENERAL
Be sure to cover:
- the disorder, diagnosis, and treatment
- medications and potential adverse reactions
- when to notify the practitioner
- complications, such as GI bleeding, infection, and malnutrition
- recovery time.

DISCHARGE PLANNING
- Refer the patient to a pulmonary rehabilitation program if indicated.

RESOURCES
Organizations
ARDS Clinical Network: *www.ardsnet.org*
National Heart, Lung, and Blood Institute: *www.nhlbi.nih.gov*

Selected references
Sands, T.L. "Partial Liquid Ventilation: A Breath of Fresh Air for ARDS Patients," *Nursing* 33(6):32cc1-32cc2, June 2003.

Acute respiratory failure LIFE-THREATENING DISORDER

OVERVIEW

- Inadequate ventilation resulting from the inability of the lungs to adequately maintain arterial oxygenation or eliminate carbon dioxide

PATHOPHYSIOLOGY

- Primarily hypercapnic respiratory failure: Results from inadequate alveolar ventilation
- Primarily hypoxemic respiratory failure: Results from inadequate exchange of oxygen between the alveoli and capillaries
- Combined hypercapnic and hypoxemic respiratory failure common

CAUSES

- Accumulated secretions secondary to cough suppression
- Airway irritants
- Any condition that increases the work of breathing and decreases the respiratory drive of patients with chronic obstructive pulmonary disease
- Bronchospasm
- Central nervous system depression
- Endocrine or metabolic disorders
- Gas exchange failure
- Heart failure
- Myocardial infarction (MI)
- Pulmonary emboli
- Respiratory tract infection
- Thoracic abnormalities
- Ventilatory failure

INCIDENCE

- Acute respiratory failure occurs in patients with hypercapnia or hypoxemia.
- The disorder occurs in patients who have an acute deterioration in arterial blood gas (ABG) values.

COMPLICATIONS

- Tissue hypoxia
- Chronic respiratory acidosis
- Metabolic alkalosis
- Respiratory and cardiac arrest

ASSESSMENT

HISTORY
Precipitating events
- Infection
- Accumulated pulmonary secretions secondary to cough suppression
- Trauma
- MI
- Heart failure
- Pulmonary emboli
- Exposure to irritants (smoke or fumes)
- Myxedema
- Metabolic acidosis

PHYSICAL FINDINGS
- Cyanosis of the oral mucosa, lips, and nail beds
- Yawning and use of accessory muscles
- Pursed-lip breathing
- Nasal flaring
- Ashen skin
- Rapid breathing
- Cold, clammy skin
- Asymmetrical chest movement
- Decreased tactile fremitus over obstructed bronchi or a pleural effusion
- Increased tactile fremitus over consolidated lung tissue
- Hyperresonance
- Diminished or absent breath sounds
- Wheezes (in asthma)
- Rhonchi (in bronchitis)
- Crackles (in pulmonary edema)

DIAGNOSTIC TEST RESULTS

LABORATORY
- ABG analysis reveals hypercapnia and hypoxemia.
- Serum white blood cell count is increased in bacterial infections.
- Serum hemoglobin and hematocrit show decreased oxygen-carrying capacity.
- Serum electrolyte results reveal hypokalemia and hypochloremia.
- Blood cultures, Gram stain, and sputum cultures show the pathogen. (See *Identifying respiratory failure*.)

IMAGING
- Chest X-rays may show underlying pulmonary diseases or conditions, such as emphysema, atelectasis, lesions, pneumothorax, infiltrates, and effusions.

DIAGNOSTIC PROCEDURES
- Electrocardiography may show arrhythmias, cor pulmonale, or myocardial ischemia.
- Pulse oximetry may show decreased arterial oxygen saturation.
- Pulmonary artery catheterization may show pulmonary or cardiovascular causes of acute respiratory failure.

Identifying respiratory failure

Use these measurements to identify respiratory failure:
- vital capacity less than 15 cc/kg
- tidal volume less than 3 cc/kg
- negative inspiratory force less than −25 cm H_2O
- respiratory rate more than twice the normal rate
- diminished partial pressure of arterial oxygen despite increased fraction of inspired oxygen
- elevated partial pressure of arterial carbon dioxide, with pH lower than 7.25.

TREATMENT

GENERAL
- Mechanical ventilation with an endotracheal or a tracheostomy tube
- High-frequency ventilation if the patient doesn't respond to conventional mechanical ventilation

DIET
- Fluid restriction (heart failure)

ACTIVITY
- As tolerated

MEDICATIONS
- Cautious oxygen therapy to increase partial pressure of arterial oxygen
- Antacids
- Histamine-receptor antagonists as ordered
- Antibiotics
- Bronchodilators
- Corticosteroids
- Positive inotropic agents
- Vasopressors
- Diuretics

SURGERY
- Possible tracheostomy

NURSING CONSIDERATIONS

NURSING DIAGNOSES
- Anxiety
- Fatigue
- Fear
- Imbalanced nutrition: Less than body requirements
- Impaired gas exchange
- Impaired skin integrity
- Impaired verbal communication
- Ineffective breathing pattern
- Ineffective coping
- Ineffective tissue perfusion: Cardiopulmonary

EXPECTED OUTCOMES
The patient will:
- express feelings of comfort and decreased anxiety
- express feelings of energy and decreased fatigue
- verbalize feelings of anxiety and fear
- consume required caloric intake
- maintain a patent airway
- maintain skin integrity
- develop alternate means of communication to express self
- maintain adequate ventilation
- cope effectively
- maintain hemodynamic stability.

NURSING INTERVENTIONS
- Give prescribed drugs.
- Orient the patient frequently.
- Administer oxygen as ordered.
- Maintain a patent airway.
- Encourage pursed-lip breathing.
- Encourage the use of an incentive spirometer.
- Reposition the patient every 1 to 2 hours.
- Help clear the patient's secretions with postural drainage and chest physiotherapy.
- Assist with or perform oral hygiene.
- Position the patient for comfort and optimal gas exchange.
- Maintain normothermia.
- Schedule care to provide frequent rest periods.

For mechanical ventilation
- Obtain blood samples for ABG analysis as ordered.
- Suction the trachea after hyperoxygenation as needed.
- Provide humidification.
- Secure the endotracheal (ET) tube per facility policy.
- Prevent infection.
- Prevent tracheal erosion.
- Maintain skin integrity.
- Provide alternative communication means.
- Provide sedation as necessary.

MONITORING
- Vital signs and pulse oximetry
- Intake and output
- Laboratory studies
- Daily weight
- Cardiac rate and rhythm
- Respiratory status (breath sounds and ABG results)
- Chest X-ray results
- Complications
- Sputum quality, consistency, and color
- Signs and symptoms of infection

For mechanical ventilation
- Ventilator settings
- Cuff pressures
- Complications of mechanical ventilation
- ET tube position and patency
- Signs and symptoms of stress ulcer

PATIENT TEACHING

GENERAL
Be sure to cover:
- the disorder, diagnosis, and treatment
- drugs and potential adverse reactions
- when to notify the practitioner
- smoking cessation, if appropriate
- communication techniques, if intubated
- signs and symptoms of respiratory infection.

DISCHARGE PLANNING
- Refer the patient to a smoking-cessation program, if applicable.

RESOURCES
Organizations
National Lung Health Education Program: *www.nlhep.org*

Selected references
Paus-Jenssen, E.S., et al. "The Use of Noninvasive Ventilation in Acute Respiratory Failure at a Tertiary Care Center," *Chest* 126(1):165-72, July 2004.
Simmons, P., and Simmons, M. "Informed Nursing Practice: The Administration of Oxygen to Patients with COPD," *MedSurg Nursing* 13(2):82-85, April 2004.

Acute tubular necrosis

- Injury to the nephron's tubular segment resulting from ischemic or nephrotoxic injury and causing renal failure and uremic syndrome
- Also known as *intrinsic renal azotemia*

PATHOPHYSIOLOGY

- In ischemic injury, circulatory collapse, severe hypotension, trauma, hemorrhage, dehydration, cardiogenic or septic shock, surgery, anesthetics, and reactions to transfusions may cause disruption of blood flow to the kidneys.
- Nephrotoxic injury may follow ingestion of certain chemical agents, such as contrast medium or antibiotics, or result from a hypersensitive reaction of the kidneys.

CAUSES

- Diseased tubular epithelium
- Ischemic or toxic injury to glomerular epithelial cells or vascular endothelium
- Obstructed urine flow

INCIDENCE

- Acute tubular necrosis accounts for about 75% of acute renal failure cases.
- This disorder is the most common cause of acute renal failure in critically ill patients.

COMPLICATIONS

- Heart failure
- Uremic pericarditis
- Pulmonary edema
- Uremic lung
- Anemia
- Anorexia, intractable vomiting
- Poor wound healing due to debilitation

⚡ **WARNING** *Fever and chills may signal the onset of an infection, the leading cause of death in acute tubular necrosis.*

- Diagnosis usually delayed until the condition has progressed to an advanced stage

HISTORY

- Ischemic or nephrotoxic injury
- Urine output less than 400 ml/24 hours
- Fever and chills

PHYSICAL FINDINGS

- Evidence of bleeding abnormalities, such as petechiae and ecchymosis
- Dry, pruritic skin
- Dry mucous membranes
- Uremic breath
- Cardiac arrhythmia, if hyperkalemic
- Muscle weakness

LABORATORY

- Urinary sediment contains red blood cells (RBCs) and casts.
- Urine specific gravity is 1.010.
- Urine osmolality is less than 400 mOsm/kg.
- Urine sodium level is 40 to 60 mEq/L.
- Blood urea nitrogen and serum creatinine levels are elevated.
- Anemia is present.
- Platelet adherence is defective.
- Metabolic acidosis is present.
- Hyperkalemia is found.

DIAGNOSTIC PROCEDURES

- Electrocardiography may show arrhythmias and, with hyperkalemia, a widening QRS complex, disappearing P waves, and tall, peaked T waves.
- Renal ultrasound, computed tomography scanning, or magnetic resonance imaging measures kidney size and excludes obstruction.

TREATMENT

GENERAL
Acute phase
- Vigorous supportive measures until normal kidney function resumes

Long-term management
- Daily replacement of projected and calculated fluid loss (including insensible loss)
- Peritoneal dialysis or hemodialysis if the patient is catabolic or if hyperkalemia and fluid volume overload aren't controlled by other measures

DIET
- Fluid restriction
- Low-sodium, low-potassium

ACTIVITY
- Rest periods when fatigued

MEDICATIONS
- Diuretics
- Transfusion of packed RBCs
- Epoetin alfa
- Antibiotics
- Emergency I.V. administration of 50% glucose, regular insulin, and sodium bicarbonate (for hyperkalemia)
- Sodium polystyrene sulfonate with sorbitol by mouth or by enema (for hyperkalemia)

NURSING CONSIDERATIONS

NURSING DIAGNOSES
- Acute pain
- Decreased cardiac output
- Excess fluid volume
- Fatigue
- Imbalanced nutrition: Less than body requirements
- Ineffective tissue perfusion: Renal
- Risk for infection
- Risk for injury

EXPECTED OUTCOMES
The patient will:
- express feelings of comfort and decreased pain
- maintain hemodynamic stability
- maintain fluid balance
- demonstrate energy conservation skills
- consume required caloric intake
- maintain urine specific gravity within the designated limits and have improved kidney function
- remain free from all signs and symptoms of infection
- remain free from injury.

NURSING INTERVENTIONS
- Give prescribed drugs and blood products.
- Restrict food containing high sodium and potassium levels.
- Use aseptic technique, particularly when handling catheters.
- Perform passive range-of-motion exercises.
- Provide meticulous skin care.

MONITORING
- Intake and output
- Vital signs
- Laboratory studies
- Complications

PATIENT TEACHING

GENERAL
Be sure to cover:
- the disorder, diagnosis, and treatment
- signs of infection and when to report them to the practitioner
- dietary restrictions
- how to set goals that are realistic for the patient's prognosis.

DISCHARGE PLANNING
- Refer the patient to appropriate supportive resources or social services.

RESOURCES
Organizations
American Association of Kidney Patients: *www.aakp.org*
National Institute of Diabetes & Digestive & Kidney Diseases: *www.niddk.nih.gov*

Selected references
Dirkes, S.M., and Kozlowski, C. "Renal Assist Device Therapy for Acute Renal Failure," *Nephrology Nursing Journal* 30(6):611-14, December 2003.

Adrenal hypofunction

- Primary adrenal hypofunction or insufficiency (Addison's disease) originating within the adrenal gland and characterized by the decreased secretion of mineralocorticoids, glucocorticoids, and androgens
- Secondary adrenal hypofunction due to a disorder outside the gland such as impaired pituitary secretion of corticotropin and characterized by decreased glucocorticoid secretion
- Adrenal crisis (addisonian crisis), a critical deficiency of mineralocorticoids and glucocorticoids generally following acute stress, sepsis, trauma, surgery, or the omission of steroid therapy in patients who have chronic adrenal insufficiency; a medical emergency that needs immediate, vigorous treatment

PATHOPHYSIOLOGY

- Results from the partial or complete destruction of the adrenal cortex
- Manifests as a clinical syndrome in which the symptoms are associated with deficient production of the adrenocortical hormones cortisol, aldosterone, and androgen
- Results in high levels of corticotropin and corticotropin-releasing hormone
- Secondary adrenal hypofunction: Involves all zones of the cortex, causing deficiencies of the adrenocortical hormones, glucocorticoids, androgens, and mineralocorticoids
- Cortisol deficiency: Causes decreased liver gluconeogenesis (the formation of glucose from molecules that aren't carbohydrates); resulting low blood glucose levels can become dangerously low in patients who take insulin routinely
- Aldosterone deficiency: Causes increased renal sodium loss and enhances potassium reabsorption
- Hypotension due to sodium excretion
- Increased production of angiotensin II due to low plasma volume and arteriolar pressure

- Androgen deficiency: May decrease hair growth in axillary and pubic areas (less noticeable in men) as well as on the extremities of women

CAUSES

Primary hypofunction

- Autoimmune process in which circulating antibodies react specifically against the adrenal tissue
- Bilateral adrenalectomy
- Family history of autoimmune disease (may predispose the patient to Addison's disease and other endocrinopathies)
- Hemorrhage into the adrenal gland
- Infection (histoplasmosis, cytomegalovirus)
- Neoplasm
- Tuberculosis (once the chief cause, now responsible for less than 20% of adult cases)

Secondary hypofunction

- Abrupt withdrawal of long-term corticosteroid therapy
- Hypopituitarism
- Removal of a corticotropin-secreting tumor

Adrenal crisis

- Exhausted body stores of glucocorticoids in a patient with adrenal hypofunction after trauma, surgery, or other physiologic stress

INCIDENCE

Primary hypofunction

- Primary adrenal hypofunction is relatively uncommon.
- This disorder can occur at any age and in both sexes.

Autoimmune Addison's disease

- Autoimmune Addison's disease is most common in white females (genetic predisposition is likely).
- This disorder is more common in patients with a familial predisposition to autoimmune endocrine diseases.

AGE FACTOR *Most people with Addison's disease are diagnosed in their 20s to 40s.*

COMPLICATIONS

- Hyperpyrexia
- Psychotic reactions
- Deficient or excessive steroid treatment
- Shock
- Profound hypoglycemia
- Ultimate vascular collapse, renal shutdown, coma, and death (if untreated)

HISTORY

- Synthetic steroid use, adrenal surgery, or recent infection
- Muscle weakness
- Fatigue
- Weight loss
- Craving for salty food
- Decreased tolerance for stress
- GI disturbances
- Dehydration
- Amenorrhea (in women)
- Impotence (in men)

PHYSICAL FINDINGS

- Poor coordination
- Decreased axillary and pubic hair (in women)
- Bronze coloration of the skin and darkening of scars
- Areas of vitiligo
- Increased pigmentation of mucous membranes
- Weak, irregular pulse
- Hypotension

LABORATORY

- Rapid corticotropin stimulation test: Low corticotropin level indicates a secondary disorder; elevated level indicates a primary disorder.
- Plasma cortisol level is less than 10 mcg/dl in the morning and even lower in the evening.
- Serum sodium and fasting blood glucose levels are decreased.
- Serum potassium, calcium, and blood urea nitrogen levels are increased.
- Hematocrit is elevated; lymphocyte and eosinophil counts are increased.

IMAGING

- Chest X-ray shows a small heart.
- Computed tomography scan of the abdomen show adrenal calcification (if the cause is infectious).

TREATMENT

GENERAL

- I.V. fluids

DIET

- Small, frequent, high-protein meals

ACTIVITY

- Periods of rest

MEDICATIONS

- Lifelong corticosteroid replacement, usually with cortisone or hydrocortisone
- Oral fludrocortisone
- Hydrocortisone
- I.V. saline and glucose solutions (for adrenal crisis)
- I.V. hydrocortisone replacement (for adrenal crisis)

NURSING DIAGNOSES

- Activity intolerance
- Deficient fluid volume
- Disturbed body image
- Imbalanced nutrition: Less than body requirements
- Ineffective coping
- Risk for imbalanced body temperature
- Risk for impaired skin integrity
- Risk for infection

EXPECTED OUTCOMES

The patient will:
- maintain joint mobility and range of motion
- maintain an adequate fluid balance
- verbalize feelings about changed body image
- consume required caloric intake
- develop effective coping skills
- remain normothermic
- maintain skin integrity
- remain free from signs and symptoms of infection.

NURSING INTERVENTIONS

- Until onset of mineralocorticoid effect, encourage fluids to replace excessive fluid loss.
- Arrange for a diet that maintains sodium and potassium balances; if the patient is anorexic, suggest six small meals per day to increase caloric intake.
- Observe for cushingoid signs such as fluid retention around the eyes and face.
- Check for petechiae.
- If the patient receives glucocorticoids alone, observe for orthostatic hypotension or electrolyte abnormalities.

MONITORING

- Vital signs
- Signs of shock (decreased level of consciousness and urine output)
- Hyperkalemia before treatment; hypokalemia after treatment
- Cardiac rhythm
- Blood glucose levels
- Daily weight
- Intake and output

GENERAL

Be sure to cover:
- lifelong steroid therapy requirement
- symptoms of steroid overdose (swelling, weight gain) and steroid underdose (lethargy, weakness)
- possible need for dosage to be increased during times of stress or illness (when the patient has a cold, for example)
- possibility of adrenal crisis being precipitated by infection, injury, or profuse sweating in hot weather
- importance of carrying a medical identification card that states the patient is on steroid therapy (drug name and dosage should be included on the card)
- how to give a hydrocortisone injection and to keep an emergency kit containing hydrocortisone in a prepared syringe available for use in times of stress
- stress management techniques.

DISCHARGE PLANNING

- Refer the patient to the National Adrenal Diseases Foundation for support and information.

RESOURCES

Organizations

National Adrenal Diseases Foundation: *www.medhelp.org/nadf*

Selected references

Becker, K.L., et al. *Principles and Practice of Endocrinology and Metabolism*, 3rd ed. Philadelphia: Lippincott Williams & Wilkins, 2004.

Greenspan, F.S., and Gardner, D.G. *Basic and Clinical Endocrinology*, 7th ed. New York: McGraw-Hill Book Co., 2003.

Adrenogenital syndrome

- A group of disorders resulting from hyperplasia of the adrenal cortex
- May be inherited (congenital adrenal hyperplasia [CAH]) or acquired, usually as a result of an adrenal tumor (adrenal virilism)
- May be autosomal recessive, resulting in complete or partial delivery of an enzyme involved in cortisol or aldosterone synthesis
- May cause fatal adrenal crisis in neonates (salt-losing CAH)

PATHOPHYSIOLOGY

- Deficiencies occur in the enzymes needed for adrenocortical secretion of cortisol and, possibly, aldosterone.
- Compensatory secretion of corticotropin produces varying degrees of adrenal hyperplasia.

Simple virilizing CAH (most common)

- Underproduction of cortisol because of deficiency of the enzyme 21-hydroxylase
- This cortisol deficiency stimulates increased secretion of corticotropin, producing large amounts of cortisol precursors and androgens that don't require 21-hydroxylase for synthesis

Salt-losing CAH

- 21-hydroxylase almost completely absent
- Corticotropin secretion increased, causing excessive production of cortisol precursors, including salt-wasting compounds
- Plasma cortisol and aldosterone levels — both dependent on 21-hydroxylase — falling precipitously and, in combination with the excessive production of salt-wasting compounds, precipitating acute adrenal crisis
- Corticotropin hypersecretion stimulates adrenal androgens and produces masculinization

CAUSES

- Transmitted as an autosomal recessive disorder

INCIDENCE

- Acquired adrenal virilism is rare and affects twice as many females as males.
- **AGE FACTOR** *CAH is the most prevalent adrenal disorder in infants and children; simple virilizing CAH and salt-losing CAH are the most common forms.*

COMPLICATIONS

- Hypertension
- Hyperkalemic infertility
- Adrenal tumor
- Adrenal crisis
- Altered growth, external genitalia, and sexual maturity

Salt-losing CAH

- Cardiovascular collapse
- Cardiac arrest

HISTORY
Simple virilizing CAH

- Failure to begin menstruation (in girls)
- Frequent erections at an early age (in boys)

Salt-losing CAH

- Apathy, failure to eat, and diarrhea (in infants)
- Symptoms of adrenal crisis in the first week of life (vomiting, dehydration from hyponatremia, hyperkalemia)

PHYSICAL FINDINGS
Simple virilizing CAH

- Pseudohermaphroditism in females or precocious puberty in both sexes strongly suggests CAH

Salt-losing CAH

- Signs of progressive virilization at an early age: Early appearance of pubic and axillary hair, deep voice, acne, facial hair
- Small testes
- Possibly taller than other children of the same age

LABORATORY

- Plasma 17-ketosteroid (17-KS) levels are elevated; this result can be suppressed by administering oral dexamethasone.
- Urinary hormone metabolite levels, particularly pregnanetriol, are elevated.
- Plasma 17-hydroxyprogesterone level is elevated.
- Urinary 17-hydroxycorticosteroid level is normal or decreased.
- **AGE FACTOR** *Adrenal hypofunction or adrenal crisis in the first week of life suggests salt-losing CAH. Hyperkalemia, hyponatremia, and hypochloremia, with excessive urinary 17-KS and pregnanetriol and decreased urinary aldosterone levels, confirm it.*

DIAGNOSTIC PROCEDURES

- Gonadal biopsy and chromosomal studies confirm hermaphroditism.

OTHER

- Sex chromatin and karyotype studies determine the genetic sex of patients with ambiguous external genitalia.

TREATMENT

DIET
◆ Well-balanced

ACTIVITY
◆ No restriction

MEDICATIONS
Simple virilizing CAH
◆ Daily administration of cortisone or hydrocortisone

Salt-losing CAH with patient in adrenal crisis
◆ Immediate I.V. sodium chloride and glucose infusion
◆ Desoxycorticosterone I.M. and hydrocortisone I.V.
◆ Maintenance includes mineralocorticoid (desoxycorticosterone, fludrocortisone, or both) and glucocorticoid (cortisone or hydrocortisone) replacement

SURGERY
◆ Reconstructive surgery based on the determined sex and external genitalia

NURSING CONSIDERATIONS

NURSING DIAGNOSES
◆ Delayed growth and development
◆ Disturbed body image
◆ Ineffective coping
◆ Risk for deficient fluid volume

EXPECTED OUTCOMES
The patient will:
◆ express understanding of norms for growth and development
◆ verbalize feelings about changed body image
◆ demonstrate effective coping skills
◆ maintain an adequate fluid balance.

NURSING INTERVENTIONS
◆ Maintain I.V. access, infuse fluids, and give steroids as ordered.
◆ Watch for cyanosis, hypotension, tachycardia, tachypnea, and signs of shock.
◆ Minimize external stressors.
◆ If a child is receiving maintenance therapy with steroid injections, rotate I.M. injection sites to prevent atrophy; tell the parents to do the same.

MONITORING
◆ Body weight
◆ Blood pressure
◆ Serum electrolyte levels
◆ Edema, weakness, and hypertension for the patient receiving desoxycorticosterone or fludrocortisone

PATIENT TEACHING

GENERAL
Be sure to cover:
◆ possible adverse effects (cushingoid symptoms) of long-term therapy (lifelong maintenance therapy with hydrocortisone, cortisone, or the mineralocorticoid fludrocortisone is essential)
◆ importance of not withdrawing therapeutic drugs suddenly because potentially fatal adrenal hypofunction will result
◆ need to report stress and infection, which require increased steroid doses
◆ importance of carrying a medical identification card that states the patient is on steroid therapy (drug name and dosage should be included on the card).

DISCHARGE PLANNING
◆ Refer the patient for psychological counseling for help in accepting this disorder, as indicated.

RESOURCES
Organizations
National Adrenal Diseases Foundation: *www.medhelp.org/nadf*

Selected references
Becker, K.L., et al. *Principles and Practice of Endocrinology and Metabolism*, 3rd ed. Philadelphia: Lippincott Williams & Wilkins, 2004.
Greenspan, F.S., and Gardner, D.G. *Basic and Clinical Endocrinology*, 7th ed. New York: McGraw-Hill Book Co., 2003.

Age-related macular degeneration

- Deterioration of the macular portion of the retina, which is responsible for detailed vision
- May be atrophic, also called *involutional* or *dry*
- May be exudative, also called *hemorrhagic* or *wet*
- No cure for atrophic form
- Commonly affects both eyes
- Also known as *AMD*

PATHOPHYSIOLOGY

- Pathologic changes occur primarily in the retinal pigment epithelium, Bruch's membrane, and choriocapillaries in the macular region that result from the hardening and obstruction of retinal arteries.
- Formation of new blood vessels in the macular area obscures central vision. (See *How AMD affects central vision.*)
- Vision loss occurs as the retinal pigment epithelium detaches and becomes atrophic.
- Exudative macular degeneration develops as new blood vessels in the choroid project through abnormalities in Bruch's membrane, invading the potential space underneath the retinal pigment epithelium.
- The vessels leak, and fluid in the retinal pigment epithelium increases, resulting in blurry vision.

CAUSES

- Unknown
- Genetic in origin

RISK FACTORS

- Smoking
- Older age
- High blood pressure
- Vascular disease
- High intake of saturated fat and cholesterol
- Farsightedness
- Exposure to sunlight

INCIDENCE

- Age-related macular degeneration affects more than 10 million Americans.
- This disorder is the leading cause of blindness in people older than age 55 in the United States.
- Irreversible central vision loss occurs in at least 10% of elderly people.
- The atrophic form affects about 70% of patients.
- The disorder is most common in whites but affects all races.

COMPLICATIONS

- Blindness
- Nystagmus

How AMD affects central vision

Central vision occurs in the macula and involves the ability to perceive sharp, detailed images. At the center of the macula is the fovea — which contains the highest concentration of rods and cones — and the most light-sensitive portion of the macula.

Light entering the cornea and lens is focused on the fovea. If any part of the macula deteriorates, the eye must rely on the less-sensitive, outer portion of the retina, which is responsible for peripheral vision.

With age-related macular degeneration (AMD), grayness, haziness, or a blind spot may appear in the area of central vision. Words may be blurred on a page, straight lines may appear to have kinks in them, and colors may seem dimmer.

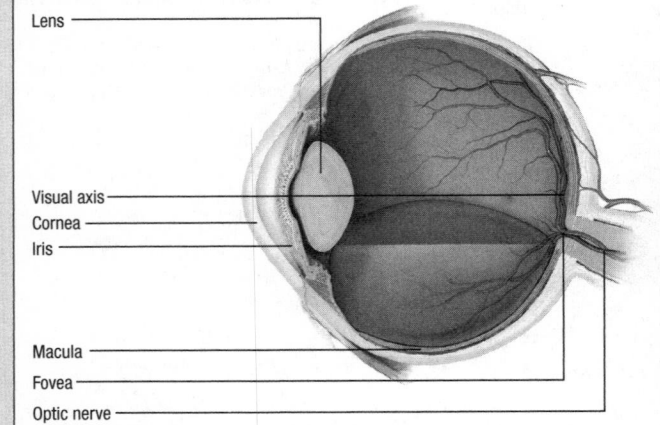

Lens
Visual axis
Cornea
Iris
Macula
Fovea
Optic nerve

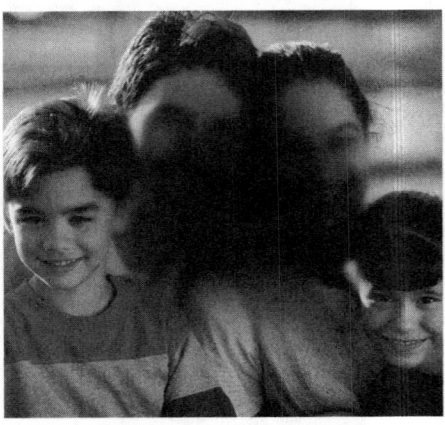

HISTORY
- Sees blank spot (scotoma) in the center of a page when reading
- Central vision blurs intermittently and has gradually worsened
- Straight lines appear distorted
- Letters appear fragmented

PHYSICAL FINDINGS
- Tiny yellowish spots (drusen) beneath retina

DIAGNOSTIC TEST RESULTS

DIAGNOSTIC PROCEDURES
- Indirect ophthalmoscopy may show changes in the macular region of the fundus.
- Amsler grid test may detect visual distortion.

IMAGING
- Fluorescein angiography may show leaking vessels in subretinal neovascular net.

TREATMENT

GENERAL
- Laser treatment, if leaking blood vessels have developed away from the fovea

DIET
- High in vitamins A, C, and E; beta-carotene; and zinc

ACTIVITY
- Restrictions based on visual acuity

MEDICATIONS
- Zinc supplements
- Lutein, vitamins C and E, and beta-carotene (investigational)

SURGERY
- Argon laser photocoagulation in exudative form (may slow the progression of severe visual loss)

NURSING CONSIDERATIONS

NURSING DIAGNOSES
- Disturbed sensory perception (visual)
- Fear
- Risk for injury
- Social isolation

EXPECTED OUTCOMES
The patient will:
- maintain optimal visual function or adapt as necessary
- express feelings of fear and verbalize concerns over diminishing eyesight
- sustain no harm or injury
- maintain social interaction to the extent possible.

NURSING INTERVENTIONS
- Help the patient to obtain optical aids such as magnifiers.
- Offer the patient emotional support.
- Encourage expression of fears and concerns.

MONITORING
- Visual acuity
- Environment (for safety purposes)

PATIENT TEACHING

GENERAL
Be sure to cover:
- ways to modify the home environment for safety
- affects on peripheral vision.

DISCHARGE PLANNING
- Refer the patient to the American Foundation for the Blind or Associated Services for the Blind & Visually Impaired as indicated.
- Refer the patient to a local support group.

RESOURCES
Organizations
American Academy of Ophthalmology: *www.aao.org*
American Foundation for the Blind: *www.afb.org*
Associated Services for the Blind & Visually Impaired: *www.asb.org*
National Eye Institute: *www.nei.nih.gov*

Selected references
Seppa, N. "Blindness Hazard: Gene Variant Tied to Macular Degeneration," *Science News* 167(11):163, March 2005.

Alcoholism

- Chronic disorder of uncontrolled intake of alcoholic beverages
- Interferes with physical and mental health, social and familial relationships, and occupational responsibilities

PATHOPHYSIOLOGY

- Alcohol: soluble in water and lipids; permeates all body tissues
- The liver, which metabolizes 90% of alcohol absorbed, most severely affected organ; hepatic steatosis, followed by hepatic fibrosis, evident days after heavy drinking
- Causes Laënnec's cirrhosis after inflammatory response (alcoholic hepatitis) or, in the absence of inflammation, from direct activation of lipocytes (Ito cells)
- Promotes lactic acidosis and excess uric acid; opposes gluconeogenesis, beta-oxidation of fatty acids, and the Krebs cycle; and results in hypoglycemia and hyperlipidemia
- Cell toxicity through reduction of mitochondrial oxygenation, depletion of deoxyribonucleic acid, and other actions

CAUSES

- Biological factors
- Psychological factors
- Sociocultural factors

RISK FACTORS

- Male gender
- Low socioeconomic status
- Family history
- Depression
- Anxiety
- History of other substance abuse disorders

INCIDENCE

- Alcoholism affects all social and economic groups.
- Ten percent of the population accounts for 50% of all alcohol consumed.
- About 13% of all adults older than age 18 have suffered from alcohol abuse or dependence.

- Men are two to five times more likely to abuse alcohol than women.
- Alcoholism occurs at all stages of the life cycle, beginning as early as elementary school age.
- Alcoholism is prevalent in 20% of adult hospital inpatients.

  AGE FACTOR *Prevalence of drinking is highest between ages 21 and 34, but current statistics show that up to 19% of 12- to 17-year-olds have serious drinking problems. Research also suggests that alcoholism affects 2% to 10% of adults older than age 60.*

COMPLICATIONS

- Cardiomyopathy
- Pneumonia
- Cirrhosis
- Esophageal varices
- Pancreatitis
- Alcoholic dementia
- Wernicke's encephalopathy
- Seizure disorder
- Depression
- Multiple substance abuse
- Hypoglycemia
- Leg and foot ulcers
- Suicide and homicide
- Death

HISTORY

- Need for daily or episodic alcohol use for adequate function
- Inability to discontinue or reduce alcohol intake
- Episodes of anesthesia or amnesia during intoxication
- Episodes of violence during intoxication
- Interference with social and familial relationships and occupational responsibilities
- Malaise, dyspepsia, mood swings or depression, and an increased incidence of infection
- Secretive behavior

PHYSICAL FINDINGS

- Poor personal hygiene
- Unusually high tolerance for sedatives and opioids
- Signs of nutritional deficiency
- Signs of injury
- Withdrawal signs and symptoms
- Major motor seizures

DSM-IV-TR *criteria*

A diagnosis is confirmed when the patient exhibits at least three of these signs and symptoms:

- more alcohol ingested than intended
- persistent desire or efforts to diminish alcohol use
- excessive time spent obtaining alcohol
- frequent intoxication or withdrawal symptoms
- impairment of social, occupational, or recreational activities
- continued alcohol consumption despite knowledge of a social, psychological, or physical problem that's caused or exacerbated by alcohol use
- marked tolerance
- characteristic withdrawal symptoms
- use of alcohol to relieve or avoid withdrawal symptoms
- persistent symptoms for at least 1 month or recurrence over a longer time.

DIAGNOSTIC TEST RESULTS

LABORATORY
- Blood alcohol tests show levels of 0.10% weight/volume (200 mg/dl) or higher.
- Serum electrolyte levels are abnormal.
- Serum ammonia levels are increased.
- Serum amylase levels are increased.
- Urine toxicology may show abuse of other drugs.
- Liver function study results are abnormal.

OTHER
- CAGE screening test: Two affirmative responses make patient seven times more likely to be alcohol dependent.
- Alcohol Use Disorders Identification Test: Score greater than 8 indicates alcohol dependency.
- Michigan Alcohol Screening Test: Score greater than 5 indicates alcohol dependency.

TREATMENT

GENERAL
Immediate
- Respiratory support
- Prevention of aspiration of vomitus
- Replacement of fluids
- I.V. glucose administration
- Correction of hypothermia or acidosis
- Treatment of trauma, infection, or GI bleeding

Long-term
- Total abstinence
- Detoxification, rehabilitation, and aftercare program
- Supportive counseling
- Individual, group, or family psychotherapy
- Ongoing support group participation
- Safety precautions, including preventing aspiration of vomitus
- Seizure precautions

DIET
- Well-balanced

MEDICATIONS
- Anticonvulsants
- Antiemetics
- Antidiarrheals
- Tranquilizers, particularly benzodiazepines
- Naltrexone
- Antipsychotics
- Daily oral disulfiram
- Vitamin supplements

NURSING CONSIDERATIONS

NURSING DIAGNOSES
- Anxiety
- Bathing or hygiene self-care deficit
- Compromised family coping
- Dressing or grooming self-care deficit
- Dysfunctional family processes: Alcoholism
- Imbalanced nutrition: Less than body requirements
- Impaired social interaction
- Risk for injury
- Risk for other-directed violence

EXPECTED OUTCOMES
The patient (or his family) will:
- verbalize feelings of anxiety and fear
- demonstrate improved hygiene and other self-care measures
- express feelings and concerns
- demonstrate improved grooming and other self-care measures
- express understanding of the disorder and treatment modality, as will his family
- consume required caloric intake
- engage in appropriate social interaction with others
- remain free from injury
- inflict no harm upon others.

NURSING INTERVENTIONS
- Institute seizure precautions.
- Give prescribed drugs.
- Orient the patient to reality.
- Maintain a calm environment, minimizing noise and shadows.
- Avoid restraints, unless necessary for protection.
- Use a nonthreatening approach.

MONITORING
- Mental status
- Vital signs
- Safety measures
- Nutritional and hydration status
- Intake and output

PATIENT TEACHING

GENERAL
Be sure to cover:
- the disorder, diagnosis, and treatment
- alcohol abstinence
- plan for relapse prevention
- drug administration, dosage, and possible adverse effects
- effects of disorder on significant others.

DISCHARGE PLANNING
- Refer the patient to a rehabilitation program.
- Refer the patient to social services.
- Refer the patient to support group services.
- Refer the patient to personal and family counseling.

RESOURCES
Organizations
Al-Anon: *www.al-anon.alateen.org*
Alateen: *www.al-anon.alateen.org/alateen.html*
Alcoholics Anonymous: *www.alcoholics-anonymous.org*
National Association for Children of Alcoholics: *www.nacoa.net*

Selected references
Blondell, R.D. "Ambulatory Detoxification of Patients with Alcohol Dependence," *American Family Physician* 71(3):495-502, February 2005.
Holbert, K.R., and Tueth, M.J. "Alcohol Abuse and Dependence: A Clinical Update on Alcoholism in the Older Population," *Geriatrics* 56(9):38-40, September 2004.

Allergic purpura

- An acute or chronic vascular inflammation affecting the skin, joints, and GI and genitourinary (GU) tracts, in association with allergy symptoms
- Purpura associated with other conditions such as erythema nodosum
- A nonthrombocytopenic purpura
- Known as Henoch-Schönlein syndrome or anaphylactoid purpura when it primarily affects the GI tract and is accompanied by joint pain

PATHOPHYSIOLOGY

- An autoimmune reaction directed against vascular walls, triggered by a bacterial infection
- An inflammation of the veins and capillaries disrupting the vascular wall, resulting in loss of red blood cells and bleeding and leakage into the skin and mucous membranes

CAUSES

- Allergic reaction to some drugs and vaccines, insect bites, and foods (such as wheat, eggs, milk, and chocolate)
- Bacterial infection (particularly streptococcal infection)

INCIDENCE

- Allergic purpura affects more males than females.
- The disorder is most prevalent in children ages 3 to 7.

COMPLICATIONS

- Renal disease (renal failure and acute glomerulonephritis)
- Hypertension

ASSESSMENT

HISTORY

- Bacterial infection or exposure to allergen
- Moderate and irregular fever
- Headache
- Anorexia
- Pruritus and paresthesia in areas of lesions

PHYSICAL FINDINGS

- Characteristic lesions that usually appear in symmetric patterns on the arms, legs, and buttocks (see *Identifying purpuric lesions*)
- In children, urticarial skin lesions that expand and become hemorrhagic
- Possibly scattered petechiae on the legs, buttocks, and perineum
- Localized edema of the hands, feet, or scalp

DIAGNOSTIC TEST RESULTS

LABORATORY

- Urine and stool tests may be positive for blood.
- Increased blood urea nitrogen and creatinine levels may indicate renal involvement.
  WARNING No laboratory test clearly identifies allergic purpura (although white blood cell count and erythrocyte sedimentation rate are elevated).

IMAGING

- Small-bowel X-rays may reveal areas of transient edema.

OTHER

- Clinical evaluation of lesions

Identifying purpuric lesions

Lesions of allergic purpura, such as those shown on the leg and foot below, characteristically vary in size.

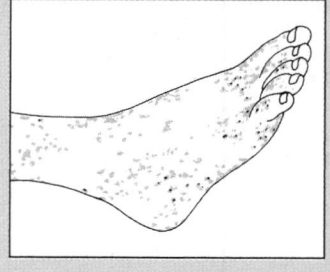

TREATMENT

GENERAL
◆ Symptomatic

MEDICATIONS
◆ Steroids
◆ Analgesics

NURSING CONSIDERATIONS

NURSING DIAGNOSES
◆ Acute pain
◆ Anxiety
◆ Disturbed body image
◆ Impaired skin integrity
◆ Ineffective tissue perfusion: Renal, GI
◆ Risk for deficient fluid volume
◆ Risk for infection

EXPECTED OUTCOMES
The patient will:
◆ express feelings of comfort and relief of pain
◆ verbalize feelings of anxiety and fear
◆ verbalize feelings about changed body image
◆ exhibit improved or healed lesions, and demonstrate appropriate skin care regimen
◆ demonstrate improved renal and GI functioning
◆ maintain an adequate fluid balance
◆ develop no signs or symptoms of infection.

NURSING INTERVENTIONS
◆ Encourage maintenance of an elimination diet to help identify specific allergenic foods.
◆ Provide analgesics as needed.
◆ Provide passive range-of-motion exercises, if appropriate.
◆ Provide emotional support and reassurance, especially if the patient is temporarily disfigured by florid skin lesions.

MONITORING
◆ Condition and number of skin lesions
◆ Level of pain
◆ GI and GU complications

PATIENT TEACHING

GENERAL
Be sure to cover:
◆ need for the patient to immediately report any recurrence of symptoms (most common about 6 weeks after initial symptoms)
◆ importance of returning for follow-up urinalysis as scheduled.

RESOURCES
Organizations
Asthma and Allergy Foundation of America: *www.aafa.org*
National Institute of Allergy and Infectious Diseases: *www3.niaid.nih.gov*

Selected references
Diseases, 4th ed. Philadelphia: Lippincott Williams & Wilkins, 2006.

Allergic rhinitis

OVERVIEW

- An immune response of the upper airways triggered by inhaled airborne allergens
- Seasonal allergic rhinitis is an immunoglobulin (Ig) E-mediated type I hypersensitivity response to an environmental antigen (allergen) in a genetically susceptible person
- In perennial allergic rhinitis, inhaled allergens provoke antigen responses that produce signs and symptoms year-round

PATHOPHYSIOLOGY

- The body's immune system overresponds to common allergens in the nose.
- Antibodies attach to mast cells, which release several chemicals, including histamine, that cause dilation of blood vessels, skin redness, and swollen membranes in the nose.

CAUSES
Seasonal allergic rhinitis

- Grass and weed pollens (in summer)
- Mold spores (occasionally, in summer and fall)
- Tree pollens (in spring)
- Weed pollens (in fall)

Perennial allergic rhinitis

- Animal dander
- House dust and dust mites
- Molds
- Processed materials or industrial chemicals
- Tobacco smoke

INCIDENCE

- Allergic rhinitis affects more than 20 million Americans.
- This disorder can affect anyone at any age.
- Allergic rhinitis is most prevalent in young children and adolescents.

COMPLICATIONS

- Nasal polyps
- Secondary sinus and middle ear infections

ASSESSMENT

HISTORY
Seasonal allergic rhinitis

- Paroxysmal sneezing, profuse watery rhinorrhea
- Nasal obstruction or congestion
- Pruritus of the nose and eyes
- Headache or sinus pain
- Itchy throat, malaise, and fever

Perennial allergic rhinitis

- Chronic and extensive nasal obstruction or stuffiness

PHYSICAL FINDINGS
Seasonal allergic rhinitis

- Pale, cyanotic, edematous nasal mucosa
- Red and edematous eyelids and conjunctivae
- Excessive lacrimation

Perennial allergic rhinitis

- Nasal polyps
- Dark circles under the eyes (allergic shiners)

DIAGNOSTIC TEST RESULTS

LABORATORY

- Eosinophil count is elevated in sputum and nasal secretions.
- IgE levels are normal or elevated.

TREATMENT

GENERAL
◆ Eliminate environmental antigens, if possible

DIET
◆ Increased fluid intake to loosen secretions

ACTIVITY
◆ Restrict activities in areas of allergen exposure

MEDICATIONS
◆ Antihistamines
◆ Intranasal corticosteroids
◆ Nasal decongestants

Long-term management
◆ Immunotherapy or desensitization with injections of allergen extracts administered before or during the allergy season or perennially

NURSING CONSIDERATIONS

NURSING DIAGNOSES
◆ Acute pain
◆ Impaired skin integrity
◆ Ineffective airway clearance
◆ Ineffective breathing pattern
◆ Ineffective health maintenance
◆ Risk for infection

EXPECTED OUTCOMES
The patient (or his family) will:
◆ express feeling of comfort and relief from pain
◆ maintain skin integrity
◆ maintain a patent airway
◆ maintain effective breathing pattern
◆ maintain current health status
◆ avoid infection and other complications.

NURSING INTERVENTIONS
◆ Implement measures to relieve signs and symptoms and increase the patient's comfort.
◆ Encourage increased fluid intake to loosen secretions.
◆ Elevate the head of the bed and provide humidification to ease breathing.

WARNING *Before giving a desensitization injection, assess the patient's symptoms. After giving the injection, observe him for 30 minutes to detect adverse reactions, including anaphylaxis and severe localized erythema. Make sure epinephrine and emergency resuscitation equipment are available.*

MONITORING
◆ Compliance with the prescribed drug regimen
◆ Changes in control of signs and symptoms
◆ Indications of drug misuse

PATIENT TEACHING

GENERAL
Be sure to cover:
◆ importance of calling the practitioner if the patient experiences a delayed reaction to the desensitization injections
◆ reduction of environmental exposure to airborne allergens
◆ skin protectant applications
◆ possible lifestyle changes, such as relocation to a pollen-free area either seasonally or year-round, in severe and resistant allergic rhinitis
◆ medication administration, dosage, and adverse effects.

RESOURCES
Organizations
Asthma and Allergy Foundation of America: *www.aafa.org*
National Institute of Allergy and Infectious Diseases: *www3.niaid.nih.gov*

Selected references
Gelfand, E.W. "Pediatric Allergic Rhinitis: Factors Affecting Treatment Choice," *Ear Nose & Throat Journal* 84(3):163-68, March 2005.
Hayden, M.L. "Allergic Rhinitis: Proper Management Benefits Concomitant Diseases," *Nurse Practitioner* 29(12): 26-30, 35-37, December 2004.
Kasper, D.L., et al, eds. *Harrison's Principles of Internal Medicine*, 16th ed. New York: McGraw-Hill Book Co., 2005.

Alopecia

- More commonly known as hair loss, typically occurring on the scalp; less common and conspicuous elsewhere on the body
- Can be irreversible in scarring alopecia, which usually destroys hair follicle
- Hair can generally regrow in nonscarring alopecia (noncicatricial alopecia)
- Most common form of nonscarring alopecia known as male pattern alopecia or androgenetic alopecia
- Telogen effluvium: A diffuse alopecia in which numerous hair follicles simultaneously change from the growing anagen phase to the resting telogen phase of the hair growth cycle
- Alopecia areata (idiopathic form): A generally reversible and self-limiting disorder most prevalent in young and middle-age adults of both sexes
- Genetic predisposition commonly influences time of onset, degree of baldness, speed with which it spreads, and pattern of hair loss
- Poor prognosis for regrowth with hair loss that persists for more than 1 year

PATHOPHYSIOLOGY
- In male pattern alopecia, a genetically predisposed response to androgens causes transformation of the androgen-sensitive follicles into vellus follicles; normal hair is shed and replaced by fine, light, short hair.
- In female pattern alopecia, serum adrenal androgen dehydroepiandrosterone sulfate is commonly elevated.

CAUSES
Nonscarring alopecia
- Aging
- Androgen response
- Bacterial and fungal infections
- Chemotherapy
- Drugs (see *Cancer drugs that cause alopecia*)
- Endocrine disorders
- Excess vitamin A
- Genetic predisposition
- Psoriasis
- Radiation
- Seborrhea

Scarring alopecia
- Chemotherapy
- Chronic tension on a hair shaft
- Destructive skin tumors
- Follicular lichen planus
- Granulomas
- Lupus erythematosus
- Physical or chemical trauma
- Radiation
- Scleroderma
- Severe bacterial or viral infections

INCIDENCE
- Alopecia affects men more than women.
- Male pattern alopecia occurs most frequently in men older than age 50.
- Incidence rises with increasing age in male pattern alopecia.
- Alopecia occurs to some degree in 37% of postmenopausal women.

COMPLICATIONS
- Impaired self-image

HISTORY
Male pattern alopecia
- Presence of predisposing factors
- Family history of hair loss
- Gradual onset of hair loss
- Typically describes hairline as receding and crown becoming bald

Female pattern alopecia
- Typically describes a widening of the part and increasing visibility of the front scalp or crown

Telogen effluvium
- Loss of about 400 hairs per day, which is four to five times greater than the normal daily hair loss

Alopecia areata
- Sudden loss of hair

PHYSICAL FINDINGS
- Small patches of visible scalp or the entire scalp may be visible (alopecia totalis); hair loss may involve the entire body (alopecia universalis)
- Although mild erythema may occur initially, affected areas of scalp or skin appear normal
- "Exclamation point" hairs (loose hairs with dark, rough, brushlike tips on narrow, less-pigmented shafts) occur at the periphery of new patches
- Regrowth initially appears as fine, white, downy hair that's replaced by normal hair

---

Cancer drugs that cause alopecia

Certain cancer drugs can cause hair loss that ranges from sporadic thinning to complete baldness. Some drugs damage hair follicles and cause hair roots to atrophy.

MILD ALOPECIA	MODERATE ALOPECIA	SEVERE ALOPECIA
• bleomycin	• busulfan	• cyclophosphamide
• carmustine	• etoposide	• daunorubicin
• fluorouracil	• floxuridine	• doxorubicin
• hydroxyurea	• methotrexate	• vinblastine
• melphalan	• mitomycin	• vincristine

LABORATORY
- Direct microscopic examination of a hair sample shows structural abnormalities or signs of infection.

DIAGNOSTIC PROCEDURES
Telogen effluvium
- Pluck or pull test reveals positive results if more than four hairs come out.
- Wood's lamp examination shows presence of fungal infection.
- Trichogram shows abnormal ratio of anagen to telogen hairs.
- Scalp biopsy shows hair phase and the extent of structural damage.

TREATMENT

GENERAL
- Identification and treatment of underlying cause
- Cosmetic interventions, such as hairpieces, weaving, or bonding
- Occlusive dressing promotes normal hair growth by protecting the site of hair loss (in trichotillomania)
- Cold cap application and use of scalp tourniquet to reduce the blood supply to the scalp and thereby preserve more hair structure

MEDICATIONS
- Topical application of minoxidil (Rogaine)
- Oral finasteride (Propecia)

   WARNING *Finasteride is contraindicated in women of childbearing age.*
- Corticosteroids
- Photochemotherapy with methoxsalen and ultraviolet light
- Dermatomucosal agents
- Antibiotics
- Antifungal agents

SURGERY
- Surgical redistribution of hair follicles by autografting
- Hair transplantation and tunnel grafting

NURSING DIAGNOSES
- Disturbed body image
- Risk for impaired skin integrity
- Risk for infection
- Situational low self-esteem

EXPECTED OUTCOMES
The patient will:
- verbalize feelings about changed body image
- maintain skin integrity
- remain free from all signs and symptoms of infection
- voice feelings related to self-esteem.

NURSING INTERVENTIONS
- Give prescribed drugs.
- Reassure the patient with female pattern alopecia that hair thinning doesn't lead to total baldness. Suggest that she use a wig or hairpiece.
- For the patient undergoing radiation therapy or chemotherapy with drugs that cause alopecia, suggest selecting a hair replacement option before treatment.
- Encourage the patient to express his feelings. Help him develop interests that contribute to a positive self-image.

MONITORING
- Complications
- Response to treatment

GENERAL
Be sure to cover:
- the disorder, diagnosis, and treatment
- medications and potential adverse reactions
- when to notify the practitioner
- familial link in male pattern alopecia
- well-balanced diet with adequate protein
- avoidance of excess vitamin A
- myths concerning commercial preparations
- signs and symptoms of skin infection
- possibility that hair may grow back in a different color or type, such as curly or straight.

RESOURCES
Organizations
American Cancer Society: *www.cancer.org*
National Alopecia Areata Foundation: *www.naaf.org*

Selected references
Prickitt, J., et al. "Helping Patients Cope with Chronic Alopecia Areata," *Dermatology Nursing* 16(3):237-41, June 2004.
Thiedke, C.C. "Alopecia in Women — Problem-Oriented Diagnosis," *American Family Physician* 65(5):1007-1014, March 2003.

Alzheimer's disease

OVERVIEW

- Degenerative disorder of the cerebral cortex (especially the frontal lobe), which accounts for more than 50% of all cases of dementia
- Poor prognosis
- No cure or definitive treatment

PATHOPHYSIOLOGY

- Initially involves the parts of the brain that control thought, memory, and language
- Brain damage caused by genetic substance (amyloid)
- Three distinguishing features of brain tissue: Neurofibrillary tangles, neuritic plaques, and granulovascular degeneration

CAUSES

- Unknown

RISK FACTORS

Neurochemical
- Risk factor gene identified for late-onset Alzheimer's disease

Environmental
- Aluminum and manganese
- Trauma
- Slow-growing central nervous system viruses

INCIDENCE

- The severe form of Alzheimer's disease usually occurs in patients older than age 65.
- Mild to moderate dementia occurs in 12% of patients.
- Alzheimer's disease may affect up to 5 million U.S. residents and more than 30 million people worldwide.

COMPLICATIONS

- Injury from violent behavior, wandering, or unsupervised activity
- Pneumonia and other infections
- Malnutrition and dehydration

ASSESSMENT

HISTORY

- History obtained from a family member or caregiver
- Insidious onset: Initial changes almost imperceptible
- Forgetfulness and subtle memory loss; difficulty learning and remembering new information
- Loss of short-term (recent) memory but retention of long-term (early life) memory
- General deterioration in personal hygiene
- Inability to concentrate
- Tendency to perform repetitive actions and experience restlessness
- Personality changes (irritability, depression, paranoia, hostility, apathy, anxiety, fear)
- Nocturnal awakening
- Disorientation
- Suspicion and fear of imaginary people and situations
- Misperceptions about own environment
- Misidentification of objects and people (inability to recognize family and friends)
- Complaints of stolen or misplaced objects
- Labile emotions
- Mood swings, sudden angry outbursts, and sleep disturbances

PHYSICAL FINDINGS

- Impaired sense of smell (usually an early symptom)
- Impaired stereognosis
- Gait disorders
- Tremors
- Loss of recent memory
- Positive snout reflex
- Organic brain disease in adults
- Urinary or fecal incontinence
- Seizures

DIAGNOSTIC TEST RESULTS

- Diagnosis is by exclusion; tests are performed to rule out other diseases.
- Positive diagnosis is made on autopsy.

IMAGING

- Positron emission tomography reveals metabolic activity of the cerebral cortex.
- Computed tomography scan shows excessive and progressive brain atrophy and rules out other neurologic problems.
- Magnetic resonance imaging rules out intracranial lesions and detects biochemical and anatomic changes.
- Cerebral blood flow studies reveal abnormalities in blood flow to the brain.

DIAGNOSTIC PROCEDURES

- Cerebrospinal fluid analysis shows chronic neurologic infection.
- EEG evaluates the brain's electrical activity and may show slowing of the brain waves in late stages of the disease.

OTHER

- Neuropsychological tests may show impaired cognitive ability and reasoning.

GENERAL
◆ Behavioral interventions (patient-centered or caregiver training) focused on managing cognitive and behavioral changes

DIET
◆ Well-balanced (may need to be monitored)

ACTIVITY
◆ Safe activities as tolerated (may need to be monitored)

MEDICATIONS
◆ Cerebral vasodilators
◆ Psychostimulators
◆ Antidepressants
◆ Anxiolytics
◆ Neurolytics
◆ Anticonvulsants (experimental)
◆ Anti-inflammatories (experimental)
◆ Anticholinesterase agents
◆ Vitamin E

NURSING CONSIDERATIONS

NURSING DIAGNOSES
◆ Bathing or hygiene self-care deficit
◆ Compromised family coping
◆ Constipation
◆ Dressing or grooming self-care deficit
◆ Feeding self-care deficit
◆ Imbalanced nutrition: Less than body requirements
◆ Impaired verbal communication
◆ Ineffective coping
◆ Risk for infection
◆ Risk for injury
◆ Toileting self-care deficit

EXPECTED OUTCOMES
The patient (or his family) will:
◆ perform self-care activities related to bathing and hygiene
◆ use support systems and develop adequate coping behaviors
◆ have normal bowel movements
◆ perform self-care activities related to dressing and grooming
◆ perform self-care activities related to feeding
◆ consume required caloric intake
◆ develop alternate means of communication to express self
◆ demonstrate effective coping skills
◆ remain free from all signs and symptoms of infection
◆ remain free from injury
◆ perform self-care activities related to toileting.

NURSING INTERVENTIONS
◆ Provide an effective communication system.
◆ Use soft tones and a slow, calm manner when speaking to the patient.
◆ Allow the patient sufficient time to answer questions.
◆ Protect the patient from injury.
◆ Provide rest periods.
◆ Provide an exercise program.
◆ Encourage independence.
◆ Offer frequent toileting.
◆ Assist with hygiene and dressing.
◆ Give prescribed drugs.
◆ Provide familiar objects to help with orientation and behavior control.
◆ Frequently remind the patient of the day and hour.
◆ Place familiar objects in the patient's easy reach and view.
◆ Be consistent and give simple step-by-step instructions.

MONITORING
◆ Response to medications
◆ Fluid intake and nutrition status
◆ Environment (for safety purposes)
◆ Follow-up visits with practitioner

GENERAL
Be sure to cover:
◆ the disease process
◆ exercise regimen
◆ aids in dressing and grooming
◆ importance of cutting food and providing finger foods, if indicated
◆ use of plates with rim guards, built-up utensils, and cups with lids
◆ independence
◆ home safety precautions.

DISCHARGE PLANNING
◆ Refer the patient (and his family or caregivers) to the Alzheimer's Association.
◆ Refer the patient (and his family or caregivers) to a local support group.
◆ Refer the patient (and his family or caregivers) to social services for additional support.

RESOURCES
Organizations
Alzheimer's Association: *www.alz.org*
National Institutes of Health: *www.nih.gov*

Selected references
Diseases, 4th ed. Philadelphia: Lippincott Williams & Wilkins, 2006.
Handbook of Pathophysiology, 2nd ed. Philadelphia: Lippincott Williams & Wilkins, 2005.
Xiong, G., and Doraiswamy, P.M. "Combination Drug Therapy for Alzheimer's Disease: What Is Evidence-based, and What Is Not?" *Geriatrics* 60(6):22-26, June 2005.

Amebiasis

OVERVIEW

- An acute or chronic protozoal infection caused by *Entamoeba histolytica*
- Produces varying degrees of illness, from no symptoms to mild diarrhea to fulminant dysentery
- Extraintestinal type can induce hepatic abscess and infections of the lungs, pleural cavity, pericardium, peritoneum and, rarely, the brain
- Also known as *amebic dysentery*

PATHOPHYSIOLOGY

- *E. histolytica* exists in two forms — as a cyst (which can survive outside the body) and a trophozoite (which can't survive outside the body).
- The ingested cysts pass through the intestine, where digestive secretions break them down and liberate the motile trophozoites within.
- The trophozoites multiply and either invade and ulcerate the mucosa of the large intestine or simply feed on intestinal bacteria.
- As the trophozoites are carried slowly toward the rectum, they're encysted and then excreted in feces.

CAUSES

- Ingestion of feces-contaminated food or water

INCIDENCE

- Amebiasis occurs worldwide but is most common in the tropics, subtropics, and other areas with poor sanitation and health practices.
- Incidence in the United States is between 1% and 3% and may be higher among homosexuals and institutionalized people, in whom fecal-oral contamination is common.

COMPLICATIONS

- Subacute appendicitis
- Perforation of the intestinal wall, with spread to the liver, lungs, pleural cavity, peritoneum, and brain

ASSESSMENT

HISTORY
Acute amebic dysentery

- Fever, chills
- Abdominal cramping
- Profuse, bloody, mucoid diarrhea

Chronic amebic dysentery

- Multiple (4 to 18) foul-smelling mucus- and blood-tinged stools daily
- Mild fever
- Vague abdominal cramps
- Possible weight loss

PHYSICAL FINDINGS
Acute amebic dysentery

- Diffuse abdominal tenderness

Chronic amebic dysentery

- Tenderness over the cecum and ascending colon
- Hepatomegaly (occasionally)

DIAGNOSTIC TEST RESULTS

LABORATORY

- Stool or aspirates from abscesses, ulcers, or tissue show *E. histolytica*.
- Positive indirect hemagglutination test result with current or previous infection.
- Positive complement fixation test result (usually only during active disease).

IMAGING

- Barium studies rule out nonamebic causes of diarrhea, such as polyps and cancer.

DIAGNOSTIC PROCEDURES

- Sigmoidoscopy detects rectosigmoid ulceration.

TREATMENT

GENERAL
◆ Avoidance of enemas

DIET
◆ Small, frequent meals
◆ Increased fluid intake

ACTIVITY
◆ Frequent rest periods

MEDICATIONS
◆ Metronidazole
◆ Emetine hydrochloride
◆ Iodoquinol (diiodohydroxyquin)
◆ Chloroquine
◆ Tetracycline (in combination with emetine hydrochloride, metronidazole, or paromomycin)

SURGERY
◆ Exploratory surgery hazardous; can lead to peritonitis, perforation, and pericecal abscess

NURSING CONSIDERATIONS

NURSING DIAGNOSES
◆ Acute pain
◆ Deficient fluid volume
◆ Diarrhea
◆ Fatigue
◆ Hyperthermia
◆ Imbalanced nutrition: Less than body requirements
◆ Impaired skin integrity
◆ Risk for infection

EXPECTED OUTCOMES
The patient will:
◆ express feelings of increased comfort and relief from pain
◆ have balanced intake and output
◆ return to a normal elimination pattern
◆ express feelings of energy and decreased fatigue
◆ remain afebrile
◆ consume required caloric intake
◆ maintain skin integrity
◆ develop no signs or symptoms of infection.

NURSING INTERVENTIONS
◆ Encourage adequate fluid intake.
◆ Give prescribed drugs.
◆ Apply perirectal protective cream to prevent excoriation and skin breakdown.

MONITORING
◆ Vital signs, especially temperature
◆ Fluid and electrolyte balance
◆ Daily weight
◆ Frequency, amount, and character of stools
◆ Skin integrity

PATIENT TEACHING

GENERAL
Be sure to cover:
◆ need for avoiding alcohol ingestion when taking metronidazole, the combination of which can cause nausea, vomiting, and headache
◆ importance of returning for follow-up appointments
◆ need to advise family and sexual partners to seek medical attention for amebiasis
◆ how to handle infectious material and perform proper hand washing
◆ safe sex practices
◆ boiling untreated or contaminated water when traveling to endemic areas.

RESOURCES
Organizations
Centers for Disease Control and Prevention: *www.cdc.gov*

Selected references
Ressel, G.W. "CDC Issues Recommendations for Diagnosing, Managing, and Reporting Foodborne Illnesses," *American Family Physician* 86:981-85, September 2004.

Amenorrhea

- The abnormal absence or suppression of menstruation
- Primary amenorrhea: The absence of menarche in an adolescent (age 16 and older)
- Secondary amenorrhea: The failure of menstruation for at least 3 months after the normal onset of menarche

PATHOPHYSIOLOGY

Primary amenorrhea
- The hypothalamic-pituitary-ovarian axis is dysfunctional.
- Anatomic defects of the central nervous system cause the ovary not to receive the hormonal signals that normally initiate the development of secondary sex characteristics and the beginning of menstruation.

Secondary amenorrhea
- The endometrium is sufficiently scarred and no functional endometrium exists.

CAUSES
- Absence of a uterus
- Constant presence of progesterone or other endocrine abnormalities
- Emotional disorders
- Endometrial damage
- Hormonal abnormalities
- Lack of ovarian response to gonadotropins
- Malnutrition and intense exercise
- Ovarian, adrenal, or pituitary tumors
- Pregnancy

INCIDENCE
- Primary amenorrhea occurs in 0.3% of women.
- Secondary amenorrhea occurs in 5% of women.

COMPLICATIONS
- Endometrial adenocarcinoma
- Estrogen deficiency syndrome
- Infertility
- Osteoporosis

HISTORY
- Failure to menstruate in women ages 16 and older
- Absence of menstruation for 3 months in a previously established menstrual pattern
- Change in menstrual pattern
- Dependent on cause of amenorrhea: May include headaches, hot flashes, nausea, weight gain or loss, emotional upset, trauma, extreme exercise, prolonged use of hormonal contraceptives

PHYSICAL FINDINGS
- Dependent on cause of amenorrhea: may include hirsutism, acne, abdominal mass, signs of malnutrition

LABORATORY
- Pregnancy test result is positive (when pregnancy is the cause).
- Pituitary gonadotropin levels may be elevated or low.
- Serum thyroid levels are abnormal.
- Serum progesterone levels are abnormal.
- Serum androgen levels are abnormal.
- Urinary 17-ketosteroid levels are elevated, with excessive androgen secretions.
- Plasma follicle-stimulating hormone (FSH) level is more than 50 IU/L, depending on the laboratory (suggests primary ovarian failure).
- FSH levels are normal or low (possible hypothalamic or pituitary abnormality, depending on the clinical situation).

IMAGING
- X-rays identify ovarian, adrenal, and pituitary tumors.

DIAGNOSTIC PROCEDURES
- Cervical mucus shows ferning on microscopic examination (an estrogen effect).
- Vaginal cytologic examination rules out carcinoma.
- Endometrial biopsy rules out endometrial hyperplasia or carcinoma.

OTHER
- Pelvic examination reveals anatomic abnormalities.

TREATMENT

GENERAL
◆ Based on cause

DIET
◆ Well-balanced

ACTIVITY
◆ Moderate exercise

MEDICATIONS
◆ Progestational agents (to stimulate menstruation)
◆ Calcium supplement (if cause is hypoestrogenism)
◆ Clomiphene citrate (may induce ovulation in women with amenorrhea caused by gonadotropin deficiency, polycystic ovarian disease, or excessive weight loss or gain)
◆ FSH and human menopausal gonadotropins for women with pituitary disease

SURGERY
◆ Removal of tumor or obstruction

NURSING CONSIDERATIONS

NURSING DIAGNOSES
◆ Anxiety
◆ Deficient fluid volume
◆ Delayed growth and development
◆ Disturbed body image
◆ Imbalanced nutrition: Less than body requirements
◆ Risk for situational low self-esteem

EXPECTED OUTCOMES
The patient will:
◆ verbalize feelings of anxiety and fear
◆ maintain adequate fluid balance
◆ express understanding of norms for growth and development
◆ verbalize feelings about changed body image
◆ consume required caloric intake
◆ voice feelings related to self-esteem.

NURSING INTERVENTIONS
◆ Provide reassurance and emotional support.
◆ Give prescribed drugs.

MONITORING
◆ Signs and symptoms
◆ Intake and output
◆ Laboratory test results

PATIENT TEACHING

GENERAL
Be sure to cover:
◆ the disorder, diagnosis, and treatment
◆ how to keep an accurate record of menstrual cycles to aid in early detection of recurrent amenorrhea.

DISCHARGE PLANNING
◆ Refer the patient for psychological counseling, if appropriate.

RESOURCES
Organizations
Association of Reproductive Health Professionals: *www.arhp.org*
Mayo Clinic: *www.mayoclinic.com*

Selected references
Kirn, T.F. "Delay Oral Contraceptive Use: Improve Diet First in Athletic Amenorrhea," *OB/GYN News* 39(15):18, August 2004.

Amyotrophic lateral sclerosis LIFE-THREATENING DISORDER

OVERVIEW

- Chronic, rapidly progressive, and debilitating neurologic disease that's incurable and invariably fatal
- Attacks neurons responsible for controlling involuntary movements
- Characterized by weakness that begins in upper extremities and progressively involves neck and throat, eventually leading to disability, respiratory failure, and death
- Also known as *ALS* or *Lou Gehrig disease*

PATHOPHYSIOLOGY

- An excitatory neurotransmitter accumulates to toxic levels.
- Motor units no longer innervate.
- Progressive degeneration of axons causes loss of myelin.
- Progressive degeneration of upper and lower motor neurons occurs.
- Progressive degeneration of motor nuclei in the cerebral cortex and corticospinal tracts results.

CAUSES

- Exact cause unknown
- Immune complexes such as those formed in autoimmune disorders
- Inherited as an autosomal dominant trait by 10% of patients
- Virus that creates metabolic disturbances in motor neurons

Precipitating factors that cause acute deterioration

- Severe stress such as myocardial infarction
- Traumatic injury
- Viral infections
- Physical exhaustion

INCIDENCE

- ALS is three times more common in men than in women.
- It affects people ages 40 to 70.

COMPLICATIONS

- Respiratory tract infections and respiratory failure
- Complications of immobility
- Aspiration
- Injury

ASSESSMENT

HISTORY

- Mental function intact
- Family history of ALS
- Asymmetrical weakness first noticed in one limb
- Easy fatigue and easy cramping in the affected muscles

PHYSICAL FINDINGS

- Location of the affected motor neurons
- Severity of the disease
- Fasciculations in the affected muscles
- Progressive weakness in muscles of the arms, legs, and trunk
- Brisk and overactive stretch reflexes
- Difficulty talking, chewing, swallowing, and breathing
- Shortness of breath and occasional drooling

DIAGNOSTIC TEST RESULTS

LABORATORY

- Protein in cerebrospinal fluid (CSF) is increased.

IMAGING

- Computed tomography scan rules out other disorders.

DIAGNOSTIC PROCEDURES

- Muscle biopsy discloses atrophic fibers.
- EEG rules out other disorders.

OTHER

- Electromyography shows the electrical abnormalities of involved muscles.
- Nerve conduction study results appear normal.
- Lumbar puncture and CSF analysis may be performed.

TREATMENT

GENERAL

- Rehabilitative measures
- Occupational and physical therapy
- Oxygen support

DIET

- May need tube feedings

ACTIVITY

- As tolerated

MEDICATIONS

- Muscle relaxants
- Antidepressants
- Benadryl (for excessive salivation)
- Dantrolene
- Baclofen
- I.V. or intrathecal administration of thyrotropin-releasing hormone
- Riluzole (Rilutek) (slows progression)

NURSING DIAGNOSES
- Anticipatory grieving
- Anxiety
- Bathing or hygiene self-care deficit
- Compromised family coping
- Dressing or grooming self-care deficit
- Feeding self-care deficit
- Imbalanced nutrition: Less than body requirements
- Impaired physical mobility
- Impaired verbal communication
- Ineffective airway clearance
- Ineffective breathing pattern
- Ineffective coping
- Risk for impaired skin integrity
- Risk for infection

EXPECTED OUTCOMES
The patient will:
- demonstrate adaptive coping behaviors
- verbalize feelings of anxiety and fear
- perform self-care activities related to bathing and hygiene
- develop adequate coping mechanisms and support systems
- perform self-care activities related to dressing and grooming
- perform self-care activities related to feeding
- consume required caloric intake
- maintain joint mobility and range of motion (ROM)
- develop alternate means of communication to express self
- maintain a patent airway and adequate ventilation
- maintain effective breathing pattern
- seek support systems and exhibit adequate coping behaviors
- maintain skin integrity
- remain free from all signs and symptoms of infection.

NURSING INTERVENTIONS
- Provide emotional and psychological support.
- Promote independence.
- Turn and reposition the patient frequently.
- Give prescribed drugs.
- Provide airway and respiratory management.
- Promote nutrition.
- Maintain aspiration precautions.

MONITORING
- Muscle weakness
- Respiratory status
- Speech
- Swallowing ability
- Skin integrity
- Nutritional status
- Environment (for safety purposes)
- Response to treatment
- Complications
- Signs and symptoms of infection

GENERAL
Be sure to cover:
- the disorder, diagnosis, and treatment
- swallowing therapy regimen
- medications and adverse effects
- skin care
- ROM exercises
- deep-breathing and coughing exercises
- safety in the home. (See *Modifying the home for a patient with ALS.*)

DISCHARGE PLANNING
- Refer the patient to a local ALS support group.
- Refer the patient to consult with a mental health counselor.

RESOURCES
Organizations
ALS Association: *www.alsa.org*
National Institutes of Health: *www.nih.gov*

Selected references
Diseases, 4th ed. Philadelphia: Lippincott Williams & Wilkins, 2006.
Handbook of Pathophysiology, 2nd ed. Philadelphia: Lippincott Williams & Wilkins, 2005.

Modifying the home for a patient with ALS

To help the patient with amyotrophic lateral sclerosis (ALS) live safely at home, follow these guidelines:
- Explain basic safety precautions, such as keeping stairs and pathways free from clutter; using nonskid mats in the bathroom and in place of loose throw rugs; keeping stairs well lit; installing handrails in stairwells and the shower, tub, and toilet areas; and removing electrical and telephone cords from traffic areas.
- Discuss the need for rearranging the furniture, moving items in or out of the patient's care area, and obtaining a hospital bed, a commode, or oxygen equipment.
- Recommend devices to ease the patient's and caregiver's work, such as extra pillows or a wedge pillow to help the patient sit up, a draw sheet to help him move up in bed, a lap tray for eating, and a bell for calling the caregiver.
- Help the patient adjust to changes in the environment. Encourage independence.
- Advise the patient to keep a suction machine handy to reduce the fear of choking due to secretion accumulation and dysphagia. Teach him how to suction himself when necessary.

Anaphylaxis LIFE-THREATENING DISORDER

OVERVIEW

- Dramatic, acute atopic reaction to an allergen
- Marked by sudden onset of rapidly progressive urticaria and respiratory distress
- More severe the sooner signs and symptoms appear after exposure to the antigen
- Severe reactions may initiate vascular collapse, leading to systemic shock and, possibly, death

PATHOPHYSIOLOGY

- After initial exposure to an antigen, the immune system produces specific immunoglobulin (Ig) antibodies in the lymph nodes. Helper T cells enhance the process.
- The antibodies (IgE) then bind to membrane receptors located on mast cells and basophils.
- After the body reencounters the antigen, the IgE antibodies, or cross-linked IgE receptors, recognize the antigen as foreign; this activates the release of powerful chemical mediators.
- IgG or IgM enters into the reaction and activates the release of complement factors.

CAUSES

- Systemic exposure to sensitizing drugs, foods, insect venom, or other specific antigens

INCIDENCE

- The most common anaphylaxis-causing antigen is penicillin, which induces a reaction in 1 to 4 of every 10,000 patients treated.

COMPLICATIONS

- Respiratory obstruction
- Systemic vascular collapse
- Death

ASSESSMENT

HISTORY

- Immediately after exposure, complaints of a feeling of impending doom or fright and exhibition of apprehension, restlessness, cyanosis, cool and clammy skin, erythema, edema, tachypnea, weakness, sweating, sneezing, dyspnea, nasal pruritus, and urticaria
- A "lump" in the patient's throat caused by angioedema
- Dyspnea and complaints of chest tightness

PHYSICAL FINDINGS

- Hives
- Hoarseness or stridor, wheezing
- Severe abdominal cramps, nausea, diarrhea
- Urinary urgency and incontinence
- Dizziness, drowsiness, headache, restlessness, and seizures
- Hypotension, shock; sometimes, angina and cardiac arrhythmias
- Angioedema

DIAGNOSTIC TEST RESULTS

- No tests are required to identify anaphylaxis. The patient's history and signs and symptoms establish the diagnosis.

LABORATORY

- Skin testing may help to identify a specific allergen.

TREATMENT

GENERAL

- Maintaining a patent airway
- Cardiopulmonary resuscitation, if cardiac arrest occurs

DIET

- Nothing by mouth until stable

ACTIVITY

- Bed rest until stable

MEDICATIONS

- Immediate injection of epinephrine 1:1,000 aqueous solution, 0.1 to 0.5 ml subcutaneously or I.V.
- Corticosteroids
- Diphenhydramine (Benadryl) I.V.
- Volume expander infusions as needed
- Vasopressors
- Norepinephrine (Leophed)
- Dopamine (Intropin)
- Aminophylline (Truphylline) I.V.
- Antihistamines

NURSING DIAGNOSES

- Anxiety
- Decreased cardiac output
- Deficient fluid volume
- Impaired gas exchange
- Impaired skin integrity
- Ineffective breathing pattern
- Powerlessness

EXPECTED OUTCOMES

The patient will:

- express feelings of decreased anxiety
- maintain normal cardiac output and normal heart rate
- maintain an adequate fluid balance
- maintain a patent airway and adequate ventilation
- maintain skin integrity
- maintain effective breathing pattern
- express feelings of having greater control over the current situation.

NURSING INTERVENTIONS

- Provide supplemental oxygen, and prepare to assist with insertion of an endotracheal tube, if necessary.
- Insert a peripheral I.V. line.
- Continually reassure the patient, and explain all tests and treatments.
- If the patient undergoes skin or scratch testing, monitor for signs of a serious allergic response. Keep emergency resuscitation equipment readily available.

WARNING *If a patient must receive a drug to which he's allergic, prevent a severe reaction by making sure he receives careful desensitization with gradually increasing doses of the antigen or with advance administration of corticosteroids. Closely monitor the patient during testing, and have resuscitation equipment and epinephrine readily available.*

MONITORING

- Vital signs
- Adverse reactions from radiographic contrast media
- Respiratory status
- Serious allergic response after skin or scratch testing
- Neurologic status
- Response to treatment
- Complications
- Degree of edema

GENERAL

Be sure to cover:

- risk of delayed symptoms and importance of reporting them immediately
- avoidance of exposure to known allergens
- importance of carrying and becoming familiar with an anaphylaxis kit and learning to use it before the need arises
- need for medical identification jewelry to identify allergy.

RESOURCES

Organizations

American Academy of Allergy, Asthma, and Immunology: w*ww.aaaai.org*
Mayo Clinic Allergy and Asthma Center: *www.mayoclinic.com/health/allergy/AA99999*
The Food Allergy & Anaphylaxis Network: *www.foodallergy.org*

Selected references

Burns, A. "Anaphylaxis," *Nursing* 34(3):88, March 2004.
Kasper, D., et al., eds. *Harrison's Principles of Internal Medicine*, 16th ed. New York: McGraw-Hill Book Co., 2005.
Nettina, S.M. *Lippincott Manual of Nursing Practice*, 8th ed. Philadelphia: Lippincott Williams & Wilkins, 2005.

Anemia, aplastic

OVERVIEW

- Potentially fatal marrow failure syndrome resulting from injury to or destruction of stem cells in bone marrow or the bone marrow matrix
- Causes pancytopenia (anemia, leukopenia, thrombocytopenia) and bone marrow hypoplasia

PATHOPHYSIOLOGY

- Usually develops when damaged or destroyed stem cells inhibit red blood cell (RBC) production
- Less commonly, develops when damaged bone marrow microvasculature creates an unfavorable environment for cell growth and maturation

CAUSES

- Congenital hypoplastic anemia, also known as anemia of Blackfan and Diamond, which develops between ages 2 and 3 months, and Fanconi's syndrome, developing between birth and age 10
- Idiopathic in some cases
- Immunologic factors; severe disease, especially hepatitis; viral infection, especially in children; and preleukemic and neoplastic infiltration of bone marrow
- Result of adverse drug reaction

INCIDENCE

- Aplastic anemia is more common in children and young adults than in other age populations.

COMPLICATIONS

- Hemorrhage
- Infection
- Heart failure

ASSESSMENT

HISTORY

- Fatigue
- Weakness
- Weight loss
- Dizziness
- Syncope
- Bruising
- Nosebleeds
- Shortness of breath

PHYSICAL FINDINGS

- Pallor, ecchymosis, petechiae, retinal hemorrhage
- Alterations in level of consciousness, weakness, fatigue
- Bibasilar crackles, tachycardia, and a gallop murmur
- Fever, oral and rectal ulcers, sore throat
- Nausea
- Decreased hair and skin quality
- Petechial rash

DIAGNOSTIC TEST RESULTS

LABORATORY

- RBC count is 1 million/mm^3 or less, usually with normochromic and normocytic cells; absolute reticulocyte count is very low.
- Serum iron levels are elevated (unless bleeding occurs), but total iron-binding capacity is normal or slightly reduced.
- Serum platelet and white blood cell counts are decreased.

DIAGNOSTIC PROCEDURES

- Bone marrow biopsies performed at several sites may yield a dry tap or show severely hypocellular or aplastic marrow, with a varying amount of fat, fibrous tissue, or gelatinous replacement; absence of tagged iron and megakaryocytes; and depression of erythroid elements.

TREATMENT

GENERAL

- Vigorous supportive measures, such as packed RBCs, platelets, and experimental histocompatibility antigen-matched leukocyte transfusions
- Respiratory support with oxygen
- Prevention of infection ranging from frequent hand washing to filtered airflow
- Neutropenic precautions, if appropriate

DIET

- Well-balanced

MEDICATIONS

- Antibiotics
- Corticosteroids
- Marrow-stimulating agents, such as androgens, antilymphocyte globulin (experimental), and immunosuppressant agents
- Granulocyte colony-stimulating factor, granulocyte-macrophage colony-stimulating factor, and erythropoietic-stimulating factor

SURGERY

- Bone marrow transplantation (for severe aplasia and patients who need continual RBC transfusions)

NURSING DIAGNOSES

- Activity intolerance
- Acute pain
- Ineffective tissue perfusion: Cerebral, cardiopulmonary
- Decreased cardiac output
- Fatigue
- Impaired gas exchange
- Impaired physical mobility
- Ineffective thermoregulation
- Risk for infection

EXPECTED OUTCOMES

The patient will:
- state the need to increase activity level gradually
- express feelings of increased comfort and decreased pain
- maintain vital signs within prescribed limits during activity
- maintain normal cardiac output
- express feelings of energy and decreased fatigue
- exhibit adequate ventilation
- maintain joint mobility and range of motion
- remain normothermic
- avoid infection and other complications.

NURSING INTERVENTIONS

- Help the patient to prevent or manage hemorrhage, infection, adverse effects of drug therapy, and blood transfusion reaction.
- If the patient's platelet count is low (less than 20,000/mm^3), prevent hemorrhage by avoiding I.M. injections by and suggesting the use of an electric razor and a soft toothbrush. Apply pressure to venipuncture sites until bleeding stops.
- Follow neutropenic precautions.
- Make sure throat, urine, nasal, stool, and blood cultures are tested regularly and correctly to check for infection.
- Schedule frequent rest periods.
- Administer oxygen therapy.
- Ensure a comfortable environmental temperature.

- If blood transfusions are necessary, administer according to facility policy and assess for transfusion reactions.

MONITORING

- Blood studies in patients receiving anemia-inducing drugs
- Early detection of bleeding

GENERAL

Be sure to cover:
- avoidance of contact with potential sources of infection, such as crowds, soil, and standing water that can harbor organisms
- disorder and its treatment
- prescribed drugs; possible adverse reactions and when to report them
- normal lifestyle with appropriate restrictions until remission occurs (for the patient who doesn't require hospitalization).

DISCHARGE PLANNING

- Refer the patient to the Aplastic Anemia Foundation of America for additional information, assistance, and support.

RESOURCES

Organizations

Aplastic Anemia & MDS International Foundation: *www.aamds.org/aplastic*
National Institutes of Health: *www.nih.gov*

Selected references

Kasper, D., et al., eds. *Harrison's Principles of Internal Medicine*, 16th ed. New York: McGraw-Hill Book Co., 2005.
Tierney, L., et al. *Current Medical Diagnosis and Treatment*. New York: McGraw-Hill Book Co., 2005.

Anemia, folic acid (folate) deficiency

OVERVIEW

- A common, slowly progressive megaloblastic anemia
- Caused by a deficiency of the vitamin folate

PATHOPHYSIOLOGY

- When folic acid stores in the body are low or diet is deficient in folic acid, the bone marrow produces large red blood cells or megaloblasts, resulting in anemia.

CAUSES

- Alcohol abuse
- Bacteria competing for available folic acid
- Excessive cooking of foods, which destroys the available nutrient
- Impaired absorption from small intestine
- Increased folic acid requirements during pregnancy; during rapid growth periods in infancy, childhood, and adolescence; and in patients with neoplastic diseases or some skin diseases such as exfoliative dermatitis
- Limited storage capacity in infants
- Poor diet
- Prolonged therapy with such drugs as anticonvulsants, estrogens, and methotrexate

INCIDENCE

- Folate deficiency anemia is most prevalent in infants, adolescents, pregnant and lactating women, alcoholics, elderly people, and people with malignant or intestinal diseases.

COMPLICATIONS

- Pregnant women with folic acid deficiency associated with increased risk of giving birth to a neonate with a neural tube defect

ASSESSMENT

HISTORY

- Severe, progressive fatigue — the hallmark of folic acid deficiency
- Diarrhea
- Nausea
- Anorexia
- Headaches
- Forgetfulness
- Irritability

PHYSICAL FINDINGS

- Shortness of breath
- Palpitations
- Weakness and light-headedness
- Generalized pallor and jaundice
- Wasted or malnourished appearance
- Possible cheilosis and glossitis
- Red, swollen, smooth, shiny, and tender tongue (glossitis)
- Reduced sense of taste

DIAGNOSTIC TEST RESULTS

LABORATORY

- Folic acid deficiency anemia and pernicious anemia are distinguished by the Schilling test and a therapeutic trial of vitamin B_{12} injections.
- Macrocytosis, decreased reticulocyte count, increased mean corpuscular volume, abnormal platelets, and serum folate levels less than 4 mg/ml are diagnostic.

TREATMENT

GENERAL
◆ Elimination of contributing causes

DIET
◆ Well-balanced; high in folic acid (see *Foods high in folic acid*)

ACTIVITY
◆ Frequent rest periods during activity as needed

MEDICATIONS
◆ Folic acid supplements
◆ Vitamin supplementation (women planning to become pregnant should begin at least 3 months before conception)
◆ Blood transfusions in severe cases

Foods high in folic acid

The body needs folic acid to develop healthy red blood cells and synthesize deoxyribonucleic acid. Although body stores are comparatively small (about 70 mg), this vitamin is plentiful in most well-balanced diets. However, because folic acid is water-soluble and heat-labile, it's easily destroyed by cooking. Also, about 20% of folic acid intake is excreted unabsorbed. Folic acid intake of less than 50 mcg/day usually induces folic acid deficiency within 4 months. Below is a list of foods high in folic acid.

FOOD	mcg/100 g
Asparagus spears	109
Beef liver	294
Broccoli spears	54
Collards (cooked)	102
Mushrooms	24
Oatmeal	33
Peanut butter	57
Red beans	180
Wheat germ	305

NURSING CONSIDERATIONS

NURSING DIAGNOSES
◆ Activity intolerance
◆ Deficient fluid volume
◆ Delayed growth and development
◆ Diarrhea
◆ Imbalanced nutrition: Less than body requirements
◆ Impaired gas exchange
◆ Impaired oral mucous membranes

EXPECTED OUTCOMES
The patient will:
◆ state the need to increase activity level gradually
◆ maintain an adequate fluid balance
◆ express understanding of norms for growth and development
◆ have normal bowel movements
◆ consume required caloric intake
◆ maintain adequate ventilation
◆ exhibit improved or healed wounds or lesions.

NURSING INTERVENTIONS
◆ Plan activities, rest periods, and necessary diagnostic tests to conserve energy.
◆ Advise the patient to report signs and symptoms of decreased perfusion to vital organs (dyspnea, chest pain, dizziness).
◆ If the patient has glossitis, emphasize the importance of good oral hygiene.
◆ Ask the dietitian to give the patient nonirritating foods, because a sore mouth and tongue make eating painful. If these symptoms make talking difficult, supply a pad and pencil or some other aid to facilitate communication.
◆ To ensure accurate Schilling test results, make sure that all urine excreted over a 24-hour period is collected and that the specimens remain uncontaminated by bacteria.
◆ Provide a well-balanced diet, including foods high in folate, such as dark green leafy vegetables, organ meats, eggs, milk, oranges, bananas, dry beans, and whole-grain breads.

MONITORING
◆ Vital signs
◆ Fluid and electrolyte balance

PATIENT TEACHING

GENERAL
Be sure to cover:
◆ importance of a well-balanced diet high in folic acid
◆ use of commercially prepared formulas for mothers who aren't breast-feeding
◆ daily folic acid requirements and the need to keep taking the supplements even when the patient begins to feel better
◆ importance of guarding against infections and reporting signs of infection promptly.

RESOURCES
Organizations
Iron Disorders Institute: *www.irondisorders.org*
Mayo Clinic: *www.mayoclinic.com*

Selected references
Kasper, D., et al., eds. *Harrison's Principles of Internal Medicine*, 16th ed. New York: McGraw-Hill Book Co., 2005.
Koren, G. "Folic Acid — Drugs, Pregnancy and Lactation," *OB/GYN News* 39(3):14, February 2004.
Koren, G. "Low-Carb Diets and Folic Acid Intake," *OB/GYN News* 39(16):9, August 2004.
Tierney, L., et al. *Current Medical Diagnosis and Treatment*. New York: McGraw-Hill Book Co., 2005.

Anemia, iron deficiency

- Decreased total iron body content, leading to diminished erythropoiesis
- Produces smaller (microcytic) cells with less color on staining (hypochromia)

PATHOPHYSIOLOGY

- Body stores of iron, including plasma iron, decrease.
- Transferrin, which binds with and transports iron, also decreases.
- Insufficient body stores of iron lead to a depleted red blood cell (RBC) mass and a decreased hemoglobin (Hb) concentration.
- Results in decreased oxygen-carrying capacity of the blood. (See *Iron absorption and storage.*)

CAUSES

- Blood loss secondary to drug-induced GI bleeding or due to heavy menses, hemorrhage from trauma, GI ulcers, malignant tumors, and varices
- Inadequate dietary intake of iron
- Intravascular hemolysis-induced hemoglobinuria or paroxysmal nocturnal hemoglobinuria
- Iron malabsorption
- Lead poisoning, in children
- Mechanical erythrocyte trauma caused by a prosthetic heart valve or vena cava filter
- Pregnancy

INCIDENCE

- Iron deficiency anemia is common worldwide.
- This type of anemia affects 10% to 30% of the adult population of the United States.
- This disorder is most prevalent among premenopausal women, infants, children, adolescents, alcoholics, and elderly people.

COMPLICATIONS

- Infection
- Organ and joint damage from overreplacement of oral or I.M. iron supplements
- Pneumonia

AGE FACTOR *In a child, iron deficiency anemia can cause pica, which may lead to eating lead-based paint, resulting in lead poisoning.*

ASSESSMENT

HISTORY

- Can persist for years without signs or symptoms
- Fatigue
- Inability to concentrate
- Headache, shortness of breath (especially on exertion)
- Increased frequency of infections
- Pica, an uncontrollable urge to eat strange things, such as clay, starch, ice and, in children, lead
- Menorrhagia
- Dysphagia
- Vasomotor disturbances
- Numbness and tingling of the extremities
- Neuralgic pain

PHYSICAL FINDINGS

- Red, swollen, smooth, shiny, and tender tongue (glossitis)
- Corners of the mouth may be eroded, tender, and swollen (angular stomatitis)
- Spoon-shaped, brittle nails
- Tachycardia

DIAGNOSTIC TEST RESULTS

LABORATORY

- Serum Hb levels are decreased (men, less than 12 g/dl; women, less than 10 g/dl) or mean corpuscular Hb levels are decreased in severe anemia.
- Serum hematocrit is decreased (men, less than 47 ml/dl; women, less than 42 ml/dl).
- Serum iron levels are decreased with high binding capacity.
- Serum ferritin levels are decreased.
- Serum RBC count is decreased, with microcytic and hypochromic cells (in early stages, RBC count may be normal, except in infants and children).

DIAGNOSTIC PROCEDURES

- Bone marrow studies reveal depleted or absent iron stores (done by staining) as well as normoblastic hyperplasia.
- GI studies, such as guaiac stool tests, barium swallow and enema, endoscopy, and sigmoidoscopy, rule out or confirm the diagnosis of bleeding causing the iron deficiency.

Iron absorption and storage

Found in abundance throughout the body, iron is needed for erythropoiesis. Two-thirds of total body iron is found in hemoglobin (Hb); the other third is found mostly in the reticuloendothelial system (liver, spleen, and bone marrow), with small amounts in muscle, serum, and body cells.

Adequate iron in the diet and recirculation of iron released from disintegrating red blood cells maintain iron supplies. The duodenum and upper part of the small intestine absorb dietary iron. Such absorption depends on the gastric acid content, the amount of reducing substances (ascorbic acid, for example) present in the alimentary canal, and the amount of iron intake. If iron intake is deficient, the body gradually depletes its iron stores, causing decreased Hb levels and, eventually, signs and symptoms of iron deficiency anemia.

GENERAL
◆ Based on underlying cause

DIET
◆ Nutritious, nonirritating foods

ACTIVITY
◆ Planned rest periods during activity

MEDICATIONS
◆ Oral preparation of iron or a combination of iron and ascorbic acid
◆ I.M. iron in rare cases
◆ Total-dose I.V. infusions of supplemental iron for pregnant and elderly patients with severe disease

NURSING CONSIDERATIONS

NURSING DIAGNOSES
◆ Activity intolerance
◆ Delayed growth and development
◆ Fatigue
◆ Imbalanced nutrition: Less than body requirements
◆ Impaired gas exchange
◆ Impaired oral mucous membranes
◆ Ineffective tissue perfusion: Cerebral, cardiopulmonary

EXPECTED OUTCOMES
The patient will:
◆ express feelings of increased energy
◆ express understanding of norms for growth and development
◆ express feelings of energy and decreased fatigue
◆ maintain weight without further loss
◆ maintain adequate ventilation
◆ exhibit improved or healed wounds or lesions
◆ maintain vital signs within prescribed limits during activity.

NURSING INTERVENTIONS
◆ Note the patient's signs or symptoms of decreased perfusion to vital organs.
◆ Provide oxygen therapy as necessary.
◆ Assess the family's dietary habits for iron intake, noting the influence of childhood eating patterns, cultural food preferences, and family income on adequate nutrition.
◆ Ask the dietitian to give the patient nonirritating foods.
◆ Give prescribed analgesics for headache and other discomfort.
◆ Evaluate the patient's drug history. Certain drugs, such as pancreatic enzymes and vitamin E, can interfere with iron metabolism and absorption; aspirin, steroids, and other drugs can cause GI bleeding.
◆ Provide frequent rest periods.
◆ If the patient receives iron I.V., monitor the infusion rate carefully and observe for an allergic reaction.
◆ Use the Z-track injection method when administering iron I.M. to prevent skin discoloration, scarring, and irritating iron deposits in the skin.
◆ Provide good nutrition and meticulous care of I.V. sites.

MONITORING
◆ Vital signs
◆ Compliance with prescribed iron supplement therapy
◆ Iron replacement overdose (see *Recognizing iron overdose*)

Recognizing iron overdose

Excessive iron replacement may produce signs and symptoms, such as diarrhea, fever, severe stomach pain, nausea, and vomiting.

When these signs and symptoms occur, notify the physician and give prescribed treatment, which may include chelation therapy, vigorous I.V. fluid replacement, gastric lavage, whole-bowel irrigation, and supplemental oxygen.

GENERAL
Be sure to cover:
◆ the disorder, diagnosis, and treatment
◆ dangers of lead poisoning, especially if the patient reports a history of pica
◆ importance of continuing therapy, even after the patient begins to feel better
◆ absorption interference of iron supplementation with milk or antacid
◆ increased absorption with vitamin C
◆ avoidance of staining teeth by drinking liquid iron supplement through a straw
◆ when to report adverse effects of iron therapy
◆ basics of a nutritionally balanced diet
◆ importance of avoiding infection and when to report signs of infection
◆ need for regular checkups
◆ compliance with prescribed treatment.

RESOURCES
Organizations
Iron Disorders Institute: *www.irondisorders.org*
Mayo Clinic: *www.mayoclinic.com*

Selected references
Kasper, D., et al., eds. *Harrison's Principles of Internal Medicine*, 16th ed. New York: McGraw-Hill Book Co., 2005.
Tierney, L., et al. *Current Medical Diagnosis and Treatment*. New York: McGraw-Hill Book Co., 2005.

Anemia, pernicious

- Deficiency of vitamin B_{12} causing serious neurologic, psychological, gastric, and intestinal abnormalities
- Characterized by decreased gastric production of hydrochloric acid and deficiency of intrinsic factor, essential for vitamin B_{12} absorption
- Also known as *Addison's anemia*

PATHOPHYSIOLOGY

- An inherited autoimmune response may cause gastric mucosal atrophy and resultant decreased production of hydrochloric acid and intrinsic factor, a substance normally secreted by the parietal cells of the gastric mucosa.
- Intrinsic factor deficiency impairs vitamin B_{12} absorption.
- Vitamin B_{12} deficiency inhibits the growth of all cells, particularly red blood cells (RBCs), leading to insufficient and deformed RBCs with poor oxygen-carrying capacity.

CAUSES

- Chronic gastric inflammation
- Genetic predisposition
- Secondary pernicious anemia results from partial removal of the stomach

INCIDENCE

- Pernicious anemia is common in Northern Europeans of fair complexion.
- In the United States, pernicious anemia is most common in New England and the Great Lakes region because of the heavy concentration of Northern Europeans in these areas.
- This type of anemia is rare in children, Blacks, and Asians.
- The onset of pernicious anemia is typically between ages 50 and 60; incidence increases with advancing age.

COMPLICATIONS

- Heart failure with severe anemia
- Myocardial ischemia
- Paralysis

- Psychotic behavior
- Loss of sphincter control of bowel and bladder
- Peptic ulcer disease

ASSESSMENT

HISTORY

- Characteristic triad of symptoms: Weakness; a beefy red, sore tongue; and numbness and tingling in the extremities
- GI disturbance: Nausea, vomiting, anorexia, weight loss, flatulence, diarrhea, and constipation
- Peripheral numbness and paresthesia
- Light-headedness
- Headache
- Diplopia and blurred vision
- Loss of taste
- Tinnitus

PHYSICAL FINDINGS

- Smooth, beefy red, painful tongue
- Slightly jaundiced sclera and pale to bright yellow skin
- Tachycardia
- Systolic murmur
- Enlarged liver and spleen
- Weakness in the extremities
- Disturbed position sense
- Lack of coordination
- Impaired fine finger movement
- Loss of bowel and bladder control
- Impotence (in men)
- Irritability, depression, delirium, and ataxia
- Memory loss
- Positive Babinski's and Romberg's signs
- Optic muscle atrophy

DIAGNOSTIC TEST RESULTS

LABORATORY

- Hemoglobin (Hb) level is decreased (4 to 5 g/dl).
- RBC count is decreased.
- Mean corpuscular volume is increased (less than 120 mm^3); mean corpuscular Hb concentration is increased.
- White blood cell and platelet counts may be decreased, and large, malformed platelets may appear.
- Serum vitamin B_{12} tests may show levels less than 0.1 mcg/ml.
- Serum lactate dehydrogenase levels may be elevated.

DIAGNOSTIC PROCEDURES

- Bone marrow studies reveal erythroid hyperplasia with increased numbers of megaloblasts but few normally developing RBCs.
- Gastric analysis shows an absence of free hydrochloric acid after histamine or pentagastrin injection.
- Schilling test may reveal a urinary excretion of less than 3% in the first 24 hours in patients with pernicious anemia; it may reveal normal excretion of vitamin B_{12} when repeated with intrinsic factor added.

TREATMENT

GENERAL
◆ Based on underlying cause

DIET
◆ Well-balanced, including foods high in vitamin B_{12}
◆ Sodium and fluid restriction for heart failure

ACTIVITY
◆ If anemia causes extreme fatigue, bed rest until Hb level increases

MEDICATIONS
◆ Early I.M. vitamin B_{12} replacement
◆ Maintenance levels (monthly) of vitamin B_{12} doses after the patient's condition improves

NURSING CONSIDERATIONS

NURSING DIAGNOSES
◆ Activity intolerance
◆ Fatigue
◆ Imbalanced nutrition: Less than body requirements
◆ Impaired gas exchange
◆ Impaired oral mucous membranes
◆ Impaired physical mobility
◆ Ineffective tissue perfusion: Cardiopulmonary
◆ Risk for infection
◆ Risk for injury

EXPECTED OUTCOMES
The patient will:
◆ state an understanding of the need to increase activity level gradually
◆ express feelings of energy and decreased fatigue
◆ consume required caloric intake
◆ maintain adequate ventilation
◆ exhibit improved or healed wounds or lesions
◆ maintain joint mobility and range of motion
◆ modify lifestyle to minimize risk of decreased tissue perfusion
◆ remain free from all signs and symptoms of infection
◆ remain free from injury.

NURSING INTERVENTIONS
◆ If the patient has severe anemia, plan activities, rest periods, and necessary diagnostic tests to conserve his energy.
◆ To ensure accurate Schilling test results, make sure that all urine excreted over a 24-hour period is collected.
◆ Provide a well-balanced diet, including foods high in vitamin B_{12}.
◆ Institute safety precautions to prevent falls.

MONITORING
◆ Vital signs
◆ Mental and neurologic status
◆ Environment (for safety purposes)

PATIENT TEACHING

GENERAL
Be sure to cover:
◆ protection against infections and when to report signs of infection
◆ when to report signs and symptoms of decreased perfusion to vital organs and symptoms of neuropathy
◆ avoidance of irritating foods
◆ avoidance of exposure to extreme heat or cold on the extremities
◆ continuation of vitamin B_{12} replacement even after symptoms subside
◆ proper injection techniques
◆ observance of symptoms of confusion and irritability and when to report them
◆ prevention of pernicious anemia by taking vitamin B_{12} supplements, in patients who have had extensive gastric resections or who follow strict vegetarian diets.

RESOURCES
Organizations
Mayo Clinic: *www.mayoclinic.com*
National Institutes of Health: *www.nih.gov*

Selected references
Kasper, D., et al., eds. *Harrison's Principles of Internal Medicine*, 16th ed. New York: McGraw-Hill Book Co., 2005.
Oh, R., and Brown D.L. "Vitamin B_{12} Deficiency," *American Family Physician* 67(5):979-86, March 2003.
Tierney, L., et al. *Current Medical Diagnosis and Treatment*. New York: McGraw-Hill Book Co., 2005.

Anemia, sickle cell

OVERVIEW

- Congenital hemolytic disease that results from a defective hemoglobin (Hb) molecule (HbS) that causes red blood cells (RBCs) to become sickle shaped
- Sickle-shaped cells impair circulation, resulting in chronic ill health (fatigue, dyspnea on exertion, swollen joints), periodic crises, long-term complications, and premature death
- No cure

PATHOPHYSIOLOGY

- The abnormal HbS found in the patient's RBCs becomes insoluble whenever hypoxia occurs.
- The RBCs become rigid, rough, and elongated, forming a crescent or sickle shape.
- Sickling can produce hemolysis (cell destruction).
- The altered cells accumulate in capillaries and smaller blood vessels, making the blood more viscous.
- Normal circulation is impaired, causing pain, tissue infarctions, and swelling.

CAUSES

- Homozygous inheritance of the HbS-producing gene (defective Hb gene from each parent)

INCIDENCE

- Sickle cell anemia is most common in tropical Africans and in people of African descent.
- About 1 in 10 blacks carry the abnormal gene; if two such carriers have offspring, each child has a 1 in 4 chance of developing the disease.
- One in every 500 blacks in the United States has sickle cell anemia.
- This type of anemia also occurs in Puerto Rico, Turkey, India, the Middle East, and the Mediterranean area.

COMPLICATIONS

- Chronic obstructive pulmonary disease
- Heart failure
- Retinopathy
- Nephropathy

ASSESSMENT

HISTORY

- Signs and symptoms usually don't develop until after age 6 months
- Chronic fatigue
- Unexplained dyspnea or dyspnea on exertion
- Joint swelling
- Aching bones
- Chest pain
- Ischemic leg ulcers
- Increased susceptibility to infection
- Pulmonary infarctions and cardiomegaly

PHYSICAL FINDINGS

- Jaundice or pallor
- Small in stature for age
- Delayed growth and puberty
- Spiderlike body build (narrow shoulders and hips, long extremities, curved spine, and barrel chest) in adult
- Tachycardia
- Hepatomegaly and, in children, splenomegaly
- Systolic and diastolic murmurs
- Sleepiness, with difficulty awakening
- Hematuria
- Pale lips, tongue, palms, and nail beds
- Body temperature greater than 104° F (40° C) or a temperature of 100° F (37.8° C) that persists for 2 or more days

In painful crisis

- Most common crisis and the hallmark of the disease, usually appears periodically after age 5, characterized by severe abdominal, thoracic, muscle, or bone pain and, possibly, increased jaundice, dark urine, and a low-grade fever

In aplastic crisis

- Pallor, lethargy, sleepiness, dyspnea, possible coma, markedly decreased bone marrow activity, and RBC hemolysis

In acute splenic sequestration crisis

- Occurs in infants between ages 8 months and 2 years; causes lethargy and pallor and, if untreated, progresses to hypovolemic shock and death

In hemolytic crisis

- Liver congestion and hepatomegaly

DIAGNOSTIC TEST RESULTS

LABORATORY

- Stained blood smear shows sickle cells; Hb electrophoresis shows HbS. (Electrophoresis should be done on umbilical cord blood samples of all neonates at risk to provide sickle cell disease screening at birth.)
- RBC counts are decreased, white blood cell and platelet counts are elevated, erythrocyte sedimentation rate is decreased, and serum iron levels are increased.
- RBC survival is decreased, and reticulocytosis is present; Hb levels are normal or low.

IMAGING

- A lateral chest X-ray detects the characteristic "Lincoln log" deformity. (This spinal abnormality develops in many adults and in some adolescents with sickle cell anemia, leaving the vertebrae resembling logs that form the corner of a cabin.)

DIAGNOSTIC PROCEDURES

- Ophthalmoscopic examination reveals corkscrew-shaped or comma-shaped vessels in the conjunctivae.

TREATMENT

GENERAL

- Avoidance of extreme temperatures
- Avoidance of stress

DIET

- Well-balanced
- Adequate amounts of folic acid-rich foods
- Adequate fluid intake

ACTIVITY
◆ Bed rest in crisis
◆ As tolerated

MEDICATIONS
◆ Vaccines, such as polyvalent pneumococcal vaccine and *Haemophilus influenzae* type B vaccine
◆ Anti-infectives
◆ Analgesics
◆ Iron supplements
◆ Transfusion of packed RBCs, if Hb level decreases suddenly or if condition deteriorates rapidly
◆ Sedation and administration of analgesics, blood transfusion, oxygen therapy, and large amounts of oral or I.V. fluids, in an acute sequestration crisis

NURSING CONSIDERATIONS

NURSING DIAGNOSES
◆ Acute pain
◆ Delayed growth and development
◆ Disturbed body image
◆ Fatigue
◆ Hyperthermia
◆ Impaired gas exchange
◆ Impaired tissue integrity
◆ Ineffective tissue perfusion: Peripheral
◆ Risk for deficient fluid volume

EXPECTED OUTCOMES
The patient will:
◆ express feelings of increased comfort and decreased pain
◆ demonstrate age-appropriate skills and behaviors to the extent possible
◆ verbalize feelings about changed body image
◆ express feelings of energy and decreased fatigue
◆ remain afebrile
◆ exhibit adequate ventilation
◆ maintain normal skin color and temperature
◆ maintain normal peripheral pulses
◆ maintain balanced fluid volume in which input equals output.

NURSING INTERVENTIONS
◆ Encourage the patient to talk about his fears and concerns.

◆ If a male patient develops sudden, painful priapism, reassure him that such episodes are common and have no permanent harmful effects.
◆ Ensure that the patient receives adequate amounts of folic acid-rich foods, such as green leafy vegetables.
◆ Encourage adequate fluid intake.
◆ Apply warm compresses, warmed thermal blankets, and warming pads or mattresses to painful areas of the patient's body, unless he has neuropathy.
◆ Administer analgesics and antipyretics as necessary.
◆ When culture specimens demonstrate the presence of infection, give prescribed antibiotics.
◆ Give prescribed prophylactic antibiotics.
◆ Use strict sterile technique when performing treatments.
◆ Encourage bed rest, with the head of the bed elevated to decrease tissue oxygen demand.
◆ Administer oxygen as needed.
◆ Administer blood transfusions.
◆ If the patient requires general anesthesia for surgery, help ensure that he receives adequate ventilation to prevent hypoxic crisis.

MONITORING
◆ Vital signs
◆ Intake and output
◆ Complete blood count and other laboratory study results

PATIENT TEACHING

GENERAL
Be sure to cover:
◆ avoidance of tight clothing that restricts circulation
◆ conditions that provoke hypoxia, such as strenuous exercise, use of vasoconstricting medications, cold temperatures, unpressurized aircraft, and high altitude
◆ importance of normal childhood immunizations, meticulous wound care, good oral hygiene, regular dental checkups, and a balanced diet as safeguards against infection

◆ need for prompt treatment of infection
◆ need to increase fluid intake to prevent dehydration, which can cause increased blood viscosity
◆ symptoms of vaso-occlusive crisis
◆ need for hospitalization in a vaso-occlusive crisis in which I.V. fluids, parenteral analgesics, oxygen therapy, and blood transfusions may be necessary
◆ need to inform all health care providers that the patient has this disease before undergoing any treatment, especially major surgery
◆ pregnancy and the disease
◆ balanced diet, including folic acid supplements during pregnancy.

DISCHARGE PLANNING
◆ Refer parents of children with sickle cell anemia for genetic counseling to answer their questions about the risk for future offspring.
◆ Refer other family members for genetic counseling to determine if they're carriers of the defective Hb gene.
◆ If necessary, refer the patient for psychological counseling to help him cope.
◆ Refer women with sickle cell anemia for birth control counseling.

RESOURCES
Organizations
Sickle Cell Disease Association of America: *www.sicklecelldisease.org*
U.S. Food and Drug Administration: *www.fda.gov*

Selected references
Kasper, D., et al., eds. *Harrison's Principles of Internal Medicine*, 16th ed. New York: McGraw-Hill Book Co., 2005.
Pinckney, R.B., and Stuart, G.W. "Adjustment Difficulties of Adolescents with Sickle Cell Disease," *Journal of Child and Adolescent Psychiatric Nursing* 17(1):5-12, January-March 2004.

Anemia, sideroblastic

- A group of heterogeneous disorders with a common defect that causes the failure to use iron in hemoglobin (Hb) synthesis despite the availability of adequate iron stores
- Can be acquired or hereditary; the acquired form, in turn, can be primary or secondary

PATHOPHYSIOLOGY

- Normoblasts fail to use iron to synthesize Hb.
- Iron is deposited in the mitochondria of normoblasts rather than in the Hb molecules.
- Iron toxicity can cause organ damage.

CAUSES

- Unknown (primary form)
- Acquired form may be secondary to ingestion of or exposure to toxins, such as alcohol and lead, or to drugs, such as isoniazid and chloramphenicol
- Complication of neoplastic and inflammatory diseases, such as lymphoma, rheumatoid arthritis, lupus erythematosus, multiple myeloma, tuberculosis, and severe infections
- Hereditary; may be due to a rare genetic defect on the X chromosome

INCIDENCE

- Sideroblastic anemia is most prevalent in young men.
- This disorder appears to be transmitted by X-linked inheritance; women are carriers and usually show no signs of this disorder.
- The primary acquired form is most common in elderly people but occasionally develops in young people.

COMPLICATIONS

- Severe cardiac, hepatic, splenic, and pancreatic disease
- Acute myelogenous leukemia

HISTORY

- Anorexia
- Fatigue
- Weakness
- Dizziness
- Dyspnea

PHYSICAL FINDINGS

- Pale skin and oral mucous membranes
- Slight jaundice
- Petechiae or bruises
- Enlarged lymph nodes
- Hepatosplenomegaly

LABORATORY

- Red blood cell (RBC) indices revealed by microscopic examination show erythrocytes to be hypochromic or normochromic and slightly macrocytic; RBC precursors may be megaloblastic, with anisocytosis (abnormal variation in RBC size) and poikilocytosis (abnormal variation in RBC shape).
- Vitamin B_{12} and folic acid levels are normal, unless combined anemias are present.
- Serum reticulocyte count is low because young cells die in the marrow.

DIAGNOSTIC PROCEDURES

- Ringed sideroblasts on microscopic examination of bone marrow aspirate stained with Prussian blue dye confirms the diagnosis (see *Ringed sideroblast*).

Ringed sideroblast

Electron microscopy shows large iron deposits in the mitochondria that surround the nucleus, forming the characteristic ringed sideroblast.

TREATMENT

GENERAL
- Based on underlying cause
- Possible phlebotomy

DIET
- Well-balanced

ACTIVITY
- Frequent rest periods

MEDICATIONS
In hereditary sideroblastic anemia
- High doses of pyridoxine

In primary acquired anemia
- Transfusion or high doses of androgens

In chronic iron overload
- Deferoxamine

NURSING CONSIDERATIONS

NURSING DIAGNOSES
- Decreased cardiac output
- Fatigue
- Impaired oral mucous membranes
- Impaired skin integrity
- Risk for infection
- Risk for injury

EXPECTED OUTCOMES
The patient will:
- maintain adequate cardiac output
- express feelings of increased energy
- show improvement or healing in lesions or wounds
- maintain skin integrity
- remain free from all signs and symptoms of infection
- remain free from injury.

NURSING INTERVENTIONS
- Provide frequent rest periods. Plan activities and diagnostic tests so the patient can rest in between.
- Institute safety measures to prevent falls.
- Give prescribed drugs.
- Provide comfort measures; have the patient perform relaxation techniques to facilitate coping.
- Administer blood transfusions. Notify the practitioner if signs of a transfusion reaction occur.
- If the patient has jaundice or pruritus, provide meticulous skin care.
- Inquire about possible exposure to lead in the home (especially for children) or on the job.

MONITORING
- Vital signs
- Complications
- Response to treatment
- Signs and symptoms of neuropathy
- Signs and symptoms of decreased perfusion

PATIENT TEACHING

GENERAL
Be sure to cover:
- prescribed treatment and possible complications
- importance of continuing prescribed therapy, even after the patient begins to feel better
- precautions for parents about house paint and not allowing children to eat paint chips because of the possibility of lead
- recognition of adrenergic adverse effects and when to report them, if androgens are used as part of the treatment
- phlebotomy (if scheduled)
- recognition of signs and symptoms of heart failure and when to report them
- need for proper hygiene and other measures to guard against infections and when to report signs and symptoms of infection.

DISCHARGE PLANNING
- Identify patients who abuse alcohol and refer them for appropriate therapy.

RESOURCES
Organizations
Iron Disorders Institute: *www.irondisorders.org*
Mayo Clinic: *www.mayoclinic.com*

Selected references
Kasper, D., et al., eds. *Harrison's Principles of Internal Medicine*, 16th ed. New York: McGraw-Hill Book Co., 2005.
Tierney, L., et al. *Current Medical Diagnosis and Treatment*. New York: McGraw-Hill Book Co., 2005.

Aneurysm, abdominal aortic

OVERVIEW

- Abnormal dilation in the arterial wall of the aorta, commonly between the renal arteries and iliac branches
- Can be fusiform (spindle-shaped), saccular (pouchlike), or dissecting

PATHOPHYSIOLOGY

- Focal weakness in the tunica media layer of the aorta due to degenerative changes that allows the tunica intima and tunica adventitia layers to stretch outward
- Increasing blood pressure within the aorta that progressively weakens vessel walls and enlarges aneurysm

CAUSES

- Arteriosclerosis or atherosclerosis (95%)
- Syphilis; other infections
- Trauma

INCIDENCE

- Abdominal aortic aneurysm is seven times more common in hypertensive men than in hypertensive women.
- This disorder is most common in whites ages 50 to 80.

COMPLICATIONS

- Hemorrhage
- Shock
- Dissection

ASSESSMENT

HISTORY

- Asymptomatic until the aneurysm enlarges and compresses surrounding tissue
- Syncope when aneurysm ruptures
- When clot forms and bleeding stops, the patient may again be asymptomatic or have abdominal pain because of bleeding into the peritoneum

PHYSICAL FINDINGS
Intact aneurysm

- Gnawing, generalized, steady abdominal pain
- Lower back pain unaffected by movement
- Gastric or abdominal fullness
- Sudden onset of severe abdominal pain or lumbar pain, with radiation to flank and groin
- May note a pulsating mass in the periumbilical area: don't palpate

Ruptured aneurysm

- Severe, persistent abdominal and back pain for rupture into the peritoneal cavity
- GI bleeding with massive hematemesis and melena for rupture into the duodenum
- Mottled skin; poor distal perfusion
- Absent peripheral pulses distally
- Decreased level of consciousness
- Diaphoresis
- Hypotension
- Tachycardia
- Oliguria
- Distended abdomen
- Ecchymosis or hematoma in the abdominal, flank, or groin area
- Paraplegia if aneurysm rupture reduces blood flow to the spine
- Systolic bruit over the aorta
- Tenderness over affected area

DIAGNOSTIC TEST RESULTS

IMAGING

- Abdominal ultrasonography or echocardiography determines the size, shape, and location of the aneurysm
- Anteroposterior and lateral abdominal X-rays detect aortic calcification, which outlines the mass, at least 75% of the time.
- Computed tomography scan can visualize an aneurysm's effect on nearby organs.
- Aortography shows condition of vessels proximal and distal to the aneurysm and extent of aneurysm; aneurysm diameter may be underestimated because only the flow channel, and not the surrounding clot, is shown.

TREATMENT

GENERAL

- If the aneurysm is small and asymptomatic, surgery delayed
- Careful control of hypertension
- Fluid and blood replacement

DIET

- Weight reduction, if appropriate
- Low-fat diet

ACTIVITY

- As tolerated

MEDICATIONS

- Beta-adrenergic blockers
- Antihypertensives
- Analgesics
- Antibiotics

SURGERY

- Endovascular grafting or resection of large aneurysms or those that produce symptoms (see *Endovascular grafting for repair of AAA*)
- Bypass procedures for poor perfusion distal to aneurysm
- Repair of ruptured aneurysm with a graft replacement

NURSING DIAGNOSES

- Acute pain
- Anxiety
- Decreased cardiac output
- Deficient fluid volume
- Impaired gas exchange
- Impaired physical mobility
- Impaired skin integrity
- Ineffective tissue perfusion: Cardio-pulmonary, renal

EXPECTED OUTCOMES

The patient will:
- express feelings of increased comfort and decreased pain
- express feelings of decreased anxiety
- maintain adequate cardiac output
- maintain adequate urine output (output equivalent to intake)
- maintain adequate ventilation
- maintain optimal mobility within the confines of the disorder
- maintain skin integrity
- maintain palpable pulses distal to the aneurysm site and hemodynamic stability.

NURSING INTERVENTIONS

For an intact aneurysm
- Allow the patient to express his fears and concerns and identify effective coping strategies.
- Offer the patient and his family psychological support.
- Before elective surgery, weigh the patient, insert an indwelling urinary catheter and an I.V. line, and assist with insertion of the arterial line and pulmonary artery catheter to monitor hemodynamic balance.
- Give prescribed preventive antibiotics.

For a ruptured aneurysm
- Insert an I.V. line with at least a 14G needle to facilitate blood replacement.
- Obtain blood samples for laboratory tests as ordered.
- Give prescribed drugs.

⚡ **WARNING** *Be alert for signs of rupture, which may be immediately fatal. If rupture does occur, surgery needs to be immediate. Medical antishock trousers may be used while transporting the patient to surgery.*

After surgery
- Assess peripheral pulses for graft failure or occlusion.
- Watch for signs of bleeding retroperitoneally from the graft site.
- Maintain blood pressure in prescribed range with fluids and medications.

⚡ **WARNING** *Assess the patient for severe back pain, which can indicate that the graft is tearing.*

- Have the patient cough, or suction the endotracheal tube, as needed.
- Provide frequent turning, and assist with ambulation as soon as the patient is able.

MONITORING

- Cardiac rhythm and hemodynamics
- Vital signs, intake and output hourly, neurologic status, and pulse oximetry
- Respirations and breath sounds at least every hour
- Arterial blood gas values as ordered
- Daily weight
- Fluid status
- Nasogastric intubation for patency, amount, and type of drainage
- Laboratory studies
- Abdominal dressings
- Wound site for infection

GENERAL

Be sure to cover:
- surgical procedure and the expected postoperative care
- importance of taking all medications as prescribed and carrying a list of medications at all times, in case of an emergency
- physical activity restrictions until medically cleared by the practitioner
- need for regular examination and ultrasound checks to monitor progression of the aneurysm, if surgery wasn't performed.

RESOURCES

Organizations
American Heart Association: *www.americanheart.org*
National Heart, Lung, and Blood Institute: *www.nhlbi.nih.gov*

Selected references
Alspach, J., ed. *AACN Core Curriculum for Critical Care Nursing*, 6th ed. Philadelphia: W.B. Saunders Co., 2006.
Beese-Bjurstrom, S. "Hidden Danger: Aortic Aneurysms & Dissections," *Nursing* 34(2):36-41, February 2004.
Dambro, M.R. *Griffith's Five-Minute Clinical Consult 2006*. Philadelphia: Lippincott Williams & Wilkins, 2006.
Risser, N., and Murphy, M. "Screening for Abdominal Aortic Aneurysms," *Nurse Practitioner* 28(12):56-57, December 2003.

Endovascular grafting for repair of AAA

Endovascular grafting is a minimally invasive procedure for the patient who requires repair of an abdominal aortic aneurysm (AAA). Endovascular grafting reinforces the walls of the aorta to prevent rupture and prevents expansion of the size of the aneurysm.

The procedure is performed with fluoroscopic guidance, whereby a delivery catheter with an attached compressed graft is inserted through a small incision into the femoral or iliac artery over a guide wire. The delivery catheter is advanced into the aorta, where it's positioned across the aneurysm. A balloon on the catheter expands the graft and affixes it to the vessel wall. The procedure usually takes 2 to 3 hours to perform. Patients are instructed to walk the first day after surgery and are discharged from the hospital in 1 to 3 days.

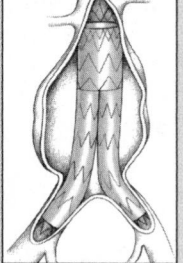

Aneurysm, femoral and popliteal

OVERVIEW

- Progressive atherosclerotic changes occurring in the walls (medial layer) of the femoral and popliteal arteries, resulting in a dilation or outpouching (see *Arteries of the leg*)
- May be fusiform (spindle-shaped) or saccular (pouchlike)
- Usually progressive, eventually ending in thrombosis, embolization, and gangrene

PATHOPHYSIOLOGY

- Atherosclerotic plaque formation or loss of elastin and collagen in the vessel wall causes localized outpouching or dilation of a weakened arterial wall.

CAUSES

- Atherosclerosis
- Bacterial infection
- Congenital weakness in the arterial wall (rare)
- Peripheral vascular reconstructive surgery (which causes a suture line or false aneurysm, whereby a blood clot forms a second lumen)
- Trauma (blunt or penetrating)

INCIDENCE

- This kind of aneurysm is most common in men older than age 50.

COMPLICATIONS

- Gangrene

ASSESSMENT

HISTORY

- Pain in affected extremity

PHYSICAL FINDINGS

- Loss of pulse and color; coldness in the affected leg or foot
- Distal petechial hemorrhages (from aneurysmal emboli)
- Pulsating mass above or below the inguinal ligament
- Firm, nonpulsating mass above or below the inguinal ligament when thrombosis has occurred

DIAGNOSTIC TEST RESULTS

IMAGING

- Arteriography or ultrasonography reveals aneurysm.

OTHER

- Physical examination reveals signs and symptoms of aneurysm.

Arteries of the leg

The illustrations below show the arteries of the anterior and posterior leg.

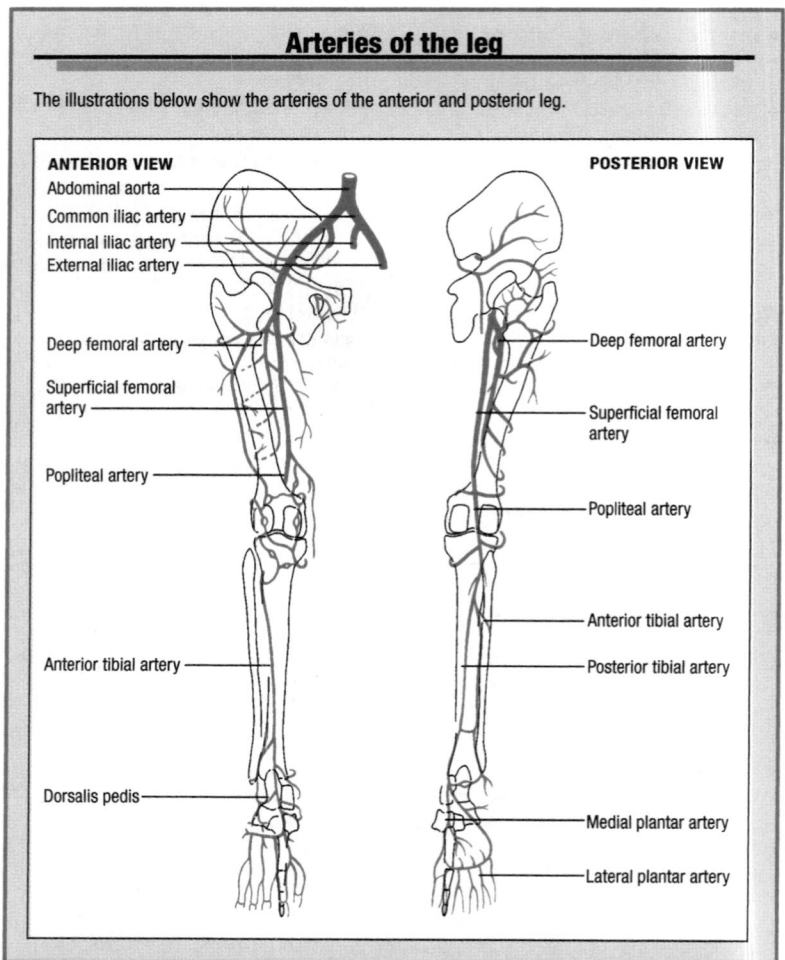

ANTERIOR VIEW
- Abdominal aorta
- Common iliac artery
- Internal iliac artery
- External iliac artery
- Deep femoral artery
- Superficial femoral artery
- Popliteal artery
- Anterior tibial artery
- Dorsalis pedis

POSTERIOR VIEW
- Deep femoral artery
- Superficial femoral artery
- Popliteal artery
- Anterior tibial artery
- Posterior tibial artery
- Medial plantar artery
- Lateral plantar artery

TREATMENT

DIET
◆ Nothing by mouth before surgery

ACTIVITY
◆ Limited movement of the affected extremity

MEDICATIONS
◆ Analgesics
◆ Antibiotics (before surgery)
◆ Anticoagulants

SURGERY
◆ Surgical bypass and reconstruction of the artery, usually with an autogenous saphenous vein graft replacement
◆ Leg amputation, if arterial occlusion causes severe ischemia and gangrene

NURSING CONSIDERATIONS

NURSING DIAGNOSES
◆ Activity intolerance
◆ Acute pain
◆ Impaired physical mobility
◆ Impaired skin integrity
◆ Ineffective tissue perfusion: Peripheral
◆ Risk for infection
◆ Risk for peripheral neurovascular dysfunction

EXPECTED OUTCOMES
The patient will:
◆ carry out activities of daily living without excess fatigue or exhaustion
◆ express feelings of increased comfort and decreased pain
◆ maintain optimal mobility within the confines of the disorder
◆ maintain skin integrity
◆ maintain normal peripheral pulses
◆ avoid infection and other complications
◆ maintain pulses and adequate circulation to damaged aneurysm site.

NURSING INTERVENTIONS
Before corrective surgery, perform the following:
◆ Evaluate the patient's circulatory status, noting the location and quality of peripheral pulses in the affected arm or leg.
◆ Administer a prophylactic antibiotic or anticoagulant as needed.
◆ Discuss expected postoperative procedures with the patient, and review the surgical procedure.
    After surgery, perform the following:
◆ Correlate condition of extremity with preoperative circulatory assessment. Mark the sites on the patient's skin where pulses are palpable, to facilitate repeated checks.
◆ Help the patient walk soon after surgery, to prevent venostasis and thrombus formation.
◆ Check vein donor site for warmth, color, sensation, and pulses.

MONITORING
◆ Neurovascular condition of affected extremity (pulse, temperature, sensation, color)
◆ Vital signs
◆ Pain control

PATIENT TEACHING

GENERAL
Be sure to cover:
◆ importance of immediately informing the practitioner of any recurrence of symptoms
◆ how to apply antiembolism stockings (Warn the patient against wearing constrictive clothing.)
◆ measures to prevent bleeding (if an anticoagulant is prescribed), such as using an electric razor
◆ importance of reporting signs of bleeding immediately (bleeding gums; easy bruising; or black, tarry stools)
◆ importance of follow-up blood studies to monitor anticoagulant therapy.

RESOURCES
Organizations
American Heart Association: *www.americanheart.org*
National Heart, Lung, and Blood Institute: *www.nhlbi.nih.gov*

Selected references
Diseases, 4th ed. Philadelphia: Lippincott Williams & Wilkins, 2006.

Aneurysm, intracranial LIFE-THREATENING DISORDER

OVERVIEW

- Weakness in the wall of a cerebral artery that causes localized dilation
- Most common form is the berry aneurysm, a saclike outpouching in a cerebral artery
- Usually occur at an arterial junction in the circle of Willis, the circular anastomosis forming the major cerebral arteries at the base of the brain
- Often rupture and cause subarachnoid hemorrhage

PATHOPHYSIOLOGY

- Blood flow exerts pressure against a congenitally weak arterial wall, stretching it like an overblown balloon and making it likely to rupture.
- Such a rupture is followed by a subarachnoid hemorrhage, in which blood spills into the space normally occupied by cerebrospinal fluid.
- Blood spills into brain tissue, where a clot can cause potentially fatal increased intracranial pressure and brain tissue damage.

CAUSES

- Combination of congenital defect and degenerative process
- Congenital defect
- Degenerative process
- Trauma

INCIDENCE

- Intracranial aneurysm has a slightly higher incidence in women than in men, especially those in their late 40s or early- to mid-50s.
- This disorder may occur at any age in either sex.

COMPLICATIONS

- Neurologic deficits
- Rebleeding
- Vasospasm
- Death

ASSESSMENT

HISTORY

- Headache
- Intermittent nausea
- Seizure
- Photophobia
- Blurred vision

PHYSICAL FINDINGS

Typically, the severity of a ruptured intracranial aneurysm is graded according to the patient's signs and symptoms. (See *Determining severity of an intracranial aneurysm rupture*.)

- Nuchal rigidity
- Back and leg pain
- Fever
- Restlessness
- Irritability
- Hemiparesis
- Hemisensory defects
- Dysphagia
- Visual defects (diplopia, ptosis, dilated pupil, and inability to rotate the eye caused by compression on the oculomotor nerve, if aneurysm is near the internal carotid artery)

DIAGNOSTIC TEST RESULTS

IMAGING

- Computed tomography scan reveals subarachnoid or ventricular bleeding, with blood in subarachnoid space and displaced midline structures.
- Magnetic resonance imaging shows a cerebral blood flow void.
- Skull X-rays may reveal calcified wall of the aneurysm and areas of bone erosion.
- Cerebral angiography reveals altered cerebral blood flow, vessel lumen dilation, and differences in arterial filling.

Determining severity of an intracranial aneurysm rupture

The severity of symptoms varies from patient to patient, depending on the site and amount of bleeding. Five grades characterize a ruptured intracranial aneurysm:

- *Grade I:* minimal bleeding — The patient is alert with no neurologic deficit; he may have a slight headache and nuchal rigidity.
- *Grade II:* mild bleeding — The patient is alert, with a mild to severe headache and nuchal rigidity; he may have third-nerve palsy.
- *Grade III:* moderate bleeding — The patient is confused or drowsy, with nuchal rigidity and, possibly, a mild focal deficit.
- *Grade IV:* severe bleeding — The patient is stuporous, with nuchal rigidity and, possibly, mild to severe hemiparesis.
- *Grade V:* moribund (often fatal) — If the rupture is nonfatal, the patient is in a deep coma or decerebrate.

TREATMENT

DIET
◆ Avoidance of coffee, other stimulants, and aspirin

ACTIVITY
◆ Bed rest in a quiet, darkened room with minimal stimulation

MEDICATIONS
◆ Analgesics
◆ Antihypertensive agents
◆ Sedatives
◆ Calcium channel blockers
◆ Corticosteroids
◆ Anticonvulsants
◆ Aminocaproic acid

SURGERY
◆ Surgical repair by clipping, ligation, or wrapping (before or after rupture)

NURSING CONSIDERATIONS

NURSING DIAGNOSES
◆ Acute pain
◆ Anxiety
◆ Imbalanced nutrition: Less than body requirements
◆ Impaired gas exchange
◆ Impaired physical mobility
◆ Ineffective breathing pattern
◆ Ineffective tissue perfusion: Cerebral
◆ Risk for imbalanced fluid volume
◆ Risk for impaired skin integrity
◆ Risk for injury

EXPECTED OUTCOMES
The patient will:
◆ express feeling of comfort and relief from pain
◆ express feelings of decreased anxiety
◆ consume required caloric intake
◆ maintain adequate ventilation
◆ maintain optimal mobility within the confines of the disorder
◆ maintain effective breathing pattern
◆ maintain or improve level of consciousness
◆ maintain an adequate fluid balance
◆ maintain skin integrity
◆ remain free from injury.

NURSING INTERVENTIONS
◆ Establish and maintain a patent airway.
◆ Position the patient to promote pulmonary drainage and prevent upper airway obstruction.
◆ Impose aneurysm precautions (bed rest in a quiet, darkened room, keeping the head of the bed flat or elevated less than 30 degrees, as ordered; limited visitation; avoidance of strenuous physical activity and straining with bowel movements; and restricted fluid intake).
◆ Assist with active range-of-motion (ROM) exercises; if the patient is paralyzed, perform regular passive ROM exercises.
◆ If the patient has facial weakness, assess the gag reflex and assist him during meals, placing food in the unaffected side of his mouth. If he can't swallow, insert a nasogastric tube, as ordered, and administer tube feedings.
◆ If the patient can't speak, establish a simple means of communication or use cards or a notepad. Encourage his family to speak to him in a normal tone, even if he doesn't seem to respond.
◆ Provide emotional support, and include the patient's family in his care as much as possible. Encourage family members to adopt a realistic attitude, but don't discourage hope.

MONITORING
◆ Vital signs
◆ Neurologic status
◆ Arterial blood gases
◆ Intake and output

PATIENT TEACHING

GENERAL
Be sure to cover:
◆ the disorder, diagnosis, and treatment
◆ how to recognize signs of rebleeding.

DISCHARGE PLANNING
◆ Refer the patient to a visiting nurse or a rehabilitation center when necessary.

RESOURCES
Organizations
American Academy of Neurology: *www.aan.com*
American Heart Association: *www.americanheart.org*

Selected references
Nettina, S.M. *Lippincott Manual of Nursing Practice*, 8th ed. Philadelphia: Lippincott Williams & Wilkins, 2005.
Walling, A.D. "Management of Unruptured Intracranial Aneurysms — Tips," *American Family Physician* 69(4):939, February 2004.
Zhang, J.H. "Introduction: Experimental Therapies for Cerebral Vascular Diseases," *Neurological Research* 27(3):227-28, April 2005.

Aneurysm, thoracic aortic

OVERVIEW

- Abnormal widening of the ascending, transverse, or descending part of the aorta
- May be saccular (outpouching), fusiform (spindle-shaped), or dissecting

PATHOPHYSIOLOGY

- Circumferential or transverse tear of the aortic wall intima, usually within the medial layer
- Occurs in about 60% of patients with aneurysms; usually an emergency; poor prognosis

CAUSES

- Atherosclerosis
- Bacterial infections, usually at an atherosclerotic plaque
- Blunt chest trauma
- Coarctation of the aorta
- Marfan syndrome
- Rheumatic vasculitis
- Syphilis infection

RISK FACTORS

- Cigarette smoking
- Hypertension

INCIDENCE

- The ascending thoracic aorta is the most common site of thoracic aortic aneurysm.
- Thoracic aortic aneurysms occur predominantly in men younger than age 60 who have coexisting hypertension.
- Descending thoracic aortic aneurysms are most common in younger patients who have had chest trauma.

COMPLICATIONS

- Cardiac tamponade
- Dissection

ASSESSMENT

HISTORY

- No signs and symptoms until aneurysm expands and begins to dissect
- Sudden pain and possibly syncope

PHYSICAL FINDINGS

- Pallor
- Diaphoresis
- Dyspnea
- Cyanosis
- Leg weakness
- Transient paralysis
- Abrupt onset of intermittent neurologic deficits
- Abrupt loss of radial and femoral pulses and right and left carotid pulses
- Increasing area of flatness over the heart, suggesting cardiac tamponade and hemopericardium

In dissecting ascending aneurysm

- Pain with a boring, tearing, or ripping sensation in the thorax or the right anterior chest; may extend to the neck, shoulders, lower back, and abdomen
- Pain most intense at onset
- Diastolic murmur of aortic insufficiency
- Pericardial friction rub (if hemopericardium present)
- Blood pressure may be normal or significantly elevated, with a large difference in systolic blood pressure between the right and left arms

In dissecting transverse aneurysm

- Sharp, boring, and tearing pain that radiates to the shoulders
- Hoarseness
- Dyspnea
- Throat pain
- Dysphagia
- Dry cough

In dissecting descending aneurysm

- Sharp, tearing pain located between the shoulder blades that usually radiates to the chest
- Carotid and radial pulses present and equal bilaterally
- Systolic blood pressure is equal

- May detect bilateral crackles and rhonchi if pulmonary edema is present

DIAGNOSTIC TEST RESULTS

LABORATORY

- Normal or decreased hemoglobin levels from blood loss are caused by a leaking aneurysm.

IMAGING

- Posteroanterior and oblique chest X-rays show widening of the aorta and mediastinum.
- Aortography shows lumen of the aneurysm and its size and location.
- Magnetic resonance imaging and computed tomography scan help confirm and locate the presence of aortic dissection.

DIAGNOSTIC PROCEDURES

- Electrocardiography helps rule out the presence of myocardial infarction.
- Echocardiography may help identify dissecting aneurysm of the aortic root.
- Transesophageal echocardiography can be used to measure the aneurysm in the ascending and descending aorta.

GENERAL
- I.V. fluids and whole blood transfusions, if needed
- Weight reduction, if appropriate

DIET
- Low-fat

ACTIVITY
- No restrictions unless surgery performed

MEDICATIONS
- Beta-adrenergic blockers
- Antihypertensives
- Negative inotropic agents
- Analgesics
- Antibiotics

SURGERY
- Surgical resection with a Dacron or Teflon graft replacement

NURSING CONSIDERATIONS

NURSING DIAGNOSES
- Acute pain
- Anxiety
- Decreased cardiac output
- Hopelessness
- Ineffective breathing pattern
- Ineffective tissue perfusion: Cardiopulmonary, renal
- Risk for deficient fluid volume
- Risk for infection

EXPECTED OUTCOMES
The patient will:
- express feelings of increased comfort and decreased pain
- express feelings of decreased anxiety
- maintain adequate cardiac output and hemodynamic stability
- express feelings of having greater control over the current situation
- maintain an effective breathing pattern
- maintain tissue perfusion and oxygenation
- maintain adequate fluid volume
- show no signs or symptoms of infection

NURSING INTERVENTIONS
- In a nonemergency situation, allow the patient to express his fears and concerns and to identify and use effective coping strategies.
- Offer the patient and his family psychological support.
- Give prescribed analgesics to relieve pain.

After repair of thoracic aneurysm
- Maintain blood pressure in prescribed range with fluids and medications.
- Give prescribed analgesics.
- After stabilization of vital signs, encourage and assist the patient in turning, coughing, and deep breathing.
- Help the patient walk as soon as he's able.
- Assist the patient with range-of-motion leg exercises.

MONITORING
- Vital signs and hemodynamics
- Chest tube drainage
- Heart and lung sounds
- Laboratory results
- Distal pulses
- Level of consciousness and pain
- Signs of infection
- I.V. therapy and intake and output

WARNING *After surgical repair, monitor for signs that resemble those of the initial dissecting aneurysm, suggesting a tear at the graft site.*

PATIENT TEACHING

GENERAL
Be sure to cover:
- the diagnosis
- procedure and expected postoperative care, if surgery is scheduled
- compliance with antihypertensive therapy, including the need for such drugs and the expected adverse effects
- monitoring of blood pressure
- need to call the practitioner if the patient has any sharp pain in the chest or back of the neck

DISCHARGE PLANNING
- Refer the patient to a smoking-cessation program if indicated.

RESOURCES
Organizations
American Heart Association: *www.americanheart.org*

Selected references
Alspach, J., ed. *AACN Core Curriculum for Critical Care Nursing*, 6th ed. Philadelphia: W.B. Saunders Co., 2006.
Beese-Bjurstrom, S. "Hidden Danger: Aortic Aneurysms & Dissections," *Nursing* 34(2):36-41, February 2004.
Kasper, D., et al., eds. *Harrison's Principles of Internal Medicine*, 16th ed. New York: McGraw-Hill Book Co., 2005.

Aneurysm, ventricular

- An outpouching, almost always of the left ventricle, that produces ventricular wall dysfunction
- May develop within days to weeks after myocardial infarction (MI) or may be delayed for years

PATHOPHYSIOLOGY

- When MI destroys a large muscular section of the left ventricle, necrosis reduces the ventricular wall to a thin sheath of fibrous tissue.
- Under intracardiac pressure, the thin sheath stretches and forms a separate noncontractile sac (aneurysm).
- Abnormal muscle wall movement accompanies ventricular aneurysm.
- During systolic ejection, the abnormal muscle wall movements cause the remaining normally functioning myocardial fibers to increase the force of contraction to maintain stroke volume and cardiac output.
- At the same time, a portion of the stroke volume is lost to passive distention of the noncontractile sac.

CAUSES

- MI

INCIDENCE

- Ventricular aneurysm occurs in about 20% of patients after MI.

COMPLICATIONS

- Ventricular arrhythmias
- Cerebral embolization
- Heart failure

HISTORY

- Previous MI
- Dyspnea
- Fatigue

PHYSICAL FINDINGS

- Edema
- Visible or palpable systolic precordial bulge
- Distended jugular veins, if heart failure is present
- Irregular peripheral pulse rhythm
- Arrhythmias, such as premature ventricular contractions
- Pulsus alternans
- Double, diffuse, or displaced apical impulse
- Gallop rhythm
- Crackles and rhonchi

IMAGING

- Two-dimensional echocardiography demonstrates abnormal motion in the left ventricular wall.
- Left ventriculography reveals left ventricular enlargement, with an area of akinesia or dyskinesia (during cineangiography) and diminished cardiac function.
- Chest X-rays may disclose an abnormal bulge distorting the heart's contour if the aneurysm is large; X-rays may be normal if the aneurysm is small.
- Noninvasive nuclear cardiology scan may indicate the site of infarction and suggest the area of aneurysm.

DIAGNOSTIC PROCEDURES

- Electrocardiography may show persistent ST-T segment elevations.

TREATMENT

GENERAL
- Determined by the size of the aneurysm and the presence of complications
- May require only routine medical examination to follow the patient's condition
- May require aggressive measures, such as cardioversion, defibrillation, and endotracheal intubation
- Weight reduction, if appropriate

DIET
- Low-fat

ACTIVITY
- No restrictions unless surgery performed

MEDICATIONS
- Antiarrhythmics
- Cardiac glycosides
- Diuretics
- Fluid and electrolyte replacement
- Analgesics
- Antihypertensives
- Nitrates
- Anticoagulation

SURGERY
- Embolectomy
- Aneurysmectomy with myocardial revascularization

NURSING CONSIDERATIONS

NURSING DIAGNOSES
- Activity intolerance
- Anxiety
- Decreased cardiac output
- Excess fluid volume
- Fatigue
- Fear
- Impaired gas exchange
- Ineffective breathing pattern
- Ineffective tissue perfusion: Cardiopulmonary
- Risk for infection

EXPECTED OUTCOMES
The patient will:
- carry out activities of daily living without excess fatigue or exhaustion
- express feelings of decreased anxiety
- maintain adequate cardiac output
- maintain adequate fluid balance
- express feelings of increased energy and decreased fatigue
- express feelings of decreased fear
- maintain adequate ventilation
- maintain an effective breathing pattern
- maintain hemodynamic stability
- remain free from signs and symptoms of infection.

NURSING INTERVENTIONS
- Give prescribed drugs.
- Prepare for surgery, if indicated.

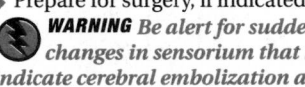 **WARNING** *Be alert for sudden changes in sensorium that may indicate cerebral embolization and for signs that suggest renal failure or MI.*

- Provide psychological support for the patient and his family.

MONITORING
Heart failure
- Vital signs and heart sounds
- Cardiac rhythm, especially for ventricular arrhythmias
- Intake and output; fluid and electrolyte balance
- Blood urea nitrogen and serum creatinine levels

After surgery
- Pulmonary artery catheter pressures
- Signs and symptoms of infection
- Type and amount of chest tube drainage

PATIENT TEACHING

GENERAL
Be sure to cover:
- the disorder, diagnosis, and treatment
- medications and potential adverse reactions
- when to notify the practitioner
- expected postoperative care, if the patient is scheduled to undergo resection
- monitoring of pulse irregularity and rate changes.

DISCHARGE PLANNING
- Refer the patient (or his family) to a community-based cardiopulmonary resuscitation training program.
- Refer the patient to a weight-reduction program, if indicated.
- Refer the patient to a smoking-cessation program, if indicated.

RESOURCES
Organizations
American Heart Association: *www.americanheart.org*

Selected references
Kasper, D., et al., eds. *Harrison's Principles of Internal Medicine*, 16th ed. New York: McGraw-Hill Book Co., 2005.
The Merck Manual of Diagnosis & Therapy, 18th ed. Whitehouse Station, N.J.: Merck & Co., Inc., 2006.

Ankylosing spondylitis

OVERVIEW

- Rheumatoid disease primarily affecting sacroiliac, apophyseal, and costocervical joints and adjacent ligamentous or tendinous attachments to bone
- Usually occurs as a primary disorder; may occur secondary to Reiter syndrome, psoriatic arthritis, or inflammatory bowel disease
- Also called *rheumatoid spondylitis* or *Marie-Strümpell disease*

PATHOPHYSIOLOGY

- Begins in the sacroiliac; gradually progresses to the lumbar, thoracic, and cervical spine
- Less frequently involves large synovial joint
- Bone and cartilage deterioration that leads to fibrous tissue formation and eventual fusion of the spine or peripheral joints

CAUSES

- Unknown
- Familial tendency
- Initial inflammation may result from immune system activation by bacterial infection

INCIDENCE

- Ankylosing spondylitis affects men two to three times more often than women.
- The disorder is well recognized in men but commonly overlooked or missed in women.
- Ankylosing spondylitis is diagnosed most frequently in early and middle adulthood.
- Women with the disorder have more peripheral joint involvement.

COMPLICATIONS

- Atlantoaxial subluxation
- Deposits of amyloid material in the kidneys, which may lead to renal impairment or failure
- Respiratory compromise

ASSESSMENT

HISTORY

- Intermittent lower back pain most severe in the morning or after inactivity and relieved by exercise
- Mild fatigue, fever, anorexia, and weight loss
- Possible description of pain in shoulders, hips, knees, and ankles
- Pain over the symphysis pubis, which may lead to its being mistaken for pelvic inflammatory disease (see *Detecting ankylosing spondylitis in women*)

PHYSICAL FINDINGS

- Stiffness or limited motion of the lumbar spine
- Pain and limited chest expansion
- Kyphosis
- Iritis
- Warmth, swelling, or tenderness of affected joints
- Small joints such as toes may become sausage-shaped
- Aortic murmur caused by regurgitation
- Cardiomegaly
- Upper lobe pulmonary fibrosis, which mimics tuberculosis, that may reduce vital capacity to 70% or less of predicted volume

---

Detecting ankylosing spondylitis in women

Because ankylosing spondylitis seldom occurs in women, diagnosticians typically overlook it when a woman's symptoms include pelvic pain and instead suspect pelvic imflammatory disease. However, it's important to carefully assess a female patient with apparent pelvic disease — especially if culture results identify no apparent cause for her discomfort. Otherwise, misdiagnosis can lead to unwarranted invasive tests and treatments, and cause the patient needless anxiety related to contracting a sexually transmitted disease. Asking the patient if there's a family history of ankylosing spondylitis and performing a thorough health and social history are advisable.

DIAGNOSTIC TEST RESULTS

- Diagnosis of primary ankylosing spondylitis requires meeting established criteria (see *Diagnosing primary ankylosing spondylitis*).

LABORATORY

- Human leukocyte antigen (HLA) typing test results show serum findings that include HLA-B27 in about 95% of patients with primary ankylosing spondylitis and in up to 80% of patients with secondary disease.
- Serum rheumatoid factor test results show the absence of rheumatoid factor, which helps to rule out rheumatoid arthritis, a disease with similar symptoms.
- Serum alkaline phosphate and creatine kinase test results show slightly elevated erythrocyte sedimentation rate, serum alkaline phosphate levels, and creatine kinase levels in active disease.
- Serum immunoglobulin (Ig) profile shows elevated serum IgA levels.

IMAGING

- X-ray studies define characteristic changes, such as bilateral sacroiliac involvement (the hallmark of the disease); blurring of the joints' bony margins in early disease; patchy sclerosis with superficial bony erosions; eventual squaring of vertebral bodies; and "bamboo spine" with complete ankylosis.

TREATMENT

GENERAL
- Good posture; stretching and deep-breathing exercises
- Braces and lightweight supports, if appropriate
- Heat, warm showers, baths, and ice
- Nerve stimulation

DIET
- Nutritious

ACTIVITY
- As tolerated

MEDICATIONS
- Nonsteroidal anti-inflammatory drugs

SURGERY
- Hip replacement surgery in the case of severe hip involvement
- Spinal wedge osteotomy in the case of severe spinal involvement

---

Diagnosing primary ankylosing spondylitis

For a reliable diagnosis, the patient must meet:
- criterion 7 and any one of criteria 1 through 5, or
- any five of criteria 1 through 6 if the patient doesn't have criterion 7.

SEVEN CRITERIA
1. Axial skeleton stiffness for at least 3 months that's relieved by exercise
2. Lumbar pain that persists at rest
3. Thoracic cage pain of at least 3 months' duration that persists at rest
4. Past or current iritis
5. Decreased lumbar range of motion
6. Decreased chest expansion (age-related)
7. Bilateral, symmetrical sacroiliitis demonstrated by radiographic studies

---

NURSING CONSIDERATIONS

NURSING DIAGNOSES
- Activity intolerance
- Chronic pain
- Disturbed body image
- Fatigue
- Impaired gas exchange
- Impaired physical mobility
- Powerlessness
- Risk for injury

EXPECTED OUTCOMES
The patient will:
- express feelings of increased energy
- express feelings of increased comfort and decreased pain
- verbalize feelings about changed body image
- express feelings of energy and decreased fatigue
- maintain adequate ventilation
- maintain optimal mobility within the confines of the disorder
- recognize limitations imposed by illness and express feelings about these limitations
- identify factors that increase the potential for injury.

NURSING INTERVENTIONS
- Keep in mind the patient's limited range of motion (ROM) when planning self-care tasks and activities.
- Offer support and reassurance.
- Give prescribed analgesics.
- Apply heat locally and massage as indicated.
- Have the patient perform active ROM exercises.
- Pace periods of exercise and rest to help the patient achieve comfortable energy levels and lung oxygenation.
- If treatment includes surgery, ensure proper body alignment and positioning.
- Involve other caregivers, such as a social worker, visiting nurse, and dietitian.

MONITORING
- Mobility and comfort level
- Respiratory status
- Heart sounds

PATIENT TEACHING

GENERAL
Be sure to cover:
- avoidance of physical activity that places stress on the back such as lifting heavy objects
- importance of standing upright; sitting upright in a high, straight-back chair; and avoiding leaning over a desk
- importance of sleeping in a prone position on a hard mattress and avoiding using pillows under the neck or knees
- avoidance of prolonged walking, standing, sitting, or driving
- regular stretching and deep-breathing exercises; swimming on a regular basis, if possible
- measurement of patient's height every 3 to 4 months to detect kyphosis
- nutrition and weight maintenance.

DISCHARGE PLANNING
- Refer the patient to physical therapy as needed.
- Refer the patient to the Spondylitis Association of America or the Arthritis Foundation for additional support and information.

RESOURCES
Organizations
Arthritis Foundation: *www.arthritis.org*
Spondylitis Association of America: *www.spondylitis.org*

Selected references
Kasper, D., et al., eds. *Harrison's Principles of Internal Medicine*, 16th ed. New York: McGraw-Hill Book Co., 2005.
Kataria, R.K., and Brent, L.H. "Spondylo-arthropathies," *American Family Physician* 69(12):2853-860, June 2004.
The Merck Manual of Diagnosis & Therapy, 18th ed. Whitehouse Station, N.J.: Merck & Co., Inc., 2006.

Anorexia nervosa

- Psychological disorder of self-imposed starvation resulting from a distorted body image and an intense and irrational fear of gaining weight
- Actual loss of appetite, which is rare
- May occur simultaneously with bulimia nervosa

PATHOPHYSIOLOGY

- Decreased calorie intake depletes body fat and protein stores.
- In women: Estrogen deficiency occurs due to lack of lipid substrate for synthesis, causing amenorrhea.
- In men: Testosterone levels fluctuate, and decreased erectile function and sperm count occur.
- Ketoacidosis occurs from increased use of fat as energy fuel.

CAUSES

- Exact cause unknown
- Achievement pressure
- Dependence and independence issues
- Elaborate food preparation and eating rituals
- History of sexual abuse
- Social attitudes that equate slimness with beauty
- Stress caused by multiple responsibilities
- Subconscious effort to exert personal control over life or to protect oneself from dealing with issues surrounding sexuality

RISK FACTORS

- Low self-esteem
- Compulsive personality
- High achievement goals

INCIDENCE

- Anorexia nervosa affects 5% to 10% of the general population; more than 90% of those affected are females.
- **AGE FACTOR** *Anorexia nervosa occurs primarily in adolescents young adults but may also affect older women and, occasionally, males.*

COMPLICATIONS

- Death
- Suicide
- Electrolyte imbalances
- Malnutrition
- Dehydration
- Esophageal erosion, ulcers, tears, and bleeding
- Tooth and gum erosion and dental caries
- Decreased left ventricular muscle mass and chamber size
- Decreased cardiac output
- Hypotension
- Electrocardiogram (ECG) changes
- Heart failure
- Increased susceptibility to infection
- Amenorrhea
- Anemia

ASSESSMENT

HISTORY

- 15% or greater weight loss for no organic reason
- Morbid fear of being fat
- Compulsion to be thin
- Angry disposition
- Tendency to minimize weight loss
- Ritualistic behaviors
- Amenorrhea
- Infertility
- Loss of libido
- Fatigue
- Sleep alterations
- Intolerance to cold
- Constipation or diarrhea

PHYSICAL FINDINGS

- Hypotension
- Bradycardia
- Emaciated appearance
- Skeletal muscle atrophy
- Loss of fatty tissue
- Atrophy of breast tissue
- Blotchy or sallow skin
- Lanugo on the face and body
- Dryness or loss of scalp hair
- Calluses on the knuckles
- Abrasions and scars on the dorsum of the hand
- Dental caries
- Oral or pharyngeal abrasions
- Painless salivary gland enlargement
- Bowel distention
- Slowed reflexes

DSM-IV-TR *criteria*

These criteria must be documented:

- Refusal to maintain or achieve normal weight for age and height
- Intense fear of gaining weight or becoming fat, even though underweight
- Disturbance in perception of body weight, size, or shape
- Absence of at least three consecutive menstrual cycles when otherwise expected to occur (in females).

DIAGNOSTIC TEST RESULTS

LABORATORY

- Hemoglobin level, platelet count, and white blood cell count are decreased.
- Bleeding time is prolonged.
- Erythrocyte sedimentation rate is decreased.
- Levels of serum creatinine, blood urea nitrogen, uric acid, cholesterol, total protein, albumin, sodium, potassium, chloride, calcium, and fasting blood glucose are decreased.
- Levels of serum alanine aminotransferase and aspartate aminotransferase are elevated in severe starvation.
- Serum amylase levels are elevated.
- In women, levels of serum luteinizing hormone and follicle-stimulating hormone are decreased.
- Triiodothyronine levels are decreased.
- Urinalysis shows dilute urine.

DIAGNOSTIC PROCEDURES

- ECG may show nonspecific ST segment, T-wave changes, and prolonged PR interval; ventricular arrhythmias may also be present

TREATMENT

GENERAL
- Behavior modification
- Group, family, or individual psychotherapy (see *Criteria for hospitalizing a patient with anorexia nervosa*)

DIET
- Balanced, with a normal eating pattern
- Parenteral nutrition, if necessary

ACTIVITY
- Gradual increase in physical activity when weight gain and stabilization occur
- Curtailed activity for cardiac arrhythmias

MEDICATIONS
- Vitamin and mineral supplements

Criteria for hospitalizing a patient with anorexia nervosa

A patient with anorexia nervosa can be successfully treated on an outpatient basis. However, if the patient displays any of the signs listed here, hospitalization is mandatory:
- rapid weight loss equal to 15% or more of normal body mass
- persistent bradycardia (50 beats/minute or less)
- hypotension with a systolic reading of less than or equal to 90 mm Hg
- hypothermia (core body temperature of less than or equal to 97° F (36.5° C)
- presence of medical complications; suicidal ideation
- persistent sabotage or disruption of outpatient treatment — resolute denial of condition and the need for treatment.

NURSING CONSIDERATIONS

NURSING DIAGNOSES
- Chronic low self-esteem
- Constipation
- Delayed growth and development
- Disturbed body image
- Imbalanced nutrition: Less than body requirements

EXPECTED OUTCOMES
The patient will:
- express positive feelings about self
- regain normal bowel function
- express understanding of norms for growth and development
- acknowledge change in body image
- achieve and maintain expected body weight.

NURSING INTERVENTIONS
- Support the patient's efforts to achieve target weight.
- Negotiate an adequate food intake with the patient.
- Supervise the patient one-on-one during meals and for 1 hour afterward.

MONITORING
- Vital signs
- Intake and output
- Electrolyte and complete blood count levels
- Weight on a regular schedule
- Activity (for compulsive exercise)

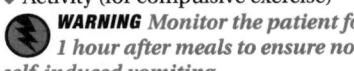 **WARNING** *Monitor the patient for 1 hour after meals to ensure no self-induced vomiting.*

PATIENT TEACHING

GENERAL
Be sure to cover:
- nutrition
- importance of keeping a food journal
- avoidance of discussions about food between the patient and her family.

DISCHARGE PLANNING
- Refer the patient to support services.

RESOURCES
Organizations
American Anorexia Bulimia Association: *www.nationaleatingdisorders.org*
National Association of Anorexia Nervosa and Associated Disorders: *www.anad.org*
Overeaters Anonymous: *www.oa.org*

Selected references
Diseases, 4th ed. Philadelphia: Lippincott Williams & Wilkins, 2006.
Harris, M., et al. "Helping Teenagers with Eating Disorders," *Nursing* 34(10):24-25, October 2004.
Nettina, S.M. *Lippincott Manual of Nursing Practice*, 8th ed. Philadelphia: Lippincott Williams & Wilkins, 2005.
Nix, S. *Williams' Basic Nutrition and Diet Therapy*, 12th ed. St. Louis: Mosby–Year Book, Inc., 2005.

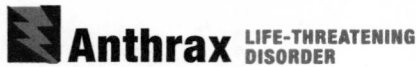

Anthrax LIFE-THREATENING DISORDER

OVERVIEW

- An acute bacterial infection occurring most commonly in herbivorous animals; the natural resistance of humans to anthrax is greater than that of these animals
- Also known as a potential agent for use in bioterrorism and biological warfare; classified as a category A biological disease
- Human cases classified as either agricultural or industrial
- In humans, occurs in three forms, depending on the mode of transmission: Cutaneous, inhalation (wool-sorter's disease), and GI
- Cutaneous anthrax most common form
- Without treatment, mortality from cutaneous anthrax 20%; mortality less than 1% with treatment
- Even with treatment, inhalation anthrax usually fatal
- With treatment, mortality from GI anthrax 25% to 60%
- No screening test available

PATHOPHYSIOLOGY

- *Bacillus anthracis* is an encapsulated, chain-forming, aerobic, gram-positive rod that forms oval spores; spores are hardy and can survive for years under adverse conditions.
- *B. anthracis*, an extracellular pathogen, evades phagocytosis, invades the bloodstream, and multiplies rapidly.
- In cutaneous anthrax, spores enter the body through abraded or broken skin or by biting flies; the spores germinate within hours, the vegetative cells multiply, and anthrax toxin is produced.
- In inhalation anthrax, spores are deposited directly into the alveoli and phagocytized by macrophages; some are carried to and germinate in mediastinal nodes. This may result in overwhelming bacteremia, hemorrhagic mediastinitis, and secondary pneumonia.
- In GI anthrax, primary infection can be caused in the intestine by organisms that survive passage through the stomach; acute inflammation of the intestinal tract results.

CAUSES

- Bacterial infection with *B. anthracis*

Human cases

- Contact with infected animals or contaminated animal products
- Ingestion
- Inhalation
- Insect bites

Agricultural cases

- Bites of contaminated or infected flies
- Consumption of contaminated meat
- Contact with animals that have anthrax

Industrial cases

- Animal hides
- Bones
- Goat's hair
- Wool

RISK FACTORS

- Laboratory and industrial workers at risk for occupational exposure

INCIDENCE

- Anthrax occurs worldwide.
- The disease is most common in developing countries.
- Anthrax is most common in domestic herbivores, including sheep, cattle, horses, and goats, and in wild herbivores.
- An estimated 20,000 to 100,000 cases of anthrax occur per year. (Approximately 95% of human anthrax cases are the cutaneous form; about 5% are the inhalation form; GI anthrax is rare.)

COMPLICATIONS

- Septicemia
- Hemorrhagic mediastinitis
- Pneumonia
- Respiratory failure
- Hemorrhagic thoracic lymphadenitis
- Meningitis
- Death

ASSESSMENT

HISTORY
Cutaneous anthrax

- Contact with animals or animal products
- Painless ulcer
- Mild or no constitutional symptoms

Inhalational anthrax

- Initial prodromal flulike symptoms
- Malaise; dry cough
- Mild fever; chills
- Headache; myalgia
- Severe respiratory distress
- Chest pain

GI anthrax

- Nausea; vomiting
- Decreased appetite
- Fever
- Abdominal pain
- Vomiting blood
- Severe bloody diarrhea

PHYSICAL FINDINGS
Cutaneous anthrax

- Initially, a small, papular, pruritic lesion that resembles an insect bite
- Lesion that develops into a vesicle in 1 to 2 days
- Lesion that finally becomes a small, painless ulcer with a necrotic center, surrounded by nonpitting edema
- Smaller secondary vesicles that may surround some lesions
- Lesions that are generally located on exposed areas of the skin
- Painful, regional, nonspecific lymphadenitis

Inhalational anthrax

- Increasing fever
- Dyspnea; stridor
- Hypoxia; cyanosis
- Hypotension; shock

GI anthrax

- Fever
- Rapidly developing ascites

DIAGNOSTIC TEST RESULTS

LABORATORY
- Gram stain, direct fluorescent antibody staining, and culture show presence of *B. anthracis.*
- Blood cultures show presence of *B. anthracis.*
- Cerebrospinal fluid analysis reveals presence of *B. anthracis.*
- Complete blood count shows polymorphonuclear leukocytosis in severe disease.
- Serum antibody tests reveal the specific antibody to *B. anthracis.*

IMAGING
- Chest X-ray shows symmetric mediastinal widening in hemorrhagic mediastinitis.

TREATMENT

GENERAL
- Initiated as soon as exposure to anthrax is suspected

DIET
- No restrictions
- Adequate fluid intake

ACTIVITY
- As tolerated

MEDICATIONS
- Antibiotics
- Oxygen as needed

SURGERY
- May be necessary for complications such as hemorrhagic mediastinitis

NURSING CONSIDERATIONS

NURSING DIAGNOSES
- Anxiety
- Diarrhea
- Fear
- Imbalanced nutrition: Less than body requirements
- Impaired physical mobility
- Ineffective breathing pattern
- Risk for deficient fluid volume

EXPECTED OUTCOMES
The patient will:
- verbalize feelings of anxiety
- regain normal bowel function
- verbalize feelings of fear
- maintain adequate nutrition and hydration
- maintain joint mobility and range of motion
- maintain effective ventilation
- have balanced intake and output.

NURSING INTERVENTIONS
- Give prescribed drugs.
- Maintain patent airway and adequate ventilation.
- Report any case of anthrax in either livestock or humans to the local board of health.
- Maintain standard precautions.
- Encourage verbalization of fears and concerns.
- Provide adequate hydration.
- Provide a well-balanced diet.
- Assist the patient in the development of effective coping mechanisms.
- Provide adequate rest periods.

MONITORING
- Vital signs
- Intake and output
- Respiratory status
- Neurologic status
- Cardiovascular status
- Skin lesions
- GI status
- Complications
- Response to treatment
- Progression of infection

PATIENT TEACHING

GENERAL
Be sure to cover:
- the disorder, diagnosis, and treatment
- medications and potential adverse reactions
- when to notify the practitioner
- anthrax prevention.

⚡ **WARNING** *An anthrax vaccine is available, but because of limited supplies, it's now given only to U.S. military personnel and isn't for routine civilian use.*

RESOURCES
Organizations
Centers for Disease Control and Prevention: *www.cdc.gov*
National Center for Infectious Diseases: *www.cdc.gov/ncidod*

Selected references
Kimmel, S.R., et al. "Vaccines and Bioterrorism: Smallpox and Anthrax," *Journal of Family Practice* 52(1 suppl): S56-61, January 2003.

Pourbohloul, B., et al. "Modeling Control Strategies of Respiratory Pathogens," *Emerging Infectious Diseases* 11(8): 1249-256, August 2005.

Seppa, N. "Anthrax Vaccine Gets Makeover — Double Shot," *Science News* 164(10):145, September 2003.

Aortic insufficiency

OVERVIEW

- A heart condition in which blood flows back into the left ventricle, causing excess fluid volume
- Also called *aortic regurgitation*

PATHOPHYSIOLOGY

- Blood flows back into the left ventricle during diastole, causing increased left ventricular diastolic pressure.
- This pressure results in volume overload, dilation and, eventually, hypertrophy of the left ventricle.
- Excess fluid volume also eventually results in increased left atrial pressure and increased pulmonary vascular pressure.

CAUSES

- Aortic aneurysm
- Aortic dissection
- Connective tissue diseases
- Hypertension
- Idiopathic valve calcification
- Infective endocarditis
- Primary disease of the aortic valve leaflets, the wall or the aortic root, or both
- Rheumatic fever
- Trauma

INCIDENCE

- Aortic insufficiency occurs most commonly among men.
- When associated with mitral valve disease, it's more common among women.

COMPLICATIONS

- Left-sided heart failure
- Pulmonary edema
- Myocardial ischemia

ASSESSMENT

HISTORY

- Exertional dyspnea, orthopnea, paroxysmal nocturnal dyspnea
- Sensation of a forceful heartbeat, especially in supine position
- Angina, especially nocturnal
- Fatigue
- Palpitations, head pounding
- Symptoms of heart failure, in late stages

PHYSICAL FINDINGS

- Corrigan's pulse
- Bisferious pulse
- Pulsating nail beds and Quincke's sign
- Wide pulse pressure
- Diffuse, hyperdynamic apical impulse, displaced laterally and inferiorly
- Systolic thrill at base or suprasternal notch
- S_3 gallop with increased left ventricular end-diastolic pressure
- High-frequency, blowing, early-peaking, diastolic decrescendo murmur best heard with the patient sitting, leaning forward, and in deep fixed expiration (see *Identifying the murmur of aortic insufficiency*)
- Austin Flint murmur
- Head bobbing with each heartbeat
- Tachycardia, peripheral vasoconstriction, and pulmonary edema if aortic insufficiency is severe

DIAGNOSTIC TEST RESULTS

IMAGING

- Chest X-rays may show left ventricular enlargement and pulmonary vein congestion.
- Echocardiography may show left ventricular enlargement, increased motion of the septum and posterior wall, thickening of valve cusps, prolapse of the valve, flail leaflet, vegetations, or dilation of the aortic root.

DIAGNOSTIC PROCEDURES

- Electrocardiography shows sinus tachycardia, left axis deviation, left ventricular hypertrophy, and left atrial hypertrophy in severe disease.
- Cardiac catheterization shows presence and degree of aortic insufficiency, left ventricular dilation and function, and coexisting coronary artery disease.

TREATMENT

GENERAL

- Periodic noninvasive monitoring of aortic insufficiency and left ventricular function with echocardiogram
- Medical control of hypertension

DIET

- Low-sodium

ACTIVITY

- Planned rest periods to avoid fatigue

MEDICATIONS

- Cardiac glycosides
- Diuretics
- Vasodilators
- Antihypertensives
- Antiarrhythmics
- Infective endocarditis prophylaxis
- ⚡ **WARNING** *Avoid using beta-adrenergic blockers due to their negative inotropic effects.*

SURGERY

- Valve replacement

Identifying the murmur of aortic insufficiency

A high-pitched, blowing decrescendo murmur that radiates from the aortic valve area to the left sternal border characterizes aortic insufficiency.

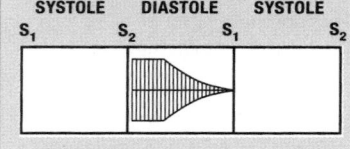

| SYSTOLE | DIASTOLE | SYSTOLE | |
| S_1 | S_2 | S_1 | S_2 |

NURSING DIAGNOSES

◆ Activity intolerance
◆ Decreased cardiac output
◆ Excess fluid volume
◆ Fatigue
◆ Impaired gas exchange
◆ Impaired physical mobility
◆ Ineffective coping
◆ Ineffective tissue perfusion: Cardiopulmonary

EXPECTED OUTCOMES

The patient will:
◆ carry out activities of daily living without excess fatigue or decreased energy
◆ maintain cardiac output, demonstrate hemodynamic stability, and not develop arrhythmias
◆ maintain adequate fluid balance
◆ express feelings of energy and decreased fatigue
◆ maintain adequate ventilation
◆ maintain optimal mobility within the confines of the disorder
◆ demonstrate effective coping skills
◆ maintain tissue perfusion and oxygenation.

NURSING INTERVENTIONS

◆ Give prescribed drugs.
◆ If the patient needs bed rest, stress its importance; provide a bedside commode.
◆ Alternate periods of activity and rest.
◆ Allow the patient to express his concerns about the effects of activity restrictions on his responsibilities and routines.
◆ Keep the patient's legs elevated while he sits in a chair.
◆ Place the patient in an upright position, if necessary, and administer oxygen.
◆ Keep the patient on a low-sodium diet. Consult a dietitian.
◆ Following surgery, watch for hypotension, arrhythmias, and thrombus formation.

MONITORING

◆ Signs and symptoms of heart failure
◆ Pulmonary edema
◆ Adverse reactions to drug therapy
◆ Complications

After surgery

◆ Vital signs and cardiac rhythm
◆ Heart sounds
◆ Chest tube drainage
◆ Neurologic status
◆ Arterial blood gas levels
◆ Intake and output; daily weight
◆ Blood chemistry studies, prothrombin time, and International Normalized Ratio values
◆ Chest X-ray results
◆ Pulmonary artery catheter pressures

GENERAL

Be sure to cover:
◆ the disorder, diagnosis, and treatment
◆ medications and potential adverse reactions
◆ when to notify the practitioner
◆ periodic rest periods in the patient's daily routine
◆ leg elevation when the patient sits
◆ dietary restrictions
◆ signs and symptoms of heart failure
◆ importance of consistent follow-up care
◆ monitoring of pulse rate and rhythm
◆ blood pressure control.

DISCHARGE PLANNING

◆ Refer the patient to an outpatient cardiac rehabilitation program if indicated.
◆ Refer the patient to a smoking-cessation program if indicated.
◆ Refer the patient to a weight-reduction program if indicated.

RESOURCES

Organizations

American Heart Association: *www.americanheart.org*
Mayo Clinic: *www.mayoclinic.com*

Selected references

Goldman, L., and Ausiello, D. *Cecil Textbook of Medicine*, 22nd ed. Philadelphia: W.B. Saunders Co., 2004.
Kasper, D., et al., eds. *Harrison's Principles of Internal Medicine*, 16th ed. New York: McGraw-Hill Book Co., 2005.
The Merck Manual of Diagnosis & Therapy, 18th ed. Whitehouse Station, N.J.: Merck & Co., Inc., 2006.

Aortic stenosis

- Narrowing of the aortic valve that affects blood flow in the heart
- Classified as either acquired or rheumatic

PATHOPHYSIOLOGY

- Stenosis of the aortic valve results in impedance to forward blood flow.
- The left ventricle requires greater pressure to open the aortic valve.
- Added workload increases myocardial oxygen demands.
- Diminished cardiac output reduces coronary artery blood flow.
- Left ventricular hypertrophy and failure result.

CAUSES

- Atherosclerosis
- Congenital aortic bicuspid valve
- Idiopathic fibrosis and calcification
- Rheumatic fever

RISK FACTORS

- Diabetes mellitus
- Hypercholesterolemia

INCIDENCE

- Symptoms may not appear until ages 50 to 70, even though stenosis has been present since childhood.
- About 80% of patients are men.

COMPLICATIONS

- Left-sided heart failure
- Right-sided heart failure
- Infective endocarditis
- Cardiac arrhythmias, especially atrial fibrillation
- Sudden death
- Left ventricular hypertrophy

HISTORY

- May be asymptomatic
- Dyspnea on exertion
- Angina
- Exertional syncope
- Fatigue
- Palpitations
- Paroxysmal nocturnal dyspnea

PHYSICAL FINDINGS

- Small, sustained arterial pulses that rise slowly
- Distinct lag between carotid artery pulse and apical pulse
- Orthopnea
- Prominent jugular vein *a* waves
- Peripheral edema
- Diminished carotid pulses with delayed upstroke
- Apex of the heart may be displaced inferiorly and laterally
- Suprasternal thrill
- **AGE FACTOR** *An early systolic ejection murmur may be present in children and adolescents who have noncalcified valves. The murmur is low-pitched, rough, and rasping and is loudest at the base in the second intercostal space.*
- Split S_2 develops as stenosis becomes more severe
- Prominent S_4
- Harsh, rasping, mid- to late-peaking systolic murmur that's best heard at the base and commonly radiates to carotids and apex (see *Identifying the murmur of aortic stenosis*)

Identifying the murmur of aortic stenosis

A low-pitched, harsh crescendo-decrescendo murmur that radiates from the aortic valve area to the carotid artery characterizes aortic stenosis.

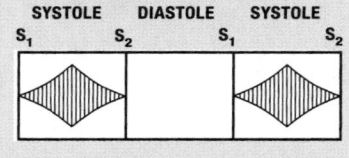

SYSTOLE	DIASTOLE	SYSTOLE
S_1 S_2	S_1	S_2

IMAGING

- Chest X-ray shows valvular calcification, left ventricular enlargement, pulmonary vein congestion, and in later stages, left atrial, pulmonary artery, right atrial, and right ventricular enlargement.
- Echocardiography shows decreased valve area, increased gradient, and increased left ventricular wall thickness.

DIAGNOSTIC PROCEDURES

- Cardiac catheterization shows increased pressure gradient across the aortic valve, increased left ventricular pressures, and presence of coronary artery disease.
- Electrocardiography may show left ventricular hypertrophy, atrial fibrillation, or other arrhythmia.

TREATMENT

GENERAL
- Periodic noninvasive evaluation of the severity of valve narrowing
- Lifelong treatment and management of congenital aortic stenosis

DIET
- Low-sodium, low-fat, low-cholesterol

ACTIVITY
- Planned rest periods

MEDICATIONS
- Cardiac glycosides
- Antibiotic infective endocarditis prophylaxis

  WARNING *The use of diuretics and vasodilators may lead to hypotension and inadequate stroke volume.*

SURGERY
- In adults, valve replacement after they become symptomatic with hemodynamic evidence of severe obstruction
- Percutaneous balloon aortic valvuloplasty
- In children without calcified valves, simple commissurotomy under direct visualization
- Ross procedure may be performed in patients younger than age 5

NURSING CONSIDERATIONS

NURSING DIAGNOSES
- Activity intolerance
- Decreased cardiac output
- Excess fluid volume
- Fatigue
- Impaired gas exchange
- Impaired physical mobility
- Ineffective coping
- Ineffective tissue perfusion: Cardiopulmonary

EXPECTED OUTCOMES
The patient will:
- carry out activities of daily living without excess fatigue or decreased energy
- maintain cardiac output, demonstrate hemodynamic stability, and not develop arrhythmias
- maintain adequate fluid balance
- express feelings of energy and decreased fatigue
- maintain adequate ventilation
- maintain optimal mobility within the confines of the disorder
- demonstrate effective coping skills
- maintain tissue perfusion and oxygenation.

NURSING INTERVENTIONS
- Give prescribed drugs.
- Maintain a low-sodium diet. Consult with a dietitian.
- If the patient requires bed rest, stress its importance. Provide a bedside commode.
- Alternate periods of activity and rest.
- Allow the patient to voice concerns about the effects of activity restrictions.
- Keep the patient's legs elevated while he sits in a chair.
- Place the patient in an upright position and administer oxygen as needed.
- Allow the patient to express his fears and concerns.

MONITORING
- Vital signs
- Intake and output
- Signs and symptoms of heart failure
- Signs and symptoms of progressive aortic stenosis
- Daily weight
- Arrhythmias
- Respiratory status

After surgery
- Signs and symptoms of thrombus formation
- Hemodynamics
- Arterial blood gas results
- Blood chemistry results
- Chest X-ray results

PATIENT TEACHING

GENERAL
Be sure to cover:
- the disorder, diagnosis, and treatment
- medications and potential adverse reactions
- when to notify the practitioner
- periodic rest in the patient's daily routine
- leg elevation whenever the patient sits in a chair
- dietary and fluid restrictions
- importance of consistent follow-up care
- signs and symptoms of heart failure
- infective endocarditis prophylaxis
- pulse rate and rhythm
- monitoring for atrial fibrillation and other arrhythmias.

DISCHARGE PLANNING
- Refer the patient to a weight-reduction program if indicated.
- Refer the patient to a smoking-cessation program if indicated.

RESOURCES
Organizations
American Heart Association: *www.americanheart.org*
Mayo Clinic: *www.mayoclinic.com*

Selected references
Dambro, M.R. *Griffith's Five-Minute Clinical Consult 2006*. Philadelphia: Lippincott Williams & Wilkins, 2006.
Goldman, L., and Ausiello, D. *Cecil Textbook of Medicine*, 22nd ed. Philadelphia: W.B. Saunders Co., 2004.
Kasper, D., et al., eds. *Harrison's Principles of Internal Medicine*, 16th ed. New York: McGraw-Hill Book Co., 2005.
The Merck Manual of Diagnosis & Therapy, 18th ed. Whitehouse Station, N.J.: Merck & Co., Inc., 2006.

Appendicitis

OVERVIEW

- Inflammation of the vermiform appendix
- Most common major abdominal surgical disease
- Fatal if left untreated; gangrene and perforation develop within 36 hours

PATHOPHYSIOLOGY

- Mucosal ulceration triggers inflammation, which temporarily obstructs the appendix.
- Obstruction causes mucus outflow, increasing pressure in the distended appendix; the appendix then contracts.
- Bacteria multiply and inflammation and pressure increase, restricting blood flow and causing thrombus and abdominal pain.

CAUSES

- Barium ingestion
- Fecal mass
- Foreign body
- Mucosal ulceration
- Neoplasm
- Stricture
- Viral infection

RISK FACTORS

- Adolescent male

INCIDENCE

- Appendicitis can occur at any age; however, the majority of cases occur between ages 11 and 20.
- The disorder affects both sexes; however, between puberty and age 25, it's more prevalent in men.

COMPLICATIONS

- Wound infection
- Intra-abdominal infection
- Fecal fistula
- Intestinal obstruction
- Incisional hernia
- Peritonitis (most common)
- Death

ASSESSMENT

HISTORY

- Abdominal pain that's initially generalized, then localizes in the right lower abdomen (McBurney's point)
- Anorexia
- Nausea, vomiting

PHYSICAL FINDINGS

- Low-grade fever, tachycardia
- Adjusting posture to decrease pain
- Guarding
- Normoactive bowel sounds, with possible constipation or diarrhea
- Rebound tenderness and spasm of the abdominal muscles
- Rovsing sign (pain in right lower quadrant that occurs with palpation of left lower quadrant)
- Psoas sign (abdominal pain that occurs when the patient flexes his hip when pressure applied to his knee)
- Obturator sign (abdominal pain that occurs when the hip is rotated)
- Absent abdominal tenderness or flank tenderness in patient with a retrocele or pelvic appendix

DIAGNOSTIC TEST RESULTS

LABORATORY

- White blood cell count is moderately elevated, with increased numbers of immature cells.

IMAGING

- Abdominal or transvaginal ultrasound shows appendiceal inflammation.
- Barium enema reveals nonfilling appendix.
- Abdominal computed tomography scan demonstrates suspected perforation or abscess.

TREATMENT	NURSING CONSIDERATIONS	PATIENT TEACHING

TREATMENT

GENERAL
◆ Incentive spirometry

DIET
◆ Nothing by mouth until after surgery, then gradual return to regular diet

ACTIVITY
◆ Early postoperative ambulation

MEDICATIONS
◆ I.V. fluids
◆ Analgesics
◆ Antibiotics preoperatively and if peritonitis develops

SURGERY
◆ Appendectomy
◆ In suspected abcess, surgery delayed until antibiotic therapy initiated

NURSING CONSIDERATIONS

NURSING DIAGNOSES
◆ Acute pain
◆ Imbalanced nutrition: Less than body requirements
◆ Impaired skin integrity
◆ Ineffective tissue perfusion: GI
◆ Risk for deficient fluid volume
◆ Risk for infection

EXPECTED OUTCOMES
The patient will:
◆ express feelings of increased comfort and decreased pain
◆ maintain calorie requirement
◆ maintain skin integrity
◆ maintain adequate GI tissue perfusion
◆ maintain normal fluid volume
◆ exhibit no signs of infection and avoid complications.

NURSING INTERVENTIONS
◆ Maintain nothing-by-mouth status until surgery is performed.
◆ Administer I.V. fluids.
◆ Avoid administering analgesics until the diagnosis is confirmed.
◆ Avoid administering cathartics or enemas that may rupture the appendix.
◆ Place the patient in Fowler's position to decrease pain.

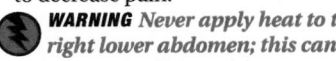 **WARNING** *Never apply heat to the right lower abdomen; this can cause the appendix to rupture.*

◆ Administer prescribed preoperative drugs.

MONITORING
After surgery
◆ Vital signs
◆ Intake and output
◆ Pain control
◆ Bowel sounds, passing of flatus, and bowel movements
◆ Wound healing

PATIENT TEACHING

GENERAL
Be sure to cover:
◆ the disorder
◆ preoperative teaching
◆ possible complications
◆ appropriate wound care
◆ prescribed medications, administration, and possible adverse reactions
◆ postoperative activity limitations.

DISCHARGE PLANNING
◆ Refer the patient to a follow-up appointment with the surgeon or practitioner.

RESOURCES
Organizations
National Digestive Diseases Information Clearinghouse: *www.niddk.nih.gov/index.htm*

Selected references
Handbook of Diseases, 3rd ed. Philadelphia: Lippincott Williams & Wilkins, 2004.
Tierney, L., et al. *Current Medical Diagnosis and Treatment.* New York: McGraw-Hill Book Co., 2005.
Yamada, T., et al. *Atlas of Gastroenterology*, 3rd ed. Philadelphia: Lippincott Williams & Wilkins, 2003.

Arterial occlusive disease

OVERVIEW

- An obstruction or narrowing of the lumen of the aorta and its major branches
- May affect arteries, including the carotid, vertebral, innominate, subclavian, femoral, iliac, renal, mesenteric, and celiac
- Prognosis depends on location of the occlusion and development of collateral circulation that counteracts reduced blood flow

PATHOPHYSIOLOGY

- Narrowing of vessel leads to interrupted blood flow, usually to the legs and feet.
- During times of increased activity or exercise, blood flow to surrounding muscles can't meet the metabolic demand.
- Process results in pain in affected areas.

CAUSES

- Atheromatous debris (plaques)
- Atherosclerosis
- Direct blunt or penetrating trauma
- Embolism
- Fibromuscular disease
- Immune arteritis
- Indwelling arterial catheter
- Raynaud's disease
- Thromboangiitis obliterans
- Thrombosis

RISK FACTORS

- Smoking
- Hypertension
- Dyslipidemia
- Diabetes mellitus
- Advanced age

INCIDENCE

- Arterial occlusive disease is more common in men than in women.
- The disorder usually occurs in people older than age 50.
- The disorder has a higher incidence in patients with diabetes.
- Arteries in the legs are more commonly affected than other arteries.

COMPLICATIONS

- Severe ischemia
- Skin ulceration
- Gangrene
- Limb loss

ASSESSMENT

HISTORY

- One or more risk factors
- Family history of vascular disease
- Intermittent claudication
- Rest pain
- Poor healing of wounds or ulcers
- Impotence
- Dizziness or near syncope
- Transient ischemic attack symptoms

PHYSICAL FINDINGS

- Trophic changes of involved arm or leg
- Diminished or absent pulses in arm or leg
- Presence of ischemic ulcers
- Pallor with elevation of arm or leg
- Dependent rubor
- Arterial bruit
- Hypertension
- Pain
- Pallor
- Pulselessness distal to the occlusion
- Paralysis and paresthesia occurring in the affected arm or leg
- Poikilothermy

DIAGNOSTIC TEST RESULTS

IMAGING

- Arteriography shows type, location, and degree of obstruction, and the establishment of collateral circulation.
- Ultrasonography and plethysmography show decreased blood flow distal to the occlusion.
- Doppler ultrasonography shows a relatively low-pitched sound and a monophasic waveform.
- EEG and computed tomography scan may show the presence of brain lesions.

DIAGNOSTIC PROCEDURES

- Segmental limb pressures and pulse volume measurements show location and extent of the occlusion.
- Ophthalmodynamometry shows degree of obstruction in the internal carotid artery.
- Electrocardiogram may show presence of cardiovascular disease.

TREATMENT

GENERAL

- Smoking cessation
- Hypertension, diabetes, and dyslipidemia control
- Foot and leg care
- Weight control

DIET

- Low-fat, low-cholesterol, high-fiber

ACTIVITY

- Regular walking program

MEDICATIONS

- Antiplatelets
- Lipid-lowering agents
- Hypoglycemic agents
- Antihypertensives
- Thrombolytics
- Anticoagulation
- Niacin or vitamin B complex

SURGERY

- Embolectomy
- Endarterectomy
- Atherectomy
- Laser angioplasty
- Endovascular stent placement
- Percutaneous transluminal angioplasty
- Laser surgery
- Patch grafting
- Bypass graft
- Lumbar sympathectomy
- Amputation
- Bowel resection

NURSING CONSIDERATIONS

NURSING DIAGNOSES

- Activity intolerance
- Chronic pain
- Impaired physical mobility
- Impaired skin integrity
- Ineffective coping
- Ineffective tissue perfusion: Peripheral
- Risk for infection

EXPECTED OUTCOMES

The patient will:

- carry out activities of daily living without excess fatigue or exhaustion
- report increased comfort and decreased pain
- maintain joint mobility and range of motion
- maintain skin integrity
- demonstrate effective coping skills
- maintain normal peripheral pulses and collateral circulation
- develop no signs or symptoms of infection.

NURSING INTERVENTIONS

For chronic arterial occlusive disease

- Use preventive measures, such as minimal pressure mattresses, heel protectors, a foot cradle, or a footboard.
- Avoid using restrictive clothing such as antiembolism stockings.
- Give prescribed drugs.
- Allow the patient to express fears and concerns.

For preoperative care during an acute episode

- Assess the patient's circulatory status.
- Give prescribed analgesics.
- Give prescribed heparin or thrombolytics.
- Wrap the patient's affected foot in soft cotton batting, and reposition it frequently to prevent pressure on any one area.
- Strictly avoid elevating or applying heat to the affected leg.

For postoperative care

- Watch the patient closely for signs of hemorrhage.
- In mesenteric artery occlusion, connect a nasogastric tube to low intermittent suction.
- Give prescribed analgesics.
- Assist with early ambulation, but don't allow the patient to sit for an extended period.
- If amputation has occurred, check the stump carefully for drainage and note and record its color and amount, and the time.
- Elevate the stump as ordered.

MONITORING

- Signs and symptoms of fluid or electrolyte imbalance or renal failure
- Signs and symptoms of stroke
- Vital signs
- Intake and output
- Distal pulses
- Neurologic status
- Bowel sounds

PATIENT TEACHING

GENERAL

Be sure to cover:

- the disorder, diagnosis, and treatment
- medications and potential adverse reactions
- when to notify the practitioner
- dietary restrictions
- regular exercise program
- foot care
- signs and symptoms of graft occlusion
- signs and symptoms of arterial insufficiency and occlusion
- avoidance of wearing constrictive clothing, crossing legs, or wearing garters
- risk factor modification
- avoidance of temperature extremes.

DISCHARGE PLANNING

- Refer the patient to a physical and occupational therapist as indicated.
- Refer the patient to a podiatrist for foot care as needed.
- Refer the patient to an endocrinologist for glucose control as indicated.
- Refer the patient to a smoking-cessation program as indicated.

RESOURCES

Organizations

American Heart Association: *www.americanheart.org*
Mayo Clinic: *www.mayoclinic.com*

Selected references

Day, M.W. "Acute Peripheral Arterial Occlusion," *Nursing* 34(1):88, January 2004.

Kasper, D., et al., eds. *Harrison's Principles of Internal Medicine*, 16th ed. New York: McGraw-Hill Book Co., 2005.

The Merck Manual of Diagnosis & Therapy, 18th ed. Whitehouse Station, N.J.: Merck & Co., Inc., 2006.

Arteriovenous malformations

- Tangled masses of thin-walled, dilated blood vessels between arteries and veins that don't connect by capillaries
- Common in the brain, primarily in the posterior portion of the cerebral hemispheres
- Adequate perfusion of brain tissue prevented due to abnormal channels between arterial and venous system mixing oxygenated and unoxygenated blood
- Range in size from a few millimeters to large malformations extending from the cerebral cortex to the ventricles
- Commonly more than one arteriovenous malformation (AVM) present

PATHOPHYSIOLOGY
- Typical structural characteristics of the blood vessels aren't present.
- Vessels of an AVM are very thin. (One or more arteries feed into the AVM, causing it to appear dilated and torturous.)
- Typically, high-pressured arterial flow moves into the venous system through the connecting channels to increase venous pressure, engorging and dilating the venous structures.
- If the AVM is large enough, the shunting can deprive the surrounding tissue of adequate blood flow.
- Thin-walled vessels may ooze small amounts of blood or actually rupture, causing hemorrhage into the brain or subarachnoid space.

CAUSES
- Congenital (hereditary)
- Penetrating injuries such as trauma

INCIDENCE
- Men and women are affected equally.
- Evidence exists that AVMs run in families.
- Most AVMs are present at birth; however, symptoms typically don't occur until ages 10 to 20.

COMPLICATIONS
- Aneurysm development and subsequent rupture
- Hemorrhage (intracerebral, subarachnoid, or subdural, depending on the location of the AVM)
- Hydrocephalus

ASSESSMENT

HISTORY
- Chronic headache
- Seizures
- Change in mental status

PHYSICAL FINDINGS
- Systolic carotid bruit
- Neurologic deficits

DIAGNOSTIC TEST RESULTS

IMAGING
- Cerebral arteriography confirms the presence of AVMs and evaluates blood flow.
- Doppler ultrasonography of cerebrovascular system indicates abnormal, turbulent blood flow.

TREATMENT

GENERAL
◆ Support measures, including aneurysm precautions (placing the patient on bed rest or with limited activity, maintaining a quiet atmosphere, and keeping the patient calm [with sedatives, if needed]) to prevent possible rupture

DIET
◆ Nothing by mouth, if scheduled for surgery

ACTIVITY
◆ Limited

MEDICATIONS
◆ I.V. fluid
◆ Analgesics
◆ Sedatives
◆ Stool softener

SURGERY
◆ Block dissection, laser surgery, or ligation to repair the communicating channels and remove the feeding vessels

OTHER
◆ Embolization or radiation therapy, if surgery isn't possible, to close the communicating channels and feeder vessels, thus reducing the blood flow to the AVM

NURSING CONSIDERATIONS

NURSING DIAGNOSES
◆ Acute pain
◆ Disturbed sensory perception (visual, tactile)
◆ Ineffective tissue perfusion: Cerebral
◆ Risk for deficient fluid volume

EXPECTED OUTCOMES
The patient will:
◆ express feeling of comfort and relief from pain
◆ maintain stable neurologic status
◆ maintain tissue perfusion and oxygenation
◆ maintain an adequate fluid balance.

NURSING INTERVENTIONS
◆ Control hypertension and seizure activity.
◆ Maintain a quiet atmosphere and provide relaxation techniques.
◆ If the AVM has ruptured, work to control elevated intracranial pressure and intracranial hemorrhage.

MONITORING
◆ Vital signs
◆ Neurologic status

PATIENT TEACHING

GENERAL
Be sure to cover:
◆ the disorder, diagnosis, and treatment
◆ importance of reporting any signs of intracranial bleeding immediately (sudden severe headache, vision changes, decreased movement in extremities, change in level of consciousness).

DISCHARGE PLANNING
◆ Refer patient to social services for support services if neurologic deficits have occurred from a ruptured AVM.

RESOURCES
Organizations
Mayo Clinic: *www.mayoclinic.com*

Selected references
Al-Shanti, R. and Stapf, C. "The Prognosis and Treatment of Arteriovenous Malformations of the Brain." *Practical Neurology* 5(4):194-205, August 2005.
Morrell, N.W. "Screening for Pulmonary Arteriovenous Malformations," *American Journal of Respiratory and Critical Care Medicine* 169(9):978-79, May 2004.

Asbestosis

OVERVIEW

- Lung disease characterized by diffuse interstitial pulmonary fibrosis resulting from prolonged exposure to airborne asbestos particles
- May develop many years (about 15 to 20) after regular exposure to asbestos ceases
- Exposure causes pleural plaques and mesotheliomas of the pleura and the peritoneum
- A form of pneumoconiosis
- Also known as *mesothelioma*

PATHOPHYSIOLOGY

- Inhaled asbestos fibers travel down the airway and penetrate respiratory bronchioles and alveolar walls.
- Mucus production and goblet cell formation are stimulated to protect the airway and aid in expectoration.
- Fibers become encased in a brown, iron-rich, proteinlike sheath called asbestosis bodies.
- Chronic irritation by the fibers continues, causing edema of the airways.
- Fibrosis develops in response to the chronic irritation.

CAUSES

- Exposure to fibrous dust or waste piles from nearby asbestos plants
- Exposure to fibrous dust shaken off workers' clothing
- Involvement in production of paints, plastics, and brake and clutch linings
- Prolonged inhalation of asbestos fibers from industries, such as mining, milling, construction, fireproofing, and textile

INCIDENCE

- Asbestosis commonly occurs between ages 40 and 75.
- Asbestosis affects men more commonly than women.

COMPLICATIONS

- Pulmonary fibrosis
- Respiratory failure
- Pulmonary hypertension
- Cor pulmonale

ASSESSMENT

HISTORY

- Exposure to asbestos fibers
- Exertional or rest dyspnea
- Cough
- Chest pain
- Recurrent respiratory tract infections

PHYSICAL FINDINGS

- Tachypnea
- Clubbing of the fingers
- Characteristic dry crackles in the lung bases

DIAGNOSTIC TEST RESULTS

LABORATORY

- Arterial blood gas (ABG) analysis shows decreased partial pressures of arterial oxygen and carbon dioxide.

IMAGING

- Chest X-rays may show fine, irregular, and linear diffuse infiltrates; a honeycomb or ground-glass appearance to lungs; and pleural thickening and pleural calcification, bilateral obliteration of costophrenic angles, and an enlarged heart with "shaggy" border.

OTHER

- Pulmonary function tests may show decreased vital capacity, forced vital capacity (FVC), and total lung capacity; decreased or normal forced expiratory volume in 1 second (FEV_1) and a normal ratio of FEV_1 to FVC; and reduced diffusing capacity for carbon monoxide.

TREATMENT

GENERAL
◆ Controlled coughing
◆ Postural drainage with chest percussion and vibration

DIET
◆ At least 3 qt (3 L) of fluids daily
◆ High-calorie, high-protein, low-sodium

ACTIVITY
◆ As tolerated

MEDICATIONS
◆ Inhaled mucolytics
◆ Supplemental oxygen
◆ Diuretics
◆ Cardiac glycosides
◆ Antibiotics

SURGERY
◆ Lung transplantation in severe cases

NURSING CONSIDERATIONS

NURSING DIAGNOSES
◆ Anxiety
◆ Fatigue
◆ Fear
◆ Imbalanced nutrition: Less than body requirements
◆ Impaired gas exchange
◆ Ineffective breathing pattern
◆ Interrupted family processes

EXPECTED OUTCOMES
The patient will:
◆ express feelings of decreased anxiety
◆ identify measures to prevent or reduce fatigue
◆ express feelings of decreased fear
◆ maintain adequate calorie intake
◆ maintain adequate ventilation
◆ maintain effective breathing pattern
◆ express understanding of the disorder and treatment modality, as will his family.

NURSING INTERVENTIONS
◆ Give prescribed drugs.
◆ Provide supportive care.
◆ Provide chest physiotherapy.
◆ Provide high-calorie, high-protein, low-sodium foods in small, frequent meals.
◆ Encourage oral fluid intake.
◆ Provide frequent rest periods.

MONITORING
◆ Vital signs
◆ Intake and output
◆ Daily weight
◆ Respiratory status (breath sounds, ABG results)
◆ Sputum production
◆ Mentation
◆ Complications

PATIENT TEACHING

GENERAL
Be sure to cover:
◆ the disorder, diagnosis, and treatment
◆ medications and potential adverse reactions
◆ transtracheal catheter care, if applicable
◆ prevention of infection; to avoid crowds and people with infection
◆ signs and symptoms of infection
◆ influenza and pneumococcus immunizations
◆ home oxygen therapy, if required
◆ importance of follow-up care
◆ chest physiotherapy
◆ high-calorie, high-protein, low-sodium diet
◆ adequate oral fluid intake
◆ energy conservation techniques.

DISCHARGE PLANNING
◆ Refer the patient to a smoking-cessation program if indicated.

RESOURCES
Organizations
National Institute for Occupational Safety and Health: *www.cdc.gov/niosh*
The Asbestos Institute, Inc.: *www.taiinfo.com*

Selected references
American Thoracic Society. "Diagnosis and Initial Management of Nonmalignant Diseases Related to Asbestos," *American Journal of Respiratory and Critical Care Medicine* 170(6):691-715, September 2004.

Ascariasis

- Intestinal infection caused by the parasitic worm *Ascaris lumbricoides*, a large roundworm resembling an earthworm
- Never passes directly from person to person
- Also known as *roundworm infection*

PATHOPHYSIOLOGY

- After ingestion, *A. lumbricoides* ova hatch and release larvae, which penetrate the intestinal wall and reach the lungs through the bloodstream.
- After about 10 days in pulmonary capillaries and alveoli, the larvae migrate to the bronchioles, bronchi, trachea, and epiglottis.
- From the epiglottis, the larvae are swallowed and return to the intestine to mature into worms.

CAUSES

- Ingestion of food, drink, or soil contaminated with *A. lumbricoides* ova

INCIDENCE

- Ascariasis occurs worldwide but is most common in tropical areas with poor sanitation and in Asia, where farmers use human stool as fertilizer.
- In the United States, this disorder is more prevalent in the South, particularly among younger children.

COMPLICATIONS

- Intestinal obstruction
- Pneumonitis

ASSESSMENT

HISTORY

- Stomach discomfort or pain
- Nausea and vomiting
- Recent travel to endemic area
- Restlessness
- Disturbed sleep

PHYSICAL FINDINGS

- Abdominal tenderness
- Dehydration
- Rales, wheezing, and tachypnea (if migrated to the lungs)

DIAGNOSTIC TEST RESULTS

LABORATORY

- Microscopic examination identifies ova in the stool or observation of adult worm in emesis.
- Complete blood count shows eosinophilia.

IMAGING

- Abdominal X-rays show whirlpool pattern of intraluminal worms. (Intestinal obstruction may be noted.)
- Chest X-rays show characteristic bronchovascular markings — infiltrates, patchy areas of pneumonitis, and widening of hilar shadows (if migrated to the lungs).

TREATMENT

GENERAL
◆ Nasogastric (NG) suctioning (with intestinal obstruction)

DIET
◆ Nothing by mouth until stable

ACTIVITY
◆ Rest as needed

MEDICATIONS
◆ I.V. fluids
◆ Mebendazole and albendazole
◆ Anthelmintic therapy (pyrantel or piperazine) (Avoid use if intestinal obstruction is present.)

⚡ **WARNING** *Piperazine is contraindicated in patients with seizure disorders and may cause stomach upset, dizziness, and urticaria. Pyrantel produces red stool and vomitus and may cause stomach upset, headache, dizziness, and rash. Albendazole and mebendazole may cause abdominal pain and diarrhea.*

SURGERY
◆ Intestinal surgery to relieve obstruction, if necessary

NURSING CONSIDERATIONS

NURSING DIAGNOSES
◆ Acute pain
◆ Constipation
◆ Hyperthermia
◆ Imbalanced nutrition: Less than body requirements
◆ Ineffective breathing pattern
◆ Risk for deficient fluid volume
◆ Risk for infection

EXPECTED OUTCOMES
The patient will:
◆ express feeling of comfort and relief from pain
◆ regain normal intestinal function
◆ remain afebrile
◆ maintain daily calorie requirements
◆ maintain effective breathing pattern
◆ maintain adequate fluid balance
◆ express understanding of proper sanitation of food and hands and avoid infection.

NURSING INTERVENTIONS
◆ Isolation is unnecessary; proper disposal of stool and soiled linen, using standard precautions, should be adequate.
◆ If the patient is receiving NG suctioning, provide good mouth care.

MONITORING
◆ Vital signs
◆ Intake and output
◆ Appearance of stools (for worms)

PATIENT TEACHING

GENERAL
Be sure to cover:
◆ proper hand washing, especially before eating and after defecating
◆ bathing and changing underwear and bed linens daily
◆ adverse effects of medications prescribed for the patient.

DISCHARGE PLANNING
◆ Refer the patient to social services if living conditions are questionable regarding cleanliness.

RESOURCES
Organizations
Centers for Disease Control and Prevention — Division of Parasitic Diseases: *www.cdc.gov/ncidod/dpd*

Selected references
Diseases, 4th ed. Philadelphia: Lippincott Williams & Wilkins, 2006.
Watts, S. "Women, Water Management and Health," *Emerging Infectious Diseases* 10(11):2025-2026, November 2004.

Aspergillosis LIFE-THREATENING DISORDER

OVERVIEW

- An opportunistic, sometimes life-threatening infection, growth, or allergic response caused by fungi of the species *Aspergillus*, usually *A. fumigatus*, *A. flavus*, or *A. niger*
- Four major forms:
- Aspergilloma produces a fungus ball in the lungs (called a mycetoma)
- Allergic aspergillosis is a hypersensitive asthmatic reaction to *Aspergillus* antigens
- Aspergillosis endophthalmitis is an infection of the anterior and posterior chambers of the eye that can lead to blindness
- Invasive aspergillosis is an acute infection that produces septicemia, thrombosis, and infarction of virtually any organ, especially the heart, lungs, brain, and kidneys
- The prognosis varies with each form; occasionally, aspergilloma causes fatal hemoptysis

PATHOPHYSIOLOGY

- Conidia (asexual spores) travel into the alveoli via inhalation or, in aspergillosis endophthalmitis, through a wound or other tissue injury.
- Pulmonary macrophages may or may not be able to kill the conidia.
- The alternative complement pathway is activated, resulting in recruitment of neutrophils and monocytes.
- The disease may be accompanied by hyphal invasion of the blood vessels in the involved tissues.
- In aspergilloma, colonization of the bronchial tree with *Aspergillus* produces plugs and atelectasis and forms a tangled ball of hyphae (fungal filaments), fibrin, and exudate in a cavity left by a previous illness such as tuberculosis.

CAUSES

- Contact with *Aspergillus*, which is commonly found growing on dry leaves, stored grain, compost piles, or decaying vegetation

RISK FACTORS

- Excessive or prolonged use of antibiotics, glucocorticoids, or other immunosuppressants
- Radiation therapy
- Acquired immunodeficiency syndrome
- Hodgkin's disease
- Leukemia
- Azotemia
- Alcoholism
- Sarcoidosis
- Bronchitis and bronchiectasis
- Organ transplants
- Tuberculosis or another cavitary lung disease (in aspergilloma)

INCIDENCE

- Aspergillosis is found worldwide, commonly in fermenting compost piles and damp hay.

COMPLICATIONS

- Infection of the ear (otomycosis), cornea (mycotic keratitis), or prosthetic heart valve (endocarditis)
- Pneumonia (especially in those receiving an immunosuppressant such as an antineoplastic drug or high-dose steroid therapy)
- Sinusitis
- Brain abscesses
- Life-threatening hemoptysis
- Septicemia

ASSESSMENT

HISTORY

Aspergilloma and allergic aspergillosis
- Immunosuppression
- Dyspnea
- Cough with sputum production

Aspergillosis endophthalmitis
- Eye pain
- Vision changes
- Recent eye injury or surgery

Invasive aspergillosis
- History based on infected organ

PHYSICAL FINDINGS

Aspergilloma and allergic aspergillosis
- Diminished breath sounds
- Adventitious breath sounds
- Cough with sputum production

Aspergillosis endophthalmitis
- Reddened conjunctivae
- Blurred vision

Invasive aspergillosis
- Findings based on infected organ

DIAGNOSTIC TEST RESULTS

LABORATORY
Aspergilloma
- Serum positive results for anti-*Aspergillus* antibodies are found.

Allergic aspergillosis
- Sputum culture reveals hyphae that grow *Aspergillus* and eosinophils.
- Serum positive results for immunoglobulin (Ig) E and IgG anti-*Aspergillus* antibodies are found.

Aspergillosis endophthalmitis
- Eye culture or exudate shows *Aspergillus*.

IMAGING
Aspergilloma
- Chest X-ray shows a round to oval mass with a radiolucent crescent over the upper portion of the mass (Monod's sign).

DIAGNOSTIC PROCEDURES
Invasive aspergillosis
- Bronchoscopy and open lung biopsy to obtain tissue sample confirm diagnosis.

TREATMENT

GENERAL
- Supportive therapy

MEDICATIONS
Allergic aspergillosis
- Desensitization
- Steroids

Aspergillosis endophthalmitis
- Amphotericin B (Amphocin)

Invasive aspergillosis
- Antifungal therapy

SURGERY
Aspergilloma
- Local excision of the lesion
- Lobectomy

NURSING CONSIDERATIONS

NURSING DIAGNOSES
- Acute pain
- Impaired gas exchange
- Impaired skin integrity
- Ineffective airway clearance
- Ineffective breathing pattern
- Risk for deficient fluid volume

EXPECTED OUTCOMES
The patient will:
- express feeling of comfort and relief from pain
- maintain adequate ventilation
- maintain skin integrity
- maintain a patent airway
- maintain effective breathing pattern
- maintain adequate fluid balance.

NURSING INTERVENTIONS
- Perform chest physiotherapy every 2 hours.
- Encourage coughing and deep breathing every hour.

MONITORING
- Vital signs
- Sputum production, amount, color, and character

PATIENT TEACHING

GENERAL
Be sure to cover:
- the disorder, diagnosis, and treatment
- adverse effects of medications.

RESOURCES
Organizations
Centers for Disease Control and Prevention — Division of Bacterial and Mycotic Diseases: *www.cdc.gov/ncidod/dbmd*

Selected references
Diseases, 4th ed. Philadelphia: Lippincott Williams & Wilkins, 2006.
Meersseman, W., et al. "Invasive Aspergillosis in Critically Ill Patients without Malignancy," *American Journal of Respiratory and Critical Care Medicine* 170(6):621-25, September 2004.
Zander, D.S. "Allergic Bronchopulmonary Aspergillosis: An Overview," *Archives of Pathology & Laboratory Medicine* 129(7):924-28, July 2005.

Asphyxia LIFE-THREATENING DISORDER

- A condition of insufficient oxygen and accumulating carbon dioxide in the blood and tissues
- Leads to cardiopulmonary arrest and is fatal without prompt treatment

PATHOPHYSIOLOGY

- An interference with respiration, causing insufficient oxygen intake
- Accumulation of carbon dioxide
- Hypoxemia
- Inadequate tissue perfusion

CAUSES

- Airway obstruction
- Aspiration
- Carbon monoxide poisoning
- Near drowning
- Opioid abuse
- Pulmonary edema
- Respiratory muscle paralysis
- Smoke inhalation
- Strangulation
- Trauma to airway
- Tumor

INCIDENCE

- Asphyxia can occur at any age.

COMPLICATIONS

- Neurologic damage
- Death

HISTORY

- Cause of the asphyxia may be apparent
- Causes of signs and symptoms vary

PHYSICAL FINDINGS

- Anxiousness or agitation
- Confusion
- Dyspnea
- Prominent neck muscles
- Wheezing and stridor
- Altered respiratory rate
- Little or no air movement
- Intercostal rib retractions
- Pale skin
- Cyanosis in mucous membranes, lips, and nail beds
- Erythema and petechiae on the upper chest (trauma)
- Cherry-red mucous membranes (carbon monoxide poisoning)
- Decreased or absent breath sounds

LABORATORY

- Decreased partial pressure of arterial oxygen (less than 60 mm Hg) and increased partial pressure of arterial carbon dioxide (more than 50 mm Hg) are indicated by arterial blood gas (ABG) analysis.
- Toxicology tests show drugs, chemicals, or abnormal hemoglobin level.

IMAGING

- Chest X-rays may detect a foreign body, pulmonary edema, or atelectasis.

DIAGNOSTIC PROCEDURES

- Pulmonary function tests may indicate respiratory muscle weakness.
- Bronchoscopy can locate foreign body.

TREATMENT

GENERAL
◆ Establish airway and ventilation.
◆ Treat the underlying cause.

DIET
◆ Nothing by mouth until able to protect airway

ACTIVITY
◆ Based on outcome of interventions

MEDICATIONS
◆ Oxygen
◆ Naloxone (if caused by opioid abuse)

SURGERY
◆ Tumor removal

NURSING CONSIDERATIONS

NURSING DIAGNOSES
◆ Decreased cardiac output
◆ Impaired gas exchange
◆ Ineffective airway clearance
◆ Ineffective breathing pattern
◆ Risk for aspiration
◆ Risk for suffocation

EXPECTED OUTCOMES
The patient will:
◆ maintain acceptable cardiac output
◆ maintain adequate ventilation
◆ maintain a patent airway
◆ maintain effective breathing pattern
◆ demonstrate knowledge of safety measures to prevent aspiration
◆ demonstrate knowledge of safety measures to prevent suffocation.

NURSING INTERVENTIONS
◆ Perform abdominal thrust, if obstruction is present.
◆ Maintain patent airway.
◆ Begin cardiopulmonary resuscitation, if necessary.
◆ Insert a nasogastric tube or an Ewald tube for lavage (for opioid abuse).
◆ Give prescribed drugs.
◆ Reassure the patient and his family.
◆ Ensure I.V. access.

MONITORING
◆ ABG levels, pulse oximetry
◆ Respiratory status
◆ Cardiac status
◆ Vital signs
◆ Neurologic status

PATIENT TEACHING

GENERAL
Be sure to cover:
◆ the cause of asphyxia (with the patient and his family, discuss measures to prevent recurrence, if appropriate)
◆ safety measures if the victim is a child.

DISCHARGE PLANNING
◆ Refer the patient to the proper authorities, if criminal intent was involved.
◆ Refer the patient to resource and support services, if appropriate.

RESOURCES
Organizations
American Academy of Neurology: *www.aan.com*

Selected references
Diseases, 4th ed. Philadelphia: Lippincott Williams & Wilkins, 2006.
Jenkins, J.L., and Braen, G.R. *Manual of Emergency Medicine*, 5th ed. Philadelphia: Lippincott Williams & Wilkins, 2005.
Klein, C.A. "Prenatal Asphyxia Requires Immediate Response," *Nurse Practitioner* 29(5):10, May 2004.

Asthma LIFE-THREATENING DISORDER

OVERVIEW

- A chronic reactive airway disorder involving episodic, reversible airway obstruction resulting from bronchospasms, increased mucus secretions, and mucosal edema
- Signs and symptoms that range from mild wheezing and dyspnea to life-threatening respiratory failure
- Signs and symptoms of bronchial airway obstruction that may persist between acute episodes

PATHOPHYSIOLOGY

- Tracheal and bronchial linings overreact to various stimuli, causing episodic smooth-muscle spasms that severely constrict the airways.
- Mucosal edema and thickened secretions further block the airways.
- Immunoglobulin (Ig) E antibodies, attached to histamine-containing mast cells and receptors on cell membranes, initiate intrinsic asthma attacks.
- When exposed to an antigen such as pollen, the IgE antibody combines with the antigen. On subsequent exposure to the antigen, mast cells degranulate and release mediators.
- The mediators cause the bronchoconstriction and edema of an asthma attack.
- During an asthma attack, expiratory airflow decreases, trapping gas in the airways and causing alveolar hyperinflation.
- Atelectasis may develop in some lung regions.
- The increased airway resistance causes labored breathing.

CAUSES

- Sensitivity to specific external allergens (extrinsic) or related to internal, nonallergenic factors (intrinsic)

Extrinsic asthma (atopic asthma)

- Animal dander
- Food additives containing sulfites and any other sensitizing substance
- House dust or mold
- Kapok or feather pillows
- Pollen

Intrinsic asthma (nonatopic asthma)

- Emotional stress
- Genetic factors

Bronchoconstriction

- Cold air
- Drugs, such as aspirin, beta-adrenergic blockers, and nonsteroidal anti-inflammatory drugs
- Exercise
- Hereditary predisposition
- Psychological stress
- Sensitivity to allergens or irritants such as pollutants
- Tartrazine
- Viral infections

INCIDENCE

- The disorder can occur at any age, but about 50% of all patients with asthma are under age 10; it affects twice as many boys as girls.
- About one-third of patients experience onset between ages 10 and 30.
- About one-third share the disease with at least one immediate family member.
- Intrinsic and extrinsic asthma can coexist in many patients with asthma.

COMPLICATIONS

- Status asthmaticus
- Respiratory failure
- Death

ASSESSMENT

HISTORY

- Intrinsic asthma is often preceded by severe respiratory tract infections, especially in adults
- Irritants, emotional stress, fatigue, endocrine changes, temperature and humidity variations, and exposure to noxious fumes may aggravate intrinsic asthma attacks
- An asthma attack may begin dramatically, with simultaneous onset of severe, multiple symptoms, or insidiously, with gradually increasing respiratory distress
- Exposure to a particular allergen is followed by a sudden onset of dyspnea and wheezing and by tightness in the chest accompanied by a cough that produces thick, clear, or yellow sputum

PHYSICAL FINDINGS

- Visible dyspnea
- Ability to speak only a few words before pausing for breath
- Use of accessory respiratory muscles
- Diaphoresis
- Increased anteroposterior thoracic diameter
- Hyperresonance
- Tachycardia; tachypnea; mild systolic hypertension
- Inspiratory and expiratory wheezes
- Prolonged expiratory phase of respiration
- Diminished breath sounds
- Cyanosis, confusion, and lethargy indicate the onset of life-threatening status asthmaticus and respiratory failure

DIAGNOSTIC TEST RESULTS

LABORATORY

- Arterial blood gas (ABG) analysis reveals hypoxemia.
- Increased serum IgE levels result from an allergic reaction.
- Complete blood count with differential shows increased eosinophil count.

IMAGING
◆ Chest X-rays may show hyperinflation with areas of focal atelectasis.

DIAGNOSTIC PROCEDURES
◆ Pulmonary function studies may show decreased peak flows and forced expiratory volume in 1 second, low-normal or decreased vital capacity, and increased total lung and residual capacities.
◆ Skin testing may identify specific allergens.
◆ Bronchial challenge testing shows the clinical significance of allergens identified by skin testing.

OTHER
◆ Pulse oximetry measurements may show decreased oxygen saturation.

TREATMENT

GENERAL
◆ Identification and avoidance of precipitating factors
◆ Desensitization to specific antigens
◆ Establishment and maintenance of patent airway

DIET
◆ Fluid replacement

ACTIVITY
◆ As tolerated

MEDICATIONS
◆ Bronchodilators
◆ Corticosteroids
◆ Histamine antagonists
◆ Leukotriene antagonists
◆ Anticholinergic bronchodilators
◆ Low-flow oxygen
◆ Antibiotics
◆ Heliox trial (before intubation)
◆ I.V. magnesium sulfate (controversial)

⚡ **WARNING** *The patient with increasingly severe asthma that doesn't respond to drug therapy is usually admitted for treatment with corticosteroids, epinephrine (Adrenalin), and sympathomimetic aerosol sprays. He may require endotracheal intubation and mechanical ventilation.*

NURSING CONSIDERATIONS

NURSING DIAGNOSES
◆ Anxiety
◆ Fear
◆ Impaired gas exchange
◆ Ineffective airway clearance
◆ Ineffective breathing pattern

EXPECTED OUTCOMES
The patient will:
◆ report feelings of comfort and decreased anxiety
◆ verbalize feelings of anxiety and fear
◆ maintain adequate ventilation
◆ maintain a patent airway
◆ maintain effective breathing pattern.

NURSING INTERVENTIONS
◆ Give prescribed drugs.
◆ Place the patient in high Fowler's position.
◆ Encourage pursed-lip and diaphragmatic breathing.
◆ Administer prescribed humidified oxygen.
◆ Adjust oxygen according to the patient's vital signs and ABG values.
◆ Assist with intubation and mechanical ventilation, if appropriate.
◆ Perform postural drainage and chest percussion, if tolerated.
◆ Suction an intubated patient as needed.
◆ Treat the patient's dehydration with I.V. or oral fluids as tolerated.
◆ Anticipate bronchoscopy or bronchial lavage.
◆ Keep the room temperature comfortable.
◆ Use an air conditioner or a fan in hot, humid weather.

MONITORING
◆ Vital signs
◆ Intake and output
◆ Response to treatment
◆ Signs and symptoms of theophylline toxicity
◆ Breath sounds
◆ ABG results
◆ Pulmonary function test results
◆ Pulse oximetry
◆ Complications of corticosteroid treatment
◆ Level of anxiety

PATIENT TEACHING

GENERAL
Be sure to cover:
◆ the disorder, diagnosis, and treatment
◆ medications and potential adverse reactions
◆ when to notify the practitioner
◆ avoidance of known allergens and irritants
◆ metered-dose inhaler or dry powder inhaler use
◆ pursed-lip and diaphragmatic breathing
◆ use of peak flow meter
◆ effective coughing techniques
◆ maintaining adequate hydration.

DISCHARGE PLANNING
◆ Refer the patient to a local asthma support group.

RESOURCES
Organizations
American Academy of Allergy, Asthma, and Immunology: *www.aaaai.org*
Asthma and Allergy Foundation of America: *www.aafa.org*
National Asthma Education and Prevention Program: *www.nhlbi.nih.gov/about/naepp*

Selected references
Mintz, M. "Asthma Update: Part I. Diagnosis, Monitoring, and Prevention of Disease Progression," *American Family Physician* 70(5):893-98, September 2004.
Murphy, K.R., et al. "Asthma: Helping Patients Breathe Easier," *Nurse Practitioner* 29(10):38-55, October 2004.
"Popular Asthma Remedy May Worsen Condition," *Nursing* 34(9):30, September 2004.

Atelectasis

OVERVIEW

- Incomplete expansion of alveolar clusters or lung segments leading to partial or complete lung collapse
- May be chronic or acute
- Good prognosis with prompt removal of any airway obstruction, relief of hypoxia, and reexpansion of the collapsed lung

PATHOPHYSIOLOGY

- Due to incomplete expansion, certain regions of the lung are removed from gas exchange process.
- Unoxygenated blood passes unchanged through these regions and produces hypoxia.
- Alveolar surfactant causes increased surface tension, permitting complete alveolar deflation.

CAUSES

- Bed rest in a supine position
- Bronchial occlusion
- Bronchiectasis
- Bronchogenic carcinoma
- Cystic fibrosis
- External compression
- General anesthesia
- Idiopathic respiratory distress syndrome of the neonate
- Inflammatory lung disease
- Oxygen toxicity
- Pleural effusion
- Pulmonary edema
- Pulmonary embolism
- Sarcoidosis

INCIDENCE

- Atelectasis is common in patients after upper abdominal or thoracic surgery.
- The disorder is more common in patients with prolonged immobility, on mechanical ventilation, or with central nervous system (CNS) depression.
- There's an increased predisposition in patients who smoke and those with chronic obstructive pulmonary disease (COPD).

COMPLICATIONS

- Hypoxemia
- Acute respiratory failure
- Pneumonia

ASSESSMENT

HISTORY

- Recent abdominal surgery
- Prolonged immobility
- Mechanical ventilation
- CNS depression
- Smoking
- COPD
- Rib fractures, tight chest dressings

PHYSICAL FINDINGS

- Decreased chest wall movement
- Cyanosis
- Diaphoresis
- Substernal or intercostal retractions
- Anxiety
- Decreased fremitus
- Mediastinal shift to the affected side
- Dullness or flatness over lung fields
- End-inspiration crackles
- Decreased (or absent) breath sounds
- Tachycardia

DIAGNOSTIC TEST RESULTS

LABORATORY

- Arterial blood gas (ABG) analysis shows hypoxia.

IMAGING

- Chest X-rays show characteristic horizontal lines in the lower lung zones and characteristic dense shadows.

DIAGNOSTIC PROCEDURES

- Bronchoscopy may show an obstructing neoplasm, foreign body, or pneumonia.
- Pulse oximetry shows decreased oxygen saturation.

GENERAL
- Incentive spirometry
- Chest percussion
- Postural drainage
- Frequent coughing and deep-breathing exercises
- Bronchoscopy, if above measures fail
- Humidity
- Intermittent positive-pressure breathing therapy
- Radiation may be required for obstructing neoplasm

DIET
- Based on patient's condition as tolerated
- Increased fluids

ACTIVITY
- As tolerated; discourage bed rest

MEDICATIONS
- Bronchodilators
- Analgesics after surgery

SURGERY
- May be required if obstructing neoplasm present

NURSING DIAGNOSES
- Acute pain
- Anxiety
- Fear
- Impaired gas exchange
- Ineffective airway clearance
- Ineffective breathing pattern
- Risk for infection

EXPECTED OUTCOMES
The patient will:
- report feelings of increased comfort and relief from pain
- express feelings of decreased anxiety
- use support systems to assist with anxiety and fear
- maintain adequate ventilation
- maintain a patent airway
- maintain effective breathing pattern
- avoid infection.

NURSING INTERVENTIONS
- Give prescribed drugs.
- Encourage coughing and deep breathing.
- Reposition the patient often.
- Encourage and assist with ambulation as soon as possible.
- Help the patient use an incentive spirometer.
- Humidify inspired air.
- Encourage adequate fluid intake.
- Loosen secretions with postural drainage and chest percussion.
- Provide suctioning as needed.
- Offer the patient reassurance and emotional support.

MONITORING
- Vital signs
- Intake and output
- Pulse oximetry
- Respiratory status (breath sounds, ABG results)

GENERAL
Be sure to cover:
- use of incentive spirometer
- postural drainage and percussion
- coughing and deep-breathing exercises
- importance of splinting incisions
- energy conservation techniques
- stress-reduction strategies
- importance of mobilization.

DISCHARGE PLANNING
- Refer the patient to a smoking-cessation program, if indicated.
- Refer the patient to a weight-reduction program, if indicated.

RESOURCES
Organizations
National Heart, Lung, and Blood Institute: *www.nhlbi.nih.gov*

Selected references
Diseases, 4th ed. Philadelphia: Lippincott Williams & Wilkins, 2006.
Nettina, S.M. *Lippincott Manual of Nursing Practice,* 8th ed. Philadelphia: Lippincott Williams & Wilkins, 2005.

Atopic dermatitis

- A chronic skin disorder characterized by superficial skin inflammation and intense itching

PATHOPHYSIOLOGY

- The allergic mechanism of hypersensitivity results in a release of inflammatory mediators through sensitized antibodies of the immunoglobulin (Ig) E class.
- Histamine and other cytokines induce acute inflammation.
- Abnormally dry skin and a decreased threshold for itching set up the "itch-scratch-itch" cycle, which eventually causes lesions (excoriations, lichenification).

CAUSES

- Exact etiology of atopic dermatitis is unknown; however, a genetic predisposition is likely
- Possible contributing factors:
- – Chemical irritants
- – Extremes of temperature and humidity
- – Food allergy
- – Infection
- – Psychological stress or strong emotions

WARNING *About 10% of juvenile cases of atopic dermatitis are caused by allergic reactions to certain foods, especially eggs, peanuts, milk, wheat, seafood, and soymilk.*

INCIDENCE

- Atopic dermatitis may appear at any age but typically begins during infancy or early childhood (may then subside spontaneously, followed by exacerbations in late childhood, adolescence, or early adulthood). (See *Atopic dermatitis in infants*.)
- The disorder affects less than 1% of the general population.

COMPLICATIONS

- Scarring
- Severe viral infections
- Bacterial and fungal skin infections
- Ocular disorders
- Allergic contact dermatitis

HISTORY

- Atopy, such as asthma, hay fever, or urticaria (or similar family history) (see *Factors contributing to atopy*)
- Exposure to allergen
- Pruritus

PHYSICAL FINDINGS

- Erythematous, weeping lesions (see *Signs of atopic dermatitis*)
- Pink pigmentation and swelling of the upper eyelid and a double fold under the lower lid
- Xerosis, lichenification, and eczematous lesions

LABORATORY

- Complete blood count reveals eosinophilia.
- Serum IgE level is elevated.

OTHER

- Physical examination findings help determine the diagnosis.

Atopic dermatitis in infants

Infants with atopic dermatitis have papular and vesicular skin eruptions, with surrounding erythema. The vesicles rupture and exude yellow, sticky exudate. The secretions form crusts on the skin as they dry.

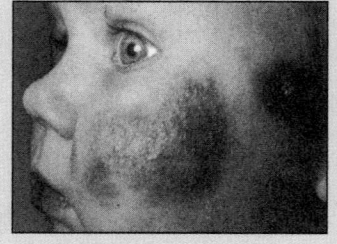

Signs of atopic dermatitis

This illustration shows the typical lesions involved in atopic dermatitis.

Edema, crusting, and scaling

Erythematous areas on dry skin

TREATMENT

GENERAL
- Meticulous skin care
- Environmental control of offending allergens
- Nonirritating topical lubricants

DIET
- Avoidance of foods that are known allergy triggers

MEDICATIONS
- Anti-inflammatories and corticosteroids
- Immunomodulators for severe disease
- Antipruritics
- Antihistamines
- Antibiotics, if secondary infection develops

NURSING CONSIDERATIONS

NURSING DIAGNOSES
- Acute pain
- Disturbed body image
- Impaired skin integrity
- Impaired tissue integrity
- Risk for infection

EXPECTED OUTCOMES
The patient will:
- express relief from itching and pain
- verbalize feelings about changed body image
- demonstrate improved skin condition and maintain skin integrity
- exhibit improved or healed wounds or lesions
- remain free from infection.

NURSING INTERVENTIONS
- Offer support to help the patient and his family cope with this chronic disorder.
- Dissuade the patient from scratching during urticaria to help prevent infection.
- Apply prescribed topical medications.

MONITORING
- Compliance with drug therapy
- Treatment of lesions
- Nutritional status

PATIENT TEACHING

GENERAL
Be sure to cover:
- when and how to apply topical corticosteroids
- importance of regular personal hygiene that involves using only water with little soap
- signs and symptoms of secondary infection
- avoidance of laundry additives, such as fragrances and dyes
- avoidance of allergens.

RESOURCES
Organizations
American Academy of Dermatology: *www.aad.org*
Dermatology Foundation: *www.dermfnd.org*

Selected references
Carter, K.F., et al. "Identifying Secondary Skin Lesions," *Nursing* 34(1):68, January 2004.
Hohwy, T., et al. "Surfactant Protein D in Atopic Dermatitis and Psoriasis," *Experimental Dermatology* 15(3):168-74, March 2006.
Holten, K.B. "How Should We Care for Atopic Dermatitis?" *Journal of Family Practice* 54(5):426-27, May 2005.

Factors contributing to atopy

- Changes associated with industrialization, such as exposure to new chemicals like diesel fumes, have increased the antigenicity of common pollens.
- Increased exposure to antigens, such as dust mites (in wall-to-wall carpets), especially at an early age, contributes to a predisposition to developing allergies.
- Cultural dietary changes and trends, such as increased fat intake and an earlier weaning from breast milk, may be contributing factors.

- Vaccination may cause a shift in T-cell function away from the normal helper T-cell (Th1) response to the Th2 allergic response by limiting early bacterial and viral infections.
- Lack of exposure to intestinal parasites may contribute to a similar shift in T-cell functioning.
- Frequent use of antibiotics, especially in early childhood, may decrease normal intestinal flora and further contribute to the shift.

Atrial fibrillation

OVERVIEW

- Rhythm disturbance of the atria
- Characterized by an irregularly irregular cardiac rate and rhythm (see *Recognizing atrial fibrillation*)

PATHOPHYSIOLOGY

- Involves rapid discharges from numerous ectopic foci in the atria
- Leads to erratic and uncoordinated atrial rhythm

CAUSES

- Atrial fibrosis
- Cardiomyopathy
- Cardiothoracic surgery
- Heart failure
- Hypersympathetic state associated with acute alcohol ingestion
- Hypertension
- Hyperthyroidism
- Myocardial infarction (MI)
- Pericarditis
- Pulmonary embolism
- Valvular disease

INCIDENCE

- Atrial fibrillation is more common in patients older than age 70.
- More men are affected than women.

COMPLICATIONS

- Transient ischemic attack
- Stroke
- Heart failure
- Thromboembolism

ASSESSMENT

HISTORY

- Palpitations
- Fatigue
- Dyspnea
- Chest pain
- Syncope

PHYSICAL FINDINGS

- Irregular pulse
- Possible tachycardia
- Hypotension
- Signs of heart failure
- Respiratory distress

DIAGNOSTIC TEST RESULTS

LABORATORY

- Cardiac enzymes show myocardial damage (with MI).
- Thyroid function studies reveal hyperthyroidism.

IMAGING

- Chest X-ray may determine if pulmonary edema is present.
- Echocardiogram or transesophageal echocardiography may help to identify valvular disease, left ventricular dysfunction, and atrial clots.

DIAGNOSTIC PROCEDURES

- Electrocardiogram may indicate irregular rhythm.
- Holter monitor may diagnose paroxysmal atrial fibrillation.

Recognizing atrial fibrillation

The following rhythm strip shows atrial fibrillation:

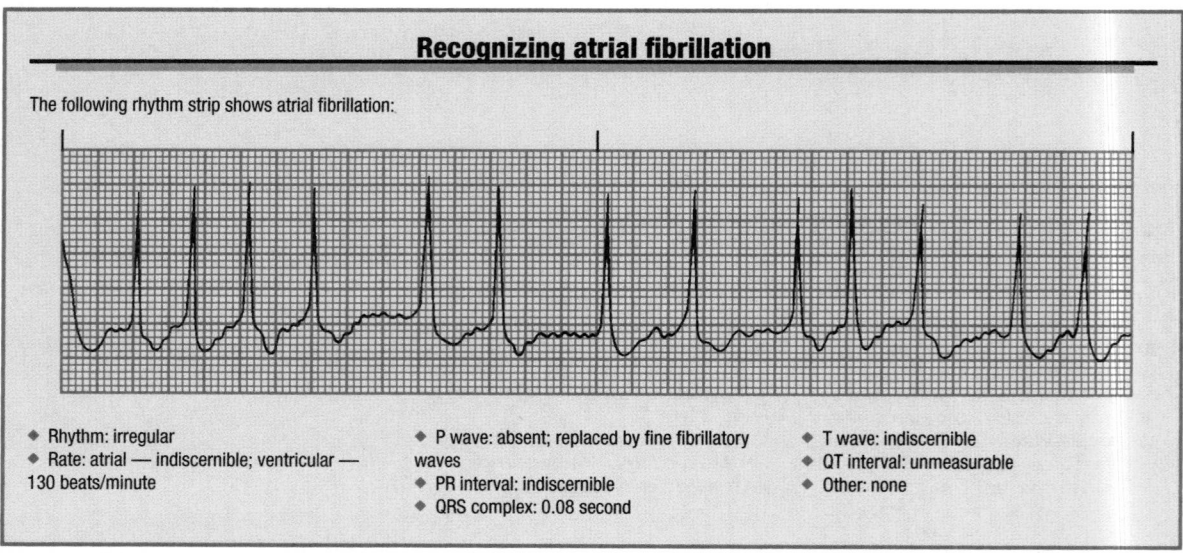

- Rhythm: irregular
- Rate: atrial — indiscernible; ventricular — 130 beats/minute
- P wave: absent; replaced by fine fibrillatory waves
- PR interval: indiscernible
- QRS complex: 0.08 second
- T wave: indiscernible
- QT interval: unmeasurable
- Other: none

TREATMENT

GENERAL
- Possible electrical cardioversion
- Atrial fibrillation suppression pacemaker
- Ablation

DIET
- Low-fat, low-sodium
- Fluid restriction, if indicated

ACTIVITY
- Planned rest periods as needed

MEDICATIONS
- Calcium channel blockers
- Beta-adrenergic blockers
- Antiarrhythmics
- Cardiac glycosides
- Anticoagulation

NURSING CONSIDERATIONS

NURSING DIAGNOSES
- Activity intolerance
- Anxiety
- Fatigue
- Noncompliance (medication regimen)

EXPECTED OUTCOMES
The patient will:
- report ways to reduce activity intolerance
- identify effective coping mechanisms to manage anxiety
- express feelings of energy and decreased fatigue
- verbalize understanding of medication regimen.

NURSING INTERVENTIONS
- Give prescribed drugs.
- Encourage the patient and his family to talk about feelings and concerns.
- Plan rest periods.

MONITORING
- Vital signs at rest and after physical activity
- Signs and symptoms of embolism
- Intake and output
- Daily weight
- Abnormal bleeding

PATIENT TEACHING

GENERAL
Be sure to cover:
- the disorder, diagnosis, and treatment
- medications and potential adverse reactions
- when to notify the practitioner
- instructions on how to monitor pulse
- anticoagulation precautions
- abnormal bleeding
- signs and symptoms of embolic events.

DISCHARGE PLANNING
- Refer the patient to programs such as "Coumadin Clinic" to monitor anticoagulant therapy.

RESOURCES
Organizations
American Heart Association:
www.americanheart.org
St. Jude Medical:
www.aboutatrialfibrillation.com

Selected references
Adkins, L. "Atrial Fibrillation," *Nursing* 33(7):46-47, July 2003.
Dambro, M.R. *Griffith's Five-Minute Clinical Consult 2006.* Philadelphia: Lippincott Williams & Wilkins, 2006.
Holten, K.B. "How Should We Manage Newly Diagnosed Atrial Fibrillation?" *Journal of Family Practice* 53(8):641-43, August 2004.

Atrial septal defect

OVERVIEW

- An acyanotic congenital heart defect featuring an opening between the left and right atria that allows blood to flow from left to right, resulting in ineffective pumping of the heart, thus increasing the risk of heart failure
- Three types: Sinus venosus, ostium secundum, and ostium primum (see *Types of atrial septal defects*)

PATHOPHYSIOLOGY

- Blood shunts from the left atrium to the right atrium because the left atrial pressure is normally slightly higher than the right atrial pressure.
- This pressure difference forces large amounts of blood through a defect.
- This shunt results in right heart volume overload, affecting the right atrium, right ventricle, and pulmonary arteries.
- Eventually, the right atrium enlarges, and the right ventricle dilates to accommodate the increased blood volume.
- If pulmonary artery hypertension develops, increased pulmonary vascular resistance and right ventricular hypertrophy follow.

- Irreversible pulmonary artery hypertension causes reversal of the shunt direction in some adults, which results in unoxygenated blood entering the systemic circulation, causing cyanosis.

CAUSES

- No known cause
- Ostium primum defects commonly occur in patients with Down syndrome

INCIDENCE

- Atrial septal defect accounts for about 10% of congenital heart defects.
- This disorder appears almost twice as commonly in females as in males, with a strong familial tendency.
- This is usually a benign defect during infancy and childhood. (Delayed development of symptoms and complications makes it one of the most common congenital heart defects diagnosed in adults.)

COMPLICATIONS

- Physical underdevelopment
- Respiratory infections
- Heart failure
- Atrial arrhythmias
- Mitral valve prolapse

ASSESSMENT

HISTORY

- Increasing fatigue
- Chest pain
- Dyspnea
- Coughing
- Dizziness or syncope

PHYSICAL FINDINGS

- Early to midsystolic murmur at the second or third left intercostal space
- Low-pitched diastolic murmur at the left lower sternal border, more pronounced on inspiration
- Fixed, widely split S_2
- Systolic click or late systolic murmur at the apex
- Peripheral edema
- Distended jugular veins
- Cyanosis

⚡ **WARNING** *An infant may be cyanotic because he has a cardiac or pulmonary disorder. Cyanosis that worsens with crying most likely has a cardiac cause because crying increases pulmonary resistance to blood flow, resulting in an increased right-to-left shunt. Cyanosis that improves with crying most likely has a pulmonary cause because deep breathing improves tidal volume.*

Types of atrial septal defects

Experts recognize three types of atrial septal defects, as shown. These defects can vary in size, but sinus venosus defects tend to be smaller than the others are.

SINUS VENOSUS

Usually located in the superior-posterior portion of the atrial septum, sinus venosus sometimes extends into the superior vena cava and is usually associated with abnormalities of the pulmonary veins as they enter the superior vena cava and the right atrium.

OSTIUM SECUNDUM

Ostium secundum, which may be single or multiple, is associated with the fossa ovalis and occasionally extends down close to the inferior vena cava.

OSTIUM PRIMUM

Ostium primum of the primitive septum occurs in the inferior portion of the septum primum and is usually associated with atrioventricular valve abnormalities (cleft mitral valve) and conduction defects.

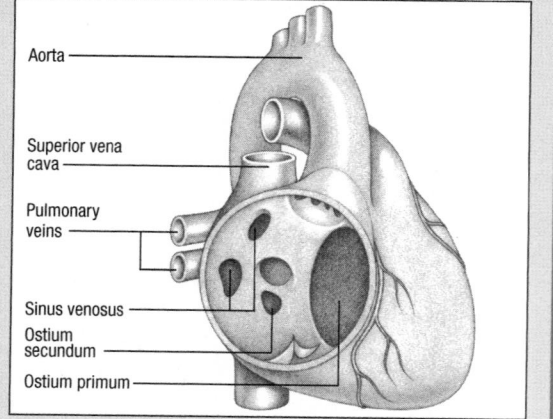

Aorta

Superior vena cava

Pulmonary veins

Sinus venosus

Ostium secundum

Ostium primum

DIAGNOSTIC TEST RESULTS

IMAGING
◆ Chest X-ray shows an enlarged right atrium and right ventricle, a prominent pulmonary artery, and increased pulmonary vascular markings.

DIAGNOSTIC PROCEDURES
◆ Electrocardiography results may be normal but commonly show right axis deviation, a prolonged PR interval, varying degrees of right bundle-branch block, right ventricular hypertrophy, atrial fibrillation (particularly in severe cases in patients older than age 30), and in ostium primum defect, left axis deviation.
◆ Echocardiography measures right ventricular enlargement, may locate the defect, and shows volume overload in the right side of the heart. It may reveal right ventricular and pulmonary artery dilation.
◆ Two-dimensional echocardiography with color flow Doppler ultrasonography, contrast echocardiography, or both has supplanted cardiac catheterization as the confirming test for atrial septal defects (ASDs). Cardiac catheterization is used if inconsistencies exist in the clinical data or if significant pulmonary hypertension is suspected.

TREATMENT

DIET
◆ Low-fat, low-cholesterol

ACTIVITY
◆ As tolerated

MEDICATIONS
◆ Diuretics
◆ Antibiotics
◆ Analgesics

SURGERY
◆ Minimally invasive heart surgery may be required for the patient with an uncomplicated ASD with evidence of significant left-to-right shunting.
◆ A large defect may need immediate surgical closure with sutures or a patch graft.
◆ Cardiac catheterization closure, involving insertion of an umbrella-like patch or septal occluder through a cardiac catheter, may be performed.

NURSING CONSIDERATIONS

NURSING DIAGNOSES
◆ Activity intolerance
◆ Decreased cardiac output
◆ Fatigue
◆ Impaired gas exchange
◆ Risk for infection

EXPECTED OUTCOMES
The patient will:
◆ express feelings of increased energy
◆ maintain an optimal cardiac output
◆ identify measures to prevent or reduce fatigue
◆ maintain adequate ventilation
◆ avoid infection.

NURSING INTERVENTIONS
◆ Encourage the child to engage in any activity he can tolerate.
◆ Give prescribed drugs.

MONITORING
◆ Vital signs
◆ Central venous and intra-arterial pressures
◆ Intake and output
◆ Cardiac rhythm
◆ Oxygenation

PATIENT TEACHING

GENERAL
Be sure to cover:
◆ pretest and posttest procedures with the child and his parents (If possible, use drawings or other visual aids to explain them to the child.)
◆ postoperative procedures, tubes, dressings, and monitoring equipment
◆ antibiotic prophylaxis to prevent infective endocarditis.

DISCHARGE PLANNING
◆ Refer the patient and his family to community resources, as needed.

RESOURCES
Organizations
American Heart Association: *www.americanheart.org*

Selected references
Diseases, 4th ed. Philadelphia: Lippincott Williams & Wilkins, 2006.
Nettina, S.M. *Lippincott Manual of Nursing Practice*, 8th ed. Philadelphia: Lippincott Williams & Wilkins, 2005.

Attention deficit hyperactivity disorder

OVERVIEW

- A behavioral problem characterized by difficulty with inattention, impulsivity, hyperactivity, and boredom
- Also called *ADHD* and *ADD*

PATHOPHYSIOLOGY
- Alleles of dopamine genes may alter dopamine transmission in the neural networks.
- During fetal development, bouts of hypoxia and hypotension could selectively damage neurons located in some of the critical regions of the anatomical networks.

CAUSES
- Limited evidence of a genetic component
- Some studies indicate that it may result from altered neurotransmitter levels in the brain
- Underlying cause unknown

RISK FACTORS
- Family history
- History of learning disability
- Mood or conduct disorder

INCIDENCE
- ADHD is present at birth, but diagnosis before age 4 or 5 is difficult; some patients aren't diagnosed until adulthood.
- The disorder occurs in 3% to 5% of school-age children.
- The disorder affects males three times more than females.

COMPLICATIONS
- Emotional and social complications
- Poor nutrition

ASSESSMENT

HISTORY
- Characterization as a fidgeter and a daydreamer
- Appearance of being inattentive and lazy
- Sporadic performance at school or work

PHYSICAL FINDINGS
Symptoms of inattention
- Making careless mistakes
- Struggling to sustain attention
- Failing to finish activities
- Difficulty with organization
- Avoiding tasks that require sustained mental effort
- Distractedness or forgetfulness

Symptoms of hyperactivity
- Fidgeting
- Inability to sit still for sustained period
- Difficulty playing quietly
- Talking excessively

Symptoms of impulsivity
- Interrupting
- Inability to wait patiently

DSM-IV-TR *criteria*
These criteria confirm a diagnosis:
- six symptoms or more from the inattention or hyperactivity-impulsivity categories
- symptoms present for at least 6 months
- symptoms evident before age 7
- impairment present in two or more settings
- symptoms aren't accounted for by another mental disorder.

DIAGNOSTIC TEST RESULTS

- Complete psychological, medical, and neurologic evaluations rule out other problems; specific tests include continuous performance test, behavior rating scales, and learning disability.

TREATMENT

GENERAL
◆ Education about the nature and effect of the disorder
◆ Behavior modification
◆ External structure
◆ Supportive psychotherapy

DIET
◆ Elimination of sugar, dyes, and additives

ACTIVITY
◆ Monitoring (for safety purposes)

MEDICATIONS
◆ Stimulants
◆ Tricyclic antidepressants
◆ Mood stabilizers
◆ Beta-adrenergic blockers

NURSING CONSIDERATIONS

NURSING DIAGNOSES
◆ Compromised family coping
◆ Impaired social interaction
◆ Ineffective family therapeutic regimen management

EXPECTED OUTCOMES
The patient (or his family) will:
◆ seek support systems and exhibit adequate coping behaviors
◆ demonstrate effective social interaction skills in one-on-one and group settings
◆ report improvement in family and social interactions.

NURSING INTERVENTIONS
◆ Set realistic expectations and limits to avoid frustrating the patient.
◆ Maintain a calm and consistent manner.
◆ Keep all instructions short and simple — make one-step requests.
◆ Provide praise, rewards, and positive feedback whenever possible.
◆ Provide diversional activities suited to a short attention span.

MONITORING
◆ Activity level
◆ Nutritional status
◆ Adverse drug reactions
◆ Response to treatment
◆ Complications
◆ Activity (for safety purposes)

PATIENT TEACHING

GENERAL
Be sure to cover:
◆ behavior therapy
◆ reinforcement of good behavior
◆ realistic expectations
◆ medication regimen and possible adverse reactions
◆ nutrition.

DISCHARGE PLANNING
◆ Refer the patient to family therapy.

RESOURCES
Organizations
ADD helpline: *www.addhelpline.org*
Children and Adults with Attention-Deficit/Hyperactivity Disorder: *www.chadd.org*
National Center for Learning Disabilities: *www.ncld.org*

Selected references
Diagnostic and Statistical Manual of Mental Disorders, Fourth Edition, Text Revision. Washington, D.C.: American Psychiatric Association, 2000.
McDonnell, M.A., and Dougherty, M. "Righting a Troubled Course. Diagnosing and Treating ADHD in Adults," *Advance for Nurse Practitioners* 13(8): 53-56, August 2005.
Wolraich, M.L., et al. "Teachers' Screening for Attention Deficit/Hyperactivity Disorder: Comparing Multinational Samples on Teacher Ratings of ADHD," *Journal of Abnormal Child Psychology* 31(4):445-55, August 2003.

Autistic disorder

OVERVIEW

- A severe, pervasive developmental disorder
- Degree of impairment varies
- Usually apparent before age 3
- Poor prognosis
- Sometimes called *Kanner's autism*

PATHOPHYSIOLOGY

- Defects in the central nervous system (CNS) that may arise from prenatal complications

CAUSES

- Exact cause unknown
- Defects in CNS from prenatal complications such as rubella
- Disease caused or triggered by immunizations
- Nutritional deficiency

RISK FACTORS

- High-risk pregnancy

INCIDENCE

- Autistic disorder affects 4 to 5 children per 10,000 births.
- The disorder is four to five times more likely in boys than in girls, usually the firstborn boy.

COMPLICATIONS

- Epileptic seizures
- Depression

During stress

- Catatonic phenomena
- Undifferentiated psychotic state

ASSESSMENT

HISTORY

- Becomes rigid or flaccid when held
- Cries when touched
- Shows little or no interest in human contact

PHYSICAL FINDINGS

- Delayed smiling response
- Severe language impairment
- Lack of socialization and imaginative play
- Echolalia
- Pronoun reversal
- Bizarre or self-destructive behavior
- Extreme compulsion for sameness
- Abnormal reaction to sensory stimuli
- Cognitive impairment
- Eating, drinking, and sleeping problems
- Mood disorders

DSM-IV-TR *criteria*
At least 6 of these 12 characteristics must be present, including at least 2 items from the first section, 1 from the second, and 1 from the third.

- Qualitative impairment in social interaction:
- Impaired nonverbal behavior
- Absence of peer relationships
- Failure to seek or share enjoyment, interests, or achievements
- Lack of social or emotional reciprocity
- Qualitative impairment in communication:
- Delay or lack of language development
- Inability to initiate or sustain conversation
- Idiosyncratic or repetitive language
- Lack of appropriate imaginative play
- Restricted repetitive and stereotyped patterns of behavior, interests, and activities:
- Abnormal preoccupation with a restricted pattern of interest
- Inflexible routines or rituals
- Repetitive motor mannerisms
- Preoccupation with parts of objects

The diagnostic criteria also include delays or abnormal functioning in at least one of these areas before age 3:

- Social interaction and language skills
- Symbolic or imaginative play

DIAGNOSTIC TEST RESULTS

- Diagnosis is made based on *DSM-IV-TR* criteria findings.

TREATMENT

GENERAL
◆ Structured treatment plan
◆ Behavioral techniques
◆ Pleasurable sensory and motor stimulation

ACTIVITY
◆ Monitoring (for safety purposes)

MEDICATIONS
◆ Haloperidol (Haldol)

NURSING CONSIDERATIONS

NURSING DIAGNOSES
◆ Delayed growth and development
◆ Disabled family coping
◆ Impaired verbal communication
◆ Interrupted family processes
◆ Risk for injury
◆ Risk for self-directed violence
◆ Social isolation

EXPECTED OUTCOMES
The patient (or his family) will:
◆ as much as possible, demonstrate age-appropriate skills and behaviors
◆ seek support systems and exhibit adequate coping behaviors
◆ develop alternate means of communication to express self
◆ identify and contact available resources as needed
◆ practice safety measures and take safety precautions in the home
◆ refrain from harming self
◆ interact with family or friends.

NURSING INTERVENTIONS
◆ Institute safety measures when appropriate.
◆ Provide positive reinforcement.
◆ Encourage development of self-esteem.
◆ Encourage self-care.
◆ Prepare the child for change by telling him about it.
◆ Assist family members in developing strong one-on-one relationships with the patient.

MONITORING
◆ Response to treatment
◆ Complications
◆ Adverse drug reactions
◆ Patterns of behavior
◆ Nutritional status
◆ Social interaction
◆ Communication skills
◆ Activity

PATIENT TEACHING

GENERAL
Be sure to cover:
◆ physical care for the child's needs
◆ importance of identifying coping skills and signs of excessive stress.

DISCHARGE PLANNING
◆ Refer the parents to resource and support services.

RESOURCES
Organizations
Autism Society of America:
www.autism-society.org
Center for the Study of Autism:
www.autism.org
National Alliance for Autism Research:
www.naar.org

Selected references
Diagnostic and Statistical Manual of Mental Disorders, Fourth Edition, Text Revision. Washington, D.C.: American Psychiatric Association, 2000.
Mohr, W.K. *Psychiatric-Mental Health Nursing,* 6th ed. Philadelphia: Lippincott Williams & Wilkins, 2006.
Schumann, C.M., et al. "The Amygdala is Enlarged in Children But Not Adolescents with Autism; the Hippocampus is Enlarged at All Ages," *Journal of Neuroscience* 24(28):6392-401, July 2004.

Avian flu

- An infectious, contagious disease caused by influenza A viruses that normally affect birds
- Carried in the intestines of wild birds worldwide without causing sickness, but highly contagious and deadly to domesticated birds (chickens, ducks, turkeys)
- Human infection caused by contact with infected poultry or contaminated surfaces
- Also called *bird flu*

PATHOPHYSIOLOGY

- After attaching to the host cell, viral ribonucleic acid enters the cell and uses host components to replicate its genetic material and protein, which are then assembled into new virus particles.
- Newly produced viruses burst forth to invade other healthy cells.
- Viral invasion destroys host cells, impairing respiratory defenses (especially the mucociliary transport system) and predisposing the patient to secondary bacterial infection.

CAUSES

- Highly pathogenic influenza A (H5N1) virus
- Isolated reports of human-to-human transmission

INCIDENCE

- Over 100 human cases of influenza infection were reported since 1997, mostly by viruses of the H5 and H7 subtypes (H5N1, H7N7, H7N3).
- Ongoing close monitoring of human infection and transmission is due to concern over potential global outbreak in humans or influenza pandemic.

COMPLICATIONS

- Conjunctivitis
- Pneumonia
- Acute respiratory distress
- Viral pneumonia
- Sepsis
- Organ failure
- Death

HISTORY

- Direct contact with infected poultry or contaminated surfaces

PHYSICAL FINDINGS

- Fever
- Cough (dry or productive)
- Sore throat
- Difficulty breathing
- Diarrhea
- Runny nose
- Headache
- Muscle aches
- Malaise

LABORATORY

- Viral culture by polymerase chain reaction is positive for H5N1 virus.

TREATMENT

GENERAL
- Fluid and electrolyte replacements
- Oxygen and assisted ventilation, if indicated

DIET
- Increased fluid intake

ACTIVITY
- Rest periods as needed

MEDICATIONS
- Oseltamivir (Tamiflu)
- Zanamivir (Relenza)
- Acetaminophen or aspirin
- Guaifenesin (Hytuss) or expectorant
- Antibiotics
- Vaccine currently under investigation

NURSING CONSIDERATIONS

NURSING DIAGNOSES
- Acute pain
- Fatigue
- Hyperthermia
- Ineffective breathing pattern
- Risk for deficient fluid volume
- Risk for infection

EXPECTED OUTCOMES
The patient will:
- express feelings of increased comfort and relief from pain
- report increased energy level
- maintain a normal temperature
- maintain respiratory rate of within 5 breaths/minute of baseline
- maintain adequate fluid volume
- avoid infection.

NURSING INTERVENTIONS
- Give prescribed drugs.
- Follow standard precautions.
- Administer oxygen therapy, if warranted.

MONITORING
- Temperature
- Signs and symptoms of dehydration
- Respiratory status
- Response to treatment
- Complications

PATIENT TEACHING

GENERAL
Be sure to cover:
- the disorder, diagnostic studies, and treatment
- importance of increased fluids to prevent dehydration.

RESOURCES
Organizations
Centers for Disease Control and Prevention: *www.cdc.gov*
U.S. Department of Agriculture: *www.usda.gov*
U.S. National Library of Medicine: *www.nlm.nih.gov*
World Health Organization: *www.who.int/en*

Selected references
Gani, R. "Potential Impact of Antiviral Drug Use during Influenza Pandemic," *Emerging Infectious Diseases* 11(9): 1355-362, September 2005.
Henley, E. "The Growing Threat of Avian Influenza," *Journal of Family Practice* 54(5):442-44, May 2005.

Basal cell carcinoma

- Slow-growing, destructive cancerous skin tumor
- Two major types: noduloulcerative and superficial
- Most common malignant tumor that affects whites (see *Identifying basal cell carcinoma*)

PATHOPHYSIOLOGY

- Although the pathogenesis is uncertain, some experts hypothesize that it originates when undifferentiated basal cells become carcinomatous instead of differentiating into sweat glands, sebum, and hair.

CAUSES

- Prolonged sun exposure (90% of tumors occur on sun-exposed areas of the body)

RISK FACTORS

- Arsenic ingestion
- Radiation exposure
- Burns
- Immunosuppression
- Vaccinations (a rare possibility)
- History of previous nonmelanoma skin cancer

INCIDENCE

- Basal cell carcinoma usually occurs in people older than age 40.
- The disease is most prevalent in blond, fair-skinned men.

COMPLICATIONS

- Disfiguring lesions of the eyes, nose, and cheeks

ASSESSMENT

HISTORY

- Odd-looking skin lesion
- Prolonged exposure to the sun
- Nonhealing sore of varying duration

PHYSICAL FINDINGS

- Lesions characterized as small, smooth, pinkish, and translucent papules (early-stage noduloulcerative)
- May be pigmented; may have telangiectatic vessels crossing the surface
- Become enlarged with depressed centers and firm and elevated borders (also called *rodent ulcers*)
- Oval or irregularly shaped, lightly pigmented plaques on chest or back
- Waxy, sclerotic, yellow to white plaques without distinct borders on head or neck

DIAGNOSTIC TEST RESULTS

DIAGNOSTIC PROCEDURES

- Incisional or excisional biopsy and histologic study may help to determine the tumor type and histologic subtype.

OTHER

- All types of basal cell carcinomas are diagnosed by clinical appearance.

Identifying basal cell carcinoma

This illustration shows an enlarged nasal nodule in basal cell carcinoma. Note its depressed center and firm, elevated border.

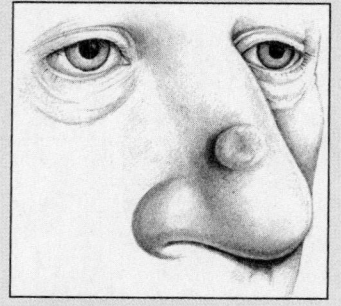

TREATMENT

GENERAL
- Depends on the size, location, and depth of the lesion
- Irradiation, if the tumor location requires it; preferred for elderly or debilitated patients who might not tolerate surgery
- Cryotherapy (liquid nitrogen that freezes the cells and kills them)

DIET
- Well-balanced; no restrictions

MEDICATIONS
- Chemotherapy, such as topical fluorouracil and topical corticosteroids

SURGERY
- Curettage and electrodesiccation
- Microscopically controlled surgical excision carefully removes recurrent lesions until a tumor-free plane is achieved (after removal of large lesions, skin grafting may be required)
- Chemosurgery

NURSING CONSIDERATIONS

NURSING DIAGNOSES
- Anxiety
- Chronic low self-esteem
- Disturbed body image
- Fear
- Imbalanced nutrition: Less than body requirements
- Impaired skin integrity
- Ineffective coping
- Risk for infection

EXPECTED OUTCOMES
The patient will:
- identify effective coping mechanisms to manage anxiety
- express positive feelings about self
- verbalize feelings about changed body image
- verbalize feelings of anxiety and fear
- maintain adequate nutrition and hydration
- exhibit improved or healed lesions or wounds
- demonstrate effective coping mechanisms
- develop no signs or symptoms of infection.

NURSING INTERVENTIONS
- Encourage verbalization and provide support.
- Provide appropriate wound care.

MONITORING
- Complications of treatment
- Response to treatment
- Signs and symptoms of infection
- Wound healing
- Skin surveillance for additional lesions

PATIENT TEACHING

GENERAL
Be sure to cover:
- the disorder, diagnosis, and treatment
- appropriate skin care.

DISCHARGE PLANNING
- Tell the patient to avoid excessive sun exposure and ultraviolet radiation and to use a strong sunscreen or sunshade to protect the skin.
- Refer the patient to resource and support services.

RESOURCES
Organizations
American Cancer Society: *www.cancer.org*
Guide to Internet Resources for Cancer: *www.cancerindex.org*
National Cancer Institute: *www.cancer.gov*

Selected references
Atlas of Pathophysiology, 2nd ed. Philadelphia: Lippincott Williams & Wilkins, 2005.

Casciato, D.A. *Manual of Clinical Oncology,* 5th ed. Philadelphia: Lippincott Williams & Wilkins, 2004.

Colvett, K.T., et al. "Atypical Presentation of Metastatic Basal Cell Carcinoma," *Southern Medical Journal* 97(3):305-307, March 2004.

Marin-Gutzke, M., et al. "Basal Cell Carcinoma in Childhood After Radiation Therapy: Case Report and Review," *Annals of Plastic Surgery* 53(6):593-95, December 2004.

Netscher, D.T., and Spira, M. "Basal Cell Carcinoma: An Overview of Tumor Biology and Treatment," *Plastic & Reconstructive Surgery* 113(5):74e-94e, April 2004.

Bell's palsy

OVERVIEW

- Rapid-onset condition in which the seventh cranial nerve impulses are blocked, causing facial muscle weakness or paralysis
- Subsides spontaneously in 80% to 90% of patients
- Usually subsides (function returns to normal) in 3 to 6 months
- Delayed recovery possible in elderly people
- In partial recovery, contracture development possible on the paralyzed side of the face
- May recur on the same or opposite side of the face

PATHOPHYSIOLOGY

- An inflammatory reaction occurs around the seventh cranial nerve (motor innervation of the facial muscles).
- Inflammation is usually at the internal auditory meatus.
- Unilateral facial weakness or paralysis results.

CAUSES

- Exact cause unknown
- Autoimmune disease
- Bacterial infection such as meningitis
- Ischemia
- Local traumatic injury
- Lyme disease
- Tumor
- Viral infection, such as herpes simplex or herpes zoster

INCIDENCE

- Bell's palsy may affect any age-group.
- The disorder most commonly occurs between ages 20 and 60.
- Bell's palsy affects males and females equally.
- The disorder affects pregnant women more often than women who aren't pregnant.

COMPLICATIONS

- Corneal ulceration and blindness
- Impaired nutrition secondary to paralysis of the lower face
- Long-term psychosocial problems

ASSESSMENT

HISTORY

- Pain on the affected side around the angle of the jaw or behind the ear for a few hours or days before onset of weakness
- Difficulty chewing on the affected side
- Difficulty speaking clearly

PHYSICAL FINDINGS

- Drooping mouth on the affected side (see *Facial paralysis in Bell's palsy*)
- Smooth forehead
- Distorted taste perception
- Inability to raise eyebrow, smile, show teeth, or puff out cheek
- Impaired ability to close eye on the weak side
- Upward eye rolling (Bell's phenomenon) during attempts to close the eye
- Excessive tearing

DIAGNOSTIC TEST RESULTS

IMAGING

- Magnetic resonance imaging rules out tumor.

OTHER

- Diagnosis is based on the clinical presentation.

Facial paralysis in Bell's palsy

Unilateral facial paralysis characterizes Bell's palsy. The paralysis produces a distorted appearance and an inability to wrinkle the forehead, close the eyelid, smile, show the teeth, or puff out the cheek

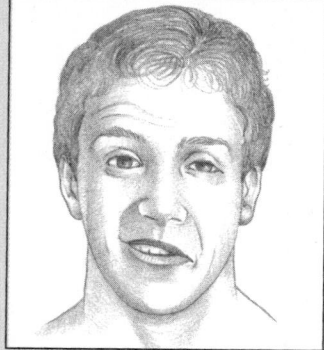

GENERAL
- Eliminating the source of damage to the nerve immediately
- Maintaining oral hygiene
- Protecting the eyes by using sunglasses and adding moisture to eyes
- Protecting the hearing
- Using moist heat
- Using physical therapy

DIET
- As tolerated

ACTIVITY
- As tolerated

MEDICATIONS
- Oral corticosteroids
- Anti-inflammatories
- Analgesics
- Antivirals
- Vitamin and mineral therapy (B_{12}, B_6, zinc)

SURGERY
- Exploration of the facial nerve
- Facial reanimation, such as direct facial nerve repair or facial nerve grafting

NURSING DIAGNOSES
- Acute pain
- Anxiety
- Disturbed body image
- Imbalanced nutrition: Less than body requirements
- Ineffective role performance
- Interrupted family processes
- Situational low self-esteem

EXPECTED OUTCOMES
The patient will:
- experience increased comfort and relief from pain
- express feelings of decreased anxiety
- verbalize feelings about changed body image
- consume an adequate number of calories daily
- express feelings about diminished capacity to perform usual roles
- report improvement in family interactions
- express positive feelings about self.

NURSING INTERVENTIONS
- Provide psychological support.
- Apply moist heat to the affected side of the face.
- Massage the patient's face with a gentle upward motion.
- Provide a facial sling.
- If the patient had surgery, provide preoperative and postoperative care.
- Administer medications, as ordered.

MONITORING
- Response to medications
- Signs and symptoms of peptic ulceration, pancreatitis, or other GI adverse effects of prednisone
- Nutritional status
- Facial muscle movement

GENERAL
Be sure to cover:
- the disorder
- medication and adverse effects
- protection of affected eye
- exercises of the facial muscles
- nutritional management program.

DISCHARGE PLANNING
- Refer the patient to physical therapy, as indicated.

RESOURCES
Organizations
National Institutes of Health: *www.nih.gov*
WebMD: *www.webmd.com*

Selected references
Ashtekar, C.S., et al. "Do We Need to Give Steroids in Children with Bell's Palsy?" *Emergency Medical Journal* 22(7):505-507, July 2005.
Diseases, 4th ed. Philadelphia: Lippincott Williams & Wilkins, 2006.
Handbook of Pathophysiology, 2nd ed. Philadelphia: Lippincott Williams & Wilkins, 2005.
Kanoh, N. et al. "Nocturnal Onset and Development of Bell's Palsy," *Laryngoscope* 115(1):99-100, January 2005.

Benign prostatic hyperplasia

- Causes prostate gland to enlarge sufficiently to compress urethra, causing overt urinary obstruction
- May be treated surgically or symptomatically, depending on the size of prostate, age and health of patient, and extent of obstruction
- Referred to as *BPH*

PATHOPHYSIOLOGY

- Changes occur in periurethral glandular tissue.
- The prostate enlarges and may extend into the bladder.
- The compression or distortion of the prostatic urethra obstructs urine outflow.
- BPH may cause a diverticulum musculature, retaining urine.

CAUSES

- Exact cause unknown
- Link to hormonal activity possible

RISK FACTORS

- Age
- Intact testes

INCIDENCE

AGE FACTOR *BPH occurs in 20% of men between ages 41 and 50, in 50% of men between 51 and 60, and in 90% of men older than age 80.*

COMPLICATIONS

- Acute or chronic renal failure
- Acute postobstructive diuresis
- Bladder diverticula and saccules
- Bladder wall trabeculation
- Detrusor muscle hypertrophy
- Hydronephrosis
- Paradoxical (overflow) incontinence
- Urethral stenosis
- Urinary stasis, urinary tract infection (UTI), or renal calculi

HISTORY

- Decreased urine stream caliber and force
- Interrupted urinary stream
- Urinary hesitancy and frequency
- Difficulty initiating urination
- Nocturia, hematuria
- Dribbling, incontinence
- Urine retention

PHYSICAL FINDINGS

- Visible midline mass above the symphysis pubis
- Distended bladder
- Enlarged prostate on digital rectal examination

LABORATORY

- Elevated blood urea nitrogen and serum creatinine levels may suggest impaired renal function.
- Bacterial count that exceeds $100,000/mm^3$ may reveal hematuria, pyuria, and UTI.

IMAGING

- Excretory urography indicates urinary tract obstruction, hydronephrosis, calculi or tumors, and bladder filling and emptying defects.

DIAGNOSTIC PROCEDURES

- Cystourethroscopy determines the best surgical intervention and shows prostate enlargement, bladder wall changes, calculi, and raised bladder.

OTHER

- International Prostate Symptom Score classifies disorder's severity.

TREATMENT

GENERAL
◆ Prostatic massage

DIET
◆ Short-term fluid restriction (prevents bladder distention)

ACTIVITY
◆ Avoidance of lifting, performing strenuous exercises, and taking long automobile rides for at least 1 month after surgery
◆ No sexual intercourse for several weeks after surgery; if surgery not indicated, sexual intercourse permitted

MEDICATIONS
◆ Antibiotics, if infection present
◆ Alpha$_1$-adrenergic blockers such as terazosin
◆ 5-alpha-reductase inhibitors such as finasteride

SURGERY
◆ For relief of acute urine retention, hydronephrosis, severe hematuria, and recurrent UTI or for palliative relief of intolerable symptoms
◆ Suprapubic (transvesical) prostatectomy
◆ Perineal prostatectomy
◆ Retropubic (extravesical) prostatectomy
◆ Transurethral resection of prostate
◆ Balloon dilatation, ultrasound needle ablation, and use of stents

NURSING CONSIDERATIONS

NURSING DIAGNOSES
◆ Acute pain
◆ Disturbed body image
◆ Impaired urinary elimination
◆ Risk for infection
◆ Sexual dysfunction

EXPECTED OUTCOMES
The patient will:
◆ express feelings of increased comfort
◆ verbalize feelings about changed body image
◆ demonstrate skill in managing urinary elimination
◆ remain free from all signs and symptoms of infection
◆ express feelings about potential or actual changes in sexual activity.

NURSING INTERVENTIONS
◆ Give prescribed drugs.
◆ Avoid giving tranquilizers, alcohol, antidepressants, or anticholinergics (which can worsen the obstruction).
◆ Provide I.V. therapy as ordered.

MONITORING
◆ Vital signs
◆ Intake and output
◆ Daily weight

WARNING *Watch for signs of postobstructive diuresis, characterized by polyuria exceeding 2 L in 8 hours and excessive electrolyte losses. Although usually self-limiting, it can result in vascular collapse and death if not promptly treated.*

After prostatic surgery
◆ Pain control
◆ Catheter function and drainage
◆ Signs of infection

PATIENT TEACHING

GENERAL
Be sure to cover:
◆ the disorder, diagnosis, and treatment
◆ signs of UTI that should be reported
◆ when to seek medical care (fever, unable to void, or passing bloody urine).

DISCHARGE PLANNING
◆ Refer the patient to support services.

RESOURCES
Organizations
American Association of Kidney Patients: *www.aakp.org*
National Institute of Diabetes & Digestive & Kidney Diseases: *www.niddk.nih.gov*

Selected references
Diseases, 4th ed. Philadelphia: Lippincott Williams & Wilkins, 2006.
Gacci, M. et al. "Urinary Symptoms, Quality of Life and Sexual Function in Patients with Benign Prostatic Hypertrophy Before and After Prostatectomy: A Prospective Study," *BJU International* 91(3):196-200, February 2003.
Gilchrist, K.L. "Twin Perils of Prostate Health," *Nursing Made Incredibly Easy!* 3(6):30-42, November-December 2005.
Tierney, L., et al., eds. *Current Medical Diagnosis and Treatment,* 45th ed. New York: McGraw-Hill Book Co., 2006.

Bipolar disorder

- Affective disorder marked by severe pathologic mood swings from hyperactivity and euphoria to sadness and depression
- Cyclothymia: Variant of bipolar disorder in which numerous episodes of hypomania and depressive symptoms are too mild to meet the criteria for major depression or bipolar disorder (see *Cyclothymic disorder*)
- Manic episodes: may emerge over a period of days to weeks or within hours
- Manic and depressive phases: If untreated, may remit in a few weeks or up to a year, with some having an unremitting course
- Rapid cycling: occurs in 15% of all patients, almost all women, when four or more episodes of either depression or mania occur in a given year
- Difficulties in work performance and psychosocial functioning common in half of patients with this disorder

PATHOPHYSIOLOGY
- Autosomal dominant inheritance has been found in genetic studies.
- Mood swings may be related to membrane changes in sodium- and potassium-activated adenosine triphosphatase involving disordered intracellular signals.

CAUSES
- Exact cause unclear
- Autosomal dominant inheritance found in genetic studies
- Imbalances in the biochemistry that controls food (biochemical) imbalances
- May be triggered by death, separation, or divorce
- Some evidence that it's linked to an X chromosome disorder

RISK FACTORS
- Family history
- Substance abuse

INCIDENCE
- Bipolar disorder affects 3 million people in the United States.
- It's equally common in women and men.
- Women are likely to have more depressive than manic episodes.
- Men experience more manic than depressive episodes.
- Incidence of this disorder is higher among relatives of affected patients than in the general population.

   AGE FACTOR *Age of onset is usually between ages 20 and 35, but 35% of patients experience onset between ages 35 and 60.*

COMPLICATIONS
- Emotional and social consequences
- Exhaustion
- Nutritional deficits
- Sexually transmitted disease
- Sleep disturbances
- Suicide

Cyclothymic disorder

A chronic mood disturbance of at least 2 years' duration, cyclothymic disorder involves numerous episodes of hypomania or depressive symptoms that aren't of sufficient severity or duration to qualify as a major depressive episode.

In the hypomanic phase, the patient may experience insomnia; hyperactivity; inflated self-esteem; increased productivity and creativity; overinvolvement in pleasurable activities, including an increased sexual drive; physical restlessness; and rapid speech. Depressive symptoms may include insomnia, feelings of inadequacy, decreased productivity, social withdrawal, loss of libido, loss of interest in pleasurable activities, lethargy, depressed speech, and crying.

A number of medical disorders (for example, endocrinopathies, such as Cushing's disease, stroke, brain tumors, head trauma, and drug overdose) can produce a similar pattern of mood alteration. These organic causes must be ruled out before making a diagnosis of cyclothymic disorder.

HISTORY
- Sleeping and eating disturbances
- Expansive, grandiose, sometimes irritable mood alternating with symptoms of depression

PHYSICAL FINDINGS
Mania
- Increased psychomotor activity
- Excessive social extroversion
- Impulsive actions
- Impaired judgment
- Delusions
- Paranoid thinking
- Limited attention span
- Inflated sense of self-esteem
- Rapid responses to external stimuli

Depression
- Slow speech and response
- No obvious disorientation or intellectual impairment
- Psychomotor retardation
- Lethargy
- Low muscle tone
- Weight loss or gain
- Slowed gait

DSM-IV-TR *criteria*
Diagnosis is confirmed when patient experiences a distinct period of abnormally and persistently elevated, expansive, or irritable mood, in which at least three of the following symptoms are present to a significant degree; four if the mood is only irritable:
- inflated self-esteem or grandiosity
- decreased need for sleep
- excessive talking
- flight of ideas
- easily distracted
- psychomotor agitation
- excessive involvement in dangerous activities
- symptoms don't meet criteria for a mixed episode
- impairment in occupational function, usual social activities, or relations with others severe enough to require hospitalization to prevent harm to self or others
- substance use or medical conditions aren't present.

DIAGNOSTIC TEST RESULTS

There are no diagnostic tests for this disorder.

TREATMENT

GENERAL
◆ Group and individual therapy

DIET
◆ No restrictions

ACTIVITY
◆ Monitoring of activity when in manic phase

MEDICATIONS
◆ Lithium (Lithobid)
◆ Antipsychotics
◆ Valproic acid (Depakene)
◆ Carbamazepine (Tegretol)
◆ Antidepressants

NURSING CONSIDERATIONS

NURSING DIAGNOSES
◆ Disturbed personal identity
◆ Impaired social interaction
◆ Ineffective coping
◆ Ineffective role performance
◆ Situational low self-esteem

EXPECTED OUTCOMES
The patient will:
◆ express positive feelings about self
◆ demonstrate effective social interaction skills
◆ identify effective coping techniques
◆ express feelings about diminished capacity to perform usual roles
◆ express feelings related to self-esteem.

NURSING INTERVENTIONS
For the manic patient
◆ Encourage activities that require gross motor movements.
◆ Assist with personal hygiene; encourage responsibility for personal care.
◆ Protect from overstimulation.
◆ Set realistic goals and limits for the patient's behavior.
◆ Provide diversional activities suited to a short attention span.
◆ Reorient to reality.
◆ Avoid power struggles.

For the depressed patient
◆ Avoid overwhelming expectations.
◆ Allow increased time for activities and responses.
◆ Provide a structured routine.
◆ Promote interaction with others.
◆ Encourage verbalization; provide support.
◆ Institute safety measures.
◆ Encourage physical activity.
◆ Limit decision making.
◆ Assess suicidal thoughts.

MONITORING
◆ Patterns of behavior
◆ Response to treatment
◆ Social interaction
◆ Complications
◆ Adverse drug reactions
◆ Nutritional status

PATIENT TEACHING

GENERAL
Be sure to cover:
◆ the disorder, diagnosis, and treatment
◆ medication administration, dosage, and possible adverse effects
◆ importance of continuing the prescribed medication regimen.

DISCHARGE PLANNING
◆ Refer the patient for psychological counseling.
◆ Refer the patient to support services.

RESOURCES
Organizations
American Psychiatric Association: *www.psych.org*
Depression and Bipolar Support Alliance: *www.dbsalliance.org*
National Alliance for the Mentally Ill: *www.nami.org*
National Mental Health Association: *www.nmha.org*

Selected references
Diagnostic and Statistical Manual of Mental Disorders, Fourth Edition, Text Revision. Washington, D.C.: American Psychiatric Association, 2000.
Schapiro, N.A. "Bipolar Disorders in Children and Adolescents," *Journal of Pediatric Health Care* 19(3):131-41, May-June 2005.
Swann, A.C., et al. "Psychosis in Mania: Specificity of Its Role in Severity and Treatment Response," *Journal of Clinical Psychiatry* 65(6):825-29, June 2004.

Bladder cancer

OVERVIEW

- Malignant tumor that develops on the bladder wall surface or grows within the wall and quickly invades underlying muscles
- Less common bladder tumors: adenocarcinomas, epidermoid carcinomas, squamous cell carcinomas, sarcomas, tumors in bladder diverticula, and carcinoma in situ
- Most common cancer of the urinary tract

PATHOPHYSIOLOGY

- About 90% of bladder cancers are transitional cell carcinomas, arising from the transitional epithelium of mucous membranes. (They may result from malignant transformation of benign papillomas.)

CAUSES

- Exact cause unknown
- Associated with chronic bladder irritation and infection in people with renal calculi, indwelling urinary catheters, chemical cystitis caused by cyclophosphamide, or pelvic irradiation

RISK FACTORS

- Certain environmental carcinogens, such as 2-naphthylamine, tobacco, nitrates, and coffee
- Occupational exposure to carcinogens, especially industrial dyes and solvents

INCIDENCE

- Bladder tumors are most prevalent in people older than age 50.
- Bladder cancer is more commonly found in men than in women.
- Bladder cancer occurs more commonly in densely populated industrial areas.

COMPLICATIONS

- Bone metastasis
- Problems resulting from tumor invasion of contiguous viscera

ASSESSMENT

HISTORY

- Gross, painless, intermittent hematuria, usually with clots
- Suprapubic pain after voiding, which suggests invasive lesions
- Bladder irritability, urinary frequency, nocturia, and dribbling
- Flank pain that may indicate an obstructed ureter

PHYSICAL FINDINGS

- Gross hematuria
- Flank tenderness if ureteral obstruction present

DIAGNOSTIC TEST RESULTS

LABORATORY

- Complete blood count helps to detect anemia.
- Urinalysis detects blood and malignant cells in the urine.

IMAGING

- Excretory urography can identify a large, early-stage tumor or an infiltrating tumor; delineate functional problems in the upper urinary tract; assess hydronephrosis; and detect rigid deformity of the bladder wall.
- Retrograde cystography evaluates bladder structure and integrity; it also helps confirm a bladder cancer diagnosis.
- Bone scan can detect metastasis.
- Computed tomography scan defines the thickness of the involved bladder wall and discloses enlarged retroperitoneal lymph nodes.
- Ultrasonography reveals metastases in tissues beyond the bladder and can distinguish a bladder cyst from a bladder tumor.

DIAGNOSTIC PROCEDURES

- Cystoscopy and biopsy confirm bladder cancer diagnosis; if the test results show cancer cells, further studies will determine the cancer stage and treatment.

OTHER

- Bimanual examination may be performed during a cystoscopy if the patient has received an anesthetic; this helps to determine whether the bladder is fixed to the pelvic wall.

TREATMENT

GENERAL
◆ Cancer's stage, patient's lifestyle, other health problems, and mental outlook influencing selection of therapy

ACTIVITY
◆ Initially postoperatively, heavy lifting and contact sports restricted
◆ After recovery, no restrictions

MEDICATIONS
◆ Intravesical chemotherapy, such as thiotepa, doxorubicin, and mitomycin
◆ Attenuated bacille Calmette-Guérin vaccine live

SURGERY
◆ Transurethral resection (cystoscopic approach) and fulguration (electrically)
◆ Segmental bladder
◆ Radical cystectomy
◆ Ureterostomy, nephrostomy, continent vesicostomy (Kock pouch), ileal bladder, and ureterosigmoidostomy

NURSING CONSIDERATIONS

NURSING DIAGNOSES
◆ Acute pain
◆ Anxiety
◆ Disabled family coping
◆ Disturbed body image
◆ Fear
◆ Impaired skin integrity
◆ Impaired urinary elimination
◆ Ineffective coping
◆ Risk for infection
◆ Sexual dysfunction

EXPECTED OUTCOMES
The patient will:
◆ express feelings of increased comfort and decreased pain
◆ express feelings of decreased anxiety
◆ seek support systems and exhibit adequate coping behaviors
◆ verbalize feelings about changed body image
◆ verbalize feelings of anxiety and fear
◆ maintain skin integrity
◆ demonstrate skill in managing urinary elimination
◆ exhibit adequate coping mechanisms
◆ avoid infection and other complications
◆ express feelings about potential or actual changes in sexual activity.

NURSING INTERVENTIONS
◆ Provide support and encourage verbalization.
◆ Give prescribed drugs.
◆ Provide preoperative teaching; discuss procedure and postoperative course.

MONITORING
◆ Wound site
◆ Postoperative complications
◆ Intake and output
◆ Pain control

PATIENT TEACHING

GENERAL
Be sure to cover:
◆ the disorder, diagnosis, and treatment
◆ stoma care
◆ skin care and evaluation
◆ avoidance of heavy lifting and contact sports (postoperatively with a urinary stoma)
◆ encouragement of participation in usual athletic and physical activities.

DISCHARGE PLANNING
◆ Before discharge, arrange for follow-up home nursing care.
◆ Refer the patient to resource and support services.
◆ Refer the patient to an enterostomal therapist and for services provided by the therapist.

RESOURCES
Organizations
American Cancer Society: *www.cancer.org*
Guide to Internet Resources for Cancer: *www.cancerindex.org*
National Cancer Institute: *www.cancer.gov*
National Institute of Diabetes & Digestive & Kidney Diseases: *www.niddk.nih.gov*
United Ostomy Association, Inc.: *www.uoa.org*

Selected references
Atlas of Pathophysiology, 2nd ed. Philadelphia: Lippincott Williams & Wilkins, 2005.
Burkhard, F.C., et al. "Continent Urinary Diversion," *Critical Reviews in Oncology/Hematology,* 57(3):255-64, March 2006.
McGrath, M., et al. "Hormonal and Reproductive Factors and the Risk of Bladder Cancer in Women," *American Journal of Epidemiology* 63(3):236-44, November 2005.
Vogelzang, N., et al. *Comprehensive Textbook of Genitourinary Oncology,* 3rd ed. Philadelphia: Lippincott Williams & Wilkins, 2006.

Blastomycosis

OVERVIEW

- Fungal infection that usually affects the lungs and produces broncho-pneumonia
- May develop into extrapulmonary disease
- Also called *Gilchrist's disease*

PATHOPHYSIOLOGY

- Inhalation of aerosolized conidial forms of the fungus from its natural soil habitat
- Transformation of the conidia to the yeast phase at body temperature (thermal dimorphism)
- Inflammatory response evoked by multiplication of organism
- Possible dissemination through the blood and lymphatics to other organs

CAUSES

- Inhalation of the yeastlike fungus *Blastomyces dermatitidis*

INCIDENCE

- Blastomycosis is usually found in North America, where *B. dermatitidis* normally inhabits the soil.
- It's endemic to the southeastern United States.
- The disorder is more commonly found in men than in women.
- The onset is most common between ages 30 and 50 but can occur at any age.

COMPLICATIONS

- Addison's disease (adrenal insufficiency)
- Arthritis
- Central nervous system, skin, and genital disorders
- Osteomyelitis
- Pericarditis

ASSESSMENT

HISTORY

- Fever, chills
- Dry, hacking, productive cough
- Weight loss
- Night sweats
- Pleuritic chest pain
- Malaise
- Myalgia

PHYSICAL FINDINGS

- Thick sputum (may contain blood)
- Bronchial breath sounds; dullness on chest percussion
- Decreased breath sounds
- Tachypnea
- Decreased pulse oximetry
- Raised and reddened lesions
- Chest pain
- Dyspnea

Extrapulmonary findings

- Skin lesions
- Osteolytic lesions
- Joint swelling

DIAGNOSTIC TEST RESULTS

LABORATORY

- Culture from skin lesions, pus, sputum, or pulmonary secretions show *B. dermatitidis*.
- White blood cell count and erythrocyte sedimentation rate are increased.
- Serum globulin levels are slightly increased, mild normochromic anemia occurs.
- Phosphatase level (with bone lesions) is increased.

IMAGING

- Chest X-ray may show pulmonary infiltrates.

DIAGNOSTIC PROCEDURES

- Biopsy of tissue from the skin or lungs or of bronchial washings, sputum, or pus shows infecting organism.

OTHER

- Immunodiffusion testing detects antibodies for the A and B antigens of blastomycosis.

TREATMENT

GENERAL
- Respiratory treatments

DIET
- Increased fluid intake

ACTIVITY
- Rest periods, as needed

MEDICATIONS
- Amphotericin B (Fungizone)
- Oral itraconazole (Sporanox)
- Fluconazole (Diflucan)
- Antipyretics

NURSING CONSIDERATIONS

NURSING DIAGNOSES
- Acute pain
- Impaired gas exchange
- Impaired physical mobility
- Impaired skin integrity
- Ineffective airway clearance
- Ineffective breathing pattern
- Ineffective coping
- Risk for injury

EXPECTED OUTCOMES
The patient will:
- report increased comfort and decreased pain
- maintain adequate ventilation
- maintain functional mobility
- maintain skin integrity
- maintain a patent airway
- maintain effective breathing pattern
- demonstrate effective coping skills
- remain free from injury.

NURSING INTERVENTIONS
- Provide a cool room; if the patient is feverish, administer a tepid sponge bath.
- Elevate painful joints and apply heat.
- Provide appropriate skin care.
- Give prescribed drugs.

MONITORING
- Vital signs
- Pulse oximetry
- Laboratory tests
- Sputum production for hemoptysis
- Level of consciousness pupil response
- Hematuria
- Lesion healing

PATIENT TEACHING

GENERAL
Be sure to cover:
- the disorder, diagnosis, and treatment
- proper administration and adverse effects of medications
- skin care.

DISCHARGE PLANNING
- Stress appropriate follow-up care.

RESOURCES
Organizations
American Lung Association: *www.lungusa.org*
Centers for Disease Control and Prevention: *www.cdc.gov*
National Lung Health Education Program: *www.nlhep.org*

Selected references
Boswell, E., and Aziz, H. "Blastomycosis: A Case Study of a Dimorphic Fungal Disease," *Clinical Laboratory Science* 17(3):145-48, Summer 2004.
Cano, M.V., et al. "Blastomycosis in Missouri: Epidemiology and Risk Factors for Endemic Disease," *Epidemiology & Infection* 131(2):907-14, October 2003.

Blepharitis

- Common inflammation of eyelash follicles and meibomian glands of the upper or lower eyelids
- May be divided into anterior (inflammation of eyelashes and follicles) and posterior (meibomian gland)
- May affect both eyes
- May affect upper and lower eyelids
- Ulcerative type may coexist with seborrheic blepharitis

PATHOPHYSIOLOGY

- Inflammatory responses of the eyelids to bacteria or seborrheic dermatitis

CAUSES

- Anterior: bacteria and scalp dandruff
- Posterior: problems with meibomian glands (oil), usually due to rosacea or scalp dandruff

Seborrheic blepharitis

- Generally results from seborrhea of the scalp, eyebrows, and ears

Ulcerative blepharitis

- Generally results from a *Staphylococcus aureus* infection
- Pediculosis

INCIDENCE

- Blepharitis occurs most commonly in elderly people.
- Blepharitis is the most common ocular disease.

COMPLICATIONS

- Ocular involvement
- Keratitis
- Stye or chalazion

HISTORY

- Eyelids itch or burn
- Feeling of foreign body
- Crusty eyelids and lashes, which stick together when awakening
- Loss of eyelashes

PHYSICAL FINDINGS

- Continual blinking
- Red-rimmed appearance to the eyelid margins
- Swelling of eyelids
- Excessive tearing

Seborrheic blepharitis

- Scales along eyelids, especially upon awakening
- Dandruff on scalp and eyebrows

Ulcerative blepharitis

- Flaky scales on eyelashes, especially in morning
- Missing eyelashes
- Ulcerations on eyelid margins

LABORATORY

- Culture of the ulcerated eyelid margin may reveal *S. aureus* in ulcerative blepharitis.

TREATMENT

GENERAL
- Early treatment to prevent recurrence or complications
- Daily shampooing (using a mild shampoo on a cotton-tipped applicator or washcloth) to remove scales from eyelid margins
- Warm eye compresses
- Removal of nits with forceps for blepharitis from pediculosis
- Avoidance of eye makeup
- Avoidance of contact lens use until resolved

MEDICATIONS
- Sulfonamide or appropriate antibiotic eye ointment for ulcerative blepharitis
- Ophthalmic physostigmine or other insecticidal ointment for blepharitis from pediculosis

NURSING CONSIDERATIONS

NURSING DIAGNOSES
- Disturbed body image
- Impaired skin integrity
- Ineffective coping
- Ineffective health maintenance
- Risk for injury

EXPECTED OUTCOMES
The patient will:
- verbalize positive feelings about self
- maintain skin integrity and wounds or lesions will heal without complications
- demonstrate appropriate coping skills
- maintain current health status
- avoid injury.

NURSING INTERVENTIONS
- Provide eyelid care at least twice daily.
- Apply warm compresses, four times daily.
- Give prescribed drugs.
- Apply ointments, as ordered. (See *Applying an ophthalmic ointment.*)

MONITORING
- Response to treatment
- Adverse reactions to medication
- Complications

PATIENT TEACHING

GENERAL
Be sure to cover:
- the disorder and treatment
- daily eyelid care
- removal of scales from eyelids
- application of warm compresses
- medications and potential adverse reactions
- potential complications.

DISCHARGE PLANNING
- Refer the patient for support services and follow-up visit with a dermatologist if he has dandruff or rosacea.

RESOURCES
Organizations
American Academy of Ophthalmology: *www.aao.org*
National Eye Institute: *www.nei.nih.gov*

Selected references
Pettinger, D. "Sodium Bicarbonate in the Treatment of Blepharitis," *Clinical & Experimental Ophthalmology* 33(4):448-49, August 2005.
Swann, P.G., and Weir, J. "Is It Blepharitis?" *Clinical & Experimental Optometry* 88(2):113-14, March 2005.

Applying an ophthalmic ointment

Follow these directions to apply an ophthalmic ointment cleanly and quickly:
- Tilt the patient's head backward and ask him to look toward the ceiling.
- Gently pull the lower eyelid down and squeeze a small ribbon of ointment along the edge of the conjunctival sac from the inner to the outer canthus.
- Take care to avoid touching the eye with the tip of the ointment tube.
- Repeat this procedure for the other eye, if ordered.

Blood transfusion reaction LIFE-THREATENING DISORDER

OVERVIEW

- A hemolytic reaction from the transfusion of mismatched blood
- Accompanies or follows I.V. administration of blood components
- Mediated by immune or nonimmune factors
- Severity from mild to severe

PATHOPHYSIOLOGY

- Recipient's antibodies, immunoglobulin (Ig) G or IgM, attach to donor red blood cells (RBCs), leading to widespread clumping and destruction of recipient's RBCs.
- Transfusion with Rh-incompatible blood triggers a less serious reaction, known as Rh isoimmunization, within several days to 2 weeks. (See *Understanding the Rh system.*)
- A febrile nonhemolytic reaction — the most common type of reaction — develops when cytotoxic or agglutinating antibodies in the recipient's plasma attack antigens on transfused lymphocytes, granulocytes, or plasma cells.

CAUSES

- Transfusion with incompatible blood

INCIDENCE

- Mild reactions occur in 1% to 2% of transfusions.

COMPLICATIONS

- Acute tubular necrosis leading to acute renal failure
- Anaphylactic shock
- Bronchospasm
- Disseminated intravascular coagulation
- Vascular collapse

ASSESSMENT

HISTORY

- Transfusion of blood product
- Chills, nausea, vomiting, chest tightness, or chest and back pain

PHYSICAL FINDINGS

- Fever, tachycardia, and hypotension
- Dyspnea and apprehension
- Urticaria and angioedema
- Wheezing
- In a surgical patient: blood oozing from mucous membranes or the incision site
- In a hemolytic reaction: fever, an unexpected decrease in serum hemoglobin (Hb) level, frank blood in urine, and jaundice

DIAGNOSTIC TEST RESULTS

LABORATORY

- Serum Hb levels are decreased.
- Serum bilirubin levels and indirect bilirubin levels are increased.
- Urinalysis may reveal hemoglobinuria.
- Indirect Coombs' test or serum antibody screen is positive for serum anti-A or anti-B antibodies.
- Prothrombin time is increased and fibrinogen level is decreased.
- Blood urea nitrogen and serum creatinine levels are increased.

Understanding the Rh system

The Rh system contains more than 30 antibodies and antigens. Of the world's population, about 85% are Rh positive, which means that their red blood cells carry the D or Rh antigen. The rest of the population are Rh negative and don't have this antigen.

EFFECTS OF SENSITIZATION

When an Rh-negative person receives Rh-positive blood for the first time, he becomes sensitized to the D antigen but shows no immediate reaction to it. If he receives Rh-positive blood a second time, he experiences a massive hemolytic reaction.

For example, an Rh-negative mother who delivers an Rh-positive baby is sensitized by the baby's Rh-positive blood. During her next Rh-positive pregnancy, her sensitized blood will cause a hemolytic reaction in the fetal circulation.

PREVENTING SENSITIZATION

To prevent the formation of antibodies against Rh-positive blood, an Rh-negative mother should receive $Rh_0(D)$ immune globulin (human) (RhoGAM) I.M. within 72 hours after delivering an Rh-positive baby.

TREATMENT

GENERAL
◆ Immediate halt of transfusion
◆ Dialysis (may be necessary if acute tubular necrosis occurs)

DIET
◆ As tolerated

ACTIVITY
◆ Bed rest

MEDICATIONS
◆ Osmotic or loop diuretics
◆ I.V. normal saline solution
◆ I.V. vasopressors
◆ Epinephrine
◆ Diphenhydramine
◆ Corticosteroids
◆ Antipyretics

NURSING CONSIDERATIONS

NURSING DIAGNOSES
◆ Acute pain
◆ Anxiety
◆ Decreased cardiac output
◆ Impaired gas exchange
◆ Impaired tissue integrity
◆ Powerlessness
◆ Risk for imbalanced body temperature
◆ Risk for injury

EXPECTED OUTCOMES
The patient will:
◆ express feelings of comfort and relief of pain
◆ verbalize measures to reduce his anxiety level
◆ maintain adequate cardiac output
◆ maintain adequate ventilation and oxygenation
◆ have reduced redness, swelling, and pain at the site of impaired tissue
◆ express feelings of control over his well-being
◆ maintain a normal body temperature
◆ remain free from complications.

NURSING INTERVENTIONS
◆ Stop blood transfusion.
◆ Maintain a patent I.V. line with normal saline solution.
◆ Insert an indwelling urinary catheter.
◆ Report early signs of complications.
◆ Cover the patient with blankets to ease chills.
◆ Administer supplemental oxygen as needed.
◆ Document the transfusion reaction on the patient's chart, noting the duration of the transfusion and the amount of blood absorbed.
◆ Follow your facility's blood transfusion policy and procedure.

WARNING Double-check the patient's name, identification number, blood type, and Rh status before administering blood. If you find any discrepancy, don't administer the blood. Notify the blood bank immediately and return the unopened unit.

MONITORING
◆ Vital signs
◆ Intake and output
◆ Signs of shock
◆ Laboratory results

PATIENT TEACHING

GENERAL
Be sure to cover:
◆ signs and symptoms of transfusion reaction
◆ type of transfusion after recovery.

RESOURCES
Organizations
National Heart, Lung, and Blood Institute: *www.nhlbi.nih.gov*
National Library of Medicine: *www.nlm.nih.gov*

Selected references
Kasper, D.L., et al., eds. *Harrison's Principles of Internal Medicine,* 16th ed. New York: McGraw-Hill Book Co., 2005.
Sapatnekar, S., et al. "Acute Hemolytic Transfusion Reaction in a Pediatric Patient Following Transfusion of Apheresis Platelets," *Journal of Clinical Apheresis* 20(4):225-29, December 2005.

Body dysmorphic disorder

OVERVIEW

- A preoccupation with an imagined (or, if present, slight) defect in physical appearance
- Characterized by patient's belief that he's hideous or grotesque despite reassurance from others that he looks fine
- Patient thinks about the defect for at least 1 hour each day

PATHOPHYSIOLOGY

- Biological theories: genetic predisposition, adolescent stressors, or imbalanced levels of serotonin or other chemicals in the brain
- Psychological theory: low self-esteem causing tendency to judge oneself almost exclusively by appearance

CAUSES

- Exact cause unknown
- Biological or psychological theories
- Perfectionism and heightened perception about appearance causing increased focus on every imperfection or slight abnormality

INCIDENCE

- Body dysmorphic disorder affects 1% to 2% of the general population in the United States.
- The disorder affects males and females equally.
- Incidence may be underestimated because the disorder frequently goes undiagnosed.
- The disorder is a chronic condition with age of onset usually in the late teens (average age 17).

COMPLICATIONS

- Obsessive-compulsive disorder
- Major depression
- Social phobia
- Suicide

ASSESSMENT

HISTORY

- Preoccupation with imagined (or, if present, slight) defect in physical appearance
- Patient thinks about defect for at least 1 hour daily

PHYSICAL FINDINGS

Suspect body dysmorphic disorder in patient who reports or exhibits any of these behaviors:

- often checks reflection in the mirror, or avoids mirrors
- frequently compares appearance against that of other people
- frequently examines the appearance of other people
- tries to cover the perceived defect with clothing, makeup, or a hat or by changing posture
- seeks corrective treatment, such as surgery or dermatologic therapy, to eradiate the perceived defect
- constantly seeks reassurance from others about the perceived flaw, or, conversely, tries to convince others of its repulsiveness
- performs long grooming rituals, such as repeatedly combing or cutting hair or applying makeup or cover-up creams
- picks at the skin or squeezes pimples or blackheads for hours
- frequently touches the perceived problem area
- measures the body part that's repulsive
- is anxious and self-conscious
- feels acute distress over appearance, causing functional impairment
- avoids social situations where the perceived defect may be exposed
- has difficulty maintaining relationships with peers, family, and spouse
- performs poorly in school, work, or takes frequent sick days
- has low self-esteem
- has suicidal thoughts or behaviors.

DSM-IV-TR *criteria*

The patient must meet all three criteria.

- Patient is preoccupied with an imagined defect in appearance; if a slight physical abnormality actually is present, concern over it is markedly excessive.
- Preoccupation causes clinically significant distress or impairment in social, occupational, or other important areas of functioning.
- Preoccupation isn't better explained by another mental disorder such as anorexia nervosa.

DIAGNOSTIC TEST RESULTS

No diagnostic test exists for this disorder.

TREATMENT

GENERAL
- Enhancement of self-esteem
- Reduce preoccupation with perceived flaw
- Eliminate harmful effects of compulsive behaviors
- Cognitive-behavioral group therapies
- Behavioral methods (aversion therapy, thought stopping, and implosion therapy)

MEDICATIONS
- Selective serotonin reuptake inhibitor
- Tricyclic antidepressants

NURSING CONSIDERATIONS

NURSING DIAGNOSES
- Chronic low self-esteem
- Disturbed body image
- Disturbed personal identity
- Impaired social interaction
- Ineffective coping
- Ineffective health maintenance
- Risk for suicide
- Social isolation

EXPECTED OUTCOMES
The patient will:
- voice feelings related to self-esteem
- express positive feelings about self
- establish a firm, positive sense of self and personal identity
- exhibit effective social interaction skills
- identify effective and ineffective coping techniques
- maintain a state of wellness
- not harm self
- maintain family and peer relationships.

NURSING INTERVENTIONS
- Approach the patient unhurriedly.
- Keep the patient's physical health in mind.
- Provide an accepting, nonjudgmental attitude.
- Let the patient see that you're aware of her behavior.
- Give the patient time to carry out ritualistic behavior.
- Impose reasonable demands.
- Set reasonable limits.
- Identify insight and improved behavior.
- Engage the patient in activities that create positive accomplishments.
- Help the patient devise new ways to solve problems.
- Listen attentively and offer feedback.
- Monitor the patient for desired effect of medications, as appropriate.

MONITORING
- Patterns of behavior
- Response to treatment
- Social interaction
- Adverse drug reactions

PATIENT TEACHING

GENERAL
Be sure to cover:
- suggesting active diversions, such as whistling or humming to divert the patient's attention away from unwanted thoughts
- helping the patient devise new ways to solve problems and develop more effective coping skills by setting limits on unacceptable behavior
- encouraging the patient to use appropriate techniques to relieve stress, loneliness, and isolation.

RESOURCES
Organizations
American Psychiatric Association: *www.psych.org*
National Mental Health Association: *www.nmha.org*

Selected references
Castle, D.J., and Rossell, S.L. "An Update on Body Dysmorphic Disorder," *Current Opinion in Psychiatry* 19(1):74-78, January 2006.
Metules, T. "Cosmetic Surgery: Is It Really Right for Your Patient?" *RN* 68(3): 32ac1-5, March 2005.
Nettina, S.M. *Lippincott Manual of Nursing Practice*, 8th ed. Philadelphia: Lippincott Williams & Wilkins, 2006.

Bone tumors, primary malignant

OVERVIEW

- Rare type of bone cancer
- Also known as *osteoblastoma*

PATHOPHYSIOLOGY

- Proliferation of cancerous cells that clump together to form a tumor
- Able to spread beyond the original site
- Osseous bone tumors
- Arise from the bony structure itself
- Include osteogenic sarcoma (most common), parosteal osteogenic sarcoma, chondrosarcoma (chondroblastic), and malignant giant cell tumor
- Nonosseous bone tumors
- Arise from hematopoietic, vascular, and neural tissues
- Include Ewing's sarcoma, fibrosarcoma (fibroblastic), and chordoma

CAUSES

- Exact cause unknown
- Exposure to carcinogens
- Genetic abnormalities (retinoblastoma, Rothmund-Thomson syndrome)
- Heredity, trauma, and excessive radiation therapy, according to theories

INCIDENCE

- Primary malignant bone tumors account for less than 0.2% of all cancers.
- This disease is more common in males than in females.
- There's a higher incidence of this disorder in children and adolescents, although some types do occur in patients between ages 35 and 60. (See *Types of primary malignant bone tumors.*)
- The most common sites are the femur, tibia, and humerus.

  AGE FACTOR *Osteogenic and Ewing's sarcomas are the most common bone tumors in children.*

  AGE FACTOR *Limb pain, refusal to walk, and limited range of motion (ROM) are common findings in children with bone tumors.*

COMPLICATIONS

- Infection
- Hemorrhage
- Local recurrence

ASSESSMENT

HISTORY

- Localized dull bone pain
- Weight loss
- Impaired mobility
- Pathological fracture

PHYSICAL FINDINGS

- Palpable mass
- Cachectic appearance
- Abnormal gait

DIAGNOSTIC TEST RESULTS

LABORATORY

- Serum alkaline phosphatase levels are elevated (with sarcoma).

IMAGING

- Bone X-rays and radioisotope bone and computed tomography (CT) scans show tumor size.
- Bone scans and CT scans of the lungs reveal metastatic disease.

DIAGNOSTIC PROCEDURES

- Incision or aspiration biopsy confirms primary malignancy.

TREATMENT

DIET

- High-protein, high-calorie

ACTIVITY

- Rest periods, as needed
- Physical therapy

MEDICATIONS

- Chemotherapy
- Analgesics

SURGERY

- Excision of the tumor
- Radical surgery, such as hemipelvectomy or interscapulothoracic amputation

NURSING CONSIDERATIONS

NURSING DIAGNOSES

- Acute pain
- Anxiety
- Disturbed body image
- Fear
- Imbalanced nutrition: Less than body requirements
- Impaired physical mobility
- Impaired tissue integrity
- Ineffective coping
- Ineffective tissue perfusion: Peripheral
- Risk for infection

EXPECTED OUTCOMES

The patient will:

- express feelings of comfort and decreased pain
- report decreased feelings of anxiety
- express positive feelings about self
- express feelings and fears
- maintain adequate nutrition and hydration
- maintain joint mobility and ROM
- experience wound healing as evidenced by the presence of granulation tissue
- demonstrate positive coping mechanisms
- exhibit signs of adequate peripheral perfusion, such as positive distal pulses and warm, pink extremities
- have no signs or symptoms of infection.

NURSING INTERVENTIONS

- Encourage communication, and help the patient set realistic goals.
- Give prescribed I.V. infusions and drugs.
- Elevate the foot of the bed or place the affected stump on a pillow for the first 24 hours. (Be careful not to leave the stump elevated for more than 48 hours because this may lead to contractures.)

MONITORING
◆ Vital signs
◆ Circulation to the affected extremity
◆ Wound dressings

PATIENT TEACHING

GENERAL
Be sure to cover:
◆ use of assistive devices
◆ wound care
◆ reporting new pain or masses
◆ need for antibiotic prophylaxis when undergoing dental procedures (with bone grafts or prosthetic implants).

DISCHARGE PLANNING
◆ Refer the patient to the American Cancer Society for information and support.

RESOURCES
Organizations
American Cancer Society:
www.cancer.org
Guide to Internet Resources for Cancer:
www.cancerindex.org
National Cancer Institute:
www.cancer.gov

Selected references
Chen, W., and Zhou, K. "High-intensity Focused Ultrasound Ablation: A New Strategy to Manage Primary Bone Tumors," *Current Opinion in Orthopedics* 16(6):494-500, December 2005.
Kirsner, K.M. "Cancer: New Therapies and New Approaches to Recurring Problems," *AANA Journal* 71(1):55-62, February 2003.

Types of primary malignant bone tumors

TYPE	CLINICAL FEATURES	TREATMENT
Osseous origin		
Chondrosarcoma	◆ Develops from cartilage ◆ Painless; grows slowly but is locally recurrent and invasive ◆ Occurs most commonly in pelvis, proximal femur, ribs, and shoulder girdle ◆ Usually in men ages 30 to 50	◆ Hemipelvectomy, surgical resection (ribs) ◆ Radiation (palliative) ◆ Chemotherapy
Malignant giant cell tumor	◆ Arises from benign giant cell tumor ◆ Found most commonly in long bones, especially in the knee area ◆ Usually in women ages 18 to 50	◆ Curettage ◆ Total excision ◆ Radiation for recurrent disease
Osteogenic sarcoma	◆ Osteoid tumor present in specimen ◆ Tumor arises from bone-forming osteoblast and bone-digesting osteoclast ◆ Occurs most commonly in femur, but also tibia and humerus; occasionally, in fibula, ileum, vertebra, or mandible ◆ Usually in men ages 10 to 30	◆ Surgery (tumor resection, high thigh amputation, hemipelvectomy, interscapulothoracic surgery) ◆ Chemotherapy
Parosteal osteogenic sarcoma	◆ Develops on surface of bone instead of interior ◆ Progresses slowly ◆ Occurs most commonly in distal femur, but also in tibia, humerus, and ulna ◆ Usually in women ages 30 to 40	◆ Surgery (tumor resection, possible amputation, interscapulothoracic surgery, hemipelvectomy) ◆ Chemotherapy ◆ Combination of the above
Nonosseous origin		
Chordoma	◆ Derived from embryonic remnants of notochord ◆ Progresses slowly ◆ Usually found at end of spinal column and in spheno-occipital, sacrococcygeal, and vertebral areas ◆ Characterized by constipation and visual disturbances ◆ Usually in men ages 50 to 60	◆ Surgical resection (often resulting in neural defects) ◆ Radiation (palliative, or when surgery not applicable, as in occipital area)
Ewing's sarcoma	◆ Originates in bone marrow and invades shafts of long and flat bones ◆ Usually affects lower extremities, most commonly femur, innominate bones, ribs, tibia, humerus, vertebra, and fibula; may metastasize to lungs ◆ Pain increasingly severe and persistent ◆ Usually in males ages 10 to 20 ◆ Prognosis poor	◆ High-voltage radiation (tumor is radiosensitive) ◆ Chemotherapy to slow growth ◆ Amputation only if there's no evidence of metastasis
Fibrosarcoma	◆ Relatively rare ◆ Originates in fibrous tissue of bone ◆ Invades long or flat bones (femur, tibia, mandible) but also involves periosteum and overlying muscle ◆ Usually in men ages 30 to 40	◆ Amputation ◆ Radiation ◆ Chemotherapy ◆ Bone grafts (with low-grade fibrosarcoma)

Botulism — LIFE-THREATENING DISORDER

OVERVIEW

- Life-threatening paralytic illness
- Results from an exotoxin produced by the gram-positive, anaerobic bacillus *Clostridium botulinum*
- Occurs as botulism food poisoning, wound botulism, and infant botulism (see *Infant botulism*)
- Mortality about 25%, with death most commonly caused by respiratory failure during the first week of illness
- Onset of disease within 24 hours after ingesting food signaling critical and potentially fatal illness

PATHOPHYSIOLOGY

- Endotoxin acts at the neuromuscular junction of skeletal muscle, preventing acetylcholine release and blocking neural transmission, eventually resulting in paralysis.

CAUSES

- *Clostridium botulinum* bacteria

RISK FACTORS

- Eating improperly preserved foods
- Using injectable street drugs

INCIDENCE

- Botulism occurs worldwide.
- There's an average annual occurrence of about 110 cases in the United States.
- Botulism affects more adults than children.

COMPLICATIONS

- Respiratory failure
- Paralytic ileus
- Death

ASSESSMENT

HISTORY

- Consumption of home-canned food 18 to 30 hours before onset of symptoms
- Vertigo
- Sore throat
- Weakness
- Nausea and vomiting
- Constipation or diarrhea
- Diplopia
- Blurred vision
- Dysarthria
- Dysphagia
- Dyspnea
- Heroin use

PHYSICAL FINDINGS

- Ptosis
- Dilated, nonreactive pupils
- Appearance of dry, red, and crusted oral mucous membranes
- Abdominal distention with absent bowel sounds
- Descending weakness or paralysis of muscles in the extremities or trunk
- Deep tendon reflexes may be intact, diminished, or absent
- Unexplained postural hypotension
- Urinary retention
- Photophobia
- Slurred speech

DIAGNOSTIC TEST RESULTS

LABORATORY

- Mouse bioassay detects toxin that's found in the patient's serum, stool, or gastric contents.

DIAGNOSTIC PROCEDURES

- Electromyography shows diminished muscle action potential after a single supramaximal nerve stimulus.

Infant botulism

Infant botulism, which usually afflicts neonates and infants between 3 and 20 weeks old, is often caused by ingesting the spores of botulinum bacteria, which then grow in the intestines and release toxin. This disorder can produce floppy infant syndrome, characterized by constipation, a feeble cry, a depressed gag reflex, and an inability to suck. The infant also exhibits a flaccid facial expression, ptosis, and ophthalmoplegia — the result of cranial nerve deficits.

As the disease progresses, the infant develops generalized weakness, hypotonia, areflexia, and sometimes a striking loss of head control. Almost 50% of affected infants develop respiratory arrest.

Intensive supportive care allows most infants to recover completely. Antitoxin therapy isn't recommended because of the risk of anaphylaxis.

TREATMENT

GENERAL
- Supportive measures
- Early tracheotomy and ventilatory assistance in respiratory failure
- Nasogastric (NG) suctioning

DIET
- Total parenteral nutrition

ACTIVITY
- Bed rest

MEDICATIONS
- I.V. or I.M. botulinum antitoxin

SURGERY
- Debridement of wounds to remove source of toxin-producing bacteria

NURSING CONSIDERATIONS

NURSING DIAGNOSES
- Acute pain
- Imbalanced nutrition: Less than body requirements
- Impaired physical mobility
- Impaired swallowing
- Impaired verbal communication
- Ineffective airway clearance
- Ineffective breathing pattern
- Risk for injury

EXPECTED OUTCOMES
The patient will:
- communicate feelings of comfort or reduced pain
- maintain daily calorie requirements
- return to his normal mobility level
- swallow without pain or difficulty
- demonstrate effective communication skills
- maintain a patent airway
- maintain tissue perfusion and cellular oxygenation
- maintain stable neurologic status.

NURSING INTERVENTIONS
- Obtain history of food intake for the past several days.
- Obtain family history of similar symptoms and food intake.
- Administer I.V. fluids as ordered.
- Administer oxygen as needed.
- Perform NG suctioning as needed.

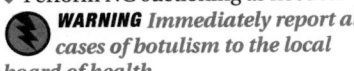 **WARNING** *Immediately report all cases of botulism to the local board of health.*

MONITORING
- Neurologic status
- Cardiac and respiratory function
- Cough and gag reflexes
- Intake and output
- Arterial blood gas levels

PATIENT TEACHING

GENERAL
Be sure to cover:
- the disorder, diagnosis, and treatment
- proper techniques in processing and preserving foods
- never tasting food from a bulging can or one with a peculiar odor
- sterilizing utensils by boiling whatever utensils touched suspected contaminated food
- not feeding honey to infants (can be fatal if contaminated).

DISCHARGE PLANNING
- Refer the patient to support services.

RESOURCES
Organizations
Centers for Diseases Control and Prevention: *www.cdc.gov*
Harvard University Consumer Health Information: *www.intelihealth.com*
National Health Information Center: *www.health.gov/nhic*
National Library of Medicine: *www.nlm.nih.gov*
National Organization for Rare Disorders: *www.rarediseases.org*

Selected references
Cherington, M. "Botulism: Update and Review," *Seminars in Neurology* 24(2):155-63, June 2004.
Gupta, A., et al. "Adult Botulism Type F in the United States, 1981-2002," *Neurology* 65(11):1694-700, December 2005.
Kasper, D.L., et al., eds. *Harrison's Principles of Internal Medicine*, 16th ed. New York: McGraw-Hill Book Co., 2005.
Sieradzan, K.A. "Wound Botulism," *Practical Neurology* 5(1):46-51, February 2005.

Brain tumor, malignant

OVERVIEW

- Abnormal growth among cells within the intracranial space
- May affect brain tissue, meninges, pituitary gland, and blood vessels
- In adults, the most common tumor types are gliomas and meningiomas, which usually occur above the covering of the cerebellum, or supratentorial tumors
- In children, the most common tumor types are astrocytomas, medulloblastomas, ependymomas, and brain stem gliomas

PATHOPHYSIOLOGY

- Tumors are classified based on histology or grade of cell malignancy.
- Central nervous system changes are caused by cancer cells invading and destroying tissues and by compression of the brain, cranial nerves, and cerebral vessels; cerebral edema; and increased intracranial pressure (ICP).

CAUSES

- Exact cause unknown

RISK FACTORS

- Preexisting cancer
- Radiation
- Chemical exposure
- Trauma

INCIDENCE

- Malignant brain tumor is slightly more common in males than in females.
- Gliomas, meningiomas, and schwannomas have an overall incidence of 4.5 per 100,000.
- Malignant brain tumor can occur at any age, but most occur in children before age 1 or between ages 2 and 12.
- In adults, incidence is highest between ages 40 and 60.

COMPLICATIONS

- Radiation encephalopathy
- Cerebral edema
- Seizures
- Neurologic deficits
- Hydrocephalus
- Brain herniation

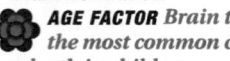 **AGE FACTOR** *Brain tumors are the most common cause of cancer death in children.*

Life-threatening complications from increased ICP

- Coma
- Respiratory or cardiac arrest
- Brain herniation

ASSESSMENT

HISTORY

- Insidious onset
- Headache
- Nausea and vomiting

PHYSICAL FINDINGS

- Signs and symptoms of increased ICP
- Vision disturbances
- Weakness, paralysis
- Aphasia, dysphagia
- Ataxia, incoordination
- Seizure (see *Brain tumors: Site-specific signs and symptoms*)

DIAGNOSTIC TEST RESULTS

IMAGING

- Skull X-rays confirm tumor.
- Brain scan confirms tumor.
- Computed tomography scan confirms tumor.
- Magnetic resonance imaging evaluates tumor location, size, and vascularity, and cerebral edema.
- Cerebral angiography confirms tumor.
- Positron emission tomography confirms tumor.

DIAGNOSTIC PROCEDURES

- Tissue biopsy confirms the type of tumor.

OTHER

- Lumbar puncture may show increased cerebrospinal fluid (CSF) pressure, which reflects ICP, increased protein levels, decreased glucose levels and, occasionally, tumor cells in CSF.

Brain tumors: Site-specific signs and symptoms

A brain tumor usually produces signs and symptoms specific to its location. Recognizing the effects helps identify the tumor site and guide treatment before and after surgery and can help you spot life-threatening complications, such as increasing intracranial pressure and imminent brain herniation. A brain tumor may cause all, some, or none of the effects shown below.

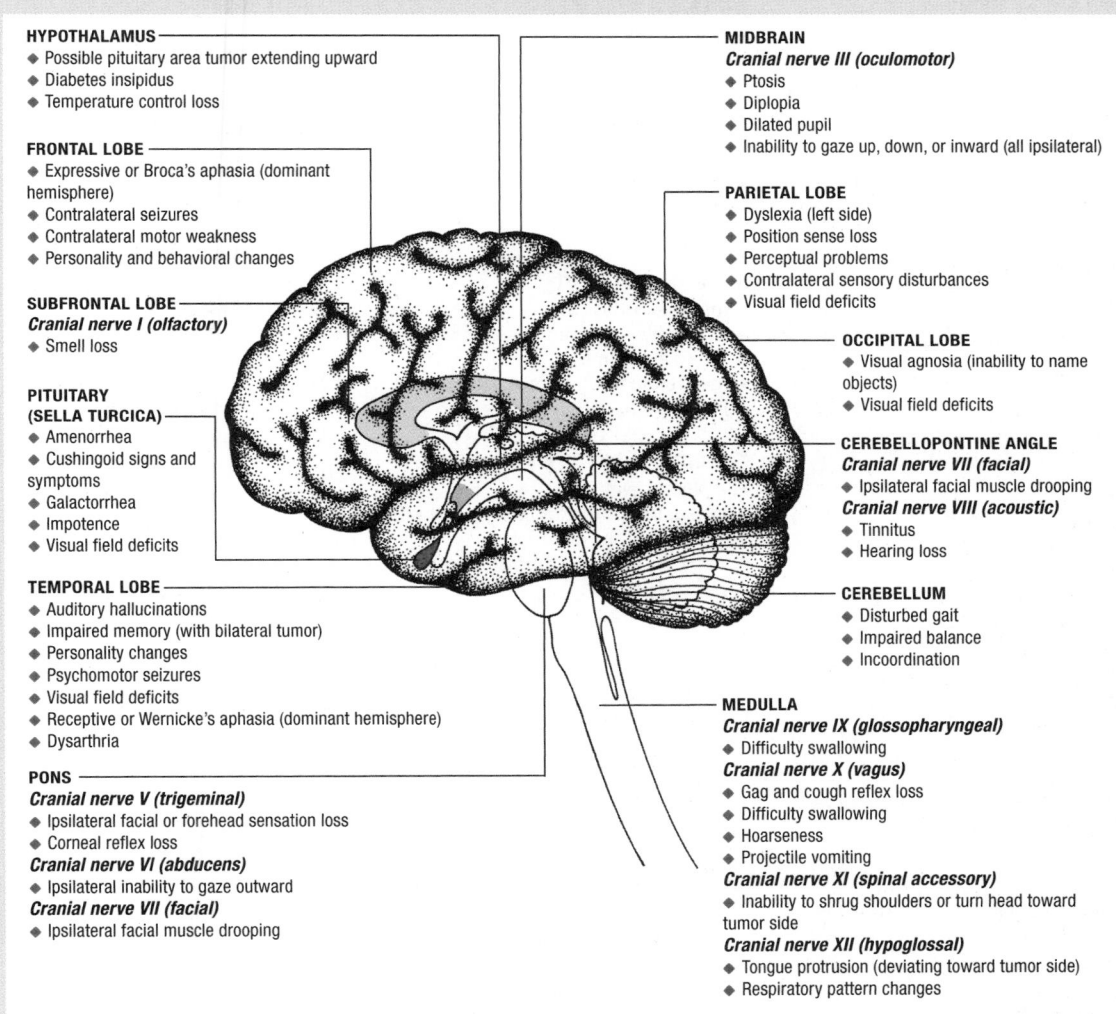

HYPOTHALAMUS
- Possible pituitary area tumor extending upward
- Diabetes insipidus
- Temperature control loss

FRONTAL LOBE
- Expressive or Broca's aphasia (dominant hemisphere)
- Contralateral seizures
- Contralateral motor weakness
- Personality and behavioral changes

SUBFRONTAL LOBE
Cranial nerve I (olfactory)
- Smell loss

PITUITARY (SELLA TURCICA)
- Amenorrhea
- Cushingoid signs and symptoms
- Galactorrhea
- Impotence
- Visual field deficits

TEMPORAL LOBE
- Auditory hallucinations
- Impaired memory (with bilateral tumor)
- Personality changes
- Psychomotor seizures
- Visual field deficits
- Receptive or Wernicke's aphasia (dominant hemisphere)
- Dysarthria

PONS
Cranial nerve V (trigeminal)
- Ipsilateral facial or forehead sensation loss
- Corneal reflex loss
Cranial nerve VI (abducens)
- Ipsilateral inability to gaze outward
Cranial nerve VII (facial)
- Ipsilateral facial muscle drooping

MIDBRAIN
Cranial nerve III (oculomotor)
- Ptosis
- Diplopia
- Dilated pupil
- Inability to gaze up, down, or inward (all ipsilateral)

PARIETAL LOBE
- Dyslexia (left side)
- Position sense loss
- Perceptual problems
- Contralateral sensory disturbances
- Visual field deficits

OCCIPITAL LOBE
- Visual agnosia (inability to name objects)
- Visual field deficits

CEREBELLOPONTINE ANGLE
Cranial nerve VII (facial)
- Ipsilateral facial muscle drooping
Cranial nerve VIII (acoustic)
- Tinnitus
- Hearing loss

CEREBELLUM
- Disturbed gait
- Impaired balance
- Incoordination

MEDULLA
Cranial nerve IX (glossopharyngeal)
- Difficulty swallowing
Cranial nerve X (vagus)
- Gag and cough reflex loss
- Difficulty swallowing
- Hoarseness
- Projectile vomiting
Cranial nerve XI (spinal accessory)
- Inability to shrug shoulders or turn head toward tumor side
Cranial nerve XII (hypoglossal)
- Tongue protrusion (deviating toward tumor side)
- Respiratory pattern changes

(continued)

GENERAL
◆ Specific treatments varying with the tumor's histologic type, radiosensitivity, and location

DIET
◆ No restrictions unless swallowing impaired

ACTIVITY
◆ Possibly altered physical ability based on neurologic status

MEDICATIONS
◆ Chemotherapy such as nitrosoureas
◆ Steroids
◆ Antacids and histamine-receptor antagonists
◆ Anticonvulsants
◆ Osmotic diuretics
◆ Antiemetics

SURGERY
For glioma
◆ Resection by craniotomy or craniectomy
◆ Radiation therapy and chemotherapy follow resection

For low-grade cystic cerebellar astrocytoma
◆ Surgical resection

For astrocytoma
◆ Repeated surgeries, radiation therapy, and shunting of fluid from obstructed CSF pathways

For oligodendroglioma and ependymoma
◆ Surgical resection and radiation therapy

For medulloblastoma
◆ Surgical resection
◆ Possibly, intrathecal infusion and methotrexate or another antineoplastic drug

For meningioma
◆ Surgical resection, including dura mater and bone

For schwannoma
◆ Microsurgical technique

NURSING DIAGNOSES
◆ Activity intolerance
◆ Acute pain
◆ Anxiety
◆ Bathing or hygiene self-care deficit
◆ Decreased intracranial adaptive capacity
◆ Disturbed body image
◆ Disturbed sensory perception (visual)
◆ Fear
◆ Hopelessness
◆ Impaired physical mobility
◆ Ineffective breathing pattern
◆ Ineffective coping
◆ Ineffective role performance
◆ Powerlessness

EXPECTED OUTCOMES
The patient will:
◆ maintain optimal mobility within the confines of the disorder
◆ verbalize feelings of comfort and decreased pain
◆ express feelings of decreased anxiety
◆ resume self-care activities to the highest level possible within the limitations of the illness
◆ exhibit signs of maintaining adequate cerebral perfusion
◆ express positive feelings about self
◆ maintain optimal functioning within the limits of the visual impairment
◆ verbalize feelings and fears about the condition
◆ make decisions about his care as appropriate
◆ maintain muscle strength and joint mobility at the highest possible level
◆ maintain respiratory rate within 5 breaths/minute of baseline
◆ demonstrate positive coping mechanisms
◆ recognize limitations imposed by the illness and express feelings about these limitations
◆ express feelings of control over his well-being.

NURSING INTERVENTIONS
◆ Maintain a patent airway.
◆ Take steps to protect the patient's safety.
◆ Give prescribed drugs.
◆ After supratentorial craniotomy, elevate the head of the bed about 30 degrees.
◆ After infratentorial craniotomy, keep the patient flat for 48 hours.
◆ As appropriate, instruct the patient to avoid Valsalva's maneuver and isometric muscle contractions when moving or sitting up in bed.
◆ Consult with occupational, speech, and physical therapists.
◆ Provide emotional support.

MONITORING
◆ Neurologic status
◆ Vital signs
◆ Wound site
◆ Postoperative complications

GENERAL
Be sure to cover:
- the disease process, diagnosis, and treatment
- signs of infection or bleeding that may result from chemotherapy
- adverse effects of chemotherapy and other treatments and actions that may alleviate them
- physical limitations that may occur
- seizure precautions
- early signs of tumor recurrence.

DISCHARGE PLANNING
- Consult with occupational and physical therapy staff for postdischarge care plan.
- Refer the patient to resource and support services.

RESOURCES
Organizations
American Brain Tumor Association:
  www.abta.org
American Cancer Society:
  www.cancer.org
Guide to Internet Resources for Cancer:
  www.cancerindex.org
National Cancer Institute:
  www.cancer.gov

Selected references
Atlas of Pathophysiology, 2nd ed. Philadelphia: Lippincott Williams & Wilkins, 2005.

Graham, C.A., and Cloughesy, T.F. "Brain Tumor Treatment: Chemotherapy and Other New Developments," *Seminars in Oncology Nursing* 20(4):260-72, November 2004.

Loghin, M., and Levin, V.A. "Headache Related to Brain Tumors," *Current Treatment Options in Neurology* 8(1):21-32, January 2006.

Lovely, M.P. "Symptom Management of Brain Tumor Patients," *Seminars in Oncology Nursing* 20(4):273-83, November 2004.

Breast cancer

- Malignant proliferation of epithelial cells lining the ducts or lobules of the breast
- Prognosis considerably influenced by early detection and treatment
- With adjunctive therapy, 10-year (or longer) survival 70% to 75% in patients with negative nodes, compared with 20% to 25% in those with positive nodes

⚡ **WARNING** *The most reliable detection method of breast cancer is regular breast self-examination, followed by an immediate professional evaluation of any abnormality. (Theoretically, slow-growing breast cancer may take up to 8 years to become palpable at 1 cm.)*

PATHOPHYSIOLOGY

- Spreads by way of the lymphatic system and the bloodstream through the right side of the heart to the lungs and to the other breast, chest wall, liver, bone, and brain
- Depends on classification:
- Adenocarcinoma (ductal) — arising from the epithelium
- Intraductal — developing within the ducts (includes Paget's disease)
- Infiltrating — occurring in the breast's parenchymal tissue
- Inflammatory (rare) — growing rapidly and causing overlying skin to become edematous, inflamed, and indurated
- Lobular carcinoma in situ — involving the lobes of glandular tissue
- Medullary or circumscribed — enlarging tumor with rapid growth rate

CAUSES

- Exact cause unknown

RISK FACTORS

- Family history of breast cancer, particularly first-degree relatives, including mother, sister, maternal grandmother, and maternal aunt
- Positive test results for genetic mutations (BRCA 1)
- Premenopausal woman older than age 45
- Long menstrual cycles
- Early onset of menses, late menopause
- Nulliparous or first pregnancy after age 30
- High-fat diet
- Endometrial or ovarian cancer
- History of unilateral breast cancer
- Radiation exposure
- Estrogen therapy
- Antihypertensive therapy
- Alcohol and tobacco use
- Preexisting fibrocystic disease

INCIDENCE

- A woman in the United States living to age 80 has a 1 in 9 chance of developing invasive breast cancer sometime during her life.
- Breast cancer is the second-leading cause of cancer death in women after lung cancer.

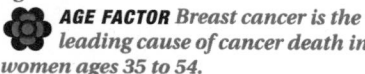 **AGE FACTOR** *Although breast cancer may develop anytime after puberty, it's most common after age 50.*

AGE FACTOR *Breast cancer is the leading cause of cancer death in women ages 35 to 54.*

- The disease seldom occurs in men.

COMPLICATIONS

- Central nervous system effects
- Distant metastasis
- Infection
- Respiratory effects

HISTORY

- Detection of a painless lump or mass in the breast
- Change in breast tissue
- History of risk factors

PHYSICAL FINDINGS

- Clear, milky, or bloody nipple discharge, nipple retraction, scaly skin around the nipple, and skin changes, such as dimpling or inflammation (see *Breast tumor sources and sites*)
- Arm edema
- Hard lump, mass, or thickening of breast tissue
- Lymphadenopathy

LABORATORY

- Alkaline phosphatase levels and liver function may reveal distant metastasis.
- Hormonal receptor assay may determine whether the tumor is estrogen or progesterone dependent; also guides decisions to use therapy that blocks the action of the estrogen hormone that supports tumor growth.

IMAGING

- Mammography can reveal a tumor that's too small to palpate.

Breast tumor sources and sites

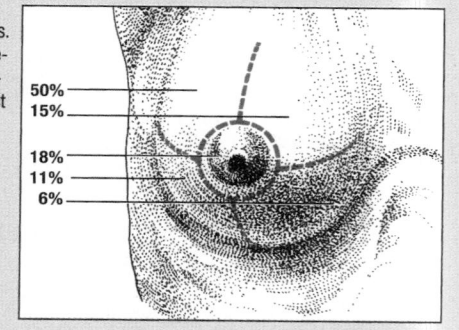

About 90% of all breast tumors arise from the epithelial cells lining the ducts. About one-half of all breast cancers develop in the breast's upper outer quadrant — the section containing the most glandular tissue.

The second most common cancer site is the nipple, where all the breast ducts converge.

The next most common site is the upper inner quadrant, followed by the lower outer quadrant and, finally, the lower inner quadrant.

50%
15%
18%
11%
6%

- Ultrasonography can distinguish between a fluid-filled cyst and solid mass.
- Chest X-rays can pinpoint metastasis in the chest.
- Scans of the bone, brain, liver, and other organs can detect distant metastasis.

DIAGNOSTIC PROCEDURES
- Fine-needle aspiration and excisional biopsy provide cells for histologic examination that may confirm the diagnosis.

TREATMENT

GENERAL
- Depends on stage and type of disease, age and menopausal status of patient, and any disfiguring effects of surgery
- Therapy including any combination of surgery, radiation, chemotherapy, and hormone therapy
- Primary radiation therapy
- Preoperative breast irradiation

ACTIVITY
- Arm-stretching exercises after surgery

MEDICATIONS
- Chemotherapy, such as a combination of drugs, including cyclophosphamide, fluorouracil, methotrexate, doxorubicin, vincristine, paclitaxel, and prednisone
- Regimen of cyclophosphamide, methotrexate, and fluorouracil, which is used in premenopausal and postmenopausal women
- Antiestrogen therapy such as tamoxifen
- Hormonal therapy, including estrogen, progesterone, androgen, or antiandrogen aminoglutethimide therapy

SURGERY
- Lumpectomy
- Partial, total, or modified radical mastectomy

NURSING CONSIDERATIONS

NURSING DIAGNOSES
- Acute pain
- Anxiety
- Disturbed body image
- Energy field disturbance
- Fear
- Imbalanced nutrition: Less than body requirements
- Impaired physical mobility
- Impaired skin integrity
- Ineffective coping
- Ineffective role performance
- Risk for infection

EXPECTED OUTCOMES
The patient will:
- communicate feelings of comfort and decreased pain
- express feelings of decreased anxiety
- express positive feelings about self
- express an increased sense of well-being
- use situational supports to reduce fear
- maintain adequate nutritional intake
- maintain optimal muscle strength and joint range of motion
- maintain skin integrity
- demonstrate adequate coping behaviors
- recognize limitations imposed by the illness and express feelings about these limitations
- remain free from signs and symptoms of infection.

NURSING INTERVENTIONS
- Provide information about the disease process, diagnostic tests, and treatment.
- Give prescribed drugs.
- Provide emotional support.

MONITORING
- Wound site
- Postoperative complications
- Vital signs
- Intake and output
- White blood cell count
- Pain control
- Psychological status

PATIENT TEACHING

GENERAL
Be sure to cover:
- procedures and treatments
- activities or exercises that promote healing
- breast self-examination
- risks and signs and symptoms of recurrence
- avoidance of venipuncture or blood pressure monitoring on the affected arm.

DISCHARGE PLANNING
- Refer the patient to local and national support groups.

RESOURCES
Organizations
American Cancer Society:
www.cancer.org
Guide to Internet Resources for Cancer:
www.cancerindex.org
National Cancer Institute:
www.cancer.gov

Selected references
Adebamowo, C.A., et al. "Dietary Patterns and the Risk of Breast Cancer," *Annals of Epidemiology* 15(10):789-95, November 2005.

Atlas of Pathophysiology, 2nd ed. Philadelphia: Lippincott Williams & Wilkins, 2005.

Leadbeater, M. "A Nurse-Led E-mail Service for Breast Cancer Information," *Nursing Times* 101(39):36-38, September-October 2005.

Perreault, A., and Bourbonnais, F.F. "The Experience of Suffering as Lived by Women with Breast Cancer," *International Journal of Palliative Nursing* 11(10):510, 512-19, October 2005.

Bronchiectasis

OVERVIEW

- Lung disease characterized by abnormal dilation of the bronchi and destruction of the bronchial walls
- Results from chronic inflammatory changes associated with repeated damage to bronchial walls and with abnormal mucociliary clearance, causing a breakdown of supporting tissue adjacent to the airways
- Can occur throughout the tracheobronchial tree, or may be confined to one segment or lobe
- Usually bilateral and involves the basilar segments of the lower lobes
- Three forms: cylindrical (fusiform), varicose, and saccular (cystic)

PATHOPHYSIOLOGY

- Hyperplastic squamous epithelium, denuded of cilia, replaces ulcerated columnar epithelia.
- Abscess formation occurs, involving all layers of the bronchial walls, which produces inflammatory cells and fibrous tissues, resulting in dilation and narrowing of the airways.
- Sputum stagnates in the dilated bronchi and leads to secondary infection, characterized by inflammation and leukocytic accumulations.
- Additional debris collects in the bronchi and occludes them.
- Building pressure from the retained secretions induces mucosal injury.
- Extensive vascular proliferation of bronchial circulation occurs and produces frequent hemoptysis.

CAUSES

- Complications of measles, pneumonia, pertussis, or influenza
- Congenital anomalies (rare) such as bronchomalacia
- Immune disorders
- Inhalation of corrosive gas
- Mucoviscidosis
- Obstruction with recurrent infection
- Recurrent bacterial respiratory tract infections
- Repeated aspiration of gastric juices
- Tuberculosis
- Various rare disorders such as immotile cilia syndrome

INCIDENCE

- Bronchiectasis affects people of both sexes and of all ages.
- Incidence has dramatically decreased over the past 20 years because of the availability of antibiotics to treat acute respiratory infections.
- Incidence is highest among Inuit populations in the northern hemisphere and the Maoris of New Zealand.

COMPLICATIONS

- Amyloidosis
- Chronic malnutrition
- Cor pulmonale
- Right-sided heart failure

ASSESSMENT

HISTORY

- Frequent bouts of pneumonia
- Coughing up of blood or blood-tinged sputum
- Chronic cough that produces copious, foul-smelling, mucopurulent secretions
- Dyspnea
- Weight loss
- Malaise

PHYSICAL FINDINGS

- Sputum may show a cloudy top layer, a central layer of clear saliva, and a heavy, thick, purulent bottom layer
- Clubbed fingers and toes
- Cyanotic nail beds
- Dullness over affected lung fields, if pneumonia or atelectasis present
- Diminished breath sounds
- Inspiratory crackles during inspiration over affected area
- Occasional wheezes
- Fever

DIAGNOSTIC TEST RESULTS

LABORATORY

- Sputum culture and Gram stain may show predominant pathogens.
- Complete blood count may reveal anemia and leukocytosis.

IMAGING

- Computed tomography scan shows bronchiectasis.
- Bronchography shows location and extent of disease.
- Chest X-rays show peribronchial thickening, atelectatic areas, and scattered cystic changes.

DIAGNOSTIC PROCEDURES

- Bronchoscopy may show the source of secretions or the bleeding site in hemoptysis.
- Pulmonary function studies show decreased vital capacity, expiratory flow, and hypoxemia.

OTHER

- A sweat electrolyte test may show cystic fibrosis as the underlying cause.

TREATMENT

GENERAL
- Postural drainage and chest percussion
- Bronchoscopy to remove secretions

DIET
- Well-balanced, high-calorie
- Adequate hydration

ACTIVITY
- As tolerated

MEDICATIONS
- Antibiotics
- Bronchodilators
- Oxygen

SURGERY
For poor pulmonary function
- Segmental resection
- Bronchial artery embolization
- Lobectomy
- Surgical removal of the affected lung portion

NURSING CONSIDERATIONS

NURSING DIAGNOSES
- Anxiety
- Fatigue
- Imbalanced nutrition: Less than body requirements
- Impaired gas exchange
- Ineffective airway clearance
- Ineffective breathing pattern
- Ineffective coping
- Risk for infection

EXPECTED OUTCOMES
The patient will:
- identify strategies to reduce anxiety
- utilize energy conservation techniques
- maintain adequate nutrition and hydration
- maintain adequate ventilation and oxygenation
- maintain a patent airway
- maintain effective breathing pattern
- demonstrate effective coping mechanisms
- avoid infection and other complications.

NURSING INTERVENTIONS
- Give prescribed drugs.
- Provide supportive care.
- Administer oxygen as needed.
- Perform chest physiotherapy.
- Provide a warm, quiet, comfortable environment.
- Alternate rest and activity periods.
- Provide well-balanced, high-calorie meals.
- Offer small, frequent meals.
- Provide adequate hydration.
- Provide frequent mouth care.

MONITORING
- Vital signs
- Intake and output
- Respiratory status
- Breath sounds
- Sputum production
- Pulse oximetry
- Arterial blood gas results
- Complications
- Chest tube drainage after surgery

PATIENT TEACHING

GENERAL
Be sure to cover:
- the disorder, diagnosis, and treatment
- medications and potential adverse reactions
- when to notify the physician
- proper disposal of secretions
- infection control techniques
- frequent rest periods
- preoperative and postoperative instructions, if surgery is required
- postural drainage and percussion
- coughing and deep-breathing techniques
- avoidance of air pollutants and people with known upper respiratory tract infections
- immunizations
- balanced, high-protein diet
- avoidance of milk products
- adequate hydration.

DISCHARGE PLANNING
- Refer the patient to a smoking-cessation program, if indicated.

RESOURCES
Organizations
American Association for Respiratory Care: *www.aarc.org*
American Lung Association: *www.lungusa.org*
National Heart, Lung, and Blood Institute: *www.nhlbi.nih.gov*

Selected references
Kasper, D.L., et al., eds. *Harrison's Principles of Internal Medicine,* 16th ed. New York: McGraw-Hill Book Co., 2005.
Pryor, J.A. "Physical Therapy for Adults with Bronchiectasis," *Clinical Pulmonary Medicine* 11(4):201-209, July 2004.
Weycker, D, et al. "Prevalence and Economic Burden of Bronchiectasis," *Clinical Pulmonary Medicine* 12(4):205-209, July 2005.

Bronchitis, chronic

OVERVIEW

- Inflammation of the lining of the bronchial tubes
- Form of chronic obstructive pulmonary disease
- Characterized by excessive production of tracheobronchial mucus with a cough for at least 3 months each year for 2 consecutive years
- Severity linked to the amount of cigarette smoke or other pollutants inhaled and inhalation duration
- Respiratory tract infections that typically worsen the cough and related symptoms
- Development of significant airway obstruction seen in few patients with chronic bronchitis
- Can occur alone or with emphysema

PATHOPHYSIOLOGY

- Hypertrophy and hyperplasia of the bronchial mucous glands, increased goblet cells, ciliary damage, squamous metaplasia of the columnar epithelium, and chronic leukocytic and lymphocytic infiltration of bronchial walls
- Additional effects: widespread inflammation, airway narrowing, and mucus within the airways — all producing resistance in the small airways and, consequently, a severe ventilation-perfusion imbalance (see *What happens in chronic bronchitis*)

CAUSES

- Cigarette smoking
- Environmental pollution
- Organic or inorganic dusts and noxious gas exposure
- Possible genetic predisposition

INCIDENCE

- About 20% of men have chronic bronchitis.
- More than 8.8 million people in the United States are diagnosed with chronic bronchitis annually.
- The disease is more prevalent in females than in males.
- Children of parents who smoke are at higher risk for contracting chronic bronchitis than children of parents who don't smoke.

COMPLICATIONS

- Cor pulmonale
- Pulmonary hypertension
- Right ventricular hypertrophy
- Acute respiratory failure

ASSESSMENT

HISTORY

- Long-time smoker
- Frequent upper respiratory tract infections
- Productive cough
- Exertional dyspnea
- Cough, initially prevalent in winter, but gradually becoming year-round
- Worsening coughing episodes
- Worsening dyspnea

PHYSICAL FINDINGS

- Cough producing copious gray, white, or yellow sputum
- Cyanosis
- Accessory respiratory muscle use
- Tachypnea
- Substantial weight gain
- Pedal edema
- Jugular vein distention
- Wheezing
- Prolonged expiratory time
- Rhonchi

DIAGNOSTIC TEST RESULTS

LABORATORY

- Arterial blood gas analysis may show decreased partial pressure of oxygen and normal or increased partial pressure of carbon dioxide.
- Sputum culture may reveal the number of microorganisms and neutrophils.

IMAGING

- Chest X-ray may show hyperinflation and increased bronchovascular markings.

DIAGNOSTIC PROCEDURES

- Pulmonary function tests may show increased residual volume, decreased vital capacity and forced expiratory flow, and normal static compliance and diffusing capacity.

What happens in chronic bronchitis

In chronic bronchitis, irritants inhaled for a prolonged period inflame the tracheobronchial tree. The inflammation leads to increased mucus production and a narrowed or blocked airway.

As inflammation continues, the mucus-producing goblet cells undergo hypertrophy, as do the ciliated epithelial cells that line the respiratory tract. Hypersecretion from the goblet cells blocks the free movement of the cilia, which normally sweep dust, irritants, and mucus from the airways.

As a result, the airway stays blocked, and mucus and debris accumulate in the respiratory tract.

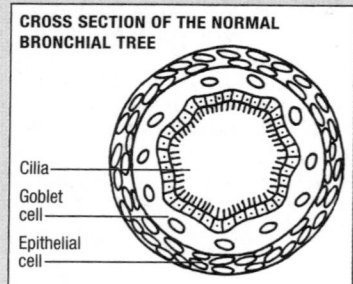

CROSS SECTION OF THE NORMAL BRONCHIAL TREE

Cilia
Goblet cell
Epithelial cell

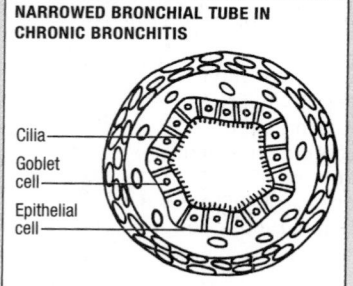

NARROWED BRONCHIAL TUBE IN CHRONIC BRONCHITIS

Cilia
Goblet cell
Epithelial cell

OTHER

- Electrocardiography may show atrial arrhythmias; peaked P waves in leads II, III, and aV_F; and right ventricular hypertrophy.

TREATMENT

GENERAL

- Smoking cessation
- Avoidance of air pollutants
- Chest physiotherapy
- Ultrasonic or mechanical nebulizer treatments

DIET

- Adequate fluid intake
- High-calorie, protein-rich

ACTIVITY

- As tolerated with frequent rest periods

MEDICATIONS

- Oxygen
- Antibiotics
- Bronchodilators
- Corticosteroids
- Diuretics

SURGERY

- Tracheostomy in advanced disease

NURSING CONSIDERATIONS

NURSING DIAGNOSES

- Anxiety
- Fatigue
- Imbalanced nutrition: Less than body requirements
- Impaired gas exchange
- Ineffective breathing pattern

EXPECTED OUTCOMES

The patient will:

- verbalize feelings of anxiety and fear
- identify measures to prevent or reduce fatigue
- maintain adequate nutrition and hydration
- maintain a patent airway and adequate ventilation
- maintain effective breathing pattern.

NURSING INTERVENTIONS

- Give prescribed drugs.
- Encourage expression of fears and concerns.
- Include the patient and his family in care decisions.
- Perform chest physiotherapy.
- Provide a high-calorie, protein-rich diet.
- Offer small, frequent meals.
- Encourage energy-conservation techniques.
- Ensure adequate oral fluid intake.
- Provide frequent mouth care.
- Encourage daily activity.
- Provide diversional activities, as appropriate.
- Provide frequent rest periods.

MONITORING

- Vital signs
- Intake and output
- Sputum production
- Respiratory status
- Breath sounds
- Daily weight
- Edema
- Response to treatment

PATIENT TEACHING

GENERAL

Be sure to cover:

- the disorder, diagnosis, and treatment
- medications and possible adverse reactions
- when to notify the physician
- infection control practices
- influenza and pneumococcus immunizations
- home oxygen therapy, if required
- postural drainage and chest percussion
- coughing and deep-breathing exercises
- inhaler use
- high-calorie, protein-rich meals
- adequate hydration
- avoidance of inhaled irritants
- prevention of bronchospasm.

DISCHARGE PLANNING

- Refer the patient to a smoking-cessation program, if indicated.
- Refer the patient to the American Lung Association for information and support.

RESOURCES

Organizations

American Lung Association: *www.lungusa.org*
Mayo Clinic: *www.mayoclinic.com*
National Heart, Lung, and Blood Institute: *www.nhlbi.nih.gov*

Selected references

Donner, C.F. "Acute Exacerbation of Chronic Bronchitis: Need for an Evidence-based Approach," *Pulmonary Pharmacology & Therapeutics* 19(Suppl 1):4-10, December 2005.

Hu, J., and Meek, P. "Health-Related Quality of Life in Individuals with Chronic Obstructive Pulmonary Disease," *Heart & Lung* 34(6):415-22, November-December 2005.

Willemse, B., et al. "High Cessation Rates of Cigarette Smoking in Subjects With and Without COPD," *Chest* 128(5): 3685-687, November 2005.

Brucellosis

OVERVIEW

- An acute febrile illness transmitted to humans from animals
- Also known as *undulant fever, Malta fever,* or *Bang's disease*

PATHOPHYSIOLOGY

- Transmitted through the consumption of unpasteurized dairy products or uncooked or undercooked contaminated meat, and through contact with infected animals or their secretions or excretions

CAUSES

- The nonmotile, non–spore-forming, gram-negative coccobacilli of the genus *Brucella*, notably *B. suis* (found in swine), *B. melitensis* (in goats), *B. abortus* (in cattle), and *B. canis* (in dogs)

INCIDENCE

- Brucellosis is most common among farmers, stock handlers, butchers, and veterinarians.
- Incidence is six times higher in men than in women.
- The disease occurs less commonly in children than in adults.
- People with chlorhydria are particularly susceptible because hydrochloric acid in gastric juices kills Brucella bacteria.
- Brucellosis is most prevalent in the Middle East, Africa, the former Soviet Union, India, South America, and Europe; it's uncommon in the United States.

COMPLICATIONS

- Abscesses in the testes, ovaries, kidneys, and brain (meningitis and encephalitis)
- Eczematous rashes, petechiae, purpura
- Orchitis
- Osteomyelitis
- Pleural effusions
- Pneumothorax
- Subacute bacterial endocarditis

ASSESSMENT

HISTORY

- Direct exposure to animals
- Ingestion of unpasteurized dairy products
- Recent travel to an endemic area
- Fatigue
- Headache
- Intermittent fever
- Profuse sweating
- Anxiety
- General aching

PHYSICAL FINDINGS

- Excessive perspiration
- Chills
- Weakness
- Lymphadenopathy
- Hepatosplenomegaly
- Tenderness in the right upper quadrant

DIAGNOSTIC TEST RESULTS

LABORATORY

- Agglutinin titers are 1:160 or more.
- Definitive diagnosis is provided by three to six cultures of blood and bone marrow and biopsies of infected tissue (for example, the spleen).
- Erythrocyte sedimentation rate is increased.
- White blood cell count is normal or reduced.

TREATMENT

GENERAL
- Secretion precautions until lesions stop draining

DIET
- High-calorie, high-protein

ACTIVITY
- Bed rest during the acute phase

MEDICATIONS
- Antibiotics
- Antipyretics
- Corticosteroids

NURSING CONSIDERATIONS

NURSING DIAGNOSES
- Acute pain
- Anxiety
- Disturbed sleep pattern
- Fatigue
- Imbalanced nutrition: Less than body requirements
- Impaired physical mobility
- Risk for infection

EXPECTED OUTCOMES
The patient will:
- experience feelings of comfort or absence of pain
- identify effective coping mechanisms to manage anxiety
- report feeling well rested
- express feelings of energy and decreased fatigue
- consume required caloric intake
- resume normal physical mobility after the recovery period
- experience no further signs or symptoms of infection.

NURSING INTERVENTIONS
- Keep suppurative granulomas and abscesses dry.
- Double-bag and properly dispose of secretions and soiled dressings.
- Reassure the patient that this infection is curable.

MONITORING
- Temperature
- Complications
- Depression and disturbed sleep pattern
- Lesion healing

PATIENT TEACHING

GENERAL
Be sure to cover:
- continuing medication for the prescribed duration
- preventing recurrence by cooking meat thoroughly and avoiding unpasteurized milk
- warning meat packers and other people at risk of occupational exposure to wear rubber gloves and goggles.

DISCHARGE PLANNING
- Refer the patient to follow-up visit with practitioner, as appropriate.

RESOURCES
Organizations
Centers for Diseases Control and Prevention: *www.cdc.gov*
National Library of Medicine: *www.nlm.nih.gov*

Selected references
Karakukcu, M., et al. "Pancytopenia, A Rare Hematologic Manifestation of Brucellosis in Children," *Journal of Pediatric Hematology/Oncology* 26(12):803-806, December 2004.
Lucero, N.E., et al. "Diagnosis of Human Brucellosis Caused by Brucella Canis," *Journal of Medical Microbiology* 54(5):457-61, May 2005.

Buerger's disease

OVERVIEW

- Inflammatory, nonatheromatous occlusive condition impairing circulation to the legs, feet and, occasionally, hands
- Sometimes called *thromboangiitis obliterans*

PATHOPHYSIOLOGY

- Polymorphonuclear leukocytes infiltrate the walls of small and medium-sized arteries and veins.
- Thrombus develops in the vascular lumen, eventually occluding and obliterating portions of the small vessels, resulting in decreased blood flow to the feet and legs.
- This diminished blood flow may produce ulceration and, eventually, gangrene.

CAUSES

- Exact cause unknown
- Linked to smoking (suggesting a hypersensitivity reaction to nicotine)

INCIDENCE

- Buerger's disease is more common in males.
- Most patients are age 20 to 45.
- The disease affects natives of India, Japan, and Korea and Ashkenazic Jews.

COMPLICATIONS

- Gangrene
- Muscle atrophy
- Ulceration

ASSESSMENT

HISTORY

- Exposure to secondhand smoke
- Use of nicotine patch
- Use of chewing tobacco
- Smoking
- Painful, intermittent claudication of the instep, aggravated by exercise and relieved by rest

PHYSICAL FINDINGS

- Feet become cold, numb, and cyanotic when exposed to low temperatures
- Digital ischemia
- Trophic nail changes
- Absent or diminished radial, ulnar, or tibial pulses
- Ischemic ulcers on the toes, feet, or fingers
- Superficial thrombophlebitis

DIAGNOSTIC TEST RESULTS

IMAGING

- Doppler ultrasonography may show diminished circulation in the peripheral vessels.
- Arteriography may locate lesions and rule out atherosclerosis.

DIAGNOSTIC PROCEDURES

- Plethysmography helps to detect decreased circulation in the peripheral vessels.

OTHER

- Allen test results may be abnormal. (See *Performing Allen's test.*)

Performing Allen's test

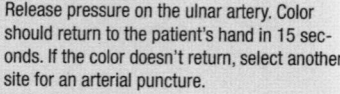

Don't obtain an arterial blood gas specimen from the radial artery until you assess collateral arterial blood supply using the Allen's test.

Direct the patient to close his hand while you occlude his radial and ulnar arteries for 10 to 30 seconds, watching for the hand to blanch.

Tell the patient to open his hand.

Release pressure on the ulnar artery. Color should return to the patient's hand in 15 seconds. If the color doesn't return, select another site for an arterial puncture.

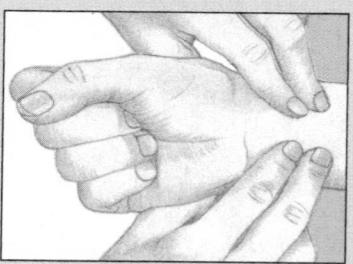
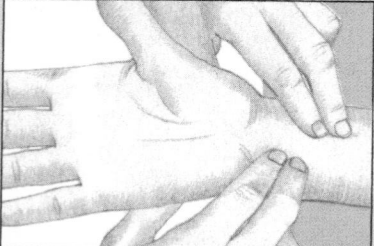
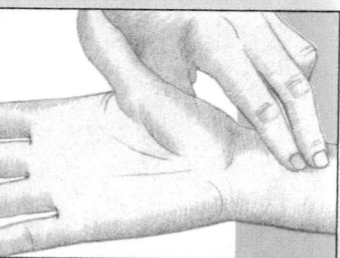

TREATMENT

GENERAL
◆ Smoking cessation

DIET
◆ Nothing by mouth, if surgery needed

ACTIVITY
◆ Exercise program that uses gravity to fill and drain the blood vessels

MEDICATIONS
◆ Antibiotics for secondary infection
◆ Analgesics

SURGERY
◆ In severe disease, a lumbar sympathectomy to increase blood supply to the skin
◆ Amputation for nonhealing ulcers, intractable pain, or gangrene

NURSING CONSIDERATIONS

NURSING DIAGNOSES
◆ Activity intolerance
◆ Acute pain
◆ Anxiety
◆ Impaired skin integrity
◆ Impaired tissue integrity
◆ Ineffective coping
◆ Ineffective role performance
◆ Ineffective thermoregulation
◆ Ineffective tissue perfusion: Peripheral
◆ Risk for infection
◆ Risk for peripheral neurovascular dysfunction

EXPECTED OUTCOMES
The patient will:
◆ maintain the ability to perform activities of daily living to the fullest extent possible
◆ express feelings of increased comfort and decreased pain
◆ verbalize strategies to reduce anxiety
◆ experience lesion and wound healing without complications
◆ maintain tissue integrity
◆ develop adequate coping mechanisms
◆ carry out previous roles within the limitations of the disease
◆ maintain a normal temperature
◆ maintain palpable pulses and warm extremities
◆ remain free from signs and symptoms of infection
◆ verbalize how to recognize peripheral neurovascular impairment.

NURSING INTERVENTIONS
◆ Provide a padded footboard or bed cradle to prevent pressure from bed linens.
◆ Protect the feet with soft padding.
◆ Provide emotional support.

MONITORING
◆ Skin integrity
◆ Peripheral circulation
◆ Infection

PATIENT TEACHING

GENERAL
Be sure to cover:
◆ avoiding precipitating factors, such as emotional stress, exposure to extreme temperatures, and trauma
◆ proper foot care, especially the importance of wearing well-fitting shoes and cotton or wool socks.

DISCHARGE PLANNING
◆ Refer the patient to a self-help group to help him stop smoking.
◆ Refer the patient for psychological counseling, if needed.
◆ If the patient has undergone amputation, refer him to physical therapists, occupational therapists, and social service agencies, as needed.

RESOURCES
Organizations
Mayo Clinic: *www.mayoclinic.com*

Selected references
Bozkurt, A.K., et al. "Surgical Treatment of Buerger's Disease," *Vascular* 12(3):192-97, May-June 2004.
Olin, J.W., and Shih, A. "Thromboangiitis Obliterans (Buerger's Disease)," *Current Opinion in Rheumatology* 18(1): 18-24, January 2006.

Bulimia nervosa

- Behavioral disorder characterized by eating binges followed by feelings of guilt, humiliation, self-deprecation, and depression
- Self-induced vomiting, the use of laxatives or diuretics, or strict dieting or fasting to overcome the effects of the binges
- Seldom incapacitating

PATHOPHYSIOLOGY
- The decreased caloric intake depletes body fat and protein stores.
- Estrogen deficiency occurs in women due to lack of lipid substrate for synthesis, causing amenorrhea.
- Testosterone levels fluctuate in men, causing decreased erectile function and sperm count.
- Ketoacidosis occurs from increased use of fat as energy fuel.

CAUSES
- Exact cause unknown

RISK FACTORS
- Cultural overemphasis on physical appearance
- Family disturbance or conflict
- Maladaptive learned behavior
- Parental obesity
- Sexual abuse
- Struggle for control or self-identity

INCIDENCE
- Bulimia nervosa affects nine females for every male.
- Between 1% and 3% of adolescent and young women meet the diagnostic criteria; 5% to 15% have some symptoms of the disorder.

 AGE FACTOR *Bulimia begins in adolescence or early adulthood.*

COMPLICATIONS
- Arrhythmias
- Cardiac failure
- Dehydration
- Dental caries
- Electrolyte imbalances
- Erosion of tooth enamel
- Esophageal tears
- Gastric ruptures
- Gum infections
- Mucosal damage to intestine
- Parotitis
- Sudden death
- Suicide

ASSESSMENT

HISTORY
- Episodic binge eating
- Continues eating until abdominal pain, sleep, or the presence of another person interrupts it
- Preferred food usually sweet, soft, and high in calories and carbohydrate content
- Exaggerated sense of guilt
- Depression
- Childhood trauma
- Parental obesity
- Unsatisfactory sexual relationships

PHYSICAL FINDINGS
- Thin or slightly overweight
- Use of diuretics, laxatives, vomiting, and exercise
- Abdominal and epigastric pain
- Amenorrhea
- Painless swelling of the salivary glands
- Unusual swelling of checks or jaw area
- Hoarseness
- Throat irritation or lacerations
- Calluses of the knuckles or abrasions and scars on the dorsum of the hand (see *Recognizing bulimic patients*)

DSM-IV-TR *criteria*
Diagnosis confirmed when two criteria are met, on average, twice a week for 3 months:
- recurrent episodes of binge eating
- repeated inappropriate behaviors (such as self-induced vomiting; misuse of diuretics, enemas, and laxatives; fasting; excessive exercise) to prevent weight gain.

DIAGNOSTIC TEST RESULTS

LABORATORY
- Serum electrolyte studies show elevated bicarbonate, decreased potassium, and decreased sodium levels.

OTHER
- The Beck Depression Inventory may identify coexisting depression.

Recognizing bulimic patients

Recognizing a bulimic patient isn't always easy. Unlike anorexic patients, bulimic patients don't deny that their eating habits are abnormal, but they commonly conceal their behavior out of shame and humiliation. If you suspect bulimia nervosa, be on the lookout for these psychological features:

- difficulties with impulse control
- distorted body image
- chronic depression
- exaggerated sense of guilt
- low tolerance for frustration
- recurrent anxiety
- feelings of alienation
- self-consciousness
- difficulty expressing feelings such as anger
- impaired social or occupational adjustment
- perfectionism.

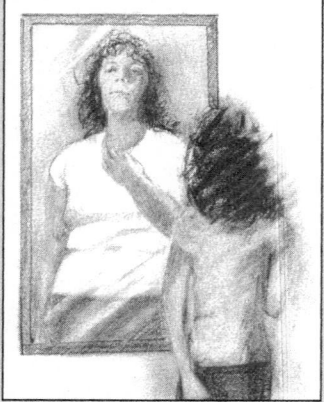

TREATMENT

GENERAL
- Inpatient or outpatient psychotherapy
- Self-help groups
- Drug rehabilitation

DIET
- Well-balanced
- Monitoring of eating pattern

ACTIVITY
- Monitoring of activity

MEDICATIONS
- Antidepressants

NURSING CONSIDERATIONS

NURSING DIAGNOSES
- Anxiety
- Chronic low self-esteem
- Constipation
- Deficient fluid volume
- Disturbed body image
- Disturbed sleep pattern
- Imbalanced nutrition: Less than body requirements
- Ineffective coping
- Social isolation

EXPECTED OUTCOMES
The patient will:
- state strategies to reduce levels of anxiety
- express positive feelings about self
- have regular bowel elimination patterns
- maintain an adequate fluid balance
- acknowledge change in body image
- verbalize feeling well rested
- display appropriate eating patterns, including regular, nutritious meals
- seek support systems and exhibit adequate coping behaviors
- interact with family or friends.

NURSING INTERVENTIONS
- Supervise mealtime and for a specified period after meals, usually up to 1 hour.
- Set a time limit for each meal.
- Provide a pleasant, relaxed environment for eating.
- Use behavior modification techniques.
- Establish a food contract, specifying the amount and type of food to be eaten at each meal.
- Encourage verbalization and provide support.

MONITORING
- Suicide potential
- Elimination patterns
- Eating patterns
- Complications
- Response to treatment
- Activity

PATIENT TEACHING

GENERAL
Be sure to cover:
- importance of keeping a food journal
- risks of laxative, emetic, and diuretic abuse
- assertiveness training
- prescribed medications, administration, dosage, and possible adverse effects.

DISCHARGE PLANNING
- Refer the patient to support services or specialized inpatient care.
- Refer the patient for psychological counseling.

RESOURCES
Organizations
National Association of Anorexia Nervosa and Associated Disorders: *www.anad.org*
National Eating Disorders Association: *www.nationaleatingdisorders.org*
Overeaters Anonymous: *www.oa.org*

Selected references
Diagnostic and Statistical Manual of Mental Disorders, Fourth Edition, Text Revision. Washington, D.C.: American Psychiatric Association, 2000.

McFarlane, T.L., et al. "Beliefs and Expectations Regarding Etiology, Treatment and Outcome in Bulimia Nervosa," *Eating and Weight Disorders* 10(3):187-92, September 2005.

Wolfe, B.E. "Reproductive Health in Women with Eating Disorders," *Journal of Obstetric, Gynecologic, and Neonatal Nursing* 34(2):255-63, March-April, 2005.

Wolfe, B.E., and Gimby, L.B. "Caring for the Hospitalized Patient with an Eating Disorder," *The Nursing Clinics of North America* 38(1):75-99, March 2003.

Burns

OVERVIEW

- Heat or chemical injury to tissue
- May be permanently disfiguring and incapacitating
- May be partial or full thickness

PATHOPHYSIOLOGY

First-degree burns (superficial, partial thickness)

- Localized injury to epidermis
- Not life-threatening

Second-degree burns (deep, partial thickness)

- Destruction of epidermis and some dermis
- Thin-walled and fluid-filled blisters
- Nerve endings exposed to air when blisters break
- Pain when nerve endings are exposed to air
- Barrier function of the skin lost

Third- and fourth-degree burns (full thickness)

- Affect every body system and organ
- Extend into the subcutaneous tissue layer
- Damage muscle, bone, and interstitial tissues
- Interstitial fluids result in edema
- Immediate immunologic response occurs
- Threat of wound sepsis
- Painless

CAUSES

- Chewing electric cords
- Child or elder abuse
- Contact with faulty electrical wiring
- Contact with high-voltage power lines
- Contact, ingestion, inhalation, or injection of acids, alkali, or vesicants
- Friction or abrasion
- Improper handling of firecrackers
- Improper use or handling of matches
- Improperly stored gasoline
- Motor vehicle accidents
- Residential fires
- Scalding accidents
- Space heater or electrical malfunctions
- Sun exposure

INCIDENCE

- Burns affect more than 2 million people each year in the United States.
- Burns cause 70,000 hospitalizations annually.
- Burns cause 20,000 specialized burn unit admissions annually.

COMPLICATIONS

- Anemia
- Hypovolemic shock
- Malnutrition
- Multiple organ dysfunction syndrome
- Respiratory collapse
- Sepsis

ASSESSMENT

HISTORY

- Cause of the burn revealed
- Preexisting medical conditions

PHYSICAL FINDINGS

- Depth and size of the burn assessed
- Severity of the burn estimated
- Major — more than 10% of the patient's body surface area (BSA); more than 20% of a child's BSA
- Moderate — 3% to 10% of a patient's BSA; 10% to 20% of a child's BSA
- Minor — less than 3% of a patient's BSA; less than 10% of a child's BSA
- Respiratory distress and cyanosis
- Edema
- Alteration in pulse rate, strength, and regularity
- Stridor, wheezing, crackles, and rhonchi
- S_3 or S_4
- Hypotension
- Soot marks on face

DIAGNOSTIC TEST RESULTS

LABORATORY

- Arterial blood gas levels may show evidence of smoke inhalation, decreased alveolar function, and hypoxia.
- Complete blood count may show decreased hemoglobin level and hematocrit, if blood loss occurs.
- Abnormal electrolyte levels may result from fluid losses and shifts.
- Blood urea nitrogen level may increase with fluid losses.
- Glucose level in children may be decreased because of limited glycogen storage.
- Urinalysis may show myoglobinuria and hemoglobinuria.
- Carboxyhemoglobin level is increased.

DIAGNOSTIC PROCEDURES

- Electrocardiography shows myocardial ischemia, injury, or arrhythmias, especially in electrical burns.
- Fiber-optic bronchoscopy shows edema of the airways.

TREATMENT

GENERAL

- Stopping the burn source
- Airway, breathing, and circulation assessed and secured
- Preventing hypoxia
- Giving I.V. fluids through a large-bore I.V. line (see *Fluid replacement after a burn*)
- Adults: maintain urine output of 30 to 50 ml/hour.
- Child weighing less than 66 lb (30 kg): maintain urine output of 1 ml/kg/hour.
- Nasogastric tube and urinary catheter insertion
- Wound care

DIET

- Nothing by mouth until severity of burn established; then high-protein, high-calorie
- Increased hydration with high-calorie, high-protein drinks, not free water
- Total parenteral nutrition if unable to take food by mouth

ACTIVITY

- With limitations based on extent and location of burn
- Physical therapy

MEDICATIONS
- Booster of tetanus toxoid
- Analgesics
- Antibiotics
- Antianxiolytics
- Osmotic diuretics

SURGERY
- Loose tissue and blister debridement
- Escharotomy
- Skin grafting

NURSING CONSIDERATIONS

NURSING DIAGNOSES
- Acute pain
- Anxiety
- Decreased cardiac output
- Deficient fluid volume
- Disturbed body image
- Hypothermia
- Imbalanced nutrition: Less than body requirements
- Impaired gas exchange
- Impaired physical mobility
- Impaired skin integrity
- Ineffective airway clearance
- Ineffective coping
- Ineffective protection
- Ineffective tissue perfusion: Peripheral
- Risk for infection
- Risk for posttraumatic stress disorder

EXPECTED OUTCOMES
The patient will:
- achieve pain relief with analgesia or other measures
- express feelings of decreased anxiety
- maintain adequate cardiac output
- maintain fluid volume within the acceptable range
- express positive feelings about self
- maintain normal body temperature
- maintain daily calorie requirements
- maintain adequate ventilation
- attain the highest degree of mobility possible within the confines of the injury
- exhibit improved or healed wounds or lesions that are clean, pink, and free of purulent drainage
- maintain a patent airway
- demonstrate effective coping mechanisms
- verbalize methods to prevent burns
- exhibit signs of adequate peripheral perfusion
- remain free from signs and symptoms of infection
- express feelings and fears about the traumatic event.

NURSING INTERVENTIONS
- Apply immediate, aggressive burn treatment.
- Use strict sterile technique.

- Remove smoldering clothing.
- Remove constricting items.
- Perform appropriate wound care.
- Provide adequate hydration.
- Weigh the patient daily.
- Encourage verbalization and provide support.

MONITORING
- Vital signs
- Respiratory status
- Signs of infection
- Intake and output
- Hydration and nutritional status
- Patient's emotional status

PATIENT TEACHING

GENERAL
Be sure to cover:
- the injury, diagnosis, and treatment
- appropriate wound care
- medications administration, dosage, and possible adverse effects
- developing a dietary plan
- signs and symptoms of complications.

DISCHARGE PLANNING
- Refer the patient to rehabilitation, if appropriate.
- Refer the patient to psychological counseling, if needed.
- Refer the patient to resource and support services.

RESOURCES
Organizations
American Burn Association: *www.ameriburn.org*
National Center for Injury Prevention and Control: *www.cdc.gov/ncipc*

Selected references
Anwar, M.U., et al. "Smoking, Substance Abuse, Psychiatric History, and Burns: Trends in Adult Patients," *Journal of Burn Care & Rehabilitation* 26(6):493-501, November-December 2005.
Atlas of Pathophysiology, 2nd ed. Philadelphia: Lippincott Williams & Wilkins, 2005.
Burd, A., and Noronha, F. "What's New in Burns Trauma?" *Surgical Practice* 9(4):126-36, November 2005.

Fluid replacement after a burn

To replace fluid in an adult with a burn, use one of the following formulas:

FIRST 24 HOURS

Evans
- 1 ml × patient's weight in kg × % total body surface area (TBSA) burn (0.9% normal saline solution)
- 1 ml × patient's weight in kg × % TBSA burn (colloid solution)

Brooke
- 1.5 ml × patient's weight in kg × % TBSA burn (lactated ringer's solution)
- 0.5 ml × patient's weight in kg × % TBSA burn (colloid solution)

Parkland
- 4 ml × patient's weight in kg × % TBSA burn (lactated Ringer's solution). Give one-half of volume in first 8 minutes; then infuse remainder over 16 minutes.

SECOND 24 HOURS

Evans
- 50% of first 24-hour replacement (0.9% normal saline solution)
- 2,000 ml (dextrose 5% in water [D_5W])

Brooke
- 50% to 75% of first 24-hour replacement (lactated Ringer's solution)
- 2,000 ml (D_5W)

Parkland
- 30% to 60% of calculated plasma volume (25% albumin)
- Volume to maintain desired urine output (D_5W)

Campylobacteriosis

OVERVIEW

- In humans and animals, intestinal infection caused by the *Campylobacter* organism, a spiral-shaped bacteria
- Signs and symptoms usually developing 2 to 5 days after exposure to *Campylobacter*
- May spread to the bloodstream in persons with compromised immune systems, causing a life-threatening infection

PATHOPHYSIOLOGY

- The organism invades and destroys the epithelial cells of the jejunum, ileum, and colon.
- The disease produces an increase in motility and secretions that results in diarrhea.

CAUSES

- Contact with an infected person's stool
- Ingestion of contaminated food or water or unpasteurized milk
- Occasionally from infected pets or wild animals

RISK FACTORS

- Occupational exposure to cattle, sheep, and other farm animals
- Laboratory workers
- Homosexual men

INCIDENCE

- Campylobacteriosis is the most common bacterial cause of diarrheal illness in the United States.
- The disease occurs most commonly in the summer months.

COMPLICATIONS

- Bacteremia
- Severe dehydration and electrolyte disturbances
- Guillain-Barré syndrome
- Reiter's syndrome

ASSESSMENT

HISTORY

- Exposure to contaminated food or water
- Acute onset of diarrhea
- Recent close contact with a person who has diarrhea

PHYSICAL FINDINGS

- Cramping abdominal pain
- Nausea and vomiting
- Fever
- Traces of blood in the stool

DIAGNOSTIC TEST RESULTS

LABORATORY

- Stool culture identifies *Campylobacter*.

TREATMENT

GENERAL
◆ Enteric and contact precautions (see *Contact precautions*)

DIET
◆ Correction of fluid and electrolyte imbalances
◆ Increased fluid intake

ACTIVITY
◆ As tolerated

MEDICATIONS
◆ Oral antibiotics

Contact precautions

In addition to standard precautions, follow these precautions:
◆ Place the patient in a private room. If a private room isn't available, consult with infection control personnel. As an alternative, place the patient in a room with a patient who has an active infection with the same microorganism.
◆ Wear gloves whenever you enter the patient's room. Always change them after contact with infected material. Remove them before leaving the room. Wash your hands immediately with an antimicrobial soap, or rub them with a waterless antiseptic. Then avoid touching contaminated surfaces.
◆ Wear a gown when entering the patient's room if you think your clothing will have extensive contact with him or anything in his room or if he has diarrhea or is incontinent. Remove the gown before leaving the room.
◆ Limit the patient's movement from the room, and check with infection control personnel whenever he must leave it.

NURSING CONSIDERATIONS

NURSING DIAGNOSES
◆ Acute pain
◆ Deficient fluid volume
◆ Diarrhea
◆ Hyperthermia
◆ Risk for infection

EXPECTED OUTCOMES
The patient will:
◆ express feelings of comfort and relief from pain
◆ regain or maintain normal fluid and electrolyte balance
◆ have an elimination pattern that returns to normal
◆ remain afebrile
◆ exhibit no further signs or symptoms of infection.

NURSING INTERVENTIONS
◆ Follow contact precautions for those with active diarrhea.
◆ Isolate a patient who can't practice good hygiene.
◆ Give prescribed drugs.
◆ Replace lost fluids and electrolytes through diet or I.V. fluids.

MONITORING
◆ Intake and output
◆ Vital signs
◆ Signs of dehydration
◆ Electrolytes
◆ Amount and characteristics of stool

PATIENT TEACHING

GENERAL
Be sure to cover:
◆ the disorder, diagnosis, and treatment
◆ proper hand-washing technique
◆ proper food-handling practices
◆ medications and potential adverse effects
◆ complications and when to notify the practitioner
◆ preventive measures.

RESOURCES
Organizations
Centers for Disease Control and Prevention: *www.cdc.gov*
U.S. Food and Drug Administration: *www.fda.gov*

Selected references
Butzler, J.P. "*Campylobacter*, From Obscurity to Celebrity," *Clinical Microbiology & Infection* 10(10):868-76, October 2004.
Gurtler, M., et al. "The Importance of *Campylobacter Coli* in Human Campylobacteriosis: Prevalence and Genetic Characterization," *Epidemiology & Infection* 133(6):1081-1087, December 2005.

Candidiasis

- Mild, superficial fungal infection
- Can lead to severe disseminated infections and fungemia in immunocompromised patient, transplant recipient, burn patient, low-birthweight neonate, or patient on hyperalimentation
- Prognosis varies, depending on patient's resistance
- Also known as *candidosis* and *moniliasis*

PATHOPHYSIOLOGY
- Change in the patient's resistance to infection, his immunocompromised state, and antibiotic use permits the sudden proliferation of *Candida albicans.*

CAUSES
- In most cases, infection with *C. albicans* or *C. tropicalis*

RISK FACTORS
- Maternal vaginitis present during vaginal delivery
- Preexisting diabetes mellitus, cancer, or immunosuppressant illness
- Immunosuppressant drug use
- Radiation
- Aging
- Irritation from dentures
- I.V. or urinary catheterization
- Drug abuse
- Total parenteral nutrition
- Surgery
- Use of antibiotic agents

INCIDENCE
- Candidiasis affects 14% of immunocompromised patients.
- The disease affects men and women equally.
- The disease can occur at any age.

COMPLICATIONS
- Dissemination with organ failure of the kidneys, brain, GI tract, eyes, lungs, and heart

HISTORY
- Underlying illness
- Recent course of antibiotic or antineoplastic therapy
- Drug abuse
- Hyperalimentation

PHYSICAL FINDINGS
- Scaly, erythematous, papular rash, possibly covered with exudate and erupting in breast folds, between fingers, and at the axillae, groin, and umbilicus
- Red, swollen, darkened nail beds; occasionally, purulent discharge; possibly nail separation from the nail bed
- Scales in the mouth and throat
- White or yellow vaginal discharge, with local excoriation; white or gray raised patches on vaginal walls, with local inflammation
- Cream-colored or bluish white lacelike patches of exudate on the tongue, mouth, or pharynx that reveal bloody engorgement when scraped (see *Identifying thrush*)
- Hemoptysis, cough; coarse breath sounds in the infected lung fields
- Flank pain, dysuria, hematuria, cloudy urine with casts
- Headache, nuchal rigidity, seizures, focal neurologic deficits
- Blurred vision, orbital or periorbital pain, eye exudate, floating scotomata, and lesions with a white, cottonball appearance seen during ophthalmoscopy
- Chest pain and arrhythmias
- Septic shock

LABORATORY
- Fungal serological panel shows the candidal organism.

Identifying thrush

Candidiasis of the oropharyngeal mucosa (thrush) causes cream-colored or bluish white pseudomembranous patches on the tongue, mouth, or pharynx (as shown). Fungal invasion may extend to circumoral tissues.

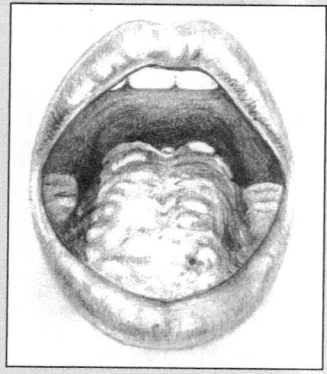

TREATMENT

GENERAL
- Treat predisposing condition

DIET
- No restrictions unless oral infection
- With oral infection, spicy food only as tolerated

ACTIVITY
- As tolerated

MEDICATIONS
- Antifungals
- Amphotericin B (Fungizone)
- Topical anesthetics

SURGERY
- Abscess drainage; surgically or percutaneously

NURSING CONSIDERATIONS

NURSING DIAGNOSES
- Acute pain
- Hyperthermia
- Impaired oral mucous membrane
- Impaired skin integrity
- Impaired urinary elimination
- Risk for aspiration
- Sexual dysfunction

EXPECTED OUTCOMES
The patient will:
- express increased comfort
- experience a normal temperature and white blood cell count
- experience lesion and wound healing without complications
- maintain skin integrity
- return to a normal elimination pattern and maintain fluid balance
- not aspirate
- express feelings about potential or actual changes in sexual activity.

NURSING INTERVENTIONS
- Follow standard precautions.
- Give prescribed drugs.
- Provide a nonirritating mouthwash to loosen tenacious secretions and a soft toothbrush to avoid irritation.
- Observe high-risk patients daily for patchy areas, irritation, sore throat, oral and gingival bleeding, and other signs of superinfection.
- Assess the patient for underlying systemic causes.

MONITORING
- Vital signs
- Intake and output
- Blood urea nitrogen, serum creatinine, and urine blood and protein levels
- Potassium levels

PATIENT TEACHING

GENERAL
Be sure to cover:
- the disorder, diagnosis, and treatment
- good oral hygiene practices
- (for a woman in her third trimester of pregnancy) the need for examination for vaginitis to protect her neonate from thrush infection at birth.

RESOURCES
Organizations
Centers for Disease Control and Prevention: *www.cdc.gov*
Harvard University Consumer Health Information: *www.intelihealth.com*
National Health Information Center: *www.health.gov/nhic*
National Library of Medicine: *www.nlm.nih.gov*

Selected references
Kasper, D.L., et al., eds. *Harrison's Principles of Internal Medicine*, 16th ed. New York: McGraw-Hill Book Co., 2005.
Spellberg, B.J., et al. "Current Treatment Strategies for Disseminated Candidiasis," *Clinical Infectious Diseases* 42(2):244-51, January 2006.
Theroux, R. "Factors Influencing Women's Decisions to Self-Treat Vaginal Symptoms," *Journal of the American Academy of Nursing Practitioners* 17(4):156-62, April 2005.

Cardiac tamponade LIFE-THREATENING DISORDER

OVERVIEW

- Rapid increase in intrapericardial pressure caused by fluid accumulation in the pericardial sac
- Impaired diastolic filling of the heart

PATHOPHYSIOLOGY

- Progressive accumulation of fluid in the pericardial sac causes compression of the heart chambers.
- Compression of the heart chambers obstructs blood flow into the ventricles and reduces the amount of blood pumped out with each contraction.
- With each contraction more fluid accumulates, decreasing cardiac output. (See *Understanding cardiac tamponade*.)

CAUSES

- Acute myocardial infarction
- Cardiac catheterization
- Cardiac surgery
- Chronic renal failure
- Connective tissue disorders
- Drug reaction
- Effusion in cancer, bacterial infections, tuberculosis and, rarely, acute rheumatic fever
- Hemorrhage from nontraumatic cause
- May be idiopathic
- Trauma
- Viral, postirradiation, or idiopathic pericarditis

INCIDENCE

- Cardiac tamponade is more common in males than in females.
- The disorder occurs with 2% of penetrating chest traumas.

COMPLICATIONS

- Cardiogenic shock
- Death

ASSESSMENT

HISTORY

- Presence of one or more causes
- Dyspnea
- Shortness of breath
- Chest pain

PHYSICAL FINDINGS

- Vary with volume of fluid and speed of fluid accumulation
- Diaphoresis
- Anxiety and restlessness
- Pallor or cyanosis
- Jugular vein distention
- Edema
- Rapid, weak pulses
- Hepatomegaly
- Decreased arterial blood pressure
- Increased central venous pressure
- Pulsus paradoxus
- Narrow pulse pressure
- Muffled heart sounds

Understanding cardiac tamponade

The pericardial sac, which surrounds and protects the heart, is composed of several layers. The fibrous pericardium is the tough outermost membrane; the inner membrane, called the *serous membrane*, consists of the visceral and parietal layers. The visceral layer clings to the heart and is also known as the *epicardial layer* of the heart. The parietal layer lies between the visceral layer and the fibrous pericardium. The pericardial space — between the visceral and parietal layers — contains 10 to 30 ml of pericardial fluid. This fluid lubricates the layers and minimizes friction when the heart contracts.

In cardiac tamponade, blood or fluid fills the pericardial space, compressing the heart chambers, increasing intracardiac pressure, and obstructing venous return. As blood flow into the ventricles falls, so does cardiac output. Without prompt treatment, low cardiac output can be fatal.

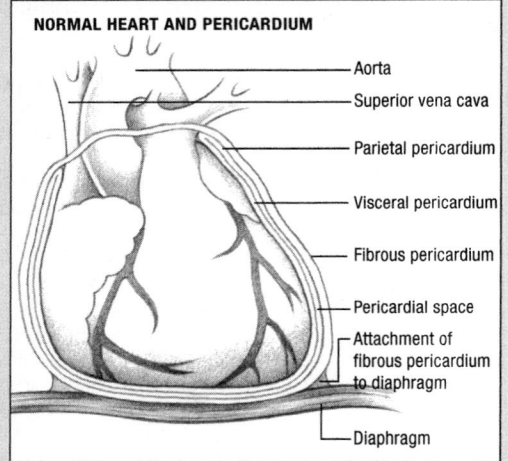

NORMAL HEART AND PERICARDIUM

- Aorta
- Superior vena cava
- Parietal pericardium
- Visceral pericardium
- Fibrous pericardium
- Pericardial space
- Attachment of fibrous pericardium to diaphragm
- Diaphragm

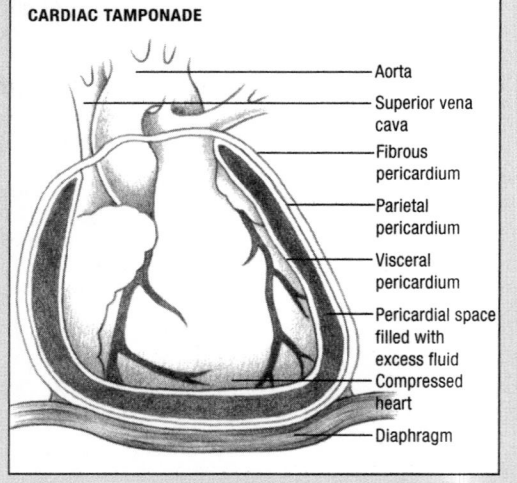

CARDIAC TAMPONADE

- Aorta
- Superior vena cava
- Fibrous pericardium
- Parietal pericardium
- Visceral pericardium
- Pericardial space filled with excess fluid
- Compressed heart
- Diaphragm

DIAGNOSTIC TEST RESULTS

IMAGING
◆ Chest X-rays show slightly widened mediastinum and enlargement of the cardiac silhouette.

DIAGNOSTIC PROCEDURES
◆ Electrocardiography may show low voltage complexes in the precordial leads.
◆ Hemodynamic monitoring shows equalization of mean right atrial, right ventricular diastolic, pulmonary artery wedge, and left ventricular diastolic pressures.
◆ Echocardiography may show an echo-free space, indicating fluid accumulation in the pericardial sac.

TREATMENT

GENERAL
◆ Pericardiocentesis, if necessary

DIET
◆ As tolerated

ACTIVITY
◆ Bed rest

MEDICATIONS
◆ Intravascular volume expansion
◆ Inotropic agents
◆ Oxygen

SURGERY
◆ Pericardiocentesis
◆ Pericardial window
◆ Subxiphoid pericardiotomy
◆ Complete pericardectomy
◆ Thoracotomy

NURSING CONSIDERATIONS

NURSING DIAGNOSES
◆ Activity intolerance
◆ Acute pain
◆ Anxiety
◆ Decreased cardiac output
◆ Deficient fluid volume
◆ Impaired gas exchange
◆ Ineffective tissue perfusion: Cardiopulmonary
◆ Risk for infection

EXPECTED OUTCOMES
The patient will:
◆ maintain his ability to perform activities of daily living to the fullest extent possible
◆ express feelings of comfort and reduced levels of pain
◆ identify strategies to reduce anxiety
◆ maintain hemodynamic stability and adequate cardiac output
◆ maintain adequate fluid volume
◆ maintain adequate ventilation and oxygenation
◆ maintain adequate cardiopulmonary perfusion
◆ remain free from signs and symptoms of infection.

NURSING INTERVENTIONS
◆ Give prescribed drugs.
◆ Provide reassurance.
◆ Assist with pericardiocentesis, if necessary.
◆ Infuse I.V. solutions, as ordered.
◆ Administer oxygen therapy as needed.
◆ Maintain the chest drainage system, if used.

MONITORING
◆ Vital signs
◆ Intake and output
◆ Signs and symptoms of increasing tamponade
◆ Cardiac rhythm
◆ Hemodynamics
◆ Arterial blood gas levels
◆ Heart and breath sounds
◆ Complications

PATIENT TEACHING

GENERAL
Be sure to cover:
◆ the disorder, diagnosis, and treatment
◆ medications and potential adverse reactions
◆ when to notify the practitioner
◆ preoperative and postoperative care
◆ emergency procedures.

RESOURCES
Organizations
American Heart Association: *www.americanheart.org*
National Heart, Lung, and Blood Institute: *www.nhlbi.nih.gov*

Selected references
Goldman, L., and Ausiello, D. *Cecil Textbook of Medicine,* 22nd ed. Philadelphia: W.B. Saunders Co., 2004.
Kasper, D.L., et al., eds. *Harrison's Principles of Internal Medicine,* 16th ed. New York: McGraw-Hill Book Co., 2005.
The Merck Manual of Diagnosis & Therapy, 18th ed. Whitehouse Station, N.J.: Merck & Co., Inc., 2006.
Shatzer, M., and Castor, A. "How Transthoracic Echocardiography Detects Cardiac Tamponade," *Nursing* 34(3):73-74, March 2004.
Wade, C.R., et al. "Postoperative Nursing Care of the Cardiac Transplant Recipient," *Critical Care Nursing Quarterly* 27(1):17-28, January-March, 2004.

Cardiomyopathy, dilated

OVERVIEW

- Disease of the heart muscle fibers
- Also called *congestive cardiomyopathy*

PATHOPHYSIOLOGY

- Extensively damaged myocardial muscle fibers reduce contractility of the left ventricle.
- As systolic function declines, cardiac output falls.
- The sympathetic nervous system is stimulated to increase heart rate and contractility.
- When compensatory mechanisms can no longer maintain cardiac output, the heart begins to fail. (See *Understanding dilated cardiomyopathy.*)

CAUSES

- Cardiotoxic effects of drugs or alcohol
- Chemotherapy
- Drug hypersensitivity
- Hypertension
- Ischemic heart disease

Understanding dilated cardiomyopathy

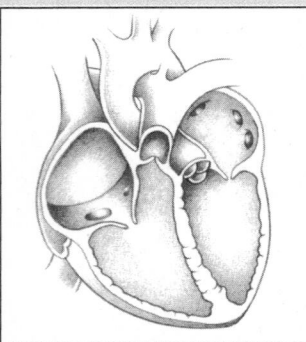

- Greatly increased chamber size
- Thinning of left ventricular muscle
- Increased atrial chamber size
- Increased myocardial mass
- Normal ventricular inflow resistance
- Decreased contractility

- Peripartum syndrome related to pre-eclampsia and eclampsia
- Valvular disease
- Viral or bacterial infections

INCIDENCE

- Most commonly affects middle-age men but can occur in any age-group.

COMPLICATIONS

- Intractable heart failure
- Arrhythmias
- Emboli

ASSESSMENT

HISTORY

- Possible history of a disorder that can cause cardiomyopathy
- Gradual onset of shortness of breath, orthopnea, dyspnea on exertion, paroxysmal nocturnal dyspnea, fatigue, dry cough at night, palpitations, and vague chest pain

PHYSICAL FINDINGS

- Peripheral edema
- Jugular vein distention
- Ascites
- Peripheral cyanosis
- Tachycardia even at rest and pulsus alternans in late stages
- Hepatomegaly and splenomegaly
- Narrow pulse pressure
- Irregular rhythms, diffuse apical impulses, pansystolic murmur
- S_3 and S_4 gallop rhythms
- Pulmonary crackles

WARNING *Dilated cardiomyopathy may need to be differentiated from other types of cardiomyopathy.* (*See* Assessment findings in cardiomyopathies.)

DIAGNOSTIC TEST RESULTS

IMAGING

- Angiography results rule out ischemic heart disease.
- Chest X-rays demonstrate moderate to marked cardiomegaly and possible pulmonary edema.
- Echocardiography may reveal ventricular thrombi, global hypokinesis, and the degrees of left ventricular dilation and systolic dysfunction.
- Gallium scans may identify patients with dilated cardiomyopathy and myocarditis.

DIAGNOSTIC PROCEDURES

- Cardiac catheterization can show left ventricular dilation and dysfunction, elevated left ventricular and, often, right ventricular filling pressures, and diminished cardiac output.
- Transvenous endomyocardial biopsy may be useful in determining the underlying disorder in some patients.
- Electrocardiography evaluates ischemic heart disease and identifies arrhythmias and intraventricular conduction defects.

TREATMENT

DIET

- Low-sodium, supplemented by vitamin therapy
- No ingestion of alcohol if cardiomyopathy caused by alcoholism

ACTIVITY

- Rest periods

AGE FACTOR *A woman of childbearing age with dilated cardiomyopathy should avoid pregnancy.*

MEDICATIONS

- Cardiac glycoside
- Diuretics
- Angiotensin-converting enzyme inhibitors
- Oxygen
- Anticoagulants
- Vasodilators
- Antiarrhythmics
- Beta-adrenergic blockers

SURGERY

- Heart transplantation
- Possible cardiomyoplasty

NURSING DIAGNOSES
- Activity intolerance
- Anxiety
- Decreased cardiac output
- Excess fluid volume
- Fatigue
- Hopelessness
- Impaired gas exchange
- Impaired physical mobility
- Ineffective breathing pattern
- Ineffective denial
- Ineffective role performance
- Ineffective tissue perfusion: Cardiopulmonary

EXPECTED OUTCOMES
The patient will:
- express feelings of increased energy and decreased fatigue
- verbalize strategies to reduce anxiety level
- maintain adequate cardiac output and hemodynamic stability
- develop no complications of excess fluid volume
- express feelings of energy and decreased fatigue

- make decisions about his care as appropriate
- maintain adequate ventilation and oxygenation
- maintain joint mobility and range of motion (ROM)
- maintain a respiratory rate within 5 breaths/minute of baseline
- recognize and accept limitations of chronic illness and the changes in lifestyle that are needed
- resume and maintain as many former roles as possible
- maintain adequate cardiopulmonary perfusion.

NURSING INTERVENTIONS
- Alternate periods of rest with required activities of daily living.
- Provide active or passive ROM exercises.
- Consult with the dietitian to provide a low-sodium diet.
- Administer oxygen as needed.
- Check serum potassium levels for hypokalemia, especially if therapy includes cardiac glycosides.
- Offer support and let the patient express his feelings.
- Allow the patient and his family to express their fears and concerns and help them identify effective coping strategies.

MONITORING
- Vital signs
- Hemodynamics
- Intake and output
- Daily weights
- Signs and symptoms of progressive heart failure

PATIENT TEACHING

GENERAL
Be sure to cover:
- the disorder, diagnosis, and treatment
- medications and potential adverse reactions
- when to notify the practitioner
- sodium and fluid restrictions
- signs and symptoms of worsening heart failure.

DISCHARGE PLANNING
- Refer family members to community cardiopulmonary resuscitation classes.

RESOURCES
Organizations
Mayo Clinic: *www.mayoclinic.com*
National Heart, Lung, and Blood Institute: *www.nhlbi.nih.gov*

Selected references
Dambro, M.R. *Griffith's Five-Minute Clinical Consult 2005.* Philadelphia: Lippincott Williams & Wilkins, 2005.
Kasper, D.L., et al., eds. *Harrison's Principles of Internal Medicine,* 16th ed. New York: McGraw-Hill Book Co., 2005.
The Merck Manual of Diagnosis & Therapy, 18th ed. Whitehouse Station, N.J.: Merck & Co., Inc., 2006.
Morooka, T., et al. "An Appropriate Indication for the Initiation of Beta-blocker Therapy in Dilated Cardiomyopathy," *Cardiology* 105(1):61-66, 2006.
Professional Guide to Diseases, 8th ed. Philadelphia: Lippincott Williams & Wilkins, 2005.

Assessment findings in cardiomyopathies

TYPE	ASSESSMENT FINDINGS
Dilated cardiomyopathy	- Generalized weakness, fatigue - Chest pain, palpitations - Syncope - Tachycardia - Narrow pulse pressure - Pulmonary congestion, pleural effusions - Jugular vein distention, peripheral edema - Paroxysmal nocturnal dyspnea, orthopnea, dyspnea on exertion
Hypertrophic cardiomyopathy	- Angina, palpitations - Syncope - Orthopnea, dyspnea with exertion - Pulmonary congestion - Loud systolic murmur - Life-threatening arrhythmias - Sudden cardiac arrest
Restrictive cardiomyopathy	- Generalized weakness, fatigue - Bradycardia - Dyspnea - Jugular vein distention, peripheral edema - Liver congestion, abdominal ascites

Cardiomyopathy, hypertrophic

OVERVIEW

OVERVIEW

- Primary disease of cardiac muscle characterized by left ventricular hypertrophy
- Also known as *idiopathic hypertrophic subaortic stenosis, hypertrophic obstructive cardiomyopathy,* and *muscular aortic stenosis*

PATHOPHYSIOLOGY

- The hypertrophied ventricle becomes stiff, noncompliant, and unable to relax during ventricular filling.
- Ventricular filling time is reduced as compensation to tachycardia.
- Reduced ventricular filling leads to low cardiac output. (See *Understanding hypertrophic cardiomyopathy.*)

CAUSES

- Associated with hypertension
- Transmission by autosomal dominant trait (about one-half of all cases)

INCIDENCE

- More common in men than women
- Affects 5 to 8 people per 100,000 in the United States
- More common in blacks than in other minority populations.

COMPLICATIONS

- Pulmonary hypertension
- Heart failure
- Ventricular arrhythmias

ASSESSMENT

HISTORY

- Generally, no visible clinical features until disease is well advanced
- Blood flow to left ventricle abruptly reduced by atrial dilation and, sometimes, atrial fibrillation
- Possible family history of hypertrophic cardiomyopathy
- Orthopnea
- Dyspnea on exertion
- Anginal pain
- Fatigue
- Syncope, even at rest

PHYSICAL FINDINGS

- Rapidly rising carotid arterial pulse possible
- Pulsus bisferiens
- Double or triple apical impulse, possibly displaced laterally
- Bibasilar crackles if heart failure is present
- Harsh systolic murmur heard after S_1 at the apex near the left sternal border
- Possible S_4

⚡ **WARNING** *Hypertrophic cardiomyopathy may need to be differentiated from other types of cardiomyopathy. (See* Assessment findings in cardiomyopathies, *page 155.)*

DIAGNOSTIC TEST RESULTS

IMAGING

- Chest X-rays may show a mild to moderate increase in heart size.
- Thallium scan usually reveals myocardial perfusion defects.
- Angiography reveals a dilated, diffusely hypokinetic left ventricle.

DIAGNOSTIC PROCEDURES

- Echocardiography shows left ventricular hypertrophy and a thick, asymmetrical intraventricular septum in obstructive hypertrophic cardiomyopathy, whereas hypertrophy affects various ventricular areas in nonobstructive hypertrophic cardiomyopathy.
- Cardiac catheterization reveals elevated left ventricular end-diastolic pressure and, possibly, mitral insufficiency.
- Electrocardiography usually shows left ventricular hypertrophy, ST-segment and T-wave abnormalities, Q waves in leads II, III, aV_F, and in V_4 to V_6 (because of hypertrophy, not infarction), left anterior hemiblock, left axis deviation, and ventricular and atrial arrhythmias.

Understanding hypertrophic cardiomyopathy

- Normal right and decreased left chamber size
- Left ventricular hypertrophy
- Thickened interventricular septum (hypertrophic obstructive cardiomyopathy)
- Atrial chamber size increased on left
- Increased myocardial mass
- Increased ventricular inflow resistance
- Increased or decreased contractility

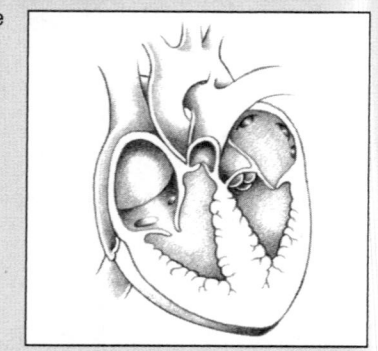

TREATMENT

GENERAL
- Cardioversion for atrial fibrillation

DIET
- Low-fat, low-salt
- Fluid restrictions
- Avoidance of alcohol

ACTIVITY
- Individualized limitations
- Bed rest, if necessary

MEDICATIONS
- Beta-adrenergic blockers
- Calcium channel blockers
- Amiodarone, unless atrioventricular block exists
- Antibiotic prophylaxis

⚡ **WARNING** *Nitrates, digoxin, angiotensin-converting enzyme inhibitors, and other beta-adrenergic blockers are contraindicated in hypertrophic cardiomyopathy.*

⚡ **WARNING** *If propranolol is to be discontinued, don't stop the drug abruptly; doing so may cause rebound effects, resulting in myocardial infarction or sudden death.*

SURGERY
- Ventricular myotomy alone or combined with mitral valve replacement
- Heart transplantation

NURSING CONSIDERATIONS

NURSING DIAGNOSES
- Activity intolerance
- Acute pain
- Decreased cardiac output
- Excess fluid volume
- Fatigue
- Ineffective coping
- Risk for infection

EXPECTED OUTCOMES
The patient will:
- carry out activities of daily living (ADLs) without excess fatigue or decreased energy
- express feelings of comfort and decreased pain
- maintain adequate cardiac output and hemodynamic stability
- develop no complications of excess fluid volume
- express feelings of energy and decreased fatigue
- develop adequate coping mechanisms
- remain free from all signs and symptoms of infection.

NURSING INTERVENTIONS
- Alternate periods of rest with required ADLs and treatments.
- Provide personal care, as needed, to prevent fatigue.
- Provide active or passive range-of-motion exercises.
- Offer support and let the patient express his feelings.
- Allow the patient and his family to express their fears and concerns and identify effective coping strategies.

MONITORING
- Vital signs
- Hemodynamics
- Intake and output

PATIENT TEACHING

GENERAL
Be sure to cover:
- that propranolol can cause depression and the need to notify the practitioner if symptoms occur
- instructions to take medication as ordered
- the need to notify any practitioner caring for the patient that he shouldn't be given nitroglycerin, digoxin, or diuretics because they can worsen obstruction
- need for antibiotic prophylaxis before dental work or surgery to prevent infective endocarditis
- warnings against strenuous activity, which may precipitate syncope or sudden death
- need to avoid Valsalva's maneuver or sudden position changes.

DISCHARGE PLANNING
- Refer family members to community cardiopulmonary resuscitation classes.

RESOURCES
Organizations
Mayo Clinic: *www.mayoclinic.com*
National Heart, Lung, and Blood Institute: *www.nhlbi.nih.gov*

Selected references
Graham-Cryan, M.A., et al. "Obstructive Hypertrophic Cardiomyopathy," *Progress in Cardiovascular Nursing* 19(4):133-40, Fall 2004.

Ivens, E. "Hypertrophic Cardiomyopathy," *Heart, Lung and Circulation* 13(Suppl 3):S48-55, 2004.

Kasper, D.L., et al., eds. *Harrison's Principles of Internal Medicine,* 16th ed. New York: McGraw-Hill Book Co., 2005.

The Merck Manual of Diagnosis & Therapy, 18th ed. Whitehouse Station, N.J.: Merck & Co., Inc., 2006.

Professional Guide to Diseases, 8th ed. Philadelphia: Lippincott Williams & Wilkins, 2005.

Steinbis, S. "Hypertrophic Obstructive Cardiomyopathy and Septal Ablation," *Critical Care Nurse* 23(3):47-50, June 2003.

Cardiomyopathy, restrictive

OVERVIEW

- Disease of the heart muscle fibers that results in restrictive filling and reduced diastolic volume of either one or both ventricles
- Irreversible if severe

PATHOPHYSIOLOGY

- Stiffness of the ventricle is caused by left ventricular hypertrophy and endocardial fibrosis and thickening, thus reducing the ventricle's ability to relax and fill during diastole.
- Failure of the rigid myocardium to contract completely during systole causes decreased cardiac output. (See *Understanding restrictive cardiomyopathy*.)

CAUSES

- Carcinoid heart disease
- Heart transplant
- Idiopathic or associated with other disease (for example, amyloidosis or endomyocardial fibrosis)
- Mediastinal radiation

INCIDENCE

- Rare; accounts for 5% of all cases of primary heart disease
- Occurs equally in men and women

COMPLICATIONS

- Heart failure
- Arrhythmias
- Systemic or pulmonary embolization
- Sudden death

ASSESSMENT

HISTORY

- Fatigue
- Viral infection
- Dyspnea
- Chest pain

PHYSICAL FINDINGS

- Peripheral edema
- Liver engorgement
- Peripheral cyanosis
- Pallor
- S_3 or S_4 gallop rhythms (due to heart failure)
- Systolic murmurs

⚡ **WARNING** *Restricted cardiomyopathy may need to be differentiated from other types of cardiomyopathy. (See* Assessment findings in cardiomyopathies, *page 155.)*

DIAGNOSTIC TEST RESULTS

LABORATORY

- Complete blood count reveals eosinophilia.

IMAGING

- Chest X-ray may reveal cardiomegaly.
- Echocardiography may reveal left ventricular muscle mass, normal or reduced left ventricular cavity size, and decreased systolic function.

DIAGNOSTIC PROCEDURES

- Electrocardiography may reveal low-voltage hypertrophy, atrioventricular conduction defects, and arrhythmias.
- Cardiac catheterization shows reduced systolic function and myocardial infiltration and increased left ventricular end-diastolic pressures.

Understanding restrictive cardiomyopathy

- Decreased ventricular chamber size
- Left ventricular hypertrophy
- Increased atrial chamber size
- Normal myocardial mass
- Increased ventricular inflow resistance
- Decreased contractility

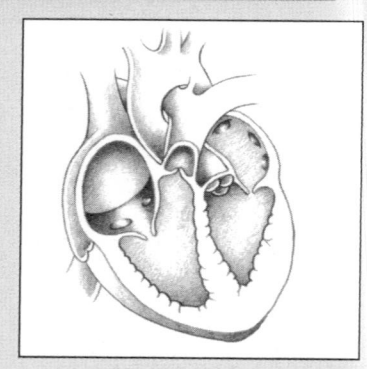

TREATMENT

GENERAL
- Treatment of underlying cause

DIET
- Low-sodium

ACTIVITY
- Initially, bed rest, then as tolerated

MEDICATIONS
- Digoxin (Lanoxin)
- Diuretics
- Vasodilators
- Angiotensin-converting enzyme inhibitors
- Anticoagulants
- Corticosteroids

SURGERY
- Permanent pacemaker
- Heart transplantation

NURSING CONSIDERATIONS

NURSING DIAGNOSES
- Activity intolerance
- Acute pain
- Decreased cardiac output
- Fatigue
- Impaired gas exchange
- Ineffective coping
- Ineffective tissue perfusion: Cardiopulmonary

EXPECTED OUTCOMES
The patient will:
- carry out activities of daily living without excess fatigue or decreased energy
- express feelings of comfort and decreased pain
- maintain adequate cardiac output and hemodynamic stability
- express feelings of energy and decreased fatigue
- maintain adequate ventilation and oxygenation
- demonstrate adaptive coping behaviors
- maintain adequate cardiopulmonary perfusion.

NURSING INTERVENTIONS
- Give prescribed drugs.
- Provide psychological support.
- Provide appropriate diversionary activities for the patient restricted to prolonged bed rest.

MONITORING
- Heart rhythm and rate
- Vital signs
- Intake and output
- Pulmonary artery pressure
- Daily weight

PATIENT TEACHING

GENERAL
Be sure to cover:
- signs of digoxin toxicity
- importance of recording daily weight and reporting weight gain of 2 lb (0.9 kg) or more
- dietary restrictions.

DISCHARGE PLANNING
- Refer for psychosocial counseling, as necessary, for assistance in coping with restricted lifestyle.

RESOURCES
Organizations
Mayo Clinic: *www.mayoclinic.com*
National Heart, Lung, and Blood Institute: *www.nhlbi.nih.gov*

Selected references
Kasper, D.L., et al., eds. *Harrison's Principles of Internal Medicine,* 16th ed. New York: McGraw-Hill Book Co., 2005.
The Merck Manual of Diagnosis & Therapy, 18th ed. Whitehouse Station, N.J.: Merck & Co., Inc., 2006.
Professional Guide to Diseases, 8th ed. Philadelphia: Lippincott Williams & Wilkins, 2005.
Russo, L.M., and Webber, S.A. "Idiopathic Restrictive Cardiomyopathy in Children," *Heart* 91(9):1199-202, September 2005.

Carpal tunnel syndrome

- Compression of the median nerve in the wrist
- Most common nerve entrapment syndrome
- May pose a serious occupational health problem

PATHOPHYSIOLOGY

- Space-occupying lesion or direct pressure within the carpal canal increases pressure on the median nerve, resulting in compression.
- Compression of the median nerve interrupts normal function. (See *The carpal tunnel.*)

CAUSES

- Exact cause unknown
- Acute sprain that may damage the median nerve
- Amyloidosis
- Dislocation
- Edema-producing conditions
- Gout
- Repetitive wrist motions involving excessive flexion or extension
- Tumors

RISK FACTORS

- Diabetes
- Pregnancy
- Alcoholism
- Hypothyroidism
- Renal failure

INCIDENCE

- Carpal tunnel syndrome is most common in women ages 30 to 60.
- This disorder occurs in people who move their wrists continuously.

COMPLICATIONS

- Tendon inflammation
- Compression
- Neural ischemia
- Permanent nerve damage with loss of movement and sensation

The carpal tunnel

The carpal tunnel is clearly visible in this palmar view and cross section of a right hand. Note the median nerve, flexor tendons of fingers, and blood vessels passing through the tunnel on their way from the forearm to the hand.

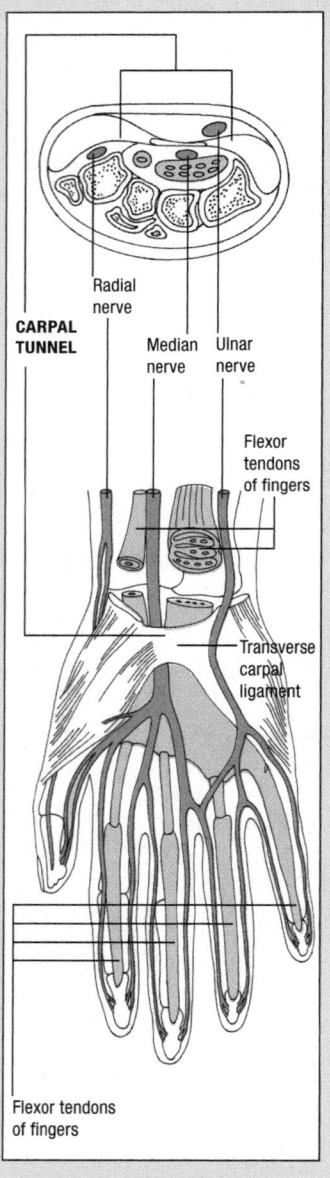

Radial nerve

CARPAL TUNNEL

Median nerve

Ulnar nerve

Flexor tendons of fingers

Transverse carpal ligament

Flexor tendons of fingers

HISTORY

- Occupation or hobby requiring strenuous or repetitive use of the hands
- Condition that causes swelling in carpal tunnel structures
- Weakness, pain, burning, numbness, or tingling that occurs in one or both hands
- Paresthesia that worsens at night and in the morning
- Pain that spreads to the forearm and, in severe cases, as far as the shoulder
- Pain that can be relieved by:
- shaking hands vigorously
- dangling the arms at sides

PHYSICAL FINDINGS

- Inability to make a fist
- Fingernails may be atrophied, with surrounding dry, shiny skin

DIAGNOSTIC TEST RESULTS

DIAGNOSTIC PROCEDURES
- Electromyography shows a median nerve motor conduction delay of more than 5 msec.
- Digital electrical stimulation shows median nerve compression by measuring the length and intensity of stimulation from the fingers to the median nerve in the wrist.

OTHER
- Compression test result supports the diagnosis.

TREATMENT

GENERAL
- Initially conservative:
- – Splinting the wrist for 1 to 2 weeks
- – Possibly changing occupation
- – Correcting any underlying disorder

ACTIVITY
- As tolerated

MEDICATIONS
- Nonsteroidal anti-inflammatory drugs (NSAIDs)
- Corticosteroids
- Vitamin B complex

SURGERY
- Decompression of the nerve
- Neurolysis

NURSING CONSIDERATIONS

NURSING DIAGNOSES
- Anxiety
- Bathing or hygiene self-care deficit
- Chronic pain
- Impaired physical mobility
- Ineffective role performance

EXPECTED OUTCOMES
The patient will:
- express reduced levels of anxiety
- perform activities of daily living within the confines of the disease process
- express feelings of increased comfort and pain relief
- maintain joint mobility and range of motion
- continue to function in usual roles as much as possible.

NURSING INTERVENTIONS
- Promote self-care.
- Give prescribed analgesics.

MONITORING
- Response to analgesia
- After surgery, vital signs
- Color, sensation, and motion of the affected hand

PATIENT TEACHING

GENERAL
Be sure to cover:
- splint application
- hand exercises in warm water
- the prescribed medication regimen
- adverse reactions to drugs
- avoidance of NSAIDs during pregnancy.

DISCHARGE PLANNING
- Refer the patient for occupational counseling if a job change is necessary.

RESOURCES
Organizations
National Institutes of Health: *www.nih.gov*
The Paget Foundation: *www.paget.org*
WebMD: *www.webmd.com*

Selected references
Caliandro, P., et al. "Distribution of Paresthesias in Carpal Tunnel Syndrome Reflects the Degree of Nerve Damage at Wrist," *Clinical Neurophysiology* 117(1):228-31 January 2006.
Diseases, 4th ed. Philadelphia: Lippincott Williams & Wilkins, 2006.
Handbook of Pathophysiology, 2nd ed. Philadelphia: Lippincott Williams & Wilkins, 2005.
Hopp, P.T., et al. "Carpal Tunnel Syndrome — The Role of Psychosocial Factors in Recovery," *AAOHN Journal* 52(11):458-60, November 2004.

Cataract

- Opacity of the lens or lens capsule of the eye
- Common cause of gradual vision loss
- Commonly affects both eyes
- Traumatic cataracts usually unilateral

PATHOPHYSIOLOGY

- The clouded lens blocks light shining through the cornea.
- Images cast onto the retina are blurred.
- A hazy image is interpreted by the brain.

CAUSES

- Classified according to cause

Senile cataracts

- Chemical changes in lens proteins in elderly patients

Congenital cataracts

- Congenital anomaly
- Genetic causes (usually autosomal dominant)
- Inborn errors of metabolism
- Maternal rubella infection during the first trimester
- Recessive cataracts may be sex linked

Traumatic cataracts

- Foreign bodies causing aqueous or vitreous humor to enter lens capsule

Complicated cataracts

- Atopic dermatitis
- Diabetes
- Glaucoma
- Hypoparathyroidism
- Ionizing radiation or infrared rays
- Retinal detachment
- Retinitis pigmentosa
- Uveitis

TOXIC CATARACTS

- Drug or chemical toxicity:
- dinitrophenol
- ergot
- naphthalene
- phenothiazines

INCIDENCE

- Cataracts are most prevalent in people older than age 70.

COMPLICATIONS

- Complete vision loss

Possible complications of surgery

- Loss of vitreous
- Wound dehiscence
- Hyphema
- Pupillary block glaucoma
- Retinal detachment
- Infection

ASSESSMENT

HISTORY

- Painless, gradual vision loss
- Blinding glare from headlights with night driving
- Poor reading vision
- Annoying glare
- Poor vision in bright sunlight
- Better vision in dim light than in bright light (central opacity)

PHYSICAL FINDINGS

- Milky white pupil on inspection with a penlight
- Grayish white area behind the pupil (advanced cataract)
- Red reflex lost (mature cataract)

DIAGNOSTIC TEST RESULTS

DIAGNOSTIC PROCEDURES

- Indirect ophthalmoscopy reveals a dark area in the normally homogeneous red reflex.
- Slit-lamp examination confirms lens opacity.
- Visual acuity test result establishes the degree of vision loss.

TREATMENT

GENERAL

- Before surgery, eyeglasses and contact lenses that may help to improve vision
- Sunglasses in bright light and lamps that provide reflected lighting rather than direct lighting, decreasing glare and aiding vision

ACTIVITY

- Restricted according to vision loss

MEDICATIONS

For cataract removal

- Nonsteroidal anti-inflammatory drugs
- Short-acting local anesthetic

SURGERY

- Lens extraction and implantation of intraocular lens (see *Comparing methods of cataract removal*)
- Extracapsular cataract extraction
- Intracapsular cataract extraction
- Phacoemulsification

NURSING DIAGNOSES
◆ Anxiety
◆ Disturbed sensory perception: Visual
◆ Risk for infection
◆ Risk for injury

EXPECTED OUTCOMES
The patient will:
◆ use support systems to assist with anxiety and fear
◆ regain normal visual functioning
◆ show no signs or symptoms of infection
◆ sustain no harm or injury.

NURSING INTERVENTIONS
◆ Perform routine postoperative care.
◆ Assist with early ambulation.
◆ Apply an eye shield or eye patch postoperatively as ordered.

MONITORING
◆ Vital signs
◆ Visual acuity
◆ Complications of surgery

GENERAL
Be sure to cover:
◆ the need to avoid activities that increase intraocular pressure, such as straining with coughing, bowel movements, or lifting
◆ the need to abstain from sexual intercourse until the patient receives practitioner's approval
◆ proper instillation of ophthalmic ointment or drops.

⚡ **WARNING** *If the patient has increased eye discharge, sharp eye pain that's unrelieved by analgesics, or deterioration in vision, instruct him to notify his practitioner immediately.*

RESOURCES
Organizations
American Academy of Ophthalmology: *www.aao.org*
National Eye Institute: *www.nei.nih.gov*

Selected references
Gallacher, R. "Understanding the Nursing Role in Patients Who Have Cataracts," *Nursing Times* 100(21):31, May 2004.
Houde, S.C., and Hugg, M.H. "Age-Related Vision Loss in Older Adults. A Challenge for Gerontological Nurses," *Journal of Gerontological Nursing* 29(4):25-33, April 2003.
Marsden, J. "Cataract: The Role of Nurses in Diagnosis, Surgery and Aftercare," *Nursing Times* 100(7):36-40, February 2004.
Robman, L., and Taylor, H. "External Factors in the Development of Cataracts," *Eye* 19(10):1074-1082, October 2005.

Comparing methods of cataract removal

Cataracts can be removed by intracapsular or extracapsular techniques.

INTRACAPSULAR CATARACT EXTRACTION
In this technique, the surgeon makes a partial incision at the superior limbus arc. He then removes the lens using specially designed forceps or a cryoprobe, which freezes and adheres to the lens to facilitate its removal.

EXTRACAPSULAR CATARACT EXTRACTION
In this technique, the surgeon may use irrigation and aspiration or phacoemulsification. In the former approach, the surgeon makes an incision at the limbus, opens the anterior lens capsule with a cystotome, and exerts pressure from below to express the lens. He then irrigates and suctions the remaining lens cortex.

In phacoemulsification, he uses an ultrasonic probe to break the lens into minute particles, which are aspirated by the probe.

Cryoprobe
Lens
Cornea

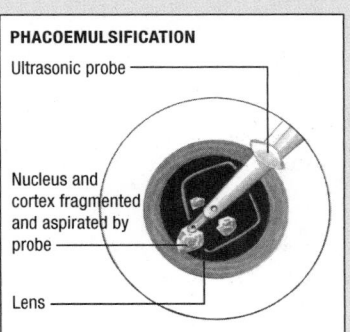

IRRIGATION AND ASPIRATION
Cystotome
Cortical and nuclear cataract material aspirated through needle
Lens

PHACOEMULSIFICATION
Ultrasonic probe
Nucleus and cortex fragmented and aspirated by probe
Lens

Cellulitis

OVERVIEW

- Acute infection of the dermis and subcutaneous tissue causing inflammation of the cells
- May follow damage to the skin, such as a bite or wound
- Prognosis usually good with timely treatment
- With other comorbidities such as diabetes, increased risk of developing or spreading cellulitis

PATHOPHYSIOLOGY

- A break in skin integrity almost always precedes infection.
- As the offending organism invades the compromised area, it overwhelms the defensive cells, including the neutrophils, eosinophils, basophils, and mast cells, that normally contain and localize the inflammation.
- As cellulitis progresses, the organism invades tissue around the initial wound site.

CAUSES

- Bacterial infections, usually by *Staphylococcus aureus* and group A beta-hemolytic streptococci
- Extension of a skin wound or ulcer
- Fungal infections
- Furuncles or carbuncles

RISK FACTORS

- Venous and lymphatic compromise
- Edema
- Diabetes mellitus
- Underlying skin lesion
- Prior trauma

INCIDENCE

- Cellulitis occurs most commonly in the lower extremities.
- The disease affects males and females equally.

  AGE FACTOR *Perianal cellulitis occurs more commonly in children, especially boys.*

COMPLICATIONS

- Sepsis
- Deep vein thrombosis (DVT)
- Progression of cellulitis
- Local abscesses
- Thrombophlebitis
- Lymphangitis
- Amputation

  AGE FACTOR *Cellulitis of the lower extremity is more likely to develop into thrombophlebitis in an elderly patient.*

ASSESSMENT

HISTORY

- Presence of one or more risk factors
- Tenderness
- Pain at the site and possibly surrounding area
- Erythema and warmth
- Edema
- Possible fever, chills, malaise

PHYSICAL FINDINGS

- Erythema with indistinct margins
- Fever
- Warmth and tenderness of the skin
- Regional lymph node enlargement and tenderness
- Red streaking visible in skin proximal to area of cellulitis

DIAGNOSTIC TEST RESULTS

LABORATORY

- White blood cell count may show mild leukocytosis.
- Erythrocyte sedimentation rate may show mild elevation.
- Culture and Gram stain may show the causative organism.

TREATMENT

GENERAL
- Immobilization and elevation of the affected extremity
- Moist heat

DIET
- Well-balanced

ACTIVITY
- Possible bed rest in severe infection

MEDICATIONS
- Antibiotics
- Topical antifungals
- Analgesics

SURGERY
- Possible tracheostomy in severe cellulitis of head and neck
- Possible abscess drainage
- Amputation (with gas-forming cellulitis [gangrene])

NURSING CONSIDERATIONS

NURSING DIAGNOSES
- Acute pain
- Fear
- Ineffective health maintenance
- Risk for infection
- Risk for injury

EXPECTED OUTCOMES
The patient will:
- express feelings of increased comfort
- verbalize feelings and concerns
- maintain current health status
- remain free from signs and symptoms of infection
- avoid injury.

NURSING INTERVENTIONS
- Give prescribed drugs.
- Elevate affected extremity.
- Apply moist heat, as ordered.
- Encourage a well-balanced diet.
- Encourage adequate fluid intake.
- Encourage verbalization of feelings and concerns.
- Institute safety precautions.

MONITORING
- Vital signs
- Pain control
- Edema
- Laboratory results
- Signs and symptoms of infection
- Complications
- Cellulitis progression

PATIENT TEACHING

GENERAL
Be sure to cover:
- the disorder, diagnosis, and treatment
- medications and possible adverse reactions
- when to notify the practitioner
- use of warm compresses
- signs and symptoms of infection
- prevention of injury and trauma
- infection control
- signs and symptoms of DVT.

DISCHARGE PLANNING
- Refer the patient for management of diabetes mellitus, if indicated.

RESOURCES
Organizations
American Academy of Dermatology: *www.aad.org*
American Diabetes Association: *www.diabetes.org*
Dermatology Foundation: *www.dermfnd.org*

Selected references
Barza, M. "Noninfectious Causes of Cellulitis," *Annals of Internal Medicine* 143(8):614, October 2005.
Donald, M., et al. "Emergency Department Management of Home Intravenous Antibiotic Therapy for Cellulitis," *Emergency Medicine Journal* 22(10):715-17, October 2005.
Williams, J.R., and Luggen, A.S. "Gerontologic Nurse Practitioner Care Guidelines: Cellulitis in the Elderly Person," *Geriatric Nursing* 25(6):373-74, November-December 2004.

Cerebral contusion

- Ecchymosis of brain tissue that results from injury to the head

PATHOPHYSIOLOGY
- Trauma to the head causes tearing or twisting of the structures and blood vessels of the brain.
- Scattered hemorrhages form over the surface.
- Functional disruption occurs and may be prolonged.

CAUSES
- Acceleration-deceleration or coup-contrecoup injuries
- Falls
- Gun-shot wounds
- Head trauma
- Motor vehicle collisions
- Stab wounds

RISK FACTORS
- Unsteady gait
- Participation in contact sports
- Receiving anticoagulant therapy

INCIDENCE
- Cerebral contusion may occur at any age.

COMPLICATIONS
- Intracranial hemorrhage
- Hematoma
- Tentorial herniation
- Respiratory failure
- Seizures
- Neurologic deficits
- Brain hemorrhage
- Increased intracranial pressure (see *What happens with increased ICP*)

ASSESSMENT

HISTORY
- Head injury or motor vehicle accident
- Loss of consciousness

PHYSICAL FINDINGS
- Unconscious patient: pale and motionless; altered vital signs
- Conscious patient: drowsy or easily disturbed
- Scalp wound
- Possible involuntary evacuation of bowel and bladder
- Hemiparesis
- Personality changes

DIAGNOSTIC TEST RESULTS

IMAGING
- Computed tomography scan shows areas of damage.
- Magnetic resonance imaging shows areas of damage.
- Electroencephalography helps confirm diagnosis.
- Cerebral angiography helps confirm diagnosis.

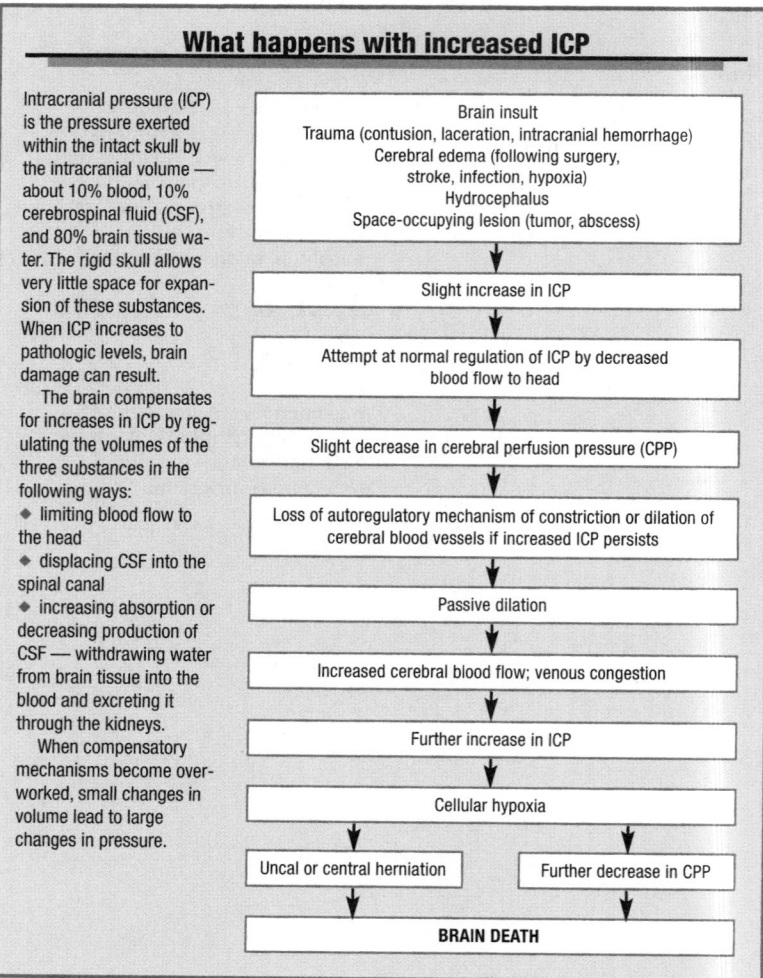

What happens with increased ICP

Intracranial pressure (ICP) is the pressure exerted within the intact skull by the intracranial volume — about 10% blood, 10% cerebrospinal fluid (CSF), and 80% brain tissue water. The rigid skull allows very little space for expansion of these substances. When ICP increases to pathologic levels, brain damage can result.

The brain compensates for increases in ICP by regulating the volumes of the three substances in the following ways:
- limiting blood flow to the head
- displacing CSF into the spinal canal
- increasing absorption or decreasing production of CSF — withdrawing water from brain tissue into the blood and excreting it through the kidneys.

When compensatory mechanisms become overworked, small changes in volume lead to large changes in pressure.

Brain insult
Trauma (contusion, laceration, intracranial hemorrhage)
Cerebral edema (following surgery, stroke, infection, hypoxia)
Hydrocephalus
Space-occupying lesion (tumor, abscess)
↓
Slight increase in ICP
↓
Attempt at normal regulation of ICP by decreased blood flow to head
↓
Slight decrease in cerebral perfusion pressure (CPP)
↓
Loss of autoregulatory mechanism of constriction or dilation of cerebral blood vessels if increased ICP persists
↓
Passive dilation
↓
Increased cerebral blood flow; venous congestion
↓
Further increase in ICP
↓
Cellular hypoxia
↓
Uncal or central herniation   Further decrease in CPP
↓
BRAIN DEATH

TREATMENT

GENERAL
- Establishment of a patent airway
- Administration of I.V. fluids
- Minimization of environmental stimuli

DIET
- Nothing by mouth until fully conscious

ACTIVITY
- Based on neurologic status
- Initially, bed rest, with proper positioning with head of bed raised to promote drainage
- Avoidance of contact sports

MEDICATIONS
- Nonopioid analgesics
- Anticonvulsants
- Antibiotics
- Corticosteroids

SURGERY
- Craniotomy
- Suturing

NURSING CONSIDERATIONS

NURSING DIAGNOSES
- Acute pain
- Anxiety
- Decreased intracranial adaptive capacity
- Disturbed sensory perception: Kinesthetic, tactile
- Impaired verbal communication
- Ineffective coping
- Risk for deficient fluid volume
- Risk for infection
- Risk for injury
- Risk for posttrauma syndrome

EXPECTED OUTCOMES
The patient will:
- express feelings of comfort and pain relief
- identify measures to reduce anxiety
- maintain a stable neurologic state
- maintain optimal functioning within the limits of the kinesthetic and tactile impairment
- use language or an alternative form of communication to communicate needs
- use support systems to assist with coping
- maintain adequate fluid volume
- remain free from signs and symptoms of infection
- remain free from injury
- express feelings and fears about the traumatic event.

NURSING INTERVENTIONS
- Perform neurologic examinations.
- Maintain a patent airway.
- Give prescribed drugs (no aspirin).
- Protect from injury.

MONITORING
- Vital signs (awaken patient every 2 hours during first 24 hours)
- Neurologic status
- Check for cerebrospinal fluid (CSF) leakage

PATIENT TEACHING

Be sure to cover:
- the need to avoid coughing, sneezing, or blowing the nose until after recovery
- observation for CSF drainage
- how to detect and report mental status changes
- importance of avoiding smoking and alcohol
- signs and symptoms of infection.

DISCHARGE PLANNING
- Refer the patient to a neurologist for follow-up, as indicated.
- Refer the patient to a social worker for further support and counseling, as needed.

RESOURCES
Organizations
American Academy of Neurology: *www.aan.com*
Brain Injury Society: *www.bisociety.org*
Head Injury Hotline: *www.headinjury.com*
Med Help International: *www.medhelp.org*

Selected references
Ahmed Bouderka, M., et al. "Early Tracheostomy versus Prolonged Endotracheal Intubation in Severe Head Injury," *Journal of Trauma-Injury Infection & Critical Care* 57(2):251-54, August 2004.

Canobbio, M. *Mosby's Handbook of Patient Teaching*, 3rd ed. St. Louis: Mosby–Year Book, Inc., 2006.

Nolan, S. "Traumatic Brain Injury: A Review," *Critical Care Nursing Quarterly* 28(2):188-94, April-June 2005.

Zink, E.K., et al. "Managing Traumatic Brain Injury," *Nursing2006* 35(9):36-43, September 2005.

Cerebral palsy

- Most common crippling neuromuscular disease in children
- Comprises several neuromuscular disorders
- Results from prenatal, perinatal, or postnatal central nervous system (CNS) damage
- Three types (sometimes occur in mixed forms):
- spastic (affecting about 70% of children with cerebral palsy)
- athetoid (affecting about 20%)
- ataxic (affecting about 10%)
- Motor impairment may be minimal or severely disabling
- Associated defects:
- seizures
- speech disorders
- mental retardation
- Prognosis varies

PATHOPHYSIOLOGY
- A lesion or an abnormality occurs in the early stages of brain development.
- Structural and functional defects occur, impairing motor or cognitive function.
- Defects may not be distinguishable until months after birth.

CAUSES
- Conditions that result in cerebral anoxia, hemorrhage, or other CNS damage

Prenatal causes
- Abnormal placental attachment
- ABO blood type incompatibility
- Anoxia
- Irradiation
- Isoimmunization
- Malnutrition
- Maternal diabetes
- Maternal infection (especially rubella in the first trimester)
- Rh factor incompatibility
- Rubella
- Toxemia

Parturition causes
- Asphyxia from the cord wrapping around the neck
- Depressed maternal vital signs from general or spinal anesthesia
- Multiple births (neonates born last in a multiple birth have an especially high rate of cerebral palsy)
- Prematurity
- Prolonged or unusually rapid labor
- Trauma during delivery

Postnatal causes
- Any condition resulting in cerebral thrombus or embolus
- Head trauma
- Infections, such as meningitis and encephalitis
- Poisoning

INCIDENCE
- Incidence of cerebral palsy is highest in premature neonates and in those who are small for gestational age.
- This disorder is slightly more common in boys than in girls.
- Cerebral palsy is more common in whites.

COMPLICATIONS
- Seizure disorders
- Speech, vision, and hearing problems
- Language and perceptual deficits
- Mental retardation (in up to 40% of patients)
- Dental problems
- Respiratory difficulties
- Poor swallowing and gag reflexes

HISTORY
- Maternal or patient history to reveal possible cause (see *When to suspect cerebral palsy*)

PHYSICAL FINDINGS
- Child with retarded growth and development
- Difficulty chewing and swallowing

Spastic cerebral palsy
- Underdevelopment of affected limbs
- Characteristic scissors gait
- Walks on toes
- Crosses one foot in front of the other
- Hyperactive deep tendon reflexes
- Increased stretch reflexes
- Rapid alternating muscle contraction and relaxation
- Muscle weakness
- Impaired fine and gross motor skills
- Contractures in response to manipulation of muscles

Athetoid cerebral palsy
- Involuntary movements
- Grimacing
- Wormlike writhing
- Dystonia
- Sharp jerks that impair voluntary movement
- Involuntary facial movements (speech difficult)
- Drooling

Ataxic cerebral palsy
- Lack of leg movement during infancy
- Wide gait when child begins to walk
- Disturbed balance

When to suspect cerebral palsy

Early detection of cerebral palsy is essential for effective treatment and requires careful clinical observation during infancy and precise neurologic assessment. Suspect cerebral palsy whenever a neonate:

- has difficulty sucking or keeping the nipple or food in his mouth
- seldom moves voluntarily or has arm or leg tremors with voluntary movement
- crosses his legs when lifted from behind rather than pulling them up or bicycling like a normal neonate
- has legs that are hard to separate, making diaper changing difficult
- persistently uses only one hand or, as he gets older, uses his hands well but not his legs.

- Incoordination (especially of the arms)
- Hypoactive reflexes
- Nystagmus
- Muscle weakness
- Tremors

DIAGNOSTIC TEST RESULTS

IMAGING
- Computed tomography scan and magnetic resonance imaging of the brain may show structural abnormalities of the brain such as cerebral atrophy.
- Electroencephalography may show the source of seizure activity.

TREATMENT

GENERAL
- Braces or splints
- Special appliances, such as adapted eating utensils and low toilet seat with arms
- Range-of-motion (ROM) exercises
- Mechanical aids

ACTIVITY
- Prescribed exercises to maintain muscle tone

MEDICATIONS
- Anticonvulsants
- Muscle relaxants
- Antianxiety agents

SURGERY
- Orthopedic surgery
- Neurosurgery

NURSING CONSIDERATIONS

NURSING DIAGNOSES
- Chronic low self-esteem
- Compromised family coping
- Delayed growth and development
- Disturbed body image
- Disturbed sensory perception (visual, auditory)
- Imbalanced nutrition: Less than body requirements
- Impaired physical mobility
- Impaired swallowing
- Interrupted family processes
- Risk for impaired parenting
- Risk for impaired skin integrity

EXPECTED OUTCOMES
The patient (or his family) will:
- verbalize feelings related to self-esteem
- develop adequate coping mechanisms
- achieve age-appropriate growth, behaviors, and skills to the fullest extent possible
- express positive feelings about self
- maintain optimal functioning within the limits of the visual or hearing impairment
- consume adequate daily calories as required
- maintain joint mobility and ROM
- swallow without pain or aspiration
- discuss how the patient's condition has affected his family's daily life
- (parents) will identify realistic goals according to the abilities of the child
- have skin that shows no signs of breakdown.

NURSING INTERVENTIONS
- Speak slowly and distinctly.
- Give all care in an unhurried manner.
- Allow participation in care decisions.
- Provide a diet with adequate calories. Stroking the throat may aid swallowing.
- Provide frequent mouth and dental care.
- Provide skin care.
- Perform prescribed exercises to maintain muscle tone.
- Care for associated hearing and vision disturbances, as necessary.
- Postoperatively, give analgesics, as ordered.
- Provide a safe physical environment.

MONITORING
- Pain relief
- Seizure activity
- Speech
- Visual and auditory acuity
- Respiratory status
- Swallowing function
- Reflexes
- Nutritional status
- Skin integrity
- Motor development
- Muscle strength

PATIENT TEACHING

GENERAL
Be sure to cover:
- prescribed medication regimen
- adverse drug reactions
- daily skin inspection and daily massage
- need to place food far back in patient's mouth to facilitate swallowing
- need to chew food thoroughly
- drinking through a straw
- sucking lollipops to develop muscle control
- proper nutrition
- opportunities for learning, such as summer camps or Special Olympics
- correct use of assistive devices.

DISCHARGE PLANNING
- Refer family members to community support groups such as the local chapter of the United Cerebral Palsy Association.

RESOURCES
Organizations
The American Academy of Pediatrics: *www.aap.org*
National Institutes of Health: *www.nih.gov*
United Cerebral Palsy Association: *www.ucpa.org*

Selected references
Handbook of Pathophysiology, 2nd ed. Philadelphia: Lippincott Williams & Wilkins, 2005.
Livinec, F., et al. "Prenatal Risk Factors for Cerebral Palsy in Very Preterm Singletons and Twins," *Obstetrics and Gynecology* 105(6):1341-347, June 2005.
McKearnan, K.A., et al. "Pain in Children with Cerebral Palsy: A Review," *Journal of Neuroscience Nursing* 36(5):252-59, October 2004.
Professional Guide to Diseases, 8th ed. Philadelphia: Lippincott Williams & Wilkins, 2005.

Cervical cancer

OVERVIEW

- Proliferation of cancer cells in the cervix
- Third most common cancer of the female reproductive system
- Classified as either preinvasive (curable in 75% to 90% of patients with early detection and proper treatment) or invasive

PATHOPHYSIOLOGY

Preinvasive cancer

- Preinvasive cancer ranges from minimal cervical dysplasia, in which the lower third of the epithelium contains abnormal cells, to carcinoma in situ, in which the full thickness of epithelium contains abnormally proliferating cells.

Invasive cancer

- Cancer cells penetrate the basement membrane and can spread directly to contiguous pelvic structures or disseminate to distant sites by way of lymphatic routes.
- Most (95%) cases are squamous cell carcinoma; 5% of cases are adenocarcinomas.

CAUSES

- Exact cause unknown

RISK FACTORS

- Frequent intercourse at a young age (under age 16)
- Multiple sexual partners
- Multiple pregnancies
- Human papillomavirus (HPV)
- Bacterial or viral venereal infections
- Exposure to diethylstilbestrol in utero
- Human immunodeficiency virus
- Smoking

INCIDENCE

- Cervical cancer typically occurs between ages 30 and 45; rarely, before age 20.

COMPLICATIONS

- Renal failure
- Distant metastasis
- Vaginal stenosis
- Ureterovaginal or vesicovaginal fistula
- Proctitis
- Cystitis
- Bowel obstruction

ASSESSMENT

HISTORY

- One or more risk factors present

Preinvasive cancer

- No symptoms or other clinical changes

Invasive cancer

- Abnormal vaginal bleeding or discharge
- Gradually increasing flank pain

PHYSICAL FINDINGS

- Vaginal discharge (may be thin and watery or bloody)
- Postcoital bleeding
- Irregular bleeding

DIAGNOSTIC TEST RESULTS

IMAGING

- Lymphangiography can show metastasis.
- Cystography can show metastasis.
- Organ and bone scans can show metastasis.

DIAGNOSTIC PROCEDURES

- Conventional or ThinPrep Papanicolaou (Pap) tests show abnormal cells, and colposcopy shows the source of the abnormal cells seen on the Pap test. (See *Testing for cervical cancer.*)
- Cone or punch biopsy is performed if endocervical curettage is positive.
- Vira Pap test (investigational) permits examination of the specimen's deoxyribonucleic acid structure to detect HPV.

TREATMENT

GENERAL

- Accurate clinical staging used to determine type of treatment (see *Staging cervical cancer*)

DIET

- Well-balanced, as tolerated

MEDICATIONS

- Multidrug chemotherapy regimens

Testing for cervical cancer

To analyze cervical cells, the ThinPrep may be collected in the same manner as a conventional Papanicolaou (Pap) test using a cytobrush and plastic spatula. The specimens are deposited in a bottle provided with a fixative and sent to the laboratory. A filter is then inserted into the bottle and excess mucus, blood, and inflammatory cells are filtered out by centrifuge. Remaining cells are then placed on a slide in a uniform, thin layer and read as a Pap test. This causes fewer slides to be classified as unreadable, significantly reducing the incidence of false-negatives and the need for repeat tests.

When the ThinPrep test is used, screening can also be easily done for the human papillomavirus (HPV), of which certain strains have been identified as the primary cause of cervical cancer. The Digene hc2 HPV deoxyribonucleic acid (DNA) test has been approved by the Food and Drug Administration to determine if those identified as high risk for developing cervical cancer have been exposed to HPV. The specimen is collected as a Pap smear but is dispersed with ThinPrep solution. Separate aliquots are used for each test, from brushings of the endocervix.

If a patient is positive for HPV, it means she has been infected with the virus. Depending on the type of HPV found through DNA testing, those harboring high-risk HPV strains have a high risk of developing cervical cancer. These patients should have a colposcopy in which the cervix is viewed under microscope and a biopsy taken from the tissue sample.

Staging cervical cancer

Treatment decisions depend on accurate staging. The International Federation of Gynecology and Obstetrics defines the following cervical cancer stages.

STAGE 0
Carcinoma in situ, intraepithelial carcinoma

STAGE I
Cancer confined to the cervix (extension to the corpus should be disregarded)
Stage IA Preclinical malignant lesions of the cervix (diagnosed only microscopically)
Stage IA1 Minimal microscopically evident stromal invasion measuring less than 3 mm deep and 7 mm wide
Stage IA2 Lesions detected microscopically, measuring 3 to 5 mm from the base of the epithelium, either surface or glandular, from which it originates; lesion width shouldn't exceed 7 mm
Stage IB Lesions measuring more than 5 mm deep and 7 mm wide, whether seen clinically or not (preformed space involvement shouldn't alter the staging but should be recorded for future treatment decisions)
Stage IB1 Visible lesions measuring less than 4 cm
Stage IB2 Visible lesions measuring more than 4 cm

STAGE II
Extension beyond the cervix but not to the pelvic wall
Stage IIA Involves the vagina but hasn't spread to the lower third
Stage IIB Obvious parametrial involvement

STAGE III
Extension to the pelvic wall; on rectal examination, no cancer-free space between the tumor and the pelvic wall; involves the lower third of the vagina; may block the ureters
Stage IIIA No extension to the pelvic wall
Stage IIIB Extension to the pelvic wall and blocked ureters

STAGE IV
Extension beyond the true pelvis or involvement of the bladder or the rectal mucosa
Stage IVA Spread to adjacent organs
Stage IVB Spread to distant organs

SURGERY
Preinvasive lesions
- Total excisional biopsy
- Cryosurgery
- Laser destruction
- Conization, with frequent Pap test follow-ups
- Hysterectomy (rare)
- Radical trachelectomy

Invasive squamous cell carcinoma
- Radical hysterectomy and radiation therapy (internal, external, or both)
- Pelvic exenteration (rare; may be performed for recurrent cervical cancer)

NURSING CONSIDERATIONS

NURSING DIAGNOSES
- Acute pain
- Anxiety
- Fear
- Impaired physical mobility
- Impaired skin integrity
- Ineffective coping
- Ineffective sexuality patterns
- Risk for infection
- Sexual dysfunction

EXPECTED OUTCOMES
The patient will:
- express increased comfort and decreased pain
- report feelings of reduced anxiety
- verbalize concerns and fears related to the diagnosis and condition
- maintain joint mobility and range of motion
- maintain skin integrity
- demonstrate adaptive coping behaviors
- resume normal sexual activity patterns to the fullest extent possible
- remain free from signs or symptoms of infection
- express feelings and perceptions about changes in sexual performance.

NURSING INTERVENTIONS
- Encourage verbalization and provide support.
- Give prescribed drugs.

MONITORING
- Vital signs
- Complications
- Pain control
- Vaginal discharge
- Renal status
- Response to treatment

PATIENT TEACHING

GENERAL
Be sure to cover:
- the disease process, diagnosis, and treatment
- importance of follow-up care
- how treatment won't radically alter the patient's lifestyle or prohibit sexual intimacy
- medication administration, dosage, and possible adverse effects.

DISCHARGE PLANNING
- Refer the patient to resource and support services.

RESOURCES
Organizations
American Cancer Society: *www.cancer.org*
Guide to Internet Resources for Cancer: *www.cancerindex.org*
National Cancer Institute: *www.nci.nih.gov*

Selected references
Atlas of Pathophysiology, 2nd ed. Philadelphia: Lippincott Williams & Wilkins, 2005.
Bertram, C.C. "Evidence for Practice: Oral Contraception and Risk of Cervical Cancer," *Journal of the American Academy of Nurse Practitioners* 16(10):455-61, October 2004.
Hilton, L.W., et al. "The Role of Nursing in Cervical Cancer Prevention and Treatment," *Cancer* 198(Suppl):2070-2074, November 2003.
Schneier, A., and Hertel H. "Surgical and Radiographic Staging in Patients with Cervical Cancer," *Current Opinion in Obstetrics & Gynecology* 16(1):11-18, February 2004.
Suprasert, P., et al. "Radical Hysterectomy for Stage IIB Cervical Cancer: A Review," *International Journal of Gynecological Cancer* 15(6):995-1001, November-December 2005.

Chalazion

OVERVIEW

- Painless, slowly growing nodule on the eyelid
- Common disorder of the sebaceous gland in the eyelid
- May become large enough to press on the eyeball, producing astigmatism
- May be chronic

PATHOPHYSIOLOGY

- A granulomatous inflammation in the upper or lower eyelid is the result of an obstruction of a duct of the meibomian or Zeis sebaceous glands (superficial chalazion).
- Edema is usually contained on the conjunctival portion of the eyelid.

CAUSES

- Chronic blepharitis
- Meibomian cancer
- Rosacea
- Seborrhea

INCIDENCE

- The incidence of chalazion is higher in fair-skinned males than in other groups, possibly because of that group's higher incidence of rosacea and blepharitis.
- This disease is more common between ages 30 and 50.

COMPLICATIONS

- Cosmetic deformity
- Bleeding after surgery
- Infection
- Vision disturbance

ASSESSMENT

HISTORY

- Nodule on eyelid
- Rosacea or blepharitis

PHYSICAL FINDINGS

- Palpable small lump in the eyelid
- Red, elevated area on the conjunctival surface (see *Recognizing chalazion*)

DIAGNOSTIC TEST RESULTS

GENERAL

- Visual examination and palpation of the eyelid reveals presence of chalazion.
- Biopsy rules out meibomian cancer.

TREATMENT

GENERAL

- Warm compresses to the affected eyelid

MEDICATIONS

- Sulfonamide eyedrops
- Steroid injection
- Tetracycline
- Antimicrobial eyedrops after surgical removal

SURGERY

- Incision and curettage under local anesthetic

Recognizing chalazion

A chalazion is a nontender, granulomatous inflammation of a meibomian or Zeis gland on the upper or lower eyelid.

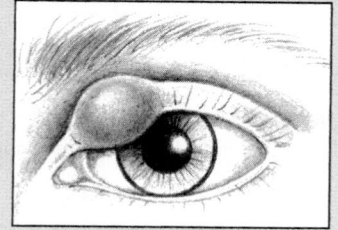

NURSING DIAGNOSES

- Anxiety
- Disturbed body image
- Disturbed sensory perception: Visual
- Ineffective health maintenance
- Risk for injury

EXPECTED OUTCOMES

The patient will:
- express feelings of decreased anxiety
- maintain positive outlook regarding body image
- regain normal visual functioning
- maintain current health status
- avoid injury.

NURSING INTERVENTIONS

- Apply warm compress after surgery.
- Apply eye patch to the affected eye for 24 hours. (See *Applying an eye patch.*)
- Instill eyedrops, as ordered.

MONITORING

- Bleeding (after surgery)
- Signs and symptoms of infection

PATIENT TEACHING

GENERAL

Be sure to cover:
- proper instillation of eyedrops
- signs and symptoms of infection
- reporting recurrence.

  WARNING *Tell the patient to start applying warm compresses at the first sign of lid irritation to increase the blood supply and keep the lumen open.*

DISCHARGE PLANNING

- Encourage follow-up care, as ordered.

RESOURCES
Organizations
American Academy of Ophthalmology: *www.aao.org*
National Eye Institute: *www.nei.nih.gov*

Selected references
Mansour, A.M., et al. "Virus-Induced Chalazion," *Eye* 18(3), March 2004.
Ozdal, P.C., et al. "Accuracy of the Clinical Diagnosis of Chalazion," *Eye* 18(2):135-38, February 2004.
Shiramizu, K.M., et al. "Severe Visual Loss Caused by Ocular Perforation During Chalazion Removal," *American Journal of Ophthalmology* 137(1):204-205, January 2004.

Applying an eye patch

You may apply an eye patch for various reasons: to protect the eye after injury or surgery, to prevent accidental damage to an anesthetized eye, to promote healing, to absorb secretions, to protect the eye from drying when the patient is comatose or unable to close the eye as in Bell's palsy, or to prevent the patient from touching or rubbing his eye.

A thicker patch, called a *pressure patch,* may be used to help corneal abrasions heal, compress postoperative edema, or control hemorrhage from traumatic injury. Application requires an ophthalmologist's prescription and supervision.

To apply a patch, choose a gauze pad of appropriate size for the patient's face, place it gently over the closed eye (as shown), and secure it with two or three strips of tape. Extend the tape from midforehead across the eye to below the earlobe.

A pressure patch, which is markedly thicker than a single-thickness gauze patch, exerts extra tension against the closed eye. After placing the initial gauze pad, build it up with additional gauze pieces. Tape it firmly so that the patch exerts even pressure against the closed eye (as shown).

For increased protection of an injured eye, place a plastic or metal shield (as shown) on top of the gauze pads and apply tape over the shield.

Occasionally, you may use a head dressing to secure a pressure patch. The dressing applies additional pressure or, in burn patients, holds the patch in place without tape.

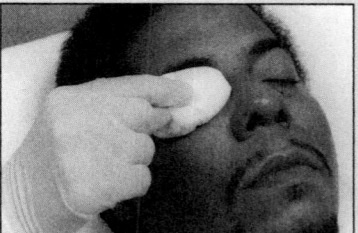

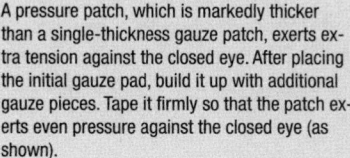

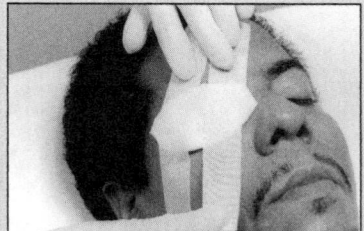

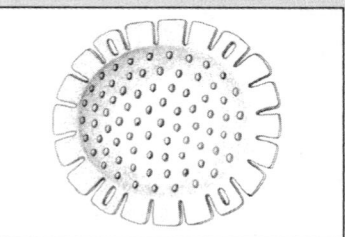

Chancroid

- Sexually transmitted disease
- Characterized by painful genital ulcers and inguinal adenitis
- Common cause of genital ulcers in patients in developing countries

PATHOPHYSIOLOGY

- Organisms are carried from the site of entry through the lymphatics to regional lymph nodes, resulting in node swelling.
- The initial lesion is a papule that ulcerates within 24 hours. (See *Chancroidal lesion.*)
- Untreated infections disseminate to other organs, causing systemic inflammation and specific organ dysfunction.

CAUSES

- *Haemophilus ducreyi*, a short, nonmotile, gram-negative bacillus

RISK FACTORS

- Poor personal hygiene
- Unprotected sex
- Multiple sex partners
- Uncircumcised males

INCIDENCE

- Incidence of chancroid is increasing in the United States.
- This disease is more common in males than in females.
- Chancroid may occur at any age but is most common among young, sexually active people.

COMPLICATIONS

- Phimosis and urethral fistulas in men
- Secondary infection
- Abscess formation
- Inguinal adenitis and formation of buboes

HISTORY

- May report unprotected sexual contact with an infected person or with unknown or multiple partners
- Pain from ulcers and lymphadenopathy
- Headaches and malaise

PHYSICAL FINDINGS

- Genital area initially with single or multiple papules surrounded by redness that rapidly become pustular and then ulcerate
- Ulcers nonindurated with ragged edges, a base of granulation tissue, and bleed easily; range from 1 to 2 mm in diameter
- Lesions on the tongue, lip, or breast
- Suppuration with bubo formation in the untreated patient; rupture of abscess may follow
- Tender, fluctuant inguinal nodes

LABORATORY

- Cultures from the lesion may show *H. ducreyi.*

Chancroidal lesion

Chancroid produces a soft, painful chancre, similar to that of syphilis. Without treatment, it may progress to inguinal adenitis and formation of buboes (enlarged, inflamed lymph nodes).

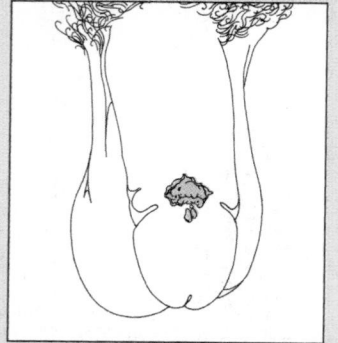

TREATMENT

GENERAL
- Aspiration of fluid-filled nodes
- Careful personal hygiene
- Evaluation of patient for syphilis, herpes simplex virus, and human immunodeficiency virus (HIV)

ACTIVITY
- Abstinence from sexual activity until genital lesions are healed

MEDICATIONS
- Antibiotics

SURGERY
- Surgical drainage for large abscess

NURSING CONSIDERATIONS

NURSING DIAGNOSES
- Acute pain
- Disturbed body image
- Impaired skin integrity
- Ineffective sexuality patterns
- Risk for infection

EXPECTED OUTCOMES
The patient will:
- report decreased levels of pain
- communicate feelings about changes in body image
- regain skin integrity with decrease in size of chancroids
- voice feelings about changes in sexual activity
- experience no further signs or symptoms of infection.

NURSING INTERVENTIONS
- Follow standard precautions.
- Give prescribed drugs.
- Wash the affected area with soap and water, followed by a bactericidal agent.
- Dry the affected area thoroughly.
- Report all cases of chancroid to the local board of health.

MONITORING
- Response to treatment
- Adverse effects of medications
- Compliance with treatment regimen
- Complications

PATIENT TEACHING

GENERAL
Be sure to cover:
- need to avoid applying creams, lotions, or oils on or near genitalia or on other lesion sites
- abstaining from sexual contact until follow up shows that healing is complete
- proper washing techniques of the genitalia
- HIV infection and recommend testing
- following safer sex practices.

DISCHARGE PLANNING
- Refer the patient and affected sexual partners for treatment.

RESOURCES
Organizations
American Social Health Association: *www.ashastd.org*
Centers for Diseases Control and Prevention: *www.cdc.gov*
Harvard University Consumer Health Information: *www.intelihealth.com*
National Health Information Center: *www.health.gov/nhic*
National Library of Medicine: *www.nlm.nih.gov*

Selected references
Kasper, D.L., et al., eds. *Harrison's Principles of Internal Medicine,* 16th ed. New York: McGraw-Hill Book Co., 2005.
Lewis, D.A. "Chancroid: Clinical Manifestations, Diagnosis, and Management," *Sexually Transmitted Infections* 79(1):68-71, February 2003.
Wu, J.J., et al. "Selected Sexually Transmitted Diseases and Their Relationship to HIV," *Clinics in Dermatology* 22(6):499-508, November-December 2004.

Chlamydial infections

OVERVIEW

- Bacterial infection that results in urethritis in men, cervicitis in women, and lymphogranuloma venereum in both sexes
- Trachoma inclusion conjunctivitis: seldom occurs in United States but is leading cause of blindness in developing countries
- Most common sexually transmitted disease (STD) in the United States

PATHOPHYSIOLOGY

- Chlamydial infections are transmitted by direct contact (such as sexual).
- Local inflammation is produced.
- Endometritis and salpingitis develop as the organism ascends the genitourinary tract.

CAUSES

- Neonatal infection caused by transport through the infected mother's birth canal
- Transmission of *Chlamydia trachomatis* by sexual contact (oral, anal, or vaginal)

RISK FACTORS

- Multiple sex partners or new sex partner
- Unprotected sex
- Coinfection with another STD

INCIDENCE

- About 4 million cases are reported annually.

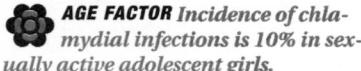 **AGE FACTOR** *Incidence of chlamydial infections is 10% in sexually active adolescent girls.*

COMPLICATIONS

- Infertility
- Pelvic inflammatory disease
- Urethral and rectal strictures
- Perihepatitis
- Cervical cancer
- Trachoma
- Urethritis and epididymitis (in males)
- Sterility
- Stillbirth, neonatal death, premature labor (with infected pregnant women)

ASSESSMENT

HISTORY

- Unprotected sexual contact with an infected person
- Previous STD

PHYSICAL FINDINGS

- Two-thirds of patients asymptomatic

Female

- Pelvic or abdominal pain
- Dyspareunia
- Cervical erosion
- Mucopurulent discharge
- Dysuria
- Urinary frequency

Male

- Dysuria
- Urinary frequency
- Pruritus
- Urethral discharge (copious and purulent)
- Meatal erythema
- Severe scrotal pain

Lymphogranuloma venereum

- Painless vesicle or nonindurated ulcer, 2 to 3 mm in diameter, on the glans or shaft of the penis; on the labia, vagina, or cervix; or in the rectum
- Enlarged inguinal lymph nodes
- Regional nodes appear as series of bilateral buboes
- Untreated buboes may rupture and form sinus tracts that discharge thick, yellow, granular secretion

DIAGNOSTIC TEST RESULTS

LABORATORY

- Swab culture of the infection site shows *C. trachomatis.* (See *Chlamydia trachomatis.*)
- Culture of aspirated blood, pus, or cerebrospinal fluid may establish epididymitis, prostatitis, and lymphogranuloma venereum.
- Serologic studies reveal previous exposure.
- Enzyme-linked immunosorbent assay may show *C. trachomatis* antibody.

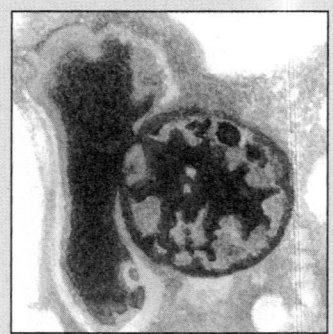

Chlamydia trachomatis

In chlamydial infections, microscopic examination reveals *Chlamydia trachomatis,* a unicellular parasite with a rigid cell wall

TREATMENT

GENERAL
◆ Symptomatic treatment (sex partners also treated)

ACTIVITY
◆ Abstinence from sexual activity until infection resolved

MEDICATIONS
◆ Antibiotics

NURSING CONSIDERATIONS

NURSING DIAGNOSES
◆ Acute pain
◆ Impaired skin integrity
◆ Impaired urinary elimination
◆ Ineffective sexuality patterns
◆ Risk for infection
◆ Sexual dysfunction
◆ Situational low self-esteem

EXPECTED OUTCOMES
The patient will:
◆ express relief from pain
◆ exhibit improved or healed lesions or wounds
◆ maintain normal urine output
◆ will state STD infection risk factors
◆ will remain free from signs or symptoms of infection
◆ voice feelings about potential or actual changes in sexuality
◆ express concern about self-concept, self-esteem, and body image.

NURSING INTERVENTIONS
◆ Follow standard precautions.
◆ Check the neonate of an infected mother for signs of infection.
◆ Give prescribed drugs.
◆ Provide appropriate skin care.
◆ If required in your state, report cases of chlamydial infection to the local board of health for follow-up on sexual contacts.

MONITORING
◆ Response to treatment
◆ Adverse effects of medication
◆ Complications

PATIENT TEACHING

GENERAL
Be sure to cover:
◆ the disorder, signs and symptoms, and treatment
◆ proper hand-washing technique
◆ abstinence from intercourse or use of condoms
◆ importance of getting tested for the human immunodeficiency virus
◆ dealing with long-term risks and complications from infection
◆ transmission of infection
◆ prevention of STDs by following safe sex practices
◆ follow-up care
◆ complications.

DISCHARGE PLANNING
◆ Refer the patient to support services.
◆ Advise rescreenings at 3 to 4 months and annual screenings for sexually active teens and females ages 20 to 25.

RESOURCES
Organizations
American Social Health Association: *www.ashastd.org*
Centers for Disease Control and Prevention: *www.cdc.gov*
Harvard University Consumer Health Information: *www.intelihealth.com*
National Health Information Center: *www.health.gov/nhic*
National Library of Medicine: *www.nlm.nih.gov*

Selected references
Kasper, D.L., et al., eds. *Harrison's Principles of Internal Medicine,* 16th ed. New York: McGraw-Hill Book Co., 2005.
Low, N., et al. "The Chlamydia Screening Studies: Rationale and Design," *Sexually Transmitted Infections* 80(5):342-48, October 2004.
Mpiga, P., and Ravaoarinoro, M. "Chlamydia Trachomatis Persistence: An Update," *Microbiological Research* 161(1):9-19, January 2006.

Cholelithiasis, cholecystitis, and related disorders

OVERVIEW

Cholelithiasis
- Leading biliary tract disease
- Formation of calculi (gallstones) in the gallbladder
- Prognosis usually good with treatment, unless infection occurs

Cholecystitis
- Related disorder that arises from formation of gallstones
- Acute or chronic inflammation of gallbladder
- Usually caused by a gallstone lodged in the cystic duct
- Acute form most common during middle age
- Chronic form most common among elderly persons
- Prognosis good with treatment

Choledocholithiasis
- Related disorder that arises from formation of gallstones
- Partial or complete biliary obstruction due to gallstones lodged in the common bile duct
- Prognosis good unless infection occurs

Cholangitis
- Related disorder that arises from formation of gallstones
- Infected bile duct
- Commonly linked to choledocholithiasis
- Rapid response of nonsuppurative type to antibiotic treatment
- Poor prognosis of suppurative type unless surgery to correct obstruction and drain infected bile performed promptly

Gallstone ileus
- Related disorder that arises from formation of gallstones
- Obstruction of the small bowel by a gallstone
- Most common in elderly persons
- Prognosis good with surgery

PATHOPHYSIOLOGY
- Calculi formation in the biliary system causes obstruction.
- Obstruction of hepatic duct leads to intrahepatic retention of bile; increased release of bilirubin into the bloodstream occurs.
- Obstruction of cystic duct leads to inflammation of the gallbladder; increased gallbladder contraction and peristalsis occurs.
- Obstruction of bile causes impairment of digestion and absorption of lipids.

CAUSES
- Acute cholecystitis also a result of conditions that alter gallbladder's ability to fill or empty (trauma, reduced blood supply to the gallbladder, prolonged immobility, chronic dieting, adhesions, prolonged anesthesia, and opioid abuse)
- Calculi formation; type of disorder that develops depends on where in the gallbladder or biliary tract the calculi collect

RISK FACTORS
- High-calorie, high-cholesterol diet
- Obesity
- Elevated estrogen levels from hormonal contraceptive use, postmenopausal hormone-replacement therapy, or pregnancy
- Diabetes mellitus, ileal disease, hemolytic disorders, hepatic disease (cirrhosis), or pancreatitis
- Rapid weight loss

INCIDENCE
- Cholelithiasis, cholecystitis, and related disorders are six times more common in females between ages 20 and 50.
- After age 50, the incidence of these disorders is equal in males and females; incidence increases with each succeeding decade.

COMPLICATIONS
Cholelithiasis
- Cholangitis
- Cholecystitis
- Choledocholithiasis
- Gallstone ileus

Cholecystitis
- Gallbladder complications, such as empyema, hydrops or mucocele, and gangrene
- Chronic cholecystitis and cholangitis

Choledocholithiasis
- Cholangitis
- Obstructive jaundice
- Pancreatitis
- Secondary biliary cirrhosis

Cholangitis
- Septic shock
- Death

Gallstone ileus
- Bowel obstruction

ASSESSMENT

HISTORY
- May be asymptomatic (even when X-rays reveal gallstones)

Gallbladder attack
- Sudden onset of severe steady or aching pain in the midepigastric region or the right upper abdominal quadrant
- Pain radiating to the back, between the shoulder blades or over the right shoulder blade, or just to the shoulder area
- Attack occurring after eating a fatty meal or a large meal after fasting for an extended time
- Attack occurring in the middle of the night
- Nausea, vomiting, and chills
- Low-grade fever
- History of milder GI symptoms that preceded the acute attack; indigestion, vague abdominal discomfort, belching, and flatulence after eating high-fat meals or snacks

PHYSICAL FINDINGS
- Severe pain
- Pallor
- Diaphoresis
- Low-grade fever (high fever in cholangitis)
- Exhaustion
- Jaundice (chronic)

- Dark-colored urine and clay-colored stools
- Tachycardia
- Tenderness over the gallbladder, which increases on inspiration (Murphy's sign)
- Palpable, painless, sausagelike mass (calculus-filled gallbladder without ductal obstruction)
- Hypoactive bowel sounds

DIAGNOSTIC TEST RESULTS

LABORATORY
- Blood studies may reveal, during a cholecystitis attack, elevated levels of serum alkaline phosphatase, lactate dehydrogenase, aspartate aminotransferase, icteric index, and total bilirubin; and a slightly increased white blood cell count.

IMAGING
- Plain abdominal X-rays show gallstones if they contain enough calcium to be radiopaque. X-rays are also helpful in identifying porcelain gallbladder, limy bile, and gallstone ileus.
- Ultrasonography of the gallbladder confirms cholelithiasis in most patients and distinguishes between obstructive and nonobstructive jaundice; calculi as small as 2 mm can be detected.
- Oral cholecystography confirms the presence of gallstones, although this test is gradually being replaced by ultrasonography.
- Technetium-labeled iminodiacetic acid scan of the gallbladder indicates cystic duct obstruction and acute or chronic cholecystitis if the gallbladder can't be seen.
- Percutaneous transhepatic cholangiography, imaging performed under fluoroscopic guidance, supports the diagnosis of obstructive jaundice and is used to visualize calculi in the ducts.

TREATMENT

GENERAL
- Endoscopic retrograde cholangiopancreatography to visualize and remove calculi
- Lithotripsy

DIET
- Low-fat
- Nothing by mouth if surgery required

ACTIVITY
- As tolerated

MEDICATIONS
- Gallstone dissolution therapy
- Bile salts
- Analgesics
- Antispasmodics
- Anticholinergics
- Antiemetics
- Antibiotics

SURGERY
- Cholecystectomy (laparoscopic or abdominal), cholecystectomy with operative cholangiography, choledochostomy, or exploration of the common bile duct

NURSING CONSIDERATIONS

NURSING DIAGNOSES
- Acute pain
- Imbalanced nutrition: Less than body requirements
- Ineffective tissue perfusion: GI
- Risk for deficient fluid volume
- Risk for infection

EXPECTED OUTCOMES
The patient will:
- express feelings of increased comfort
- achieve adequate caloric and nutritional intake
- maintain adequate GI perfusion
- maintain an adequate fluid balance
- remain free from signs and symptoms of infection.

NURSING INTERVENTIONS
- Give prescribed drugs.

MONITORING
- Vital signs
- Intake and output
- Pain control

After surgery
- Signs and symptoms of bleeding, infection, or atelectasis
- Wound site
- T-tube patency and drainage

PATIENT TEACHING

GENERAL
Be sure to cover:
- the disease, diagnosis, and treatment
- how to breathe deeply, cough, expectorate, and perform leg exercises that are necessary after surgery
- dietary modifications
- medication administration, dosage, and possible adverse effects
- wound care.

RESOURCES
Organizations
Digestive Disease National Coalition: *www.ddnc.org*
National Institute of Diabetes & Digestive & Kidney Diseases: *www.niddk.nih.gov*

Selected references
Handbook of Diseases, 3rd ed. Philadelphia: Lippincott Williams & Wilkins, 2004.
Kaaja, R.J., and Greer, I.A. "Manifestations of Chronic Disease During Pregnancy," *JAMA* 294(21):2751-757, December 2005.
Lammert, F., and Sauerbruch, T. "Mechanisms of Disease: The Genetic Epidemiology of Gallbladder Stones," *National Clinical Practice Gastroenterology and Hepatology* 2(9):423-33, September 2005.

Cholera

- Acute enterotoxin-mediated GI infection
- Transmitted through food and water contaminated with fecal material from carriers or people with active infections
- Food poisoning caused by *Vibrio parahaemolyticus*, a similar bacterium (see Vibrio parahaemolyticus *food poisoning*)
- Also known as *Asiatic cholera* or *epidemic cholera*

PATHOPHYSIOLOGY

- Humans are the only hosts and victims of *V. cholerae*, a motile, aerobic organism.

CAUSES

- The gram-negative bacillus *V. cholerae*

RISK FACTORS

- Deficiency or absence of hydrochloric acid

INCIDENCE

- Although most common in Africa, southern and Southeast Asia, and the Middle East, cholera outbreaks have also occurred in Japan, Australia, and Europe.
- The disease occurs during the warmer months and is most prevalent among lower socioeconomic groups.
- Cholera is common among children ages 1 to 5 in India but it's equally distributed among all age-groups in other endemic areas.

COMPLICATIONS

- Dehydration
- Hypovolemic shock
- Metabolic acidosis
- Uremia
- Coma and death

HISTORY

- Profuse, watery diarrhea
- Vomiting
- Intense thirst
- Weakness
- Muscle cramps (especially in the extremities)

PHYSICAL FINDINGS

- Stools containing white flecks of mucus (rice-water stools)
- Loss of skin turgor, wrinkled skin, sunken eyes
- Pinched facial expression
- Cyanosis
- Tachycardia, tachypnea
- Thready or absent peripheral pulses
- Decreased blood pressure
- Fever
- Inaudible, hypoactive bowel sounds

LABORATORY

- A culture of *V. cholerae* from feces or vomitus indicates cholera.
- Microscopic examination of fresh feces shows rapidly moving bacilli (like shooting stars).
- Agglutination reveals reactions to group- and type-specific antisera.

OTHER

- In endemic areas or during epidemics, typical clinical features strongly suggest cholera.

Vibrio parahaemolyticus food poisoning

Vibrio parahaemolyticus is a common cause of gastroenteritis in Japan. Outbreaks also occur on American cruise ships and in the eastern and southeastern coastal areas of the United States, especially during the summer.

V. parahaemolyticus, which thrives in a salty environment, is transmitted through the ingestion of uncooked or undercooked contaminated shellfish, particularly crab and shrimp. After an incubation period of 2 to 48 hours, *V. parahaemolyticus* causes watery diarrhea, moderately severe cramps, nausea, vomiting, headache, weakness, chills, and fever. Food poisoning is usually self-limiting and subsides spontaneously within 2 days. Occasionally, however, it's more severe, and may even be fatal in debilitated or elderly persons.

Diagnosis requires bacteriologic examination of vomitus, blood, stool smears, or fecal specimens collected by rectal swab. Diagnosis must rule out not only other causes of food poisoning but also other acute GI disorders.

Treatment is supportive, consisting primarily of bed rest and oral fluid replacement. I.V. replacement therapy is seldom necessary but oral tetracycline may be prescribed. Thorough cooking of seafood prevents this infection.

TREATMENT

GENERAL
◆ Enteric precautions
◆ Supportive care

DIET
◆ Increased fluid intake

MEDICATIONS
◆ Rapid I.V. infusion of large amounts (50 to 100 ml/minute) of isotonic saline solution, alternating with isotonic sodium bicarbonate or sodium lactate
◆ Tetracycline

NURSING CONSIDERATIONS

NURSING DIAGNOSES
◆ Deficient fluid volume
◆ Diarrhea
◆ Fatigue
◆ Ineffective tissue perfusion: Cardiopulmonary, renal
◆ Risk for infection

EXPECTED OUTCOMES
The patient will:
◆ regain and maintain adequate fluid and electrolyte balance
◆ have normal elimination patterns
◆ express feelings of energy and decreased fatigue
◆ maintain tissue perfusion and cellular oxygenation
◆ experience no further signs or symptoms of infection.

NURSING INTERVENTIONS
◆ Wear a gown and gloves when handling feces-contaminated articles.
◆ Carefully observe jugular veins.
◆ Auscultate the lungs frequently.

MONITORING
◆ Vital signs
◆ Intake and output
◆ Laboratory values
◆ I.V. infusion
◆ Jugular veins

PATIENT TEACHING

GENERAL
Be sure to cover:
◆ administration of cholera vaccine to travelers in endemic areas
◆ proper hand-washing technique
◆ need for increased fluid intake.

DISCHARGE PLANNING
◆ Explain the use of oral tetracycline to family members.
◆ If the practitioner orders a cholera vaccine, tell the patient that he'll need a booster 3 to 6 months later for continuing protection.

RESOURCES
Organizations
Centers for Disease Control and Prevention: *www.cdc.gov*
National Organization for Rare Disorders: *www.rarediseases.org*

Selected references
Diseases, 4th ed. Philadelphia: Lippincott Williams & Wilkins, 2006.
Kabir, S., "Cholera Vaccines: The Current Status and Problems," *Reviews in Medical Microbiology* 16(3):101-16, August 2005.

Chronic fatigue and immune dysfunction syndrome

OVERVIEW

- Characterized by prolonged overwhelming fatigue
- Also called *chronic fatigue syndrome, chronic Epstein-Barr virus,* and *myalgic encephalomyelitis*

PATHOPHYSIOLOGY

- Infectious agents or environmental factors trigger an abnormal immune response and hormonal alterations.

CAUSES

- Exact cause unknown
- Possibly cytomegalovirus, Epstein-Barr virus, herpes simplex virus types 1 and 2, human herpesvirus 6, Inoue-Melnick virus, human adenovirus 2, enteroviruses, measles virus, or a retrovirus that resembles human T-cell lymphotropic virus type II
- May result from overactive immune system

RISK FACTORS

- Genetic predisposition
- Hormonal balance
- Neuropsychiatric factors
- Gender
- Previous illness
- Stressful environment

INCIDENCE

- Chronic fatigue and immune dysfunction syndrome affects people of all ages, occupations, and income levels.
- It's more common in women than in men or children, especially women younger than age 45.
- Sporadic incidence and epidemic clusters have been observed.
- The disease is estimated to affect about 200 out of every 100,000 persons in the United States.

  AGE FACTOR *Chronic fatigue and immune dysfunction syndrome is most prevalent among professionals in their 20s and 30s.*

COMPLICATIONS

- Social and occupational impairment

ASSESSMENT

HISTORY

- Characteristic complaints of prolonged, overwhelming fatigue (see *Diagnosing chronic fatigue syndrome*)

PHYSICAL FINDINGS

- Myalgia
- Cognitive dysfunction

DIAGNOSTIC TEST RESULTS

LABORATORY

- Lymphocyte differential may reveal reduced natural killer cell cytotoxicity, abnormal CD4+:CD8+ T-cell ratios, and mild lymphocytosis.
- Immunoglobulin profile may show decreased immunoglobulin subclasses.
- Immune complex profile may reveal circulating immune complexes.
- Antimicrosomal antibody testing may reveal increased levels of antimicrosomal antibodies.

Diagnosing chronic fatigue syndrome

Chronic fatigue and immune dysfunction syndrome is defined by:
- New or relapsing fatigue that isn't the result of ongoing exertion or alleviated by rest and reduces occupational, educational, social, or personal activities or efforts.
- Four or more of the following symptoms, occurring for 6 months or more:
  – self-reported impairment in short-term memory or concentration
  – sore throat
  – tender cervical or axillary nodes
  – muscle pain
  – multiple joint pain without redness or swelling
  – headaches of a new pattern or severity
  – nonrefreshing sleep
  – postexertional malaise lasting 24 hours or longer.

TREATMENT

GENERAL
- Focus on supportive care
- Psychiatric evaluation
- Behavioral therapy
- Massage therapy
- Chiropractic and therapeutic touch

DIET
- Well-balanced, high in vitamins and minerals

ACTIVITY
- Physical therapy
- Frequent rest periods, as needed
- Avoidance of strenuous activities

MEDICATIONS
- Nonsteroidal anti-inflammatory drugs
- Antidepressants
- Antihistamines
- Anxiolytics
- Stimulants

NURSING CONSIDERATIONS

NURSING DIAGNOSES
- Activity intolerance
- Fatigue
- Ineffective coping
- Ineffective role performance
- Powerlessness

EXPECTED OUTCOMES
The patient will:
- verbalize the importance of balancing activity, as tolerated, with rest
- verbally report having an increased energy level
- use support systems to help with coping
- express feelings about diminished capacity to perform usual roles
- participate in self-care and decision-making process.

NURSING INTERVENTIONS
- Provide emotional support.
- Begin a graded exercise program.

MONITORING
- Response to treatment
- Adverse effects of medication
- Complications

PATIENT TEACHING

GENERAL
Be sure to cover:
- need for daily routine including moderate levels of exercise
- need to avoid bed rest, which has no proven therapeutic value
- medication administration, dosage, and possible adverse effects
- appropriate activity planning.

DISCHARGE PLANNING
- Refer the patient to support services.

RESOURCES
Organizations
Centers for Disease Control and Prevention: *www.cdc.gov*
CFIDS Association of America: *www.cfids.org*
Harvard University Consumer Health Information: *www.intelihealth.com*
National Health Information Center: *www.health.gov/nhic/*
National Library of Medicine: *www.nlm.nih.gov*

Selected references
Aylett, E., and Fawcett, T.N. "Chronic Fatigue Syndrome: The Nurse's Role," *Nursing Standard* 17(35):33-37, May 2003.
Kasper, D.L., et al., eds. *Harrison's Principles of Internal Medicine,* 16th ed. New York: McGraw-Hill Book Co., 2005.
Shaver, J.L. "Fibromyalgia Syndrome in Women," *The Nursing Clinics of North America* 39(1):195-204, viii, March 2004.
Viner, R., et al. "Outpatient Rehabilitative Treatment of Chronic Fatigue Syndrome," *Archives of Disease in Childhood* 89(7):615-19, July 2004.

Cirrhosis

OVERVIEW

- Chronic hepatic disease
- Several types

PATHOPHYSIOLOGY

- Diffuse destruction and fibrotic regeneration of hepatic cells occurs.
- Necrotic tissue yields to fibrosis.
- Liver structure and normal vasculature are altered.
- Blood and lymph flow are impaired.
- Hepatic insufficiency occurs.

CAUSES

Laënnec's or micronodular cirrhosis
- Chronic alcoholism
- Malnutrition

Postnecrotic or macronodular cirrhosis
- Complication of viral hepatitis
- Possible after exposure to such liver toxins as arsenic, carbon tetrachloride, and phosphorus

Biliary cirrhosis
- Prolonged biliary tract obstruction or inflammation

Idiopathic cirrhosis (cryptogenic)
- Chronic inflammatory bowel disease
- Sarcoidosis

RISK FACTORS

- Alcoholism
- Toxins
- Biliary obstruction
- Hepatitis
- Metabolic disorders

INCIDENCE

- Cirrhosis is the tenth most common cause of death in the United States.
- Cirrhosis is most common among those ages 45 to 75.
- The disease occurs in twice as many men as women.

COMPLICATIONS

- Portal hypertension
- Bleeding esophageal varices
- Hepatic encephalopathy
- Hepatorenal syndrome
- Death

ASSESSMENT

HISTORY

- Chronic alcoholism
- Malnutrition
- Viral hepatitis
- Exposure to liver toxins, such as arsenic and certain medications
- Prolonged biliary tract obstruction or inflammation

Early stage
- Vague signs and symptoms
- Abdominal pain
- Diarrhea, constipation
- Fatigue
- Nausea, vomiting
- Muscle cramps

Later stage
- Chronic dyspepsia
- Constipation
- Pruritus
- Weight loss
- Bleeding tendency, such as frequent nosebleeds, easy bruising, and bleeding gums
- Hepatic encephalopathy

PHYSICAL FINDINGS

- Telangiectasis on the cheeks
- Spider angiomas on the face, neck, arms, and trunk
- Gynecomastia
- Umbilical hernia
- Distended abdominal blood vessels
- Ascites
- Testicular atrophy
- Menstrual irregularities
- Palmar erythema
- Clubbed fingers
- Thigh and leg edema
- Ecchymosis
- Anemia
- Jaundice
- Palpable, large, firm liver with a sharp edge (early finding)
- Enlarged spleen
- Asterixis
- Slurred speech, paranoia, hallucinations

DIAGNOSTIC TEST RESULTS

LABORATORY

- Elevated levels of liver enzymes, such as alanine aminotransferase, aspartate aminotransferase, total serum bilirubin, and indirect bilirubin; decreased total serum albumin and protein levels; prolonged prothrombin time; decreased hemoglobin, hematocrit, and serum electrolyte levels; deficient vitamins A, C, and K
- Increased urine levels of bilirubin and urobilinogen; decreased fecal urobilinogen levels
- Elevated ammonia levels

IMAGING

- Abdominal X-rays show liver and spleen size and cysts or gas in the biliary tract or liver; liver calcification; and massive ascites.
- Computed tomography and liver scans determine liver size, identify liver masses, and visualize hepatic blood flow and obstruction.
- Radioisotope liver scans show liver size, blood flow, or obstruction.

DIAGNOSTIC PROCEDURES

- Liver biopsy, the definitive test for cirrhosis, reveals hepatic tissue destruction and fibrosis.
- Esophagogastroduodenoscopy reveals bleeding esophageal varices, stomach irritation or ulceration, and duodenal bleeding and irritation.

TREATMENT

GENERAL
- Removal or alleviation of underlying cause
- Paracentesis
- Esophageal balloon tamponade
- Sclerotherapy
- I.V. fluids
- Blood transfusion

DIET
- Restricted sodium consumption
- Restricted fluid intake
- No alcohol intake
- High-calorie

ACTIVITY
- Frequent rest periods, as needed

MEDICATIONS
- Vitamin and nutritional supplements
- Antacids
- Potassium-sparing diuretics
- Beta-adrenergic blockers and vasopressin
- Ammonia detoxicant
- Antiemetics

SURGERY
- May be required to divert ascites into venous circulation; if so, peritoneovenous shunt is used
- Portal-systemic shunts
- Transplantation

NURSING CONSIDERATIONS

NURSING DIAGNOSES
- Activity intolerance
- Excess fluid volume
- Hopelessness
- Imbalanced nutrition: Less than body requirements
- Risk for deficient fluid volume
- Risk for impaired skin integrity
- Risk for injury

EXPECTED OUTCOMES
The patient will:
- perform activities of daily living without fatigue or exhaustion
- maintain normal fluid volume and show no signs of circulatory overload
- participate in decisions about care
- maintain adequate caloric intake
- maintain an adequate fluid balance
- maintain skin integrity
- avoid or minimize injury or complications.

NURSING INTERVENTIONS
- Give prescribed I.V. fluids and blood products.
- Give prescribed drugs.
- Encourage verbalization and provide support.
- Provide appropriate skin care.

MONITORING
- Vital signs
- Laboratory values
- Hydration and nutritional status
- Abdominal girth
- Weight
- Bleeding tendencies
- Skin integrity
- Changes in mentation, behavior
- Ammonia level

PATIENT TEACHING

GENERAL
Be sure to cover:
- the disorder, diagnosis, and treatment
- over-the-counter medications that may increase bleeding tendencies
- dietary modifications
- need to avoid infections and abstain from alcohol
- need to avoid sedatives and acetaminophen (hepatotoxic)
- high-calorie diet and small, frequent meals.

DISCHARGE PLANNING
- Refer the patient to Alcoholics Anonymous, if appropriate.
- Refer the patient for psychological counseling, if needed.

RESOURCES
Organizations
Alcoholics Anonymous: *www.alcoholics-anonymous.org*
American Liver Foundation: *www.liverfoundation.org*
Digestive Disease National Coalition: *www.ddnc.org*
National Institute of Diabetes & Digestive & Kidney Diseases: *www.niddk.nih.gov*

Selected references
Durston, S. "Cirrhosis: Scarred for Life," *Nursing Made Incredibly Easy!* 2(6):14-24, November-December 2004.
Handbook of Diseases, 3rd ed. Philadelphia: Lippincott Williams & Wilkins, 2004.
Kasper, D.L., et al., eds. *Harrison's Principles of Internal Medicine,* 16th ed. New York: McGraw-Hill Book Co., 2005.
Randi, G., et al. "History of Cirrhosis and Risk of Digestive Tract Neoplasms," *Annals of Oncology* 16(9):1551-555, September 2005.

Cleft lip and cleft palate

- Front and sides of the face and the palatine shelves fuse imperfectly during pregnancy
- May occur separately or in combination
- Can occur unilaterally, bilaterally or, rarely, in the midline
- May affect just the lip or extend into the upper jaw or nasal cavity (see *Types of cleft deformities*)

PATHOPHYSIOLOGY

- Chromosomal abnormality, exposure to teratogens, genetic abnormality, or environmental factors cause the lip or palate to fuse imperfectly during the second month of pregnancy.
- A complete cleft includes the soft palate, the bones of the maxilla, and the alveolus on one or both sides of the premaxilla.
- A double cleft runs from the soft palate forward to either side of the nose, separating the maxilla and premaxilla into freely moving segments. The tongue and other muscles can displace the segments, enlarging the cleft.

WARNING *Isolated cleft palate occurs more commonly with congenital defects other than isolated cleft lip. The constellation of U-shaped cleft palate, mandibular hypoplasia, and glossoptosis known as Robin sequence can occur as an isolated defect or as one feature of many different syndromes. These infants should have comprehensive genetic evaluation. Because of their mandibular hypoplasia and glossoptosis, the airway in infants with Robin sequence must be carefully evaluated and managed.*

CAUSES

- Chromosomal or Mendelian syndrome (cleft defects caused by more than 300 syndromes)
- Exposure to teratogens during fetal development
- Combined genetic and environmental factors

INCIDENCE

- Cleft lip and cleft palate occur twice as commonly in males than in females.
- These disorders occur more commonly in children with a family history of cleft defects.
- Cleft lip with or without cleft palate occurs in about 1 in 1,000 births among Whites; incidence is higher in Asians (1.7 in 1,000) and Native Americans (more than 3.6 in 1,000) but lower in Blacks (1 in 2,500).

COMPLICATIONS

- Malnutrition
- Hearing impairment
- Permanent speech impediment

HISTORY

- Family history of cleft defects
- Maternal exposure to teratogens during pregnancy

PHYSICAL FINDINGS

- Cleft that runs from the soft palate forward to either side of the nose

---

Types of cleft deformities

These illustrations show variations of cleft lip and cleft palate.

NOTCH IN THE VERMILLION BORDER (JUNCTION OF THE LIP AND SURROUNDING SKIN)

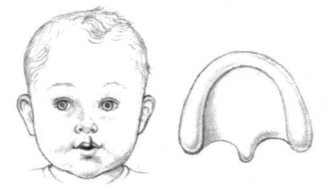
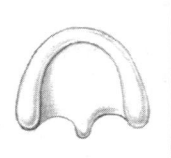

UNILATERAL CLEFT LIP AND PALATE

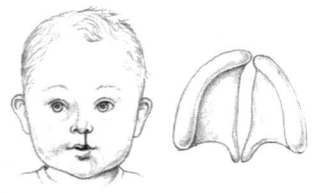

BILATERAL CLEFT LIP AND PALATE

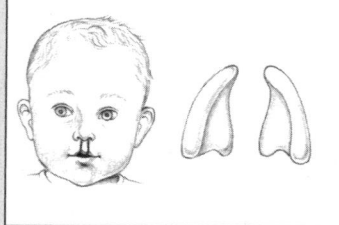

CLEFT PALATE

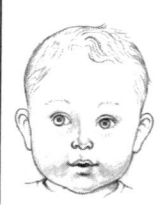
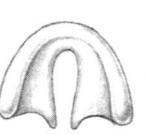

IMAGING
◆ Prenatal targeted ultrasound reveals abnormality.

OTHER
◆ Clinical presentation, obvious at birth

TREATMENT

GENERAL
◆ Orthodontic prosthesis to improve sucking
◆ Use of a contoured speech bulb attached to the posterior of a denture to occlude the nasopharynx when a wide horseshoe defect makes surgery impossible (to help the child develop intelligible speech)

DIET
◆ Use of a large, soft nipple with large holes, such as a lamb's nipple, to improve feeding patterns and promote adequate nutrition

MEDICATIONS
⚡ **WARNING** *Daily use of folic acid before conception decreases the risk for isolated (not associated with another genetic or congenital malformation) cleft lip or palate by up to 25%. Women of childbearing age should be encouraged to take a daily multivitamin containing folic acid until menopause or until they're no longer fertile.*

SURGERY
◆ Surgical correction of cleft lip in the first few days of life and again at 12 to 18 months, after the infant gains weight and is infection-free

NURSING CONSIDERATIONS

NURSING DIAGNOSES
◆ Anxiety
◆ Chronic low self-esteem
◆ Delayed growth and development
◆ Disabled family coping
◆ Disturbed body image
◆ Fear
◆ Imbalanced nutrition: Less than body requirements
◆ Impaired swallowing
◆ Risk for aspiration
◆ Risk for impaired parent/infant/child attachment
◆ Risk for injury

EXPECTED OUTCOMES
The patient (or his family) will:
◆ identify strategies to reduce anxiety
◆ express feelings related to self-esteem, when age appropriate
◆ exhibit normal growth and development
◆ seek appropriate resources to assist with coping
◆ express positive feelings about self, when age appropriate
◆ express fears and concerns
◆ maintain daily calorie requirements
◆ swallow without coughing or choking
◆ not aspirate feedings
◆ show signs of bonding with parents
◆ avoid injury.

NURSING INTERVENTIONS
◆ Encourage the mother of an infant with cleft lip to breast-feed if the cleft doesn't prevent effective sucking.
◆ Suction, as necessary.
◆ Help the parents deal with their feelings about the child's deformity.
⚡ **WARNING** *Never place a child with Robin sequence on his back because his tongue could fall back and obstruct his airway. Place the infant on his side for sleeping. Most other infants with a cleft palate can sleep on their backs without difficulty.*

MONITORING
◆ Swallowing ability
◆ Weight gain
◆ Intake and output

PATIENT TEACHING

GENERAL
Be sure to cover:
◆ treatment plan
◆ how to best feed the infant
◆ burping the infant frequently
◆ gently cleaning the palatal cleft with a cotton-tipped applicator dipped in half-strength hydrogen peroxide or water after each feeding.

DISCHARGE PLANNING
◆ Refer the patient to speech therapy to correct speech patterns.
◆ Refer the parents to a social worker who can guide them to community resources, if needed, and to a genetic counselor to determine the recurrence risk.

RESOURCES
Organizations
Cleft Palate Foundation: *www.cleftline.org*
Harvard University Consumer Health Information: *www.intelihealth.com*
Mayo Clinic: *www.mayoclinic.com*

Selected references
Diseases, 4th ed. Philadelphia: Lippincott Williams & Wilkins, 2006.
Harville, E.W., et al. "Cleft Lip and Palate versus Cleft Lip Only: Are They Distinct Defects?" *American Journal of Epidemiology* 162(5):448-53, September 2005.
Merritt, L. "Part 2. Physical Assessment of the Infant with Cleft Lip and/or Palate," *Advances in Neonatal Care* 5(3):125-34, June 2005.
Sadler, C. "Palatable Truth," *Nursing Standard* 19(43):24-26, July 2005.

Clostridium difficile infection

- A gram-positive anaerobic bacterium often resulting in antibiotic-related diarrhea
- Symptoms ranging from asymptomatic carrier states to severe pseudomembranous colitis caused by exotoxins (toxin A is an enterotoxin and toxin B is a cytotoxin)
- Within 14 to 30 days of treatment, recurrence with the same organism possible in 10% to 20% of patients

PATHOPHYSIOLOGY

- Antibiotics may trigger toxin production.
- Toxin A mediates alteration in fluid secretion, enhances inflammation, and causes leakage of albumin from the postcapillary venules.
- Toxin B causes damage and exfoliation to the superficial epithelial cells and inhibits adenosine diphosphate ribosylation of Rho proteins.
- Both toxins cause electrophysiologic alterations of colonic tissue.

CAUSES

- Antibiotics that disrupt the bowel flora
- Enemas and intestinal stimulants
- Some antifungal and antiviral agents
- Transmission from infected person

RISK FACTORS

- Contaminated equipment and surfaces
- Antibiotics
- Abdominal surgery
- Antineoplastic agents that have an antibiotic activity
- Immunocompromised state

INCIDENCE

- *C. difficile* infection is most common in people in nursing homes and day-care facilities.
- This is one of the most common nosocomial infections. (About 20% of hospitalized patients taking antibiotics contract *C. difficile* infection.)

COMPLICATIONS

- Electrolyte abnormalities
- Hypovolemic shock
- Toxic megacolon
- Colonic perforation
- Peritonitis
- Sepsis
- Hemorrhage
- Pseudomembranous colitis

ASSESSMENT

HISTORY

- Recent antibiotic therapy
- Abdominal pain
- Cramping

PHYSICAL FINDINGS

- Soft, unformed, or watery diarrhea (more than three stools in a 24-hour period) that may be foul smelling or grossly bloody
- Abdominal tenderness
- Fever

DIAGNOSTIC TEST RESULTS

LABORATORY

- Cell cytotoxin test may show toxins A and B.
- Enzyme immunoassay may identify *C. difficile*; slightly less sensitive than cell cytotoxin test but has turnaround time of only a few hours.
- Stool culture may identify *C. difficile*.

TREATMENT

GENERAL
- Withdrawal of causative antibiotic
- Avoidance of antimotility agents
- Good skin care

DIET
- Well-balanced
- Increased fluid intake, if appropriate

ACTIVITY
- Rest periods, if fatigued

MEDICATIONS
- Metronidazole
- Vancomycin
- If relapse and previous treatment was metronidazole, low-dose vancomycin may be effective
- Combination of vancomycin and rifampin
- Experimental treatments involve the administration of yeast *Saccharomyces boulardii* with metronidazole or vancomycin and biologic vaccines to restore the normal GI flora
- Lactobacillus
- Cholestyramine

NURSING CONSIDERATIONS

NURSING DIAGNOSES
- Activity intolerance
- Acute pain
- Fatigue
- Hyperthermia
- Imbalanced nutrition: Less than body requirements
- Impaired skin integrity
- Risk for deficient fluid volume

EXPECTED OUTCOMES
The patient will:
- perform activities of daily living without excess fatigue or exhaustion
- express feelings of comfort and report absence of pain
- report an increased energy level
- remain afebrile
- maintain normal electrolyte levels
- exhibit improved or healed lesions or wounds
- maintain adequate fluid volume.

NURSING INTERVENTIONS
- Give prescribed drugs.
- Institute enteric precautions for those with active diarrhea.
- Wash your hands with an antiseptic soap after direct contact with the patient or his immediate environment.
- Make sure reusable equipment is disinfected before it's used on another patient.

MONITORING
- Vital signs
- Intake and output
- Complications
- Serum electrolytes
- Adverse effects of medication
- Response to treatment
- Amount and characteristics of stools
- Skin integrity

PATIENT TEACHING

GENERAL
Be sure to cover:
- the disorder, diagnosis, and treatment
- proper hand-washing technique
- proper disinfection of contaminated clothing or household items
- adequate fluid intake
- signs and symptoms of dehydration
- medications and potential adverse reactions
- complications and when to notify the practitioner
- perirectal skin care.

RESOURCES
Organizations
Centers for Disease Control and Prevention: *www.cdc.gov*
Harvard University Consumer Health Information: *www.intelihealth.com*
National Health Information Center: *www.health.gov/nhic*
National Institute of Allergy and Infectious Diseases: *www.niaid.nih.gov*
National Library of Medicine: *www.nlm.nih.gov*

Selected references
Diseases, 4th ed. Philadelphia: Lippincott Williams & Wilkins, 2006.
Kasper, D.L., et al., eds. *Harrison's Principles of Internal Medicine,* 16th ed. New York: McGraw-Hill Book Co., 2005.
Starr, J. "*Clostridium Difficile* Associated Diarrhoea: Diagnosis and Treatment," *British Medical Journal* 331(7515):498-501, September 2005.
Tonna, I., and Welsby, P.D. "Pathogenesis and Treatment of *Clostridium Difficile* Infection," *Postgraduate Medical Journal* 81(956):367-69, June 2005.

Clubfoot

- A deformed talus and shortened Achilles' tendon give the foot a characteristic clublike appearance. In talipes equinovarus, the foot points downward (equinus) and turns inward (varus), and the front of the foot curls toward the heel (forefoot adduction).
- Clubfoot, also known as *talipes*, is the most common congenital disorder of the lower extremities.

PATHOPHYSIOLOGY
- Unknown, but contributing factors may include:
- defective cartilage with ligamentous laxity
- muscle imbalance
- abnormal intrauterine position
- central nervous system anomaly.

CAUSES
- Combination of genetic and environmental factors in utero
- Heredity
- Idiopathic
- Suspected muscle abnormalities, leading to variations in length and tendon insertions

INCIDENCE
- Clubfoot occurs in 1 of every 1,000 live births.
- This disorder usually occurs bilaterally.
- Clubfoot is twice as common in males as it is in females.
- Clubfoot may be linked to other birth defects, such as myelomeningocele, spina bifida, and arthrogryposis.

COMPLICATIONS
- Abnormal gait
- Stress changes on lateral side of the foot
- Residual deformity

HISTORY
- Family history
- Muscular atrophy or dystrophy

PHYSICAL FINDINGS
- Deformed talus with a shortened Achilles' tendon, the calcaneus somewhat shortened and flattened (see *Recognizing clubfoot*)
- Shortened, underdeveloped calf muscles, with soft tissue contractures at the site of the deformity
- Foot tight in its deformed position and resistant of manual efforts to push it back into normal position

IMAGING
- X-rays show superimposition of the talus and the calcaneus and a ladder-like appearance of the metatarsals.

OTHER
- Physical examination reveals clubfoot.

Recognizing clubfoot

Clubfoot (talipes) may have various names, depending on the orientation of the deformity, as shown in the illustrations below.

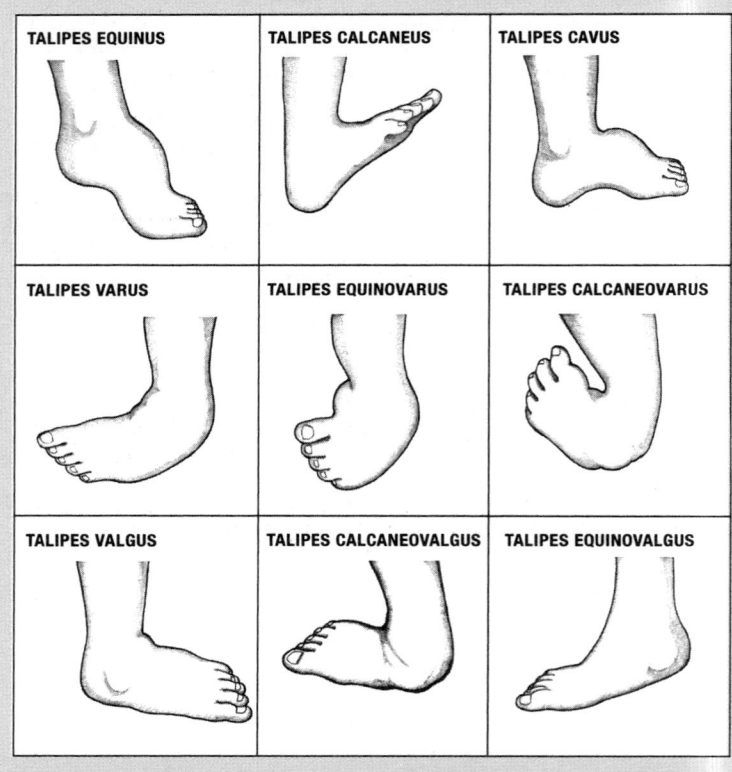

TALIPES EQUINUS   TALIPES CALCANEUS   TALIPES CAVUS

TALIPES VARUS   TALIPES EQUINOVARUS   TALIPES CALCANEOVARUS

TALIPES VALGUS   TALIPES CALCANEOVALGUS   TALIPES EQUINOVALGUS

TREATMENT

GENERAL
- Correction of the deformity
- Maintaining the correction until the foot regains normal muscle balance
- Close observation to prevent the deformity from recurring

ACTIVITY
- According to ability

Sequential correction
- Forefoot adduction; uncurling the front of the foot away from the heel (forefoot abduction)
- Varus deformity; turning the foot so the sole faces outward (eversion)
- Equinus; casting the foot with the toes pointing up (dorsiflexion)

Surgery
- Subcutaneous tenotomy of the Achilles' tendon and posterior capsulotomy of the ankle joint, with the equinus stage of correction
- In severe cases, bone surgery (wedge resections, osteotomy, or astragalectomy), with cast applied afterwards to preserve the correction

NURSING CONSIDERATIONS

NURSING DIAGNOSES
- Disturbed body image
- Fear
- Impaired physical mobility
- Risk for impaired skin integrity
- Risk for injury

EXPECTED OUTCOMES
The patient will:
- express positive feelings about self
- express fears and concerns
- maintain joint mobility, range of motion, and muscle strength
- maintain skin integrity
- show no evidence of complications, such as contractures, venous stasis, thrombus formulation, or skin breakdown.

NURSING INTERVENTIONS
- After casting, elevate the child's feet with pillows.
- Perform proper skin and cast care.

MONITORING
- Neurovascular status of affected extremity after casting or surgery
- Proper foot alignment
- Pain control

PATIENT TEACHING

GENERAL
Be sure to cover:
- the need for prompt treatment
- signs of circulatory impairment
- proper skin care
- use of exercise, night splints, and orthopedic shoes to maintain alignment.

DISCHARGE PLANNING
- Refer the parents to support services.
- Refer the parents to an orthopedic pediatrician for treatment or follow-up, as needed.
- Refer the parents to physical therapy, as needed.

RESOURCES
Organizations
American Academy of Orthopaedic Surgeons: *www.aaos.org*
American Orthopaedic Association: *www.aoassn.org*

Selected references
Diseases, 4th ed. Philadelphia: Lippincott Williams & Wilkins, 2006.
Faulks, S., and Luther, B. "Changing Paradigm for the Treatment of Clubfeet," *Orthopaedic Nursing* 24(1):25-30, January-February 2005.
Hart, E.S. "The Newborn Foot: Diagnosis and Management of Common Conditions," *Orthopaedic Nursing* 24(5):313-21, September-October 2005.
Nettina, S.M. *Lippincott Manual of Nursing Practice,* 8th ed. Philadelphia: Lippincott Williams & Wilkins, 2006.

Coarctation of the aorta

- A narrowing of the aorta, usually just below the left subclavian artery, near the site where the ligamentum arteriosum (the remnant of the ductus arteriosus, a fetal blood vessel) joins the pulmonary artery to the aorta
- May occur with aortic valve stenosis (usually of a bicuspid aortic valve) and with severe cases of hypoplasia of the aortic arch, patent ductus arteriosus (PDA), and ventricular septal defect
- Ineffective pumping of the heart and increased risk from heart failure due to the obstruction of blood flow

PATHOPHYSIOLOGY

- Coarctation of the aorta may develop as a result of spasm and constriction of the smooth muscle in the ductus arteriosus as it closes.
- This contractile tissue extends into the aortic wall, causing narrowing.
- The obstructive process causes hypertension in the aortic branches above the constriction (arteries that supply the arms, neck, and head) and diminished pressure in the vessel below the constriction.
- Restricted blood flow through the narrowed aorta increases the pressure load on the left ventricle and causes dilation of the proximal aorta and ventricular hypertrophy.
- As oxygenated blood leaves the left ventricle, a portion travels through the arteries that branch off the aorta proximal to the coarctation.
- If PDA is present, the rest of the blood travels through the coarctation, mixes with deoxygenated blood from the PDA, and travels to the legs.
- If PDA is closed, the legs and lower portion of the body must rely solely on the blood that gets through the coarctation.

CAUSES

- Exact cause unknown
- Turner's syndrome

INCIDENCE

- Coarctation of the aorta accounts for about 7% of all congenital heart defects in children.
- This disorder occurs twice as commonly in males as in females.
- In females, coarctation of the aorta is commonly linked to Turner's syndrome, a chromosomal disorder that causes ovarian dysgenesis.

COMPLICATIONS

- Heart failure
- Severe hypertension
- Cerebral aneurysms and hemorrhage
- Rupture of the aorta
- Aortic aneurysm
- Infective endocarditis

HISTORY

- Tachypnea
- Dyspnea
- Failure to thrive
- Headache
- Vertigo
- Epistaxis
- Claudication

PHYSICAL FINDINGS

- Pallor
- Hypertension
- Crackles
- Edema
- Tachycardia
- Cardiomegaly
- Hepatomegaly
- Hypertension
- Pink upper arms and cyanotic legs
- Absent or diminished femoral pulses
- Arm blood pressure greater than leg blood pressure
- Chest and arms more developed than legs

IMAGING

- Chest X-rays may show left ventricular hypertrophy, heart failure, a wide ascending and descending aorta, and notching of the ribs' undersurfaces due to erosion by collateral circulation. (See *Recognizing coarctation of the aorta*.)
- Echocardiography may show increased left ventricular muscle thickness, coexisting aortic valve abnormalities, and the coarctation site.
- Aortography locates the site and extent of coarctation.

DIAGNOSTIC PROCEDURES

- Electrocardiography may reveal left ventricular hypertrophy.
- Cardiac catheterization evaluates collateral circulation and measures pressure in the right and left ventricles and in the ascending and descending aortas (on both sides of the obstruction).

Recognizing coarctation of the aorta

Collateral circulation develops to bypass the occluded aortic lumen, and can be seen on X-ray as notching of the ribs. By adolescence, palpable, visible pulsations may be evident.

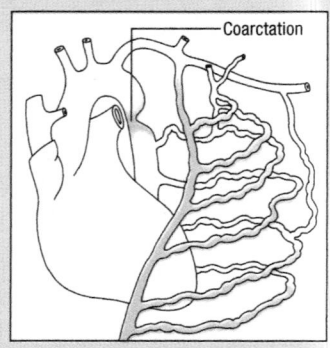

Coarctation

TREATMENT

DIET
◆ Low-sodium
◆ Fluid restrictions

ACTIVITY
◆ Limited

MEDICATIONS
◆ Digoxin
◆ Diuretics
◆ Oxygen
◆ Sedatives
◆ Prostaglandin infusion to keep the ductus open
◆ Antibiotic prophylaxis
◆ Antihypertensive therapy

SURGERY
◆ A flap of the left subclavian artery may be used to reconstruct the aorta.
◆ Balloon angioplasty or resection with end-to-end anastomosis or use of a tubular graft may also be performed.

NURSING CONSIDERATIONS

NURSING DIAGNOSES
◆ Activity intolerance
◆ Decreased cardiac output
◆ Fatigue
◆ Impaired parenting
◆ Ineffective tissue perfusion: Peripheral
◆ Risk for infection

EXPECTED OUTCOMES
The patient (or his family) will:
◆ carry out activities of daily living without weakness or fatigue
◆ maintain hemodynamic stability and cardiac output will remain adequate
◆ express feelings of energy and decreased fatigue
◆ agree to seek help from peer support groups or professional counselors to increase adaptive coping behaviors
◆ exhibit signs of adequate peripheral perfusion, such as positive distal pulses and warm extremities
◆ remain free from signs and symptoms of infection.

NURSING INTERVENTIONS
◆ Offer emotional support.
◆ Regulate environmental temperature.
◆ Give prescribed drugs.

MONITORING
◆ Vital signs
◆ Intake and output
◆ Oxygenation
◆ Blood glucose levels
◆ Postoperative pain
◆ Signs of infection

PATIENT TEACHING

GENERAL
Be sure to cover:
◆ the disorder, diagnosis, and treatment
◆ exercise restrictions
◆ endocarditis prophylaxis.

DISCHARGE PLANNING
◆ Stress the need for follow-up care, as ordered.

RESOURCES
Organizations
American Heart Association: *www.americanheart.org*
National Heart, Lung, and Blood Institute: *www.nhlbi.nih.gov*

Selected references
Kothari, S.S. "Dissection After Stent Dilatation for Coarctation of Aorta," *Catheterization and Cardiovascular Interventions* 62(3):421, July 2004.
Nettina, S.M. *Lippincott Manual of Nursing Practice,* 8th ed. Philadelphia: Lippincott Williams & Wilkins, 2006.

Coccidioidomycosis

OVERVIEW

- Fungal infection that occurs primarily as a respiratory tract infection, although generalized dissemination may occur
- Also known as *valley fever* or *San Joaquin Valley fever*

PATHOPHYSIOLOGY

- After spores are inhaled, cell activation and cytokine formation stimulate inflammatory cells and facilitate killing of the organism.
- Immunosuppression may delay resolution of the infection.

CAUSES

- Dressings or plaster casts of infected persons
- Inhaled spores of *Coccidioides immitis* found in the soil

INCIDENCE

- Disseminated illness is more common in dark-skinned men, pregnant women, and patients receiving an immunosuppressant.
- Coccidioidomycosis is endemic to the southwestern United States, especially between the San Joaquin Valley in California and southwestern Texas; it's also found in Mexico, Guatemala, Honduras, Venezuela, Colombia, Argentina, and Paraguay.
- This disease generally affects Filipino Americans, Hispanic Americans, Native Americans, and Blacks because of population distribution and an occupational link (common in migrant farm laborers).

COMPLICATIONS

- Meningitis
- Bronchiectasis
- Osteomyelitis
- Hepatosplenomegaly
- Liver failure

ASSESSMENT

HISTORY

- Living or traveling to an endemic area
- Fever
- Dry cough
- Pleuritic chest pain
- Sore throat
- Chills
- Malaise
- Headache
- Joint pain

PHYSICAL FINDINGS

- Fever
- Itchy macular rash
- Hemoptysis
- Local swelling and redness in involved sites (with musculoskeletal involvement)
- Bronchial breath sounds

DIAGNOSTIC TEST RESULTS

LABORATORY

- Complement fixation for immunoglobulin G antibodies.
- Positive serum precipitins (immunoglobulins) may be seen.
- *C. immitis* spores may be detected through immunodiffusion testing of sputum, pus from lesions, and tissue biopsy.
- Presence of antibodies in pleural and joint fluid and a rising serum or body fluid antibody titer (indicate dissemination) may be present.
- White blood cell count may be increased.
- Eosinophil count may be increased.
- Erythrocyte sedimentation rate may be increased.

IMAGING

- Chest X-ray shows bilateral diffuse infiltrates.

OTHER

- Abnormal coccidioidin skin test result

TREATMENT

GENERAL
◆ Symptomatic measures

ACTIVITY
◆ Bed rest

MEDICATIONS
◆ I.V. fluids
◆ Amphotericin B
◆ Analgesics

SURGERY
◆ Excision or drainage of lesions
◆ Lobectomy for severe pulmonary lesions

NURSING CONSIDERATIONS

NURSING DIAGNOSES
◆ Acute pain
◆ Impaired gas exchange
◆ Impaired skin integrity
◆ Ineffective airway clearance
◆ Ineffective breathing pattern
◆ Ineffective tissue perfusion: Cerebral, cardiopulmonary

EXPECTED OUTCOMES
The patient will:
◆ be free from pain
◆ maintain adequate ventilation
◆ exhibit improved or healed wounds
◆ maintain a patent airway
◆ maintain effective breathing pattern
◆ maintain tissue perfusion.

NURSING INTERVENTIONS
◆ Encourage bed rest.
◆ Encourage adequate fluid intake.
◆ Provide measures to relieve pain and increase comfort.

MONITORING
◆ Intake and output
◆ Vital signs
◆ Sputum color, consistency, and amount
◆ Respiratory status

PATIENT TEACHING

GENERAL
Be sure to cover:
◆ the disorder, diagnosis, and treatment
◆ proper hand-washing technique
◆ wound care.

RESOURCES
Organizations
Centers for Disease Control and Prevention: *www.cdc.gov*

Selected references
Diseases, 4th ed. Philadelphia: Lippincott Williams & Wilkins, 2006.

Galgiani, J.N., et al. "Coccidioidomycosis," *Clinical Infectious Diseases* 41(9):1217-223, November 2005.

Johnson, R.H., and Einstein, H.E. "Coccidioidal Meningitis," *Clinical Infectious Diseases* 42(1):103-107, January 2006.

Snyder, C.H. "Coccidioidal Meningitis Presenting as Memory Loss," *Journal of the American Academy of Nurse Practitioners* 17(5):181-86, May 2005.

Cold injuries

OVERVIEW

- Injury caused by overexposure to cold air or water
- Includes localized injuries (frostbite) and systemic injuries (hypothermia)
- Frostbite: superficial or deep; can lead to gangrene
- Hypothermia: core body temperature below 95° F (35° C)

PATHOPHYSIOLOGY

- Cold temperature causes ice crystals to form within and around tissue cells.
- Cell membranes rupture and enzymatic activities are interrupted.
- Histamine is released.
- Aggregation of red blood cells results.

CAUSES

- Administration of large amounts of cold blood
- Prolonged exposure to cold, wet environments
- Prolonged exposure to freezing temperatures

RISK FACTORS

- Lack of insulating body fat
- Substance abuse
- Cardiac disease
- Poverty, homelessness
- Immersion in cold water
- Altered mental state

INCIDENCE

- Cold injuries are more common in men than in women.

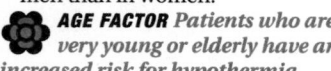 **AGE FACTOR** *Patients who are very young or elderly have an increased risk for hypothermia.*

COMPLICATIONS

- Renal failure
- Rhabdomyolysis
- Avascular necrosis
- Gangrene
- Severe infection
- Aspiration pneumonia
- Cardiac arrhythmias
- Hypoglycemia or hyperglycemia
- Metabolic acidosis
- Pancreatitis

ASSESSMENT

HISTORY

- Burning, numbness, tingling, and itching of affected area
- Paresthesia and stiffness while the part is still frozen
- Burning pain when the part thaws

PHYSICAL FINDINGS

Frostbite

- Superficial — swollen, with a mottled, blue-gray skin color
- Deep — white or yellow until thawed; then turns purplish blue
- Edema, skin blisters, and necrosis
- Skin immobility
- Presence or absence of associated peripheral pulses

Hypothermia

- Mild — severe shivering, slurred speech, and amnesia
- Moderate — unresponsive, with peripheral cyanosis and muscle rigidity
- Severe — appears dead, with no palpable pulse and no audible heart sounds

DIAGNOSTIC TEST RESULTS

LABORATORY

- Complete blood count and coagulation profile may show blood loss related to clotting abnormalities.
- Serum amylase may be elevated.
- Serum glucose may show hypoglycemia or hyperglycemia.
- Liver function studies may show hepatic failure.
- Serum corticotropin is elevated.
- Serum thyroid-stimulating hormone is elevated.
- White blood cell count is elevated.
- Arterial blood gas levels may show acid-base derangements; hypoxia.
- Serum electrolytes may show electrolyte derangements.

IMAGING

- Technetium pertechnetate scanning shows perfusion defects, deep tissue damage, and nonviable bone.
- Doppler and plethysmographic studies locate pulses and show extent of frostbite.

TREATMENT

GENERAL
Frostbite injuries
- Rapid rewarming of injured part
- Whirlpool treatments
- Elevation of extremity after rewarming

Hypothermia
- Removal of wet clothing
- Supportive measures
- Cardiopulmonary resuscitation
- Administration of warmed, humidified oxygen
- Endotracheal intubation with controlled ventilation
- Warmed I.V. fluids
- Treatment of metabolic acidosis

DIET
Hypothermia
- Nothing by mouth until fully alert
- Warmed fluids to drink
- Use of a convective air warmer

ACTIVITY
Frostbite injuries
- Active range-of-motion (ROM) exercises

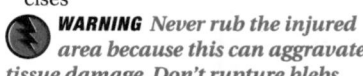 **WARNING** *Never rub the injured area because this can aggravate tissue damage. Don't rupture blebs.*

MEDICATIONS
Frostbite injuries
- Tetanus toxoid
- Antibiotics

Hypothermia
- Antiarrhythmics, as needed

SURGERY
- Fasciotomy or amputation for extensive tissue damage

NURSING CONSIDERATIONS

NURSING DIAGNOSES
- Acute pain
- Anxiety
- Decreased cardiac output
- Hypothermia
- Impaired gas exchange
- Impaired physical mobility
- Impaired skin integrity
- Ineffective tissue perfusion: Cardiopulmonary, peripheral
- Risk for disuse syndrome
- Risk for infection

EXPECTED OUTCOMES
The patient will:
- express feelings of increased comfort and relief from pain
- express feelings of decreased anxiety
- maintain adequate cardiac output
- experience a return of body temperature to normal
- maintain adequate ventilation
- attain the highest degree of mobility possible within the confines of the injury
- regain skin integrity
- exhibit signs of adequate cardiopulmonary and peripheral perfusion
- maintain muscle strength and tone and joint ROM
- remain free from signs and symptoms of infection.

NURSING INTERVENTIONS
Frostbite
- Remove constrictive clothing and jewelry.
- Perform rewarming measures.
- Give prescribed drugs.
- Never rub the injured area; this aggravates tissue damage.

Hypothermia
- Remove wet clothing.
- Maintain airway, breathing, and circulation.
- Perform rewarming measures.
- Perform supportive measures, as needed.

MONITORING
- Core body temperature
- Vital signs
- Cardiac status
- Peripheral vascular circulation

PATIENT TEACHING

GENERAL
Be sure to cover:
- the disorder, diagnosis, and treatment
- measures to avoid hypothermia
- complications and when to notify the practitioner.

DISCHARGE PLANNING
- Refer the patient to resource and support services.

RESOURCES
Organizations
National Center for Injury Prevention and Control: *www.cdc.gov/ncipc*
National Institutes of Health: *www.nih.gov*

Selected references
Davies, A. "Nursing a Patient with Frostbite," *Nursing Times* 101(46):52-54, November 2005.
McGillion, R. "Frostbite: Case Report, Practical Summary of ED Treatment," *Journal of Emergency Nursing* 31(5): 500-502, October 2005.
Neno, R. "Hypothermia: Assessment, Treatment and Prevention," *Nursing Standard* 19(20):47-52, January-February 2005.
Wolfson, A.B., et al. *Harwood-Nuss' Clinical Practice of Emergency Medicine*, 4th ed. Philadelphia: Lippincott Williams & Wilkins, 2005.

Colorectal cancer

OVERVIEW

- Malignant tumors of colon or rectum almost always adenocarcinomas (about half are sessile lesions of rectosigmoid area; all others are polypoid lesions)
- Slow progression
- Five-year survival rate 50%; potentially curable in 75% of patients if early diagnosis allows resection before nodal involvement
- Second most common visceral neoplasm in United States and Europe

PATHOPHYSIOLOGY

- Most lesions of the large bowel are moderately differentiated adenocarcinomas.
- Tumors tend to grow slowly and remain asymptomatic for long periods.
- Tumors in the sigmoid and descending colon undergo circumferential growth and constrict the intestinal lumen.
- Tumors in the ascending colon are usually large at diagnosis and are palpable on physical examination.

CAUSES

- Unknown

RISK FACTORS

- Excessive intake of saturated animal fat
- Digestive tract diseases
- Older than age 40
- History of ulcerative colitis
- Familial polyposis
- Family history of colon cancer
- High-protein, low-fiber diet

INCIDENCE

- Colorectal cancer is equally distributed among men and women.
- Incidence of this disease is greater in areas of higher economic development.

COMPLICATIONS

- Abdominal distention and intestinal obstruction as tumor growth encroaches on abdominal organs
- Anemia

ASSESSMENT

HISTORY

- Right colon tumors: no signs and symptoms in early stages because stool is liquid in that part of colon
- Black, tarry stools
- Abdominal aching, pressure, or dull cramps
- Weakness
- Diarrhea, anorexia, obstipation, weight loss, and vomiting
- Rectal bleeding
- Intermittent abdominal fullness
- Rectal pressure
- Urgent need to defecate on arising

PHYSICAL FINDINGS

- Abdominal distention or visible masses
- Enlarged abdominal veins
- Enlarged inguinal and supraclavicular nodes
- Abnormal bowel sounds
- Abdominal masses (right-side tumors that usually feel bulky; tumors of transverse portion more easily detected)
- Generalized abdominal tenderness

DIAGNOSTIC TEST RESULTS

LABORATORY

- Fecal occult blood test possibly may show blood in stools, a warning sign of rectal cancer.
- Carcinoembryonic antigen may permit patient monitoring before and after treatment to detect metastasis or recurrence.

IMAGING

- Excretory urography verifies bilateral renal function and allows inspection for displacement of the kidneys, ureters, or bladder by a tumor pressing against these structures.
- Barium enema studies use a dual contrast of barium and air and reveal the location of lesions that aren't detectable manually or visually. Barium examination shouldn't precede colonoscopy or excretory urography because barium sulfate interferes with these tests.
- Computed tomography scan allows better visualization if a barium enema yields inconclusive results or if metastasis to the pelvic lymph nodes is suspected.

DIAGNOSTIC PROCEDURES

- Proctoscopy or sigmoidoscopy permits visualization of the lower GI tract. It can detect up to 66% of colorectal cancers.
- Colonoscopy permits visual inspection and photography of the colon up to the ileocecal valve and provides access for polypectomies and biopsies of suspected lesions.

OTHER

- Digital rectal examination can be used to detect almost 15% of colorectal cancers; specifically, it can be used to detect suspicious rectal and perianal lesions.

TREATMENT

GENERAL
◆ Radiation preoperatively and postoperatively to induce tumor regression

DIET
◆ High-fiber

ACTIVITY
◆ After surgery, avoidance of heavy lifting and contact sports

MEDICATIONS
◆ Chemotherapy for metastasis, residual disease, or recurrent inoperable tumor
◆ Analgesics

SURGERY
◆ Resection or right hemicolectomy for advanced disease; surgery may include resection of the terminal segment of the ileum, cecum, ascending colon, and right half of the transverse colon with corresponding mesentery
◆ Right colectomy that includes the transverse colon and mesentery corresponding to midcolic vessels, or segmental resection of the transverse colon and associated midcolic vessels
◆ Resection surgery usually limited to the sigmoid colon and mesentery
◆ Anterior or low anterior resection (newer method, using a stapler, allows for much lower resections than previously possible)
◆ Abdominoperineal resection and permanent sigmoid colostomy required

NURSING CONSIDERATIONS

NURSING DIAGNOSES
◆ Acute pain
◆ Anxiety
◆ Constipation
◆ Deficient fluid volume
◆ Diarrhea
◆ Disturbed body image
◆ Fear
◆ Imbalanced nutrition: Less than body requirements
◆ Impaired oral mucous membrane
◆ Impaired skin integrity
◆ Ineffective coping
◆ Risk for infection
◆ Sexual dysfunction

EXPECTED OUTCOMES
The patient will:
◆ express feeling of comfort and relief from pain
◆ express feelings of decreased anxiety
◆ have soft, formed stools that are easy to pass
◆ maintain normal fluid volume
◆ resume a regular elimination pattern
◆ express positive feelings about self
◆ verbalize fears and concerns relating to the diagnosis and condition
◆ maintain adequate nutrition and hydration
◆ have mucous membranes that remain intact
◆ maintain skin integrity
◆ demonstrate adaptive coping behaviors
◆ avoid infection and other complications
◆ verbalize feelings about potential or actual changes in sexual activity.

NURSING INTERVENTIONS
◆ Provide support and encourage verbalization.
◆ Give prescribed drugs.

MONITORING
◆ Stools
◆ Diet

Postoperative
◆ Vital signs
◆ Intake and output
◆ Hydration and nutritional status
◆ Electrolyte levels
◆ Wound site
◆ Postoperative complications
◆ Bowel function
◆ Pain control
◆ Psychological status

PATIENT TEACHING

GENERAL
Be sure to cover:
◆ the disease process, treatment, and postoperative course
◆ stoma care
◆ avoidance of heavy lifting
◆ the need for keeping follow-up appointments
◆ risk factors and signs of reoccurrence.

DISCHARGE PLANNING
◆ Refer the patient to resource and support services.

RESOURCES
Organizations
American Cancer Society: *www.cancer.org*
Guide to Internet Resources for Cancer: *www.cancerindex.org*
National Cancer Institute: *www.nci.nih.gov*
United Ostomy Association, Inc.: *www.uoa.org*

Selected references
Atlas of Pathophysiology, 2nd ed. Philadelphia: Lippincott Williams & Wilkins, 2005.
Casciato, D.A. *Manual of Clinical Oncology,* 5th ed. Philadelphia: Lippincott Williams & Wilkins, 2004.
Viale, P.H., et al. "Advanced Colorectal Cancer: Current Treatment and Nursing Management with Economic Considerations," *Clinical Journal of Oncology Nursing* 9(5):541-52, October 2005.
Wilkes, G.M. "Therapeutic Options in the Management of Colon Cancer: 2005 Update," *Clinical Journal of Oncology Nursing* 9(1):31-44, February 2005.

Common cold

- Acute, usually afebrile viral infection that causes inflammation of the upper respiratory tract
- Transmission through airborne respiratory droplets or through contact with contaminated objects, including hands
- Accounts for 30% to 50% of time lost from work by adults and 60% to 80% of time lost from school by children, more than any other illness
- Communicable for 2 to 3 days after onset of symptoms
- Usually benign and self-limiting

PATHOPHYSIOLOGY

- Rhinoviruses infect cells by attaching to specific receptors.
- Infiltration with neutrophils, lymphocytes, plasma cells, and eosinophils occurs.
- Mucus-secreting glands become hyperactive and nasal turbinates become engorged. (See *What happens in the common cold.*)

CAUSES

- More than 200 viruses, including rhinoviruses, coronaviruses, myxoviruses, adenoviruses, coxsackieviruses, and echoviruses
- Mycoplasma
- Viral infection of the upper respiratory tract passages and consequent mucous membrane inflammation responsible for 90% of cases

INCIDENCE

- The cold is the most common infectious disease.
- It's more prevalent in children, adolescent boys, and women.
- In temperate climates, colds occur more often in the colder months.
- In the tropics, colds occur more often during the rainy season.

COMPLICATIONS

- Secondary bacterial infection, causing sinusitis, otitis media, pharyngitis, or lower respiratory tract infection

HISTORY

- Exposure to persons with the common cold
- Sore throat
- Fatigue
- Malaise
- Myalgia
- Fever

PHYSICAL FINDINGS

- Copious nasal discharge that often irritates the nose
- Increased erythema of nasal and pharyngeal mucous membranes
- Nasal quality to voice
- Excoriated skin around nose

There are no diagnostic tests for this disorder.

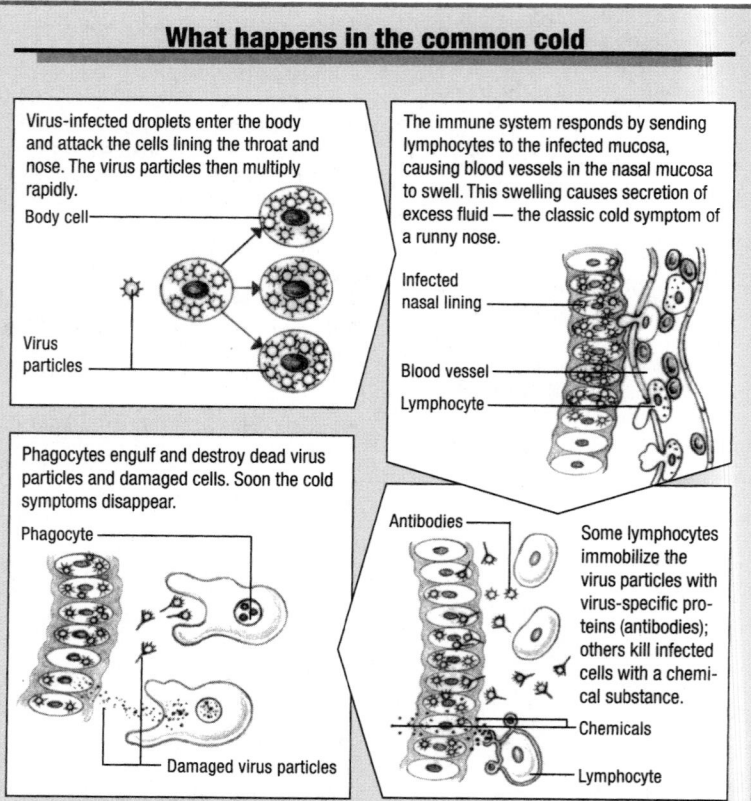

What happens in the common cold

Virus-infected droplets enter the body and attack the cells lining the throat and nose. The virus particles then multiply rapidly.

Body cell

Virus particles

The immune system responds by sending lymphocytes to the infected mucosa, causing blood vessels in the nasal mucosa to swell. This swelling causes secretion of excess fluid — the classic cold symptom of a runny nose.

Infected nasal lining

Blood vessel

Lymphocyte

Phagocytes engulf and destroy dead virus particles and damaged cells. Soon the cold symptoms disappear.

Phagocyte

Damaged virus particles

Some lymphocytes immobilize the virus particles with virus-specific proteins (antibodies); others kill infected cells with a chemical substance.

Antibodies

Chemicals

Lymphocyte

TREATMENT

GENERAL
◆ Use of humidified inspired air
◆ Prevention of chilling

DIET
◆ Increased fluid intake

ACTIVITY
◆ Rest periods, as needed

MEDICATIONS
◆ Acetylsalicylate acid
◆ Ibuprofen
◆ Acetaminophen
◆ Throat lozenges
◆ Antitussives
◆ In infants, saline nose drops and mucus aspiration with a bulb syringe
◆ Vitamin therapy, interferon administration, and experimental vaccines (under investigation)

NURSING CONSIDERATIONS

NURSING DIAGNOSES
◆ Acute pain
◆ Fatigue
◆ Hyperthermia
◆ Ineffective airway clearance
◆ Ineffective breathing pattern
◆ Risk for infection

EXPECTED OUTCOMES
The patient will:
◆ express feeling of increased comfort
◆ report increased energy
◆ remain afebrile
◆ expectorate sputum effectively and maintain a patent airway
◆ maintain effective breathing pattern and express feelings of comfort in maintaining air exchange
◆ experience no further signs or symptoms of infection.

NURSING INTERVENTIONS
◆ Give prescribed drugs.
◆ A lubricant on nostrils can decrease irritation.
◆ Relieve throat irritation with sugarless hard candy or cough drops.
◆ A warm bath or heating pad can reduce aches and pains.
◆ Suggest a hot or cold steam vaporizer to relieve nasal congestion.

MONITORING
◆ Body temperature
◆ Respiratory status
◆ Response to treatment
◆ Adverse effects of medication
◆ Complications

PATIENT TEACHING

GENERAL
Be sure to cover:
◆ advice against overuse of nose drops or sprays
◆ how to avoid spreading colds
◆ proper hand-washing technique.

DISCHARGE PLANNING
◆ Refer the patient for medical care if a high fever persists, level of consciousness changes, or significant respiratory symptoms develop.

RESOURCES
Organizations
Centers for Disease Control and Prevention: *www.cdc.gov*
Harvard University Consumer Health Information: *www.intelihealth.com*
National Health Information Center: *www.health.gov/nhic/*
National Library of Medicine: *www.nlm.nih.gov*

Selected references
Arroll, B. "Non-Antibiologic Treatments for Upper-Respiratory Tract Infections (Common Cold)," *Respiratory Medicine* 99(12):1477-484, December 2005.
Diseases, 4th ed. Philadelphia: Lippincott Williams & Wilkins, 2006.
Eccles, R. "Understanding the Symptoms of the Common Cold and Influenza," *The Lancet Infectious Diseases* 5(11): 718-25, November 2005.
Kasper, D.L., et al., eds. *Harrison's Principles of Internal Medicine,* 16th ed. New York: McGraw-Hill Book Co., 2005.
Sitzman, K. "Managing the Common Cold," *AAOHN Journal* 53(2):96, February 2005.

Complex regional pain syndrome

- A chronic pain disorder that results from abnormal healing after minor or major injury to a bone, muscle, or nerve
- Also known as *reflex sympathetic dystrophy* or *causalgia*

PATHOPHYSIOLOGY

- Abnormal functioning of the sympathetic nervous system causes development of symptoms commonly disproportionate to the injury's severity.
- Interference with normal signals for sensations, temperature, and blood flow may be caused by impaired communication between the damaged nerves of the sympathetic nervous system and the brain.

CAUSES

- Exact cause unknown

Precipitating factors

- Trauma
- Neurologic disorder
- Herpes zoster infection
- Myocardial infarction
- Musculoskeletal disorder (shoulder rotator cuff injury)
- Malignancy

INCIDENCE

- Complex regional pain syndrome may occur at any age but is less common in children.
- This syndrome is more common in women.

COMPLICATIONS

- Impaired mobility
- Depression

ASSESSMENT

HISTORY

- Injury
- Severe pain that worsens after activity

PHYSICAL FINDINGS

- Altered blood flow, feeling either warm or cool to the touch, with discoloration, sweating, or swelling to the affected extremity
- Skin, hair, and nail changes
- Impaired mobility and weakness
- Muscle wasting (see *Stages of complex regional pain syndrome*)

Stages of complex regional pain syndrome

Complex regional pain syndrome is divided into three stages. The stages aren't always distinct and not all of the signs may be present.

STAGE	DURATION	PAIN, SWELLING, AND IMMOBILITY	SKIN	HAIR AND NAILS	OSTEOPOROSIS
I (acute)	• Symptoms begin within hours, days, or weeks of the injury; this stage lasts several weeks	• Gradual or abrupt onset of severe aching, throbbing, and burning pain at site of injury • Pain may be accompanied by sensitivity to touch, swelling, muscle spasm, stiffness, and limited mobility	• Warm, red, dry skin at onset; changes to bluish and becomes cold and sweaty	• Accelerated hair and nail growth	• Early osteoporosis symptoms
II (subacute or dystrophic)	• Lasts 3 to 6 months	• Continuous burning, aching, or throbbing pain that's more severe than stage I • Swelling spreads and changes from soft to brawny and firm • Loss of range of motion, muscle wasting	• Cool, pale, bluish, sweaty	• Altered hair growth; cracked, grooved, or ridged nails	• More apparent osteoporosis
III (chronic or atrophic)	• Lasts more than 6 months	• Pain spreads proximately and may be intractable, but sometimes lessens and stabilizes • More distinct dystrophic changes and irreversible tissue damage • Muscle atrophy and contractures	• Thin, shiny	• Increasingly brittle and ridged nails	• Marked diffuse osteoporosis

DIAGNOSTIC TEST RESULTS

IMAGING
◆ Bone X-rays to rule out other conditions

TREATMENT

GENERAL
◆ Physical therapy

ACTIVITY
◆ As tolerated

MEDICATIONS
◆ Anti-inflammatories
◆ Antidepressants
◆ Vasodilators
◆ Analgesics
◆ Nerve blocks

SURGERY
◆ Surgical sympathectomy

NURSING CONSIDERATIONS

NURSING DIAGNOSES
◆ Acute pain
◆ Anxiety
◆ Impaired tissue integrity
◆ Ineffective tissue perfusion: Peripheral

EXPECTED OUTCOMES
The patient will:
◆ express increased comfort and reduced levels of pain
◆ identify strategies to reduce anxiety
◆ experience decreased redness, swelling, and pain at the site of impaired tissue
◆ have palpable peripheral pulses and warm extremities.

NURSING INTERVENTIONS
◆ Offer emotional support.
◆ Apply antiembolism stockings.
◆ Apply heat or cold therapy.

MONITORING
◆ Pain control
◆ Effects of medications
◆ Blood glucose level

PATIENT TEACHING

GENERAL
Be sure to cover:
◆ the disease and treatment
◆ relaxation techniques
◆ medication administration, dosage, and adverse effects.

DISCHARGE PLANNING
◆ Refer the patient for home therapy or for physical or occupational therapy.
◆ Refer the patient to a pain care specialist.
◆ Refer the patient for psychological counseling and support groups, as indicated.

RESOURCES
Organizations
American Chronic Pain Association: *www.theacpa.org*
American Neurological Association: *www.aneuroa.org*

Selected references
Diseases, 4th ed. Philadelphia: Lippincott Williams & Wilkins, 2006.

Greipp, M.E. "Complex Regional Pain Syndrome — Type I: Research Relevance, Practice Realities," *The Journal of Neuroscience Nursing* 35(1):16-20, February 2003.

Moseley, G.L. "Distorted Body Image in Complex Regional Pain Syndrome," *Neurology* 65(5):773, September 2005.

Schinkel, C., et al. "Inflammatory Mediators are Altered in the Acute Phase of Post-traumatic Complex Regional Pain Syndrome," *Clinical Journal of Pain* 22(3):235-39, March-April 2006.

Concussion

- Blow to the head forceful enough to jostle the brain and make it strike the skull
- Acceleration-deceleration injury
- Causes temporary (less than 48 hours) neural dysfunction

PATHOPHYSIOLOGY

- Concussion causes diffuse soft tissue damage.
- Inflammation occurs.
- Structural damage is usually minimal.

CAUSES

- Trauma to the head

INCIDENCE

- There are more than 2 million instances of concussion per year in the United States.
- Concussion may occur in up to 20% of football players.
- This disorder is more common in males than in females.
- Concussion most commonly affects those ages 15 to 24.

COMPLICATIONS

- Seizures
- Persistent vomiting
- Intracranial hemorrhage (rare)

HISTORY

- Trauma to head
- Short-term loss of consciousness
- Vomiting
- Antegrade and retrograde amnesia
- Change in level of consciousness (LOC)
- Dizziness
- Nausea
- Severe headache

PHYSICAL FINDINGS

- Tenderness or hematomas on skull palpation

IMAGING

- Computed tomography scan and magnetic resonance imaging help to rule out fractures and more serious injuries.

TREATMENT

GENERAL
- Observation for changes in mental status
- Proper positioning of head-of-bed to promote venous drainage

DIET
- Clear liquids if vomiting occurs

ACTIVITY
- Bed rest initially
- Avoidance of contact sports until fully recovered

MEDICATIONS
- Nonopioid analgesics

What to look for after a concussion

Before the patient's discharge, follow these teaching guidelines. Instruct the caregiver to awaken the patient every 2 hours through the night and to ask his name and whether he can identify the caregiver.

Advise the caregiver to return the patient to the facility immediately if he is difficult to arouse, is disoriented, has headache, forceful or constant vomiting, blurred vision, changes in personality, abnormal eye movements, a staggering gait, or twitching. If the patient is a child, explain to the parents that some children have no apparent ill effects immediately after a concussion but may grow lethargic or somnolent a few hours later. Teach the patient the signs of postconcussion syndrome — headache, vertigo, anxiety, personality changes, memory loss, and fatigue. Explain that these signs may persist for several weeks.

NURSING CONSIDERATIONS

NURSING DIAGNOSES
- Acute pain
- Anxiety
- Decreased intracranial adaptive capacity
- Ineffective coping
- Risk for deficient fluid volume
- Risk for injury
- Risk for posttrauma syndrome

EXPECTED OUTCOMES
The patient will:
- state and carry out appropriate interactions for pain relief
- report feelings of decreased anxiety
- maintain a stable neurologic state
- demonstrate effective coping mechanisms
- maintain adequate fluid volume
- identify factors that increase the potential for injury
- express feelings and fears about the traumatic event.

NURSING INTERVENTIONS
- Give prescribed drugs, and avoid opioids that may decrease LOC.
- Reorient to time and place, if needed.

MONITORING
- Vital signs
- Neurologic status
- Pain

PATIENT TEACHING

GENERAL
Be sure to cover:
- the injury, diagnosis, and treatment
- nonopioid analgesics for a headache and avoidance of products containing aspirin
- change in LOC or projectile vomiting, which requires a return to the hospital
- signs and symptoms of increased intracranial pressure
- residual effects (dizziness, headaches, and memory loss) and possibility that they may persist for up to 3 to 4 months after head injury

DISCHARGE PLANNING
- Arrange for continued observation at home. (See *What to look for after a concussion.*)

RESOURCES
Organizations
American Academy of Neurology: *www.aan.com*
Brain Injury Society: *www.bisociety.org*
Head Injury Hotline: *www.headinjury.com*
Med Help International: *www.medhelp.org*

Selected references
Collins, M., et al. "New Developments in the Management of Sports Concussion," *Current Opinion in Orthopedics* 15(2):100-107, April 2004.
Moser, R.S., et al. "Prolonged Effects of Concussion in High School Athletes," *Neurosurgery* 57(2):300-306, August 2005.
Nolan, S. "Traumatic Brain Injury: A Review," *Critical Care Nursing Quarterly* 28(2):188-94, April-June 2005.

Conduct disorder

- Aggressive behavior
- A child with this disorder fights, bullies, intimidates, and assaults others physically or sexually
- The patient typically has poor relationships with peers and adults, and violates others' rights and society's rules
- Evolves slowly over time until a consistent pattern of behavior is established

PATHOPHYSIOLOGY

- Biological (including genetic) and psychosocial components

CAUSES

- Biological (including genetic) and psychosocial
- Child abuse and neglect
- Impaired functioning of the non-adrenergic system
- Neurologic damage caused by low birth weight or birth complications
- Social risk factors that predispose a child to the disorder include: socioeconomic deprivation; harsh punitive parenting with verbal or physical aggression; separation from parents; early institutionalization; family neglect, abuse, or neglect; frequent verbal abuse; parental psychiatric illness, substance abuse, or marital discord; large family size, crowding, and poverty; and divorce with persistent hostility between the parents.
- Underarousal of the autonomic nervous system

INCIDENCE

- The prevalence of conduct disorder among children ages 9 to 17 is about 1% to 4%.
- Conduct disorder occurs in 6% to 16% of boys and 2% to 9% of girls younger than 18.

COMPLICATIONS

- Adult antisocial personality disorders (in children with early onset)
- Poor performance in school
- Substance abuse
- Injury from risk-taking behaviors
- Higher incidence of attention deficit hyperactivity disorder, mood disorders, anxiety disorders, depression, and learning difficulties

HISTORY

- Child fights, bullies, intimidates, and assaults others physically and sexually

PHYSICAL FINDINGS

- Abusing others sexually
- Cheating in school
- Cruelty to animals
- Engaging in precocious sexual activity
- Fighting with family members and peers
- Skipping classes
- Smoking cigarettes
- Speaking to others in a hostile manner
- Stealing or shoplifting
- Using drugs or alcohol
- Vandalizing or destroying property

DSM-IV-TR *criteria*

A patient with conduct disorder must meet at least three of the criteria from any of the following categories (must have been noted within the year prior to the time of examination, and at least one criterion must have been present within the past 6 months):

- Aggression to people and animals
- Destruction of property
- Deceitfulness
- Serious violations of rules
- Additional criteria:
- The behavior disturbance must cause clinically significant impairment in social, academic, or occupational functioning.
- The patient is age 18 or older and doesn't meet the criteria for antisocial personality disorder.

There are no diagnostic tests for this disorder.

TREATMENT

GENERAL
- Structured living environment
- Consistent rules and consequences

MEDICATIONS
- Antipsychotics
- Lithium
- Clonidine
- Selective serotonin reuptake inhibitors

NURSING CONSIDERATIONS

NURSING DIAGNOSES
- Disabled family coping
- Impaired adjustment
- Impaired social interaction
- Ineffective coping
- Interrupted family processes
- Risk for other-directed violence

EXPECTED OUTCOMES
The patient (or his family) will:
- attend counseling to discuss the patient's illness and learn how to handle his behavior
- develop effective coping skills to help process stressors
- develop effective social interaction and problem-solving skills
- utilize constructive channels to release anger
- express awareness of how his actions affect others
- not harm others physically or emotionally.

NURSING INTERVENTIONS
- Work to establish a trusting relationship with the child.
- Provide clear behavioral guidelines, including consequences for disruptive and manipulative behavior.
- Help the child accept responsibility for behavior rather than blaming others, becoming defensive, and wanting revenge.

MONITORING
- Patterns of behavior
- Social interaction
- Response to treatment
- Complications
- Adverse drug reactions

PATIENT TEACHING

GENERAL
Be sure to cover:
- effective coping skills, social skills, and problem-solving skills, and have the child demonstrate them in return.
- expressing anger appropriately through constructive methods to release negative feelings and frustrations.
- role-playing in order to help the child practice handling stress and gain skill and confidence in managing difficult situations.

RESOURCES
Organizations
American Psychiatric Association: *www.psych.org*
National Mental Health Association: *www.nmha.org*

Selected references
Diagnostic and Statistical Manual of Mental Disorders, Fourth Edition, Text Revision. Washington, D.C.: American Psychiatric Association, 2000.
Nettina, S.M. *Lippincott Manual of Nursing Practice,* 8th ed. Philadelphia: Lippincott Williams & Wilkins, 2006.
Thomas, C.R. "Evidence-based Practice for Conduct Disorder Symptoms," *Journal of the American Academy of Child and Adolescent Psychiatry* 45(1):109-14, January 2006.

Conjunctivitis

OVERVIEW

- Inflammation of palpebral or bulbar conjunctiva
- Characterized by hyperemia of the conjunctiva
- Usually spreads rapidly from one eye to the other
- Usually benign and self-limiting
- Seldom affects vision
- Acute bacterial conjunctivitis (pink eye): usually lasts about 2 weeks
- Viral conjunctivitis: lasts 2 to 3 weeks, is chronic, and may produce severe disability
- If chronic, may signal degenerative changes or damage from repeated acute attacks

PATHOPHYSIOLOGY

- Conjunctivitis is an inflammatory response of the conjunctiva.
- Vernal conjunctivitis is associated with a severe form of immunoglobulin E–mediated mast cell hypersensitivity reaction.

CAUSES

- Allergens
- Bacteria
- Candidal infection
- Chemical irritations
- Systemic diseases, such as erythema multiforme and thyroid disease
- Transmission by contaminated towels, washcloths, or one's own hand
- Viruses

INCIDENCE

- Conjunctivitis is the most common eye disorder in the Western hemisphere.
- This disorder is responsible for about 30% of all eye complaints.

COMPLICATIONS

- Tic
- Corneal infiltrates
- Corneal ulcers
- Eye loss

ASSESSMENT

HISTORY

- Eye pain
- Photophobia
- Burning, itching, and sensation of a foreign body in the eye
- Sore throat and fever, in children

PHYSICAL FINDINGS

- Conjunctival hyperemia
- Discharge
- Tearing
- Crust of sticky, mucopurulent discharge (in bacterial conjunctivitis)
- Profuse, purulent discharge (in gonococcal conjunctivitis)
- Copious tearing and minimal discharge (in viral conjunctivitis)
- Conjunctival papillae (in vernal conjunctivitis) (see *Recognizing conjunctival papillae*)
- Ipsilateral preauricular lymph node enlargement (in viral conjunctivitis)

DIAGNOSTIC TEST RESULTS

LABORATORY

- Culture and sensitivity tests may identify the bacterial pathogen.
- Stained smears of conjunctival scrapings may show mostly monocytes with viral conjunctivitis; polymorphonuclear cells (neutrophils) predominating with bacterial conjunctivitis; and eosinophils predominating with allergic conjunctivitis.

Recognizing conjunctival papillae

If you see papillae in the conjunctiva of the upper eyelid, your patient may have vernal (allergic) conjunctivitis. These cobblestone bumps are the telltale sign. They result from swollen lymph tissue within the conjunctival membrane.

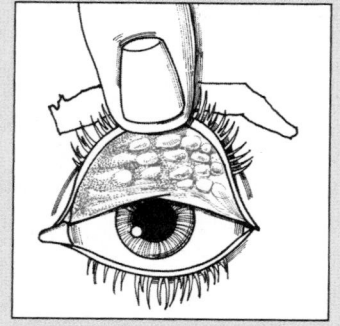

TREATMENT

GENERAL
- Warm compresses
- Depends on cause

MEDICATIONS
- Antibiotic eyedrops
- Antivirals
- Corticosteroids
- Histamine-1 receptor antagonists
- Oral antihistamines

NURSING CONSIDERATIONS

NURSING DIAGNOSES
- Anxiety
- Disturbed sensory perception: Visual
- Ineffective health maintenance
- Risk for infection
- Risk for injury

EXPECTED OUTCOMES
The patient will:
- report feeling less anxious
- regain normal visual functioning
- maintain current health status
- remain free from signs and symptoms of infection
- avoid injury.

NURSING INTERVENTIONS
- Apply warm compresses.
- Apply therapeutic ointment or eyedrops, as ordered.
- Avoid irrigating the eye to prevent the spread of infection.
- Notify public health officials if culture results identify *Neisseria gonorrhoeae.*
- Obtain culture specimens before antibiotic therapy.

MONITORING
- Response to treatment
- Signs and symptoms of complications
- Adverse reactions
- Visual acuity

PATIENT TEACHING

GENERAL
Be sure to cover:
- proper hand-washing technique
- instillation of eyedrops and ointments
- completing the prescribed antibiotics
- methods for preventing disease transmission
- importance of avoiding chemical irritants
- avoiding eye makeup and contact lens use until the infection has cleared.

WARNING *Caution the patient to avoid rubbing the infected eye so that he can prevent the spread of infection to the other eye or to other people.*

RESOURCES
Organizations
American Academy of Ophthalmology: *www.aao.org*
National Institute of Allergy and Infectious Diseases: *www.niaid.nih.gov*

Selected references
Bonini, S. "Allergic Conjunctivitis: The Forgotten Disease," *Chemical Immunology and Allergy* 91:110-20, 2006.
Khan, J. "Eye Know It's Red," *Lancet* 366(9496):1583, October-November 2005.
Professional Guide to Diseases, 8th ed. Philadelphia: Lippincott Williams & Wilkins, 2005.

Corneal abrasion

OVERVIEW

- Scratch on the epithelial surface of the cornea
- Prognosis usually good with appropriate treatment

PATHOPHYSIOLOGY

- Epithelial layers of cornea are lost due to trauma.
- Superficial abrasions don't involve the Bowman's membrane.
- Deep abrasions penetrate the Bowman's membrane.

CAUSES

- Chemicals
- Contact lenses
- Corneal or epithelial disease (dry eye)
- Dust
- Eye trauma
- Fingernails
- Foreign bodies embedded under eyelid
- Hair brushes
- Tree branches

INCIDENCE

- Corneal abrasion affects males and females equally.

COMPLICATIONS

- Corneal erosion
- Corneal ulceration
- Permanent vision loss
- Secondary infection

ASSESSMENT

HISTORY

- Eye trauma
- Prolonged contact lens wear
- Sensation of foreign body in eye
- Sensitivity to light
- Decreased visual acuity
- Eye pain

PHYSICAL FINDINGS

- Redness in eye
- Increased tearing
- Possibly a foreign object embedded under the eyelid, uncovered by eyelid eversion
- Disruption of corneal surface

DIAGNOSTIC TEST RESULTS

DIAGNOSTIC PROCEDURES

- Fluorescein staining of the injured area of the cornea appears green when illuminated.
- Slit-lamp examination discloses the depth of the abrasion.

TREATMENT

GENERAL

- Eye irrigation (see *Performing eye irrigation*)
- Removal of foreign body
- Warm compresses
- Eye patch for 24 hours
- Eye protection with potentially dangerous activities

MEDICATIONS

- Antibiotic eyedrops or ointment

SURGERY

- Surgical repair of corneal lacerations by an ophthalmologist

NURSING CONSIDERATIONS

NURSING DIAGNOSES
◆ Acute pain
◆ Disturbed sensory perception: Visual
◆ Fear
◆ Ineffective health maintenance
◆ Risk for injury

EXPECTED OUTCOMES
The patient will:
◆ express feelings of increased comfort
◆ regain normal visual functioning
◆ verbalize feelings and concerns
◆ maintain current health status
◆ avoid injury.

NURSING INTERVENTIONS
◆ Use a flashlight to inspect the cornea.
◆ Check visual acuity before treatment begins.
◆ If a foreign body is present, irrigate the eye with 0.9% sodium chloride solution.
◆ Give prescribed antibiotics and cycloplegics.
◆ Instill prescribed topical anesthetics.

 WARNING *Never give the patient topical anesthetic drops for self-administration. Abuse of this medication can delay healing, especially if the patient rubs the numb eye and further injures it.*

MONITORING
◆ Visual acuity
◆ Response to treatment

 WARNING *Pulse oximeter probes should be applied to the middle, ring, or preferably little finger, but never the index finger, in order to minimize the likelihood of corneal abrasion, especially as patients emerge from anesthesia.*

PATIENT TEACHING

GENERAL
Be sure to cover:
◆ the healing process
◆ proper instillation of antibiotic eyedrops or ointment
◆ effects of untreated corneal infection
◆ need to wear safety glasses in the workplace, if appropriate
◆ contact lens care and instructions for wear.

RESOURCES
Organizations
American Academy of Ophthalmology: *www.aao.org*
National Eye Institute: *www.nei.nih.gov*

Selected references
Mukherjee, P. and Sivakumar, A. "Tetanus Prophylaxis in Superficial Corneal Abrasions," *Emergency Medicine Journal* 20(1):62-64, January 2003.
Nettina, S.M. *Lippincott Manual of Nursing Practice,* 8th ed. Philadelphia: Lippincott Williams & Wilkins, 2006.
Professional Guide to Diseases, 8th ed. Philadelphia: Lippincott Williams & Wilkins, 2005.

Performing eye irrigation

SQUEEZE BOTTLE
For moderate-volume irrigation — to remove eye secretions, for example — apply sterile ophthalmic irrigant to the eye directly from the squeeze bottle container. Direct the stream at the inner canthus and position the patient so that the stream washes across the cornea and exits at the outer canthus.

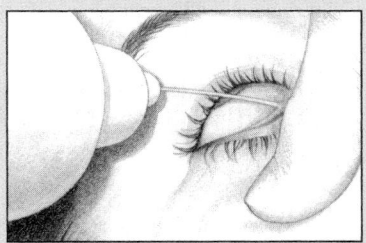

I.V. TUBE
For copious irrigation — to treat chemical burns, for example — set up an I.V. bag and tubing without a needle. Use the procedure described for moderate irrigation to flush the eye for at least 15 minutes. Alkali burns may require irrigation for several hours.

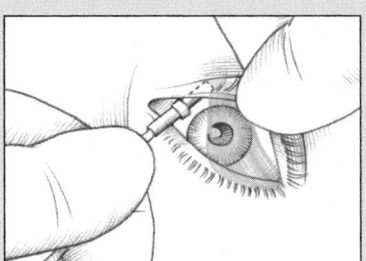

MORGAN LENS
Connected to irrigation tubing, a Morgan lens permits continuous lavage and delivers medication to the eye. Use an adapter to connect the lens to the I.V. tubing and the solution container. Begin the irrigation at the prescribed flow rate. To insert the device, ask the patient to look down as you insert the lens under the upper eyelid. Then have her look up as you retract and release the lower eyelid over the lens.

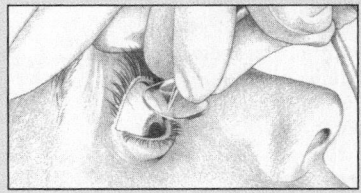

Coronary artery disease

OVERVIEW

- Heart disease that results from narrowing of coronary arteries over time due to atherosclerosis
- Primary effect: loss of oxygen and nutrients to myocardial tissue because of diminished coronary blood flow

PATHOPHYSIOLOGY

- Increased blood levels of low-density lipoprotein (LDL) irritate or damage the inner layer of coronary vessels.
- LDL enters the vessel after damaging the protective barrier, accumulates, and forms a fatty streak.
- Smooth muscle cells move to the inner layer to engulf the fatty substance, produce fibrous tissue, and stimulate calcium deposition.
- Cycle continues, resulting in transformation of the fatty streak into fibrous plaque and, eventually, a coronary artery disease (CAD) lesion evolves.
- Oxygen deprivation forces the myocardium to shift from aerobic to anaerobic metabolism, leading to accumulation of lactic acid and reduction of cellular pH.
- The combination of hypoxia, reduced energy availability, and acidosis rapidly impairs left ventricular function.
- The strength of contractions in the affected myocardial region is reduced as the fibers shorten inadequately, resulting in less force and velocity.
- Wall motion is abnormal in the ischemic area, resulting in less blood being ejected from the heart with each contraction.

CAUSES

- Atherosclerosis
- Dissecting aneurysm
- Infectious vasculitis
- Syphilis
- Congenital defects
- Coronary artery spasm

RISK FACTORS

- Family history
- High cholesterol level
- Smoking
- Diabetes
- Hormonal contraceptives
- Obesity
- Sedentary lifestyle
- Stress
- Increased homocystine levels

INCIDENCE

- CAD usually occurs after age 40.
- Men are eight times more susceptible than premenopausal women.
- Risk of developing CAD is increased by a positive family history.
- White men are more susceptible to CAD than nonwhite men, and nonwhite women are more susceptible to CAD than white women.
- CAD occurs in about 11 million Americans.

COMPLICATIONS

- Arrhythmias
- Myocardial infarction (MI)
- Heart failure

ASSESSMENT

HISTORY

- Angina that may radiate to the left arm, neck, jaw, or shoulder blade
- Commonly occurs after physical exertion but may also follow emotional excitement, exposure to cold, or a large meal
- May develop during sleep; symptoms wake the patient
- Nausea
- Vomiting
- Fainting
- Sweating
- Stable angina (predictable and relieved by rest or nitrates)
- Unstable angina (increases in frequency and duration and is more easily induced and generally indicates extensive or worsening disease and, untreated, may progress to MI)
- Crescendo angina (an effort-induced pain that occurs with increasing frequency and with decreasing provocation)
- Prinzmetal's or variant angina pectoris (severe non–effort-induced pain occurs at rest without provocation)

PHYSICAL FINDINGS

- Cool extremities
- Xanthoma
- Arteriovenous nicking of the eye
- Obesity
- Hypertension
- Positive Levine sign (holding fist to chest)
- Decreased or absent peripheral pulses

DIAGNOSTIC TEST RESULTS

IMAGING

- Myocardial perfusion imaging with thallium 201 during treadmill exercise shows ischemic areas of the myocardium, visualized as "cold spots."
- Pharmacologic myocardial perfusion imaging in arteries with stenosis shows decrease in blood flow proportional to the percentage of occlusion.
- Multiple-gated acquisition scanning demonstrates cardiac wall motion and reflects injury to cardiac tissue.
- Coronary angiography reveals the location and degree of coronary artery stenosis or obstruction, collateral circulation, and the condition of the artery beyond the narrowing.
- Stress echocardiography may show abnormal wall motion.

DIAGNOSTIC PROCEDURES

- Electrocardiography may be normal between anginal episodes. During angina, it may show ischemic changes.
- Exercise testing may be performed to detect ST-segment changes during exercise, indicating ischemia, and to determine a safe exercise prescription.

TREATMENT

GENERAL

- Stress reduction techniques essential, especially if known stressors precipitate pain

- Lifestyle modifications, such as smoking cessation and maintaining ideal body weight (see *Preventing coronary artery disease*)

DIET
- Low-fat, low-sodium

ACTIVITY
- Restrictions possible
- Regular exercise

MEDICATIONS
- Aspirin
- Nitrates
- Beta-adrenergic blockers
- Calcium channel blockers
- Antiplatelets
- Antilipemics
- Antihypertensives
- Estrogen replacement therapy

SURGERY
- Coronary artery bypass graft
- "Keyhole" or minimally invasive surgery
- Angioplasty
- Endovascular stent placement
- Laser angioplasty
- Atherectomy

Preventing coronary artery disease

Because coronary artery disease is so widespread, prevention is important. Dietary restrictions aimed at reducing the intake of calories (in obesity) and of salt, fats, and cholesterol minimize the risk, especially when supplemented with regular exercise. Abstention from smoking and reduction of stress are also essential.

Other preventive actions include control of hypertension (with diuretics or sympathetic beta-adrenergic blockers), control of elevated serum cholesterol or triglyceride levels (with antilipemics such as HMG-CoA reductase inhibitors, including atorvastatin, pravastatin, or simvastatin), and measures to minimize platelet aggregation and the danger of blood clots (with aspirin, for example).

NURSING CONSIDERATIONS

NURSING DIAGNOSES
- Activity intolerance
- Acute pain
- Anxiety
- Decreased cardiac output
- Disturbed body image
- Imbalanced nutrition: More than body requirements
- Impaired gas exchange
- Ineffective denial
- Ineffective role performance
- Ineffective sexuality patterns
- Ineffective tissue perfusion: Cardiopulmonary

EXPECTED OUTCOMES
The patient will:
- state the importance of balancing activity as tolerated with rest periods
- express feelings of increased comfort and decreased pain
- verbalize strategies to reduce anxiety
- maintain adequate cardiac output
- express concern about self-concept, esteem, and body image
- plan menus for prescribed diet
- maintain adequate ventilation and oxygenation
- recognize and accept needed lifestyle changes
- verbalize feelings about how the chronic condition affects roles and responsibilities
- identify measures to maintain sexual function as tolerated
- maintain hemodynamic stability.

NURSING INTERVENTIONS
- Ask the patient to grade the severity of his pain on a scale of 1 to 10.
- Keep nitroglycerin available for immediate use. Instruct the patient to call immediately whenever he feels pain and before taking nitroglycerin.
- Observe for signs and symptoms that may signify worsening of condition.
- Perform vigorous chest physiotherapy and guide the patient in pulmonary self-care.

MONITORING
- Vital signs
- Intake and output

- Effectiveness of pain medication during anginal episodes
- Abnormal bleeding and distal pulses following intervention procedures
- Breath sounds
- Chest tube drainage, after surgery
- Cardiac rate and rhythm

PATIENT TEACHING

GENERAL
Be sure to cover:
- risk factors for CAD
- avoidance of activities that precipitate episodes of pain
- effective coping mechanisms to deal with stress
- the need to follow the prescribed drug regimen
- low-sodium and low-calorie diet
- the importance of regular, moderate exercise.

DISCHARGE PLANNING
- Refer the patient to a weight-loss program, if needed.
- Refer the patient to a smoking-cessation program, if needed.
- Refer the patient to a cardiac rehabilitation program, if indicated.

RESOURCES
Organizations
American Heart Association: *www.americanheart.org*
Mayo Clinic: *www.mayoclinic.com*

Selected references
Casey, P.E. "Markers of Myocardial Injury and Dysfunction," *AACN Clinical Issues* 15(4):547-57, October-December 2004.
Coats, A.J. "Advances in the Non-Drug, Non-Surgical, Non-Device Management of Chronic Heart Failure," *International Journal of Cardiology* 100(1):1-4, April 2005.
Kasper, D.L., et al., eds. *Harrison's Principles of Internal Medicine*, 16th ed. New York: McGraw-Hill Book Co., 2005.
Price, J.A. "Management and Prevention of Cardiovascular Disease in Women," *The Nursing Clinics of North America* 39(4):873-84, xi, December 2004.
Professional Guide to Diseases, 8th ed. Philadelphia: Lippincott Williams & Wilkins, 2005.

Cor pulmonale

- Hypertrophy and dilation of the right ventricle secondary to disease affecting the structure or function of the lungs or their vasculature
- Can occur at the end stage of various chronic disorders of the lungs, pulmonary vessels, chest wall, or respiratory control center
- Also called *right-sided heart failure*

PATHOPHYSIOLOGY

- An occluded vessel impairs the heart's ability to generate enough pressure.
- Increased blood flow creates pulmonary hypertension.
- Pulmonary hypertension increases the heart's workload.
- To compensate, the right ventricle hypertrophies to force blood through the lungs.
- In response to hypoxia, the bone marrow produces more red blood cells, causing polycythemia.
- The blood's viscosity increases, further aggravating pulmonary hypertension. This increases the right ventricle's workload, causing heart failure. (See *Cor pulmonale pathway*.)

CAUSES

- Bronchial asthma
- Chronic obstructive pulmonary disease
- Disorders affecting the pulmonary parenchyma
- External vascular obstruction resulting from a tumor or aneurysm
- High altitude
- Kyphoscoliosis
- Muscular dystrophy
- Obesity
- Pectus excavatum (funnel chest)
- Poliomyelitis
- Primary pulmonary hypertension
- Pulmonary emboli
- Vasculitis

INCIDENCE

- Cor pulmonale accounts for 6% to 7% of all types of adult heart disease in the United States.
- The disease affects males and females equally.

COMPLICATIONS

- Right- and left-sided heart failure
- Hepatomegaly
- Edema
- Ascites
- Pleural effusions
- Thromboembolism due to polycythemia

HISTORY

- Dyspnea
- Chronic productive cough
- Fatigue
- Weakness

PHYSICAL FINDINGS

- Wheezing respirations
- Tachypnea

Cor pulmonale pathway

Although pulmonary restrictive disorders (such as fibrosis or obesity), obstructive disorders (such as bronchitis), or primary vascular disorders (such as recurrent pulmonary emboli) may cause cor pulmonale, these disorders share this common pathway.

Pulmonary disorder
↓
Anatomic alterations in the pulmonary blood vessels and functional alterations in the lung
↓
Increased pulmonary vascular resistance
↓
Pulmonary hypertension
↓
Right ventricular hypertrophy (cor pulmonale)
↓
HEART FAILURE

- Dependent edema
- Distended jugular veins
- Enlarged, tender liver
- Hepatojugular reflux
- Tachycardia
- Pansystolic murmur at the lower left sternal border

LABORATORY

- Arterial blood gas analysis detects decreased partial pressure of arterial oxygen (usually less than 70 mm Hg and rarely more than 90 mm Hg).
- Hematocrit is typically over 50%.
- Serum hepatic tests may show an elevated level of aspartate aminotransferase levels.

IMAGING

- Echocardiography demonstrates right ventricular enlargement.
- Angiography shows right ventricular enlargement.
- Chest X-rays reveal large central pulmonary arteries and right ventricular enlargement.
- Magnetic resonance imaging measures the right ventricular mass, wall thickness, and ejection fraction.

DIAGNOSTIC PROCEDURES

- Cardiac catheterization measures pulmonary vascular pressures.
- Electrocardiography shows arrhythmias, such as premature atrial and ventricular contractions and atrial fibrillation during severe hypoxia, and also right bundle-branch block, right axis deviation, prominent P waves, and an inverted T wave in right precordial leads.
- Pulmonary function studies reflect underlying pulmonary disease.

OTHER

- Pulmonary artery catheterization shows increased right ventricular and pulmonary artery pressures.
- Hemodynamic profile shows increased pulmonary vascular resistance.

TREATMENT

GENERAL
- Phlebotomy, if necessary

DIET
- Low-sodium
- Fluid restrictions

ACTIVITY
- Limited or bed rest

MEDICATIONS
- Digoxin
- Antibiotics
- Vasodilators
- Oxygen

NURSING CONSIDERATIONS

NURSING DIAGNOSES
- Activity intolerance
- Acute pain
- Anxiety
- Decreased cardiac output
- Excess fluid volume
- Fatigue
- Impaired gas exchange
- Ineffective airway clearance
- Ineffective breathing pattern

EXPECTED OUTCOMES
The patient will:
- carry out activities of daily living without excess fatigue or exhaustion
- report feelings of comfort and reduced levels of pain
- verbalize strategies to reduce anxiety
- maintain adequate cardiac output
- maintain normal fluid balance
- verbalize the importance of balancing activity with adequate rest periods
- maintain adequate ventilation and oxygenation
- maintain a patent airway
- maintain an effective breathing pattern.

NURSING INTERVENTIONS
- Reposition the patient often.
- Give prescribed drugs.

MONITORING
- Vital signs
- Oxygenation
- Intake and output
- Laboratory values
- Respiratory status

PATIENT TEACHING

GENERAL
Be sure to cover:
- the disorder, diagnosis, and treatment
- dietary restrictions
- medication administration and potential adverse reactions.

DISCHARGE PLANNING
- Refer the patient for home services, as indicated.

RESOURCES
Organizations
American Heart Association: *www.americanheart.org*
National Heart, Lung, and Blood Institute: *www.nhlbi.nih.gov*

Selected references
Budev, M.M., et al. "Cor Pulmonale: An Overview," *Seminars in Respiratory & Critical Care Medicine* 24(3):233-43, June 2003.
Kingman, M.S., et al. "Nesiritide for Pulmonary Arterial Hypertension with Decompensated Cor Pulmonale," *Progress in Cardiovascular Nursing* 20(4):168-72, Fall 2005.
Nettina, S.M. *Lippincott Manual of Nursing Practice,* 8th ed. Philadelphia: Lippincott Williams & Wilkins, 2006.

Creutzfeldt-Jakob disease LIFE-THREATENING DISORDER

OVERVIEW

- Rapidly progressive prion disease that attacks the central nervous system (CNS)
- Manifested by progressive dementia, tremors, and muscle wasting
- Always fatal
- Not transmitted by normal casual contact (although iatrogenic transmission can occur)
- Has a 15- to 20-month incubation period
- Typical duration 6 months
- New variant of Creutzfeldt-Jakob disease in Europe in 1996 (see *Understanding new-variant Creutzfeldt-Jakob disease*)
- No cure and progress can't be slowed
- Also known as *CJD*

PATHOPHYSIOLOGY

- CJD is caused by the abnormal accumulation or metabolism of prion proteins (isoform).
- These modified proteins are resistant to proteolytic digestion and aggregate in the brain to produce rodlike particles.
- The accumulation of these modified cellular proteins results in neuronal degeneration and spongiform changes in brain tissue.

CAUSES

- Familial or genetically inherited form
- Iatrogenic or acquired form due to inadvertent exposure to CJD-contaminated equipment or material as a result of brain surgery, corneal grafts, or use of human pituitary-derived growth hormones or gonadotropin
- Sporadic form of unknown etiology

INCIDENCE

- One case of CJD occurs in 1 million people worldwide annually.
- About 85% of cases are sporadic.
- About 5% to 15% of cases are familial, with an autosomal dominant pattern of inheritance.
- CJD usually affects patients over age 55; the median age of death from CJD in the United States is 68.
- CJD affects men and women of diverse ethnic backgrounds.
- Most cases occur in Libya, North Africa, and Slovakia.

COMPLICATIONS

- Severe, progressive dementia
- CNS abnormalities
- Death

Understanding new-variant Creutzfeldt-Jakob disease

Like conventional Creutzfeldt-Jakob disease (CJD), new-variant CJD (nvCJD) is a rare, fatal neurodegenerative disease. Most cases have been reported in the United Kingdom, and it's most likely caused by exposure to bovine spongiform encephalopathy (BSE), a fatal brain disease in cattle also known as *mad cow disease*. Ingestion of beef products from cattle with BSE is the most probable route of exposure.

NvCJD affects patients at a much younger age than CJD, and the duration of the illness is much longer (14 months versus 6 months).

Regulations have been established in Europe to control outbreaks of BSE in cattle and to prevent contaminated meat from entering the food supply. NvCJD and its relationship with BSE are still being explored by the Centers for Disease Control and Prevention, and World Health Organization.

A European commission report released in 2000 placed Canada in the second rank of risk for mad cow disease.

ASSESSMENT

HISTORY

- Mood changes
- Emotional lability
- Poor concentration
- Lethargy
- Impaired judgment
- Memory loss
- Involuntary muscle movements
- Vision disturbances or other types of hallucinations
- Gait disturbances

PHYSICAL FINDINGS

- Dementia
- Myoclonus
- Spasticity
- Agitation
- Tremor
- Clumsiness
- Ataxia
- Hypokinesis and rigidity
- Hyperreflexia

DIAGNOSTIC TEST RESULTS

LABORATORY
- Cerebral spinal fluid (CSF) immuno-assay may show abnormal protein species.
- CSF analysis may show mildly elevated protein level.

IMAGING
- Computed tomography scan and magnetic resonance imaging of the brain may show evidence of generalized cortical atrophy.

DIAGNOSTIC PROCEDURES
- Electroencephalography may show burst suppression changes in brain wave activity.
- Brain biopsy may show spongiform changes.

OTHER
- Autopsy of brain tissue allows definitive diagnosis.

TREATMENT

GENERAL
- No specific treatment
- Palliative care to make the patient comfortable and to ease symptoms

DIET
- Well-balanced
- Adequate fluid intake

ACTIVITY
- As tolerated

MEDICATIONS
- Amantadine

SURGERY
- Possible brain biopsy for diagnosis

NURSING CONSIDERATIONS

NURSING DIAGNOSES
- Anticipatory grieving
- Compromised family coping
- Dressing or grooming self-care deficit
- Risk for injury

EXPECTED OUTCOMES
The patient will:
- appropriately express feelings related to grief, anger, and sorrow
- use support services and demonstrate adequate coping behaviors
- participate in self-care activities to the fullest extent possible
- remain free from injury and family members will identify strategies to make the patient's environment safe.

NURSING INTERVENTIONS
- Assist the patient and his family through the grieving process.
- Follow standard precautions.
- Encourage verbalization of concerns and fears.
- Encourage involvement of the patient and his family in care decisions.

MONITORING
- Vital signs
- Intake and output
- Neurologic status
- Mental status

PATIENT TEACHING

GENERAL
Be sure to cover:
- the disorder, diagnosis, and supportive treatment
- prevention of disease transmission
- effective coping strategies
- safety precautions.

DISCHARGE PLANNING
- Refer the patient and his family to CJD support groups.
- Refer the patient for hospice care, as appropriate.

RESOURCES
Organizations
Centers for Disease Control and Prevention: *www.cdc.gov*
National Center for Infectious Diseases: *www.cdc.gov/ncidod*
National Prion Disease Pathology Surveillance Center: *www.cjdsurveillance.com*

Selected references
Bosque, P. "Molecular Types of Creutzfeldt-Jakob Disease: The Strange Diversity of Prions," *Neurology* 65(10):1520-521, November 2005.
Smith-Bathgate, B. "Creutzfeldt-Jakob Disease: Diagnosis and Nursing Care Issues," *Nursing Times* 101(20):52-53, May 2005.
Sperling, R., et al. "Creutzfeldt-Jakob Disease in the Obstetric Patient," *Journal of Obstetric, Gynecologic, and Neonatal Nursing* 34(5):546-50, September-October 2005.

Crohn's disease

- Inflammatory bowel disease that may affect any part of the GI tract but commonly involves the terminal ileum
- Fifty percent of cases involving colon and small bowel; 33%, terminal ileum; 10% to 20%, only colon
- Extends through all layers of the intestinal wall; may involve regional lymph nodes and mesentery

PATHOPHYSIOLOGY

- Crohn's disease involves slow, progressive inflammation of the bowel.
- Lymphatic obstruction is caused by enlarged lymph nodes.
- Edema, mucosal ulceration, fissures, and abscesses occur.
- Elevated patches of closely packed lymph follicles (Peyer's patches) develop in the small intestinal lining.
- Fibrosis occurs, thickening the bowel wall and causing stenosis.
- Inflamed bowel loops adhere to other diseased or normal loops.
- The diseased bowel becomes thicker, shorter, and narrower.

CAUSES

- Exact cause unknown
- Lymphatic obstruction and infection among contributing factors

RISK FACTORS

- History of allergies
- Immune disorders
- Genetic predisposition — 10% to 20% of patients having one or more affected relatives; sometimes occurring in monozygotic twins

INCIDENCE

- Crohn's disease occurs equally in males and females.
- Crohn's disease more commonly occurs in Jewish people.
- Onset is usually before age 30.

COMPLICATIONS

- Anal fistula
- Perineal abscess
- Fistulas of the bladder or vagina or to the skin in an old scar area
- Intestinal obstruction
- Perforation
- Nutritional deficiencies caused by malabsorption and maldigestion

ASSESSMENT

HISTORY

- Gradual onset of signs and symptoms, marked by periods of remission and exacerbation
- Fatigue and weakness
- Fever, flatulence, nausea
- Steady, colicky, or cramping abdominal pain that usually occurs in the right lower abdominal quadrant
- Diarrhea that may worsen after emotional upset or ingestion of poorly tolerated foods, such as milk, fatty foods, and spices
- Weight loss

PHYSICAL FINDINGS

- Possible soft or semiliquid stool, usually without gross blood
- Right lower abdominal quadrant tenderness or distention
- Possible abdominal mass, indicating adherent loops of bowel
- Hyperactive bowel sounds
- Bloody diarrhea
- Perianal and rectal abscesses

DIAGNOSTIC TEST RESULTS

LABORATORY

- Occult blood in stools may be present.
- Hemoglobin (Hb) level and hematocrit may be decreased.
- White blood cell count and erythrocyte sedimentation rate may be increased.
- Serum potassium, calcium, magnesium, and Hb levels may be decreased.
- Hypoglobulinemia from intestinal protein loss may occur.
- Vitamin B_{12} and folate deficiency may occur.

IMAGING

- Small bowel X-rays may show irregular mucosa, ulceration, and stiffening.
- Barium enema reveals the string sign (segments of stricture separated by normal bowel) and may also show fissures and narrowing of the lumen.

DIAGNOSTIC PROCEDURES

- Sigmoidoscopy and colonoscopy show patchy areas of inflammation and may also reveal the characteristic coarse irregularity (cobblestone appearance) of the mucosal surface.
- Biopsy reveals granulomas in up to 50% of all specimens.

TREATMENT

GENERAL
◆ Stress reduction

DIET
◆ Avoidance of foods that worsen diarrhea
◆ Avoidance of raw fruits and vegetables if blockage occurs
◆ Adequate caloric, protein, and vitamin intake
◆ Parenteral nutrition, if necessary

ACTIVITY
◆ Reduced

MEDICATIONS
◆ Corticosteroids
◆ Immunosuppressants
◆ Sulfonamides
◆ Anti-inflammatories
◆ Antibacterials and antiprotozoals
◆ Antidiarrheals
◆ Opioids
◆ Vitamin supplements
◆ Antispasmodics

SURGERY
◆ Indicated for acute intestinal obstruction
◆ Colectomy with ileostomy

NURSING CONSIDERATIONS

NURSING DIAGNOSES
◆ Acute pain
◆ Diarrhea
◆ Disturbed body image
◆ Imbalanced nutrition: Less than body requirements
◆ Ineffective coping
◆ Ineffective tissue perfusion: GI
◆ Risk for deficient fluid volume
◆ Risk for impaired skin integrity
◆ Risk for injury

EXPECTED OUTCOMES
The patient will:
◆ express feelings of comfort and decreased pain
◆ regain normal intestinal function
◆ express positive feelings about self
◆ maintain adequate caloric intake
◆ exhibit adequate coping mechanisms and seek appropriate sources of support
◆ exhibit signs of adequate GI perfusion
◆ maintain normal fluid volume
◆ maintain skin integrity
◆ avoid or minimize complications.

NURSING INTERVENTIONS
◆ Provide emotional support to the patient and his family.
◆ Provide meticulous skin care after each bowel movement.
◆ Schedule patient care to include rest periods throughout the day.
◆ Assist with dietary modification.
◆ Give prescribed iron supplements and blood transfusions.
◆ Give prescribed analgesics.

MONITORING
◆ Abdominal pain and distention
◆ Vital signs
◆ Intake and output, including amount of stool
◆ Daily weight
◆ Serum electrolytes and glucose, Hb, and stools for occult blood
◆ Signs of infection or obstruction
◆ Bleeding, especially with steroid use

PATIENT TEACHING

GENERAL
Be sure to cover:
◆ information about the disease, symptoms, and complications
◆ ordered diagnostic tests and pretest guidelines
◆ the importance of adequate rest
◆ how the patient can identify and reduce sources of stress
◆ prescribed dietary changes
◆ prescribed medications, administration, and possible adverse reactions.

DISCHARGE PLANNING
◆ Refer the patient to a smoking-cessation program, if appropriate.
◆ Refer the patient to an enterostomal therapist, if indicated.

RESOURCES
Organizations
Crohn's and Colitis Foundation of America: *www.ccfa.org*
United Ostomy Association, Inc.: *www.uoa.org*

Selected references
Beeb, J.R., and Scott, B.B. "How Effective are the Usual Treatments for Crohn's Disease?" *Alimentary Pharmacology & Therapeutics* 20(2):151-59, July 2004.

Freeman, H.J. "Comparison of Long-standing Pediatric-Onset and Adult-Onset Crohn's Disease," *Journal of Pediatric Gastroenterology & Nutrition* 39(2):183-86, August 2004.

Ghosh, S., et al. "Is Thiopurine Therapy in Ulcerative Colitis as Effective as in Crohn's Disease?" *Gut* 55(1):6-8, January 2006.

Handbook of Diseases, 3rd ed. Philadelphia: Lippincott Williams & Wilkins, 2004.

Homan, M., et al. "Managing Complicated Crohn's Disease in Children and Adolescents," *Nature Clinical Practice – Gastroenterology & Hepatology* 2(12): 572-79, December 2005.

Croup

OVERVIEW

- Viral infection causing severe inflammation and obstruction of the upper airway
- Childhood disease manifested by acute laryngotracheobronchitis (most commonly), laryngitis, acute spasmodic laryngitis, and febrile rhinitis
- Incubation period about 3 to 6 days; contagious while febrile
- Recovery usually complete

PATHOPHYSIOLOGY

- Viral invasion of the laryngeal mucosa leads to inflammation, hyperemia, edema, epithelial necrosis, and shedding.
- This leads to irritation and cough, reactive paralysis and continuous stridor, or collapsible supraglottic or inspiratory stridor and respiratory distress.
- A thin, fibrinous membrane covers the mucosa of the epiglottis, larynx, and trachea. (See *How croup affects the upper airways.*)

CAUSES

- Adenoviruses
- Bacteria (pertussis and diphtheria)
- Influenza viruses
- Measles viruses
- Parainfluenza viruses
- Respiratory syncytial virus

INCIDENCE

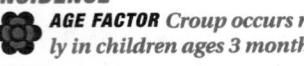 **AGE FACTOR** *Croup occurs mainly in children ages 3 months to 5 years.*
- Croup affects boys more commonly than girls.
- Croup usually occurs in late autumn and early winter.

AGE FACTOR *Acute spasmodic laryngitis affects children between ages 1 and 3, particularly those with allergies.*

COMPLICATIONS

- Airway obstruction
- Respiratory failure
- Dehydration
- Ear infection
- Pneumonia
- Hypoxia
- Hypercapnia

ASSESSMENT

HISTORY

- Recent upper respiratory infection

Laryngotracheobronchitis

- Fever and breathing problems that usually occur at night
- Difficulty exhaling

Laryngitis in children

- Mild sore throat
- Cough
- Marked hoarseness (rare)
- No respiratory distress

Laryngitis in infants

- Respiratory distress

Acute spasmodic laryngitis

- Mild to moderate hoarseness
- Nasal discharge
- Characteristic cough and noisy inspiration
- Anxiety
- Increased dyspnea
- Transient cyanosis

PHYSICAL FINDINGS

- Rhinorrhea
- Use of accessory muscles
- Nasal flaring
- Barklike cough
- Hoarse, muffled vocal sounds
- Inspiratory stridor
- Diminished breath sounds

Laryngotracheobronchitis

- Edema of bronchi and bronchioles
- Decreased breath sounds
- Expiratory rhonchi
- Scattered crackles

Laryngitis

- Suprasternal and intercostal retractions
- Inspiratory stridor
- Dyspnea, tachypnea
- Diminished breath sounds
- Severe dyspnea and exhaustion in later stages

How croup affects the upper airways

In croup, inflammatory swelling and spasms constrict the larynx, thereby reducing airflow. This cross-sectional drawing (from chin to chest) shows the upper airway changes caused by croup. Inflammatory changes almost completely obstruct the larnyx (which includes the epiglottis) and significantly narrow the trachea.

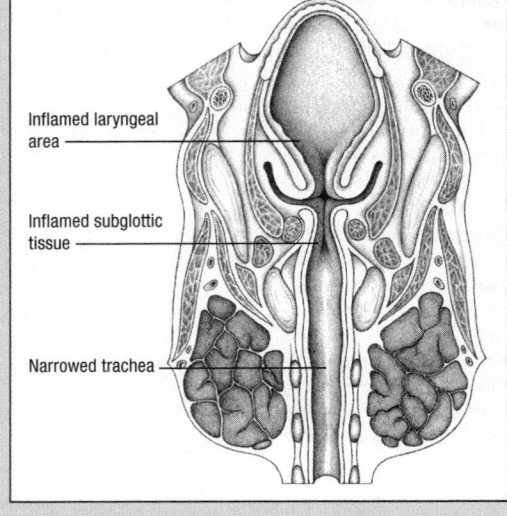

Inflamed laryngeal area

Inflamed subglottic tissue

Narrowed trachea

Acute spasmodic laryngitis
- Labored breathing with retractions
- Clammy skin
- Rapid pulse rate

DIAGNOSTIC TEST RESULTS

LABORATORY
- Throat cultures show bacteria and sensitivity to antibiotics.

IMAGING
- Neck X-ray may show upper airway narrowing and edema in subglottic folds; helps to differentiate croup from bacterial epiglottitis.
- Computed tomography scan helps differentiate among croup, epiglottitis, and noninfection.

DIAGNOSTIC PROCEDURES
- Laryngoscopy may reveal inflammation and obstruction in epiglottal and laryngeal areas.

TREATMENT

GENERAL
- Home or hospitalized care
- Humidification during sleep
- Intubation as needed

DIET
- As tolerated
- Parenteral fluids, if required

ACTIVITY
- Rest periods

MEDICATIONS
- Oxygen therapy, as needed
- Antipyretics
- Antibiotics if cause is bacterial
- Aerosolized racemic epinephrine for moderately severe croup
- Corticosteroids for acute laryngotracheobronchitis (controversial)

SURGERY
- Tracheostomy (rare)

NURSING CONSIDERATIONS

NURSING DIAGNOSES
- Anxiety
- Disabled family coping
- Fear
- Hyperthermia
- Impaired gas exchange
- Ineffective airway clearance

EXPECTED OUTCOMES
The patient will:
- verbalize strategies to reduce anxiety
- use available support systems to assist with coping
- verbalize fears and concerns
- have a temperature within the normal range
- maintain adequate ventilation and oxygenation
- maintain a patent airway.

NURSING INTERVENTIONS
- Give prescribed drugs.
- Provide quiet diversional activities.
- Engage parents in the care of the infant or child.
- Position an infant in an infant seat or prop him up with a pillow.
- Position an older child in Fowler's position.
- Provide humidification.
- Avoid milk-based fluids if the patient has thick mucus or swallowing difficulties.
- Provide frequent mouth care.
- Isolate patients for respiratory syncytial virus and parainfluenza infections.
- Use sponge baths and hypothermia blanket, as ordered, for temperatures above 102° F (38.9° C).

MONITORING
- Vital signs
- Intake and output
- Respiratory status
- Signs and symptoms of dehydration

PATIENT TEACHING

GENERAL
Be sure to cover:
- the disorder, diagnosis, and treatment
- medications and possible adverse reactions
- when to notify the practitioner
- humidification
- hydration
- signs and symptoms of ear infection
- signs and symptoms of pneumonia.

RESOURCES
Organizations
American Academy of Pediatrics: *www.aap.org*

Selected references
Bjornson, C.L., and Johnson, D.W. "Croup — Treatment Update," *Pediatric Emergency Care* 21(12):863-70, December 2005.
Diseases, 4th ed. Philadelphia: Lippincott Williams & Wilkins, 2006.
Kline, A. "Pinpointing the Cause of Pediatric Respiratory Distress," *Nursing2004* 33(9):58-63, September 2003.
Savoy, N.B. "Differentiating Stridor in Children at Triage: It's Not Always Croup," *Journal of Emergency Nursing* 31(5):503-505, October 2005.

Cryptococcosis

- Yeast infection that usually begins as asymptomatic pulmonary infection in patient who presents with meningoencephalitis on diagnosis
- Fungal infection also known as *torulosis* and *European blastomycosis*

PATHOPHYSIOLOGY

- Small granulomas and cysts in the cerebral cortex and, later, in deep cerebral tissues produce a minimal inflammatory response.
- In chronic cases, dense basilar arachnoiditis occurs.
- Lung lesions with intense granulomatous inflammation occur.

CAUSES

- Airborne fungus *Cryptococcus neoformans* found in dust particles contaminated by pigeon stool
- Transmission by inhalation of cryptococci

INCIDENCE

- Cryptococcosis is prevalent in immunocompromised patients and those taking immunosuppressant drugs.
- Incidence rate is increasing, especially in patients with acquired immunodeficiency syndrome.

COMPLICATIONS

- Optic atrophy
- Ataxia
- Hydrocephalus
- Deafness
- Paralysis
- Organic mental syndrome
- Personality changes
- Coma
- Death

HISTORY

- Human immunodeficiency virus infection or another immunosuppressive disorder
- Usually asymptomatic but patient may complain of dull chest pain and cough producing slight amount of white, blood-streaked sputum

PHYSICAL FINDINGS

- Progressively severe frontal and temporal headache
- Diplopia, blurred vision, papilledema
- Tinnitus, dizziness, ataxia, and aphasia
- Vomiting
- Memory changes, inappropriate behavior, irritability, and psychosis
- Facial weakness
- Hyperactive reflexes and seizures in the late stage
- Pain in the long bones, skull, spine, and joints
- Red facial papules and other skin abscesses, with or without ulceration
- Rarely, pleural friction rub or crackles
- Photophobia

IMAGING

- Chest X-ray or computed tomography scan of the chest reveals lesions in pulmonary cryptococcosis.

LABORATORY

- Analysis or cultures of the sputum, urine, prostatic secretions, or bone marrow aspirate show *C. neoformans.*
- Tissue or neural biopsy shows myriad cryptococci.
- India ink preparation of cerebrospinal fluid (CSF) diagnoses central nervous system (CNS) infection when *C. neoformans* is detected.
- Blood cultures are positive only in severe infection.
- Antigen titer is elevated in serum and CSF in disseminated infection.
- Protein levels and white blood cell count are elevated in CNS infection.
- CSF glucose levels are moderately decreased in about 50% of patients.

OTHER

- Lumbar puncture shows increased CSF pressure.

TREATMENT

GENERAL
◆ Early treatment for cryptococcal disease

MEDICATIONS
◆ Combination of antifungal antibiotics amphotericin B and flucytosine, or amphotericin B alone

NURSING CONSIDERATIONS

NURSING DIAGNOSES
◆ Acute pain
◆ Impaired gas exchange
◆ Impaired physical mobility
◆ Ineffective breathing pattern
◆ Ineffective tissue perfusion: Cerebral, cardiopulmonary
◆ Risk for injury

EXPECTED OUTCOMES
The patient will:
◆ be free from pain
◆ maintain a patent airway and adequate ventilation
◆ maintain joint mobility and muscle strength
◆ maintain an effective breathing pattern
◆ maintain tissue perfusion and cellular oxygenation and maintain or improve current level of consciousness
◆ remain free from injury or complications.

NURSING INTERVENTIONS
◆ Before therapy, draw serum for testing to determine electrolyte levels and baseline renal status.
◆ Give prescribed drugs.
◆ Observe for adverse effects such as diarrhea.
◆ Evaluate the need for long-term venous access for administering amphotericin B.
◆ Encourage verbalization and provide psychological support to help the patient cope with long-term treatment.
◆ If vision loss occurs, provide a safe environment.

MONITORING
◆ Vital signs
◆ Neurologic checks
◆ Headache, vomiting, and nuchal rigidity
◆ Urine output
◆ Blood urea nitrogen, creatinine levels, and complete blood count results
◆ Urinalysis results
◆ Magnesium and potassium levels and hepatic function test results
◆ Blood levels of flucytosine

PATIENT TEACHING

GENERAL
Be sure to cover:
◆ the disorder and treatment
◆ medication therapy, including dosage, desired drug actions, adverse effects, and need for long-term treatment.

DISCHARGE PLANNING
◆ Urge the patient to return for follow-up care and evaluation every few months for 1 year.
◆ Refer the patient for resource and support services, as needed.

RESOURCES
Organizations
Centers for Disease Control and Prevention: *www.cdc.gov*
Harvard University Consumer Health Information: *www.intelihealth.com*
National Health Information Center: *www.health.gov/nhic*
National Library of Medicine: *www.nlm.nih.gov*

Selected references
Kasper, D.L., et al., eds. *Harrison's Principles of Internal Medicine*, 16th ed. New York: McGraw-Hill Book Co., 2005.
Kiertiburanakul, S., et al. "Cryptococcosis in Human Immunodeficiency Virus-Negative Patients," *International Journal of Infectious Diseases* 10(1):72-78, January 2006.
Lortholary, O., et al. "Pulmonary Cryptococcosis," *Seminars in Respiratory & Critical Care Medicine* 25(2):145-57, April 2004.

Cryptorchidism

- Congenital disorder in which one or both testes fail to descend into the scrotum, remaining in the abdomen or inguinal canal or at the external ring
- May be bilateral, but more commonly affects the right testis (see *Varieties of cryptorchidism*)

PATHOPHYSIOLOGY

- In the male fetus, testosterone normally stimulates the formation of the gubernaculum. A fibromuscular band connects the testes to the scrotal floor.
- This band probably helps pull the testes into the scrotum by shortening as the fetus grows.
- Thus, cryptorchidism may result from inadequate testosterone levels or a defect in the testes or the gubernaculum.
- Because the testis is maintained at a higher temperature, spermatogenesis is impaired, leading to reduced fertility.
- True undescended testes remain along the path of normal descent, while ectopic testis deviates from that path.

CAUSES

- Genetic predisposition
- Hormonal factors
- Structural factors
- Testosterone deficiency

INCIDENCE

- Cryptorchidism occurs in 30% of premature male neonates but in only 3% of those born at term.
- In about 80% of affected infants, the testes descend spontaneously during the first year; in the rest, the testes may descend later.

COMPLICATIONS

- Sterility
- Increased risk for testicular cancer
- Increased vulnerability of the testes to trauma

ASSESSMENT

PHYSICAL FINDINGS
- Nonpalpable testes
- Underdeveloped scrotum

DIAGNOSTIC TEST RESULTS

LABORATORY
- Buccal smear (cells from oral mucosa) determines genetic sex (a male sex chromatin pattern).
- Serum gonadotropin confirms the presence of testes by showing presence of circulating hormone.

OTHER
- Physical examination may be performed.

Varieties of cryptorchidism

Descent interrupted beyond external inguinal ring

Partially descended

Testis retained in abdomen

Descended but not to bottom of scrotum

Normal

TREATMENT

MEDICATIONS
◆ Human chorionic gonadotropin

SURGERY
◆ Orchiopexy

NURSING CONSIDERATIONS

NURSING DIAGNOSES
◆ Acute pain
◆ Anxiety
◆ Disabled family coping
◆ Risk for injury
◆ Situational low self-esteem

EXPECTED OUTCOMES
The patient will:
◆ express or demonstrate feelings of comfort
◆ express feelings about the condition
◆ develop adequate coping mechanisms
◆ be free from complications
◆ express positive feelings about self.

NURSING INTERVENTIONS
◆ Encourage the parents of the child with undescended testes to express their concern about his condition.
◆ Tell the parents that a rubber band may be taped to the patient's thigh for about 1 week after surgery to keep the testis in place. Explain that his scrotum may swell but shouldn't be painful.

MONITORING
After surgery
◆ Vital signs
◆ Intake and output
◆ Operative site

PATIENT TEACHING

GENERAL
Be sure to cover:
◆ the disorder, treatment, and effect on reproduction
◆ surgery or medications prescribed.

RESOURCES
Organizations
American Society for Reproductive Medicine: *www.asrm.org*
Harvard University Consumer Health Information: *www.intelihealth.com*

Selected references
Diseases, 4th ed. Philadelphia: Lippincott Williams & Wilkins, 2006.
Lee, P.A. "Fertility After Cryptorchidism: Epidemiology and Other Outcome Studies," *Urology* 66(2):427-31, August 2005.
Yalcin, B., et al. "Vascular Anatomy of Normal and Undescended Testes: Surgical Assessment of Anastomotic Channels Between Testicular and Deferential Arteries," *Urology* 66(4):854-57, October 2005.

Cushing's syndrome

OVERVIEW

- Clinical manifestations of glucocorticoid excess, particularly cortisol
- May also reflect excess secretion of mineralocorticoids and androgens
- Classified as primary, secondary, or iatrogenic, depending on etiology
- Prognosis dependent on early diagnosis, identification of underlying cause, and effective treatment

PATHOPHYSIOLOGY

- A loss of normal feedback inhibition by cortisol occurs.
- Elevated levels of cortisol don't suppress hypothalamic and anterior pituitary secretion of corticotropin-releasing hormone and adrenocorticotropic hormone (ACTH).
- The result is excessive levels of circulating cortisol.

CAUSES

- Corticotropin-producing tumor in another organ
- Cortisol-secreting adrenal tumor
- Excess production of corticotropin
- Pituitary microadenoma
- Prolonged exposure to elevated levels of endogenous or exogenous glucocorticoids

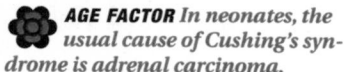 **AGE FACTOR** *In neonates, the usual cause of Cushing's syndrome is adrenal carcinoma.*

INCIDENCE

- Cushing's syndrome is more common in females than in males.
- This syndrome can occur at any age.

COMPLICATIONS

- Osteoporosis and pathologic fractures
- Peptic ulcer
- Dyslipidemia
- Impaired glucose tolerance
- Diabetes insipidus
- Diabetes mellitus
- Frequent infections
- Slow wound healing
- Suppressed inflammatory response
- Hypertension
- Ischemic heart disease; heart failure
- Menstrual disturbances
- Sexual dysfunction
- Psychiatric problems, ranging from mood swings to frank psychosis

ASSESSMENT

HISTORY

- Use of synthetic steroids
- Fatigue
- Muscle weakness
- Sleep disturbances
- Polyuria
- Thirst
- Frequent infections (immunosuppression)
- Water retention
- Amenorrhea
- Decreased libido
- Irritability; emotional instability
- Symptoms resembling those of hyperglycemia
- Impotence
- Headache

PHYSICAL FINDINGS

- Thin hair
- Moon-shaped face
- Hirsutism
- A buffalo-hump–like back
- Thin extremities
- Muscle wasting and muscle weakness
- Petechiae, ecchymoses, and purplish striae
- Delayed wound healing
- Swollen ankles
- Hypertension
- Central obesity
- Acne
- Osteopenic growth retardation in children

DIAGNOSTIC TEST RESULTS

LABORATORY

- Salivary free cortisol is elevated.
- ACTH in adrenal disease is decreased and excess pituitary or ectopic secretion of ACTH is increased.
- Blood chemistry may show hypernatremia, hypokalemia, hypocalcemia, and elevated blood glucose.
- Urinary free cortisol is elevated.
- Serum cortisol is elevated in the morning.
- Glycosuria occurs.

IMAGING

- Ultrasonography, computed tomography scan, and magnetic resonance imaging may show the location of a pituitary or adrenal tumor.

DIAGNOSTIC PROCEDURES

- A low-dose dexamethasone suppression test shows failure of plasma cortisol levels to be suppressed.

TREATMENT

GENERAL

- Management to restore hormone balance and reverse Cushing's syndrome, including radiation, drug therapy, or surgery

DIET

- High-protein, high-potassium, low-calorie, low-sodium

ACTIVITY

- As tolerated

MEDICATIONS

- Aminoglutethimide
- Antifungals
- Antihypertensives
- Diuretics
- Potassium supplements
- Antineoplastics, antihormonals

◆ Glucocorticoids

WARNING *Glucocorticoid administration on the morning of surgery can help prevent acute adrenal insufficiency during surgery. Cortisol therapy is essential during and after surgery to help the patient tolerate the physiologic stress caused by removal of the pituitary or adrenal glands.*

SURGERY
◆ Possible hypophysectomy or pituitary irradiation
◆ Bilateral adrenalectomy
◆ Excision of nonendocrine corticotropin-producing tumor, followed by drug therapy

NURSING CONSIDERATIONS

NURSING DIAGNOSES
◆ Activity intolerance
◆ Disturbed body image
◆ Excess fluid volume
◆ Impaired skin integrity
◆ Ineffective coping
◆ Risk for infection
◆ Risk for injury
◆ Sexual dysfunction

EXPECTED OUTCOMES
The patient will:
◆ perform activities of daily living as tolerated within the confines of the disorder
◆ express positive feelings about self
◆ maintain normal fluid volume
◆ maintain skin integrity
◆ demonstrate adaptive coping behaviors
◆ remain free from signs and symptoms of infection
◆ avoid complications
◆ verbalize feelings related to sexual impairment.

NURSING INTERVENTIONS
◆ Give prescribed drugs.
◆ Consult a dietitian.
◆ Use protective measures to reduce the risk of infection.
◆ Use meticulous hand-washing technique.
◆ Schedule adequate rest periods.
◆ Institute safety precautions.
◆ Provide meticulous skin care.
◆ Encourage verbalization of feelings.
◆ Offer emotional support.
◆ Help to develop effective coping strategies.

With transsphenoidal approach to hypophysectomy
◆ Keep the head of the bed elevated at least 30 degrees.
◆ Maintain nasal packing.
◆ Provide frequent mouth care.
◆ Avoid activities that increase intracranial pressure (ICP).

MONITORING
◆ Vital signs
◆ Intake and output
◆ Daily weights
◆ Serum electrolyte results

After bilateral adrenalectomy and hypophysectomy
◆ Neurologic and behavioral status
◆ Severe nausea, vomiting, and diarrhea
◆ Bowel sounds
◆ Adrenal hypofunction
◆ Increased ICP
◆ Hypopituitarism
◆ Transient diabetes insipidus
◆ Hemorrhage and shock

After transsphenoidal approach to hypophysectomy
◆ Cerebrospinal fluid leak

PATIENT TEACHING

GENERAL
Be sure to cover:
◆ the disorder, diagnosis, and treatment
◆ medications and potential adverse reactions
◆ when to notify the practitioner
◆ lifelong steroid replacement
◆ signs and symptoms of adrenal crisis
◆ medical identification bracelet
◆ prevention of infection
◆ signs and symptoms of adrenal crisis
◆ stress-reduction strategies.

DISCHARGE PLANNING
◆ Refer the patient to a mental health professional for additional counseling, if necessary.

RESOURCES
Organizations
Addison and Cushing International Federation:
   www.nvacp.nl/page.php?main=5
Cushing's Support and Research Foundation, Inc.: *www.csrf.net*
Endocrine Society: *www.endo-society.org*
National Adrenal Diseases Foundation:
   www.medhelp.org/www/nadf.htm

Selected references
De, P., et al. "'Osler's Phenomenon': Misdiagnosing Cushing's Syndrome," *Postgraduate Medical Journal* 79(936):594-96, October 2003.
Nettina, S.M. *Lippincott Manual of Nursing Practice*, 8th ed. Philadelphia: Lippincott Williams & Wilkins, 2006.

Cystic fibrosis

- Chronic, progressive, inherited, incurable disease affecting exocrine (mucus-secreting) glands
- Transmitted as an autosomal recessive trait
- Genetic mutation that involves chloride transport across epithelial membranes (more than 100 specific mutations of the gene identified)
- Characterized by major aberrations in sweat gland, respiratory, and GI functions
- Accounts for almost all cases of pancreatic enzyme deficiency in children
- Clinical effects apparent soon after birth or take years to develop
- Death typically from pneumonia, emphysema, or atelectasis

PATHOPHYSIOLOGY

- The viscosity of bronchial, pancreatic, and other mucous gland secretions increases, obstructing glandular ducts.
- The accumulation of thick, tenacious secretions in the bronchioles and alveoli causes respiratory changes, eventually leading to severe atelectasis and emphysema.
- The disease also causes characteristic GI effects in the intestines, pancreas, and liver.
- Obstruction of the pancreatic ducts results in a deficiency of trypsin, amylase, and lipase. This prevents the conversion and absorption of fat and protein in the intestinal tract and interferes with the digestion of food and absorption of fat-soluble vitamins.
- In the pancreas, fibrotic tissue, multiple cysts, thick mucus, and fat replace the acini, producing signs of pancreatic insufficiency.

CAUSES

- Autosomal recessive mutation of gene on chromosome 7
- Causes of symptoms: increased viscosity of bronchial, pancreatic, and other mucous gland secretions and consequent destruction of glandular ducts

INCIDENCE

- Cystic fibrosis is the most common fatal genetic disease of white children.
- A 25% chance of transmission exists with each pregnancy when both parents are carriers of the recessive gene.
- Incidence is highest in people of northern European ancestry.
- The disease is less common in Blacks, Native Americans, and people of Asian ancestry.
- Cystic fibrosis is equally common in both sexes.

COMPLICATIONS

- Bronchiectasis
- Pneumonia
- Atelectasis
- Dehydration
- Distal intestinal obstructive syndrome
- Malnutrition
- Gastroesophageal reflux
- Cor pulmonale
- Hepatic disease
- Diabetes
- Arthritis
- Biliary disease
- Clotting problems
- Retarded bone growth
- Delayed sexual development
- Azoospermia in males
- Secondary amenorrhea in females
- Electrolyte imbalances
- Cardiac arrhythmias
- Potentially fatal shock
- Death

HISTORY

- Recurring bronchitis and pneumonia
- Nasal polyps and sinusitis
- Wheezing
- Dry, nonproductive cough
- Shortness of breath
- Abdominal distention, vomiting, constipation
- Frequent, bulky, foul-smelling, and pale stool with a high fat content
- Poor weight gain
- Poor growth
- Ravenous appetite

- Hematemesis

AGE FACTOR *Neonates may exhibit meconium ileus and develop symptoms of intestinal obstruction: abdominal distention, vomiting, constipation, dehydration, and electrolyte imbalance.*

PHYSICAL FINDINGS

- Wheezy respirations
- Dry, nonproductive, paroxysmal cough
- Dyspnea
- Tachypnea
- Bibasilar crackles and hyperresonance
- Barrel chest
- Cyanosis, and clubbing of the fingers and toes
- Distended abdomen
- Thin extremities
- Sallow skin with poor turgor
- Delayed sexual development
- Neonatal jaundice
- Hepatomegaly
- Rectal prolapse
- Failure to thrive

LABORATORY

- Sweat tests using pilocarpine solution reveals sodium and chloride values.
- Stool specimen analysis shows absence of trypsin.
- Deoxyribonucleic acid testing shows presence of the delta F 508.
- Liver enzyme tests may show hepatic insufficiency.
- Sputum culture may show such organisms as *Pseudomonas* and *Staphylococcus*.
- Serum albumin level is decreased.
- Serum electrolytes may show hypochloremia and hyponatremia.
- Arterial blood gas analysis shows hypoxemia.

IMAGING

- Chest X-rays may show early signs of lung obstruction.
- High-resolution chest computed tomography scan shows bronchial wall

thickening, cystic lesions, and bronchiectasis.

DIAGNOSTIC PROCEDURES
◆ Pulmonary function tests show decreased vital capacity, elevated residual volume, and decreased forced expiratory volume in 1 second.

TREATMENT

GENERAL
◆ Based on organ systems involved
◆ Chest physiotherapy, nebulization, and breathing exercises several times per day
◆ Postural drainage
◆ Gene therapy (experimental)
◆ Annual influenza vaccination

DIET
◆ Salt supplements
◆ High-fat, high-protein, high-calorie

ACTIVITY
◆ As tolerated

MEDICATIONS
◆ Dornase alfa, a pulmonary enzyme given by aerosol nebulizer
◆ Antibiotics
◆ Oxygen therapy, as needed
◆ Oral pancreatic enzymes
◆ Bronchodilators
◆ Prednisone
◆ Vitamin A, D, E, and K supplements

SURGERY
◆ Heart-lung transplantation

NURSING CONSIDERATIONS

NURSING DIAGNOSES
◆ Anxiety
◆ Delayed growth and development
◆ Disabled family coping
◆ Fear
◆ Imbalanced nutrition: Less than body requirements
◆ Impaired gas exchange
◆ Ineffective airway clearance
◆ Ineffective breathing pattern
◆ Ineffective coping

EXPECTED OUTCOMES
The patient (or his family) will:
◆ identify strategies to reduce anxiety
◆ achieve age-appropriate growth to the fullest extent possible
◆ express concerns about coping with the illness
◆ discuss fears and concerns
◆ consume adequate calories daily
◆ maintain adequate ventilation and oxygenation
◆ maintain a patent airway
◆ maintain an effective breathing pattern
◆ use a support system to assist with coping.

NURSING INTERVENTIONS
◆ Give prescribed drugs.
◆ Administer pancreatic enzymes with meals and snacks.
◆ Perform chest physiotherapy and postural drainage.
◆ Administer oxygen therapy, as needed.
◆ Provide a well-balanced, high-protein, high-calorie diet; include adequate fats.
◆ Provide vitamin A, D, E, and K supplements, if indicated.
◆ Ensure adequate oral fluid intake.
◆ Provide exercise and activity periods.
◆ Encourage breathing exercises.
◆ Provide the young child with play periods.
◆ Enlist the help of the physical therapy department and play therapists, if available.
◆ Provide emotional support.
◆ Include family members in all phases of the child's care.

MONITORING
◆ Vital signs
◆ Intake and output
◆ Daily weight
◆ Hydration
◆ Pulse oximetry
◆ Respiratory status

PATIENT TEACHING

GENERAL
Be sure to cover:
◆ the disorder, diagnosis, and treatment
◆ medications and potential adverse reactions
◆ when to notify the practitioner
◆ aerosol therapy
◆ chest physiotherapy
◆ signs and symptoms of infection
◆ complications.

DISCHARGE PLANNING
◆ Refer family members for genetic counseling, as appropriate.
◆ Refer the patient and his family to a local support group such as the Cystic Fibrosis Foundation.

RESOURCES
Organizations
American Academy of Pediatrics: *www.aap.org*
Cystic Fibrosis Foundation: *www.cff.org*
National Institute of Diabetes & Digestive & Kidney Diseases: *www.niddk.nih.gov*

Selected references
Aronson, B.S., and Marquis, M. "Care of the Adult Patient with Cystic Fibrosis," *Medical-Surgical Nursing* 13(3):143-54, June 2004.
Diseases, 4th ed. Philadelphia: Lippincott Williams & Wilkins, 2006.
Grossman, S., and Grossman, L.C. "Pathophysiology of Cystic Fibrosis: Implications for Critical Care Nurses," *Critical Care Nurse* 25(4):46-51, August 2005.
Rinaldi, C.D., and Narsavage, G.L. "One Breath at a Time: Living with Cystic Fibrosis," *Journal of Pediatric Nursing* 19(1):25-32, February 2004.

Cytomegalovirus infection

OVERVIEW

- A member of the herpesvirus group
- Also called *generalized salivary gland disease, cytomegalic inclusion disease,* and *CMV*

PATHOPHYSIOLOGY

- CMV is found in the saliva, urine, semen, breast milk, feces, blood, and vaginal and cervical secretions of infected people. It can be detected in body fluids for weeks or months after infection.
- CMV usually remains latent, but when T-lymphocyte–mediated immunity is compromised (as in organ transplantation, lymphoid neoplasms, and certain acquired immunodeficiencies), CMV is reactivated.
- CMV spreads through the body in lymphocytes or mononuclear cells to the lungs, liver, GI tract, eyes, and central nervous system (CNS), typically producing inflammatory reactions.

CAUSES

- May be transmitted in semen during homosexual activity (such transmission not yet proven in heterosexual men)
- Results from a deoxyribonucleic acid virus belonging to the herpes family
- Transmission through direct contact with secretions and excretions, through blood transfusions, transplacentally, and through transplanted organs
- Transmitted by human contact; once infected, a person carries CMV for life

INCIDENCE

- This infection occurs worldwide.
- It occurs in about 30% to 50% of acquired immunodeficiency syndrome patients.
- CMV is one of the most opportunistic pathogens in patients infected with human immunodeficiency virus.

COMPLICATIONS

- Pneumonia
- Hepatitis
- Ulceration of the GI tract and esophagus
- Retinitis
- Encephalopathy

Neonatal complications

- Stillbirth
- Neonatal retinitis
- Microcephaly
- Mental retardation
- Seizures
- Hearing loss
- Thrombocytopenia
- Hemolytic anemia

ASSESSMENT

HISTORY

- Immunosuppressive condition

PHYSICAL FINDINGS

- Fever common
- Lethargy
- In immunocompetent patient with CMV mononucleosis, 3 or more weeks of irregular high fever may be the only finding
- Tachypnea
- Dyspnea
- Cyanosis
- Cough
- Jaundice
- Spider angiomas
- Hepatomegaly
- Splenomegaly
- In infants, CNS damage (mental retardation, hearing loss, seizures), jaundice, petechial rash, respiratory distress

DIAGNOSTIC TEST RESULTS

LABORATORY

- Isolating the virus or demonstrating increasing serologic titers by complement fixation studies, hemagglutination inhibition antibody tests and, in congenital infections, indirect immunofluorescent tests for CMV immunoglobulin M antibody allowing diagnosis.

IMAGING

- Chest X-ray reveals bilateral, diffuse, white infiltrates.
- Computed tomography scan or magnetic resonance imaging shows CNS involvement.

DIAGNOSTIC PROCEDURES

- Endoscopy shows GI involvement.
- Funduscopy may show retinitis.

TREATMENT

GENERAL

- Currently no treatment for CMV infection in the healthy individual
- Antiviral therapy that's now being evaluated in neonates
- Vaccines that are still in the research and development stage

ACTIVITY

- Rest, as needed

MEDICATIONS

- Antivirals
- Immune serums

NURSING DIAGNOSES

- Activity intolerance
- Acute pain
- Compromised family coping
- Diarrhea
- Fatigue
- Hyperthermia
- Impaired gas exchange
- Ineffective breathing pattern
- Risk for infection

EXPECTED OUTCOMES

The patient will:

- demonstrate skill in conserving energy while carrying out daily activities to tolerance level
- articulate factors that intensify pain and modify behavior accordingly
- develop effective coping behaviors (family)
- return to a normal elimination pattern
- report having an increased energy level
- remain afebrile
- maintain adequate ventilation and oxygenation
- maintain an effective breathing pattern
- experience no further signs or symptoms of infection.

NURSING INTERVENTIONS

- Institute standard precautions.
- Give prescribed drugs.
- If vision impairment occurs, provide a safe environment and encourage optimal independence.

MONITORING

- Intake and output
- Ventilation and oxygenation if the respiratory system is involved

GENERAL

Be sure to cover:

- proper hand-washing technique
- need for parents to wear gloves when in contact with secretions or changing diapers and to dispose of diapers or soiled articles properly and wash hands thoroughly
- need for female health care workers trying to get pregnant to have CMV titers drawn to identify their risk of contracting the infection
- need for an immunosuppressed or pregnant patient to avoid contact with any person who has confirmed or suspected CMV infection
- need for an immunosuppressed patient who's CMV-seronegative to carry this information with him so he won't be given CMV-positive blood.

DISCHARGE PLANNING

- Provide emotional support and counseling to the parents of a child with severe CMV infection. Help them find support systems, and coordinate referrals to other health care professionals.
- For information and support, refer the patient and his family to a local chapter of the National Center for Infectious Diseases.

RESOURCES

Organizations

Centers for Disease Control and Prevention — National Center for Infectious Diseases: *www.cdc.gov/ncidod*

Harvard University Consumer Health Information: *www.intelihealth.com*

National Health Information Center: *www.health.gov/nhic*

National Library of Medicine: *www.nlm.nih.gov*

Selected references

Diseases, 4th ed. Philadelphia: Lippincott Williams & Wilkins, 2006.

Jim, W.T., et al. "Transmission of Cytomegalovirus from Mothers to Preterm Infants by Breast Milk," *The Pediatric Infectious Disease Journal* 23(9):848-51, September 2004.

Kasper, D.L., et al., eds. *Harrison's Principles of Internal Medicine,* 16th ed. New York: McGraw-Hill Book Co., 2005.

Lawson, C.A. "Cytomegalovirus After Kidney Transplantation: A Case Review," *Progress in Transplantation* 15(2):157-60, June 2005.

Dacryocystitis

- Infection of the lacrimal sac resulting from obstruction of the nasolacrimal duct
- Acute or chronic

PATHOPHYSIOLOGY

- The lacrimal excretory system is a mucous membrane–lined tract that's contiguous with conjunctival and nasal mucosa.
- Conjunctival and nasal mucosa are normally colonized with bacteria.
- Inability to drain tears due to a blocked lacrimal drainage system results in infection. (See *A close look at tears.*)

CAUSES

Acute form

- Beta-hemolytic streptococci
- Nasal disease
- *Staphylococcus aureus*

Chronic form

- Chronic mucosal degeneration
- Fungus, such as *Actinomyces* or *Candida albicans*
- *Streptococcus pneumoniae*

INCIDENCE

- Dacryocystitis is most common in adults older than age 40.
- This disease occurs more commonly on the left side than the right side.
- It occurs rarely in blacks.
- Dacryocystitis affects females more commonly than males.

COMPLICATIONS

- Hemorrhage
- Infection
- Cerebrospinal fluid leakage

HISTORY

- Eye pain
- Fever

PHYSICAL FINDINGS

- Severe erythematous swelling around nasal aspect of lower eyelid
- Tenderness of eyelid
- Tearing
- Conjunctival injection
- Palpable mass inferior to the medial canthal tendon
- Decreased visual acuity
- Orbital cellulitis

LABORATORY

- Culture of discharge demonstrates organism.
- White blood cell count is elevated.

IMAGING

- X-ray after injection of radiopaque medium locates atresia.
- Dacryocystography and dacryoscintigraphy identify anatomical abnormalities of the nasolacrimal drainage system.

OTHER

- Physical examination reveals erythematous swelling around nasal side of lower eyelid.

A close look at tears

Tears begin in the lacrimal gland and drain through the nasolacrimal duct into the nose.

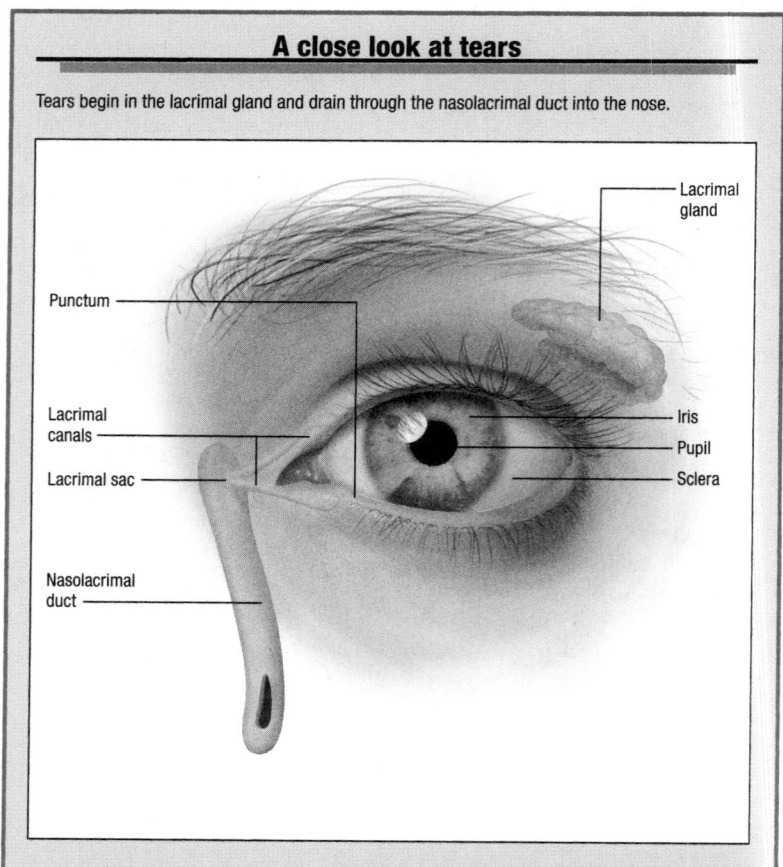

Labels: Punctum, Lacrimal canals, Lacrimal sac, Nasolacrimal duct, Lacrimal gland, Iris, Pupil, Sclera

TREATMENT

GENERAL
◆ Warm compresses

ACTIVITY
◆ As tolerated

MEDICATIONS
◆ Topical polymyxin/trimethoprim eyedrops
◆ Systemic amoxicillin
◆ I.V. antibiotics

SURGERY
◆ Incision and drainage
◆ Dacryocystorhinostomy (chronic cases)

NURSING CONSIDERATIONS

NURSING DIAGNOSES
◆ Acute pain
◆ Anxiety
◆ Impaired tissue integrity
◆ Ineffective health maintenance
◆ Risk for infection

EXPECTED OUTCOMES
The patient will:
◆ express feelings of increased comfort
◆ express feelings of decreased anxiety
◆ have reduced swelling, redness, and pain
◆ maintain current health status
◆ remain free from signs and symptoms of infection.

NURSING INTERVENTIONS
◆ Give prescribed antibiotics.
◆ Apply compresses.

MONITORING
◆ Bleeding
◆ Pain

PATIENT TEACHING

GENERAL
Be sure to cover:
◆ the disorder, diagnosis, and treatment
◆ applying warm compresses and eyedrops
◆ reporting signs of worsening infection.

RESOURCES
Organizations
American Academy of Ophthalmology: *www.aao.org*
Harvard University Consumer Health Information: *www.intelihealth.com*
The Merck Manuals Online Medical Library: *www.merck.com/mmhe*
National Eye Institute: *www.nei.nih.gov*

Selected references
Kotlus, B.S., et al. "Dacryocystitis Caused by Community-onset Methicillin-resistant *Staphylococcus aureus*," *Ophthalmic Plastic and Reconstructive Surgery* 21(5):371-75, September 2005.

Morgan, S., et al. "The Treatment of Acute Dacryocystitis Using Laser Assisted Endonasal Dacryocystorhinostomy," *British Journal of Ophthalmology* 88(1):139-41, January 2004.

Sun, X., et al. "Microbiological Analysis of Chronic Dacryocystitis," *Ophthalmic & Physiological Optics* 25(3):261-63, May 2005.

Dermatophytosis

OVERVIEW

- A group of superficial fungal infections usually classified according to their anatomic location
- May affect the scalp (tinea capitis), the bearded skin of the face (tinea barbae), the body (tinea corporis, occurring mainly in children), the groin (tinea cruris, or jock itch), the nails (tinea unguium, also called onychomycosis), and the feet (tinea pedis, or athlete's foot)
- May vary from mild inflammations to acute vesicular reactions

PATHOPHYSIOLOGY

- Tinea infections result from dermatophytes (fungi) of the genera *Trichophyton*, *Microsporum*, and *Epidermophyton*.

CAUSES

- Contact with contaminated animals or soil
- Direct transmission (through contact with infected lesions) or indirect transmission (through contact with contaminated articles, such as shoes, towels, or shower stalls)
- Warm weather, humidity, and tight clothing, which encourage fungus growth

INCIDENCE

- Tinea infections are prevalent in the United States.
- Dermatophytosis is more common in males than in females.
- Remissions and exacerbations are common.
- Cure rate is high with effective treatment.
- About 20% of infected people develop chronic conditions.

COMPLICATIONS

- Hair or nail loss and secondary bacterial infections, resulting in inflammation, itching, tenderness, and maceration

ASSESSMENT

HISTORY

- With tinea capitis: small, spreading papules on the scalp that may progress to inflamed, pus-filled lesions (kerions) or patchy hair loss with scaling
- With tinea corporis: flat skin lesions at any site except the scalp, bearded skin, or feet that are dry and scaly or moist and crusty; as they enlarge, their centers heal, producing the classic ring-shaped appearance
- With tinea cruris: raised, sharply defined, itchy red lesions in the groin that may extend to the buttocks, inner thighs, and external genitalia
- With tinea unguium: gradual thickening, discoloration, and crumbling of the nail, with accumulation of subungual debris; the nail may eventually be completely destroyed
- With tinea pedis: extreme itching and pain on walking with scaling and blisters between the toes, and possibly, a dry, squamous inflammation that affects the entire sole

PHYSICAL FINDINGS

- Tinea capitis: small papules on scalp, pus-filled lesions, or patchy hair loss with scaling
- Tinea barbae: pustular follicles
- Tinea corporis: flat skin lesions (dry and scaly or moist and crusty) and classic ring-shaped appearance
- Tinea cruris: sharply defined, itchy red lesions in groin, buttocks, inner thighs, and external genitalia
- Tinea unguium: thick, discolored, crumbling nail
- Tinea pedis: scaling and blisters between toes or dry, squamous inflammation on the sole

DIAGNOSTIC TEST RESULTS

LABORATORY

- Culture of the affected area may help to identify the infecting organism.

DIAGNOSTIC PROCEDURES

- Potassium hydroxide test and microscopic examination of lesion scrapings help confirm tinea infection.

OTHER

- Wood's light examination may help confirm some types of tinea capitis.

TREATMENT

GENERAL

- Application of open, wet dressings
- Removal of scabs and scales
- Administration of a keratolytic (salicylic acid) to soften and remove hyperkeratotic lesions of the heels or soles

MEDICATIONS

- Topical antifungal (imidazole cream)
- Other antifungals: naftifine (Naftin), ciclopirox (Loprox), terbinafine (Lamisil), tolnaftate (Tinactin)
- Oral griseofulvin (Gris-Peg) for infections of the skin and hair
- Oral terbinafine or itraconazole (Sporanox) for nail infections
- Oral griseofulvin (for 1 to 3 months) for tinea capitis

NURSING DIAGNOSES
◆ Acute pain
◆ Disturbed body image
◆ Impaired skin integrity
◆ Risk for infection

EXPECTED OUTCOMES
The patient will:
◆ report feelings of increased comfort
◆ voice feelings about his changed body image
◆ exhibit improved or healed wounds or lesions
◆ avoid or minimize the risk of secondary infection.

NURSING INTERVENTIONS
◆ Nursing interventions are guided by the type of tinea infection.
◆ Assist with daily skin care.
◆ Encourage verbalization of feelings.
◆ Offer emotional support and reassurance.

MONITORING
◆ Adverse reactions
◆ Response to treatment
◆ Liver function
◆ Complications
◆ Wound site

GENERAL
Be sure to cover:
◆ the disorder, diagnosis, and treatment
◆ skin care
◆ prescribed drugs and potential adverse reactions
◆ adverse reactions to griseofulvin therapy, including sensitivity reactions, GI disturbances, headaches, photosensitivity, and possibly, liver damage
◆ careful hand-washing technique
◆ sitz baths for tinea cruris to relieve itching
◆ avoidance of sharing clothing, hats, towels, bed linens, or pillows with others, and the need to keep lesions covered
◆ avoidance of scratching because scarring and secondary infection may occur.

DISCHARGE PLANNING
◆ Teach the patient and his family about transmission and recurrence of the infection.
◆ For tinea capitis, suggest that other family members be checked for the disorder.
◆ Instruct the patient with tinea cruris to dry the affected area thoroughly after bathing and to dust evenly with antifungal powder. Suggest sitz baths to relieve itching.
◆ Recommend that the patient with tinea barbae let his beard grow and trim his whiskers with scissors, not a razor. If he insists that he must shave, advise him to use an electric razor instead of a blade.
◆ Encourage the patient with tinea pedis to expose his feet to air whenever possible and to wear sandals or leather shoes and clean cotton socks. Tell him to wash his feet twice daily and, after drying them thoroughly, to dust them evenly with an antifungal powder to absorb perspiration and prevent excoriation.
◆ Refer the patient to the American Academy of Dermatology.

RESOURCES
Organizations
American Academy of Dermatology: *www.aad.org*
Dermatology Foundation: *www.dermfnd.org*

Selected references
Borgers, M., et al. "Fungal Infections of the Skin: Infection Process and Antimycotic Therapy," *Current Drug Targets* 6(8):849-62, December 2005.
Gupta, A.K., et al. "Optimal Management of Fungal Infections of the Skin, Hair, and Nails," *American Journal of Clinical Dermatology* 5(4):225-37, 2004.
Tosanger, M., and Crutchfield, C.E. "Tinea Corporis," *Dermatology Nursing* 16(5):453, October 2004.

Developmental dysplasia of the hip

OVERVIEW

- An abnormality of the hip joint present at birth
- The most common disorder affecting the hip joints in children younger than age 3
- Can be unilateral or bilateral
- Occurs in three forms of varying severity (see *Degrees of hip dysplasia*)
- Also known as *DDH*

PATHOPHYSIOLOGY

- Excessive or abnormal movement of the joint during a traumatic birth may cause dislocation.
- Displacement of bones within the joint may damage joint structures, including articulating surfaces, blood vessels, tendons, ligaments, and nerves.
- Disruption of blood flow to the joint may lead to ischemic necrosis.

CAUSES

- Exact cause unknown

RISK FACTORS

- Breech delivery
- Elevated maternal relaxin level (hormone secreted by the corpus luteum during pregnancy that causes relaxation of pubic symphysis and cervical dilation)
- Large neonates and twins

INCIDENCE

- About 85% of affected infants are females.

COMPLICATIONS

- Degenerative hip changes
- Abnormal acetabular development
- Lordosis (abnormally increased concave curvature of the lumbar and cervical spine)
- Joint malformation
- Sciatic nerve injury (paralysis)
- Avascular necrosis of femoral head
- Soft tissue damage
- Permanent disability

ASSESSMENT

HISTORY

- Traumatic birth
- Large birth size
- Twin

PHYSICAL FINDINGS

- Extra fold on the thigh of the affected side
- Limited abduction on the dislocated side
- Level of knees uneven
- Swaying from side to side ("duck waddle") because of uncorrected bilateral dysplasia
- Limp due to uncorrected unilateral dysplasia

Degrees of hip dysplasia

Normally, the head of the femur fits snugly into the acetabulum, allowing the hip to move properly. In congenital hip dysplasia, flattening of the acetabulum prevents the head of the femur from rotating adequately. The child's hip may be unstable, subluxated (partially dislocated), or completely dislocated, with the femoral head lying totally outside the acetabulum. The degree of dysplasia and the child's age are considered in determining the treatment choice.

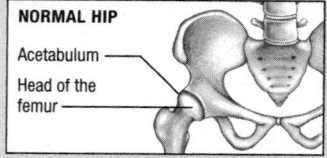

NORMAL HIP

Acetabulum
Head of the femur

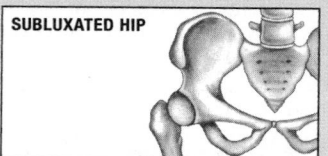

SUBLUXATED HIP

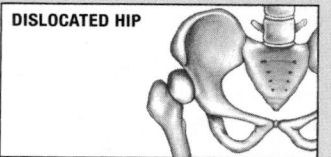

DISLOCATED HIP

DIAGNOSTIC TEST RESULTS

IMAGING

- X-rays show the location of the femur head and a shallow acetabulum.
- Sonography and magnetic resonance imaging assess reduction.

OTHER

- Physical examination (see *Ortolani's and Trendelenburg's signs of DDH*)

Ortolani's and Trendelenburg's signs of DDH

A positive Ortolani's or Trendelenburg's sign confirms developmental dysplasia of the hip (DDH).

ORTOLANI'S SIGN

- Place the infant on his back, with hip flexed and in abduction. Adduct the hip while pressing the femur downward. This will dislocate the hip.
- Next, abduct the hip while moving the femur upward. A click or a jerk (produced by the femoral head moving over the acetabular rim) indicates subluxation in an infant younger than age 1 month. The sign indicates subluxation or complete dislocation in an older infant.

TRENDELENBURG'S SIGN

- When the child rests his weight on the side of the dislocation and lifts his other knee, the pelvis drops on the normal side because abductor muscles in the affected hip are weak.
- However, when the child stands with his weight on the normal side and lifts the other knee, the pelvis remains horizontal.

TREATMENT

GENERAL

✿ **AGE FACTOR** *Treatment of DDH varies with the patient's age.*

◆ *Younger than age 3 months:*
- *Gentle manipulation to reduce the dislocation, followed by splint-brace or harness*
- *Splint-brace or harness worn continuously for 2 to 3 months, then a night splint for another month*

◆ *Older than age 3 months:*
- *Bilateral skin traction (in infants) or skeletal traction (in children who have started walking)*
- *Bryant's traction or divarication traction (both extremities placed in traction, even if only one is affected, to help maintain immobilization) for children younger than 3 years and weighing less than 35 lb (15.9 kg) for 2 to 3 weeks*
- *Immobilization in a spica cast for about 3 months for children ages 6 to 12 months*

✿ **AGE FACTOR** *Treatment begun after age 5 rarely restores satisfactory hip function.*

DIET
◆ No restriction

ACTIVITY
◆ As tolerated

SURGERY
◆ Gentle closed reduction under general anesthesia to further abduct the hips, followed by a spica cast for 3 months (if traction fails)
◆ In children older than age 18 months, open reduction and pelvic or femoral osteotomy to correct bony deformity followed by immobilization in a spica cast for 6 to 8 weeks
◆ In children ages 2 to 5 years, skeletal traction and subcutaneous adductor tenotomy (surgical cutting of the tendon)

NURSING CONSIDERATIONS

NURSING DIAGNOSES
◆ Deficient fluid volume
◆ Disturbed body image
◆ Fear
◆ Impaired physical mobility
◆ Risk for impaired skin integrity
◆ Risk for injury

EXPECTED OUTCOMES
The patient (and his family) will:
◆ maintain adequate fluid volume
◆ maintain positive outlook about body image
◆ verbalize fears or concerns
◆ achieve the highest level of mobility possible within the confines of the disease
◆ maintain intact skin
◆ show no evidence of complications, such as contractures, venous stasis, thrombus formation, or skin breakdown.

NURSING INTERVENTIONS
◆ Provide reassurance to the parents.
◆ Turn the child every 2 hours.
◆ Provide appropriate cast care.

MONITORING
◆ Parental care of cast or equipment
◆ Skin integrity
◆ Color, sensation, and motion of the infant's legs and feet
◆ Comfort

PATIENT TEACHING

GENERAL
Be sure to cover:
◆ how to correctly splint or brace the hips, as ordered
◆ good hygiene
◆ signs and symptoms of cast compression (cyanosis, cool extremities, or pain).

DISCHARGE PLANNING
◆ Stress the need for frequent check-ups.
◆ Refer the child and parents to a child life specialist to ensure continued developmental progress.

RESOURCES
Organizations
American Academy of Pediatrics: *www.aap.org*
American Orthopaedic Association: *www.aoassn.org*

Selected references
Kamath, S.U., and Benniet, G.C. "Does Developmental Dysplasia of the Hip Cause a Delay in Walking?" *Journal of Pediatric Orthopedics* 24(3):265, May 2004.
Kim, Y.H., and Kim, J.S. "Total Hip Arthroplasty in Adult Patients who had Developmental Dysplasia of the Hip," *The Journal of Arthroplasty* 20(8):1029-1036, December 2005.
Roovers, E.A., et al. "The Natural History of Developmental Dysplasia of the Hip: Sonographic Findings in Infants of 1-3 Months of Age," *Journal of Pediatric Orthopaedics Part B* 14(5):325-30, September 2005.

Diabetes insipidus

OVERVIEW

- Disorder of water balance regulation characterized by decreased secretion of antidiuretic hormone, resulting in excessive fluid intake and hypotonic polyuria
- Two types: primary and secondary
- May occur transiently during pregnancy, usually after the 5th or 6th month of gestation
- Impaired or absent thirst mechanism increases risk of complications
- If uncomplicated, prognosis good
- If complicated by underlying disorder, such as cancer, prognosis is variable
- Also referred to as *DI*

PATHOPHYSIOLOGY

- Vasopressin (antidiuretic hormone) is synthesized in the hypothalamus and stored by the posterior pituitary gland.
- Once released into the general circulation, vasopressin acts on the distal and collecting tubules of the kidneys.
- Vasopressin increases the water permeability of the tubules and causes water reabsorption.
- The absence of vasopressin allows filtered water to be excreted in the urine instead of being reabsorbed.

CAUSES

- Certain medications such as lithium
- Congenital malformation of the central nervous system (CNS)
- Damage to hypothalamus or pituitary gland
- Failure of the kidneys to respond to vasopressin, called *nephrogenic DI*
- Failure of vasopressin secretion in response to normal physiologic stimuli
- Familial
- Granulomatous disease
- Idiopathic
- Infection
- Neurosurgery, skull fracture, or head trauma
- Pregnancy (gestational DI)
- Psychogenic
- Trauma
- Tumors
- Vascular lesions

INCIDENCE

- DI affects men and women equally.
- Primary DI occurs in 50% of patients.

COMPLICATIONS

- Hypovolemia
- Hyperosmolality
- Circulatory collapse
- Loss of consciousness
- CNS changes
- Bladder distention
- Hydroureter
- Hydronephrosis

ASSESSMENT

HISTORY

- Abrupt onset of extreme polyuria
- Extreme thirst
- Extraordinarily large oral fluid intake
- Weight loss
- Dizziness; weakness; fatigue
- Constipation
- Nocturia

AGE FACTOR *In children, reports of enuresis, sleep disturbances, irritability, anorexia, thirst, and decreased weight gain and linear growth are common.*

PHYSICAL FINDINGS

- Signs of dehydration
- Fever
- Dyspnea
- Pale, voluminous urine
- Poor skin turgor
- Tachycardia
- Decreased muscle strength
- Hypotension
- Hypernatremia

DIAGNOSTIC TEST RESULTS

LABORATORY

- Urinalysis shows colorless urine with low osmolality and specific gravity.
- Serum sodium level is increased.
- Serum osmolality is increased.
- Serum vasopressin level is decreased.
- 24-hour urine test shows decreased specific gravity and increased volume.
- Blood urea nitrogen (BUN) and creatinine levels are elevated.

DIAGNOSTIC PROCEDURES

- Dehydration test or water deprivation test shows an increase in urine osmolality after vasopressin administration exceeding 9%.

TREATMENT

GENERAL
- Identification and treatment of underlying cause

DIET
- Control of fluid balance
- Dehydration prevention
- Free access to oral fluids
- With nephrogenic DI, low-sodium

MEDICATIONS
- Vasopressin (Pitressin)
- Synthetic vasopressin analogue
- Vasopressin stimulant
- Thiazide diuretics in nephrogenic DI
- I.V. fluids:
- If serum sodium level greater than 150: 5% dextrose in water
- If serum sodium level less than 150: normal saline solution

SURGERY
- Not indicated, unless required to treat underlying cause such as a tumor

NURSING CONSIDERATIONS

NURSING DIAGNOSES
- Anxiety
- Deficient fluid volume
- Delayed growth and development
- Disabled family coping
- Energy field disturbance
- Fear
- Impaired oral mucous membrane
- Impaired urinary elimination
- Ineffective coping
- Risk for injury

EXPECTED OUTCOMES
The patient (and his family) will:
- identify strategies to reduce anxiety
- demonstrate balanced fluid volume
- demonstrate age-appropriate skills and behavior to the extent possible
- develop adequate coping mechanisms and support systems
- verbalize having an increased sense of well-being
- discuss fears and concerns
- maintain intact oral mucous membranes
- have balanced intake and output
- display adaptive coping behaviors
- avoid complications.

NURSING INTERVENTIONS
- Administer medications, as ordered.
- Provide meticulous skin and mouth care.

WARNING *Use caution when administering vasopressin to a patient with coronary artery disease because it can cause coronary artery constriction.*

- Encourage verbalization of feelings.
- Offer encouragement while providing a realistic assessment of the situation.
- Help the patient develop effective coping strategies.

MONITORING
- Intake and output
- Vital signs
- Daily weight
- Urine specific gravity
- Serum electrolytes and BUN
- Signs and symptoms of hypovolemic shock
- Changes in mental or neurologic status
- Cardiac rhythm

PATIENT TEACHING

GENERAL
Be sure to cover:
- the disorder, diagnosis, and treatment
- medication and potential adverse reactions
- when to notify the practitioner
- signs and symptoms of dehydration
- daily weight
- intake and output
- use of a hydrometer to measure urine specific gravity
- need for medical identification jewelry
- need for ongoing medical care.

DISCHARGE PLANNING
- Refer the patient to a mental health professional for additional counseling as indicated.

RESOURCES
Organizations
American Association of Clinical Endocrinologists: *www.aace.com*
Diabetes Insipidus Foundation, Inc.: *www.diabetesinsipidus.org*
Endocrine Society: *www.endo-society.org*

Selected references
Brewster, U.C., and Hayslett, J.P. "Diabetes Insipidus in the Third Trimester of Pregnancy," *Obstetrics & Gynecology* 105(5 Part 2) Supplement:1173-176, May 2005.
Davies, J.H., et al. "Clinical Features, Diagnosis and Molecular Studies of Familial Central Diabetes Insipidus," *Hormone Research* 64(5):231-37, Epub October 2005.
Jani, R., et al. "Heparin-induced Thrombocytopenia Presenting as Central Diabetes Insipidus," *Endocrinologist* 15(6):374-76, November-December 2005.

Diabetes mellitus

OVERVIEW

- Chronic disease of absolute or relative insulin deficiency or resistance
- Characterized by disturbances in carbohydrate, protein, and fat metabolism
- Two primary forms:
- Type 1, characterized by absolute insulin insufficiency
- Type 2, characterized by insulin resistance with varying degrees of insulin secretory defects

PATHOPHYSIOLOGY

- The effects of diabetes mellitus (DM) result from insulin deficiency or resistance to endogenous insulin.
- Insulin allows glucose transport into the cells for use as energy or storage as glycogen.
- Insulin also stimulates protein synthesis and free fatty acid storage in the adipose tissues.
- Insulin deficiency compromises the body tissues' access to essential nutrients for fuel and storage.

CAUSES

- Autoimmune disease (type 1)
- Genetic factors

RISK FACTORS

- Viral infections (type 1)
- Obesity (type 2)
- Physiologic or emotional stress
- Sedentary lifestyle (type 2)
- Pregnancy
- Medication, such as thiazide diuretics, adrenal corticosteroids, and hormonal contraceptives

INCIDENCE

- Type 1 diabetes usually occurs before age 30, although it may occur at any age.
- DM is more common in men.
- Type 2 diabetes usually occurs in obese adults after age 30, although it may be seen in obese North American youths of African-American, Native American, or Hispanic descent.
- DM affects about 8% of the population of the United States.
- About one-third of patients with DM are undiagnosed.
- Incidence of type 2 diabetes increases with age.

COMPLICATIONS

- Ketoacidosis
- Hyperosmolar hyperglycemic nonketotic syndrome
- Cardiovascular disease
- Peripheral vascular disease
- Retinopathy, blindness
- Nephropathy
- Diabetic dermopathy
- Impaired resistance to infection
- Cognitive depression

 AGE FACTOR *Neonates of diabetic mothers have a two to three times greater incidence of congenital malformations and fetal distress unless the mothers' blood glucose levels are well-controlled before conception and during pregnancy.*

ASSESSMENT

HISTORY

- Polyuria, nocturia
- Dehydration
- Polydipsia
- Dry mucous membranes
- Poor skin turgor
- Weight loss and hunger
- Weakness; fatigue
- Vision changes
- Frequent skin and urinary tract infections
- Dry, itchy skin
- Sexual problems
- Numbness or pain in the hands or feet
- Postprandial feeling of nausea or fullness
- Nocturnal diarrhea

Type 1
- Rapidly developing symptoms

Type 2
- Vague, long-standing symptoms that develop gradually
- Family history of DM
- Pregnancy
- Severe viral infection
- Other endocrine diseases

- Recent stress or trauma
- Use of drugs that increase blood glucose levels

PHYSICAL FINDINGS

- Retinopathy or cataract formation
- Skin changes, especially on the legs and feet
- Muscle wasting and loss of subcutaneous fat (type 1)
- Obesity, particularly in the abdominal area (type 2)
- Poor skin turgor
- Dry mucous membranes
- Decreased peripheral pulses
- Cool skin temperature
- Diminished deep tendon reflexes
- Orthostatic hypotension
- Characteristic "fruity" breath odor in ketoacidosis
- Possible hypovolemia and shock in ketoacidosis and hyperosmolar hyperglycemic state

DIAGNOSTIC TEST RESULTS

LABORATORY

- Fasting plasma glucose level is greater than or equal to 126 mg/dl on at least two occasions.
- Random blood glucose level is greater than or equal to 200 mg/dl.
- Two-hour postprandial blood glucose level is greater than or equal to 200 mg/dl.
- Glycosylated hemoglobin (HbA_{1C}) is increased.
- Urinalysis may show acetone or glucose.

DIAGNOSTIC PROCEDURES

- Ophthalmologic examination may show diabetic retinopathy.

TREATMENT

GENERAL

- American Diabetes Association recommendations to reach target glucose, HbA_{1C} lipid, and blood pressure levels
- Exercise and diet control
- Tight glycemic control for prevention of complications

DIET
◆ Modest caloric restriction for weight loss or maintenance

ACTIVITY
◆ Regular aerobic exercise

MEDICATIONS
◆ Exogenous insulin (type 1 or possibly type 2)
◆ Oral antihyperglycemic drugs (type 2)

SURGERY
◆ Pancreas transplantation

NURSING CONSIDERATIONS

NURSING DIAGNOSES
◆ Deficient fluid volume
◆ Disabled family coping
◆ Disturbed sensory perception: Visual, tactile
◆ Imbalanced nutrition: Less than body requirements
◆ Imbalanced nutrition: More than body requirements
◆ Impaired skin integrity
◆ Impaired urinary elimination
◆ Ineffective coping
◆ Ineffective tissue perfusion: Renal, cardiopulmonary, peripheral
◆ Risk for infection
◆ Risk for injury
◆ Sexual dysfunction

EXPECTED OUTCOMES
The patient will:
◆ maintain adequate fluid balance
◆ develop adequate coping mechanisms and support systems
◆ maintain optimal functioning within the confines of the visual and tactile impairment
◆ maintain daily calorie requirements
◆ maintain weight within an acceptable range
◆ maintain skin integrity
◆ have balanced intake and output
◆ demonstrate adaptive coping behaviors
◆ exhibit signs of adequate renal, cardiopulmonary, and peripheral perfusion

◆ remain free from signs and symptoms of infection
◆ avoid injury and complications
◆ discuss feelings about sexual impairment.

NURSING INTERVENTIONS
◆ Give prescribed drugs.
◆ Give rapidly absorbed carbohydrates for hypoglycemia or, if the patient is unconscious, glucagon or I.V. dextrose, as ordered.
◆ Administer I.V. fluids and insulin replacement for hyperglycemic crisis, as ordered.
◆ Provide meticulous skin care, especially to the feet and legs.
◆ Treat all injuries, cuts, and blisters immediately.
◆ Avoid constricting hose, slippers, or bed linens.
◆ Encourage adequate fluid intake.
◆ Encourage verbalization of feelings.
◆ Offer emotional support.
◆ Help to develop effective coping strategies.

MONITORING
◆ Vital signs
◆ Intake and output
◆ Daily weight
◆ Serum glucose
◆ Urine acetone
◆ Renal status
◆ Cardiovascular status
◆ Signs and symptoms of:
– Hypoglycemia
– Hyperglycemia
– Hyperosmolar coma
– Urinary tract and vaginal infections
– Diabetic neuropathy

PATIENT TEACHING

GENERAL
Be sure to cover:
◆ disorder, diagnosis, and treatment
◆ medication and potential adverse reactions
◆ when to notify the practitioner
◆ prescribed meal plan
◆ prescribed exercise program
◆ signs and symptoms of:
– infection
– hypoglycemia

– hyperglycemia
– diabetic neuropathy
◆ self-monitoring of blood glucose
◆ complications of hyperglycemia
◆ foot care
◆ annual regular ophthalmologic examinations
◆ safety precautions
◆ management of diabetes during illness.

DISCHARGE PLANNING
◆ Refer the patient to a dietitian.
◆ Refer the patient to a podiatrist if indicated.
◆ Refer the patient to an ophthalmologist.
◆ Refer adult diabetic patients who are planning families for preconception counseling.
◆ Refer the patient to the Juvenile Diabetes Research Foundation, the American Association of Diabetes Educators, and the American Diabetes Association to obtain additional information.

RESOURCES
Organizations
American Diabetes Association: *www.diabetes.org*
Juvenile Diabetes Research Foundation International: *www.jdf.org*
National Institute of Diabetes, Digestive, and Kidney Diseases: *www.niddk.nih.gov*

Selected references
Sieggreen, M.Y. "Stepping Up Care for Diabetic Foot Ulcers," *Nursing* 35(10):36-41, October 2005.
Sperling, M.A. "Neonatal Diabetes Mellitus: From Understudy to Center Stage," *Current Opinion in Pediatrics* 17(4):512-18, August 2005.
Stuebe, A.M., et al. "Duration of Lactation and Incidence of Type 2 Diabetes," *JAMA* 294(20):2601-610, November 2005.
Watkinson, S., and Chetram, N. "A Nurse-led Approach to Diabetic Retinal Screening," *Nursing Times* 101(36):32-34, September 2005.

Diphtheria

OVERVIEW

- Acute, highly contagious, toxin-mediated infection that usually infects the respiratory tract — primarily the tonsils, nasopharynx, and larynx
- GI and urinary tracts, conjunctivae, and ears rarely involved

PATHOPHYSIOLOGY
- Proliferation of organism at site of implantation
- Endotoxin: produced, absorbed by the blood, and transported to the heart and central nervous system

CAUSES
- *Corynebacterium diphtheriae,* a gram-positive rod
- Transmission usually through intimate contact, airborne respiratory droplets, or a break in the skin

INCIDENCE
- The disease is more prevalent during the colder months.
- Diphtheria is rare in many parts of the world, including the United States.
- The incidence of cutaneous diphtheria has been rising since 1972, especially in the Pacific Northwest and the Southwest.
- The disease is more prevalent in children younger than age 15.

COMPLICATIONS
- Thrombocytopenia
- Myocarditis
- Neurologic involvement (primarily affecting motor fibers but possibly also sensory neurons)
- Renal involvement
- Pulmonary involvement (bronchopneumonia)

ASSESSMENT

HISTORY
- Fever
- Sore throat
- Rasping cough
- Malaise
- Vomiting
- Dysphagia

PHYSICAL FINDINGS
- Hoarseness or stridor
- Thick, patchy, grayish green membrane over the mucous membranes of the pharynx, larynx, tonsils, soft palate, and nose
- Swelling of the palate
- Yellow spots or lesions (cutaneous)

DIAGNOSTIC TEST RESULTS

LABORATORY
- Throat culture or culture of other suspect lesions grows *C. diphtheriae.*

TREATMENT

GENERAL
- Symptomatic
- Droplet precautions (see *Droplet precautions*)

DIET
- As tolerated

ACTIVITY
- As tolerated

MEDICATIONS
- Diphtheria antitoxin
- Antibiotics

SURGERY
- Tracheotomy if airway obstruction occurs

Droplet precautions

Droplet precautions prevent the spread of infectious diseases transmitted by contact with nasal or oral secretions (droplets arising from coughing or sneezing) from the infected patient with the mucous membranes of the susceptible host.

Effective droplet precautions require a single room (not necessarily a negative-pressure room) and the door doesn't need to be closed. People having direct contact with, or who will be within 3' (1 m) of, the patient should wear a surgical mask covering the nose and mouth.

When handling infants or young children who require droplet precautions, you may also need to wear gloves and a gown to prevent soiling of clothing with nasal and oral secretions.

NURSING CONSIDERATIONS

NURSING DIAGNOSES
- Hyperthermia
- Imbalanced nutrition: Less than body requirements
- Impaired skin integrity
- Ineffective airway clearance
- Ineffective breathing pattern
- Risk for imbalanced fluid volume
- Risk for infection
- Risk for injury

EXPECTED OUTCOMES
The patient will:
- remain afebrile
- maintain a healthy nutritional status
- remain free from lesions or wounds
- maintain a patent airway
- maintain effective breathing pattern
- maintain an adequate fluid balance
- remain free from signs and symptoms of infection
- remain free from injury.

NURSING INTERVENTIONS
- Enforce strict isolation techniques.
- Give prescribed drugs.
- Obtain cultures, as ordered.
- Report all cases to local public health authorities.

MONITORING
- Pulse oximetry
- Airway
- Signs of shock
- Cardiac rhythm

PATIENT TEACHING

GENERAL
Be sure to cover:
- proper disposal of nasopharyngeal secretions
- maintaining infection precautions until after two consecutive negative nasopharyngeal cultures — at least 1 week after drug therapy stops.

DISCHARGE PLANNING
- Stress the need for childhood immunizations to all parents.

RESOURCES
Organizations
Centers for Disease Control and Prevention: *www.cdc.gov*
National Library of Medicine: *www.nlm.nih.gov*

Selected references
Raucci, J., et al. "Childhood Immunizations (part one)," *Journal of Pediatric Health Care* 18(2):95-101, March-April 2004.
Trollfors, B., et al. "Reduced Immunogenicity of Diphtheria and Tetanus Toxoids when Combined with Pertussis Toxoid," *Pediatric Infectious Disease Journal* 24(1):85-86, January 2005.

Dislocations and subluxations

- Dislocation — displacement of joint bones so that articulating surfaces totally lose contact (see *Common dislocation*)
- Subluxation — partial displacement of articulating surfaces
- May accompany fractures of joints

PATHOPHYSIOLOGY

- Trauma causes displacement of the joint.
- Joint structures (blood vessels, ligaments, tendons, and nerves) are damaged.
- Injuries may result in deposition of fracture fragments between joint surfaces, damaging surrounding structures.
- Joint function is impaired.

CAUSES

- Congenital
- Paget's disease of surrounding joint tissues
- Trauma

RISK FACTORS

- Participation in contact sports

INCIDENCE

- Shoulder dislocations account for more than one-half of dislocations seen in emergency departments.
- Hip dislocations from trauma are more common in those younger than age 35; from falls they're more common in those older than age 65.

COMPLICATIONS

- Avascular necrosis
- Bone necrosis

ASSESSMENT

HISTORY

- Trauma or fall
- Extreme pain at injury site
- Participation in contact sports

PHYSICAL FINDINGS

- Joint surface fractures
- Deformity around the joint
- Change in the length of the involved extremity
- Impaired joint mobility
- Point tenderness

DIAGNOSTIC TEST RESULTS

IMAGING

- X-rays confirm the diagnosis and show any associated fractures.

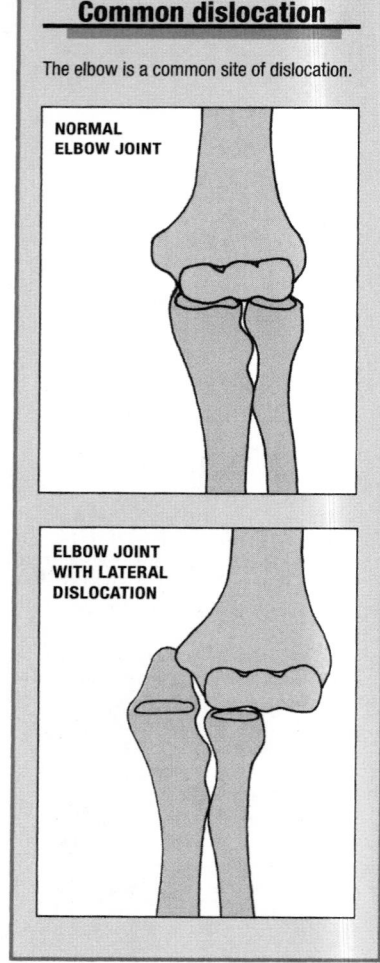

Common dislocation

The elbow is a common site of dislocation.

NORMAL ELBOW JOINT

ELBOW JOINT WITH LATERAL DISLOCATION

TREATMENT

GENERAL
◆ Immediate reduction and immobilization

DIET
◆ Nothing by mouth if surgery scheduled

ACTIVITY
◆ Limitations based on injury
◆ Active range-of-motion (ROM) exercises for adjacent joints not immobilized

MEDICATIONS
◆ Sedatives
◆ Analgesics
◆ Muscle relaxants

SURGERY
◆ Open reduction
◆ Skeletal traction
◆ Ligament repair

NURSING CONSIDERATIONS

NURSING DIAGNOSES
◆ Acute pain
◆ Disturbed body image
◆ Dressing or grooming self-care deficit
◆ Impaired physical mobility
◆ Ineffective tissue perfusion: Peripheral
◆ Risk for disuse syndrome

EXPECTED OUTCOMES
The patient will:
◆ articulate factors that intensify pain and will modify behavior accordingly
◆ express positive feelings about self
◆ perform self-care activities at the highest level possible
◆ attain the highest degree of mobility possible within the confines of the injury
◆ show signs of adequate peripheral perfusion
◆ maintain joint ROM and muscle strength.

NURSING INTERVENTIONS
◆ Give prescribed drugs.
◆ Provide proper positioning of the affected area.
◆ Apply ice, as ordered.
◆ Encourage ROM exercises, as ordered, for adjacent nonmobilized joints.
◆ Provide meticulous skin care.
  ⚡ **WARNING** *Immediately report signs and symptoms of severe vascular compromise, such as pallor, pain, loss of pulse, paralysis, and paresthesia; the patient needs an immediate orthopedic examination and emergency reduction.*

MONITORING
◆ Respiratory status when I.V. sedatives used
◆ Neurovascular status of involved extremity
◆ Integrity of skin

PATIENT TEACHING

GENERAL
Be sure to cover:
◆ the need to report numbness, pain, cyanosis, and coldness of the extremity below the cast or splint
◆ how to evaluate skin integrity
◆ how to assess neurovascular status
◆ the use of assistive devices
◆ the importance of follow-up visits
◆ drug administration, dosage, and possible adverse effects.

DISCHARGE PLANNING
◆ Refer the patient to a rehabilitation program if appropriate.
◆ Refer the patient for home health care if appropriate.

RESOURCES
Organizations
American Academy of Neurology: *www.aan.com*
Southern California Orthopedic Institute: *www.scoi.com*

Selected references

Flanigan, D.C., and Kaplan, L.D. "Elbow Dislocations and Instability," *Current Opinion in Orthopedics* 15(4):280-85, August 2004.

Shinoda-Tagawa, T., et al. "Resident-to-resident Violent Incidents in Nursing Homes," *JAMA* 291(17):2074-2075, May 2004.

Yasukawa, A., et al. "Shoulder Support for Children with Subluxation: A Case Study," *JPO: Journal of Prosthetics & Orthotics* 17(3):74-79, July 2005.

Disseminated intravascular coagulation LIFE-THREATENING DISORDER

OVERVIEW

◆ Syndrome of activated coagulation characterized by bleeding or thrombosis
◆ Complicates diseases and conditions that accelerate clotting, causing occlusion of small blood vessels, organ necrosis, depletion of circulating clotting factors and platelets, and activation of the fibrinolytic system
◆ Also known as *DIC, consumption coagulopathy,* and *defibrination syndrome*

PATHOPHYSIOLOGY

◆ Typical accelerated clotting results in generalized activation of prothrombin and a consequent excess of thrombin. (See *Three mechanisms of DIC.*)
◆ Excess thrombin converts fibrinogen to fibrin, producing fibrin clots in the microcirculation.
◆ This process consumes exorbitant amounts of coagulation factors (especially platelets, factor V, prothrombin, fibrinogen, and factor VIII), causing thrombocytopenia, deficien-

cies in factors V and VIII, hypoprothrombinemia, and hypofibrinogenemia.
◆ Circulating thrombin activates the fibrinolytic system, which lyses fibrin clots into fibrinogen degradation products (FDPs).
◆ The hemorrhage that occurs may be due largely to the anticoagulant activity of FDPs and depletion of plasma coagulation factors.

CAUSES

◆ Disorders that produce necrosis, such as extensive burns and trauma
◆ Infection, sepsis
◆ Neoplastic disease
◆ Obstetric complications
◆ Other disorders, such as heatstroke, shock, incompatible blood transfusion, drug reactions, cardiac arrest, surgery necessitating cardiopulmonary bypass, acute respiratory distress syndrome, diabetic ketoacidosis, pulmonary embolism, and sickle cell anemia

INCIDENCE

◆ Incidence depends on the cause.

COMPLICATIONS

◆ Renal failure
◆ Hepatic damage
◆ Stroke
◆ Ischemic bowel
◆ Respiratory distress
◆ Death (mortality is greater than 50%)

ASSESSMENT

HISTORY

◆ Abnormal bleeding without a history of a serious hemorrhagic disorder; bleeding may occur at all bodily orifices
◆ Possible presence of one of the causes of DIC
◆ Possible signs of bleeding into the skin, such as cutaneous oozing, petechiae, ecchymoses, and hematomas
◆ Possible bleeding from surgical or invasive procedure sites, such as incisions or venipuncture sites
◆ Possible nausea and vomiting; severe muscle, back, and abdominal pain; chest pain; hemoptysis; epistaxis; seizures; and oliguria
◆ Possible GI bleeding, hematuria

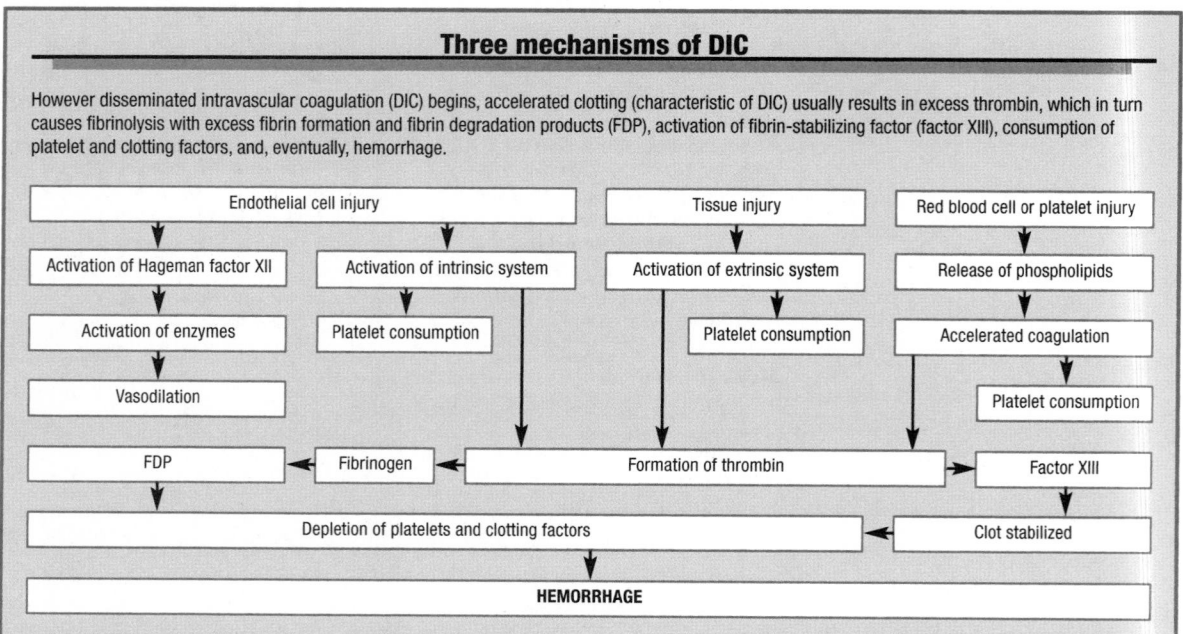

Three mechanisms of DIC

However disseminated intravascular coagulation (DIC) begins, accelerated clotting (characteristic of DIC) usually results in excess thrombin, which in turn causes fibrinolysis with excess fibrin formation and fibrin degradation products (FDP), activation of fibrin-stabilizing factor (factor XIII), consumption of platelet and clotting factors, and, eventually, hemorrhage.

Endothelial cell injury → Activation of Hageman factor XII → Activation of enzymes → Vasodilation

Endothelial cell injury → Activation of intrinsic system → Platelet consumption

Tissue injury → Activation of extrinsic system → Platelet consumption

Red blood cell or platelet injury → Release of phospholipids → Accelerated coagulation → Platelet consumption

FDP ← Fibrinogen ← Formation of thrombin → Factor XIII

Depletion of platelets and clotting factors ← Clot stabilized

HEMORRHAGE

PHYSICAL FINDINGS
◆ Petechiae
◆ Acrocyanosis
◆ Dyspnea, tachypnea
◆ Mental status changes, including confusion

DIAGNOSTIC TEST RESULTS

LABORATORY
◆ Serum platelet count is decreased (less than 150,000/µl).
◆ Serum fibrinogen level is decreased (less than 170 mg/dl).
◆ Prothrombin time is prolonged (more than 19 seconds).
◆ Partial thromboplastin time is prolonged (more than 40 seconds).
◆ FDPs are increased (commonly greater than 45 mcg/ml, or positive at less than 1:100 dilution).
◆ Result of D-dimer test (specific fibrinogen test for DIC) is positive at less than 1:8 dilution.
◆ Thrombin time is prolonged.
◆ Blood clotting factors V and VIII are diminished.
◆ Complete blood count shows hemoglobin levels less than 10 g/dl.
◆ Blood urea nitrogen level is elevated (greater than 25 mg/dl) and serum creatinine levels are elevated (greater than 1.3 mg/dl).

TREATMENT

GENERAL
◆ Treatment of the underlying condition
◆ Possibly supportive care alone if the patient isn't actively bleeding

ACTIVITY
◆ As tolerated

MEDICATIONS
If the patient is actively bleeding
◆ Administration of blood, fresh frozen plasma, platelets, or packed red blood cells
◆ Cryoprecipitate
◆ Antithrombin III
◆ Fluid replacement

NURSING CONSIDERATIONS

NURSING DIAGNOSES
◆ Acute pain
◆ Anxiety
◆ Fatigue
◆ Fear
◆ Impaired gas exchange
◆ Impaired physical mobility
◆ Impaired tissue integrity
◆ Ineffective tissue perfusion: Renal, cerebral, GI
◆ Risk for deficient fluid volume
◆ Risk for injury

EXPECTED OUTCOMES
The patient will:
◆ express feelings of increased comfort and decreased pain
◆ verbalize strategies to reduce anxiety level
◆ express feelings of energy and decreased fatigue
◆ use available support systems to assist in coping with fears
◆ maintain adequate ventilation and oxygenation
◆ perform activities of daily living with the maximum level of mobility and independence
◆ have reduced redness, swelling, and pain at the site of impaired tissue
◆ maintain a blood pressure high enough to maintain cerebral, GI, and renal perfusion pressure but low enough to prevent intracranial bleeding and cerebral swelling
◆ maintain fluid balance
◆ remain free from injury or complications.

NURSING INTERVENTIONS
⚡ **WARNING** *Focus on early recognition of signs of abnormal bleeding, prompt treatment of the underlying disorders, and prevention of further bleeding.*
◆ Provide emotional support.
◆ Provide adequate rest periods.
◆ Give prescribed analgesics as necessary.
◆ Reposition the patient every 2 hours and provide meticulous skin care.
◆ Give prescribed oxygen therapy.

⚡ **WARNING** *To prevent clots from dislodging and causing fresh bleeding, don't vigorously rub the affected areas when bathing.*
◆ Protect the patient from injury.
◆ If bleeding occurs, use pressure and topical hemostatic agents to control bleeding.
◆ Limit venipunctures whenever possible.
◆ Watch for transfusion reactions and signs of fluid overload.
◆ Measure the amount of blood lost, weigh dressings and linen and record drainage.
◆ Weigh the patient daily, particularly in renal involvement.

MONITORING
◆ Vital signs
◆ Results of serial blood studies
◆ Signs of shock
◆ Intake and output, especially when administering blood products

PATIENT TEACHING

GENERAL
Be sure to cover (with the patient and his family):
◆ an explanation of the disorder
◆ signs and symptoms of the problem, diagnostic procedures required, and treatment that the patient will receive.

RESOURCES
Organizations
American Heart Association: *www.americanheart.org*
Mayo Clinic: *www.mayoclinic.com*

Selected references
Backhouse, R. "Understanding Disseminated Intravascular Coagulation," *Nursing Times* 100(36): 38-42, September 2004.
Kasper, D.L., et al., eds. *Harrison's Principles of Internal Medicine,* 16th ed. New York: McGraw-Hill Book Co., 2005.
Toh, C., and Downey, C. "Back to the Future: Testing in Disseminated Intravascular Coagulation," *Blood Coagulation & Fibrinolysis* 16(8):535-42, November 2005.

Diverticular disease

- Bulging pouches (diverticula) in GI wall pushing the mucosal lining through surrounding muscle
- Sigmoid colon: most common site, but may develop anywhere, from proximal end of the pharynx to the anus
- Other typical sites:
- The duodenum, near the pancreatic border or the ampulla of Vater
- The jejunum
- Diverticular disease of the ileum (Meckel's diverticulum) — most common congenital anomaly of the GI tract (see *Meckel's diverticulum*)
- Two clinical forms:
- Diverticulosis: diverticula are present but don't cause symptoms
- Diverticulitis: diverticula become inflamed and may cause complications

PATHOPHYSIOLOGY

- Pressure in the intestinal lumen is exerted on weak areas, such as points where blood vessels enter the intestine, causing a break in the muscular continuity of the GI wall, creating a diverticulum.
- Diverticulitis occurs when retained undigested food mixed with bacteria accumulates in the diverticulum, forming a hard mass (fecalith). This substance cuts off the blood supply to the diverticulum's thin walls, increasing its susceptibility to attack by colonic bacteria.
- Inflammation follows bacterial infection, causing abdominal pain.

CAUSES

- Defects in colon wall strength
- Diminished colonic motility and increased intraluminal pressure

RISK FACTORS

- Age
- Low-fiber diet

INCIDENCE

- Diverticular disease is most common in adults age 45 and older.
- The disease affects 30% of adults older than age 60.

- Diverticular disease is more common in women than in men.

COMPLICATIONS

- Ruptured diverticula that cause abdominal abscesses or peritonitis
- Intestinal obstruction
- Rectal hemorrhage
- Portal pyemia
- Fistula

HISTORY
Diverticulosis
- May be symptom-free

Meckel's diverticulum

Meckel's diverticulum is a congenital abnormality that occurs when a blind tube like the appendix opens into the distal ileum near the ileocecal valve. This disorder results when the intra-abdominal portion of the yolk sac fails to close completely during fetal development. It occurs in about 2% of the population, mostly in males.

COMPLICATIONS

Uncomplicated Meckel's diverticulum produces no symptoms, but complications cause melena and abdominal pain, especially around the umbilicus. The lining of the diverticulum may be either gastric mucosa or pancreatic tissue. This disorder can lead to peptic ulceration, perforation, and peritonitis and may resemble acute appendicitis.

Meckel's diverticulum can also cause bowel obstruction when a fibrous band that connects the diverticulum to the abdominal wall, the mesentery, or other structures snares a loop of the intestine. This can cause intussusception into the diverticulum or volvulus near the diverticular attachment to the back of the umbilicus or another intra-abdominal structure.

Meckel's diverticulum should be considered in patients with GI obstruction or hemorrhage, especially when routine GI X-rays are negative.

TREATMENT

Treatment involves surgical resection of the inflamed bowel and antibiotic therapy, if infection occurs.

- Occasional intermittent pain in the left lower abdominal quadrant, which may be relieved by defecation or the passage of flatus
- Alternating bouts of constipation and diarrhea

Diverticulitis
- History of diverticulosis
- Low fiber consumption
- Recent consumption of foods containing seeds or kernels or indigestible roughage, such as celery and corn
- Complaints of moderate dull or steady pain in the left lower abdominal quadrant, aggravated by straining, lifting, or coughing
- Mild nausea, gas, diarrhea, or intermittent bouts of constipation, sometimes accompanied by rectal bleeding

PHYSICAL FINDINGS
Diverticulitis
- Distressed appearance
- Left lower quadrant abdominal tenderness
- Low-grade fever
- Palpable mass

Acute diverticulitis
- Muscle spasms
- Signs of peritoneal irritation
- Guarding and rebound tenderness

LABORATORY

- Complete blood count reveals leukocytosis.
- Erythrocyte sedimentation rate is elevated in diverticulitis.
- Stool test is positive for occult blood in 25% of patients with diverticulitis.

IMAGING

- Barium studies reveal barium filled diverticula or outlines, but barium doesn't fill diverticula blocked by impacted stools. This procedure isn't performed for acute diverticulitis due to potential rupture.
- Radiography may reveal colonic

spasm if irritable bowel syndrome accompanies diverticular disease.

♦ Abdominal X-rays rule out perforation.

♦ Computed tomography scan of the abdomen evaluates the presence of abscess.

DIAGNOSTIC PROCEDURES

♦ Colonoscopy or flexible sigmoidoscopy shows diverticula or inflamed mucosa. It isn't usually performed in the acute phase.

♦ Biopsy results may rule out cancer.

TREATMENT

GENERAL
♦ No treatment for asymptomatic diverticulosis required

♦ Nasogastric (NG) decompression for severe diverticulitis

ACTIVITY
♦ Bed rest

DIET
For diverticulosis

♦ Liquid or low-residue diet (if experiencing pain)

♦ Increased water consumption if appropriate

♦ High-residue diet (if not in pain)

For severe diverticulitis

♦ Nothing by mouth

MEDICATIONS
For diverticulosis

♦ Stool softeners

♦ Bulk medication

For diverticulitis

♦ Antibiotics

♦ Analgesics

♦ Antispasmodics

♦ I.V. therapy for severe diverticulitis

SURGERY
♦ Colon resection

♦ May require temporary colostomy to drain abscesses or to rest the colon for 6 to 8 weeks

♦ Needed for rupture or to correct cases refractory to medical treatment

NURSING CONSIDERATIONS

NURSING DIAGNOSES
♦ Acute pain

♦ Anxiety

♦ Constipation

♦ Deficient fluid volume

♦ Diarrhea

♦ Ineffective tissue perfusion: GI

EXPECTED OUTCOMES
The patient will:

♦ express feelings of increased comfort

♦ identify strategies to reduce anxiety

♦ have stools that are soft and pass easily

♦ maintain normal fluid volume

♦ have bowel movements that return to normal

♦ exhibit signs of adequate GI perfusion.

NURSING INTERVENTIONS
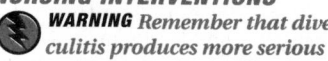 **WARNING** *Remember that diverticulitis produces more serious signs and symptoms as well as complications, and requires more interventions than diverticulosis.*

♦ If the patient is anxious, provide psychological support.

♦ Give prescribed drugs.

♦ Maintain bed rest for acute diverticulitis.

♦ Maintain the prescribed diet.

♦ If surgery is scheduled, provide routine preoperative care.

After colon resection

♦ Provide meticulous wound care.

♦ Encourage coughing and deep breathing.

♦ Give I.V. fluids and prescribed drugs.

♦ Provide colostomy care if appropriate.

MONITORING
♦ Pain control

♦ Stools for color, consistency, and frequency

♦ NG drainage if appropriate

♦ Signs and symptoms of complications

After colon resection

♦ Signs of infection and postoperative bleeding

♦ Intake and output

♦ Vital signs

PATIENT TEACHING

GENERAL
Be sure to cover:

♦ bowel and dietary habits (in uncomplicated diverticulosis)

♦ the disorder, diagnosis, and treatment

♦ preoperative teaching (for a patient needing surgery)

♦ postoperative teaching (for a patient who must care for his colostomy as needed)

♦ the desired actions and possible adverse effects of prescribed medications.

DISCHARGE PLANNING
♦ Refer the patient to an enterostomal therapist if appropriate.

♦ Refer the patient to a dietitian if needed.

RESOURCES
Organizations

Digestive Disease National Coalition: *www.ddnc.org*

National Digestive Diseases Information Clearinghouse: *www.niddk.nih.gov/ health/digest/nddic.htm*

Selected references

Burch, J. "Exploring the Conditions Leading to Stoma-forming Surgery," *British Journal of Nursing* 14(2):94-98, January-February 2005.

Clemens, C.H.M., et al. "Colorectal Visceral Perception in Diverticular Disease," *Gut* 53(5):717-22, May 2004.

Handbook of Diseases, 3rd ed. Philadelphia: Lippincott Williams & Wilkins, 2004.

Yamada, T., et al. *Atlas of Gastroenterology,* 3rd ed. Philadelphia: Lippincott Williams & Wilkins, 2003.

Down syndrome

- A chromosomal aberration that results in mental retardation, abnormal facial features, and other distinctive physical abnormalities
- Commonly associated with heart defects and other congenital disorders
- Average IQ between 30 and 50 (some higher)
- Also known as *mongolism* and *trisomy 21 syndrome*

PATHOPHYSIOLOGY

- Down syndrome is an aberration in which chromosome 21 has three copies instead of the normal two because of faulty meiosis (nondisjunction) of the ovum or, sometimes, the sperm.
- There's unbalanced translocation, in which the long arm of chromosome 21 breaks and attaches to another chromosome.
- The result is a karyotype of 47 chromosomes instead of the normal 46.

CAUSES

- Deterioration of the oocyte resulting from age or cumulative effects of radiation and viruses
- Trisomy 21

RISK FACTORS

AGE FACTOR *Maternal age, especially if the mother is older than age 35.*

INCIDENCE

- Down syndrome occurs in 1 per 800 to 1,000 live births.
- The incidence of Down syndrome increases with maternal age, especially after age 35.

COMPLICATIONS

- Death
- Congenital heart defects
- Premature senile dementia
- Leukemia
- Acute and chronic infections
- Diabetes mellitus
- Thyroid disorders

HISTORY

- Neonate lethargic and a poor feeder

PHYSICAL FINDINGS

- Slanting, almond-shaped eyes
- Small, open mouth, protruding tongue
- Single transverse palmar crease
- Brushfield's spots on the iris
- Small skull
- Flat bridge across the nose
- Flattened face
- Small external ears
- Short neck with excess skin
- Dry, sensitive skin with decreased elasticity
- Umbilical hernia
- Short stature
- Short extremities with broad, flat, and squarish hands and feet
- Dysplastic middle phalanx of the fifth finger
- Wide space between the first and second toes
- Abnormal fingerprints and footprints
- Impaired reflex development
- Absent Moro reflex and hyperextensible joints
- Impaired posture, coordination, and balance
- Clubfoot
- Imperforate anus
- Cleft lip and palate
- Pelvic bone abnormalities

LABORATORY

- Karyotype analysis or chromosome mapping shows the chromosomal abnormality and confirms the diagnosis of Down syndrome.
- Serum alpha-fetoprotein reveals reduced levels of alpha-fetoprotein prenatally.

IMAGING

- Prenatal ultrasonography can suggest Down syndrome if a duodenal obstruction or an atrioventricular canal defect is present.

OTHER

- Developmental screening tests show severity and progress of retardation.
- Amniocentesis allows prenatal diagnosis.

TREATMENT

GENERAL
- Early intervention
- Special education programs
- Special athletic programs
- Maximal environmental simulation for infants
- Safety precautions for children and adults in a controlled environment

MEDICATIONS
- Antibiotic therapy for recurrent infections
- Thyroid hormone replacement for hypothyroidism

SURGERY
- Open-heart surgery to correct cardiac defects, such as ventricular septal defects or atrial septal defects
- Plastic surgery to correct congenital abnormalities, such as protruding tongue, cleft lip, and cleft palate

NURSING CONSIDERATIONS

NURSING DIAGNOSES
- Bathing or hygiene self-care deficit
- Compromised family coping
- Delayed growth and development
- Dressing or grooming self-care deficit
- Ineffective health maintenance
- Risk for impaired parenting

EXPECTED OUTCOMES
The patient (and his family) will:
- perform bathing and hygiene activities of daily living (ADLs) to the fullest extent possible
- demonstrate adaptive coping behaviors
- demonstrate age-appropriate skills and behaviors to the extent possible
- perform dressing and grooming ADLs to the fullest extent possible
- perform health maintenance activities according to level of ability
- express understanding of norms for growth and development (parents).

NURSING INTERVENTIONS
- Establish a trusting relationship with the child's parents.
- Encourage verbalization and provide support.
- Encourage the parents to hold and nurture their child.

MONITORING
- Response to treatment
- Signs and symptoms of infection
- Complications
- Nutritional status
- Growth and development
- Thyroid function test results
- Heart sounds

PATIENT TEACHING

GENERAL
Be sure to cover:
- the need for adequate exercise and maximal environmental stimulation
- realistic goals for the parents and child
- information about a balanced diet
- the importance of remembering the emotional needs of other children in the family.

DISCHARGE PLANNING
- Refer the parents to infant stimulation classes.
- Refer the parents and older siblings for genetic and psychological counseling, as appropriate.
- Refer the patient and his parents to support services.

RESOURCES
Organizations
National Association for Down Syndrome: *www.nads.org*
National Down Syndrome Congress: *www.ndsccenter.org*
National Down Syndrome Society: *www.ndss.org*

Selected references
Diagnostic and Statistical Manual of Mental Disorders, Fourth Edition, Text Revision. Washington, D.C.: American Psychiatric Association, 2000.
Egan, J.F.X., et al. "Down Syndrome Births in the United States from 1989-2001," *American Journal of Obstetrics & Gynecology* 191(3):1044-48, September 2004.
Harvey, B. "Down's Syndrome: A Biopsychosocial Perspective," *Nursing Standard* 18(30):43-45, April 2004.
Kasper, D.L., et al., eds. *Harrison's Principles of Internal Medicine,* 16th ed. New York: McGraw-Hill Book Co., 2005.
Zindler, L. "Ethical Decision Making in First Trimester Pregnancy Screening," *Journal of Perinatal & Neonatal Nursing* 19(2): 122-31, April-June 2005.

Dysmenorrhea

- Painful menstruation associated with ovulation that isn't related to pelvic disease
- Most common gynecologic complaint
- Leading cause of absenteeism from school and work
- A primary disorder or secondary to an underlying disease

CAUSES
Primary
- Unrelated to an identifiable cause

Secondary
- Cervical stenosis
- Endometriosis
- Pelvic inflammatory disease
- Pelvic tumors (see *Causes of pelvic pain*)
- Uterine leiomyomas (benign fibroid tumors)

RISK FACTORS
Primary
- Hormonal imbalance
- Psychogenic factors

PATHOPHYSIOLOGY
- Pain may result from increased prostaglandin secretion in menstrual blood, which intensifies normal uterine contractions.
- Prostaglandins intensify myometrial smooth-muscle contraction and uterine blood vessel constriction, thereby worsening the uterine hypoxia normally associated with menstruation.
- Intense muscle contractions and hypoxia cause the intense pain of dysmenorrhea.

INCIDENCE
- Dysmenorrhea affects 10% of high school girls each month.
- Incidence usually peaks in the early 20s and then slowly decreases.
- Dysmenorrhea usually results from another condition when it occurs after age 20.

- The condition may improve or disappear after childbirth.

COMPLICATIONS
- Dehydration

ASSESSMENT

HISTORY
- Pelvic disease
- Urinary frequency
- Nausea
- Vomiting
- Diarrhea
- Headache
- Backache
- Chills
- Depression
- Irritability

PHYSICAL FINDINGS
- Abdominal bloating
- Painful breasts

DIAGNOSTIC TEST RESULTS

IMAGING
- Pelvic ultrasonography, laparoscopy, and hysteroscopy help to diagnose underlying disorders in secondary dysmenorrhea.

OTHER
- Pelvic examination and a detailed patient history help to identify causation.

Causes of pelvic pain

The characteristic pelvic pain of dysmenorrhea must be distinguished from the acute pain caused by many other disorders, such as:
- GI disorders: appendicitis, acute diverticulitis, acute or chronic cholecystitis, chronic cholelithiasis, acute pancreatitis, peptic ulcer perforation, intestinal obstruction
- urinary tract disorders: cystitis, renal calculi
- reproductive disorders: acute salpingitis, chronic inflammation, degenerative fibroid, ovarian cyst torsion
- pregnancy disorders: impending abortion (pain and bleeding early in pregnancy), ectopic pregnancy, abruptio placentae, uterine rupture, leiomyoma degeneration, toxemia
- emotional conflicts: psychogenic (functional) pain.

Other conditions that may mimic dysmenorrhea include ovulation and normal uterine contractions experienced in pregnancy.

TREATMENT

GENERAL
◆ Heat applied locally to the lower abdomen

DIET
◆ Increased fluid intake

ACTIVITY
◆ As tolerated

MEDICATIONS
◆ Analgesics
◆ Prostaglandin inhibitors
◆ Sex steroids (primary)

SURGERY
◆ Surgical treatment of underlying disorders, such as endometriosis or uterine leiomyomas (secondary)

NURSING CONSIDERATIONS

NURSING DIAGNOSES
◆ Acute pain
◆ Disturbed body image

EXPECTED OUTCOMES
The patient will:
◆ remain free from pain
◆ express positive feelings about self.

NURSING INTERVENTIONS
◆ Provide emotional support.
◆ Give prescribed analgesics.

MONITORING
◆ Depression
◆ Hydration
◆ Pain control

PATIENT TEACHING

GENERAL
Be sure to cover:
◆ explanation of normal female anatomy and physiology as well as the nature of dysmenorrhea
◆ information on pregnancy and contraception
◆ keeping a detailed record of menstrual cycle and symptoms
◆ seeking medical care if symptoms persist.

DISCHARGE PLANNING
◆ Refer the patient for psychological counseling, if appropriate.

RESOURCES
Organizations
American College of Obstetricians and Gynecologists: *www.acog.com*
Mayo Clinic: *www.mayoclinic.com*
National Library of Medicine: *www.nlm.nih.gov*

Selected references
Davis, A.R., et al. "Oral Contraceptives for Dysmenorrhea in Adolescent Girls: A Randomized Trial," *Obstetrics & Gynecology* 106(1):97-104, July 2005.
Durain, D. "Primary Dysmenorrhea: Assessment and Management Update," *Journal of Midwifery & Women's Health* 49(6):520-28, November-December 2004.

Ebola virus infection LIFE-THREATENING DISORDER

OVERVIEW

- An unclassified ribonucleic acid virus that results in bleeding
- Four known strains: *Ebola* Zaire, *Ebola* Sudan, *Ebola* Ivory Coast, and *Ebola* Reston (affects only monkeys)
- Poor prognosis

PATHOPHYSIOLOGY

- Transmitted by direct contact with infected blood, body secretions, or organs
- Nosocomial and community-acquired transmission
- Viral replication (causes focal tissue necrosis, most severely in the liver)
- Microvasculature damage (causes increased vascular permeability and bleeding)
- Remains contagious even after the patient has died

CAUSES

- Infection with one of three subtypes of *Ebola* virus: EBO-Z, EBO-S, and EBO-C

INCIDENCE

- *Ebola* virus isn't endemic to the United States.
- The virus affects men and women of all ages.

COMPLICATIONS

- Liver and kidney dysfunction
- Dehydration
- Hemorrhage
- Abortion

ASSESSMENT

HISTORY

- Contact with an infected person
- Headache
- Malaise
- Myalgia
- Fever
- Cough
- Sore throat

PHYSICAL FINDINGS

- Conjunctival injection
- Bruising
- Maculopapular eruptions
- Melena
- Hematemesis
- Bleeding gums

DIAGNOSTIC TEST RESULTS

LABORATORY

- Blood studies reveal specific antigens or antibodies and may show the isolated virus.
- Blood studies reveal neutrophil leukocytosis, hypofibrinogenemia, thrombocytopenia, and microangiopathic hemolytic anemia.

TREATMENT

GENERAL
- Supportive care
- Strict isolation (see *Preventing the spread of* Ebola *virus*)

DIET
- As tolerated or total parental nutrition

ACTIVITY
- Bed rest or limited

MEDICATIONS
- I.V. fluids
- Blood transfusions

Preventing the spread of *Ebola* virus

The Centers for Disease Control and Prevention recommends the following guidelines to help prevent the spread of this deadly disease:
- Keep the patient in isolation throughout the course of the disease.
- If possible, place the patient in a negative-pressure room at the beginning of hospitalization to avoid the need for transfer as the disease progresses.
- Restrict nonessential staff members from entering the patient's room.
- Make sure that anyone who enters the patient's room wears gloves and a gown to prevent contact with any surface in the room that may have been soiled.
- Use barrier precautions to prevent skin and mucous membrane exposure to blood or other body fluids, secretions, or excretions when caring for the patient.
- If you must come within 3′ (1 m) of the patient, also wear a face shield or a surgical mask and goggles or eyeglasses with side shields.
- Don't reuse gloves or gowns unless they have been completely disinfected.
- Make sure any patient who dies of the disease is promptly buried or cremated. Precautions to avoid contact with the patient's body fluids and secretions should continue even after the patient's death.

NURSING CONSIDERATIONS

NURSING DIAGNOSES
- Acute pain
- Fatigue
- Hyperthermia
- Impaired gas exchange
- Ineffective airway clearance
- Ineffective breathing pattern
- Risk for deficient fluid volume
- Risk for infection

EXPECTED OUTCOMES
The patient will:
- report decreased levels or absence of pain
- report an increased energy level
- remain afebrile
- maintain adequate ventilation
- maintain a patent airway
- maintain effective breathing pattern
- maintain adequate fluid balance
- experience no further signs or symptoms of infection.

NURSING INTERVENTIONS
- Enforce strict isolation.
- Provide emotional support.
- Give prescribed I.V. solutions and blood products.
- Provide safety precautions.

MONITORING
- Vital signs
- Signs of bleeding
- Intake and output
- Laboratory studies

PATIENT TEACHING

GENERAL
Be sure to cover:
- the disorder, diagnosis, and treatment
- signs of bleeding
- isolation precautions.

DISCHARGE PLANNING
- Refer the patient for home care if appropriate.
- Stress to the patient the need for continued follow-up care.

RESOURCES
Organizations
Centers for Disease Control and Prevention: *www.cdc.gov*
World Health Organization: *www.who.int*

Selected references
Hampton, T. "Vaccines Against *Ebola* and Marburg Viruses Show Promise in Primate Studies," *JAMA* 294(2): 163-64, July 2005.
Kawaoka, Y. "How *Ebola* Virus Infects Cells," *New England Journal of Medicine* 352(25):2645-646, June 2005.

Ectopic pregnancy

- Implantation of a fertilized ovum outside the uterine cavity, most commonly in the fallopian tube (see *Implantation sites of ectopic pregnancy*)
- Prognosis good with prompt diagnosis, appropriate surgical intervention, and control of bleeding
- Very few fetuses carried to term; rarely, with abdominal implantation, fetus survives to term

PATHOPHYSIOLOGY

- Transport of a blastocyst to the uterus is delayed.
- The blastocyst implants at another available vascularized site, usually the fallopian tube lining.
- Normal signs of pregnancy may initially be present.
- Uterine enlargement occurs in about 25% of cases.
- Human chorionic gonadotropin (hCG) hormonal levels are lower than in uterine pregnancies.
- If not interrupted, internal hemorrhage occurs with rupture of the fallopian tube.

CAUSES

- Congenital defects in reproductive tract
- Diverticula
- Ectopic endometrial implants in the tubal mucosa
- Endosalpingitis
- History of multiple elective abortions
- Intrauterine device
- Previous surgery, such as tubal ligation or resection
- Sexually transmitted tubal infection
- Transmigration of the ovum
- Tumors pressing against the tube

INCIDENCE

- In whites, ectopic pregnancies occur in about 1 in 200 pregnancies.
- In nonwhites, ectopic pregnancies occur in about 1 in 120 pregnancies.

COMPLICATIONS

- Rupture of fallopian tube
- Hemorrhage
- Shock
- Peritonitis
- Infertility
- Disseminated intravascular coagulation
- Death

HISTORY

- Amenorrhea
- Abnormal menses (after fallopian tube implantation)
- Slight vaginal bleeding
- Unilateral pelvic pain over the mass
- With ruptured fallopian tube, sharp lower abdominal pain, possibly radiating to the shoulders and neck
- GI disturbances

> **WARNING** *Ectopic pregnancy sometimes produces symptoms of normal pregnancy or no symptoms other than mild abdominal pain (especially in abdominal pregnancy), making diagnosis difficult.*

PHYSICAL FINDINGS

- Extreme pain possible when cervix is moved and adnexa palpated
- Boggy and tender uterus
- Enlarged adnexa possible
- Pain radiating to neck and shoulder

LABORATORY

- Serum hCG level is abnormally low; when test is repeated in 48 hours, level remains lower than those found in a normal (intrauterine) pregnancy.

IMAGING

- Real-time ultrasonography shows intrauterine pregnancy or ovarian cyst.

DIAGNOSTIC PROCEDURES

- Culdocentesis shows free blood in the peritoneum.
- Laparoscopy may reveal pregnancy outside the uterus.

Implantation sites of ectopic pregnancy

In approximately 95% of patients with ectopic pregnancy, the ovum implants in part of the fallopian tube: the fimbria, ampulla, or isthmus. Other possible abnormal sites of implantation include the interstitium, ovarian ligament, ovary, abdominal viscera, and internal cervical os.

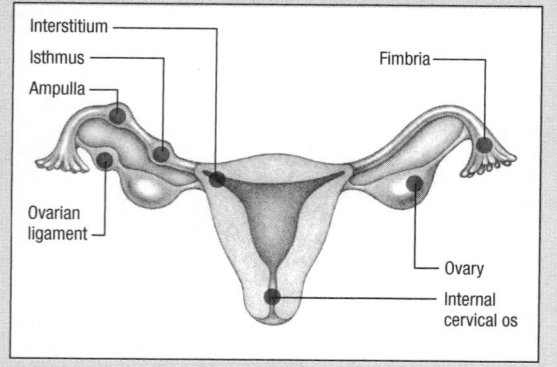

Interstitium
Isthmus
Ampulla
Fimbria
Ovarian ligament
Ovary
Internal cervical os

TREATMENT

GENERAL
◆ Initially, in the event of pelvic-organ rupture, management of shock

DIET
◆ Determined by clinical status

ACTIVITY
◆ Determined by clinical status

MEDICATIONS
◆ Transfusion with whole blood or packed red blood cells
◆ Broad-spectrum I.V. antibiotics
◆ Supplemental iron
◆ Methotrexate (Trexall)

SURGERY
◆ Laparotomy and salpingectomy if culdocentesis shows blood in the peritoneum; possibly after laparoscopy to remove affected fallopian tube and control bleeding
◆ Microsurgical repair of the fallopian tube for patients who wish to have children
◆ Oophorectomy for ovarian pregnancy
◆ Hysterectomy for interstitial pregnancy
◆ Laparotomy to remove the fetus for abdominal pregnancy

NURSING CONSIDERATIONS

NURSING DIAGNOSES
◆ Anxiety
◆ Deficient fluid volume
◆ Dysfunctional grieving
◆ Fear
◆ Ineffective coping

EXPECTED OUTCOMES
The patient will:
◆ express feelings of reduced anxiety
◆ maintain adequate fluid volume
◆ express feelings about the current situation
◆ discuss fears and concerns
◆ use available support systems, such as family and friends, to aid in coping.

NURSING INTERVENTIONS
◆ Prepare the patient with excessive blood loss for emergency surgery.
◆ Give prescribed blood transfusions.
◆ Provide emotional support.
◆ Give prescribed analgesics.
◆ Administer $Rh_o(D)$ immune globulin (RhoGAM), as ordered, if the patient is Rh negative.
◆ Determine the date and description of her last menstrual period.
◆ Provide a quiet, relaxing environment.
◆ Encourage the patient to express her feelings of fear, loss, and grief.
◆ Help the patient to develop effective coping strategies.

MONITORING
◆ Vital signs
◆ Vaginal bleeding
◆ Pain
◆ Intake and output
◆ Signs of hypovolemia
◆ Signs of impending shock

PATIENT TEACHING

GENERAL
Be sure to cover:
◆ the disorder, diagnosis, and treatment
◆ postoperative care
◆ prevention of recurrent ectopic pregnancy
◆ prompt treatment of pelvic infections
◆ risk factors for ectopic pregnancy, including surgery involving the fallopian tubes and pelvic inflammatory disease.

DISCHARGE PLANNING
◆ Refer the patient to a mental health professional for additional counseling, if necessary.

RESOURCES
Organizations
American College of Obstetricians and Gynecologists: *www.acog.org*
American Society for Reproductive Medicine: *www.asrm.org*

Selected references
Kirk, E., et al. "The Non-surgical Management of Ectopic Pregnancy," *Ultrasound in Obstetrics & Gynecology* 27(1):91-100, January 2006.
Latchaw, G., et al. "Risk Factors Associated with the Rupture of Tubal Ectopic Pregnancy," *Gynecologic and Obstetric Investigation* 60(3):177-80, 2005.
Lozeau, A.M., and Potter, B. "Diagnosis and Management of Ectopic Pregnancy," *American Family Practitioner* 72(9):1707-714, November 2005.

Electric shock LIFE-THREATENING DISORDER

OVERVIEW

- Electric current passing through body
- Physical damage depending on the intensity of the current, resistance of the tissues it passes through, type of current, and frequency and duration of current flow
- Classified as lightning, low-voltage (less than 600 V), and high-voltage (greater than 600 V)

PATHOPHYSIOLOGY

- Electrical energy results in altered cell membrane resting potential, causing depolarization in muscles and nerves.
- Electric shock alters normal electrical activity of the heart and brain.
- Electric shock resulting from a high-frequency current generates more heat in tissues than a low-frequency current, resulting in burns and local tissue coagulation and necrosis.
- Muscle tetany is elicited.
- Tissue destruction and coagulative necrosis occurs.

CAUSES

- Accidental contact with an exposed part of an electrical appliance or wiring
- Flash of electric arcs from high-voltage power lines or machines
- Lightning

INCIDENCE

- Electric shock causes more than 500 deaths annually.
- Electric shock is more common in men ages 20 to 40.

COMPLICATIONS

- Sepsis
- Neurologic dysfunction
- Cardiac dysfunction
- Psychiatric dysfunction
- Renal failure
- Electrolyte abnormalities
- Peripheral nerve injuries
- Vascular disruption
- Thrombi
- Death

ASSESSMENT

HISTORY

- Exposure to electricity or lightning
- Loss of consciousness
- Muscle pain
- Fatigue
- Headache
- Nervous irritability

PHYSICAL FINDINGS

- Determined by voltage exposure
- Burns
- Local tissue coagulation
- Entrance and exit injuries
- Cyanosis
- Apnea
- Markedly decreased blood pressure
- Cold skin
- Unconsciousness
- Numbness or tingling or sensorimotor deficits

DIAGNOSTIC TEST RESULTS

LABORATORY

- Urinalysis shows evidence of myoglobin.

IMAGING

- Computed tomography or magnetic resonance imaging may rule out intracranial bleeding or contusion of the brain if the patient is unresponsive or unconscious.
- Chest X-rays reveal internal damage such as fractures or dislocations.

OTHER

- Electrocardiogram (ECG) reveals cardiac arrhythmias.

GENERAL

◆ Separation of victim from current source
◆ Stabilization of cervical spine
◆ Emergency measures
◆ Treatment of acid-base imbalance
◆ Vigorous fluid replacement

DIET

◆ No restrictions if swallowing ability intact

ACTIVITY

◆ Based on outcome of interventions

MEDICATIONS

◆ Osmotic diuretics
◆ Tetanus prophylaxis

NURSING CONSIDERATIONS

NURSING DIAGNOSES

◆ Acute pain
◆ Anxiety
◆ Decreased cardiac output
◆ Impaired skin integrity
◆ Impaired spontaneous ventilation
◆ Ineffective tissue perfusion: Cardiopulmonary
◆ Risk for injury
◆ Risk for posttrauma syndrome

EXPECTED OUTCOMES

The patient will:
◆ report pain relief with analgesic or other measures
◆ express feelings of decreased anxiety
◆ maintain cardiac output
◆ regain skin integrity
◆ maintain adequate ventilation either spontaneously or with assisted ventilation
◆ exhibit signs of adequate cardiopulmonary perfusion
◆ verbalize methods to prevent future injury from electric shock
◆ express feelings and fears about the traumatic event.

NURSING INTERVENTIONS

◆ Separate the victim from the current source.
◆ Provide emergency treatment.
◆ Give rapid I.V. fluid infusion.
◆ Obtain a 12-lead ECG.
◆ Give prescribed drugs.

MONITORING

◆ Cardiac rhythm (continuously)
◆ Intake and output (hourly)
◆ Neurologic status
◆ Sensorimotor deficits
◆ Peripheral neurovascular status

Preventing electric shock

Take the following steps to help prevent electric shock in your facility:

◆ Regularly check for cuts, cracks, or frayed insulation on electric cords, call bells (also check for warm call bells), and electrical devices attached to the patient's bed. Report any problems to maintenance personnel.

◆ Keep electrical devices away from hot or wet surfaces and sharp corners. Don't set glasses of water, damp towels, or other wet items on electrical equipment. Wipe up accidental spills before they leak into electrical equipment.

◆ Avoid using extension cords because they may circumvent the ground. If they're necessary, don't place them under carpeting or where they'll be walked on.

◆ Make sure ground connections on electrical equipment are intact. Line cord plugs should have three prongs; the prongs should be straight and firmly fixed. Check that prongs fit wall outlets properly and that outlets aren't loose or broken. Don't use adapters on plugs.

◆ If a machine sparks, smokes, seems unusually hot, or gives you or your patient a slight shock, unplug it immediately, if doing so won't endanger the patient's life. Promptly report such equipment to maintenance personnel. Check inspection labels and report equipment that's overdue for inspection.

◆ Be especially careful when using electrical equipment near a patient with a pacemaker or direct cardiac line because a cardiac catheter or pacemaker can create a direct, low-resistance path to the heart; even a small shock could cause ventricular fibrillation.

PATIENT TEACHING

GENERAL

Be sure to cover:
◆ information about the injury, diagnosis, and treatment
◆ how to avoid electrical hazards at home and at work (see *Preventing electric shock*)
◆ electrical safety regarding children.

RESOURCES

Organizations

Harborview Injury Prevention and Research Center: *www.depts.washington.edu/hiprc*
National Center for Injury Prevention and Control: *www.cdc.gov/ncipc*

Selected references

Diseases, 4th ed. Philadelphia: Lippincott Williams & Wilkins, 2006.
Hendler, N. "Overlooked Diagnoses in Chronic Pain: Analysis of Survivors of Electric Shock and Lightning Strike," *Journal of Occupational & Environmental Medicine* 47(8):796-805, August 2005.

Emphysema

OVERVIEW

- Chronic lung disease characterized by permanent enlargement of air spaces distal to the terminal bronchioles and by exertional dyspnea
- One of several diseases usually labeled collectively as chronic obstructive pulmonary disease or chronic obstructive lung disease

PATHOPHYSIOLOGY

- Recurrent inflammation associated with the release of proteolytic enzymes from lung cells causes abnormal, irreversible enlargement of the air spaces distal to the terminal bronchioles.
- This enlargement leads to the destruction of alveolar walls, which results in a breakdown of elasticity. (See *What happens in emphysema*.)

CAUSES

- Cigarette smoking
- Genetic deficiency of $alpha_1$-antitrypsin

INCIDENCE

- Emphysema is the most common cause of death from respiratory disease in the United States.
- Emphysema is more prevalent in men than in women.
- About 2 million Americans are affected.
- The disease affects 1 in 3,000 neonates.

COMPLICATIONS

- Recurrent respiratory tract infections
- Cor pulmonale
- Respiratory failure
- Peptic ulcer disease
- Spontaneous pneumothorax
- Pneumomediastinum

ASSESSMENT

HISTORY

- Smoking
- Shortness of breath
- Chronic cough
- Anorexia and weight loss
- Malaise

PHYSICAL FINDINGS

- Barrel chest
- Pursed-lip breathing
- Use of accessory muscles
- Cyanosis
- Clubbed fingers and toes
- Tachypnea
- Decreased tactile fremitus
- Decreased chest expansion
- Hyperresonance
- Decreased breath sounds
- Crackles
- Inspiratory wheeze
- Prolonged expiratory phase with grunting respirations
- Distant heart sounds

DIAGNOSTIC TEST RESULTS

LABORATORY

- Arterial blood gas analysis shows decreased partial pressure of oxygen; partial pressure of carbon dioxide is normal until late in the disease.
- Red blood cell count shows an increased hemoglobin level late in the disease.

IMAGING

- Chest X-ray may show:
- a flattened diaphragm
- reduced vascular markings at the lung periphery
- overaeration of the lungs
- a vertical heart
- enlarged anteroposterior chest diameter
- large retrosternal air space.

DIAGNOSTIC PROCEDURES

- Pulmonary function tests typically show:
- increased residual volume and total lung capacity
- reduced diffusing capacity

What happens in emphysema

In normal, healthy breathing, air moves in and out of the lungs to meet metabolic needs. A change in airway size compromises the lungs' ability to circulate sufficient air.

In a patient with emphysema, recurrent pulmonary inflammation damages and eventually destroys the alveolar walls, creating large air spaces. This breakdown leaves the alveoli unable to recoil normally after expanding and results in bronchiolar collapse on expiration. This traps air within the lungs.

Associated pulmonary capillary destruction usually allows a patient with severe emphysema to match ventilation to perfusion and thus avoid cyanosis.

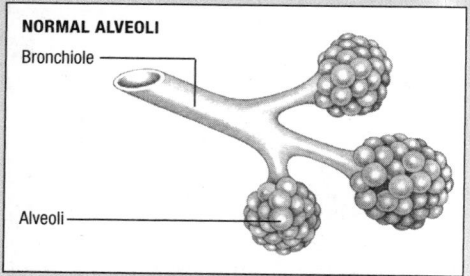

NORMAL ALVEOLI
Bronchiole
Alveoli

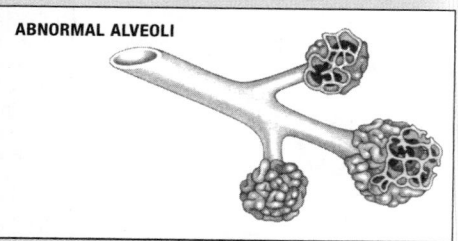

ABNORMAL ALVEOLI

- increased inspiratory flow.
- Electrocardiography may show tall, symmetrical P waves in leads II, III, and aV_F; a vertical QRS axis; and signs of right ventricular hypertrophy late in the disease.

TREATMENT

GENERAL
- Chest physiotherapy
- Possible transtracheal catheterization and home oxygen therapy
- Mechanical ventilation (in acute exacerbations)

DIET
- Adequate hydration
- High-protein, high-calorie

ACTIVITY
- As tolerated

MEDICATIONS
- Bronchodilators
- Anticholinergics
- Mucolytics
- Corticosteroids
- Antibiotics
- Oxygen

SURGERY
- Chest tube insertion for pneumothorax

NURSING CONSIDERATIONS

NURSING DIAGNOSES
- Anxiety
- Fatigue
- Fear
- Impaired gas exchange
- Ineffective airway clearance
- Ineffective breathing pattern
- Interrupted family processes
- Risk for infection

EXPECTED OUTCOMES
The patient will:
- identify strategies to reduce anxiety
- verbalize the importance of balancing activity with adequate rest periods

- discuss fears and concerns
- maintain adequate ventilation and oxygenation
- maintain a patent airway
- maintain effective breathing pattern
- along with family members identify and contact available support systems as needed
- remain free from signs or symptoms of infection.

NURSING INTERVENTIONS
- Give prescribed drugs.
- Provide supportive care.
- Help the patient adjust to lifestyle changes necessitated by a chronic illness.
- Encourage the patient to express his fears and concerns.
- Perform chest physiotherapy.
- Provide a high-calorie, protein-rich diet.
- Give small, frequent meals.
- Encourage daily activity and diversional activities.
- Provide frequent rest periods.

MONITORING
- Vital signs
- Intake and output
- Daily weight
- Complications
- Respiratory status
- Activity tolerance

PATIENT TEACHING

GENERAL
Be sure to cover:
- the disorder, diagnosis, and treatment
- medication and potential adverse reactions
- when to notify the practitioner
- energy conservation techniques
- the importance of receiving an influenza vaccine yearly
- avoidance of smoking and areas where smoking is permitted
- avoidance of crowds and people with known infections
- home oxygen therapy, if indicated
- transtracheal catheter care, if needed
- coughing and deep breathing exercises

- the proper use of handheld inhalers
- the need for a high-calorie, protein-rich diet
- adequate oral fluid intake
- avoidance of respiratory irritants
- signs and symptoms of pneumothorax.

WARNING *Urge the patient to notify the practitioner if he experiences a sudden onset of worsening dyspnea or sharp pleuritic chest pain exacerbated by chest movement, breathing, or coughing.*

DISCHARGE PLANNING
- Refer the patient to a smoking-cessation program if indicated.
- Refer the patient for influenza and pneumococcal pneumonia immunizations as needed.
- Refer the family of patients with familial emphysema for $alpha_1$-antitrypsin deficiency screening.

RESOURCES
Organizations
National Emphysema Foundation: *www.emphysemafoundation.org*
National Institute of Drug Abuse: *www.nida.nih.gov*
Tobacco Information and Prevention Source: *www.cdc.gov/tobacco*

Selected references
Burton, S. "Early Discharge of People with Chronic Obstructive Pulmonary Disease," *Nursing Times* 100(6):65-67, February 2004.
Nettina, S.M. *Lippincott Manual of Nursing Practice,* 8th ed. Philadelphia: Lippincott Williams & Wilkins, 2006.
Wisniewski, A. "Chronic Bronchitis and Emphysema: Clearing the Air," *Nursing* 33(5):46-49, May 2003.

Encephalitis

◆ Severe inflammation of the brain

PATHOPHYSIOLOGY

◆ Intense lymphocytic infiltration of brain tissues and the leptomeninges results in:
– cerebral edema
– degeneration of the brain's ganglion cells
– diffuse nerve cell destruction (gray matter more than white).

CAUSES

◆ Adenoviruses
◆ Enteroviruses in urban areas (coxsackievirus, poliovirus, and echovirus)
◆ Herpesvirus
◆ Human immunodeficiency virus
◆ Measles, varicella, or rubella vaccination
◆ Mosquito- or tick-borne arboviruses specific to rural areas
◆ Mumps virus
◆ Swimming in fresh water (amebic)
◆ Systemic viral infection

INCIDENCE

◆ Determining true incidence is nearly impossible because reporting policies differ.

COMPLICATIONS

◆ Bronchial pneumonia
◆ Urine retention and urinary tract infection
◆ Paralysis
◆ Pressure ulcers
◆ Coma
◆ Epilepsy
◆ Parkinsonism
◆ Mental deterioration

ASSESSMENT

HISTORY

◆ Systemic symptoms:
– Headache
– Muscle stiffness and malaise
– Sore throat and upper respiratory tract symptoms
– Sudden onset of altered levels of consciousness
– Seizures

PHYSICAL FINDINGS

◆ Confusion, disorientation, or hallucinations
◆ Tremors
◆ Cranial nerve palsies
◆ Exaggerated deep tendon reflexes and absent superficial reflexes
◆ Paresis or paralysis of the extremities
◆ Stiff neck when the head is bent forward
◆ Fever
◆ Nausea and vomiting
◆ Cerebral hemispheres
◆ Aphasia
◆ Involuntary movements
◆ Ataxia
◆ Sensory defects

DIAGNOSTIC TEST RESULTS

LABORATORY

◆ Blood analysis identifies the virus.
◆ Serologic studies in herpes encephalitis show rising titers of complement-fixing antibodies.

IMAGING

◆ Computed tomography scan rules out cerebral hematoma.

DIAGNOSTIC PROCEDURES

◆ Cerebrospinal fluid (CSF) analysis identifies the virus.
◆ Lumbar puncture discloses CSF pressure.

OTHER

◆ EEG shows slowing of waveforms.
◆ Diagnosis is readily made from the clinical findings and patient history.

TREATMENT

GENERAL
- Supportive measures
- Airway maintenance
- Oxygen administration

DIET
- Adequate fluid and electrolyte intake
- As tolerated

ACTIVITY
- As tolerated

MEDICATIONS
- Osmotic diuretics
- Corticosteroids
- Anticonvulsants
- Aspirin or acetaminophen
- Antibiotics
- Vidarabine, an antiviral
- Immunologic agents

NURSING CONSIDERATIONS

NURSING DIAGNOSES
- Acute pain
- Anxiety
- Hyperthermia
- Imbalanced nutrition: Less than body requirements
- Impaired gas exchange
- Impaired physical mobility
- Risk for deficient fluid volume
- Risk for impaired skin integrity

EXPECTED OUTCOMES
The patient will:
- verbalize feelings of increased comfort and relief from pain
- identify strategies to reduce anxiety
- maintain a normal temperature
- consume adequate calorie requirements daily
- maintain adequate ventilation and oxygenation
- maintain joint mobility and muscle strength
- exhibit fluid balance within normal limits
- maintain intact skin with no signs of breakdown.

NURSING INTERVENTIONS
- Make sure the patient has adequate fluid intake.
- Give prescribed drugs.
- Position and turn the patient often.
- Assist with range-of motion exercises.
- Maintain adequate nutrition.
- Administer laxatives or stool softeners.
- Administer mouth care.
- Maintain a quiet environment.
- Start seizure precautions if necessary.
- Reorient the patient often if necessary.

MONITORING
- Neurologic function (continuous) for cranial nerve involvement
- Intake and output
- Response to medications
- Intracranial pressure (severe cases)

PATIENT TEACHING

GENERAL
Be sure to cover:
- the disorder, diagnosis, and treatment
- transient behavior changes
- the medication regimen
- adverse effects of medication
- the importance of immediately reporting worsening of symptoms
- follow-up care.

DISCHARGE PLANNING
- Refer the patient to an outpatient rehabilitation program as indicated.
- Stress the importance of following up with the practitioner or with a pulmonary care physician.

RESOURCES
Organizations
National Institutes of Health: *www.nih.gov*
WebMD: *www.webmd.com*

Selected references
De Tiege, X., et al. "Herpes Simplex Encephalitis: Diagnostic Problems and Late Relapse," *Developmental Medicine and Child Neurology* 48(1):60-63, January 2006.
Diseases, 4th ed. Philadelphia: Lippincott Williams & Wilkins, 2006.
Handbook of Pathophysiology, 2nd ed. Philadelphia: Lippincott Williams & Wilkins, 2005.

Endocarditis

- Infection of the endocardium, heart valves, or cardiac prosthesis
- Includes three types: native valve (acute and subacute) endocarditis, prosthetic valve (early and late) endocarditis, and endocarditis related to I.V. drug abuse (usually involving the tricuspid valve)

PATHOPHYSIOLOGY

- Fibrin and platelets cluster on valve tissue and engulf circulating bacteria or fungi. (See *Degenerative changes in endocarditis.*)
- This produces vegetation, which in turn may cover the valve surfaces, causing deformities and destruction of valvular tissue and may extend to the chordae tendineae, causing them to rupture, leading to valvular insufficiency.
- Vegetative growth on the heart valves, endocardial lining of a heart chamber, or the endothelium of a blood vessel may embolize to the spleen, kidneys, central nervous system, and lungs.

CAUSES

Native valve endocarditis

- Alpha-hemolytic *Streptococcus* or enterococci (subacute form)
- Group B hemolytic *Streptococcus*
- *Staphylococcus aureus*

Prosthetic valve

- Alpha-hemolytic *Streptococcus*, enterococci, and *Staphylococcus* (late; 60 days or more after implant)
- *Staphylococcus*, gram-negative bacilli, and *Candida* (early; within 60 days after implant)

Related to I.V. drug abuse

- *S. aureus*

INCIDENCE

- Up to 40% of affected patients have no underlying heart disease.
- This disease is more common in males than in females.
- Most patients are older than age 50.

- The disease is uncommon in children.
- Rheumatic valvular disease occurs in about 25% of all cases.
- The mitral valve is the most commonly involved valve.
- Drug abusers with endocarditis are commonly young males.

COMPLICATIONS

- Left-sided heart failure
- Valve stenosis or insufficiency
- Myocardial erosion
- Embolic debris lodged in the small vasculature of the visceral tissue

ASSESSMENT

HISTORY

- Predisposing condition such as heart failure
- Nonspecific symptoms, such as weakness, fatigue, weight loss, anorexia, arthralgia, night sweats, and intermittent fever that may recur for weeks
- Dyspnea and chest pain common with I.V. drug abusers

Degenerative changes in endocarditis

This illustration shows typical vegetations on the endocardium produced by fibrin and platelet deposits on infection sites.

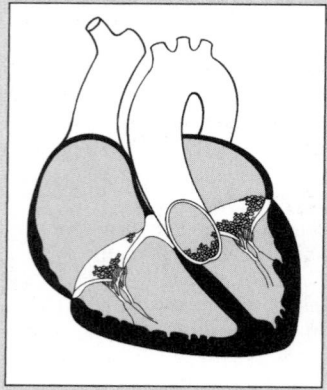

PHYSICAL FINDINGS

- Petechiae on the skin (especially common on the upper anterior trunk) and on the buccal, pharyngeal, or conjunctival mucosa
- Splinter hemorrhages under the nails
- Clubbing of the fingers in patients with long-standing disease
- Heart murmur in all patients except those with early acute endocarditis and I.V. drug users with tricuspid valve infection
- Osler's nodes
- Roth's spots
- Janeway lesions
- A murmur that changes suddenly or a new murmur that develops in the presence of fever (classic physical sign)
- Splenomegaly in long-standing disease
- Dyspnea, tachycardia, and bibasilar crackles possible with left-sided heart failure
- Splenic infarction causing pain in the upper left quadrant, radiating to the left shoulder, and abdominal rigidity
- Renal infarction causing hematuria, pyuria, flank pain, and decreased urine output
- Cerebral infarction causing hemiparesis, aphasia, and other neurologic deficits
- Pulmonary infarction causing cough, pleuritic pain, pleural friction rub, dyspnea, and hemoptysis
- Peripheral vascular occlusion causing numbness and tingling in arm, leg, finger, or toe or signs of impending peripheral gangrene

DIAGNOSTIC TEST RESULTS

LABORATORY

- Three or more blood cultures during a 24- to 48-hour period identify the causative organism (in up to 90% of patients).
- White blood cell count and differential is normal or elevated.
- Complete blood count and anemia panel show normocytic, normochromic anemia in subacute native valve endocarditis.

- Erythrocyte sedimentation rate and serum creatinine levels are elevated.
- Serum rheumatoid factor is positive in about 50% of all patients with endocarditis longer than 6 weeks.
- Urinalysis shows proteinuria and microscopic hematuria.

IMAGING
- Echocardiography may identify valvular damage in up to 80% of patients with native valve disease.

DIAGNOSTIC PROCEDURES
- Electrocardiography reading may show atrial fibrillation and other arrhythmias that accompany valvular disease.

TREATMENT

GENERAL
- Prompt therapy that continues for several weeks
- Selection of anti-infective drug based on type of infecting organism and sensitivity studies
- If blood cultures negative (10% to 20% of subacute cases), possible I.V. antibiotic therapy (usually for 4 to 6 weeks) against probable infecting organism

DIET
- Sufficient fluid intake

ACTIVITY
- Bed rest

MEDICATIONS
- Aspirin
- Antibiotics

SURGERY
- With severe valvular damage, especially aortic insufficiency or infection of a cardiac prosthesis, possible corrective surgery if refractory heart failure develops or if an infected prosthetic valve must be replaced

NURSING CONSIDERATIONS

NURSING DIAGNOSES
- Activity intolerance
- Decreased cardiac output
- Deficient diversional activity
- Impaired gas exchange
- Impaired physical mobility
- Ineffective role performance
- Risk for infection

EXPECTED OUTCOMES
The patient will:
- carry out activities of daily living without weakness or fatigue
- maintain hemodynamic stability with adequate cardiac output
- express interest in using leisure time meaningfully
- maintain adequate ventilation
- maintain joint mobility and muscle strength
- express feelings about diminished capacity to perform usual roles
- show no further signs or symptoms of infection.

NURSING INTERVENTIONS
- Stress the importance of bed rest.
- Provide a bedside commode.
- Allow the patient to express his concerns.
- Obtain a history of allergies.
- Administer antibiotics on time.
- Administer oxygen.

MONITORING
WARNING *Watch for signs of embolization, a common occurrence during the first 3 months of treatment. Tell the patient to watch for and report these signs.*
- Renal status
- Frequent cardiovascular status assessment
- Arterial blood gas analysis as needed

PATIENT TEACHING

GENERAL
Be sure to cover:
- the disorder, diagnosis, and treatment
- anti-infectives the patient needs to continue taking
- the need to watch closely for fever, anorexia, and other signs of relapse about 2 weeks after treatment stops
- the need for prophylactic antibiotics before dental work and some surgical procedures
- proper dental hygiene and avoiding flossing the teeth
- how to recognize symptoms of endocarditis and to notify the practitioner immediately if such symptoms occur.

DISCHARGE PLANNING
- Encourage follow-up care with cardiologist.
- Refer I.V. drug abuser to rehabilitation programs and support services.

RESOURCES
Organizations
American Heart Association: *www.americanheart.org*
Mayo Clinic: *www.mayoclinic.com*
National Heart, Lung and Blood Institute: *www.nhlbi.nih.gov/nhlbi/cardio*

Selected references
Eftychiou, C., et al. "Factors Associated with Non-bacterial Thrombotic Endocarditis: Case Report and Literature Review," *Journal of Heart Valve Disease* 14(6):859-62, November 2005.
Habib, G. "Management of Infective Endocarditis," *Heart* 92(1):124-30, January 2006.
Kasper, D.L., et al., eds. *Harrison's Principles of Internal Medicine*, 16th ed. New York: McGraw-Hill Book Co., 2005.
The Merck Manual of Diagnosis & Therapy, 18th ed., Whitehouse Station, N.J.: Merck & Co., Inc., 2006.
Wisniewski, A. "Identifying Infective Endocarditis," *Nursing* 33(12):30, December 2003.

Endometriosis

OVERVIEW

- Poorly understood gynecologic condition characterized by pain that occurs with menstruation
- Endometrial tissue: appears outside uterine cavity lining
- Ectopic tissue: generally confined to the pelvic area, but can appear anywhere in the body

PATHOPHYSIOLOGY

- Endometrial cells respond to estrogen and progesterone with proliferation and secretion.
- During menstruation, ectopic tissue bleeds and causes inflammation of the surrounding tissues.
- Inflammation leads to fibrosis.
- Fibrosis leads to adhesions that produce pain and infertility.

CAUSES

- Direct cause unknown
- Direct implantation
- Environmental contaminants
- Familial susceptibility
- Formation in situ
- Immune system defects
- Induction
- Inflammatory influence
- Lymphatic spread theory
- Transportation (retrograde menstruation)

INCIDENCE

- Endometriosis usually occurs between ages 20 and 40.
- The condition is more common in women who postpone childbearing.
- Endometriosis is uncommon before age 20.

COMPLICATIONS

- Infertility
- Spontaneous abortion
- Anemia secondary to excessive bleeding
- Emotional problems secondary to infertility
- Pelvic adhesions
- Severe dysmenorrhea
- Ovarian cyst

ASSESSMENT

HISTORY

- Cyclic pelvic pain that peaks 5 to 7 days before menses and lasts 2 to 3 days
- Infertility
- Acquired dysmenorrhea
- Pain in lower abdomen, vagina, posterior pelvis and back; commonly radiates down legs
- Additional symptoms depending on site of involvement:
  - Abdominal cramps (small bowel and appendix)
  - Deep thrust dyspareunia (ovaries and cul-de-sac)
  - Dyschezia, rectal bleeding with menses, and pain in the coccyx or sacrum (rectovaginal septum and colon)
  - Hypermenorrhea (oviducts and ovaries)
  - Nausea and vomiting that worsen before menses (small bowel and appendix)
  - Suprapubic pain, dysuria, and hematuria (bladder)

PHYSICAL FINDINGS

- Multiple tender nodules on uterosacral ligaments or rectovaginal septum
- Enlarged nodules (tender during menses)
- Ovarian enlargement with endometrial cysts on the ovaries
- Thickened, nodular adnexa

DIAGNOSTIC TEST RESULTS

DIAGNOSTIC PROCEDURES

- A scoring and staging system created by the American Fertility Society quantifies endometrial implants according to size, character, and location:
  - Stage I indicates minimal disease (1 to 5 points).
  - Stage II indicates mild disease (6 to 15 points).
  - Stage III indicates moderate disease (16 to 40 points).
  - Stage IV indicates severe disease (more than 40 points).
- Laparoscopy results confirm the diagnosis and identify the disease stage.

TREATMENT

GENERAL
- Determined by stage of disease, patient's age, and desire to have children
- Pregnancy, if possible: temporary treatment

ACTIVITY
- As tolerated

MEDICATIONS
- Progestins
- Hormonal contraceptives
- Gonadotropin releasing analogues
- Androgens
- Analgesics

SURGERY
- Laparoscopy to lyse adhesions, remove small implants, and cauterize implants; for laser vaporization of implants; usually followed by hormonal therapy to suppress return of endometrial implants
- Total abdominal hysterectomy with bilateral salpingo-oophorectomy in stages III and IV

NURSING CONSIDERATIONS

NURSING DIAGNOSES
- Anxiety
- Chronic pain
- Disturbed body image
- Fear
- Ineffective coping
- Risk for infection
- Sexual dysfunction

EXPECTED OUTCOMES
The patient will:
- identify strategies to reduce anxiety
- express feelings of increased comfort
- express positive feelings about self
- discuss fears and concerns
- develop adequate coping behaviors
- remain free from signs and symptoms of infection
- verbalize feelings about sexual impairment.

NURSING INTERVENTIONS
- Encourage the patient to express her feelings about the disorder.
- Offer the patient emotional support.
- Encourage using open communication before and during intercourse.
- Help the patient to develop effective coping strategies.

MONITORING
- Effect of treatment
- Complications
- Adverse drug reactions
- Coping ability

PATIENT TEACHING

GENERAL
Be sure to cover:
- the disorder, diagnosis, and treatment
- associated complications
- avoiding minor gynecologic procedures immediately before and during menstruation
- not postponing childbearing because of potential for infertility
- annual pelvic examination and Papanicolaou test.

DISCHARGE PLANNING
- Refer the patient and her partner to a mental health professional for additional counseling if necessary.
- Refer the patient to a support group such as the Endometriosis Association.

RESOURCES
Organizations
American College of Obstetricians and Gynecologists: *www.acog.org*
American Society for Reproductive Medicine: *www.asrm.org*
Endometriosis Association: *www.endometriosisassn.org*

Selected references
Huntington, A., and Gilmour, J.A. "A Life Shaped by Pain: Women and Endometriosis," *Journal of Clinical Nursing* 14(9):1124-132, October 2005.
Jackson, L.W., et al. "Oxidative Stress and Endometriosis," *Human Reproduction* 20(7):2014-2020, July 2005.
Taylor, M.M. "Endometriosis — A Missed Malady," *AORN Journal* 77(2):298, 301-309, 312-13, February 2003.

Enterobacteriaceae infections

- Variety of infections caused by a family of mostly aerobic, gram-negative bacilli
- Cause local and systemic infections, including invasive diarrhea resembling shigellosis and noninvasive, toxin-mediated diarrhea resembling cholera
- *Escherichia coli:* the cause of most nosocomial infections

PATHOPHYSIOLOGY

- When a patient becomes infected, incubation takes 12 to 72 hours.
- Noninvasive diarrhea results from two toxins produced by enterotoxigenic or enteropathogenic strains of *E. coli.*
- Toxins interact with intestinal juices and promote excessive loss of chloride and water.
- The invasive form directly attacks the intestinal mucosa without producing enterotoxins, causing local irritation, inflammation, and diarrhea. This form produces sporadic and outbreak-associated bloody diarrhea from hemorrhagic colitis, which can be life-threatening in infants and elderly people.

CAUSES

- Enterotoxigenic *E. coli* (major cause of diarrhea among those who travel from industrialized to developing regions)
- Infection usually from nonindigenous strains
- Ingestion of contaminated food or water or contact with contaminated utensils
- Most common food source: chopped beef
- Some strains of *E. coli* that are part of normal GI flora but cause infection in immunocompromised patients
- Transmission directly from an infected person

INCIDENCE

- *Enterobacteriaceae* infections may be the major cause of diarrheal illness in children in United States.
- Incidence is highest among travelers returning from abroad, especially Mexico (noninvasive form), Southeast Asia (noninvasive form), and South America (invasive form).

COMPLICATIONS

- Bacteremia
- Severe dehydration and life-threatening electrolyte disturbances
- Acidosis
- Shock

HISTORY

- Recent travel to another country
- Ingestion of contaminated food or water
- Recent close contact with a person who has diarrhea
- Abrupt onset of watery diarrhea

PHYSICAL FINDINGS

- Cramping abdominal pain with hyperactive bowel sounds
- Blood and pus in infected stools
- Vomiting and anorexia
- Low-grade fever
- Signs of dehydration, especially in children
- Signs and symptoms of hyponatremia, hypokalemia, hypomagnesemia, and hypocalcemia from electrolyte losses
- Orthostatic hypotension
- Rapid, thready pulse
- Initially in infants, loose, watery stools that change from yellow to green and contain little mucus or blood
- Listlessness and irritability in infants

DIAGNOSTIC TEST RESULTS

LABORATORY
◆ Cultures — growth of *E. coli* in a normally sterile location, including the bloodstream, cerebrospinal fluid, biliary tract, pleural fluid, or peritoneal cavity — suggest *E. coli* infection at that site.

TREATMENT

GENERAL
◆ Enteric precautions

DIET
◆ Correction of fluid and electrolyte imbalances
◆ Initially, nothing by mouth
◆ Increased fluid intake (if appropriate)
◆ Avoidance of foods that cause diarrhea
◆ Small frequent meals until bowel function returns to normal

ACTIVITY
◆ As tolerated

MEDICATIONS
◆ I.V. antibiotics
◆ Bismuth subsalicylate or tincture of opium

NURSING CONSIDERATIONS

NURSING DIAGNOSES
◆ Acute pain
◆ Deficient fluid volume
◆ Diarrhea
◆ Imbalanced nutrition: Less than body requirements
◆ Ineffective tissue perfusion: Cardiopulmonary, GI
◆ Risk for infection

EXPECTED OUTCOMES
The patient will:
◆ report feelings of comfort and reduced pain
◆ regain and maintain normal fluid and electrolyte balance
◆ have an elimination pattern that returns to normal
◆ show no further evidence of weight loss
◆ maintain normal cardiac output and GI perfusion
◆ remain free from all signs and symptoms of infection.

NURSING INTERVENTIONS
◆ Institute contact precautions and use proper hand-washing technique.
◆ Replace fluids and electrolytes as needed.
◆ Clean the perianal area and lubricate it after each episode of diarrhea.
◆ Give prescribed antibiotics.
◆ During epidemics, screen all facility personnel and visitors for diarrhea, and prevent people with the disorder from having direct patient contact.

MONITORING
◆ Intake and output
◆ Stool volume measurement and presence of blood and pus
◆ Serum electrolyte results
◆ Signs and symptoms of gram-negative septic shock
◆ Signs and symptoms of dehydration
◆ Vital signs

PATIENT TEACHING

GENERAL
Be sure to cover:
◆ the disorder, diagnosis, and treatment
◆ proper hand-washing technique
◆ the need to avoid unbottled water, ice, unpeeled fruit, and uncooked vegetables in other countries
◆ signs of dehydration and seeking prompt medical attention if these occur (if the patient is to be cared for at home).

RESOURCES
Organizations
Centers for Disease Control and Prevention: *www.cdc.gov*
Harvard University Consumer Health Information: *www.intelihealth.com*
National Health Information Center: *www.health.gov/nhic*
National Library of Medicine: *www.nlm.nih.gov*

Selected references
Kasper, D.L., et al., eds. *Harrison's Principles of Internal Medicine,* 16th ed. New York: McGraw-Hill Book Co., 2005.
Mylotte, J.M. "Nursing Home-acquired Bloodstream Infection," *Infection Control and Hospital Epidemiology* 26(10):833-37, October 2005.

Epididymitis

- Infection of the epididymis (cordlike excretory duct of the testis)
- One of most common infections of the male reproductive tract

PATHOPHYSIOLOGY

- Organisms enter the epididymis by the vas deferens or lymphatics.
- Inflammation occurs.
- Other organs, such as the testes and prostate, may be affected.

CAUSES

- Brucellosis
- Certain drugs (such as amiodarone [Cordarone])
- Leprosy
- Obstruction
- Pyogenic organisms, such as staphylococci, *Escherichia coli*, streptococci, chlamydia, *Neisseria gonorrhoeae*, and *Treponema pallidum*
- Sarcoidosis
- Trauma
- Tuberculosis

RISK FACTORS

- Urinary tract infection
- Unprotected sex
- Prostatitis
- Trauma

INCIDENCE

- Epididymitis usually affects boys and men ages 15 to 30 or older than 60.
- The disease affects 1 in 1,000 men annually.
- The disease rarely occurs before puberty.

COMPLICATIONS

- Orchitis (see *Understanding orchitis*)
- Infertility
- Abscess
- Atrophy
- Pyocele
- Infarction

HISTORY

- Unilateral, dull, aching scrotal pain and swelling
- Pain that radiates to spermatic cord, lower abdomen, and flank
- Extremely heavy feeling in scrotum
- Dysuria, frequency, urgency
- Mild scrotal cellulitis

PHYSICAL FINDINGS

- Erythema
- Mild scrotal cellulitis
- High fever
- Characteristic waddle (attempt to protect groin and scrotum while walking)
- Urethral discharge
- Prehn's sign: elevation of hemiscrotum relieves pain
- Tenderness and induration in the epididymal tail

LABORATORY

- Urinalysis shows an increased white blood cell (WBC) count, indicating infection.
- Urine culture and sensitivity tests may show the causative organism.
- Serum WBC count is greater than 10,000/µl, indicating infection.

IMAGING

- Ultrasonography shows enlarged epididymis (larger than 17 mm); can rule out testicular torsion

Understanding orchitis

Orchitis, an infection of the testes, is a serious complication of epididymitis. It may also result from mumps, which can lead to sterility or, less commonly, another systemic infection.

SIGNS AND SYMPTOMS

Typical effects of orchitis include unilateral or bilateral tenderness and redness, sudden onset of pain, and swelling of the scrotum and testes. Nausea and vomiting also occur. Sudden cessation of pain indicates testicular ischemia, which can cause permanent damage to one or both testes. Hydrocele may also be present.

TREATMENT

Appropriate treatment consists of immediate antibiotic therapy in bacterial infection or, in mumps orchitis, injection of 20 ml of lidocaine (Xylocaine) near the spermatic cord of the affected testis, which may relieve swelling and pain. Severe orchitis may require surgery to incise and drain the hydrocele and to improve testicular circulation. Other treatments are similar to those for epididymitis.

To prevent mumps orchitis, suggest that prepubertal males receive the mumps vaccine (or gamma globulin injection after contracting mumps).

TREATMENT

GENERAL
- Scrotal elevation
- Ice bag to groin
- Use of an athletic supporter until recovered

DIET
- Increased oral fluids

ACTIVITY
- Bed rest until condition improves

MEDICATIONS
- Broad spectrum antibiotics
- Analgesics
- Antipyretics
- Anti-inflammatories

SURGERY
- Scrotal exploration for complications of acute epididymitis
- Epididymectomy under local anesthesia when disease is refractory to antibiotic therapy

NURSING CONSIDERATIONS

NURSING DIAGNOSES
- Acute pain
- Disturbed body image
- Hyperthermia
- Impaired urinary elimination
- Ineffective sexuality patterns
- Risk for infection
- Risk for injury
- Sexual dysfunction

EXPECTED OUTCOMES
The patient will:
- express feelings of increased comfort
- express positive feelings about self-concept and body image
- maintain a normal body temperature
- demonstrate skill in managing the urinary elimination problem
- express feelings about potential or actual changes in sexual activity
- exhibit no signs or symptoms of infection
- avoid or minimize complications
- resume sexual activity to the fullest extent possible.

NURSING INTERVENTIONS
- Give prescribed drugs.
- Apply ice packs for comfort.

MONITORING
- Signs of abscess formation
- Vital signs
- Pain control
- Intake and output

PATIENT TEACHING

GENERAL
Be sure to cover:
- the disorder, diagnosis, and treatment
- drug administration, dosage, and possible adverse effects
- the use of a scrotal support while sitting, standing, or walking
- safer sex practices.

RESOURCES
Organizations
American Association of Kidney Patients: *www.aakp.org*
National Institute of Diabetes & Digestive & Kidney Diseases: *www.niddk.nih.gov*

Selected references
Brisson, P., et al. "Torsion of the Epididymis," *Journal of Pediatric Surgery* 40(11):1795-797, November 2005.
Diseases, 4th ed. Philadelphia: Lippincott Williams & Wilkins, 2006.
Somekh, E., et al. "Acute Epididymitis in Boys: Evidence of a Post-Infectious Etiology," *Journal of Urology* 171(1):391-94, January 2004.

Epidural hematoma LIFE-THREATENING DISORDER

- Acceleration-deceleration or coup-contrecoup injuries that disrupt normal nerve functions in bruised area and cause intracranial bleeding

PATHOPHYSIOLOGY

- Injury is directly beneath the site of impact when the brain rebounds against the skull from the force of a blow (a beating with a blunt instrument, for example), when the force of the blow drives the brain against the opposite side of the skull, or when the head is hurled forward and stopped abruptly (as in an automobile accident when a driver's head strikes the windshield).
- Brain continues moving and slaps against the skull (acceleration), then rebounds (deceleration). Brain may strike bony prominences inside the skull (especially the sphenoidal ridges), causing intracranial hemorrhage or hematoma that may result in tentorial herniation.

CAUSES

- Anticoagulation
- Coagulopathy or bleeding diathesis
- Disk herniation
- Epidural anesthesia
- Hepatic disease with portal hypertension
- Hypertension
- Lumbar puncture
- Paget's disease of bone
- Skull fracture
- Thrombolysis
- Trauma
- Valsalva's maneuver
- Vascular malformation

INCIDENCE

- Epidural hematoma is rare in patients younger than age 2 or older than age 60.
- It's four times more common in men than in women.

COMPLICATIONS

- Increased intracranial pressure (ICP)
- Seizures
- Respiratory depression and failure

ASSESSMENT

HISTORY

- Injury to head
- Headache
- Nausea, vomiting
- Change in mental status

PHYSICAL FINDINGS

- Head wound
- Neurologic signs based on the extent of bleeding — dilated pupils, weakness, sensory deficits, alterations in reflexes, alterations in bladder or anal sphincter tone
- Bradycardia and hypertension (with increased ICP)

DIAGNOSTIC TEST RESULTS

LABORATORY

- Coagulation studies show clotting abnormalities (if cause is anticoagulation).

IMAGING

- Computed tomography scan or magnetic resonance imaging identifies abnormal masses or structural shifts within the cranium.

TREATMENT

GENERAL
- Supportive: airway, breathing, circulation
- Wound care
- Head of the bed elevated 30 degrees with intracerebral injury

DIET
- Based on extent of injury
- Nothing by mouth if surgery necessary

ACTIVITY
- Bed rest initially, then as tolerated

MEDICATIONS
- Vitamin K, fresh frozen plasma, platelets, or clotting products (if coagulation study results are abnormal)
- Analgesics (after extent of injury is determined)
- Osmotic diuretics
- Anticonvulsants
- Prophylactic antibiotics
- Corticosteroids

SURGERY
- Placement of burr holes
- Evacuation of the hematoma
- Craniotomy

NURSING CONSIDERATIONS

NURSING DIAGNOSES
- Acute pain
- Compromised family coping
- Decreased cardiac output
- Impaired physical mobility
- Impaired skin integrity
- Impaired tissue integrity
- Ineffective coping
- Ineffective tissue perfusion: Cerebral
- Posttrauma syndrome
- Risk for injury

EXPECTED OUTCOMES
The patient will:
- express feelings of increased comfort and pain relief
- use support systems to assist with coping
- maintain adequate cardiac output and hemodynamic stability
- recover or be rehabilitated from physical injuries to the greatest extent possible
- experience lesion and wound healing without complications
- maintain tissue integrity
- demonstrate adaptive coping behaviors
- exhibit signs of maintaining adequate cerebral perfusion
- express feelings and fears about the traumatic event
- sustain no further harm or injury.

NURSING INTERVENTIONS
- Provide appropriate wound care.
- Give prescribed drugs.
- Provide emotional support.
- Institute seizure precautions.

MONITORING
- Vital signs
- Neurologic status
- Wound healing
- Seizure activity
- Respiratory status

PATIENT TEACHING

GENERAL
Be sure to cover:
- reporting changes in neurologic status
- avoiding aspirin as a pain treatment
- observing for cerebrospinal fluid drainage and signs of infection.

DISCHARGE PLANNING
- Refer the patient to physical, occupational, and speech therapy, as appropriate.
- Refer the patient to social service for extended services, as appropriate.

RESOURCES
Organizations
American Academy of Neurology: *www.aan.com*
Brain Injury Society: *www.bisociety.org*
Head Injury Hotline: *www.headinjury.com*
National Center for Injury Prevention and Control: *www.cdc.gov/ncipc*

Selected references
Day, M.W. "Epidural Hematoma," *Nursing* 33(8):96, August 2003.
Qureshi, A.A., et al. "Are We Able to Comply with the NICE Head Injury Guidelines?" *Emergency Medicine Journal* 22(12):861-62, December 2005.
Zink, E.K., and McQuillan, K. "Managing Traumatic Brain Injury," *Nursing* 35(9):36-43, September 2005.

◼ Epiglottiditis LIFE-THREATENING DISORDER

OVERVIEW

- Acute inflammation of the epiglottis and surrounding area
- Life-threatening emergency that rapidly causes edema and induration
- If untreated, results in complete airway obstruction
- Mortality 8% to 12%, typically in children ages 2 to 8

PATHOPHYSIOLOGY

- An infection of the epiglottis and surrounding area leads to intense inflammation of the supraglottic region.
- Swelling of the epiglottis, aryepiglottic folds, arytenoid cartilage, and ventricular bands leads to acute airway obstruction.

CAUSES

- Bacterial infection, usually *Haemophilus influenzae* type B
- Pneumococci or group A streptococci
- Thermal injuries

INCIDENCE

- Epiglottiditis may occur from infancy to adulthood.
- The disease may occur in any season.
- Males account for 60% of cases of epiglottiditis.

COMPLICATIONS

- Airway obstruction
- Death

ASSESSMENT

HISTORY

- Recent upper respiratory tract infection
- Sore throat
- Dysphagia
- Sudden onset of high fever

PHYSICAL FINDINGS

- Red and inflamed throat
- Fever
- Cyanosis
- Stridor
- Drooling
- Pale or cyanotic skin
- Restlessness and irritability
- Nasal flaring
- Patient sitting in tripod position
- Thick, muffled voice sounds

DIAGNOSTIC TEST RESULTS

LABORATORY

- Arterial blood gas (ABG) analysis may show hypoxia.

IMAGING

- Lateral neck X-rays show an enlarged epiglottis and distended hypopharynx.

DIAGNOSTIC PROCEDURES

- Direct laryngoscopy shows swollen, beefy red epiglottis.

OTHER

- Pulse oximetry may show decreased oxygen saturation.

TREATMENT

GENERAL
- Emergency hospitalization
- Humidification of airway
- Parenteral fluids

ACTIVITY
- As tolerated

MEDICATIONS
- Parenteral antibiotics
- Corticosteroids
- Oxygen therapy

SURGERY
- Possible tracheotomy

Airway crisis

Epiglottiditis can progress to complete airway obstruction within minutes. To prepare for this medical emergency, keep these tips in mind:

- Watch for the inability to speak; weak, ineffective cough; high-pitched sounds or no sounds while inhaling; increased difficulty breathing; and possible cyanosis. These are warning signs of total airway obstruction and the need for an emergency tracheotomy.
- Keep the following equipment available at the patient's bedside in case of sudden, complete airway obstruction: a tracheotomy tray, endotracheal tubes, a handheld resuscitation bag, oxygen equipment, and a laryngoscope with blades of various sizes.
- Remember that using a tongue blade or throat culture swab can initiate sudden, complete airway obstruction.
- Before examining the patient's throat, request trained personnel, such as an anesthesiologist, to stand by if emergency airway insertion is needed.

NURSING CONSIDERATIONS

NURSING DIAGNOSES
- Anxiety
- Deficient fluid volume
- Disabled family coping
- Fear
- Imbalanced nutrition: Less than body requirements
- Impaired gas exchange
- Impaired verbal communication
- Ineffective airway clearance

EXPECTED OUTCOMES
The patient (and his family) will:
- express reduced levels of anxiety
- maintain adequate fluid volume
- use support systems to assist with coping
- discuss fears and concerns
- show no signs of malnutrition
- maintain adequate ventilation
- use alternate means of communication
- maintain a patent airway (see *Airway crisis*).

NURSING INTERVENTIONS
- Give prescribed drugs.
- Place the patient in a sitting position.
- Place the patient in a cool mist tent.
- Encourage the parents to remain with their child.
- Offer reassurance and support.
- Ensure adequate fluid intake.
- Minimize external stimuli.

MONITORING
- Vital signs
- Intake and output
- Respiratory status
- ABG results
- Pulse oximetry
- Signs and symptoms of secondary infection
- Signs and symptoms of dehydration

PATIENT TEACHING

GENERAL
Be sure to cover:
- the disorder, diagnosis, and treatment
- prescribed drugs and potential adverse effects
- when to call the practitioner
- humidification
- signs and symptoms of respiratory distress
- signs and symptoms of dehydration.

DISCHARGE PLANNING
- Refer the patient for *H. influenzae* b conjugate vaccine, preferably at age 2 months, if indicated.

RESOURCES
Organizations
American Academy of Pediatrics: *www.aap.org*

Selected references
Diseases, 4th ed. Philadelphia: Lippincott Williams & Wilkins, 2006.
Katori, H. and Tsukuda, M. "Acute Epiglottitis: Analysis of Factors Associated with Airway Intervention," *Journal of Laryngology and Otology* 119(12):967-72, December 2005.

Erectile dysfunction

OVERVIEW

- Inability to attain or maintain penile erection long enough to complete intercourse
- Classified as primary or secondary:
- Primary impotence — never achieving sufficient erection
- Secondary impotence — patient has achieved erection and completed intercourse in the past
- Also called *impotence*

PATHOPHYSIOLOGY

- A lack of autonomic signal or impairment of perfusion may interfere with arteriolar dilation because of inappropriate adrenergic stimulation.
- The sacs of the corpus cavernosum collapse prematurely.
- Pelvic steal syndrome can cause loss of erection before ejaculation because of increased blood flow to pelvic muscles.

CAUSES

- Organic cause, such as vascular insufficiency and veno-occlusive dysfunction (80% of cases)
- Psychogenic cause (20% of cases)

RISK FACTORS

- Medication
- Pelvic injury or surgery
- Alcohol use
- Increasing age
- Smoking
- Obesity
- Hypertension
- Diabetes mellitus
- Scleroderma
- Renal failure
- Cancer treatment
- Stroke
- Multiple sclerosis
- Alzheimer's disease
- Depression
- Atherosclerosis
- Cardiovascular disease
- Performance anxiety

INCIDENCE

- Erectile dysfunction affects men of all age-groups, but incidence increases with age.

COMPLICATIONS

- Serious disruption of marital or other sexual relationships

ASSESSMENT

HISTORY

- Long-standing inability to achieve erection
- Sudden loss of erectile function
- Gradual decline in sexual function
- Medical disorders, drug therapy, or psychological trauma
- Achievement of erection through masturbation but not with a partner

PHYSICAL FINDINGS

- Anxious appearance
- Signs of depression

DSM-IV-TR *criteria*

- Diagnosis confirmed when patient meets either of two criteria:
- Persistent or recurrent partial or complete failure to attain or maintain erection until completion of sexual activity
- Marked distress or interpersonal difficulty occurs as a result of erectile dysfunction
- Disorder doesn't occur only during course of other Axis I disorder such as major depression

DIAGNOSTIC TEST RESULTS

LABORATORY

- Serum testosterone levels may be decreased.
- Glycosylated hemoglobin level may be elevated, indicating uncontrolled diabetes mellitus.
- Urinalysis results may be abnormal, indicating kidney damage or diabetes mellitus.
- Lipid profiles may be increased, indicating atherosclerosis.
- Blood glucose levels may be increased, indicating diabetes mellitus.
- Serum creatinine levels may be elevated, indicating kidney damage.
- Prostate-specific antigen results help rule out prostate cancer.

IMAGING

- Ultrasonography evaluates vascular function.
- Angiography evaluates vaso-occlusive disease.

OTHER

- Direct injection of alprostadil (Caverject) into the corpora evaluates the quality of erection.
- Nocturnal penile tumescence testing helps distinguish psychogenic impotence from organic impotence.

GENERAL
- Sex therapy for psychogenic impotence
- Treatment of underlying cause for organic impotence
- Psychological counseling
- External vacuum device

DIET
- Avoidance of alcohol

MEDICATIONS
- Intracavernosal injection therapy
- Medication Urethral System for Erections intraurethral suppository
- Sildenafil (Viagra)
- Vardenafil (Levitra)

SURGERY
- Surgically inserted inflatable or semirigid penile prosthesis

NURSING DIAGNOSES
- Anxiety
- Chronic low self-esteem
- Ineffective coping
- Ineffective sexuality patterns
- Interrupted family processes
- Sexual dysfunction

EXPECTED OUTCOMES
The patient will:
- have reduced levels of anxiety
- voluntarily discuss the condition
- acknowledge a problem in sexual function
- agree to obtain sexual evaluation and therapy if needed
- discuss feelings and perceptions with partner about changes in sexual performance
- develop and maintain a positive attitude toward sexuality and sexual performance.

NURSING INTERVENTIONS
- Encourage verbalization and provide support.
- Refer the patient to a practitioner, nurse, psychologist, social worker, or counselor trained in sex therapy as needed.

After penile prosthesis surgery
- Apply ice packs to the penis for 24 hours.
- Empty the drainage device when it's full.
- If the patient has an inflatable prosthesis, provide instructions for use.

MONITORING
- Response to treatment
- Adverse effects of medication
- Complications
- Postoperative bleeding
- Postoperative infection

GENERAL
Be sure to cover:
- the disorder, diagnosis, and treatment
- the anatomy and physiology of the reproductive system and the human sexual response cycle
- the need to avoid intercourse until the incision heals, usually 6 weeks after penile implant surgery
- signs of infection.

DISCHARGE PLANNING
- Refer the patient to support services.

RESOURCES
Organizations
American Association of Sex Educators, Counselors, and Therapists: *www.aasect.org*
American Psychiatric Association: *www.psych.org*
American Urological Association: *www.auanet.org*
National Cancer Institute: *www.nci.nih.gov*

Selected references
Diagnostic and Statistical Manual of Mental Disorders, Fourth Edition, Text Revision. Washington, D.C.: American Psychiatric Association, 2000.
Lewis, J.H. "Challenges in the Assessment of Erectile Dysfunction and Treatment with Oral Therapies: Review with Case Examples," *Journal of the American Academy of Nurse Practitioners* 16(10):428-40, October 2004.
Lewis, J.H., et al. "Erectile Dysfunction in Primary Care," *Nurse Practitioner* 29(12):42-46, 48-50, 55, December 2004.
Montosori, P., et al. "Common Grounds for Erectile Dysfunction and Coronary Artery Disease," *Current Opinion in Urology* 14(6):361-65, November 2004.

Erythroblastosis fetalis LIFE-THREATENING DISORDER

- Hemolytic disease of the fetus and neonate
- Stems from an incompatibility of fetal and maternal blood
- Also known as *hemolytic disease of the newborn*

PATHOPHYSIOLOGY
ABO incompatibility

- Each blood group has specific antigens on red blood cells (RBCs) and specific antibodies in the serum.
- The maternal immune system forms antibodies against fetal cells when blood groups differ.
- This can cause hemolytic disease even if fetal erythrocytes don't escape into the maternal circulation during pregnancy.

Rh incompatibility

- During her first pregnancy, an Rh-negative female becomes sensitized (during delivery or abortion) by exposure to Rh-positive fetal blood antigens inherited from the father.
- A female may also become sensitized from receiving blood transfusions with alien Rh antigens; from inadequate doses of $Rh_o(D)$ (RhoGAM); or from failure to receive $Rh_o(D)$ after significant fetal-maternal leakage during abruptio placentae (premature detachment of the placenta).
- A subsequent pregnancy with an Rh-positive fetus provokes maternal production of agglutinating antibodies, which cross the placental barrier, attach to Rh-positive cells in the fetus, and cause hemolysis and anemia.
- To compensate, the fetal blood-forming organs step up the production of RBCs, and erythroblasts (immature RBCs) appear in the fetal circulation.
- Extensive hemolysis releases more unconjugated bilirubin than the liver can conjugate and excrete, causing hyperbilirubinemia and hemolytic anemia.

CAUSES

- ABO incompatibility — commonly occurs during first pregnancy; present in about 12% of pregnancies
- Rh isoimmunization (see *What happens in Rh isoimmunization*)
- Rh negativity — more common in Whites than Blacks and rare in Asians
- Rh sensitization — 11 cases per 10,000 births

COMPLICATIONS

- Fetal death in utero
- Severe anemia
- Heart failure
- Kernicterus

HISTORY

- Mother Rh-positive; father Rh-negative
- Antigen-antibody response developed during previous pregnancy
- Blood transfusion
- Maternal history (for erythroblastotic stillbirths, abortions, previously affected children, previous anti-Rh titers)

PHYSICAL FINDINGS

- Pallor
- Edema
- Petechiae
- Bile-stained umbilical cord
- Yellow- or meconium-stained amniotic fluid
- Mild to moderate hepatosplenomegaly
- Pulmonary crackles
- Heart murmur
- Jaundice

What happens in RH isoimmunization

Rh-negative woman before pregnancy

↓

Pregnancy with Rh-positive fetus

↓

Placental separation

↓

Maternal sensitization to Rh-positive blood

↓

Maternal development of anti-Rh-positive antibodies

↓

Next pregnancy with Rh-positive fetus

↓

Maternal anti-Rh antibodies enter fetal circulation

↓

Anti-Rh antibody to fetal Rh-positive red blood cells (RBCs)

↓

HEMOLYSIS OF FETAL RBCS

LABORATORY

- Paternal blood typing is positive for ABO and Rh.
- Amniotic fluid analysis shows increased bilirubin and anti-Rh titers.
- Direct Coombs' test of umbilical cord blood measures RBC (Rh-positive) antibodies in the neonate (positive only when the mother is Rh negative and the fetus is Rh positive).
- Neonatal cord hemoglobin level less than 10 g indicates severe disease.
- Many nucleated peripheral RBCs are present.

IMAGING

- Radiologic studies show edema and, in hydrops fetalis, the halo sign (edematous, elevated, subcutaneous fat layers) and the Buddha position (fetus's legs are crossed).

TREATMENT

GENERAL

- Phototherapy (exposure to ultraviolet light to reduce bilirubin levels)
- Intubation of neonate
- Removal of excess fluid
- Maintenance of body temperature

MEDICATIONS

- Intrauterine-intraperitoneal transfusion (if amniotic fluid analysis suggests the fetus is severely affected and isn't mature enough to deliver)
- Exchange transfusion
- Albumin infusion
- Gamma globulin containing anti-Rh antibody ($Rh_o[D]$)

SURGERY

- Planned delivery (usually 2 to 4 weeks before term date, depending on maternal history, serologic test results, and amniocentesis)

NURSING DIAGNOSES

- Impaired gas exchange
- Impaired tissue integrity
- Ineffective breathing pattern
- Ineffective tissue perfusion: Cardiopulmonary
- Risk for deficient fluid volume
- Risk for imbalanced body temperature
- Risk for impaired parent/infant/child attachment
- Risk for impaired skin integrity

EXPECTED OUTCOMES

The patient will:

- exhibit adequate ventilation and oxygenation
- have reduced redness, swelling, and pain at the site of impaired tissue
- maintain effective breathing pattern
- remain hemodynamically stable
- maintain fluid balance within normal limits
- maintain normal temperature
- demonstrate eye, voice, and touch contact with the infant
- maintain skin integrity.

NURSING INTERVENTIONS

- Encourage expression of fears by parents concerning possible complications of treatment.
- Promote normal parental bonding.
- Administer $Rh_o(D)$ I.M., as ordered.

MONITORING

- Cardiac rhythm and rate
- Temperature
- Airway and ventilation
- Transfusion complications
- Intake and output

GENERAL

Be sure to cover:

- the disorder, diagnosis, and treatment
- medications, drug routes, and administration
- preventive measures for reoccurrence.

DISCHARGE PLANNING

- Encourage follow-up appointments.

RESOURCES

Organizations

American Academy of Pediatrics: *www.aap.org*
National Library of Medicine: *www.nlm.nih.gov*

Selected references

Colyar, M. "Newborn Screening Tests," *Advance for Nurse Practitioners* 12(10):22, October 2004.

Green, T.P. "The Treatment of Erythroblastosis Fetalis with Replacement Transfusion," *Journal of Pediatrics* 144(3):357, March 2004.

Queenan, J.T. "Noninvasive Fetal Rh Genotyping: The Time Has Come," *Obstetrics and Gynecology* 106(4):682-83, October 2005.

Esophageal cancer

OVERVIEW

- Esophageal tumors usually fungating and infiltrating and nearly always fatal
- Liver and lungs: common sites of metastasis
- If symptom-producing, cancer usually already spread to lymph nodes
- Includes two types of malignant tumors: squamous cell carcinoma and adenocarcinoma
- Grim prognosis (5-year survival rates in less than 5% of cases; most patients die within 6 months of diagnosis)

PATHOPHYSIOLOGY

- Esophageal cancer begins in the mucosa and then invades the submucosal and muscular layers of the esophagus.
- Regional metastasis occurs early by way of submucosal lymphatics, commonly fatally invading adjacent vital intrathoracic organs. (If the patient survives primary extension, the liver and lungs are the usual sites of distant metastasis; unusual metastasis sites include the bone, kidneys, and adrenal glands.)

CAUSES

- Alcohol use
- Chronic exposure of the esophageal mucosa to noxious or toxic stimuli, resulting in dysplasia
- Chronic gastroesophageal reflux
- Tobacco use

RISK FACTORS

- Chronic irritation from heavy smoking
- Excessive use of alcohol
- Stasis-induced inflammation, as in achalasia or stricture
- Previous head and neck tumors
- Nutritional deficiency, such as in untreated sprue and Plummer-Vinson syndrome

INCIDENCE

- Cancer of the esophagus is most common in men older than age 60.
- Although it occurs worldwide, esophageal cancer is most common in Japan, Russia, China, the Middle East, and the Transkei region of South Africa.

COMPLICATIONS

- Direct invasion of adjoining structures
- Inability to control secretions
- Obstruction of the esophagus
- Loss of lower esophageal sphincter control (may result in aspiration pneumonia)

ASSESSMENT

HISTORY

- Feeling of fullness, pressure, indigestion, or substernal burning
- Dysphagia and weight loss; the degree of dysphagia varies, depending on the extent of disease
- Hoarseness
- Pain on swallowing or pain that radiates to the back
- Anorexia, vomiting, and regurgitation of food

PHYSICAL FINDINGS

- Chronic cough (possibly from aspiration)
- Cachexia and dehydration

DIAGNOSTIC TEST RESULTS

IMAGING

- X-rays of the esophagus, with barium swallow and motility studies, delineate structural and filling defects and reduced peristalsis.
- Computed tomography scan helps to diagnose and monitor esophageal lesions.
- Magnetic resonance imaging permits evaluation of the esophagus and adjacent structures.

DIAGNOSTIC PROCEDURES

- Esophagoscopy, punch and brush biopsies, and exfoliative cytologic tests confirm esophageal tumors.
- Bronchoscopy (usually performed after an esophagoscopy) may reveal tumor growth in the tracheobronchial tree.
- Endoscopic ultrasonography of the esophagus combines endoscopy and ultrasound technology to measure the depth of penetration of the tumor.

TREATMENT

GENERAL
- Surgery and other treatments to relieve disease effects
- Palliative therapy used to keep esophagus open:
  - Dilatation of the esophagus
  - Laser therapy
  - Radiation therapy
  - Installation of prosthetic tubes (such as Celestin's tube)

DIET
- Liquid to soft, as tolerated
- High-calorie supplements

MEDICATIONS
- Chemotherapy and radiation therapy
- Analgesics

SURGERY
- Radical surgery to excise tumor and resect esophagus or stomach and esophagus
- Gastrostomy or jejunostomy

OTHER
- Endoscopic laser treatment and bipolar electrocoagulation

NURSING CONSIDERATIONS

NURSING DIAGNOSES
- Acute pain
- Anxiety
- Deficient fluid volume
- Fatigue
- Fear
- Imbalanced nutrition: Less than body requirements
- Impaired swallowing
- Risk for aspiration
- Risk for infection

EXPECTED OUTCOMES
The patient will:
- express feelings of increased comfort and decreased pain
- express feelings of decreased anxiety
- maintain fluid volumes within the normal range
- express feelings of energy and decreased fatigue
- express concerns and fears related to his diagnosis and condition
- maintain weight within an acceptable range
- swallow without coughing or choking
- not aspirate
- show no evidence of infection.

NURSING INTERVENTIONS
- Provide support and encourage verbalization.
- Position the patient properly to prevent food aspiration.
- Provide tube feedings, as ordered.
- Give prescribed drugs.

MONITORING
- Vital signs
- Hydration and nutritional status
- Electrolyte levels
- Intake and output
- Postoperative complications
- Swallowing ability
- Pain control

PATIENT TEACHING

GENERAL
Be sure to cover:
- the disease process, treatment, and postoperative course
- dietary needs
- the need for rest between activities.

DISCHARGE PLANNING
- Arrange for home care follow-up after discharge.
- Refer the patient to the American Cancer Society.
- Arrange for a referral to hospice and support services.

RESOURCES
Organizations
American Cancer Society:
www.cancer.org
Guide to Internet Resources for Cancer:
www.cancerindex.org
National Cancer Institute:
www.cancer.gov

Selected references
Atlas of Pathophysiology, 2nd ed. Philadelphia: Lippincott Williams & Wilkins, 2005.
Mackenzie, D.J., et al. "Care of Patients after Esophagectomy," *Critical Care Nurse* 24(1):16-29, February 2004.
Odelli, C., et al. "Nutrition Support Improves Patient Outcomes, Treatment Tolerance and Admission Characteristics in Oesophageal Cancer," *Clinical Oncology* 17(8):639-45, December 2005.

Exophthalmos

OVERVIEW

- Unilateral or bilateral bulging or protrusion of the eyeballs or their apparent forward displacement (with lid retraction)
- Also called *proptosis*

PATHOPHYSIOLOGY

- Increase in volume within the fixed bony orbital confines displaces the globular orbit anteriorly.

CAUSES

- Edema
- Hemorrhage
- Infection
- Ophthalmic Graves' disease
- Orbital cellulitis
- Panophthalmitis
- Thrombosis
- Trauma
- Tumors and neoplastic diseases
- Varicosities

INCIDENCE

- Exophthalmos is more common in women than in men.
- The disorder can occur at any age, but it's more common between ages 30 and 50.

COMPLICATIONS

- Vision changes

ASSESSMENT

HISTORY

- Vision changes
- Eye trauma

PHYSICAL FINDINGS

- Eye protrusion (see *Detecting unilateral exophthalmos*)
- Visible rim of the sclera
- Infrequent blinking
- Limited ocular movement
- Ocular tenderness

DIAGNOSTIC TEST RESULTS

LABORATORY

- Culture of discharge determines the infecting organism.
- Sensitivity testing indicates appropriate antibiotic therapy.

IMAGING

- Computed tomography scan detects swollen extraocular muscles or lesions within the orbit.

DIAGNOSTIC PROCEDURES

- Exophthalmometer readings confirm diagnosis by showing the degree of anterior projection and asymmetry between the eyes. (Normal bar readings range from 12 to 20 mm.)

OTHER

- Physical examination indicates the presence of exophthalmos. (See *Recognizing exophthalmos.*)

Detecting unilateral exophthalmos

If one of the patient's eyes seems more prominent than the other, examine both eyes from above the patient's head. Look down across his face, gently draw his lids up, and compare the relationship of the corneas to the lower lids. Abnormal protrusion of one eye suggests unilateral exophthalmos.

Don't perform this test if you suspect eye trauma.

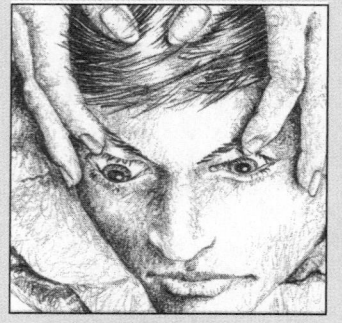

Recognizing exophthalmos

This photo shows the characteristic forward protrusion of the eyes from the orbit associated with exophthalmos.

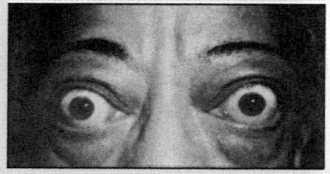

TREATMENT

GENERAL
◆ Cold and warm compresses (trauma)

ACTIVITY
◆ As tolerated

MEDICATIONS
◆ Antibiotics (infection)
◆ Antithyroid therapy (Graves' disease)
◆ Corticosteroids (optic neuropathy)
◆ Eye lubricants

SURGERY
◆ Orbital decompression (removal of the superior and lateral orbital walls) if vision is threatened, followed by lid (blepharoplasty) and muscle surgery
◆ Surgical exploration of the orbit and excision of the tumor

NURSING CONSIDERATIONS

NURSING DIAGNOSES
◆ Anxiety
◆ Disturbed body image
◆ Disturbed sensory perception: Visual
◆ Ineffective coping
◆ Risk for injury

EXPECTED OUTCOMES
The patient will:
◆ express feelings of decreased anxiety
◆ express positive feelings about self
◆ maintain functional eyesight
◆ demonstrate effective coping skills
◆ remain free from injury.

NURSING INTERVENTIONS
◆ Give prescribed drugs.
◆ Apply cold and warm compresses, as ordered, for fracture or other trauma.
◆ Provide postoperative care.
◆ Provide emotional support.
◆ Protect the exposed cornea with lubricants to prevent corneal drying.

MONITORING
◆ Response to therapy
◆ Visual acuity

PATIENT TEACHING

GENERAL
Be sure to cover:
◆ the disorder, diagnosis, and treatment.

DISCHARGE PLANNING
◆ Encourage follow-up care.

RESOURCES
Organizations
American Academy of Ophthalmology: *www.aao.org*
Endocrine Society: *www.endo-society.org*
Merck Manuals Online Medical Library: *www.merck.com/mmhe*
National Eye Institute: *www.nei.nih.gov*

Selected references
Bonavolonta, G., et al. "Unilateral Exophthalmos Associated with Ipsilateral Mucosal Turbinate Hypertrophy: Benign Exophthalmos Syndrome (BEDS). A Description of a New Clinical Condition," *European Journal of Ophthalmology* 15(6):800-803, November-December 2005.
Kubo, T., et al. "An Infant Case of Graves' Disease with Ophthalmopathy," *Endocrine Journal* 52(5):647-50, October 2005.

Fibromyalgia syndrome

- ◆ A diffuse pain syndrome
- ◆ Formerly known as fibrositis
- ◆ Also called *FMS*

PATHOPHYSIOLOGY

- ◆ Several theories describe FMS:
- – Blood flow to the muscle is decreased (due to poor muscle aerobic conditioning, rather than other physiologic abnormalities).
- – Blood flow in the thalamus and caudate nucleus is decreased, leading to a lowered pain threshold.
- – Endocrine dysfunction — such as abnormal pituitary-adrenal axis responses or abnormal levels of the neurotransmitter serotonin in brain centers — affects pain and sleep.
- – The functioning of other pain-processing pathways is abnormal.

CAUSES

- ◆ Unknown
- ◆ May be multifactorial and influenced by stress, physical conditioning, abnormal-quality sleep, and neuroendocrine, psychiatric, or hormonal factors
- ◆ May be primary disorder or associated with underlying disease such as infection

INCIDENCE

- ◆ FMS is observed in up to 15% of patients seen in general rheumatology practice and 5% of general medicine clinic patients.
- ◆ The disease affects 90% more women than men.
- ◆ FMS may occur at almost any age, but incidence peaks between ages 20 and 60.

COMPLICATIONS

- ◆ Pain
- ◆ Depression
- ◆ Sleep deprivation

HISTORY

- ◆ Diffuse, dull, aching pain across neck and shoulders and in lower back and proximal limbs
- ◆ Pain typically worse in the morning, sometimes with stiffness; can be exacerbated by stress, lack of sleep, weather changes, and inactivity
- ◆ Sleep disturbances with frequent arousal and fragmented sleep or frequent waking throughout night (patient unaware of arousals)
- ◆ Possible report of irritable bowel syndrome, tension headaches, puffy hands, and paresthesia

PHYSICAL FINDINGS

- ◆ Tender points elicited by applying a moderate amount of pressure to a specific location. (See *Tender points of fibromyalgia*.)

GENERAL

- ◆ Diagnostic testing in FMS not associated with an underlying disease is generally negative for significant abnormalities.

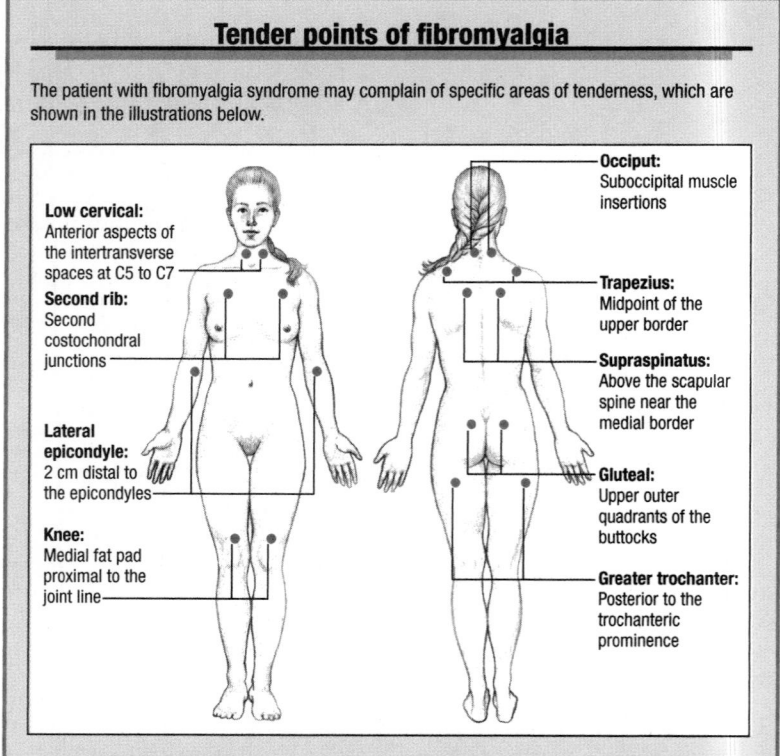

Tender points of fibromyalgia

The patient with fibromyalgia syndrome may complain of specific areas of tenderness, which are shown in the illustrations below.

Low cervical: Anterior aspects of the intertransverse spaces at C5 to C7

Second rib: Second costochondral junctions

Lateral epicondyle: 2 cm distal to the epicondyles

Knee: Medial fat pad proximal to the joint line

Occiput: Suboccipital muscle insertions

Trapezius: Midpoint of the upper border

Supraspinatus: Above the scapular spine near the medial border

Gluteal: Upper outer quadrants of the buttocks

Greater trochanter: Posterior to the trochanteric prominence

TREATMENT

GENERAL
- Massage therapy
- Ultrasound treatments

ACTIVITY
- Regular, low-impact aerobic exercise program such as water aerobics
- Preexercise and postexercise stretching to minimize injury

MEDICATIONS
- Amitriptyline, nortriptyline, or cyclobenzaprine
- Tricyclic antidepressants and serotonin reuptake inhibitors
- Nonsteroidal anti-inflammatory drugs
- Magnesium supplements
- Steroid or lidocaine injections
- Pramipexole (Mirapex), a dopamine agonist (possibly helpful in some patients)

NURSING CONSIDERATIONS

NURSING DIAGNOSES
- Activity intolerance
- Chronic pain
- Disturbed sleep pattern
- Energy field disturbance
- Fatigue
- Hopelessness
- Impaired physical mobility
- Ineffective coping
- Ineffective health maintenance
- Ineffective role performance
- Powerlessness

EXPECTED OUTCOMES
The patient will:
- verbalize the importance of balancing activity, as tolerated, with rest
- express feelings of increased comfort and decreased pain
- express feelings of being well rested or will appear well rested
- express an increased sense of well-being
- verbalize feelings of increased energy
- make decisions on her own behalf
- attain the highest degree of mobility possible within the confines of the disease
- demonstrate effective coping behaviors
- continue to receive treatments that help promote relaxation and inner well-being
- recognize limitations imposed by the illness and express feelings about these limitations
- express feelings of control over the pain.

NURSING INTERVENTIONS
- Give prescribed drugs.
- Provide emotional support.
- Encourage the patient to perform regular stretching exercises safely and effectively.
- Provide reassurance that FMS can be treated.

MONITORING
- Sensory disturbances
- Level of pain
- Response to treatment
- Fatigue
- Depression

PATIENT TEACHING

GENERAL
Be sure to cover:
- the disorder, diagnosis, and treatment
- the importance of exercise in maintaining muscle conditioning, improving energy and, possibly, improving sleep quality
- the importance of taking the tricyclic antidepressant dose 1 to 2 hours before bedtime, which can improve sleep benefits while reducing the morning-after effect
- the avoidance of decongestants and caffeine before bedtime
- the need for a low-fat diet, high in complex carbohydrates, to decrease symptoms.

DISCHARGE PLANNING
- Refer the patient to appropriate counseling as needed.

RESOURCES
Organizations
American Fibromyalgia Syndrome Association, Inc.: *www.afsafund.org*
Arthritis Foundation: *www.arthritis.org*

Selected references
D'Arcy, Y. "Following New Guidelines to Treat Fibromyalgia Pain," *Nursing* 35(10):17-18, October 2005.
Schultz, M.A., et al. "Help Patients Cope with Fibromyalgia," *RN* 67(9):46-48, 50, September 2004.

Folliculitis, furunculosis, and carbunculosis

OVERVIEW

- Folliculitis
- Superficial bacterial infection of hair follicles that usually heals without scarring
- Characterized by the formation of pustules
- Typically a localized eruption
- Predilection for perifollicular (hairy) areas and flexural surfaces
- May occur in the beard region (sycosis barbae)
- May occur in the scalp or on extremities (follicular impetigo)
- May lead to the development of furuncles (furunculosis) or carbuncles
- Prognosis dependant on severity, the patient's physical condition, and ability to resist infection
- Furunculosis
- Deeper infections characterized by deeper, more tender, and erythematous nodules or "boils"
- Worsened by irritation, friction, or perspiration
- Carbunculosis
- Abscess of adjacent furuncles
- Slower development

PATHOPHYSIOLOGY
- The infecting organism invades the hair follicle.
- An inflammatory reaction within the hair follicle results. (See *Hair follicles and bacterial infection*.)

CAUSES
- Bacterial infection, typically coagulase-positive *Staphylococcus aureus*
- Contamination from an infected wound elsewhere on the body

RISK FACTORS
- Poor personal hygiene
- Debilitation
- Immunosuppression
- Diabetes mellitus
- Occlusive agents or chemicals such as cosmetics
- Tight-fitting clothing
- Improper shaving technique
- Occlusive therapy, using steroids
- Obesity
- Chronic colonization of *S. aureus* in nares or perineum

INCIDENCE
Folliculitis
- Folliculitis is a common infection.
- The infection affects all ages.
- Folliculitis affects males more commonly than females.

Furunculosis
- Furunculosis is uncommon in children unless they're immunocompromised.
- Furunculosis occurs more frequently after puberty.
- The disease is more common in adolescents and young adults.
- Furunculosis affects males and females equally.

Carbunculosis
- Carbunculosis affects males more commonly than females.
- It isn't uncommon for several family members to be affected at the same time.
- The disease is more common in patients with diabetes and in those who are immunocompromised.

COMPLICATIONS
- Cellulitis
- Septicemia
- Hematogenous seeding to heart valves, joints, and other organs
- Residual scarring

ASSESSMENT

HISTORY
- Presence of risk factors
- Pain and erythema for several days or more
- Malaise

PHYSICAL FINDINGS
Folliculitis
- Localized pustules, usually on the scalp or extremities
- Pustules possibly also in beard area or on eyelids (styes)

Furunculosis
- Hard, painful, or fluctuant nodules usually on neck, face, axillae, or buttocks
- If nodules enlarge and rupture, pus and necrotic material on the skin surface
- Erythema that may persist for days or weeks after nodule rupture

Carbunculosis
- Fever
- Extremely painful, deep abscesses
- Abscesses drain through multiple openings onto the skin surface
- Pain, tenderness, and edema around pustule sites
- Hard or fluctuant nodules under skin surface
- Localized lymphadenopathy

DIAGNOSTIC TEST RESULTS

LABORATORY
- Wound culture and sensitivity results show the infecting organism.
- Complete blood count possibly reveals leukocytosis.

TREATMENT

GENERAL
- Thorough cleaning of infected area with soap and water
- Avoidance of occlusive agents
- Application of warm, moist compresses

MEDICATIONS
- Topical or systemic antibiotics

SURGERY
- Possible incision and drainage in patients with furunculosis or carbunculosis

---

Hair follicles and bacterial infection

The degree of hair follicle involvement in bacterial skin infection ranges from superficial folliculitis (erythema and a pustule in a single follicle) to deep folliculitis (extensive follicle involvement), to furunculosis (red, tender nodules that surround follicles with a single draining point) and, finally, to carbunculosis (deep abscesses that involve several follicles with multiple draining points).

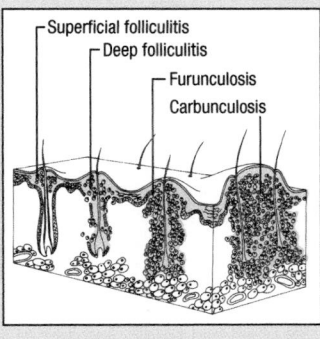

- Superficial folliculitis
- Deep folliculitis
- Furunculosis
- Carbunculosis

NURSING CONSIDERATIONS

NURSING DIAGNOSES
- Acute pain
- Disturbed body image
- Impaired skin integrity
- Impaired tissue integrity
- Risk for infection

EXPECTED OUTCOMES
The patient will:
- report feelings of increased comfort
- voice feelings about his changed body image
- exhibit improved or healed wounds or lesions
- will have reduced redness, swelling, and pain at the site of impaired tissue
- show no signs or symptoms of infection.

NURSING INTERVENTIONS
- Perform wound care.
- Properly dispose of contaminated dressings.
- Follow standard precautions.
- Apply warm, moist compresses.
- Assist with general hygiene and comfort measures as needed.
- Give prescribed pain medications and antibiotics.

MONITORING
- Adverse drug reactions
- Response to treatment
- Level of comfort
- Complications

PATIENT TEACHING

GENERAL
Be sure to cover:
- the disorder, diagnosis, and treatment
- meticulous hand-washing technique
- good personal hygiene
- how to prevent the spread of the infection
- lesion care
- the prescribed medication and potential adverse reactions.

DISCHARGE PLANNING
- Refer patients with recurrent furunculosis for a physical examination to assess for underlying diseases.

RESOURCES
Organizations
American Academy of Dermatology: *www.aad.org*
Dermatology Foundation: *www.dermfnd.org*

Selected references
Ladhani, S., and Garbash, M. "Staphylococcal Skin Infections in Children: Rational Drug Therapy Recommendations," *Paediatric Drugs* 7(2):77-102, 2005.

Nettina, S.M. *Lippincott Manual of Nursing Practice,* 8th ed. Philadelphia: Lippincott Williams & Wilkins, 2006.

Rosen, T. "Update on Treating Uncomplicated Skin and Skin Structure Infections," *Journal of Drugs in Dermatology* 4(6 Suppl):s9-14, November-December 2005.

Fragile X syndrome

OVERVIEW

- Most common inherited cause of mental retardation
- Clinical features demonstrated in about 85% of males and 50% of females who inherit the fragile X mental retardation-1 (FMR1) gene
- Distinct physical features, behavioral difficulties, and cognitive impairment typically seen in postpubescent males
- More subtle symptoms in females

PATHOPHYSIOLOGY

- This X-linked condition doesn't follow a simple X-linked inheritance pattern.
- Full mutation typically causes abnormal methylation (methyl groups attach to components of the gene) of FMR1.
- Methylation inhibits gene transcription and, thus, protein production.
- The reduced or absent protein production leads to the clinical features of fragile X syndrome.

CAUSES

- Gene alteration on the X chromosome
- Well-defined mutation at a specific location on the FMR1 gene

INCIDENCE

- Fragile X syndrome is estimated to occur in about 1 in 4,000 males and 1 in 6,000 females.
- Fragile X syndrome occurs in almost all races and ethnic groups.
- The syndrome is more common in blacks than in whites.

COMPLICATIONS

- Behavioral or learning difficulties
- Cognitive impairment
- Connective tissue abnormalities

ASSESSMENT

HISTORY

- Average IQ between 30 and 70
- Hyperactivity, speech difficulties, language delay, and autistic-like behaviors
- Excessive shyness or social anxiety

PHYSICAL FINDINGS

- A prominent jaw and forehead in postpubertal males
- Head circumference exceeding the 90th percentile
- Long, narrow face with long or large ears that may be posteriorly rotated
- Hyperextension of the fingers
- Unusually large testes

DIAGNOSTIC TEST RESULTS

LABORATORY

- Positive result of genetic test, preferably DNA analysis of blood or buccal samples, detects the size of the cytosine-guanine-guanine repeat and the methylation status of FMR1.

TREATMENT

GENERAL
◆ Controlling individual symptoms

ACTIVITY
◆ As tolerated

MEDICATIONS
◆ Anticonvulsants
◆ Antidepressants
◆ Sedatives

SURGERY
◆ Mitral valve repair

NURSING CONSIDERATIONS

NURSING DIAGNOSES
◆ Bathing or hygiene self-care deficit
◆ Compromised family coping
◆ Delayed growth and development
◆ Dressing or grooming self-care deficit
◆ Ineffective health maintenance
◆ Risk for impaired parenting

EXPECTED OUTCOMES
The patient (and his family) will:
◆ perform bathing and hygiene activities of daily living (ADLs) to the fullest extent possible
◆ demonstrate adaptive coping behaviors
◆ demonstrate age-appropriate skills and behaviors to the extent possible
◆ perform dressing and grooming ADLs to the fullest extent possible
◆ perform health maintenance activities according to level of ability
◆ express understanding of norms for growth and development (parents).

NURSING INTERVENTIONS
◆ Give prescribed drugs.
◆ Provide emotional support to the patient and his family.
◆ Encourage appropriate activities for the patient's ability.

MONITORING
◆ Language development
◆ Seizures
◆ Hyperactivity

PATIENT TEACHING

GENERAL
Be sure to cover:
◆ drug administration and adverse effects.

DISCHARGE PLANNING
◆ Refer the patient and his family for genetic counseling.
◆ Refer the family to a support group.
◆ Advocate for special education services and individualized speech, language, and occupational therapy services during the patient's schooling.

RESOURCES
Organizations
The Fragile X Research Foundation: *www.fraxa.org*
The National Fragile X Foundation: *www.fragilex.org*
National Institute of Child Health & Human Development: *www.nichd.nih.gov*

Selected references
Cronister, A., et al. "Fragile X Syndrome Carrier Screening in the Prenatal Genetic Counseling Setting," *Genetics in Medicine* 7(4):246-50, April 2005.
Sherman, S., et al. "Fragile X Syndrome: Diagnostic and Carrier Testing," *Genetics in Medicine* 7(8):584-87, October 2005.

Gas gangrene

OVERVIEW

- Rare condition caused by local infection with an anaerobic, spore-forming, gram-positive, rod-shaped bacillus *Clostridium perfringens* or another clostridial species
- Occurs in devitalized tissues and results from compromised arterial circulation

PATHOPHYSIOLOGY

- Incubation is 1 to 4 days but can vary from 3 hours to 6 weeks or longer.
- *C. perfringens* invades soft tissues, producing thrombosis of regional blood vessels, tissue necrosis, and localized edema. (See *Effects of* Clostridium perfringens.)
- Necrosis releases carbon dioxide and hydrogen subcutaneously, producing interstitial gas bubbles.

CAUSES

- Infection with *C. perfringens*
- Trauma or surgery, allowing organism to enter body

RISK FACTORS

- Diabetes mellitus

INCIDENCE

- The condition is rare, although more than 30% of deep wounds are infected with clostridia.
- It's most common in deep wounds, especially when tissue necrosis further reduces the oxygen supply.
- It's most common in extremities and abdominal wounds and less common in the uterus.

COMPLICATIONS

- Renal failure
- Hypotension and shock
- Hemolytic anemia
- Tissue death requiring amputation of the affected body part

ASSESSMENT

HISTORY

- Recent surgery (within 72 hours)
- Traumatic injury
- Septic abortion
- Delivery

PHYSICAL FINDINGS

- Normothermia, followed by a moderate increase, usually not above 101° F (38.3° C)
- Toxemia (hypotension, tachycardia, tachypnea)
- Localized swelling and discoloration (usually dusky brown or reddish)
- Bullae and tissue necrosis
- Dark red or black necrotic muscle
- Foul-smelling, watery or frothy discharge
- Subcutaneous emphysema (hallmark of gas gangrene)
- In later stages, altered level of consciousness that may deteriorate to delirium and coma

DIAGNOSTIC TEST RESULTS

LABORATORY

- Anaerobic cultures of wound drainage show *C. perfringens*.
- Gram stain of wound drainage shows large, gram-positive, rod-shaped bacteria.
- Blood studies show leukocytosis and, later, hemolysis.

IMAGING

- X-rays reveal gas in tissues.

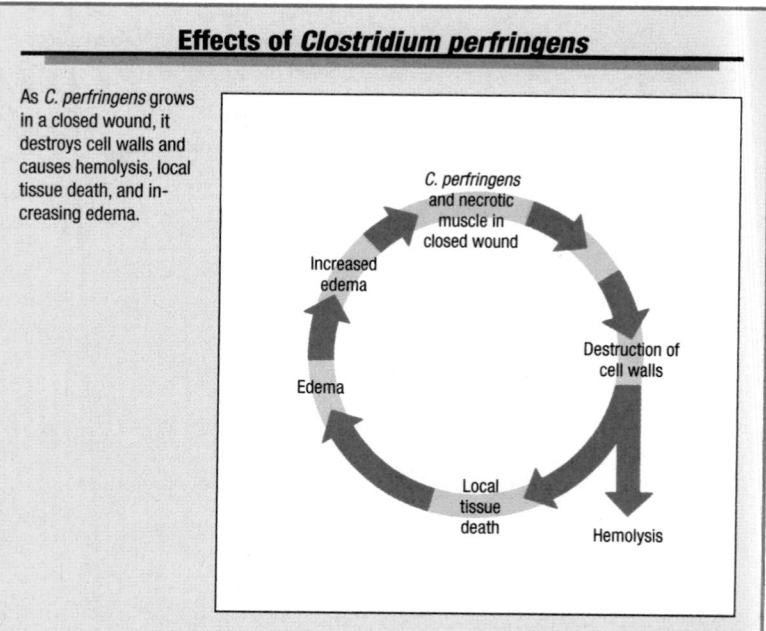

Effects of *Clostridium perfringens*

As *C. perfringens* grows in a closed wound, it destroys cell walls and causes hemolysis, local tissue death, and increasing edema.

- C. perfringens and necrotic muscle in closed wound
- Destruction of cell walls
- Hemolysis
- Local tissue death
- Edema
- Increased edema

TREATMENT

GENERAL
◆ Hyperbaric oxygenation

DIET
◆ Adequate hydration
◆ Nothing by mouth if surgery planned

ACTIVITY
◆ Bed rest until recovery begins

MEDICATIONS
◆ I.V. antibiotics
◆ Analgesics

SURGERY
◆ Immediate wide surgical excision of all affected tissues and necrotic muscle in myositis
◆ Amputation of the affected part

NURSING CONSIDERATIONS

NURSING DIAGNOSES
◆ Acute pain
◆ Anxiety
◆ Decreased cardiac output
◆ Fear
◆ Impaired skin integrity
◆ Impaired tissue integrity
◆ Ineffective tissue perfusion: Cardiopulmonary, peripheral
◆ Risk for infection

EXPECTED OUTCOMES
The patient will:
◆ express feelings of increased comfort and relief from pain
◆ identify measures to reduce anxiety
◆ maintain adequate cardiac output
◆ verbalize feelings of anxiety and fear
◆ have skin that remains warm, dry, and intact
◆ exhibit improved or healed lesions or wounds
◆ maintain hemodynamic stability and collateral circulation
◆ experience no further signs or symptoms of infection.

NURSING INTERVENTIONS
◆ Give prescribed analgesics.
◆ Prepare for surgery, if indicated.
◆ Provide adequate fluid replacement.
◆ Maintain the airway and ventilation.
◆ Provide appropriate skin care and meticulous wound care; place the patient on an air mattress or an air-fluidized bed.
◆ Encourage verbalization and provide support.

MONITORING
◆ Vital signs
◆ Intake and output
◆ Pulmonary and cardiac function
◆ Wound site

PATIENT TEACHING

GENERAL
Be sure to cover:
◆ the disorder, diagnosis, and treatment
◆ the need to report severe pain at the wound site immediately
◆ the need to report foul odor or drainage from the wound site.

DISCHARGE PLANNING
◆ After recovery, refer the patient for physical rehabilitation as necessary.
◆ After extensive surgery, such as amputation, refer the patient for psychological support as necessary.

RESOURCES
Organizations
Centers for Disease Control and Prevention: *www.cdc.gov*
Harvard University Consumer Health Information: *www.intelihealth.com*
National Health Information Center: *www.health.gov/nhic*
National Library of Medicine: *www.nlm.nih.gov*

Selected references
Kasper, D.L., et al., eds. *Harrison's Principles of Internal Medicine,* 16th ed. New York: McGraw-Hill Book Co., 2005.
Titball, R.W. "Gas Gangrene: An Open and Closed Case," *Microbiology* 151(Pt 9):2821-828, September 2005.
Yildiz, T., et al. "Spontaneous, Nontraumatic Gas Gangrene Due to Clostridium Perfringens," *International Journal of Infectious Diseases* 10(1):83-85, January 2006.

Gastric cancer

- Cancer of the GI tract classified according to gross appearance (polypoid, ulcerating, ulcerating and infiltrating, or diffuse)
- Prognosis dependent on the stage of the disease at the time of diagnosis (5-year survival rate is about 15%)

PATHOPHYSIOLOGY

- The most commonly affected areas of the stomach are the pylorus and antrum.
- The remaining areas affected, in order of most common to least common, are the lesser curvature of the stomach, the cardia, the body of the stomach, and the greater curvature of the stomach.
- Rapid metastasis occurs to the regional lymph nodes, omentum, liver, and lungs.

CAUSES

- Unknown

RISK FACTORS

- Gastritis with gastric atrophy
- Type A blood (10% increased risk)
- Family history of gastric cancer
- Smoked foods, pickled vegetables, and salted fish and meat
- High alcohol consumption
- Smoking

INCIDENCE

- The second most common cancer-related death in the world is by gastric cancer.
- Gastric cancer is the 17th most common cancer and the 7th leading cause of cancer death in the United States.
- Gastric cancer is slightly more common in men than women and usually occurs between ages 40 and 70.

COMPLICATIONS

- Malnutrition
- GI obstruction
- Iron deficiency anemia
- Metastasis

HISTORY

- Back, epigastric, or retrosternal pain not relieved with nonprescription medications
- Vague feeling of fullness, heaviness, and moderate abdominal distention after meals
- Weight loss, nausea, vomiting
- Weakness and fatigue
- Dysphagia

PHYSICAL FINDINGS

- Abdominal distention
- Palpable mass
- Palpable lymph nodes, especially the supraclavicular and axillary nodes
- Other assessment findings that depend on extent of disease and location of metastasis

LABORATORY

- Complete blood count may reveal iron deficiency anemia.
- Liver function study results may be elevated with metastatic spread of tumor to liver.
- Carcinoembryonic antigen radioimmunoassay result may be elevated.

IMAGING

- Barium X-rays of the GI tract with fluoroscopy show changes that suggest gastric cancer, including a tumor or filling defect in the outline of the stomach, loss of flexibility and distensibility, and abnormal gastric mucosa with or without ulceration.

DIAGNOSTIC PROCEDURES

- Gastroscopy with fiber-optic endoscope helps rule out other diffuse gastric mucosal abnormalities by allowing direct visualization.
- Gastroscopic biopsy permits evaluation of gastric mucosal lesions.

OTHER

- Gastric acid stimulation test discloses whether the stomach secretes acid properly.

GENERAL
- Radiation therapy combined with chemotherapy (not indicated preoperatively because it may damage viscera and impede healing)

DIET
- Based on the extent of the disorder and the patient's condition
- Parenteral feeding, if patient can't consume adequate calories

MEDICATIONS
- Chemotherapy
- Antiemetics
- Sedatives and tranquilizers
- Opioid analgesics

SURGERY
- Excision of lesion with appropriate margins (in more than one-third of patients)
- Gastroduodenostomy
- Gastrojejunostomy
- Partial gastric resection
- Total gastrectomy (with metastasis, omentum and spleen may have to be removed)

NURSING DIAGNOSES
- Acute pain
- Anxiety
- Diarrhea
- Fatigue
- Fear
- Imbalanced nutrition: Less than body requirements
- Impaired gas exchange
- Impaired oral mucous membrane
- Impaired skin integrity
- Impaired swallowing
- Risk for aspiration

EXPECTED OUTCOMES
The patient will:
- report feelings of pain relief
- express feelings of decreased anxiety
- return to a normal elimination pattern
- express feelings of increased energy
- verbalize feelings and concerns about his diagnosis and condition
- maintain weight within an acceptable range
- maintain adequate ventilation
- maintain intact oral mucous membranes
- maintain skin integrity
- be able to swallow without coughing or choking
- not aspirate.

NURSING INTERVENTIONS
- Provide a high-protein, high-calorie diet with dietary supplements.
- Give prescribed drugs.
- Provide parenteral nutrition as appropriate.
- After surgery, provide supportive care.

MONITORING
- Pain control
- Vital signs
- Hydration and nutritional status
- Nasogastric tube function and drainage
- Wound site
- Postoperative complications
- Effects of medication

GENERAL
Be sure to cover (with the patient or his family):
- the disorder, diagnosis, and treatment
- the dietary plan
- effective pulmonary toileting
- avoidance of crowds and people with known infection
- relaxation techniques
- all drugs, including administration, dosage, and possible adverse effects.

DISCHARGE PLANNING
- Direct the patient and his family to support services.
- Refer the patient for home services as necessary.
- Refer the patient for physical or occupational therapy as necessary.
- Refer the patient to hospice and supportive services.

RESOURCES
Organizations
American Cancer Society: *www.cancer.org*
Guide to Internet Resources for Cancer: *www.cancerindex.org*
National Cancer Institute: *www.cancer.gov*
National Institute of Diabetes & Digestive & Kidney Diseases: *www.niddk.nih.gov*

Selected references
Ajani, J.A. "Evolving Chemotherapy for Advanced Gastric Cancer," *The Oncologist* 10 (Suppl 3):49-58, 2005.
Atlas of Pathophysiology, 2nd ed. Philadelphia: Lippincott Williams & Wilkins, 2005.
Leong, T. "Chemotherapy and Radiotherapy in the Management of Gastric Cancer," *Current Opinion in Gastroenterology* 21(6):673-78, November 2005.

Gastritis

- Inflammation of the gastric mucosa
- May be acute or chronic
- Most common stomach disorder (acute)

PATHOPHYSIOLOGY
Acute gastritis
- The protective mucosal layer is altered.
- Acid secretion produces mucosal reddening, edema, and superficial surface erosion.

Chronic gastritis
- Gastric mucosa progressively thins and degenerates.

CAUSES
Acute gastritis
- Chronic ingestion of irritating foods and alcohol
- Complication of acute illness
- Drugs such as aspirin and other non-steroidal anti-inflammatory agents (in large doses), cytotoxic agents, caffeine, corticosteroids, antimetabolites, and indomethacin
- Endotoxins released from infecting bacteria, such as staphylococci, *Escherichia coli,* and salmonella
- Ingested poisons, especially dichloro-diphenyl-trichloroethane, ammonia, mercury, carbon tetrachloride, or corrosive substances

Chronic gastritis
- *Helicobacter pylori* infection (common cause of nonerosive gastritis)
- Pernicious anemia, renal disease, or diabetes mellitus
- Recurring exposure to irritating substances, such as drugs, alcohol, cigarette smoke, and environmental agents

RISK FACTORS
- Patient older than age 60
- Exposure to toxic substances
- Hemodynamic disorder

INCIDENCE
- Gastritis may occur at any age, although incidence of *H. pylori* increases in people older than 60.
- Gastritis occurs equally in men and women.
- Acute gastritis occurs in 8 of 1,000 people; chronic gastritis, in 2 of 10,000 people.

COMPLICATIONS
- Hemorrhage
- Obstruction
- Perforation
- Peritonitis
- Gastric cancer

HISTORY
- One or more causative agents revealed by patient
- Rapid onset of symptoms (acute gastritis)
- Epigastric discomfort
- Indigestion
- Cramping
- Anorexia
- Nausea, hematemesis, and vomiting
- Coffee-ground emesis or melena if GI bleeding is present

PHYSICAL FINDINGS
- Possible normal appearance
- Grimacing
- Restlessness
- Pallor
- Tachycardia
- Hypotension
- Abdominal distention, tenderness, and guarding
- Normoactive to hyperactive bowel sounds

LABORATORY
- Occult blood found in vomitus or stools (or both) indicates gastric bleeding.
- Hemoglobin (Hb) level and hematocrit are decreased.
- Urea breath test shows *H. pylori.*

DIAGNOSTIC PROCEDURES
- Upper GI endoscopy reveals gastritis when it's performed within 24 hours of bleeding.
- Biopsy reveals inflammatory process.

TREATMENT

GENERAL
- Elimination of cause
- For massive bleeding:
- Blood transfusion
- Iced saline lavage
- Angiography with vasopressin

DIET
- Nothing by mouth if bleeding occurs
- Elimination of irritating foods

ACTIVITY
- As tolerated (encourage mobilization)

MEDICATIONS
- Histamine antagonists
- Antacids
- Proton pump inhibitors
- Prostaglandins
- Vitamin B_{12}
- Dual therapy — antibiotic and proton pump inhibitor
- Triple therapy — two antibiotics and bismuth subsalicylate

SURGERY
- When conservative treatment fails
- Vagotomy, pyloroplasty
- Partial or total gastrectomy (rarely)

NURSING CONSIDERATIONS

NURSING DIAGNOSES
- Acute pain
- Imbalanced nutrition: Less than body requirements
- Ineffective coping
- Risk for deficient fluid volume

EXPECTED OUTCOMES
The patient will:
- express feelings of increased comfort
- maintain weight
- express concerns about current condition
- maintain normal fluid volume.

NURSING INTERVENTIONS
- Provide physical and emotional support.
- Give prescribed drugs and I.V. fluids.
- Assist the patient with diet modification.
- If surgery is necessary, prepare the patient preoperatively and provide appropriate postoperative care.
- Consult a dietitian as necessary.

MONITORING
- Vital signs
- Fluid intake and output
- Electrolyte and Hb levels
- Returning symptoms as food is reintroduced
- Response to medication
- Pain control

PATIENT TEACHING

GENERAL
Be sure to cover:
- the disorder, diagnosis, and treatment
- lifestyle and diet modifications
- preoperative teaching if surgery is necessary
- stress reduction techniques
- drug administration and possible adverse effects.

DISCHARGE PLANNING
- Refer the patient to a smoking-cessation program if indicated.

RESOURCES
Organizations
The National Digestive Diseases Information Clearinghouse: *www.niddk.nih.gov/health/digest/nddic.htm*

Selected references
Handbook of Diseases, 3rd ed. Philadelphia: Lippincott Williams & Wilkins, 2004.
Krumberger, J.M. "How to Manage an Acute Upper GI Bleed," *RN* 68(3):34-39, March 2005.
Rugge, M, and Genta, R.M. "Staging Gastritis: An International Proposal," *Gastroenterology* 129(5):1807-808, November 2005.
Yamada, T., et al. *Atlas of Gastroenterology,* 3rd ed. Philadelphia: Lippincott Williams & Wilkins, 2003.

Gastroenteritis

OVERVIEW

- Self-limiting inflammation of the stomach and small intestine
- Intestinal flu, traveler's diarrhea, viral enteritis, and food poisoning

PATHOPHYSIOLOGY

- The bowel reacts to the various causes of gastroenteritis with increased luminal fluid that can't be absorbed.
- This results in abdominal pain, vomiting, severe diarrhea (primarily), and secondary depletion of intracellular fluid.
- Dehydration and electrolyte loss occur.

CAUSES

- Amebae, especially *Entamoeba histolytica*
- Bacteria, such as *Staphylococcus aureus, Salmonella, Shigella, Clostridium botulinum, Clostridium perfringens,* and *Escherichia coli*
- Drug reactions from antibiotics
- Enzyme deficiencies
- Food allergens
- Ingestion of toxins, such as poisonous plants and toadstools
- Parasites, such as *Ascaris, Enterobius,* and *Trichinella spiralis*
- Viruses, such as adenoviruses, echoviruses, and coxsackieviruses

INCIDENCE

- Gastroenteritis occurs at any age.
- This disorder is the major cause of morbidity and mortality in underdeveloped nations.
- Gastroenteritis ranks second to common cold as cause of lost work time in the United States.
- Gastroenteritis is the fifth most common cause of death among young children.
- The disorder can be life-threatening in elderly and debilitated patients.

COMPLICATIONS

- Severe dehydration
- Electrolyte imbalance

ASSESSMENT

HISTORY

- Acute onset of diarrhea
- Abdominal pain and discomfort
- Nausea, vomiting
- Malaise and fatigue
- Exposure to contaminated food
- Recent travel (see *Preventing traveler's diarrhea*)

PHYSICAL FINDINGS

- Slight abdominal distention
- Poor skin turgor (with dehydration)
- Hyperactive bowel sounds
- Decreased blood pressure
- Nausea
- Vomiting
- Diarrhea

DIAGNOSTIC TEST RESULTS

LABORATORY

- Gram stain, stool culture (by direct rectal swab), or blood culture shows the causative bacteria.

Preventing traveler's diarrhea

If the patient travels, especially to developing nations, discuss precautions that he can take to reduce his chances of getting traveler's diarrhea. Explain that traveler's diarrhea is caused by inadequate sanitation and occurs after bacteria-contaminated food or water is ingested. These organisms attach to the lining of the small intestine, where they release a toxin that causes diarrhea and cramps. To minimize this risk, advise him to:

- drink water (or brush his teeth with water) only if it's chlorinated or bottled (Chlorination protects the water supply from bacterial contaminants such as *Escherichia coli.*)
- avoid beverages in glasses that may have been washed in contaminated water
- refuse ice cubes that may have been made from contaminated water
- drink only beverages made with boiled water, such as coffee and tea, or those in bottles or cans
- sanitize impure water by adding 2% tincture of iodine (5 drops/L of clear water, 10 drops/L of cloudy water) or by adding liquid laundry bleach (about 2 drops/L of clear water; 4 drops/L of cloudy water)
- avoid uncooked vegetables, unpeeled fresh fruits, salads, unpasteurized milk, and other dairy products
- beware of foods from street vendors.

If traveler's diarrhea occurs despite precautions, bismuth subsalicylate (Pepto-Bismol), diphenoxylate with atropine (Lomotil), or loperamide (Imodium) can be used to relieve symptoms.

TREATMENT

GENERAL
- Supportive treatment for nausea, vomiting, and diarrhea

DIET
- Rehydration
- Initially, clear liquids as tolerated
- Electrolyte solutions
- Avoidance of milk products

ACTIVITY
- As tolerated (encourage mobilization)

MEDICATIONS
- Antidiarrheal therapy
- Antiemetics
- Antibiotics
- I.V. fluids

NURSING CONSIDERATIONS

NURSING DIAGNOSES
- Acute pain
- Diarrhea
- Imbalanced nutrition: Less than body requirements
- Risk for deficient fluid volume

EXPECTED OUTCOMES
The patient will:
- express feelings of increased comfort
- return to a normal elimination pattern
- maintain weight without further loss
- maintain adequate fluid volume.

NURSING INTERVENTIONS
- Allow uninterrupted rest periods.
- Replace lost fluids and electrolytes through diet or I.V. fluids.
- Give prescribed drugs.

MONITORING
- Intake and output
- Vital signs
- Signs of dehydration
- Electrolytes

PATIENT TEACHING

GENERAL
Be sure to cover:
- the disorder, diagnosis, and treatment
- dietary modifications
- all prescribed drugs, including administration and possible adverse effects
- preventive measures
- how to perform warm sitz baths three times per day to relieve anal irritation.

RESOURCES
Organizations
The National Digestive Diseases Information Clearinghouse: *www.niddk.nih.gov/health/digest/nddic.htm*

Selected references
Handbook of Diseases, 3rd ed. Philadelphia: Lippincott Williams & Wilkins, 2004.

Jones, S. "A Clinical Pathway for Pediatric Gastroenteritis," *Gastroenterology Nursing* 26(1):7-18, January-February 2003.

Neville, K.A., et al. "High Antidiuretic Hormone Levels and Hyponatremia in Children with Gastroenteritis," *Pediatrics* 116(6):1401-407, December 2005.

Winter, G. "Gut Reaction," *Nursing Standard* 20(11):26-27, November 2005.

Yamada, T., et al. *Atlas of Gastroenterology,* 3rd ed. Philadelphia: Lippincott Williams & Wilkins, 2003.

Gastroesophageal reflux disease

- Backflow of gastric or duodenal contents, or both, into the esophagus and past the lower esophageal sphincter (LES), without associated belching or vomiting
- Reflux of gastric acid, causing acute epigastric pain, usually after a meal
- Popularly called heartburn
- Also called *GERD*

PATHOPHYSIOLOGY
- Reflux occurs when LES pressure is deficient or pressure in the stomach exceeds LES pressure. The LES relaxes, and gastric contents regurgitate into the esophagus.
- The degree of mucosal injury is based on the amount and concentration of refluxed gastric acid, proteolytic enzymes, and bile acids.

CAUSES
- Any condition or position that increases intra-abdominal pressure
- Hiatal hernia with incompetent sphincter
- Pyloric surgery (alteration or removal of the pylorus), which allows reflux of bile or pancreatic juice

RISK FACTORS
- Any agent that lowers LES pressure: acidic and fatty food, alcohol, cigarettes, anticholinergics (atropine, belladonna, propantheline) or other drugs (morphine, diazepam, calcium channel blockers, meperidine)
- Nasogastric (NG) intubation for more than 4 days

INCIDENCE
- GERD affects about 7 million U.S. residents.
- GERD affects all ethnic groups and socioeconomic classes.
- GERD is most common in people ages 45 to 64.

COMPLICATIONS
- Reflux esophagitis
- Esophageal stricture
- Esophageal ulcer
- Barrett's esophagus (metaplasia and possible increased risk of neoplasm)
- Anemia from esophageal bleeding
- Reflux aspiration leading to chronic pulmonary disease

HISTORY
- Minimal or no symptoms in one-third of patients
- Heartburn typically occurring 1½ to 2 hours after eating
- Heartburn worsening with vigorous exercise, bending, lying down, wearing tight clothing, coughing, constipation, and obesity
- Reported relief by using antacids or sitting upright
- Regurgitation without nausea or belching
- Feeling of fluid accumulation in the throat without a sour or bitter taste
- Chronic pain radiating to the neck, jaws, and arms that may mimic angina pectoris
- Nocturnal hypersalivation and wheezing
- Chronic cough

PHYSICAL FINDINGS
- Odynophagia (sharp substernal pain on swallowing), possibly followed by a dull substernal ache
- Bright red or dark brown blood in vomitus
- Laryngitis and morning hoarseness
- Chronic cough

IMAGING
- Barium swallow with fluoroscopy shows evidence of recurrent reflux.

DIAGNOSTIC PROCEDURES
- Esophageal acidity test reveals degree of gastroesophageal reflux.
- Gastroesophageal scintillation testing shows reflux.
- Esophageal manometry reveals abnormal LES pressure and sphincter incompetence.
- Acid perfusion (Bernstein) test result confirms esophagitis.
- Esophagoscopy and biopsy results confirm pathologic changes in the mucosa.

TREATMENT

GENERAL
- Modification of lifestyle
- Positional therapy
- Removal of cause
- Weight reduction, if appropriate

DIET
- Avoidance of acidic or fatty foods
- Avoidance of eating 2 hours before sleep (see *Factors affecting LES pressure*)
- Parenteral nutrition or tube feedings

ACTIVITY
- No restrictions for medical treatment
- Lifting restrictions for surgical treatment

MEDICATIONS
- Antacids
- Cholinergics
- Histamine-2 receptor antagonists
- Proton pump inhibitors

SURGERY
- Hiatal hernia repair
- Vagotomy or pyloroplasty
- Esophagectomy

NURSING CONSIDERATIONS

NURSING DIAGNOSES
- Acute pain
- Anxiety
- Imbalanced nutrition: Less than body requirements
- Risk for aspiration

EXPECTED OUTCOMES
The patient will:
- express feelings of increased comfort
- identify strategies to reduce anxiety
- achieve adequate caloric and nutritional intake
- not aspirate.

NURSING INTERVENTIONS
- Offer emotional and psychological support.
- Assist with diet modification.
- Perform chest physiotherapy.
- Use semi-Fowler's position for the patient with an NG tube.

MONITORING
After surgery
- Respiratory status
- Pain control
- Intake and output
- Vital signs
- Chest tube drainage
- Bowel function

PATIENT TEACHING

GENERAL
Be sure to cover:
- the disorder, diagnosis, and treatment
- causes of gastroesophageal reflux
- prescribed antireflux regimen of medication, diet, and positional therapy
- developing a dietary plan
- the need to identify situations or activities that increase intra-abdominal pressure
- the need to refrain from using substances that reduce sphincter control
- signs and symptoms to watch for and report.

RESOURCES
Organizations
American Gastroenterological Association: *www.gastro.org*
The National Digestive Diseases Information Clearinghouse: *www.niddk.nih. gov/health/digest/nddic.htm*
Pediatric/Adolescent Gastroesophageal Reflux Association, Inc.: *www.reflux.org*

Selected references
Chen, Y.K. "Endoscopic Approaches to the Treatment of Gastroesophageal Reflux Disease," *Current Opinion in Internal Medicine* 4(6):643-48, December 2005.
Handbook of Diseases, 3rd ed. Philadelphia: Lippincott Williams & Wilkins, 2004.
Henry, S.M. "Discerning Differences: Gastroesophageal Reflux and Gastroesophageal Reflux Disease in Infants," *Advances in Neonatal Care* 4(4):235-47, August 2004.
Simpson, T., and Ivey, J. "Pediatric Management Problems. GERD." *Pediatric Nursing* 31(3):214-15, May-June 2005.
Yamada, T., et al. *Atlas of Gastroenterology,* 3rd ed. Philadelphia: Lippincott Williams & Wilkins, 2003.

Factors affecting LES pressure

Various dietary and lifestyle elements can increase or decrease lower esophageal sphincter (LES) pressure. Consider these as you plan the patient's treatment program.

WHAT INCREASES LES PRESSURE
- Protein
- Carbohydrates
- Nonfat milk
- Low-dose ethanol

WHAT DECREASES LES PRESSURE
- Fat
- Whole milk
- Orange juice
- Tomatoes
- Antiflatulent (simethicone)
- Chocolate
- High-dose ethanol
- Cigarette smoking
- Lying on right or left side
- Sitting

Generalized anxiety disorder

OVERVIEW

- Feeling of apprehension sometimes described as an exaggerated feeling of impending doom, dread, or uneasiness
- Reaction to an internal threat
- Uncontrollable, unreasonable worry that persists for at least 6 months and narrows perceptions or interferes with normal functioning

PATHOPHYSIOLOGY

- Few physiologic data
- Aberration in benzodiazepine receptor regulation

CAUSES

- Conflict

INCIDENCE

- Generalized anxiety disorder can begin at any age but typically begins between ages 20 and 40.
- The disorder is equally common in men and women.

COMPLICATIONS

- Impaired social or occupational functioning
- Substance abuse

ASSESSMENT

HISTORY

- Muscle aches and spasms
- Headaches
- Inability to relax
- Apprehension
- Fear
- Anger
- Difficulty concentrating, eating, and sleeping

PHYSICAL FINDINGS

- Trembling
- Shortness of breath
- Tachycardia
- Sweating

DSM-IV-TR *criteria*

Diagnosis is confirmed when the patient's symptoms match the following criteria:

- Excessive anxiety and worry about a number of events or activities occur more days than not for at least 6 months.
- The person finds it difficult to control the worry.
- The anxiety and worry are associated with at least three of the following six symptoms:
- restlessness or feeling keyed up or on edge
- being easily fatigued
- difficulty concentrating or mind going blank
- irritability
- muscle tension
- sleep disturbances (difficulty falling or staying asleep, or restless, unsatisfying sleep).
- The focus of the anxiety and worry isn't confined to features of an axis disorder.
- The anxiety, worry, or physical symptoms cause clinically significant distress or impairment in social, occupational, or other important areas of functioning.

- The disturbance isn't due to the direct physiologic effects of a substance or a general medical condition and doesn't occur exclusively during a mood disorder, a psychotic disorder, or a pervasive, developmental disorder.

DIAGNOSTIC TEST RESULTS

LABORATORY

- Tests, such as cardiac enzymes, troponin level, and thyroid studies, rule out organic causes of symptoms.

DIAGNOSTIC PROCEDURES

- Electrocardiography excludes myocardial ischemia.

OTHER

- Psychiatric evaluation confirms diagnosis.

TREATMENT

GENERAL
- Psychotherapy
- Relaxation techniques
- Stress management

MEDICATIONS
- Benzodiazepines
- Tricyclic antidepressants
- Selective serotonin reuptake inhibitors

NURSING CONSIDERATIONS

NURSING DIAGNOSES
- Anxiety
- Chronic low self-esteem
- Decisional conflict (excessive worry)
- Impaired social interaction
- Ineffective coping
- Social isolation

EXPECTED OUTCOMES
The patient will:
- experience reduced anxiety by identifying internal precipitating situation
- express positive feelings about self
- maintain autonomy and independence without handicapping fears and use of phobic behavior
- demonstrate effective social interaction skills
- develop effective coping mechanisms
- maintain family and peer relationships.

NURSING INTERVENTIONS
- Give prescribed drugs.
- Reduce environmental stimuli.
- Help identify triggers to anxiety.
- Provide emotional support.

MONITORING
- Response to therapy

PATIENT TEACHING

GENERAL
Be sure to cover:
- prescribed drugs
- relaxation techniques
- effective coping strategies
- stress management techniques.

DISCHARGE PLANNING
- Refer the patient for psychological counseling.

RESOURCES
Organizations
Anxiety Disorders Association of America: *www.adaa.org*
National Mental Health Association: *www.nmha.org*

Selected references
Cottraux, J. "Recent Developments in the Research on Generalized Anxiety Disorder," *Current Opinion in Psychiatry* 17(1):49-52, January 2004.
Diseases, 4th ed. Philadelphia: Lippincott Williams & Wilkins, 2006.
Masi, G., et al. "Generalized Anxiety Disorder in Referred Children and Adolescents," *Journal of the American Academy of Child & Adolescent Psychiatry* 43(6):752-60, June 2004.
Mathew, S.J., et al. "Open-label Trial of Riluzole in Generalized Anxiety Disorder," *American Journal of Psychiatry* 162(12):2379-381, December 2005.

Genital herpes

OVERVIEW

- Acute inflammatory disease of the genitalia
- Usually self-limiting but may cause painful local or systemic disease (see *Understanding the herpes cycle*)

PATHOPHYSIOLOGY
- Virus invades and replicates in neurons and epidermal and dermal cells.
- Virions travel to sensory dorsal root ganglion.
- Replication in the sensory ganglia leads to recurrent clinical outbreaks.

CAUSES
- Herpes simplex virus (HSV), type 1 or type 2
- Typically transmitted through sexual intercourse, orogenital sexual activity, kissing, hand-to-body contact, and vaginal delivery

INCIDENCE
- One in five adults is serologically positive for HSV infection in the United States.

COMPLICATIONS
- Herpetic keratitis, which may lead to blindness
- Herpetic encephalitis

ASSESSMENT

HISTORY
- Intimate contact with an infected person
- Fever
- Malaise
- Dysuria
- Leukorrhea (females)

PHYSICAL FINDINGS
- Shallow, reddened, painful ulcers with yellow, oozing centers usually on the cervix (the primary infection site) and possibly on the labia, perianal skin, vulva, or vagina of the female and on the glans penis, foreskin, or penile shaft of the male
- Extragenital lesions, possibly on the mouth or anus
- Marked edema
- Tender inguinal lymph nodes

DIAGNOSTIC TEST RESULTS

LABORATORY
- Vesicular fluid reveals HSV.
- Antigen testing identifies specific antigens.

OTHER
- Physical examination and patient history help to confirm the diagnosis.

Understanding the herpes cycle

After a patient is infected with herpes, a latency period follows. The virus takes up permanent residence in the nerve cells surrounding the lesions, and intermittent viral shedding may take place.

Repeated outbreaks may develop at any time, again followed by a latent stage during which the lesions heal completely. Outbreaks may recur as often as three to eight times yearly.

Although the cycle continues indefinitely, some people remain symptom-free for years.

INITIAL INFECTION
Highly infectious period marked by fever, aches, adenopathy, pain, and ulcerated skin and mucous membranes

↓

LATENCY
Intermittently infectious period marked by viral dormancy or viral shedding and no disease symptoms

RECURRENT INFECTION
Highly infectious period similar to initial infection with milder symptoms that resolve faster

---

TREATMENT

GENERAL
◆ Standard precautions

ACTIVITY
◆ Adequate rest periods

MEDICATIONS
◆ Acyclovir (Zovirax)
◆ Famciclovir (Famvir)
◆ Valacyclovir (Valtrex)

NURSING CONSIDERATIONS

NURSING DIAGNOSES
◆ Acute pain
◆ Impaired oral mucous membranes
◆ Impaired skin integrity
◆ Impaired social interaction
◆ Ineffective sexuality patterns
◆ Powerlessness
◆ Risk for infection
◆ Risk for injury
◆ Social isolation

EXPECTED OUTCOMES
The patient will:
◆ report feelings of increased comfort and relief from pain
◆ remain free from complications related to trauma to oral mucous membranes
◆ exhibit improved or healed lesions or wounds
◆ resume effective communication patterns with spouse or partner
◆ voice feelings about potential or actual changes in sexuality
◆ verbalize feelings of control and hope regarding his medical condition
◆ experience no further signs or symptoms of infection
◆ remain free from complications
◆ maintain relationships with family and friends.

NURSING INTERVENTIONS
◆ Encourage expression of feelings and concerns.
◆ Keep lesions dry.
◆ Follow standard precautions.

MONITORING
◆ Response to treatment
◆ Skin integrity
◆ Wound healing

PATIENT TEACHING

GENERAL
Be sure to cover:
◆ avoiding sexual intercourse during the active stage of this disease (while lesions are present)
◆ using condoms during all sexual encounters
◆ urging sexual partners to seek medical examination
◆ having a Papanicolaou test every 6 months (females).

DISCHARGE PLANNING
◆ Refer the patient to the Herpes Resource Center for support.

RESOURCES
Organizations
American Social Health Association: *www.ashastd.org*
Centers for Disease Control and Prevention: *www.cdc.gov*
National Health Information Center: *www.health.gov/nhic*
National Institute of Allergy and Infectious Diseases: *www.niaid.nih.gov*
National Library of Medicine: *www.nlm.nih.gov*

Selected references
Brown, Z.A., et al. "Genital Herpes Complicating Pregnancy," *Obstetrics & Gynecology* 106(4):845-56, October 2005.
Nettina, S.M. *Lippincott Manual of Nursing Practice,* 8th ed. Philadelphia: Lippincott Williams & Wilkins, 2006.
Perfect, M.M., et al. "Use of Complementary and Alternative Medicine for the Treatment of Genital Herpes," *Herpes* 12(2):38-41, October 2005.
Roe, V.A. "Living with Genital Herpes: How Effective is Antiviral Therapy?" *Journal of Perinatal & Neonatal Nursing* 18(3):206-15, July-September 2004.

Genital warts

- Papillomas that consist of fibrous tissue overgrowth from the dermis and thickened epithelial coverings
- Also known as *venereal warts* and *condylomata acuminata*

PATHOPHYSIOLOGY

- Infection is transmitted by sexual contact and incubates for 1 to 6 months (2 months, average) before warts erupt.
- Infection of the basal cells occurs, with proliferation of all epidermal layers, producing acanthosis, parakeratosis, and hyperkeratosis.

CAUSES

- Infection with one of more than 60 known strains of human papillomavirus
- Possibly receptive anal intercourse

INCIDENCE

- Genital warts is one of the most common sexually transmitted diseases (STDs) in the United States.

COMPLICATIONS

- During pregnancy, genital warts in the vaginal and cervical walls that grow large enough to impede vaginal delivery
- Genital tract dysplasia
- Cervical and vulvar cancer in women, penile cancer in men, and some rectal carcinomas in both genders

HISTORY

- Unprotected sexual contact with a new partner, with many partners, or with a partner with a known infection

PHYSICAL FINDINGS

- Warts on moist genital surfaces (subpreputial sac, urethral meatus, penile shaft, scrotum, vulva, vaginal and cervical walls)
- Red or pink, possibly pedunculated swellings that may be tiny or may grow as large as 10 cm (see *Recognizing genital warts*)
- Infected lesions that become malodorous

LABORATORY

- Dark-field microscopy of wart cell scrapings shows marked epidermal cell vascularization.
- Application of 5% acetic acid (white vinegar) turns warts white if they're papillomas.

Recognizing genital warts

Genital warts are marked by clusters of flesh-colored papillary growths that may be barely visible or several inches in diameter.

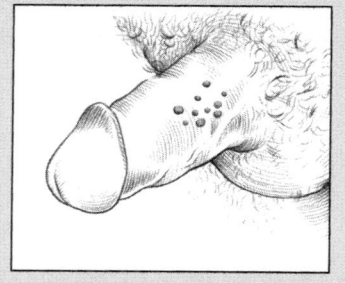

GENERAL
◆ Circumcision, which may prevent recurrence

MEDICATIONS
◆ Topical antimetabolites
◆ Topical podophyllum resin
◆ Topical interferon
◆ Vaccine preparations

SURGERY
◆ Cryosurgery
◆ Electrodesiccation
◆ Surgical excision
◆ Laser ablation

NURSING DIAGNOSES
◆ Acute pain
◆ Disturbed body image
◆ Impaired skin integrity
◆ Ineffective coping
◆ Ineffective sexuality patterns
◆ Risk for infection
◆ Risk for injury

EXPECTED OUTCOMES
The patient will:
◆ express feelings of increased comfort and decreased pain
◆ acknowledge the change in body image
◆ exhibit improved or healed lesions or wounds
◆ resume effective communication patterns with spouse or partner
◆ voice feelings about potential or actual changes in sexuality
◆ experience no further signs or symptoms of infection
◆ remain free from complications.

NURSING INTERVENTIONS
◆ Use standard precautions.
◆ Provide a nonthreatening, nonjudgmental atmosphere that encourages verbalization, and provide support.
◆ Remove podophyllum resin with soap and water 4 to 6 hours after applying it to warts.

MONITORING
◆ Response to treatment
◆ Adverse effects of medication
◆ Signs and symptoms of infection (postoperative)
◆ Concomitant STDs or infections
◆ Papanicolaou (Pap) test results

GENERAL
Be sure to cover:
◆ the disorder, diagnosis, and treatment
◆ the need for sexual abstinence or condom use during intercourse until healing is complete
◆ evaluation of the patient's sexual partners
◆ the importance of testing for human immunodeficiency virus infection and other STDs
◆ the emphasis that genital warts can recur and that the virus can mutate, causing infection with warts of a different strain
◆ recommendation that female patients have a Pap test every 6 months.

RESOURCES
Organizations
Centers for Disease Control and Prevention: *www.cdc.gov*
Harvard University Consumer Health Information: *www.intelihealth.com*
National Health Information Center: *www.health.gov/nhic*
National Institute of Allergy and Infectious Diseases: *www.niaid.nih.gov*
National Library of Medicine: *www.nlm.nih.gov*

Selected references
Kahn, J.A., and Bernstein, D.I. "Human Papillomavirus Vaccines and Adolescents," *Current Opinion in Obstetrics & Gynecology* 17(5):476-82, October 2005.
Kasper, D.L., et al., eds. *Harrison's Principles of Internal Medicine,* 16th ed. New York: McGraw-Hill Book Co., 2005.
O'Mahony, C. "Genital Warts: Current and Future Management Options," *American Journal of Clinical Dermatology* 6(4):239-43, 2005.

Giardiasis

- Infection of the small bowel by *Giardia lamblia,* a symmetrical flagellate protozoan
- Reinfection possible because infection doesn't confer immunity
- Also called *lambliasis* and *giardia enteritis infection*

PATHOPHYSIOLOGY

- Cysts enter the small bowel and release trophozoites, which attach to the bowel's epithelial surface.
- Attachment causes superficial mucosal invasion and destruction, inflammation, and irritation.
- Trophozoites become encysted again, travel down the colon, and are excreted. (Unformed stools may contain trophozoites as well as cysts.)

CAUSES

- Ingestion of *G. lamblia* cysts in stool-contaminated water
- Oral-anal transfer of cysts from an infected person

INCIDENCE

- Giardiasis occurs worldwide but is most common in developing countries and other areas where sanitation and hygiene are poor. (*G. lamblia* has been found in municipal water sources, nursing homes, and day care centers.)
- Children are generally more likely to develop giardiasis than adults.
- In the United States, the disease is most common in travelers who have recently returned from endemic areas, campers who drink water from contaminated streams, male homosexuals, patients with congenital immunoglobulin A deficiency, and children in day care centers.

COMPLICATIONS

- Malabsorption
- Dehydration
- Lactose intolerance
- Death, in hypogammaglobulinemia

HISTORY

- Recent travel to an area with poor sanitation
- Sexual practices that involve oral-anal contact
- Drinking of suspect water
- Institutionalization

PHYSICAL FINDINGS

- Possibly, no intestinal symptoms in mild infection
- Abdominal cramps, bloating
- Belching, flatus
- Nausea, vomiting
- Explosive pale, loose, greasy, malodorous, frequent stools (occurring 2 to 10 times daily)
- Fatigue, weight loss
- Hyperactive bowel sounds in the right upper and left lower quadrants just before bowel movements
- General upper and right lower quadrant discomfort and guarding

LABORATORY

- Examination of a fresh stool specimen shows cysts or examination of duodenal aspirate or biopsy shows trophozoites.

GENERAL
- Examination of people who have had sexual contact with or live with an infected person, for possible testing and treatment
- Parenteral fluid replacement to prevent dehydration

MEDICATIONS
- Metronidazole (Flagyl)

NURSING DIAGNOSES
- Acute pain
- Deficient fluid volume
- Diarrhea
- Fatigue
- Imbalanced nutrition: Less than body requirements
- Impaired skin integrity
- Risk for infection

EXPECTED OUTCOMES
The patient will:
- express feelings of increased comfort and relief from pain
- maintain normal electrolyte levels
- have an elimination pattern that returns to normal
- report an increased energy level
- experience no further weight loss
- avoid skin breakdown
- experience no further signs or symptoms of infection.

NURSING INTERVENTIONS
- Institute enteric precautions, and quickly dispose of all fecal material.
- Place a child or incontinent adult in a private room.
- Keep the perianal area clean, especially after each bowel movement.
- Administer I.V. fluid therapy, as needed.
- Provide nutritionally adequate foods.
- Give prescribed drugs.
- Report epidemic situations to public health authorities.

MONITORING
- Frequency and characteristics of bowel movements
- Nutritional intake (to prevent malnutrition)
- Adverse drug effects
- Skin integrity
- Signs and symptoms of dehydration

GENERAL
Be sure to cover:
- prescribed drugs, including precautions and adverse effects
- need for a patient taking metronidazole to avoid alcohol while taking the drug and for 3 days after completing treatment
- need for the family and others in contact with the patient to have their stools tested for *G. lamblia* cysts
- need for good personal hygiene, especially proper hand washing as well as correct handling of infectious material by the patient and his family
- importance of safer sex practices
- need for campers to purify all stream and lake water before drinking it
- need for travelers to endemic areas to avoid drinking tap or suspect water and to avoid eating uncooked and unpeeled fruits or vegetables.

DISCHARGE PLANNING
- Encourage the patient to return for follow-up appointments because relapses can occur.

RESOURCES
Organizations
Centers for Disease Control and Prevention: *www.cdc.gov*
Harvard University Consumer Health Information: *www.intelihealth.com*
National Health Information Center: *www.health.gov/nhici*
National Library of Medicine: *www.nlm.nih.gov*

Selected references
Dawson, D. "Foodborne Protozoan Parasites," *International Journal of Food Microbiology* 103(2):207-27, August 2005.
Diseases, 4th ed. Philadelphia: Lippincott Williams & Wilkins, 2006.
Kasper, D.L., et al., eds. *Harrison's Principles of Internal Medicine*, 16th ed. New York: McGraw-Hill Book Co., 2005.

Glaucoma

- Eye disorder characterized by high intraocular pressure (IOP) and optic nerve damage
- Two forms:
- Open-angle (also known as *chronic, simple,* or *wide-angle*) glaucoma, which begins insidiously and progresses slowly
- Angle-closure (also known as *acute* or *narrow-angle*) glaucoma, which occurs suddenly and can cause permanent vision loss in 48 to 72 hours

PATHOPHYSIOLOGY

Open-angle glaucoma

- Degenerative changes in the trabecular meshwork block the flow of aqueous humor from the eye, increasing IOP and resulting in optic nerve damage.

Angle-closure glaucoma

- Obstruction to the outflow of aqueous humor is caused by an anatomically narrow angle between the iris and the cornea.
- IOP increases suddenly.

CAUSES

Open-angle glaucoma

- Degenerative changes

Angle-closure glaucoma

- Anatomically narrow angle between the iris and the cornea
- Attacks triggered by trauma, pupillary dilation, stress, or ocular changes that push the iris forward

RISK FACTORS

Open-angle glaucoma

- Family history
- Myopia
- Ethnic origin

Angle-closure glaucoma

- Family history
- Cataracts
- Hyperopia

INCIDENCE

- Glaucoma is a leading cause of blindness, accounting for about 12% of newly diagnosed blindness in the United States.
- The highest incidence is in males and among Black and Asian populations.
- Incidence is highest in Blacks older than age 40 and in everyone, especially Mexican Americans, older than age 60.

COMPLICATIONS

- Varying degrees of vision loss
- Total blindness

HISTORY

Open-angle glaucoma

- Possibly no symptoms
- Dull, morning headache
- Mild aching in the eyes
- Loss of peripheral vision
- Halos around lights
- Reduced visual acuity (especially at night) not corrected by glasses

Angle-closure glaucoma

- Pain and pressure over the eye
- Blurred vision
- Decreased visual acuity
- Halos around lights
- Nausea and vomiting (from increased IOP)

PHYSICAL FINDINGS

- Unilateral eye inflammation
- Cloudy cornea
- Moderately dilated pupil, nonreactive to light
- With gentle fingertip pressure to the closed eyelids, one eye feels harder than the other (in angle-closure glaucoma)

DIAGNOSTIC PROCEDURES

- Tonometry measurement shows increased IOP.
- Slit-lamp examination shows effects of glaucoma on the anterior eye structures.
- Gonioscopy shows angle of the eye's anterior chamber.
- Ophthalmoscopy aids visualization of the fundus. (See *Optic disk changes.*)
- Perimetry or visual field tests show extent of peripheral vision loss.
- Fundus photography shows optic disk changes.

Optic disk changes

Ophthalmoscopy and slit-lamp examination show cupping of the optic disk, which is characteristic of glaucoma.

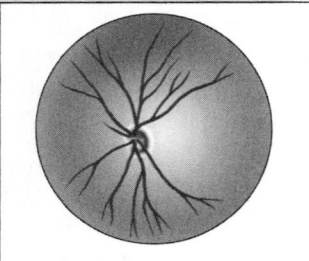

TREATMENT

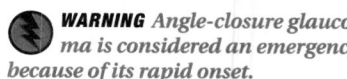 **WARNING** *Angle-closure glaucoma is considered an emergency because of its rapid onset.*

GENERAL
◆ Reduction of IOP by decreasing aqueous humor production with medications

ACTIVITY
◆ Bed rest (with acute angle-closure glaucoma)

MEDICATIONS
◆ Topical adrenergic agonists
◆ Cholinergic agonists
◆ Beta-adrenergic blockers
◆ Topical or oral carbonic anhydrase inhibitors

 WARNING *Occasionally, systemic absorption of a beta-adrenergic blocker from eyedrops may be enough to cause bradycardia, hypotension, heart block, bronchospasm, impotence, or depression.*

SURGERY
For glaucoma nonrefractive to drug therapy
◆ Argon laser trabeculoplasty
◆ Trabeculectomy

For angle-closure glaucoma
◆ Laser iridectomy
◆ Surgical peripheral iridectomy
◆ In end-stage glaucoma, tube shunt or valve

NURSING CONSIDERATIONS

NURSING DIAGNOSES
◆ Acute pain
◆ Anxiety
◆ Disturbed sensory perception: Visual
◆ Fear
◆ Risk for injury

EXPECTED OUTCOMES
The patient will:
◆ express feelings of increased comfort
◆ identify strategies to reduce anxiety
◆ regain normal visual functioning
◆ express fears and concerns
◆ avoid injury.

NURSING INTERVENTIONS
◆ Give prescribed drugs.
◆ Prepare for surgery, if indicated.
◆ After surgery, protect the affected eye.
◆ Encourage ambulation immediately after surgery.
◆ Encourage the patient to express his concerns related to the chronic condition.

MONITORING
◆ Vital signs
◆ Response to treatment
◆ Visual acuity

PATIENT TEACHING

GENERAL
Be sure to cover:
◆ the disorder, diagnosis, and treatment
◆ need for meticulous compliance with prescribed drug therapy
◆ all procedures and treatments, especially surgery
◆ the fact that lost vision can't be restored but treatment can usually prevent further loss
◆ modification of the patient's environment for safety
◆ signs and symptoms that require immediate medical attention, such as sudden vision change or eye pain
◆ the importance of glaucoma screening for early detection and prevention.

RESOURCES
Organizations
Glaucoma Research Foundation: *www.glaucoma.org*
Prevent Blindness America: *www.preventblindness.org*

Selected references
Grieshaber, M.C., and Flammer, J. "Blood Flow in Glaucoma," *Current Opinion in Ophthalmology* 16(2):79-83, April 2005.
Jonas, J.B., et al. "Central Corneal Thickness and Development of Glaucomatous Optic Disk Hemorrhages," *American Journal of Ophthalmology* 140(6):1139-141, December 2005.
Marquis, R.E., and Whitson, J.T. "Management of Glaucoma: Focus on Pharmacological Therapy," *Drugs & Aging* 22(1):1-21, 2005.

Glomerulonephritis

OVERVIEW

- Bilateral inflammation of the glomeruli, usually after a streptococcal infection
- Also called *acute poststreptococcal glomerulonephritis*

PATHOPHYSIOLOGY

- The epithelial or podocyte layer of the glomerular membrane is disturbed.
- Acute poststreptococcal glomerulonephritis results from antigen-antibody complexes becoming trapped and collecting in the glomerular capillary membranes, after infection with group A beta-hemolytic streptococcus.
- Antigens stimulate the formation of antibodies.
- Circulating antigen-antibody complexes become lodged in the glomerular capillaries.
- Complement activation is initiated and immunologic substances are released that lyse cells and increase membrane permeability.
- Antibody damage to basement membranes causes crescent formation.
- Antibody or antigen-antibody complexes in the glomerular capillary wall activate biochemical mediators of inflammation — complement, leukocytes, and fibrin.
- Lysosomal enzymes are released that damage the glomerular cell walls and cause a proliferation of the extracellular matrix, affecting glomerular blood flow.
- Membrane permeability increases and protein filtration is enhanced.
- Membrane damage leads to platelet aggregation, and platelet degranulation releases substances that increase glomerular permeability.

CAUSES

- Immunoglobulin A nephropathy (Berger's disease)
- Impetigo
- Lipoid nephrosis
- Streptococcal infection of the respiratory tract

Chronic glomerulonephritis

- Focal glomerulosclerosis
- Goodpasture's syndrome
- Hemolytic uremic syndrome
- Membranoproliferative glomerulonephritis
- Membranous glomerulopathy
- Poststreptococcal glomerulonephritis
- Rapidly progressive glomerulonephritis (RPGN)
- Systemic lupus erythematosus

INCIDENCE

- Acute glomerulonephritis is most common in boys ages 3 to 7, but it can occur at any age.
- RPGN most commonly occurs between ages 50 and 60.

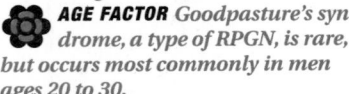 **AGE FACTOR** *Goodpasture's syndrome, a type of RPGN, is rare, but occurs most commonly in men ages 20 to 30.*

WARNING *A child with glomerulonephritis may initially experience encephalopathy with seizures and local neurologic deficits. An elderly patient with glomerulonephritis may report vague, nonspecific symptoms, such as nausea, malaise, and arthralgia.*

COMPLICATIONS

- Pulmonary edema
- Heart failure
- Sepsis
- Renal failure
- Severe hypertension
- Cardiac hypertrophy

ASSESSMENT

HISTORY

- Sudden onset of proteinuria
- Sudden onset of red blood cells (RBCs) and casts in urine
- Decreased urination
- Recent streptococcal infection of the respiratory tract

PHYSICAL FINDINGS

- Smoky or coffee-colored urine
- Dyspnea
- Periorbital edema
- Increased blood pressure

DIAGNOSTIC TEST RESULTS

LABORATORY

- Throat culture shows group A beta-hemolytic streptococcus.
- Electrolyte, blood urea nitrogen, and creatinine levels are increased.
- Serum protein level is decreased.
- Hemoglobin level (chronic glomerulonephritis) is decreased.
- Antistreptolysin-O titers are elevated.
- Streptozyme and anti-DNase B levels are elevated.
- Serum complement levels are abnormally low.
- Urinalysis shows RBCs, white blood cells, mixed cell casts, protein, fibrin-degradation products, and C3 protein.

IMAGING

- Kidney-ureter-bladder X-ray shows bilateral kidney enlargement (acute glomerulonephritis).
- X-ray reveals symmetrical contraction with normal pelves and calyces (chronic glomerulonephritis).

DIAGNOSTIC PROCEDURES

- Renal biopsy confirms diagnosis.

TREATMENT

GENERAL
- Treatment of the primary disease
- Correction of electrolyte imbalance
- Dialysis
- Plasmapheresis

DIET
- Fluid restriction
- Sodium restriction

ACTIVITY
- Bed rest

MEDICATIONS
- Antibiotics
- Anticoagulants
- Diuretics
- Vasodilators
- Corticosteroids

SURGERY
- Kidney transplant

NURSING CONSIDERATIONS

NURSING DIAGNOSES
- Acute pain
- Decreased cardiac output
- Excess fluid volume
- Fatigue
- Imbalanced nutrition: Less than body requirements
- Impaired physical mobility
- Ineffective health maintenance
- Ineffective role performance
- Risk for infection
- Risk for injury

EXPECTED OUTCOMES
The patient will:
- report increased comfort
- maintain hemodynamic stability
- maintain adequate fluid balance
- verbalize the importance of balancing activity with adequate rest periods
- verbalize appropriate food choices for his diet plan
- maintain joint mobility and muscle strength
- identify risk factors that exacerbate the condition, and modify lifestyle accordingly
- resume regular roles and responsibilities to the fullest extent possible
- remain free from signs or symptoms of infection
- avoid or minimize complications.

NURSING INTERVENTIONS
- Provide appropriate skin care and oral hygiene.
- Encourage the patient to express his feelings about the disorder.
- Give prescribed drugs.

MONITORING
- Vital signs
- Intake and output
- Daily weight
- Laboratory studies
- Signs of renal failure

PATIENT TEACHING

GENERAL
Be sure to cover:
- taking prescribed drugs
- how to assess ankle edema
- reporting signs of infection
- recording daily weight.

RESOURCES
Organizations
American Academy of Pediatrics: *www.aap.org*
American Association of Kidney Patients: *www.aakp.org*
Harvard University Consumer Health Information: *www.intelihealth.com*
National Institute of Diabetes & Digestive & Kidney Diseases: *www.niddk.nih.gov*

Selected references
Javaid, B., and Quigg, R.J. "Treatment of Glomerulonephritis: Will We Ever Have Options Other than Steroids and Cytotoxics?" *Kidney International* 67(5):1692-703, May 2005.
Nettina, S.M. *Lippincott Manual of Nursing Practice,* 8th ed. Philadelphia: Lippincott Williams & Wilkins, 2006.
Vinen, C.S., and Oliveira, D.B.G. "Acute Glomerulonephritis," *Postgraduate Medical Journal* 79(930):206-13, April 2003.

Goiter

- Thyroid gland enlargement not caused by inflammation or a neoplasm
- Commonly classified as toxic (associated with hyperthyroidism) or nontoxic (not associated with hyperthyroidism or hypothyroidism)

PATHOPHYSIOLOGY

- Thyroid gland can't produce enough thyroid hormone to meet metabolic requirements.
- Thyroid gland enlarges to compensate for inadequate hormone synthesis.

CAUSES

- Inadequate dietary intake of iodine
- Ingestion of large amounts of goitrogenic foods (such as rutabagas, cabbage, soybeans, peanuts, peaches, peas, strawberries, spinach, and radishes) or the use of goitrogenic drugs (such as propylthiouracil, methimazole, iodides, and lithium)
- Inherited defects
- Thyroid growth-stimulating immunoglobulins

INCIDENCE

- The incidence of goiter decreases with age.
- More women than men commonly have goiter.

COMPLICATIONS

- Tracheal compression
- Hyperthyroidism
- Lymphoma
- Abscess

ASSESSMENT

HISTORY

- Respiratory distress
- Dysphagia

PHYSICAL FINDINGS

- Swelling and distention of the neck, which may be mildly to massively enlarged (see *Understanding simple goiter*)

Understanding simple goiter

A simple (nontoxic) goiter is any enlargement of the thyroid gland not caused by inflammation or neoplasm. The thyroid mass increases to compensate for inadequate hormone synthesis. It's most common in females, occurring when thyroid hormone secretion fails to meet metabolic needs.

Sporadic goiter follows ingestion of goitrogenic drugs (such as propylthiouracil) and iodides or foods (such as rutabagas and cabbage). Endemic goiter results from geographically related nutritional factors such as iodine-depleted soil. Inherited defects may contribute to either type of goiter.

The patient may report respiratory distress and dysphagia from compression of the trachea and esophagus and dizziness or syncope when raising her arms over her head. A firm, irregular enlargement and stridor caused by tracheal compression may be found.

Diagnostic tests reveal normal serum thyroid hormone levels; abnormalities rule out this diagnosis. Thyroid antibody titers are usually normal. Iodine-131 uptake is usually normal but may increase with iodine deficiency or a biosynthetic defect. Urinalysis may show low urinary excretion of iodine.

Treatment to reduce thyroid hyperplasia involves thyroid hormone replacement. Iodide administration commonly relieves goiters caused by iodine deficiency. Sporadic goiter requires avoidance of goitrogenic drugs and food. Radioiodine ablation therapy aids some patients. Rarely, partial thyroidectomy is needed to relieve pressure on the surrounding structures.

DIAGNOSTIC TEST RESULTS

LABORATORY

- Thyroid-stimulating hormone level is high or normal.
- Serum thyroxine level is low-normal or normal.
- Iodine-131 uptake is normal or increased (50% of the dose at 24 hours).

OTHER

- Patient history and physical examination help to confirm the diagnosis.

TREATMENT

GENERAL
◆ Avoidance of known goitrogenic drugs and foods

MEDICATIONS
◆ Thyroid hormone replacement
◆ Small doses of iodine

SURGERY
◆ Subtotal thyroidectomy

NURSING CONSIDERATIONS

NURSING DIAGNOSES
◆ Decreased cardiac output
◆ Disturbed body image
◆ Imbalanced nutrition: Less than body requirements
◆ Impaired swallowing
◆ Ineffective coping
◆ Risk for aspiration
◆ Risk for deficient fluid volume

EXPECTED OUTCOMES
The patient will:
◆ remain hemodynamically stable
◆ have a reduced goiter
◆ consume required daily caloric intake
◆ swallow without coughing or choking
◆ demonstrate effective coping skills
◆ not aspirate
◆ have balanced intake and output.

NURSING INTERVENTIONS
◆ Give prescribed drugs.
◆ Encourage the patient to express feelings and concerns.

MONITORING
◆ Neck circumference
◆ Response to therapy
◆ Blood test to regulate thyroid replacement medication

PATIENT TEACHING

GENERAL
Be sure to cover:
◆ drug administration and dosage
◆ symptoms of thyroid toxicosis
◆ use of iodized salt.

RESOURCES
Organizations
Endocrine Society: *www.endo-society.org*
Mayo Clinic: *www.mayoclinic.com*

Selected references
Nettina, S.M. *Lippincott Manual of Nursing Practice,* 8th ed. Philadelphia: Lippincott Williams & Wilkins, 2006.

Nieuwlaat, W., et al. "Nontoxic, Nodular Goiter: New Management Paradigms," *Endocrinologist* 13(1):31-37, January-February 2003.

Gonadotropin deficiency

- Lack of follicle-stimulating hormone (FSH) and luteinizing hormone (LH), which stimulate the sex glands, primarily the testes and ovaries
- If chronic and untreated, can cause infertility and osteopenia

PATHOPHYSIOLOGY

- Gonadotropin-releasing hormone (Gn-RH) is secreted by the hypothalamus and causes the anterior pituitary to secrete the gonadotropins — testosterone, estrogen, FSH, and LH.
- Estrogen, progesterone, and testosterone, produced by the gonads, function in a negative-feedback loop that regulates Gn-RH secretion.
- Mechanisms that cause Gn-RH deficiency include:
- pituitary tumors, which produce another hormone that impairs Gn-RH biosynthesis
- medical treatments such as radiation, which impairs cells that produce Gn-RH
- oversecretion of estrogen, progesterone, or testosterone by dysfunctional target glands, causing Gn-RH inhibition through the negative-feedback loop
- prolactin-secreting tumors, reducing pituitary secretion of Gn-RH
- the hypothalamus' response to physical stress, obesity, or starvation, reducing Gn-RH secretion.

CAUSES

- Genetics
- Mechanisms that reduce Gn-RH

INCIDENCE

- Gonadotropin deficiency can occur at any age.
- The disorder affects men more commonly than women.

COMPLICATIONS

- Infertility
- Sexual dysfunction

HISTORY

- Illness that affects testes
- Underdeveloped secondary sex characteristics
- Mood and behavior changes
- Sexual dysfunction
- Infertility

PHYSICAL FINDINGS

- Testicular atrophy
- Underdeveloped secondary characteristics
- Decreased body hair
- Fine wrinkles around eyes and lips

LABORATORY

- Testosterone level is low and Gn-RH level is high, in primary testicular failure).
- Estrogen level is low and Gn-RH level is high, in primary ovarian failure.
- Gn-RH and testosterone or estrogen levels are low, in hypothalamic or pituitary dysfunction.
- Human chorionic gonadotropin stimulation test result is abnormal.
- Gn-RH stimulation test reveals insufficient elevation of LH or FSH levels.

GENERAL
◆ Stress reduction
◆ Strategies to gain or lose weight

MEDICATIONS
◆ Gonadotropin, estrogen, or testosterone replacement

SURGERY
◆ Removal of tumors

NURSING DIAGNOSES
◆ Disturbed body image
◆ Ineffective coping
◆ Ineffective sexuality patterns
◆ Sexual dysfunction

EXPECTED OUTCOMES
The patient will:
◆ express positive feelings regarding body image
◆ seek support systems and exhibit adequate coping behaviors
◆ voice his feelings about potential or actual changes in sexual activity
◆ identify measures to maintain sexual function as tolerated.

NURSING INTERVENTIONS
◆ Give prescribed drugs.
◆ Provide emotional support.

MONITORING
◆ Laboratory results

GENERAL
Be sure to cover:
◆ the disorder and treatment
◆ taking prescribed drugs.

DISCHARGE PLANNING
◆ Stress to the patient the importance of obtaining ongoing follow-up care.

RESOURCES
Organizations
Endocrine Society: *www.endo-society.org*
National Library of Medicine: *www.nlm.nih.gov*

Selected references
Lazarou, S., and Morgentaler, A. "Hypogonadism in the Man with Erectile Dysfunction: What to Look for and When to Treat," *Current Urology Reports* 6(6):476-81, November 2005.
Nettina, S.M. *Lippincott Manual of Nursing Practice,* 8th ed. Philadelphia: Lippincott Williams & Wilkins, 2006.

Gonorrhea

- Common venereal disease that usually starts as infection of the genitourinary tract; can also begin in rectum, pharynx, or eyes
- Left untreated, spreads through the blood to the joints, tendons, meninges, and endocardium
- In women, can lead to chronic pelvic inflammatory disease (PID) and sterility

PATHOPHYSIOLOGY

- Gonococci infect mucus-secreting epithelial surfaces and penetrate through or between the cells to the connective tissue.
- Inflammation and spread of the infection results.

CAUSES

- Acquisition of gonococcal conjunctivitis by touching the eyes with a contaminated hand
- For a child born to an infected mother, acquisition of gonococcal ophthalmia neonatorum during passage through the birth canal
- Transmission of *Neisseria gonorrhoea*, the causative organism, through sexual contact with an infected person

INCIDENCE

- Among sexually active individuals, incidence is highest in those with multiple partners, teenagers, nonwhites, the poor, the poorly educated, city dwellers, and unmarried people who live alone.
- Reinfection is common.

COMPLICATIONS

- PID
- Acute epididymitis
- Proctitis
- Salpingitis
- Septic arthritis
- Dermatitis
- Perihepatitis
- Corneal ulceration
- Blindness
- Meningitis
- Osteomyelitis

- Pneumonia
- Acute respiratory distress syndrome

ASSESSMENT

HISTORY

- Unprotected sexual contact (vaginal, oral, or anal) with an infected person, an unknown partner, or multiple sex partners
- History of sexually transmitted disease

PHYSICAL FINDINGS

- Fever
- Purulent discharge from urethral meatus
- Female urethral meatus possibly red and edematous
- Friable cervix and a greenish yellow discharge
- Engorged, red, swollen vagina with profuse purulent discharge
- Rectal infection
- Ocular infection
- Pharyngeal infection
- Papillary skin lesions on hands and feet
- PID
- Perihepatitis
- Pain and a cracking noise when moving an involved joint

DIAGNOSTIC TEST RESULTS

LABORATORY

- Culture from the infection site of the urethra, cervix, rectum, or pharynx, usually establishes the diagnosis.
- Culture of conjunctival scrapings confirms gonococcal conjunctivitis.
- In males, a Gram stain showing gram-negative diplococci may confirm the diagnosis.
- Gonococcal arthritis requires identification of gram-negative diplococci on smear from joint fluid and skin lesions.
- Complement fixation and immunofluorescent assays of serum reveal antibody titers four times the normal rate.
- Venereal Disease Research Laboratories test result may be reactive (false-positive) in a patient with syphilis.
- Rapid plasma reagin test may be reactive (false-positive) in a patient with syphilis.

TREATMENT

GENERAL

- Follow-up cultures 4 to 7 days after treatment and again in 6 months
- For a pregnant patient, final follow-up before delivery
- Effective therapy (ends communicability within hours)

ACTIVITY

- Abstinence from sexual activity until infection treated

MEDICATIONS

- Ceftriaxone plus doxycycline
- Azithromycin (Zithromax)
- In neonates, to prevent gonococcal ophthalmia neonatorum, 1% silver nitrate drops or erythromycin ointment

NURSING DIAGNOSES
- Acute pain
- Ineffective sexuality patterns
- Risk for infection
- Situational low self-esteem

EXPECTED OUTCOMES
The patient will:
- remain free from pain
- voice his feelings about potential or actual changes in sexual activity
- identify signs and symptoms of infection and experience no further signs or symptoms of infection
- express concern about self-concept, esteem, and body image.

NURSING INTERVENTIONS
- Practice standard precautions.
- Isolate the patient if his eyes are infected.
- With gonococcal arthritis, apply moist heat to ease pain in affected joints.
- Give prescribed drugs.
- Report all cases of gonorrhea to the local public health authorities as required.
- Report all cases of gonorrhea in children to child abuse authorities.
- Routinely instill prophylactic drugs, according to facility protocol, in the eyes of all neonates on admission to the nursery.
- Check the neonate of an infected mother for signs of infection, and obtain specimens for culture from the neonate's eyes, pharynx, and rectum.

MONITORING
- Response to treatment
- Adverse drug effects
- Complications
- Follow-up culture results

GENERAL
Be sure to cover:
- the disorder, diagnosis, and treatment
- informing all sexual partners of the infection so that they can seek treatment
- avoiding sexual contact until cultures are negative and infection is eradicated
- being careful when coming into contact with any bodily discharges to avoid contaminating the eyes
- safer sex practices
- taking anti-infective drugs for the time prescribed
- the importance of returning for follow-up testing. (See *Preventing gonorrhea*.)

RESOURCES
Organizations
Centers for Disease Control and Prevention: *www.cdc.gov*
Harvard University Consumer Health Information: *www.intelihealth.com*
National Health Information Center: *www.health.gov/nhic*
National Library of Medicine: *www.nlm.nih.gov*

Selected references
Kasper, D.L., et al., eds. *Harrison's Principles of Internal Medicine,* 16th ed. New York: McGraw-Hill Book Co., 2005.
Nsuami, M., et al. "Chlamydia and Gonorrhea Co-occurrence in a High School Population," *Sexually Transmitted Diseases* 31(7):424-27, July 2004.
Warner, L., et al. "Condom Use and Risk of Gonorrhea and Chlamydia: A Systemic Review of Design and Measurement Factors Assessed in Epidemiologic Studies," *Sexually Transmitted Diseases* 33(1):36-51, January 2006.

Preventing gonorrhea

To prevent gonorrhea, provide the following patient teaching:

- Tell the patient to avoid sexual contact until cultures prove negative and infection is eradicated.
- Advise the patient's partner to receive treatment even if the partner doesn't have a positive culture. Recommend that the partner avoid sexual contact with anyone until treatment is complete because reinfection is extremely common.
- Counsel the patient and all sexual partners to be tested for the human immunodeficiency virus and hepatitis B infection.
- Instruct the patient to be careful when coming into contact with any bodily discharges to avoid contaminating the eyes.
- Tell the patient to take anti-infective drugs for the time prescribed.
- To prevent reinfection, tell the patient to avoid sexual contact with anyone *suspected of* being infected, to use condoms during intercourse, to wash genitalia with soap and water before and after intercourse, and to avoid sharing washcloths or douche equipment.
- Advise returning for follow-up testing.

Goodpasture's syndrome

- Pulmonary renal syndrome characterized by hemoptysis and rapidly progressive glomerulonephritis

PATHOPHYSIOLOGY

- Abnormal production and deposition of antibodies against glomerular basement membrane (GBM) and alveolar basement membrane activate the complement and inflammatory responses.
- This results in glomerular and alveolar tissue damage.

CAUSES

- Unknown
- Possible genetic predisposition
- Possible link to exposure to hydrocarbons or with type II hypersensitivity reaction

INCIDENCE

- Goodpasture's syndrome may occur at any age, most commonly in men between the ages of 20 and 30.

COMPLICATIONS

- Renal failure
- Pulmonary edema and hemorrhage

HISTORY

- Possible malaise, fatigue, and pallor
- Possible pulmonary bleeding for months or years before developing overt hemorrhage and signs of renal disease

PHYSICAL FINDINGS

- Hematuria
- Decreased urine output
- Dyspnea, tachypnea, orthopnea
- Restlessness
- Hemoptysis, ranging from a cough with blood tinged sputum to frank pulmonary hemorrhage
- Pulmonary crackles and rhonchi

LABORATORY

- Immunofluorescence of alveolar basement membrane shows linear deposition of immunoglobulins as well as C3 and fibrinogen.
- Immunofluorescence of GBM shows linear deposition of immunoglobulins.
- Serum anti-GBM antibody test reveals the presence of circulating anti-GBM antibodies, which distinguishes Goodpasture's syndrome from other pulmonary renal syndromes, such as Wegener's granulomatosis, polyarteritis, and systemic lupus erythematosus.
- Serum creatinine and blood urea nitrogen (BUN) levels are typically increased to two to three times normal.
- Urinalysis may show red blood cells and cellular casts, which typify glomerular inflammation; it may also show granular casts and proteinuria.

IMAGING

- Chest X-rays reveal pulmonary infiltrates in a diffuse, nodular pattern.

DIAGNOSTIC PROCEDURES

- Lung biopsy shows interstitial and intra-alveolar hemorrhage with hemosiderin-laden macrophages.
- Renal biopsy usually shows focal necrotic lesions and cellular crescents.

TREATMENT

GENERAL
- Plasmapheresis
- Dialysis

DIET
- Low-protein, low-sodium

ACTIVITY
- As tolerated

MEDICATIONS
- High-dose corticosteroids
- Cyclophosphamide (Cytoxan)

SURGERY
- Kidney transplantation

NURSING CONSIDERATIONS

NURSING DIAGNOSES
- Activity intolerance
- Acute pain
- Anxiety
- Excess fluid volume
- Fatigue
- Fear
- Impaired gas exchange
- Impaired urinary elimination
- Ineffective airway clearance
- Ineffective breathing pattern
- Risk for injury

EXPECTED OUTCOMES
The patient will:
- verbalize the importance of balancing activity, as tolerated, with rest periods
- verbalize feelings of comfort and reduced levels of pain
- verbalize measures to reduce anxiety levels
- maintain adequate fluid balance
- express feelings of increased energy
- verbalize fears and concerns
- maintain adequate ventilation and oxygenation
- have adequate urine output
- maintain a patent airway
- maintain an effective breathing pattern
- develop no complications.

NURSING INTERVENTIONS
- Elevate the head of the bed and administer humidified oxygen, as ordered.
- Encourage the patient to conserve his energy.
- Assist with range-of-motion exercises.
- Assist with activities of daily living, and provide frequent rest periods.
- Transfuse blood and administer corticosteroids, as ordered. Watch closely for signs of adverse reactions.

MONITORING
- Respiratory status
- Vital signs
- Arterial blood gas levels
- Intake and output
- Daily weight
- Creatinine clearance, BUN, and serum creatinine levels
- Hematocrit and coagulation studies

PATIENT TEACHING

GENERAL
Be sure to cover:
- the disorder, diagnosis, and treatment
- the importance of conserving energy
- an explanation that fluid intake may be restricted
- the name, dosage, purpose, and adverse effects of all medications
- how to effectively deep-breathe and cough
- how to recognize the signs of respiratory or genitourinary bleeding and the need to report such signs to the practitioner at once.

DISCHARGE PLANNING
- If dialysis or kidney transplantation is required, refer the patient to a renal support group.
- Encourage regular follow-up care.

RESOURCES
Organizations
National Kidney and Urologic Diseases Information Clearinghouse: *www.niddk.nih.gov*
National Kidney Foundation: *www.kidney.org*

Selected references
Bergs, L. "Goodpasture Syndrome," *Critical Care Nurse* 25(5):50-54, 56, 57-58, October 2005.
Kasper, D.L., et al., eds. *Harrison's Principles of Internal Medicine,* 16th ed. New York: McGraw-Hill Book Co., 2005.
The Merck Manual of Diagnosis & Therapy, 18th ed., Whitehouse Station, N.J.: Merck & Co., Inc., 2006.

Gout

OVERVIEW

- Inflammatory arthritis caused by uric acid and crystal deposits
- Red, swollen, and acutely painful joints
- Mostly affects feet, great toe, ankle, and midfoot
- Patient may remain symptom-free for years between attacks
- First acute attack strikes suddenly and peaks quickly
- Delayed attacks associated with olecranon bursitis
- Chronic polyarticular gout — the final, unremitting stage of the disease marked by persistent painful polyarthritis

PATHOPHYSIOLOGY

- Uric acid crystallizes in blood or body fluids, and the precipitate accumulates in connective tissue (tophi).
- Crystals trigger an immune response.
- Neutrophils secrete lysosomes for phagocytosis.
- Lysosomes damage tissue and exacerbate the immune response.

CAUSES

- Decreased renal excretion of uric acid
- Genetic defect in purine metabolism (hyperuricemia)
- Heredity factors
- Oversecretion of uric acid
- Radical dieting practices that involve starvation
- Secondary gout associated with drugs (hydrochlorothiazide or pyrazinamide)
- Secondary gout associated with other diseases:
- Diabetes mellitus
- Hypertension
- Leukemia
- Myeloma
- Obesity
- Polycythemia
- Renal disease
- Sickle cell anemia

INCIDENCE

- Primary gout typically occurs in men older than age 30 and in postmenopausal women taking diuretics.

COMPLICATIONS

- Renal calculi
- Atherosclerotic disease
- Cardiovascular lesions
- Stroke
- Coronary thrombosis
- Hypertension
- Infection when tophi rupture

ASSESSMENT

HISTORY

- Sedentary lifestyle
- Hypertension
- Renal calculi
- Waking during the night with pain in great toe
- Alcohol ingestion
- Initial moderate pain that grows intense
- Chills, mild fever

PHYSICAL FINDINGS

- Swollen, dusky red or purple joint
- Limited movement of joint
- Tophi, especially in the outer ears, hands, and feet (see *Recognizing gouty tophi*)
- Skin over tophi that may ulcerate and release chalky white exudate or pus
- Secondary joint degeneration
- Erosions, deformity, and disability
- Warmth over joint
- Extreme tenderness
- Fever
- Hypertension

DIAGNOSTIC TEST RESULTS

LABORATORY

- Serum uric acid level is elevated during an acute gout attack.
- White blood cell count is elevated during an acute gout attack.
- Urine uric acid level is chronically elevated in 20% of patients.

IMAGING

- X-ray of the articular cartilage and subchondral bone shows evidence of chronic gout.

DIAGNOSTIC PROCEDURES

- Needle aspiration of synovial fluid shows needlelike intracellular crystals.

Recognizing gouty tophi

In advanced gout, urate crystal deposits develop into hard, irregular, yellow-white nodules called tophi. These bumps commonly protrude from the great toe and ear.

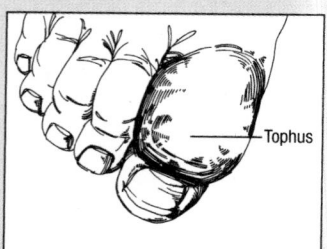

Tophus

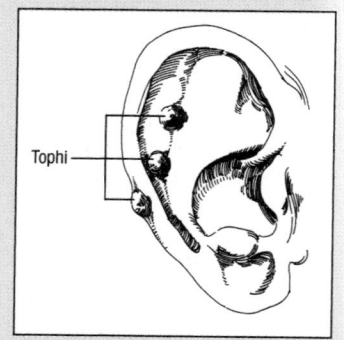

Tophi

TREATMENT

GENERAL
◆ Termination of acute attack
◆ Protection of inflamed, painful joints
◆ Treatment for hyperuricemia
◆ Local application of cold
◆ Prevention of recurrent gout
◆ Prevention of renal calculi
◆ Weight loss program, if indicated

DIET
◆ Avoidance of alcohol
◆ Sparing use of purine rich foods (such as anchovies, liver, and sardines)

ACTIVITY
◆ Bed rest (in acute attack)
◆ Immobilization of joint

MEDICATIONS
◆ Analgesics
◆ Nonsteroidal anti-inflammatory drugs
◆ Colchicine
◆ Allopurinol
◆ Probenecid or sulfinpyrazone (Anturane)
◆ Corticosteroids

NURSING CONSIDERATIONS

NURSING DIAGNOSES
◆ Activity intolerance
◆ Acute pain
◆ Anxiety
◆ Disturbed sleep pattern
◆ Impaired physical mobility
◆ Ineffective coping
◆ Risk for injury

EXPECTED OUTCOMES
The patient will:
◆ perform activities of daily living within the confines of the disease
◆ express feelings of increased comfort and decreased pain
◆ identify strategies to reduce anxiety
◆ verbalize feeling well rested
◆ maintain joint mobility and range of motion
◆ express adequate coping skills
◆ remain free from injury or complications.

NURSING INTERVENTIONS
◆ Allow adequate time for self-care.
◆ Institute bed rest.
◆ Use a bed cradle, if appropriate.
◆ Give pain medication as needed.
◆ Apply cold packs to affected areas.
◆ Identify techniques and activities that promote rest and relaxation.
◆ Administer anti-inflammatories.
◆ Provide a purine-poor diet.

MONITORING
◆ Intake and output
◆ Serum uric acid levels
◆ Acute gout attacks 24 to 96 hours after surgery

PATIENT TEACHING

GENERAL
Be sure to cover:
◆ the disorder, diagnosis, and treatment
◆ the need to drink plenty of fluids (up to 2 qt [2 L] per day)
◆ relaxation techniques
◆ compliance with the prescribed drug regimen
◆ dietary adjustments
◆ the need to control hypertension.

DISCHARGE PLANNING
◆ Refer the patient to a weight-reduction program if appropriate.

RESOURCES
Organizations
National Institutes of Health: *www.nih.gov*
WebMD: *www.webmd.com*

Selected references
Diseases, 4th ed. Philadelphia: Lippincott Williams & Wilkins, 2006.
Handbook of Pathophysiology, 2nd ed. Philadelphia: Lippincott Williams & Wilkins, 2005.
Masseoud, D., et al. "Overview of Hyperuricaemia and Gout," *Current Pharmaceutical Design* 11(32):4117-124, 2005.
Moreland, L.W. "Febuxostat — Treatment for Hyperuricemia and Gout?" *New England Journal of Medicine* 353(23):2505-507, December 2005.

Graft rejection syndrome

- Rejection of a donated organ occurring when the host's immune responses are directed against the graft
- Three subtypes based on time of onset and mechanisms involved:
 – Hyperacute rejection
 – Acute rejection
 – Chronic rejection

PATHOPHYSIOLOGY

- Hyperacute rejection occurs within minutes to hours after graft transplantation.
- Circulating host antibodies recognize and bind to graft antigens.
- Binding of these antibodies leads to initiation of the complement cascade, recruitment of neutrophils, platelet activation, damage to graft endothelial cells, and stimulation of coagulation reactions.
- Acute rejection may occur several hours to days (even weeks) after transplantation.
- Alloantigen-reactive T cells from the host infiltrate the graft and are activated by contact with foreign, graft-related proteins that are presented to them by antigen-presenting cells.
- These T cells may cause graft tissue damage.
- Chronic rejection is characterized by the development of blood vessel luminal occlusion due to progressive thickening of the intimal layers of medium and large arterial walls.
- Large amounts of intimal matrix are produced, leading to increasingly occlusive vessel wall thickening.
- A slowly progressing reduction in blood flow results in regional tissue ischemia, cell death, and tissue fibrosis.

CAUSES

- Immune system response to a graft

INCIDENCE

- Hyperacute rejection is rare, affecting less than 1% of transplant recipients.
- Acute rejection occurs in 50% of transplant patients (only 10% progress to graft loss).
- Chronic rejection occurs in 50% of transplant patients within 10 years after transplantation.

COMPLICATIONS

- Rapid thrombosis
- Loss of graft function

ASSESSMENT

HISTORY

- Signs and symptoms that vary markedly, depending on type of rejection, underlying illnesses, and type of organ transplanted

PHYSICAL FINDINGS

- Oliguria and increasing serum creatinine and blood urea nitrogen levels with kidney transplant
- Elevated transaminase levels, decreased albumin levels, and hypocoagulability with liver transplant
- Hypotension, heart failure, and edema with heart transplant

DIAGNOSTIC TEST RESULTS

DIAGNOSTIC PROCEDURES

- Biopsy of the transplanted tissue confirms rejection.
- Hyperacute rejection is characterized by large numbers of polymorphonuclear leukocytes in the graft blood vessels, widespread microthrombi, platelet accumulation, and interstitial hemorrhage. There's little or no interstitial inflammation.

TREATMENT

GENERAL

- Close monitoring of function of grafted organ
- Surveillance, with prophylactic measures against opportunistic infections

DIET

- Restrictions based on organ system affected

ACTIVITY

- As tolerated

MEDICATIONS

- Immunosuppressants
- Antirejection therapies
- Antibiotics

NURSING CONSIDERATIONS

NURSING DIAGNOSES
◆ Activity intolerance
◆ Disturbed body image
◆ Fatigue
◆ Hopelessness
◆ Hyperthermia
◆ Imbalanced nutrition: Less than body requirements
◆ Impaired skin integrity
◆ Impaired tissue integrity
◆ Ineffective coping
◆ Ineffective health maintenance
◆ Ineffective tissue perfusion: Renal, cardiopulmonary
◆ Interrupted family processes
◆ Powerlessness
◆ Risk for deficient fluid volume
◆ Risk for infection
◆ Social isolation

EXPECTED OUTCOMES
The patient will:
◆ verbalize the importance of balancing activity, as tolerated, with rest
◆ express feelings related to a changed body image
◆ express feelings of increased energy
◆ make decisions on his own behalf
◆ maintain a normal body temperature
◆ exhibit no signs of malnutrition
◆ exhibit normal healing of wounds and lesions
◆ experience decreased areas of redness, swelling, and inflammation
◆ use support systems to assist with coping
◆ perform health maintenance activities according to the level of his ability
◆ maintain adequate renal and cardiopulmonary perfusion
◆ voice feelings about the condition
◆ express feelings of control over his well-being
◆ maintain a normal fluid balance
◆ experience no fever, chills, or other signs or symptoms of illness
◆ maintain social interaction to the extent possible.

NURSING INTERVENTIONS
◆ Give prescribed immunosuppressants.
◆ Give prescribed antirejection therapies.
◆ Give prescribed antibiotics for infection.

MONITORING
◆ Vital signs
◆ Function of the transplanted organ
◆ Signs and symptoms of infection
◆ Signs and symptoms of rejection

PATIENT TEACHING

GENERAL
Be sure to cover:
◆ the disorder, diagnosis, and treatment
◆ how to recognize signs and symptoms of organ dysfunction
◆ the need to immediately report fever, chills, and other symptoms of infection
◆ the need for lifelong medication compliance.

DISCHARGE PLANNING
◆ Refer the patient and his family to social support, including psychological support services, as indicated.

RESOURCES
Organizations
Centers for Disease Control and Prevention: *www.cdc.gov*
National Institutes of Health: *www.nih.gov*

Selected references
Diseases, 4th ed. Philadelphia: Lippincott Williams & Wilkins, 2006.
Kasper, D.L., et al., eds. *Harrison's Principles of Internal Medicine*, 16th ed. New York: McGraw-Hill Book Co., 2005.
Storm, T.B. "Rejection — More than the Eye Can See," *New England Journal of Medicine* 353(22):2394-396, December 2005.

Guillain-Barré syndrome LIFE-THREATENING DISORDER

OVERVIEW

- A form of polyneuritis
- Acute, rapidly progressive, and potentially fatal
- Three phases:
- Acute: beginning from first symptom, ending in 1 to 3 weeks
- Plateau: lasting several days to 2 weeks
- Recovery: coincides with remyelination and axonal process regrowth; extends over 4 to 6 months and may take up to 2 to 3 years; recovery possibly not complete

PATHOPHYSIOLOGY

- Segmented demyelination of peripheral nerves occurs, preventing normal transmission of electrical impulses.
- Sensorimotor nerve roots are affected; autonomic nerve transmission may also be affected. (See *Understanding sensorimotor nerve degeneration.*)

CAUSES

- Unknown

RISK FACTORS

- Surgery
- Rabies or swine influenza vaccination
- Viral illness
- Hodgkin's or some other malignant disease
- Lupus erythematosus

INCIDENCE

- Guillain-Barré syndrome occurs equally in both sexes.
- The syndrome typically occurs between ages 30 and 50.

COMPLICATIONS

- Thrombophlebitis
- Pressure ulcers
- Contractures
- Muscle wasting
- Aspiration
- Respiratory tract infections
- Life-threatening respiratory and cardiac compromise

ASSESSMENT

HISTORY

- Minor febrile illness 1 to 4 weeks before current symptoms
- Tingling and numbness (paresthesia) in the legs
- Progression of symptoms to arms, trunk and, finally, the face
- Stiffness and pain in the calves

PHYSICAL FINDINGS

- Muscle weakness (the major neurologic sign)
- Sensory loss, usually in the legs (spreads to arms)
- Difficulty talking, chewing, and swallowing
- Paralysis of the ocular, facial, and oropharyngeal muscles
- Loss of position sense
- Diminished or absent deep tendon reflexes

Understanding sensorimotor nerve degeneration

Guillain-Barré syndrome attacks the peripheral nerves so that they can't transmit messages to the brain correctly. Here's what goes wrong:

The myelin sheath degenerates for unknown reasons. This sheath covers the nerve axons and conducts electrical impulses along the nerve pathways. With degeneration comes inflammation, swelling, and patchy demyelination. As this disorder destroys myelin, the nodes of Ranvier (at the junctures of the myelin sheaths) widen. This delays and impairs impulse transmission along the dorsal and ventral nerve roots.

Because the dorsal nerve roots handle sensory function, the patient may experience sensations, such as tingling and numbness, when the nerve root is impaired. Similarly, because the ventral roots are responsible for motor function, impairment causes varying weakness, immobility, and paralysis.

DIAGNOSTIC TEST RESULTS

DIAGNOSTIC PROCEDURES

- Cerebrospinal fluid (CSF) analysis may show a normal white blood cell count, an elevated protein count and, in severe disease, increased CSF pressure.

OTHER

- Electromyography may demonstrate repeated firing of the same motor unit instead of widespread sectional stimulation.
- Nerve conduction studies show marked slowing of nerve conduction velocities.

TREATMENT

GENERAL
- Supportive measures
- Emotional support
- Maintenance of skin integrity
- Possible endotracheal (ET) intubation or tracheotomy
- Fluid volume replacement
- Plasmapheresis
- Possible tube feedings with ET intubation

DIET
- Adequate caloric intake

ACTIVITY
- Exercise program to prevent contractures

MEDICATIONS
- I.V. beta-adrenergic blockers
- Parasympatholytics
- I.V. immune globulin

SURGERY
- Possible tracheostomy
- Possible gastrostomy or jejunotomy feeding tube insertion

NURSING CONSIDERATIONS

NURSING DIAGNOSES
- Anxiety
- Fear
- Imbalanced nutrition: Less than body requirements
- Impaired gas exchange
- Impaired physical mobility
- Impaired urinary elimination
- Impaired verbal communication
- Ineffective breathing pattern

EXPECTED OUTCOMES
The patient will:
- identify strategies to reduce anxiety
- express fears and concerns
- maintain required daily caloric intake
- maintain adequate ventilation and oxygenation
- maintain joint mobility and range of motion (ROM)
- establish routine urinary elimination patterns
- develop alternate means of expressing himself
- maintain effective breathing pattern.

NURSING INTERVENTIONS
- Establish a means of communication before intubation is required, if possible.
- Turn and reposition the patient.
- Encourage coughing and deep breathing.
- Provide meticulous skin care.
- Provider passive ROM exercises.
- In case of facial paralysis, provide eye and mouth care.
- Provide emotional support.
- Give prescribed drugs.

MONITORING
- Vital signs
- Respiratory status
- Arterial blood gas measurements
- Level of consciousness
- Pulse oximetry
- Signs of thrombophlebitis
- Signs of urine retention
- Response to medications
- Skin integrity

PATIENT TEACHING

GENERAL
Be sure to cover:
- the disorder, diagnosis, and treatment
- effective means of communication
- the appropriate home care plan
- instructions about medications
- adverse drug reactions.

DISCHARGE PLANNING
- Refer the patient to physical rehabilitation sources as indicated.
- Refer the patient to occupational and speech rehabilitation resources as indicated.
- Refer the patient to the Guillain-Barré Syndrome Foundation.

RESOURCES
Organizations
Guillain-Barré Syndrome Foundation, International: *www.gbsfi.com*
National Institutes of Health: *www.nih.gov*

Selected references
Diseases, 4th ed. Philadelphia: Lippincott Williams & Wilkins, 2006.

Gregory, M.A., et al. "Understanding Guillain-Barré Syndrome and Central Nervous System Involvement," *Rehabilitation Nursing* 30(5):207-12, September-October 2005.

Haldeman, D., and Zulkosky, K. "Treatment and Nursing Care for a Patient with Guillain-Barré Syndrome," *Dimensions of Critical Care Nursing* 24(6):267-72, November-December 2005.

Handbook of Pathophysiology, 2nd ed. Philadelphia: Lippincott Williams & Wilkins, 2005.

Kuwabara, S. "Guillain-Barré Syndrome: Epidemiology, Pathophysiology and Management," *Drugs* 64(6):597-610, 2004.

Haemophilus influenzae infection

- Infection that most commonly attacks respiratory system
- Common cause of epiglottiditis, laryngotracheobronchitis, pneumonia, bronchiolitis, otitis media, and meningitis
- Infrequent cause of bacterial endocarditis, conjunctivitis, facial cellulitis, septic arthritis, and osteomyelitis

PATHOPHYSIOLOGY

- An antigenic response occurs with the invasion of bacteria.
- A systemic disease results from the invasion and hematogenous spread to distant sites: bones, joints, meninges.
- Local invasion occurs on mucosal surfaces.
- Otitis media occurs when bacteria reach the middle ear through the eustachian tube.

CAUSES

- *H. influenzae*, a gram-negative, pleomorphic aerobic bacillus
- Transmission by direct contact with secretions or airborne droplets

INCIDENCE

- *H. influenzae* type B (Hib) infection predominantly affects children at a rate of 3% to 5%; incidence is lower when a vaccine is administered at ages 2, 4, 6, and 15 months.
- *H. influenzae* epiglottiditis is most common in children between ages 3 and 7 but can occur at any age.
- Meningitis due to Hib has a higher incidence rate in Black children than in White children.
- Incidence rate is 10 times higher in Native Americans, possibly due to exposure, socioeconomic conditions, and genetic differences in immune responses.

COMPLICATIONS

- Permanent neurologic sequelae from meningitis
- Complete upper airway obstruction from epiglottiditis
- Cellulitis
- Pericarditis, pleural effusion
- Respiratory failure from pneumonia

ASSESSMENT

HISTORY

- Possible report of recent viral infection
- Malaise
- Fatigue
- Fever

PHYSICAL FINDINGS
Epiglottiditis

- Restlessness and irritability
- Use of accessory muscles, inspiratory retractions, stridor
- Sitting up, leaning forward with mouth open, tongue protruding, and nostrils flaring
- Expiratory rhonchi; diminishing breath sounds as the condition worsens
- Pharyngeal mucosa that may look reddened (rarely, with soft yellow exudate)
- Epiglottis that appears cherry-red with considerable edema
- Severe pain that makes swallowing difficult or impossible

Pneumonia

- Shaking chills
- Tachypnea
- Productive cough
- Impaired or asymmetrical chest movement caused by pleuritic pain
- Dullness over areas of lung consolidation

Meningitis

- Altered level of consciousness
- Seizures and coma as disease progresses
- Positive Brudzinski's and Kernig's signs
- Exaggerated and symmetrical deep tendon reflexes
- Nuchal rigidity
- Opisthotonos

DIAGNOSTIC TEST RESULTS

LABORATORY

- Isolation of the organism in blood culture confirms infection.
- Hib meningitis is detected in cerebrospinal fluid cultures.

TREATMENT

GENERAL
◆ Airway maintenance (critical in epiglottiditis)

DIET
◆ Based on respiratory status (possible need for small, frequent meals)
◆ Nothing by mouth with inability to swallow adequately

ACTIVITY
◆ As tolerated

MEDICATIONS
◆ Cephalosporin
◆ Chloramphenicol and ampicillin (alternate regimen)
◆ Glucocorticoids

NURSING CONSIDERATIONS

NURSING DIAGNOSES
◆ Acute pain
◆ Anxiety
◆ Deficient fluid volume
◆ Imbalanced nutrition: Less than body requirements
◆ Impaired gas exchange
◆ Ineffective airway clearance
◆ Ineffective breathing pattern
◆ Risk for aspiration
◆ Risk for infection

EXPECTED OUTCOMES
The patient will:
◆ report reduced levels of pain
◆ verbalize feelings of anxiety and fear
◆ attain and maintain normal fluid and electrolyte balance
◆ maintain nutritional health through oral intake of I.V. fluids
◆ maintain adequate gas exchange
◆ maintain a patent airway
◆ maintain effective breathing pattern and not have adventitious breath sounds
◆ not aspirate
◆ remain free from signs and symptoms of infection.

NURSING INTERVENTIONS
◆ Maintain respiratory isolation.
◆ Maintain adequate respiratory function through cool humidification; oxygen, as needed; and croup or face tents.
◆ Keep emergency resuscitation equipment readily available.
◆ Suction, as needed.
◆ Give prescribed drugs.
◆ Maintain adequate nutrition and elimination.

MONITORING
◆ Pulse oximetry
◆ Arterial blood gas results
◆ Complete blood count for signs of bone marrow depression when therapy includes ampicillin or chloramphenicol
◆ Intake and output
◆ Respiratory status
◆ Neurologic status
◆ Vital signs

PATIENT TEACHING

GENERAL
Be sure to cover:
◆ the disorder, diagnosis, and treatment
◆ the importance of continuing the prescribed antibiotic until the entire prescription is finished
◆ using a room humidifier or breathing moist air from a shower or bath, as necessary, for home treatment of a respiratory infection
◆ coughing and deep-breathing exercises to clear secretions
◆ the disposal of secretions and use of proper hand-washing technique.

DISCHARGE PLANNING
◆ Refer the patient to an infectious disease specialist, if necessary.
◆ Encourage the patient to receive vaccinations to prevent future infections.

RESOURCES
Organizations
Centers for Disease Control and Prevention: *www.cdc.gov*
Harvard University Consumer Health Information: *www.intelihealth.com*
National Health Information Center: *www.health.gov/nhic/*
National Library of Medicine: *www.nlm.nih.gov*

Selected references
Heininger, U., and Zuberbuhler, M. "Immunization Rates and Timely Administration in Pre-school and School-aged Children," *European Journal of Pediatrics* 165(2):124-29, February 2006.
Kasper, D.L., et al., eds. *Harrison's Principles of Internal Medicine*, 16th ed. New York: McGraw-Hill Book Co., 2005.
Sheff, B. "*Haemophilus Influenzae* Type B (Hib)," *Nursing* 36(1):31, January 2006.

Hantavirus pulmonary syndrome

- Viral disease that causes flulike symptoms
- Rapidly progresses to respiratory failure

PATHOPHYSIOLOGY

- Rodents shed the virus in stool, urine, and saliva.
- Human infection with this disorder occurs from inhalation, ingestion (of contaminated food or water, for example), contact with rodent excrement, or rodent bites. (See *Sin Nombre virus.*)

CAUSES

- Farming, hiking, or camping in rodent-infested areas and occupying rodent-infested dwellings
- Hantaviruses
- Transmission with exposure to infected rodents: brush mice, deer mice, pinion mice, and western chipmunks

INCIDENCE

- This disease occurs mainly in the southwestern United States.
- This disease more commonly affects whites.
- This disease affects more males than females.

COMPLICATIONS

- Respiratory failure
- Death (in 80% of cases)

HISTORY

- Rodent exposure (2 weeks before symptoms)
- Fever
- Myalgia
- Abdominal discomfort
- Dizziness

PHYSICAL FINDINGS

- Cough
- Hypotension
- Tachycardia
- Tachypnea
- Severe hypoxemia and respiratory failure

GENERAL

- The Centers for Disease Control and Prevention and state health departments can perform definitive testing for hantavirus exposure and antibody formation.

LABORATORY

- White blood cell count is elevated, with a predominance of neutrophils, myeloid precursors, and atypical lymphocytes.
- Hematocrit is elevated.
- Platelet count is decreased.
- Partial thromboplastin time is elevated.
- Fibrinogen level is normal.
- Serum creatinine level is no greater than 2.5 mg/dl.

IMAGING

- Chest X-rays show bilateral diffuse infiltrates in almost all patients (findings consistent with acute respiratory distress syndrome).

Sin Nombre virus

This illustration shows the Sin Nombre virus, the most common cause of Hantavirus pulmonary syndrome in the United States and Canada. It exists primarily in western states and provinces.

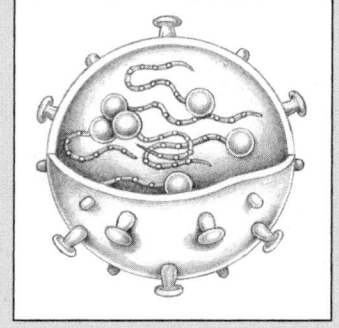

TREATMENT

GENERAL
- Intubation and aggressive respiratory management
- Adequate oxygenation
- Stabilization of heart rate and blood pressure
- Cautious fluid volume replacement

DIET
- Nothing by mouth until recovery begins

ACTIVITY
- As tolerated, with frequent rest periods

MEDICATIONS
- Vasopressors
- Ribavirin (Virazole)

NURSING CONSIDERATIONS

NURSING DIAGNOSES
- Acute pain
- Fatigue
- Hyperthermia
- Impaired gas exchange
- Ineffective airway clearance
- Ineffective breathing pattern
- Risk for deficient fluid volume
- Risk for infection

EXPECTED OUTCOMES
The patient will:
- report decreased levels or absence of pain
- report an increased energy level
- remain afebrile
- maintain adequate gas exchange
- cough effectively and maintain a patent airway
- maintain effective breathing pattern
- maintain an adequate fluid balance
- experience no further signs or symptoms of infection.

NURSING INTERVENTIONS
- Maintain a patent airway by suctioning.
- Ensure adequate humidification, and check mechanical ventilator settings frequently.
- Give prescribed drugs.
- Provide I.V. fluid therapy based on results of hemodynamic monitoring.
- Provide emotional support.
- Report cases of Hantavirus pulmonary syndrome to your state health department.

MONITORING
- Serum electrolyte levels
- Respiratory status
- Neurologic status

PATIENT TEACHING

GENERAL
Be sure to cover:
- the disorder, diagnosis, and treatment
- the importance of immediately reporting signs or symptoms of respiratory distress
- prevention guidelines, with a focus on rodent control.

DISCHARGE PLANNING
- Refer the patient for follow-up with a pulmonologist, if indicated.

RESOURCES
Organizations
Centers for Disease Control and Prevention: *www.cdc.gov*
Harvard University Consumer Health Information: *www.intelihealth.com*
National Health Information Center: *www.health.gov/nhic/*
National Library of Medicine: *www.nlm.nih.gov*

Selected references
Dara, S.I., et al. "Acute Sin Nombre Hantavirus Infection Complicated by Renal Failure Requiring Hemodialysis," *Mayo Clinic Proceedings* 80(5):703-704, May 2005.

Kasper, D.L., et al., eds. *Harrison's Principles of Internal Medicine,* 16th ed. New York: McGraw-Hill Book Co., 2005.

Miedzinski, L. "Community-acquired Pneumonia: New Facets of an Old Disease — Hantavirus Pulmonary Syndrome," *Respiratory Care Clinics of North America* 11(1):45-58, March 2005.

Overturf, G.D. "Clinical Sin Nombre Hantaviral Infections in Children," *The Pediatric Infectious Disease Journal* 24(4):373-74, April 2005.

Headache

- Head pain that may or may not be a symptom of an underlying disorder

PATHOPHYSIOLOGY
Headache
- Sustained muscle contractions directly deform pain receptors.
- Inflammation or direct pressure affects the cranial nerves.
- Pain-sensitive structures respond, including the skin; scalp; muscles; arteries; veins; cranial nerves V, VII, IX, and X; and cervical nerves 1, 2, and 3.

Migraine
- Biochemical abnormalities occur, including leakage of a vasodilator polypeptide through the dilated arteries and a decreased plasma serotonin level.

CAUSES
Headache
- Allergy
- Caffeine withdrawal
- Disorder of the scalp, teeth, extracranial arteries, or external or middle ear
- Emotional stress
- Environmental stimuli
- Fatigue
- Glaucoma
- Head trauma and tumors
- Hypertension
- Hypoxia
- Inflammation of the eyes or mucosa of the nasal or paranasal sinuses
- Intracranial bleeding, abscess, or aneurysm
- Menstruation
- Muscle spasms of the face, neck, or shoulders
- Overuse of over-the-counter headache medications (rebound headache)
- Psychological disorders
- Systemic disorder
- Tension (muscle contraction)
- Underlying intracranial disorder
- Vasodilators

Migraine
- Constriction and dilation of intracranial and extracranial arteries
- Associated with:
  - Depression
  - Epilepsy
  - Hereditary hemorrhagic telangiectasia
  - Ischemic stroke
  - Tourette syndrome

INCIDENCE
Headache
- This condition affects 60% to 80% of people in the United States at any given time.

Migraine
- Migraines first appear in childhood or adolescence.
- Migraines commonly recur throughout adulthood.
- The disorder affects 17% of females and 6% of males in the United States.
- A strong familial incidence occurs with migraines.

COMPLICATIONS
- Worsening of existing hypertension
- Photophobia
- Emotional lability
- Motor weakness
- Loss of work

HISTORY
Headache
- Location (frontal, temporal, or cervical), characteristics (frequency and intensity), onset and duration (continuous or intermittent)
- Precipitating factors: tension, menstruation, loud noises, menopause, alcohol consumption, stress, and food allergies
- Aggravating factors: coughing, sneezing, and sunlight
- Associated symptoms: nausea or vomiting, weakness, facial pain, and scotomas
- Use of headache-inducing medications
- Familial history of headaches

Migraine
- Unilateral, pulsating pain that gradually becomes more generalized
- May be preceded by scintillating scotoma, hemianopsia, unilateral paresthesias, or speech disorders
- May be accompanied by irritability, anorexia, nausea or vomiting, and photophobia

PHYSICAL FINDINGS
Headache
- Findings based on cause
- If no underlying problem, normal physical findings
- Possible crepitus or tender spots of the head and neck

Migraine
- Pallor
- Possible extraocular muscle palsies
- Possible ptosis
- Possible neurologic deficits

DIAGNOSTIC TEST RESULTS

IMAGING
- Skull X-rays show a skull fracture (with trauma).
- Sinus X-rays may show sinusitis.
- Computed tomography scan shows a tumor or subarachnoid hemorrhage or other intracranial pathology; may show pathology of sinuses.
- Magnetic resonance imaging also shows tumor.

DIAGNOSTIC PROCEDURES
- A lumbar puncture may show increased intracranial pressure, suggesting tumor, edema, or hemorrhage.
- Electroencephalography may show alterations in the brain's electrical activity, suggesting intracranial lesion, head injury, meningitis, or encephalitis.
- Patient questionnaire tool evaluates functional status and quality of life.

TREATMENT

GENERAL
- Yoga, meditation, or other relaxation therapy
- Identification and elimination of causative factors (including environmental)
- Psychotherapy, if emotional stress involved

DIET
- For migraine patient, adequate oral fluid intake and avoidance of dietary triggers

ACTIVITY
- For migraine patient, bed rest in dark, quiet room

MEDICATIONS
Headache
- Analgesics
- Tranquilizers
- Muscle relaxants

Migraine
- Ergotamine preparations
- Preventive drugs
- Triptan agents
- Serotonin receptor agonists

NURSING CONSIDERATIONS

NURSING DIAGNOSES
- Acute pain
- Anxiety
- Energy field disturbance
- Fatigue
- Hopelessness
- Interrupted family processes
- Ineffective health maintenance

EXPECTED OUTCOMES
The patient will:
- express feelings of increased comfort and decreased pain
- feel increasingly relaxed
- express an increased sense of well-being
- verbalize feeling well rested
- participate in self-care and make decisions regarding care
- use support systems to assist with coping
- demonstrate methods of promoting relaxation and inner well-being.

NURSING INTERVENTIONS
- Encourage the use of relaxation techniques.
- Keep the patient's room dark and quiet.
- Place ice packs on the patient's forehead or a cold cloth over his eyes.
- Give prescribed drugs for pain.

MONITORING
- Pain control
- Response to alternative treatment
- Vital signs, especially blood pressure
- Neurologic status

PATIENT TEACHING

GENERAL
Be sure to cover:
- the disorder, diagnosis, and treatment
- migraine prevention
- avoidance of migraine triggers
- lifestyle changes
- nonpharmacologic strategies
- monitoring of headaches with headache diary
- appropriate use of preventive medications
- potential adverse reactions to prescribed drugs.

DISCHARGE PLANNING
- Refer the patient to the National Headache Foundation.

RESOURCES
Organizations
National Headache Foundation: *www.headaches.org*
National Institutes of Health: *www.nih.gov*

Selected references
Davis, G.C., and Grassley, J.S. "Measurement of the Experience of Living with Primary Recurrent Headache," *Pain Management Nursing* 6(1):37-44, March 2005.
Diseases, 4th ed. Philadelphia: Lippincott Williams & Wilkins, 2006.
Gurney, D. "Patients with Chief Complaint of Headache: High-risk Decision-Making at Triage," *Journal of Emergency Nursing* 31(1):115-16, February 2005.
Handbook of Pathophysiology, 2nd ed. Philadelphia: Lippincott Williams & Wilkins, 2005.
Linde, K., et al. "Acupuncture for Patients with Migraine: A Randomized Controlled Trial," *JAMA* 293(17):2118-125, May 2005.

Hearing loss

- Mechanical or nervous impediment to the transmission of sound waves to the brain
- Classified as sensorineural, conductive, or central
- Presbycusis: most common type of sensorineural hearing loss
- Congenital hearing loss: may be conductive or sensorineural
- Sudden hearing loss: may be conductive, sensorineural, or mixed; usually affects only one ear
- Depending on the cause, with prompt treatment (within 48 hours), hearing possibly restored
- Noise-induced hearing loss possibly transient or permanent

PATHOPHYSIOLOGY

- In conductive hearing loss, sound wave transmission is interrupted between the external canal and the inner ear (junction of the stapes and oval window).
- In sensorineural hearing loss, sound wave transmission is interrupted between the inner ear and the brain, and there's cochlea or acoustic nerve dysfunction.
- In mixed hearing loss, a conduction dysfunction and sensorineural transmission are combined.

CAUSES

Conductive hearing loss

- Blockage of the external ear
- Cerumen impaction
- Cholesteatoma
- Otitis media, otitis externa
- Otosclerosis
- Serous otitis
- Trauma
- Tumor
- Tympanic membrane thickening, retraction, scarring, or perforation

Sensorineural hearing loss

- Acoustic neuroma
- Arteriosclerosis
- Brief exposure to extremely loud noise (greater than 90 dB)
- Drug toxicity
- Head or ear trauma
- Impairment of the cochlea, eighth cranial or acoustic nerve
- Infectious diseases
- Loss of hair cells and nerve fibers in the cochlea
- Organ of Corti degeneration
- Otospongiosis
- Perilymphatic fistula
- Prolonged exposure to loud noise (85 to 90 dB)
- Vascular occlusion of the anterior cerebellar artery

Congenital hearing loss

- May be transmitted as a dominant, autosomal dominant, autosomal recessive, or sex-linked recessive trait
- Sensorineural or conductive

Hearing loss in neonates

- Congenital abnormalities of the ears, nose, or throat
- Infection during pregnancy or delivery
- Hereditary disorders
- Maternal exposure to rubella or syphilis during pregnancy
- Prolonged fetal anoxia during delivery
- Toxicity
- Trauma during delivery
- Use of ototoxic drugs during pregnancy

Sudden hearing loss

- Acoustic neuroma
- Bacterial and viral infections
- Blood dyscrasias
- Ménière's disease
- Metabolic, vascular, or neurologic disorders
- Occlusion of internal auditory artery by spasm or thrombosis
- Ototoxic drugs
- Subclinical mumps

RISK FACTORS

AGE FACTOR *Premature or low-birth-weight neonates with congenital hearing loss are most likely to have structural or functional hearing impairments.*

- Neonates with serum bilirubin levels greater than 20 mg/dl (toxic effects on the brain)
- Erythroblastosis fetalis
- Maternal infection or drug abuse
- Frequent ear infections
- Use of headphones with loud music

INCIDENCE

- Hearing loss is the most common disability in the United States.
- It is the third most prevalent disorder in adults older than age 65.
- Presbycusis is prevalent in adults older than age 50.

COMPLICATIONS

- Tympanic membrane perforation
- Cholesteatoma
- Permanent hearing loss

HISTORY

- Deficient response to auditory stimuli within 2 to 3 days after birth
- Older child with hearing loss that impairs speech development
- Recent upper respiratory tract infection
- Use of ototoxic substances

Sudden deafness

- Recent exposure to loud noise
- Brief exposure to extremely loud noise
- Persistent tinnitus
- Transient vertigo

PHYSICAL FINDINGS

- Obvious hearing difficulty

DIAGNOSTIC TEST RESULTS

IMAGING
- Computed tomography scan shows vestibular and auditory pathways.
- Magnetic resonance imaging shows acoustic tumors and brain lesions.

DIAGNOSTIC PROCEDURES
- Auditory brain responses may show activity in the auditory nerve and the brain stem.
- Pure tone audiometry may show the presence and the degree of hearing loss.
- Electronystagmography may show the vestibular function involved with hearing loss.
- Otoscopic or microscopic examinations may show middle ear disorders and remove debris.
- Rinne and Weber's tests may show whether hearing loss is conductive or sensorineural.

OTHER
- Hearing evaluation may confirm diagnosis.

TREATMENT

GENERAL
- Varies with the type and cause of impairment
- Hearing aids or other effective means of aiding communication

ACTIVITY
- Avoidance of activities that allow water to enter ear, if eardrum perforated

MEDICATIONS
- Antibiotics
- Agents to dissolve cerumen
- Decongestants
- Analgesics
- Antipyretics
- Sedatives
- Antibiotic steroids

SURGERY
- Correction of tympanic membrane perforation

NURSING CONSIDERATIONS

NURSING DIAGNOSES
- Acute pain
- Anxiety
- Chronic low self-esteem
- Disturbed sensory perception (auditory)
- Fear
- Impaired verbal communication
- Ineffective coping
- Risk for infection
- Risk for injury

EXPECTED OUTCOMES
The patient will:
- express feelings of comfort
- identify strategies to reduce anxiety
- express positive feelings related to self-esteem
- regain hearing or develop other means of communication
- express fears and concerns
- effectively communicate feelings and needs
- express feelings about the disorder and exhibit adequate coping mechanisms
- exhibit no signs or symptoms of infection
- avoid injury.

NURSING INTERVENTIONS
- Face the patient when speaking and enunciate words clearly, slowly, and in a normal tone.
- Provide an alternative method of communication.
- Provide support to help the patient resist the urge to withdraw from social situations.

MONITORING
- Response to medications
- Progression of hearing loss
- Adaptation to hearing aid

PATIENT TEACHING

GENERAL
Be sure to cover:
- excessive noise exposure dangers
- exposure to drugs, chemicals, and infection dangers (with pregnancy)
- hearing loss, causes, and treatments
- how to instill otic medications
- lip-reading lessons
- medication use and possible adverse effects
- use and maintenance of hearing aid
- preoperative and postoperative instructions
- proper techniques for ear cleaning or irrigation
- tests and procedures
- using protective devices in a noisy environment.

DISCHARGE PLANNING
- If hearing deteriorates, refer the patient for speech and hearing rehabilitation.
- Refer a child to an audiologist or otolaryngologist for further evaluation.
- Refer the patient to special augmentation services for telephone use.
- Refer the patient to community resources, as appropriate.

RESOURCES
Organizations
Alexander Graham Bell Association for the Deaf, Inc.: *www.agbell.org*
National Institute on Deafness and Other Communication Disorders: *www.nidcd.nih.gov*

Selected references
Folmer, R.L. "Noise-induced Hearing Loss in Young People," *Pediatrics* 117(1): 248-49, January 2006.
Mamak, A., et al. "A Study of Prognostic Factors in Sudden Hearing Loss," *Ear, Nose, & Throat Journal* 84(10):641-44, October 2005.
Williams, D. "Does Irrigation of the Ear to Remove Impacted Wax Improve Hearing?" *British Journal of Community Nursing* 10(5):228-32, May 2005.
Wills, T. "Learning How to Communicate Better with Deafened Patients," *Nursing Times* 101(3):44, January 2005.

Heart failure LIFE-THREATENING DISORDER

OVERVIEW

- Fluid buildup in the heart from myo-cardium that can't provide sufficient cardiac output
- Usually occurs in a damaged left or right ventricle
- May result secondarily from left-sided heart failure

PATHOPHYSIOLOGY

Left-sided heart failure
- The pumping ability of the left ventricle fails and cardiac output falls. (See *Classifying heart failure.*)
- Blood backs up into the left atrium and lungs, causing pulmonary congestion.

Right-sided heart failure
- Ineffective contractile function of the right ventricle leads to blood backing up into the right atrium and the peripheral circulation, which results in peripheral edema and engorgement of the kidneys and other organs.

CAUSES

- Anemia
- Arrhythmias
- Atherosclerosis with myocardial infarction
- Constrictive pericarditis
- Emotional stress
- Hypertension
- Increased salt or water intake
- Infections
- Mitral or aortic insufficiency
- Mitral stenosis secondary to rheumatic heart disease, constrictive pericarditis, or atrial fibrillation
- Myocarditis
- Pregnancy
- Pulmonary embolism
- Thyrotoxicosis
- Ventricular and atrial septal defects

INCIDENCE

- Heart failure affects 1% of people older than age 50 and 10% of people older than age 80.

COMPLICATIONS

- Pulmonary edema
- Organ failure, especially the brain and kidneys
- Myocardial infarction

ASSESSMENT

HISTORY

- A disorder or condition that can precipitate heart failure
- Dyspnea or paroxysmal nocturnal dyspnea
- Peripheral edema
- Fatigue
- Weakness
- Insomnia
- Anorexia
- Nausea
- Sense of abdominal fullness (particularly in right-sided heart failure)
- Substance abuse

PHYSICAL FINDINGS

- Cough that produces pink, frothy sputum
- Cyanosis of the lips and nail beds
- Pale, cool, clammy skin
- Diaphoresis
- Jugular vein distention
- Ascites
- Tachycardia
- Pulsus alternans
- Hepatomegaly and, possibly, splenomegaly
- Decreased pulse pressure
- S_3 and S_4 heart sounds
- Moist, bibasilar crackles, rhonchi, and expiratory wheezing
- Decreased pulse oximetry
- Peripheral edema
- Decreased urinary output

DIAGNOSTIC TEST RESULTS

LABORATORY

- B-type natriuretic peptide immunoassay is elevated.

IMAGING

- Chest X-rays show increased pulmonary vascular markings, interstitial edema, or pleural effusion and cardiomegaly.

Classifying heart failure

Heart failure is classified according to its pathophysiology. It may be right- or left-sided, systolic or diastolic, and acute or chronic.

RIGHT-SIDED OR LEFT-SIDED

Right-sided heart failure is the result of ineffective right ventricular contraction. It may be caused by an acute right ventricular infarction or pulmonary embolus. However, the most common cause is profound backward flow due to left-sided heart failure.

Left-sided heart failure is the result of ineffective left ventricular contraction. It may lead to pulmonary congestion or pulmonary edema and decreased cardiac output. Left ventricular myocardial infarction, hypertension, and aortic and mitral valve stenosis or regurgitation are common causes. As the decreased pumping ability of the left ventricle persists, fluid accumulates, backing up into the left atrium and then into the lungs. If this worsens, pulmonary edema and right-sided heart failure may also result.

SYSTOLIC OR DIASTOLIC

In patients with systolic heart failure, the left ventricle can't pump enough blood out to the systemic circulation during systole and the ejection fraction falls. Consequently, blood backs up into the pulmonary circulation, pressure rises in the pulmonary venous system, and cardiac output falls.

In patients with diastolic heart failure, the left ventricle can't relax and fill properly during diastole and the stroke volume falls. Therefore, larger ventricular volumes are needed to maintain cardiac output.

ACUTE OR CHRONIC

Acute refers to the timing of the onset of symptoms and whether compensatory mechanisms kick in. Typically, fluid status is normal or low, and sodium and water retention don't occur.

In patients with chronic heart failure, signs and symptoms have been present for some time, compensatory mechanisms have taken effect, and fluid volume overload persists. Drug therapy, diet changes, and activity restrictions usually help control symptoms.

DIAGNOSTIC PROCEDURES

◆ Electrocardiography may reflect heart strain, enlargement, or ischemia. It may also reveal atrial enlargement, tachycardia, extrasystole, or atrial fibrillation.

◆ Pulmonary artery pressure monitoring typically may show elevated pulmonary artery and pulmonary artery wedge pressures, left ventricular end diastolic pressure in left-sided heart failure, and elevated right atrial or central venous pressure in right-sided heart failure.

TREATMENT

GENERAL
◆ Antiembolism stockings
◆ Elevation of lower extremities

DIET
◆ Sodium restriction
◆ Fluid restriction
◆ Calorie restriction, if indicated
◆ Low-fat, if indicated

ACTIVITY
◆ As tolerated (walking encouraged)

MEDICATIONS
◆ Diuretics
◆ Oxygen
◆ Inotropic drugs
◆ Vasodilators
◆ Angiotensin-converting enzyme inhibitors
◆ Angiotensin receptor blockers
◆ Cardiac glycosides
◆ Diuretics
◆ Potassium supplements
◆ Beta-adrenergic blockers
◆ Anticoagulants

SURGERY
◆ For valvular dysfunction with recurrent acute heart failure, surgical replacement
◆ Heart transplantation
◆ Ventricular assist device
◆ Stent placement

NURSING CONSIDERATIONS

NURSING DIAGNOSES
◆ Activity intolerance
◆ Decreased cardiac output
◆ Excess fluid volume
◆ Fatigue
◆ Imbalanced nutrition: Less than body requirements
◆ Impaired gas exchange
◆ Ineffective airway clearance
◆ Ineffective breathing pattern
◆ Ineffective tissue perfusion: Cardiopulmonary

EXPECTED OUTCOMES
The patient will:
◆ carry out activities of daily living without excess fatigue or decreased energy
◆ maintain adequate cardiac output
◆ develop no complications of fluid volume excess
◆ verbalize the importance of balancing activity with rest periods
◆ maintain adequate nutrition and hydration
◆ maintain adequate ventilation and oxygenation
◆ maintain a patent airway
◆ maintain an effective breathing pattern
◆ maintain hemodynamic stability.

NURSING INTERVENTIONS
◆ Place the patient in Fowler's position, and give supplemental oxygen.
◆ Provide continuous cardiac monitoring in acute and advanced stages.
◆ Assist the patient with range-of-motion exercises.
◆ Apply antiembolism stockings. Check for calf pain and tenderness.

MONITORING
◆ Daily weight for peripheral edema and other signs and symptoms of fluid overload
◆ Cardiac rhythm
◆ Intake and output
◆ Response to treatment
◆ Vital signs
◆ Mental status
◆ Peripheral edema

⚡ **WARNING** *Auscultate for abnormal heart and breath sounds, and report changes immediately.*

◆ Blood urea nitrogen and serum creatinine, potassium, sodium, chloride, and magnesium levels

PATIENT TEACHING

GENERAL
Be sure to cover:
◆ disorder, diagnosis, and treatment
◆ signs and symptoms of worsening heart failure
◆ when to notify the practitioner
◆ the importance of follow-up care
◆ the need to avoid high-sodium foods
◆ the need to avoid fatigue
◆ instructions about fluid restrictions
◆ the need to weigh himself every morning at the same time (before eating, after urinating); to keep record of weight, and to report weekly weight gain of 3 to 5 lb (1.5 to 2.5 kg)
◆ the importance of smoking cessation, if appropriate
◆ weight reduction, as needed
◆ medication administration, dosage, potential adverse effects, and monitoring needs.

DISCHARGE PLANNING
◆ Encourage follow-up care.
◆ Refer the patient to a smoking-cessation program, if appropriate.

RESOURCES
Organizations
American Heart Association: *www.americanheart.org*
Heart Failure Online: *www.heartfailure.org*

Selected references
D'Amico, C.L. "Cardiac Transplantation: Patient Selection in the Current Era," *Journal of Cardiovascular Nursing* 20(5 Suppl):S4-13, September-October 2005.
Jarcho, J.A. "Resynchronizing Ventricular Contraction in Heart Failure," *New England Journal of Medicine* 352(15):-1594-597, April 2005.
Tsukui, H., et al. "Biventricular Assist Device Utilization for Patients with Morbid Congestive Heart Failure: A Justifiable Strategy," *Circulation* 112(9 Suppl):I65-72, August 2005.

⚡Heat syndrome LIFE-THREATENING DISORDER

OVERVIEW

- Heat exhaustion — acute heat injury with hyperthermia caused by dehydration
- Heat stroke — extreme hyperthermia with thermoregulatory failure

PATHOPHYSIOLOGY

- Normal regulation of temperature is by evaporation (30% of body's heat loss) or vasodilation. When heat is generated or gained by the body faster than it can dissipate, the thermoregulatory mechanism is stressed and eventually fails.
- This causes hyperthermia to accelerate.
- Cerebral edema and cerebrovascular congestion occurs.
- Cerebral perfusion pressure increases and cerebral perfusion decreases.
- Tissue damage occurs when temperature exceeds 107.6° F (42° C), resulting in tissue necrosis, organ dysfunction, and failure.

CAUSES

- Behavior
- Dehydration
- Drugs, such as phenothiazines, anticholinergics, and amphetamines
- Endocrine disorders
- Excessive clothing
- Excessive physical activity
- Heart disease
- Hot environment without ventilation
- Illness
- Inadequate fluid intake
- Infection (fever)
- Lack of acclimatization
- Neurologic disorder
- Sudden discontinuation of Parkinson's disease medications

RISK FACTORS

- Obesity
- Salt and water depletion
- Alcohol use
- Poor physical condition
- Age
- Socioeconomic status

INCIDENCE

- This disorder affects men and women equally.
- Incidence rate increases among older patients and neonates during excessively hot summer days.

COMPLICATIONS

- Hypovolemic shock
- Cardiogenic shock
- Cardiac arrhythmias
- Renal failure
- Disseminated intravascular coagulation
- Hepatic failure

ASSESSMENT

HISTORY

Heat exhaustion
- Prolonged activity in a very warm or hot environment
- Muscle cramps
- Nausea and vomiting
- Thirst
- Weakness
- Headache
- Fatigue
- Sweating
- Tachycardia

Heat stroke
- Exposure to high temperature and humidity without air circulation
- Same signs as heat exhaustion
- Blurred vision
- Confusion
- Hallucinations
- Decreased muscle coordination
- Syncope

PHYSICAL FINDINGS
Heat exhaustion
- Rectal temperature greater than 100° F (37.8° C)
- Pale skin
- Thready, rapid pulse
- Cool, moist skin
- Decreased blood pressure
- Irritability
- Syncope
- Impaired judgment
- Hyperventilation

Heat stroke
- Rectal temperature of at least 104° F (40° C)
- Red, diaphoretic, hot skin in early stages
- Gray, dry, hot skin in later stages
- Tachycardia
- Slightly elevated blood pressure in early stages
- Decreased blood pressure in later stages
- Tachypnea
- Decreased level of consciousness
- Signs of central nervous system dysfunction
- Altered mental status
- Hyperpnea
- Cheyne-Stokes respirations
- Anhidrosis (late sign)

DIAGNOSTIC TEST RESULTS

LABORATORY
◆ Serum electrolytes are elevated, which may show hyponatremia and hypokalemia.
◆ Arterial blood gas levels may indicate respiratory alkalosis.
◆ Complete blood count may reveal leukocytosis and thrombocytopenia.
◆ Coagulation studies may show increased bleeding and clotting times.
◆ Urinalysis may show concentrated urine and proteinuria with tubular casts and myoglobinuria.
◆ Blood urea nitrogen may be elevated.
◆ Serum calcium level may be decreased.
◆ Serum phosphorus level may be decreased.
◆ Myoglobinuria may indicate rhabdomyolosis.

TREATMENT

GENERAL
Heat exhaustion
◆ Cool environment
◆ Oral or I.V. fluid administration

Heat stroke
◆ Lowering the body temperature as rapidly as possible
◆ Evaporation, hypothermia blankets, and ice packs to the groin, axillae, and neck
◆ Supportive respiratory and cardiovascular measures

DIET
◆ Increased hydration; cool liquids only
◆ Avoidance of caffeine and alcohol

ACTIVITY
◆ Rest periods, as needed

NURSING CONSIDERATIONS

NURSING DIAGNOSES
◆ Decreased cardiac output
◆ Deficient fluid volume
◆ Hyperthermia
◆ Impaired gas exchange
◆ Impaired home maintenance

EXPECTED OUTCOMES
The patient will:
◆ exhibit signs of adequate cardiac output
◆ express understanding of the need to maintain adequate fluid intake
◆ maintain a normal body temperature
◆ maintain adequate ventilation
◆ express understanding of how to prevent recurrent episodes of hyperthermia.

NURSING INTERVENTIONS
◆ Perform rapid cooling procedures.
◆ Provide supportive measures.
◆ Provide adequate fluid intake.
◆ Give prescribed drugs.

MONITORING
◆ Vital signs
◆ Pulse oximetry readings
◆ Complications
◆ Level of consciousness
◆ Cardiac rhythm
◆ Intake and output
◆ Myoglobin test results

PATIENT TEACHING

GENERAL
Be sure to cover:
◆ the disorder, diagnosis, and treatment
◆ how to avoid reexposure to high temperatures
◆ the need to maintain adequate fluid intake
◆ the need to wear loose clothing
◆ activity limitation in hot weather.

DISCHARGE PLANNING
◆ Refer the patient to social services, if appropriate.

RESOURCES
Organizations
National Center for Injury Prevention and Control: *www.cdc.gov/ncipc*
National Institutes of Health: *www.nih.gov*

Selected references
Auber, G. "Taking the Heat Off: How to Manage Heat Injuries," *Nursing* 34(7):50-52, July 2004.
Deleu, D., et al. "Downbeat Nystagmus Following Classical Heat Stroke," *Clinical Neurology and Neurosurgery* 108(1):102-104, December 2005.
Glazer, J.L. "Management of Heatstroke and Heat Exhaustion," *American Family Physician* 71(11):2133-140, June 2005.
Sucholeiki, R. "Heatstroke," *Seminars in Neurology: Tropical Neurology* 25(3): 307-14, September 2005.
Wolfson, A.B., et al. *Harwood-Nuss' Clinical Practice of Emergency Medicine,* 4th ed. Philadelphia: Lippincott Williams & Wilkins, 2005.

Hemophilia

OVERVIEW

- Hereditary bleeding disorder
- Characterized by greatly prolonged coagulation time
- Results from deficiency of specific clotting factors
- Hemophilia A (classic hemophilia): affects more than 80% of hemophiliacs; results from factor VIII deficiency
- Hemophilia B (Christmas disease): affects 15% of hemophiliacs; results from factor IX deficiency
- Incurable

PATHOPHYSIOLOGY

- A low level or absence of the blood protein necessary for clotting causes a disruption of the normal intrinsic coagulation cascade.
- Abnormal bleeding, which may be mild, moderate, or severe, depending on the degree of protein factor deficiency, is produced.
- After a platelet plug at a bleeding site, the lack of clotting factors impairs formation of a stable fibrin clot.
- Immediate hemorrhage isn't prevalent; delayed bleeding is common.

CAUSES

- Acquired immunologic process
- Hemophilia A and B inherited as X-linked recessive traits
- Spontaneous mutation

INCIDENCE

- This disease is the most common X-linked genetic disease.
- This disease occurs in about 1.25 of 10,000 live male births.

COMPLICATIONS

- Pain, swelling, extreme tenderness, and permanent joint and muscle deformity
- Peripheral neuropathies, pain, paresthesia, and muscle atrophy
- Ischemia and gangrene
- Shock and death

ASSESSMENT

HISTORY

- Familial history of bleeding disorders
- Prolonged bleeding with circumcision
- Concomitant illness
- Pain and swelling in a weight-bearing joint, such as the hip, knee, or ankle
- With mild hemophilia or after minor trauma, lack of spontaneous bleeding, but prolonged bleeding with major trauma or surgery
- Moderate hemophilia producing only occasional spontaneous bleeding episodes
- Severe hemophilia causing spontaneous bleeding
- Prolonged bleeding after surgery or trauma or joint pain in spontaneous bleeding into muscles or joints
- Signs of internal bleeding, such as abdominal, chest, or flank pain; episodes of hematuria or hematemesis; and tarry stools
- Activity or movement limitations and need for assistive devices, such as splints, canes, or crutches

PHYSICAL FINDINGS

- Hematomas on extremities, torso, or both
- Joint swelling in episodes of bleeding into joints
- Limited and painful joint range of motion in episodes of bleeding into joints

DIAGNOSTIC TEST RESULTS

LABORATORY

Hemophilia A
- Factor VIII assay is 25% of normal or less.
- Partial thromboplastin time (PTT) is prolonged.
- Platelet count and function, bleeding time, and prothrombin time are normal.

Hemophilia B
- Factor IX assay is deficient.
- Baseline coagulation results are similar to those of hemophilia A, but with normal factor VIII.

Hemophilia A or B
- Degree of factor deficiency defines severity:
- Mild hemophilia — factor levels 5% to 25% of normal
- Moderate hemophilia — factor levels 1% to 5% of normal
- Severe hemophilia — factor levels less than 1% of normal.

TREATMENT

GENERAL

- To quickly stop bleeding by increasing plasma levels of deficient clotting factors

DIET

- Foods high in vitamin K

ACTIVITY

- As guided by degree of factor deficiency

MEDICATIONS

- Aminocaproic acid (Amicar)

Hemophilia A
- Cryoprecipitated antihemophilic factor (AHF), lyophilized AHF, or both
- Desmopressin (Stimate)

Hemophilia B
- Factor IX concentrate

NURSING DIAGNOSES

- Activity intolerance
- Acute pain
- Anxiety
- Impaired physical mobility
- Ineffective coping
- Ineffective tissue perfusion: Cardio-pulmonary
- Powerlessness
- Risk for deficient fluid volume
- Risk for injury
- Social isolation

EXPECTED OUTCOMES

The patient will:

- verbalize the importance of balancing activity, as tolerated, with rest
- express feelings of increased comfort and decreased pain
- verbalize feelings of anxiety and fear
- maintain range of motion and joint mobility
- demonstrate adequate coping skills
- maintain hemodynamic stability
- express feelings of control over his well-being
- maintain an adequate fluid balance
- verbalize appropriate safety and preventive measures
- maintain existing social relationships.

NURSING INTERVENTIONS

- Follow standard precautions.
- Provide emotional support, and reassurance when indicated.

During bleeding episodes

- Apply pressure to bleeding sites.
- Give the deficient clotting factor or plasma, as ordered, until bleeding stops.
- Apply cold compresses or ice bags, and elevate the injured part.
- To prevent recurrence of bleeding, restrict activity for 48 hours after bleeding is under control.
- Control pain with prescribed analgesics.
- Avoid I.M. injections.
- Avoid aspirin and aspirin-containing drugs.

During bleeding into a joint

- Immediately elevate the joint.
- To restore joint mobility, begin range-of-motion exercises at least 48 hours after the bleeding is controlled.
- Restrict weight bearing until bleeding stops and swelling subsides.
- Give prescribed analgesics for pain.
- Apply ice packs and elastic bandages to alleviate pain.

MONITORING

- PTT
- Adverse reactions to blood products
- Signs and symptoms of decreased tissue perfusion
- Vital signs
- Bleeding from the skin, mucous membranes, and wounds

GENERAL

Be sure to cover:

- the benefits of regular isometric exercises
- how parents can protect their child from injury while avoiding unnecessary restrictions that impair normal development
- the avoidance of contact sports
- injury directions; for parents to apply cold compresses or ice bags and to elevate the injured part or apply light pressure to bleeding
- the need to notify the practitioner immediately after even a minor injury
- the need for parents to watch for signs of internal bleeding
- the importance of avoiding aspirin, combination medications that contain aspirin, and over-the-counter anti-inflammatory agents (use acetaminophen instead)
- the importance of good dental care and the need to check with the practitioner before dental extractions or surgery
- the need to wear medical identification at all times
- how to administer blood factor components at home, if appropriate

- the need to keep blood factor concentrate and infusion equipment available at all times
- adverse reactions that can result from replacement factor procedures
- signs, symptoms, and treatment of anaphylaxis
- the need for the patient or parents to watch for early signs of hepatitis
- the need to follow standard precautions.

DISCHARGE PLANNING

- Refer new patients to a hemophilia treatment center for evaluation.
- For more information, refer the patient's family to the National Hemophilia Foundation.

RESOURCES

Organizations

Centers for Disease Control and Prevention: *www.cdc.gov*

National Hemophilia Foundation: *www.hemophilia.org*

Selected references

Dunn, A.L. "Management and Prevention of Recurrent Hemarthrosis in Patients with Hemophilia," *Current Opinion in Hematology* 12(5):390-94, September 2005.

Kasper, D.L., et al., eds. *Harrison's Principles of Internal Medicine,* 16th ed. New York: McGraw-Hill Book Co., 2005.

Millier, K.L. "Factor Products in the Treatment of Hemophilia," *Journal of Pediatric Health Care* 18(3):156-57, May-June 2004.

Tierney, L., et al. *Current Medical Diagnosis and Treatment 2006.* New York: McGraw-Hill Book Co., 2006.

Hemorrhoids

OVERVIEW

- Varicosities found in the superior or inferior hemorrhoidal venous plexus
- Classified as first, second, third, or fourth degree, depending on their severity
- First-degree hemorrhoids: confined to the anal canal
- Second-degree hemorrhoids: prolapsed during straining but reduced spontaneously
- Third-degree hemorrhoids: prolapsed hemorrhoids that require manual reduction after each bowel movement
- Fourth-degree hemorrhoids: irreducible

PATHOPHYSIOLOGY

- Dilation and enlargement of the superior plexus of the superior hemorrhoidal veins above the dentate line cause internal hemorrhoids.
- Enlargement of the plexus of the inferior hemorrhoidal veins below the dentate line causes external hemorrhoids, which may protrude from the rectum. (See *Comparing types of hemorrhoids.*)

CAUSES

- Constipation, low-fiber diet
- Obesity
- Pregnancy
- Prolonged sitting
- Straining at defecation

INCIDENCE

- Hemorrhoids occur in both sexes.
- Most cases of hemorrhoids occur in people ages 20 to 50.

COMPLICATIONS

- Constipation
- Local infection
- Thrombosis of hemorrhoids
- Secondary anemia from severe or recurrent bleeding

ASSESSMENT

HISTORY

- Bright red blood on stool or toilet tissue
- Anal itching
- Vague feeling of anal discomfort
- Pain

PHYSICAL FINDINGS

- Prolapse of rectal mucosa
- Anal tenderness on palpation
- Internal hemorrhoids (with digital examination)

DIAGNOSTIC TEST RESULTS

DIAGNOSTIC PROCEDURES

- Anoscopy and flexible sigmoidoscopy may visualize internal hemorrhoids.

OTHER

- Physical examination findings may confirm diagnosis.

Comparing types of hemorrhoids

Covered by mucosa, internal hemorrhoids bulge into the rectal lumen and may prolapse during defecation. Covered by skin, external hemorrhoids protrude from the rectum and are more likely to thrombose than internal hemorrhoids. The illustrations below show both frontal and cross-sectional views.

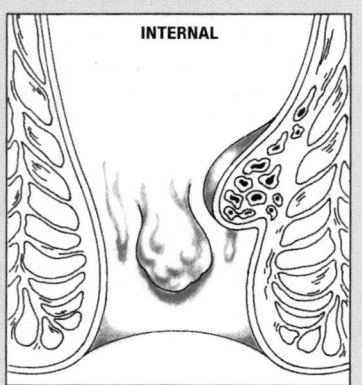

INTERNAL

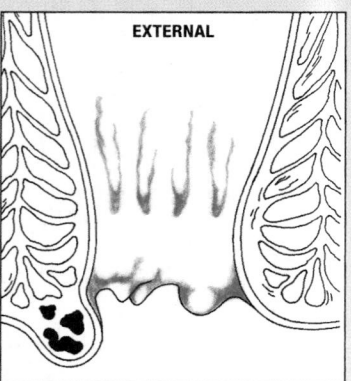

EXTERNAL

TREATMENT

GENERAL
◆ Warm sitz baths to relieve pain

DIET
◆ High-fiber, increased fluid intake

ACTIVITY
◆ Avoidance of prolonged sitting

MEDICATIONS
◆ Local anesthetic agents
◆ Hydrocortisone cream and suppositories

SURGERY
◆ Injection sclerotherapy or rubber band ligation
◆ Hemorrhoidectomy by cauterization or excision

NURSING CONSIDERATIONS

NURSING DIAGNOSES
◆ Acute pain
◆ Constipation
◆ Risk for infection

EXPECTED OUTCOMES
The patient will:
◆ express feelings of increased comfort
◆ regain normal bowel function
◆ remain free from signs and symptoms of infection.

NURSING INTERVENTIONS
◆ Give enemas preoperatively.
◆ Give prescribed drugs.
◆ Keep the wound site clean.
◆ Provide sitz baths.

MONITORING
◆ Bleeding
◆ Pain

PATIENT TEACHING

GENERAL
Be sure to cover:
◆ the importance of regular bowel habits and good anal hygiene
◆ avoiding too-vigorous wiping with washcloths and use of harsh soaps
◆ the use of medicated astringent pads and white, unscented toilet paper.

RESOURCES
Organizations
American Gastroenterological Association: *www.gastro.org*
Hemorrhoid Care Medical Clinic: *www.hemorrhoid.net*
Mayo Clinic: *www.mayoclinic.com*

Selected references

Alonso-Coello, P., et al. "Fiber for the Treatment of Hemorrhoids Complications: A Systematic Review and Meta-Analysis," *American Journal of Gastroenterology* 101(1):181-88, January 2006.

Fukuda, A., et al. "Colonoscopic Classification of Internal Hemorrhoids: Usefulness in Endoscopic Band Ligation," *Journal of Gastroenterology & Hepatology* 20(1):46-50, January 2005.

Scheyer, M., et al. "Doppler-guided Hemorrhoidal Artery Ligation," *American Journal of Surgery* 191(1):89-93, January 2006.

Hemothorax

OVERVIEW

- Blood in the pleural cavity
- May result in lung collapse

PATHOPHYSIOLOGY

- Damaged intercostal, pleural, mediastinal, and sometimes lung parenchymal vessels cause blood to enter the pleural cavity.
- The amount of bleeding and the cause is associated with varying degrees of lung collapse and mediastinal shift.

CAUSES

- Anticoagulant therapy
- Blunt or penetrating chest trauma
- Central venous catheter insertion
- Damaged intercostal, pleural, or mediastinal vessels
- Damaged parenchymal vessels
- Dissecting thoracic aneurysm
- Heart or thorax surgery
- Hereditary hemorrhagic telangiectasis
- Necrotizing infections
- Neoplasm
- Pulmonary arteriovenous fistulas
- Pulmonary infarction
- Thoracic endometriosis
- Tuberculosis

INCIDENCE

- This disease occurs in about 25% of patients with chest trauma.

COMPLICATIONS

- Mediastinal shift
- Ventilatory compromise
- Lung collapse
- Cardiopulmonary arrest
- Pneumothorax
- Empyema

ASSESSMENT

HISTORY

- Recent trauma
- Recent thoracic surgery
- Metastatic disease

PHYSICAL FINDINGS

- Tachypnea
- Dusky skin color
- Diaphoresis
- Hemoptysis
- Restlessness
- Anxiety
- Cyanosis
- Stupor
- Affected side may expand and stiffen
- Unaffected side may rise with gasping respirations
- Dullness over affected side
- Decreased or absent breath sounds over affected side
- Symptoms associated with blunt trauma
- Tachycardia
- Hypotension

DIAGNOSTIC TEST RESULTS

LABORATORY

- Pleural fluid analysis shows hematocrit greater than 50% of serum hematocrit.
- Arterial blood gas (ABG) analysis may show increased partial pressure of carbon dioxide and decreased partial pressure of oxygen.
- Serum hemoglobin level may be decreased, depending on blood loss.

IMAGING

- Chest X-rays and computed tomography scan of the thorax show presence and extent of hemothorax and helping to evaluate treatment.

DIAGNOSTIC PROCEDURES

- Thoracentesis may yield blood or serosanguineous fluid.

TREATMENT

GENERAL

- Stabilization of the patient's clinical condition
- Stoppage of bleeding
- Thoracentesis
- Insertion of chest tube
- Autotransfusion if blood loss approaches or exceeds 1 L (see *Using autotransfusion for chest wounds*)
- I.V. therapy

DIET

- As tolerated

ACTIVITY

- As tolerated

MEDICATIONS

- Oxygen
- Analgesics

SURGERY

- Thoracotomy if chest tube doesn't improve condition

NURSING CONSIDERATIONS

NURSING DIAGNOSES

- Acute pain
- Anxiety
- Deficient fluid volume
- Impaired gas exchange
- Ineffective breathing pattern
- Ineffective tissue perfusion: Cardiopulmonary
- Risk for infection

EXPECTED OUTCOMES

The patient will:

- express feelings of increased comfort and decreased pain
- express feelings of reduced anxiety
- maintain fluid volume balance
- maintain adequate ventilation and oxygenation
- maintain effective breathing pattern
- maintain adequate cardiopulmonary perfusion
- remain free from signs and symptoms of infection.

NURSING INTERVENTIONS

◆ Give prescribed drugs.
◆ Promote comfort and relaxation.
◆ Give prescribed oxygen.
◆ Give prescribed I.V. fluids and blood transfusions.
◆ Assist with thoracentesis.
◆ Prepare the patient for surgery, if needed.

◆ Change the chest tube dressing, and provide chest tube care, as needed.

MONITORING

◆ Vital signs
◆ Intake and output
◆ Chest tube drainage
◆ Central venous pressure
◆ ABG results
◆ Chest X-ray results
◆ Complete blood count results
◆ Respiratory status
◆ Complications
◆ Signs and symptoms of infection

GENERAL

Be sure to cover:
◆ the disorder, diagnosis, and treatment
◆ prescribed drugs and potential adverse effects
◆ when to notify the practitioner
◆ preoperative and postoperative care, if needed
◆ mechanical ventilation, if needed
◆ deep-breathing exercises
◆ smoking cessation, if appropriate.

RESOURCES
Organizations
American Thorax Society:
www.thoracic.org

Selected references
Mason, R.J., et al. *Murray and Nadel's Textbook of Respiratory Medicine,* 4th ed. Philadelphia: W.B. Saunders Co., 2005.
Wiklund, C.U., et al. "Misplacement of Central Vein Catheters in Patients with Hemothorax: A New Approach to Resolve the Problem," *Journal of Trauma-Injury Infection & Critical Care* 59(4):1029-1031, October 2005.
Yamamoto, L., et al. "Thoracic Trauma: The Deadly Dozen," *Critical Care Nursing Quarterly* 28(1):22-40, January-March 2005.

Using autotranfusion for chest wounds

Autotransfusion is used most often in patients with chest wounds, especially those that involve hemothorax. Through autotransfusion, a patient's own blood is collected, filtered, and reinfused. The procedure may also be used when two or three units of pooled blood can be recovered, such as in cardiac or orthopedic surgery.

Autotransfusion eliminates the patient's risk of transfusion reaction or blood-borne disease, such as cytomegalovirus, hepatitis, and human immunodeficiency virus. It's contraindicated in patients with sepsis or cancer.

HOW AUTOTRANSFUSION WORKS

A large-bore chest tube connected to a closed drainage system is used to collect the patient's blood from a wound or chest cavity. This blood passes through a filter, which catches most potential thrombi, including clumps of fibrin and damaged red blood cells (RBCs). The filtered blood passes into a collection bag. From the bag, the blood is reinfused immediately, or it may be processed in a commercial cell washer that reduces anticoagulated whole blood to washed RBCs for later infusion.

ASSISTING WITH AUTOTRANSFUSION

Set up the blood collection system as you would any closed chest drainage system. Attach the collection bag according to the manufacturer's instructions.

If ordered, inject an anticoagulant, such as heparin or acid-citrate-dextrose solution, into the self-sealing port on the connector of the patient's drainage tubing.

During reinfusion, monitor the patient for complications, such as blood clotting, hemolysis, coagulopathies, thrombocytopenia, particulate and air emboli, sepsis, and citrate toxicity (from the acid-citrate-dextrose solution).

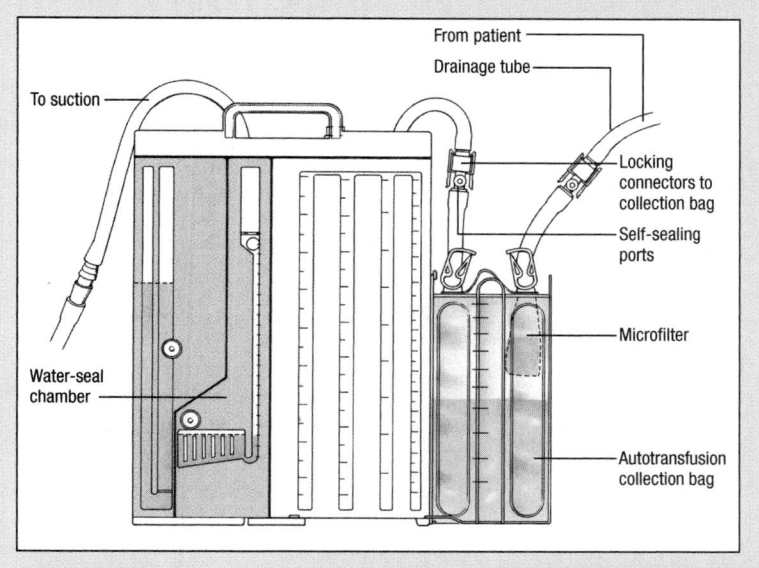

From patient
Drainage tube
To suction
Locking connectors to collection bag
Self-sealing ports
Microfilter
Water-seal chamber
Autotransfusion collection bag

⚡Hepatic encephalopathy LIFE-THREATENING DISORDER

OVERVIEW

- A neurologic syndrome that develops as a complication of aggressive fulminant hepatitis or chronic hepatic disease
- Most common in patients with cirrhosis
- In advanced stages, prognosis extremely poor despite vigorous treatment
- Acute form: occurs with acute fulminant hepatic failure, possibly fatal
- Chronic form: occurs with chronic liver disease, often reversible
- Also called *hepatic coma*

PATHOPHYSIOLOGY

- Normally, the ammonia produced by protein breakdown in the bowel is metabolized to urea in the liver. When portal blood shunts past the liver, ammonia directly enters the systemic circulation and is carried to the brain.
- Such shunting may result from the collateral venous circulation that develops in portal hypertension or from surgically created portal systemic shunts.
- Cirrhosis further compounds this problem because impaired hepatocellular function prevents conversion of ammonia that reaches the liver.

CAUSES

- Exact cause unknown
- Ammonia intoxication of the brain

RISK FACTORS

- Excessive protein intake
- Sepsis
- Excessive accumulation of nitrogenous body wastes (from constipation or GI hemorrhage)
- Bacterial action on protein and urea to form ammonia
- Hepatitis
- Diuretic therapy
- Alcoholism
- Fluid and electrolyte imbalance (especially metabolic alkalosis)
- Hypoxia
- Azotemia
- Impaired glucose metabolism

- Infection
- Use of sedatives, opioids, and general anesthetics

INCIDENCE

- This disease occurs in about 4 of 100,000 people.
- This disease is observed in 70% of patients with cirrhosis.

COMPLICATIONS

- Irreversible coma
- Death

ASSESSMENT

HISTORY
Prodromal stage

- Slight personality changes, such as agitation, belligerence, disorientation, and forgetfulness
- Trouble concentrating or thinking clearly
- Fatigue
- Mental changes, such as confusion and disorientation
- Sleep-wake reversal

Impending stage

- Mental changes, such as confusion and disorientation

Stuporous stage

- Marked mental confusion

Comatose stage

- Unable to arouse

PHYSICAL FINDINGS
Prodromal stage

- Slurred or slowed speech
- Slight tremor

Impending stage

- Tremors that have progressed to asterixis
- Lethargy
- Aberrant behavior
- Apraxia
- Possible incontinence

Stuporous stage

- Drowsy and stuporous
- Noisy and abusive when aroused
- Hyperventilation
- Muscle twitching
- Asterixis

Comatose stage

- Obtunded
- Seizures
- Hyperactive reflexes
- Positive Babinski's sign
- Fetor hepaticus (musty, sweet breath odor)

DIAGNOSTIC TEST RESULTS

LABORATORY
- Serum ammonia levels are elevated and, together with characteristic clinical features, strongly suggest hepatic encephalopathy.
- Serum bilirubin level is elevated.
- Prothrombin time is prolonged.

DIAGNOSTIC PROCEDURES
- Electroencephalography may show slowing waves as the disease progresses.

TREATMENT

GENERAL
- Elimination of underlying cause
- I.V. fluid administration
- Control of GI bleeding
- Life-support measures, if appropriate
- Bowel cleansing

DIET
- Limited protein intake
- Avoidance of alcohol
- Nothing by mouth, with decreased responsiveness
- Parenteral or enteric feedings, if appropriate

ACTIVITY
- Bed rest until condition improves

MEDICATIONS
- Lactulose (Cholac)
- Neomycin (Neo-fradin)
- Potassium supplements
- Salt-poor albumin

SURGERY
- Possible liver transplant

NURSING CONSIDERATIONS

NURSING DIAGNOSES
- Acute pain
- Anxiety
- Deficient fluid volume
- Diarrhea
- Disturbed thought processes
- Fear
- Imbalanced nutrition: Less than body requirements
- Ineffective tissue perfusion: GI, cerebral
- Risk for injury

EXPECTED OUTCOMES
The patient will:
- express feelings of increased comfort
- identify strategies to reduce anxiety
- have fluid volume return to normal parameters
- regain normal bowel function
- remain oriented to his environment
- discuss fears and concerns
- achieve adequate caloric and nutritional intake
- maintain adequate GI and cerebral perfusion
- avoid injury and complications.

NURSING INTERVENTIONS
- Promote rest, comfort, and a quiet atmosphere.
- Give prescribed drugs.
- Use appropriate safety measures to protect the patient from injury.
- Maintain skin integrity.
- Perform passive range-of-motion exercises.
- Provide emotional support.

MONITORING
- Level of consciousness
- Intake and output
- Fluid and electrolyte balance
- Weight and abdominal girth
- Signs of anemia, alkalosis, GI bleeding, and infection
- Serum ammonia level
- Changes in handwriting for progression of neurologic involvement

PATIENT TEACHING

GENERAL
Be sure to cover:
- the disorder, diagnosis, and treatment
- signs of complications or worsening symptoms
- dietary modifications
- medication administration, dosage, and possible adverse effects.

DISCHARGE PLANNING
- Refer the patient to social services, as indicated.

RESOURCES
Organizations
American Liver Foundation: *www.liverfoundation.org*
Digestive Disease National Coalition: *www.ddnc.org*
National Digestive Diseases Information Clearinghouse: *www.niddk.nih.gov/health/digest/nddic.htm*

Selected references
Amodio, P., and Gatta, A. "Neurophysiological Investigation of Hepatic Encephalopathy," *Metabolic Brain Disease* 20(4):369-79, December 2005.
Blei, A.T. "Albumin Dialysis for the Treatment of Hepatic Encephalopathy," *Journal of Gastroenterology & Hepatology* 19 (Suppl 7):S224-228, December 2004.
Handbook of Diseases, 3rd ed. Philadelphia: Lippincott Williams & Wilkins, 2004.

Hepatitis, nonviral

OVERVIEW

- Inflammation of the liver
- Classified as toxic or drug-induced (idiosyncratic)

PATHOPHYSIOLOGY

- Hepatocellular damage and necrosis are usually caused by toxins.
- Nonviral hepatitis occurs primarily in connection with acetaminophen overdose, and it's dose-dependent.

CAUSES

- Alcohol overuse
- Antibiotics
- Antidiabetic drugs
- Cholestatic reactions
- Cytotoxic drugs
- Direct hepatotoxicity
- Hormonal contraceptives or anabolic steroids
- Hypersensitivity to phenothiazine derivatives such as chlorpromazine
- Infectious agents
- Lack of bile excretion
- Metabolic and autoimmune disorders
- Thyroid medications

INCIDENCE

- Hepatitis can affect males and females (autoimmune hepatitis affects females more commonly).
- Hepatitis can occur at any age.

   WARNING *Carbon tetrachloride poisoning also produces headache, dizziness, drowsiness, and vasomotor collapse; halothane-related hepatitis produces fever, moderate leukocytosis, and eosinophilia; chlorpromazine produces a rash, abrupt fever, arthralgias, lymphadenopathy, and epigastric or right upper quadrant pain.*

COMPLICATIONS

- Fulminant hepatic failure
- Renal failure
- Liver fibrosis
- Cirrhosis

ASSESSMENT

HISTORY

- Causative agent
- Anorexia
- Nausea
- Vomiting
- Possibly abdominal pain
- Pruritus

PHYSICAL FINDINGS

- Jaundice
- Dark urine
- Hepatomegaly
- Clay-colored stools

DIAGNOSTIC TEST RESULTS

LABORATORY

- Serum aspartate aminotransferase and alanine aminotransferase levels are elevated.
- Total and direct bilirubin levels are elevated (with cholestasis).
- Alkaline phosphatase level is elevated.
- White blood cell count is elevated.
- Eosinophil count may be elevated in drug-induced nonviral hepatitis.

DIAGNOSTIC PROCEDURES

- A liver biopsy may help identify the underlying pathology.

GENERAL
◆ Removal of causative agent by lavage, catharsis, or hyperventilation, depending on the route of exposure

DIET
◆ Nutritious, with adequate fluid intake

ACTIVITY
◆ As tolerated

MEDICATIONS
◆ Acetylcysteine (Mucomyst) (acetaminophen poisoning)
◆ Corticosteroids (drug-induced hepatitis)

NURSING DIAGNOSES
◆ Acute pain
◆ Imbalanced nutrition: Less than body requirements

EXPECTED OUTCOMES
The patient will:
◆ express feelings of increased comfort and reduced levels of pain
◆ maintain adequate caloric and nutritional intake.

NURSING INTERVENTIONS
◆ Give prescribed drugs.
◆ Provide emotional support.

MONITORING
◆ Response to treatment
◆ Laboratory values
◆ Vital signs
◆ Complications

GENERAL
Be sure to cover:
◆ the disorder, diagnosis, and treatment
◆ medication administration, dosage, and possible adverse effects
◆ proper handling of cleaning agents and solvents.

DISCHARGE PLANNING
◆ Encourage follow-up care.

RESOURCES
Organizations
American Liver Foundation: *www.liverfoundation.org*
Digestive Disease National Coalition: *www.ddnc.org*
National Digestive Diseases Information Clearinghouse: *www.niddk.nih.gov/health/digest/nddic.htm*

Selected references
Diseases, 4th ed. Philadelphia: Lippincott Williams & Wilkins, 2006.
Ho, C., et al. "Side Effects Related to Cancer Treatment: CASE 1. Hepatitis Following Treatment with Gefitinib," *Journal of Clinical Oncology* 23(33): 8531-533, November 2005.
Strategies for Managing Multisystem Disorders. Philadelphia: Lippincott Williams & Wilkins, 2005.

Hepatitis, viral

- Infection and inflammation of the liver caused by a virus
- Six types recognized (A, B, C, D, E, and G) and a seventh suspected
- Marked by hepatic cell destruction, necrosis, and autolysis, leading to anorexia, jaundice, and hepatomegaly
- Recovery possible in most patients, because hepatic cells eventually regenerate with little or no residual damage
- Complications more likely with old age and serious underlying disorders
- Prognosis poor if edema and hepatic encephalopathy develop

PATHOPHYSIOLOGY

- Hepatic inflammation caused by the virus leads to diffuse injury and necrosis of hepatocytes.
- Hypertrophy and hyperplasia of Kupffer cells and sinusoidal lining cells occurs.
- Bile obstruction may occur.

CAUSES

- Infection with the causative viruses for each of six major forms of viral hepatitis

Type A

- Transmittal by the fecal-oral or parenteral route
- Ingestion of contaminated food, milk, or water

Type B

- Transmittal by contact with contaminated human blood, secretions, and stool

Type C

- Transmittal primarily through needles shared by I.V. drug users or used in tattooing, through blood transfusions, or through nose-sharing paraphernalia used for sniffing cocaine

Type D

- Found only in patients with an acute or a chronic episode of hepatitis B

Type E

- Transmittal by parenteral route and commonly water-borne

Type G

- Thought to be blood-borne, with transmission similar to that of hepatitis B and C

INCIDENCE

Hepatitis A

- Hepatitis A occurs in nationwide epidemics.

Hepatitis B

- About 1.25 million Americans are chronically infected with hepatitis B.
- The highest rate of disease occurs in people ages 20 to 49.

Hepatitis C

- About 3.9 million Americans are chronically infected with hepatitis C.

COMPLICATIONS

- Life-threatening fulminant hepatitis
- Chronic active hepatitis (in hepatitis B)
- Syndrome resembling serum sickness, characterized by arthralgia or arthritis, rash, and angioedema; can lead to misdiagnosis of hepatitis B as rheumatoid arthritis or lupus erythematosus (in hepatitis B)
- Primary liver cancer (in hepatitis B or C)
- In hepatitis D, mild or asymptomatic form of hepatitis B that flares into severe, progressive chronic active hepatitis and cirrhosis

HISTORY

- No signs or symptoms in 50% to 60% of people with hepatitis B
- No signs or symptoms in 80% of people with hepatitis C
- Revelation of a source of transmission

Prodromal stage

- Patient easily fatigued, with generalized malaise
- Anorexia, mild weight loss
- Depression
- Headache, photophobia
- Weakness
- Arthralgia, myalgia (hepatitis B)
- Nausea or vomiting
- Changes in the senses of taste and smell

Clinical jaundice stage

- Pruritus
- Abdominal pain or tenderness
- Indigestion
- Anorexia
- Possible jaundice of sclerae, mucous membranes, and skin

Posticteric stage

- Most symptoms decreasing or subsided

PHYSICAL FINDINGS

Prodromal stage

- Fever (100° to 102° F [37.8° to 38.9° C])
- Dark urine
- Clay-colored stools

Clinical jaundice stage

- Rashes, erythematous patches, or hives
- Abdominal tenderness in the right upper quadrant
- Enlarged and tender liver
- Splenomegaly
- Cervical adenopathy

Posticteric stage

- Decrease in liver enlargement

LABORATORY

- In suspected viral hepatitis, routine hepatitis profile identifies antibodies specific to the causative virus, establishing the type of hepatitis:
- – Type A — Detection of an antibody to hepatitis A confirms the diagnosis.
- – Type B — The presence of hepatitis B surface antigens and hepatitis B antibodies confirms the diagnosis.
- – Type C — The diagnosis depends on serologic testing for the specific antibody one or more months after the

onset of acute illness; until then, diagnosis is principally established by obtaining negative test results for hepatitis types A, B, and D.
–   Type D — Detection of intrahepatic delta antigens or immunoglobulin (Ig) M antidelta antigens in acute disease (or IgM and IgG in chronic disease) establishes the diagnosis.
–   Type E — Detection of hepatitis E antigens support the diagnosis.
–   Type G — Detection of hepatitis G ribonucleic acid supports the diagnosis (serologic assays are being developed).
◆   Additional findings from liver function studies support the diagnosis:
–   Serum aspartate aminotransferase and serum alanine aminotransferase levels are increased in the prodromal stage of acute viral hepatitis.
–   Serum alkaline phosphatase levels are slightly increased.
–   Serum bilirubin level is elevated; level may stay elevated late in the disease, especially with severe disease.
–   Prothrombin time is prolonged (more than 3 seconds longer than normal), indicating severe liver damage.
–   White blood cell counts commonly reveal transient neutropenia and lymphopenia, followed by lymphocytosis.

DIAGNOSTIC PROCEDURES
◆   A liver biopsy may show chronic hepatitis.

TREATMENT

GENERAL
For hepatitis C
◆   Aimed at clearing hepatitis C from the body, stopping or slowing hepatic damage, and relieving symptoms
◆   Symptomatic
◆   Parenteral feeding, if appropriate

DIET
◆   Small, high-calorie, high-protein meals (reduced protein intake if signs of precoma — lethargy, confusion, mental changes — develop)
◆   Avoidance of alcohol

ACTIVITY
◆   Frequent rest periods, as needed
◆   Avoidance of contact sports and strenuous activity

MEDICATIONS
◆   Standard immunoglobulin
◆   Vaccine
◆   Alfa-2b interferon (hepatitis B and C)
◆   Antiemetics
◆   Cholestyramine (Questran)
◆   Lamivudine (Epivir) (hepatitis B)
◆   Ribavirin (Virazole) (hepatitis C)

SURGERY
◆   Possible liver transplant (hepatitis C)

NURSING CONSIDERATIONS

NURSING DIAGNOSES
◆   Activity intolerance
◆   Anxiety
◆   Fear
◆   Imbalanced nutrition: Less than body requirements
◆   Risk for infection
◆   Risk for injury

EXPECTED OUTCOMES
The patient will:
◆   perform activities of daily living within the confines of the disease process
◆   identify strategies to reduce anxiety
◆   discuss fears and concerns
◆   achieve adequate caloric and nutritional intake
◆   remain free from signs and symptoms of infection
◆   avoid complications.

NURSING INTERVENTIONS
◆   Observe standard precautions to prevent transmission of the disease.
◆   Provide rest periods during the day.
◆   Give prescribed drugs.
◆   Encourage oral fluid intake.

MONITORING
◆   Hydration and nutritional status
◆   Daily weight
◆   Intake and output
◆   Stool for color, consistency, amount, and frequency
◆   Signs of complications

PATIENT TEACHING

GENERAL
Be sure to cover:
◆   the disorder, diagnosis, and treatment
◆   measures to prevent the spread of disease
◆   the importance of rest and a proper diet
◆   the need to abstain from alcohol
◆   medication administration, dosage, and possible adverse effects
◆   the need to avoid over-the-counter medications unless approved by the practitioner
◆   the need for follow-up care.

DISCHARGE PLANNING
◆   Refer the patient to Alcoholics Anonymous, if indicated.

RESOURCES
Organizations
Alcoholics Anonymous:
   www.alcoholics-anonymous.org
American Liver Foundation:
   www.liverfoundation.org
Digestive Disease National Coalition:
   www.ddnc.org
National Digestive Diseases Information Clearinghouse:
   www.niddk.nih.gov/health/digest/ nddic.htm

Selected references
Handbook of Diseases, 3rd ed. Philadelphia: Lippincott Williams & Wilkins, 2004.
Keller, S., et al. "Hepatitis C Prevention with Nurses," *Nursing & Health Sciences* 7(2):99-106, June 2005.
Kerbleski, M. "Hepatitis C: Are You Confused? Issues Related to Patient Education," *Gastroenterology Nursing* 28(3 Suppl):S19-23, May-June 2005.
Smith, D.R., and Leggat, P.A. "Needlestick and Sharps Injuries among Nursing Students," *Journal of Advanced Nursing* 51(5):449-55, September 2005.
Tierney, L., et al. *Current Medical Diagnosis and Treatment 2006.* New York: McGraw-Hill Book Co., 2006.

Hereditary hemorrhagic telangiectasia LIFE-THREATENING DISORDER

OVERVIEW

- Inherited vascular disorder of the blood vessels that can cause excessive bleeding
- Also called *Osler Weber-Rendu disease*

PATHOPHYSIOLOGY

- Venules and capillaries dilate to form fragile masses of thin convoluted vessels (telangiectases), resulting in an abnormal tendency to hemorrhage.

CAUSES

- Autosomal dominant inheritance

INCIDENCE

- Hereditary hemorrhagic telangiectasia occurs in 1 in 50,000 births.
- This disease affects both sexes but may cause less severe bleeding in females.

COMPLICATIONS

- Secondary iron deficiency anemia
- Vascular malformation causing pulmonary arteriovenous fistulas (rare)
- Recurring cerebral embolism and brain abscess
- Hemorrhagic shock
- Intracranial hemorrhage

ASSESSMENT

HISTORY

- Established familial pattern of bleeding disorders
- Epistaxis, hemoptysis, or tarry stools
- Appearance of telangiectasia during late childhood or adolescence

PHYSICAL FINDINGS

- Localized aggregations of dilated capillaries on the skin of the face, ears, tongue, lips, conjunctivae, scalp, hands, arms, and feet and under the nails
- Characteristic telangiectases: violet, bleed spontaneously, flat or raised, blanch on pressure, and nonpulsatile
- Signs of capillary fragility (may exist without overt telangiectasia): Spontaneous bleeding, petechiae, ecchymoses, and spider hemangiomas of varying size (see *Typical lesions of hereditary hemorrhagic telangiectasia*)
- Clubbing of the digits

DIAGNOSTIC TEST RESULTS

LABORATORY

- Platelet count may be abnormal.
- Complete blood count and anemia panel may show hypochromic, microcytic anemia.

IMAGING

- Chest X-rays may show arteriovenous malformation.
- Echocardiography may show "high-output" cardiac failure.

DIAGNOSTIC PROCEDURES

- Bone marrow aspiration may show depleted iron stores and confirms secondary iron deficiency anemia.

Typical lesions of hereditary hemorrhagic telangiectasia

These illustrations below show the commonly encountered lesions of hereditary hemorrhagic telangiectasia.

Dilated flat or raised capillaries appear in localized aggregations, as on the fingers.

On the face, spider hemangiomas reflect capillary fragility.

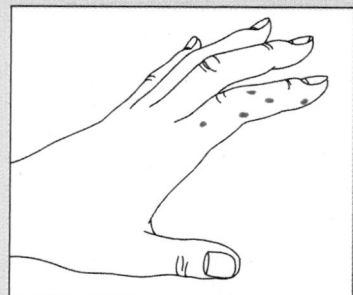
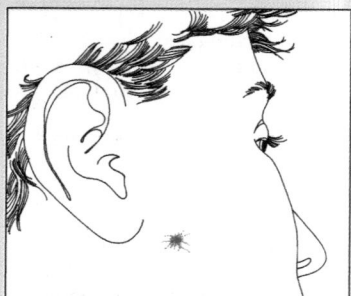

TREATMENT

GENERAL
- Supportive therapy, including blood transfusions and supplemental iron administration
- Ancillary treatment consisting of applying pressure and topical hemostatic agents to bleeding sites, cauterizing bleeding sites not readily accessible, and protecting the patient from trauma and unnecessary bleeding
- Laser treatment to destroy vessel

ACTIVITY
- Avoidance of activities with the potential for trauma

MEDICATIONS
- Parenteral iron
- Antipyretics or antihistamines

NURSING CONSIDERATIONS

NURSING DIAGNOSES
- Activity intolerance
- Anxiety
- Disturbed body image
- Impaired skin integrity
- Ineffective tissue perfusion: Cardiopulmonary
- Risk for deficient fluid volume
- Risk for infection

EXPECTED OUTCOMES
The patient will:
- verbalize the importance of balancing activity, as tolerated, with rest
- verbalize measures to reduce anxiety level
- express positive feelings about self
- experience improvement or healing of wounds and lesions
- maintain hemodynamic stability
- exhibit signs of adequate fluid balance
- remain free from signs and symptoms of infection.

NURSING INTERVENTIONS
- Provide emotional and psychological support.
- Give prescribed blood transfusions.
- Encourage fluid intake if the patient is bleeding or hypovolemic.
- Provide meticulous skin care and hygiene.
- Use aseptic technique when caring for the patient.

MONITORING
- Vital signs
- Intake and output
- Signs of febrile or allergic transfusion reaction
- Indications of GI bleeding
- Laboratory values to detect possible renal, hepatic, or respiratory failure

PATIENT TEACHING

GENERAL
Be sure to cover:
- the disorder, signs and symptoms, and treatment
- iron supplements, including the importance of following dosage instructions and of taking oral iron with meals to minimize GI irritation
- a warning that iron turns stools dark green or black and may cause constipation
- the management of minor bleeding episodes, especially recurrent epistaxis
- how to recognize major bleeding episodes that require emergency intervention.

DISCHARGE PLANNING
- Refer the patient for genetic counseling, as appropriate.

RESOURCES
Organizations
Mayo Clinic: *www.mayoclinic.com*
National Heart, Lung, and Blood Institute: *www.nhlbi.nih.gov*

Selected references
Gallitelli, M., et al. "Emergencies in Hereditary Haemorrhagic Telangiectasia," *QJM* 99(1):15-22, January 2006.

Kasper, D.L., et al., eds. *Harrison's Principles of Internal Medicine*, 16th ed. New York: McGraw-Hill Book Co., 2005.

Nguyen, N.Q. "Hereditary Hemorrhagic Telangiectasia," *Dermatology Online Journal* 11(4):19, December 2005.

Post, M.C., et al. "A Pulmonary Right-to-Left Shunt in Patients with Hereditary Hemorrhagic Telangiectasia is Associated with an Increased Prevalence of Migraine," *Chest* 128(4):2485-489, October 2005.

Tierney, L., et al. *Current Medical Diagnosis and Treatment 2006.* New York: McGraw-Hill Book Co., 2006.

Hernia, hiatal

OVERVIEW

- Defect in the diaphragm that permits a portion of the stomach to pass through the diaphragmatic opening into the chest
- Three types: sliding hernia, paraesophageal (rolling) hernia, and mixed hernia (sliding and rolling hernia)

PATHOPHYSIOLOGY

Sliding hernia

- The muscular collar around the esophageal and diaphragmatic junction loosens.
- Increased intra-abdominal pressure causes the lower portion of the esophagus and the upper portion of the stomach to rise into the chest.

Paraesophageal hernia

- The stomach isn't properly anchored below the diaphragm.
- Increased intra-abdominal pressure causes the upper portion of the stomach to slide through the esophageal hiatus.

CAUSES

Sliding hernia

- Aging
- Chronic esophagitis
- Diaphragmatic malformations that can cause congenital weakness
- Esophageal carcinoma, kyphoscoliosis, trauma, or surgery

Paraesophageal hernia

- Not fully understood

RISK FACTORS

- Obesity
- Smoking
- Pregnancy
- Presence of ascites

INCIDENCE

- The sliding hernia is 3 to 10 times more common than paraesophageal and mixed hernias combined.
- The incidence rate for this disorder increases with age.

- By age 60, 60% of people have hiatal hernias.
- This disorder is more prevalent in women than in men.

COMPLICATIONS

- Esophageal stricture
- Incarceration (with paraesophageal hernia)
- In association with gastroesophageal reflux disease:
  - Esophagitis
  - Esophageal ulceration and perforation
  - Hemorrhage
  - Peritonitis
  - Mediastinitis
  - Aspiration
  - Strangulation and gangrene of herniated portion of stomach
- Iron deficiency anemia
- Chronic cough
- Dysphagia

ASSESSMENT

HISTORY

- Heartburn 1 to 4 hours after eating; aggravated by reclining, belching, or conditions that increase intra-abdominal pressure
- Regurgitation or vomiting
- Retrosternal or substernal chest pain (typically after meals or at bedtime)
- Feeling of fullness after eating
- Feeling of breathlessness or suffocation
- Chest pain resembling angina pectoris
- Reflux
- Chronic cough
- Belching

PHYSICAL FINDINGS

- Possibly none
- Dysphagia

DIAGNOSTIC TEST RESULTS

LABORATORY

- Serum hemoglobin level and hematocrit are decreased with paraesophageal hernia, if bleeding from esophageal ulceration is present.
- Results of fecal occult blood test may be positive.
- Analysis of gastric contents may reveal blood.

IMAGING

- Chest X-rays reveal an air shadow behind the heart in a large hernia; lower lobe infiltrates with aspiration.
- Barium swallow with fluoroscopy detects a hiatal hernia and diaphragmatic abnormalities.

DIAGNOSTIC PROCEDURES

- Endoscopy and biopsy results identify the mucosal junction and the edge of the diaphragm indenting the esophagus; differentiate hiatal hernia, varices, erosions, ulcers, Barrett's esophagus, and other small gastroesophageal lesions; and rule out malignant tumors.
- Esophageal motility studies reveal esophageal motor or lower esophageal pressure abnormalities before surgical repair of the hernia.
- pH studies identify reflux of gastric contents.
- Acid perfusion (Bernstein) test identifies esophageal reflux.

TREATMENT

GENERAL
- Smoking cessation (smoking stimulates gastric acid production)
- Weight reduction, as appropriate

DIET
- Six small meals per day
- No fluids or food 1 to 2 hours before bedtime
- Elimination of spicy or irritating foods, alcohol, and coffee

ACTIVITY
- Upright posture for 2 to 3 hours after eating
- Restriction of activities that increase intra-abdominal pressure

MEDICATIONS
- Antacids
- Histamine-2 receptor antagonists
- Cholinergics
- Motility agents
- Antiemetics
- Cough suppressants

SURGERY
- Hernia repair (rare)

NURSING CONSIDERATIONS

NURSING DIAGNOSES
- Acute pain
- Imbalanced nutrition: Less than body requirements
- Impaired swallowing
- Risk for aspiration

EXPECTED OUTCOMES
The patient will:
- express feelings of increased comfort
- achieve adequate caloric and nutritional intake
- swallow without choking or coughing
- show no evidence of aspiration.

NURSING INTERVENTIONS
- Prepare the patient for diagnostic tests.
- Teach positional therapy.
- If surgery is necessary, provide appropriate preoperative and postoperative care.

MONITORING
WARNING *After endoscopy, watch for signs of perforation, including decreasing blood pressure, rapid pulse, shock, and sudden pain.*
- Patient response to prescribed antacids and other medications

PATIENT TEACHING

GENERAL
Be sure to cover:
- the disorder, diagnosis, and treatment
- developing a dietary plan
- sitting upright after meals and snacks
- situations or activities that increase intra-abdominal pressure
- desired drug actions and potential adverse effects
- sleeping with the head of the bed elevated about 6" (15 cm).

DISCHARGE PLANNING
- Refer the patient to a smoking-cessation program, if appropriate.
- Refer the patient to a weight-reduction program, if appropriate.

RESOURCES
Organizations
American Gastroenterological Association: *www.gastro.org*
International Foundation for Functional Gastrointestinal Disorders: *www.iffgd.org*
National Digestive Diseases Information Clearinghouse: *www.niddk.nih.gov/health/digest/nddic.htm*

Selected references
Agrawal, A., et al. "Identification of Hiatal Hernia by Esophageal Manometry: Is It Reliable?" *Diseases of the Esophagus* 18(5):316-19, October 2005.
Handbook of Diseases, 3rd ed. Philadelphia: Lippincott Williams & Wilkins, 2004.
Stylopoulos, N., and Rattner, D.W. "The History of Hiatal Hernia Surgery: From Bowditch to Laparoscopy," *Annals of Surgery* 241(1):185-93, January 2005.
Yamada, T., et al. *Atlas of Gastroenterology,* 3rd ed. Philadelphia: Lippincott Williams & Wilkins, 2003.

Herniated intervertebral disk

OVERVIEW

- Rupture of fibrocartilaginous material that surrounds the intervertebral disk, allowing protrusion of the nucleus pulposus
- Results in pressure on spinal nerve roots or spinal cord that causes back pain and other symptoms of nerve root irritation
- Most common site for herniation L4-L5 disk space; other sites L5-S1, L2-L3, L3-L4, C6-C7, and C5-C6
- Clinical manifestations determined by:
  - Location and size of the herniation into the spinal canal
  - Amount of space that exists inside the spinal canal
- Also known as *herniated nucleus pulposus, slipped disk*, or *ruptured disk*

PATHOPHYSIOLOGY

- The ligament and posterior capsule of the disk are usually torn, allowing the nucleus pulposus to extrude, compressing the nerve root.
- Occasionally, the injury tears the entire disk loose, causing protrusion onto the nerve root or compression of the spinal cord.
- Large amounts of extruded nucleus pulposus or complete disk herniation of the capsule and nucleus pulposus may compress the spinal cord.

CAUSES

- Degenerative disk disease
- Direct injury
- Improper lifting or twisting
- Obesity

RISK FACTORS

- Advanced age
- Congenitally small lumbar spinal canal
- Osteophytes along the vertebrae
- Work environment

INCIDENCE

- About 90% of those who have this disorder are affected in the lumbar and lumbosacral spine, 8% are affected in the cervical spine, and 1% to 2% are affected in thoracic spine.
- Lumbar herniation is more common in people ages 20 to 45.
- Cervical herniation is more common in people ages 45 and older.
- Herniated disks are more common in men than in women.

COMPLICATIONS

- Neurologic deficits
- Bowel and bladder dysfunction
- Sexual dysfunction

ASSESSMENT

HISTORY

- Previous traumatic injury or back strain
- Unilateral, lower back pain
- Pain that may radiate to the buttocks, legs, and feet
- Pain that may begin suddenly, subside in a few days, and then recur at shorter intervals with progressive intensity
- Sciatic pain beginning as a dull ache in the buttocks, worsening with Valsalva's maneuver, coughing, sneezing, or bending
- Pain that may subside with rest

Two tests for a herniated disk

The straight-leg-raising test and its variant, Lasègue's sign, are perhaps the best tests to perform when a herniated disk is suspected.

STRAIGHT-LEG-RAISING TEST

Have the patient lie in a supine position. Place one hand on the patient's ilium to stabilize the pelvis and the other hand under the patient's ankle. Slowly raise the patient's leg. If the patient complains of posterior leg (sciatic) pain — *not back pain* — suspect a herniated disk.

LASÈGUE'S SIGN

To do this test, have the patient lie in a supine position with his thigh and knee flexed (to a 90-degree angle). Resistance and pain as well as loss of ankle or knee-jerk reflex indicate spinal root compression.

- Muscle spasms
- Chronic repetitive injury

PHYSICAL FINDINGS

- Limited ability to bend forward (see *Two tests for a herniated disk*)
- Posture favoring the affected side
- Gait difficulty
- Muscle atrophy, in later stages
- Constipation or incontinence
- Urgency difficulties or incontinence
- Tenderness over the affected region
- Radicular pain with straight leg raising in lumbar herniation
- Increased pain with neck movement in cervical herniation
- Referred upper trunk pain with cervical neck compression
- Weakness in affected area

DIAGNOSTIC TEST RESULTS

IMAGING

- X-rays of the spine show degenerative changes.
- Myelography shows the level of the herniation.
- Computed tomography scan shows bone and soft-tissue abnormalities; can also show spinal canal compression.
- Magnetic resonance imaging shows soft-tissue abnormalities.

OTHER

- Electromyography measures muscle response to nerve stimulation.
- Nerve conduction studies show sensory and motor loss.

TREATMENT

GENERAL

- Initial treatment conservative and symptomatic, unless neurologic impairment progresses rapidly
- Possible traction
- Supportive devices such as a brace
- Heat or ice applications
- Transcutaneous electrical nerve stimulation
- Chemonucleolysis

DIET
◆ As tolerated

ACTIVITY
◆ Avoidance of repetitive activity
◆ Bed rest, initially
◆ Prescribed exercise program
◆ Physical therapy

MEDICATIONS
◆ Nonsteroidal anti-inflammatory drugs
◆ Steroids
◆ Muscle relaxants
◆ Analgesics

SURGERY
◆ Laminectomy
◆ Spinal fusion
◆ Microdiskectomy

NURSING CONSIDERATIONS

NURSING DIAGNOSES
◆ Activity intolerance
◆ Anxiety
◆ Chronic pain
◆ Dressing or grooming self-care deficit
◆ Fear
◆ Impaired physical mobility
◆ Risk for injury

EXPECTED OUTCOMES
The patient will:
◆ perform activities of daily living (ADLs) without excessive fatigue or pain
◆ identify strategies to reduce anxiety
◆ express feelings of comfort and decreased pain
◆ perform ADLs within the confines of the disorder
◆ discuss fears and concerns
◆ achieve the highest level of mobility possible within the confines of the disorder
◆ remain free from injury.

NURSING INTERVENTIONS
◆ Give prescribed drugs.
◆ Plan a pain-control regimen.
◆ Offer supportive care.
◆ Provide encouragement.

◆ Help the patient cope with chronic pain and impaired mobility.
◆ Include the patient and his family in all phases of his care.
◆ Encourage the patient to express his concerns.
◆ Encourage performance of self-care.
◆ Help the patient to identify activities that promote rest and relaxation.
◆ Prepare the patient for myelography, if indicated.
◆ Periodically remove traction to inspect skin.
◆ Prevent deep vein thrombosis.
◆ Prevent footdrop.
◆ Ensure a consistent regimen of leg and back-strengthening exercises.
◆ Encourage adequate oral fluid intake.
◆ Encourage coughing and deep-breathing exercises.
◆ Provide meticulous skin care.
◆ Provide a fracture bedpan for the patient on complete bed rest.

⚡ **WARNING** *During conservative treatment, watch for a deterioration in neurologic status, especially during the first 24 hours after admission, which may indicate an urgent need for surgery.*

After surgery
◆ Enforce bed rest, as ordered.
◆ Use the logrolling technique to turn the patient.
◆ Assist the patient during his first attempt to walk.
◆ Provide a straight-backed chair for the patient to sit in briefly.

MONITORING
◆ Vital signs
◆ Intake and output
◆ Pain control
◆ Mobility
◆ Motor strength
◆ Deep vein thrombosis
◆ Bowel and bladder function

After surgery
◆ Blood drainage system
◆ Drainage
◆ Incisions
◆ Dressings
◆ Neurovascular status
◆ Bowel sounds and abdominal distention

PATIENT TEACHING

GENERAL
Be sure to cover:
◆ the disorder, diagnosis, and treatment
◆ prescribed drugs and potential adverse effects
◆ when to notify the practitioner
◆ bed rest
◆ traction
◆ heat application
◆ the exercise program
◆ myelography, if indicated
◆ preoperative and postoperative care, if indicated
◆ relaxation techniques
◆ proper body mechanics
◆ skin care.

DISCHARGE PLANNING
◆ Refer the patient to physical therapy, if indicated.
◆ Refer the patient to occupational therapy, if indicated.
◆ Refer the patient to a weight-reduction program, if appropriate.

RESOURCES
Organizations
American Academy of Orthopaedic Surgeons: *www.aaos.org*
American College of Sports Medicine: *www.acsm.org*
American Physical Therapy Association: *www.apta.org*

Selected references
Jansson, K.A., et al. "Health-related Quality of Life in Patients Before and After Surgery for a Herniated Lumbar Disc," *Journal of Bone and Joint Surgery* (British volume) 87(7):959-64, July 2005.
Puschak, T.J., and Sasso, R.C. "Use of Artificial Disc Replacement in Degenerative Conditions of the Cervical Spine," *Current Opinion in Orthopedics* 15(3):175-79, June 2004.
Strayer, A. "Lumbar spine: Common Pathology and Interventions," *Journal of Neuroscience Nursing* 37(4):181-93, August 2005.

Herpes simplex

- Common viral infection that may be latent for years
- After initial herpes simplex virus (HSV) infection, causes patient to become carrier susceptible to recurrent attacks
- Recurrent infections provoked by fever, menses, stress, heat, cold, lack of sleep, sun exposure, and contact with reactivated disease (kissing, sharing cosmetics, sexual intercourse)

PATHOPHYSIOLOGY

- Virus enters mucosal surfaces or abraded skin sites and initiates replication in cells of the epidermis and dermis.
- Replication continues to permit infection of sensory or autonomic nerve endings.
- Virus enters the neuronal cell and is transported intra-axonally to nerve cell bodies in ganglia (where the virus establishes latency) and spreads by the peripheral sensory nerves. (See *Understanding the herpes cycle*, page 302.)

CAUSES

- Type 1 (HSV-1) — *Herpesvirus hominis* transmitted primarily by contact with oral secretions; mainly affects oral, labial, ocular, or skin tissues
- Type 2 (HSV-2) — *Herpesvirus hominis* transmitted primarily by contact with genital secretions; mainly affects genital structures

INCIDENCE

- This disease occurs worldwide and equally in males and females.
- Lower socioeconomic groups are infected more often, probably because of crowded living conditions.
- Infection with HSV-1 is more common and occurs earlier in life than infection with HSV-2.

COMPLICATIONS

- Primary (or initial) HSV infection during pregnancy leading to abortion, premature labor, microcephaly, and uterine growth retardation
- Congenital herpes transmitted during vaginal birth, producing a subclinical neonatal infection or severe infection with seizures, chorioretinitis, skin vesicles, and hepatosplenomegaly
- HSV-1 causing life-threatening nonepidemic encephalitis in infants
- Gingivostomatitis in children ages 1 to 3
- Blindness from ocular infection
- Increased risk for cervical cancer
- Urethral stricture from recurrent genital herpes
- Perianal ulcers
- Colitis
- Esophagitis (more frequent in the impaired host)
- Pneumonitis
- Neurologic disorders
- Uremia with multiple organ involvement

HISTORY

- Oral, vaginal, or anal sexual contact with an infected person or other direct contact with lesions
- With recurrent infection, various precipitating factors identified

PHYSICAL FINDINGS

Primary perioral HSV

- Sore throat, fever, anorexia, adenopathy
- Increased salivation
- Severe mouth pain, halitosis
- Small erythematous vesicles on pharyngeal or oral mucosa

Primary genital HSV

- Malaise, tender inguinal nodes, adenopathy
- Dysuria, leukorrhea
- Dyspareunia
- Fluid-filled vesicles on the cervix, labia, perianal skin, vulva, and vagina; glans penis, foreskin, and penile shaft
- Extragenital lesions possible on the mouth or anus

Primary ocular infection

- Photophobia, excessive tearing
- Follicular conjunctivitis, chemosis
- Blepharitis, vesicles on eyelids
- Lethargy and fever
- Regional adenopathy

LABORATORY

- Tissue culture shows isolation of virus (gold standard).
- Staining of scrapings from the base of the lesion demonstrates characteristic giant cells or intranuclear inclusions of herpes virus infection.
- Tissue analysis shows HSV antigens or DNA in scrapings from lesions.

TREATMENT

GENERAL
- Symptomatic and supportive therapy
- Ophthalmologist treatment for eye infections

DIET
- Avoidance of acidic foods (with stomatitis)

ACTIVITY
- Abstinence from sexual activity during active phase (with genital lesions)

MEDICATIONS
- Antipyretics and analgesics
- Anesthetic mouthwashes
- Bicarbonate-based mouth rinse
- Drying agents
- Ophthalmic drugs
- Antivirals
- Docosanol (Abreva)

NURSING CONSIDERATIONS

NURSING DIAGNOSES
- Acute pain
- Impaired oral mucous membrane
- Impaired skin integrity
- Impaired social interaction
- Ineffective sexuality patterns
- Powerlessness
- Risk for infection
- Risk for injury
- Social isolation

EXPECTED OUTCOMES
The patient will:
- express feelings of increased comfort and decreased pain
- exhibit no complications related to trauma to oral mucous membranes
- exhibit improved or healed lesions or wounds
- resume effective communication patterns with his spouse or partner
- voice feelings about potential or actual changes in sexuality
- verbalize feelings of control and hope about his medical condition
- experience no further signs or symptoms of infection
- remain free from complications
- maintain relationships with family and friends.

NURSING INTERVENTIONS
- Observe standard precautions.
- Give prescribed drugs.
- Encourage the patient to express his feelings, and provide support.

MONITORING
- Response to treatment
- Adverse reactions to medications
- Complications
- Lesions
- Fluid and electrolyte balance

PATIENT TEACHING

GENERAL
Be sure to cover:
- the disorder, diagnosis, and treatment
- proper hand-washing technique
- the recommended use of lip balm with sunscreen (with oral lesions)
- instructions to keep lesions dry, except for applying prescribed topical drugs
- information about medication administration, dosage, and possible adverse effects
- the use of sunscreen to prevent skin-induced recurrences
- the recommendation that sexual partners be screened for sexually transmitted diseases (with genital herpes)
- for a patient with genital herpes, the recommendation to use warm compresses or take sitz baths several times per day and avoid sexual contact during outbreaks of active infection.

DISCHARGE PLANNING
- Refer the patient with an eye infection to an ophthalmologist.
- Refer the patient to a support group such as the Herpes Resource Center, as appropriate.
- If child abuse is suspected, make a report to local authorities and social services.

RESOURCES
Organizations
Centers for Disease Control and Prevention: *www.cdc.gov*
Harvard University Consumer Health Information: *www.intelihealth.com*
The Herpes Resource Center: *www.herpesresourcecenter.com*
National Health Information Center: *www.health.gov/nhic/*
National Library of Medicine: *www.nlm.nih.gov*

Selected references
Ensor, D. "The Significance of Herpes Simplex for School Nurses," *Journal of School Nursing* 21(1):10-16, February 2005.
Novak, N., and Peng, W.M. "Dancing with the Enemy: The Interplay of Herpes Simplex Virus with Dendritic Cells," *Clinical & Experimental Immunology* 142(3):405-10, December 2005.
Rodrigues, F., et al. "Herpes Simplex Virus Esophagitis in Immunocompetent Children," *Journal of Pediatric Gastroenterology & Nutrition* 39(5):560-63, November 2004.

Herpes zoster

- Acute unilateral and segmental inflammation of dorsal root ganglia that remains in people who have had chickenpox
- Also called *shingles*

PATHOPHYSIOLOGY

- Herpes zoster erupts when the virus reactivates after dormancy in the cerebral ganglia (extramedullary ganglia of the cranial nerves) or the ganglia of posterior nerve roots.
- The virus may multiply as it reactivates, and antibodies remaining from the initial infection may neutralize it.
- Without opposition from effective antibodies, the virus continues to multiply in the ganglia, destroys neurons, and spreads down the sensory nerves to the skin, causing localized vascular eruptions.

CAUSES

- Dormant varicella zoster virus (herpesvirus that also causes chickenpox) that reactivates

INCIDENCE

- This virus is most common in adults ages 50 to 70.
- Bone marrow transplant patients are especially at risk.
- People who had chickenpox at a young age may be at a higher risk.

COMPLICATIONS

- Deafness
- Bell's palsy
- Secondary skin infection
- Postherpetic neuralgia
- Meningoencephalitis
- Cutaneous dissemination
- Ocular involvement with facial zoster
- Hepatitis
- Pneumonitis
- Peripheral motor weakness
- Guillain-Barré syndrome
- Cranial nerve syndrome

HISTORY

- Typically no history of exposure to others with the varicella zoster virus
- Fever
- Malaise
- Pain that mimics appendicitis
- Pleurisy
- Musculoskeletal pain
- Severe, deep pain
- Pruritus
- Paresthesia or hyperesthesia (usually affecting the trunk and occasionally the arms and legs)

PHYSICAL FINDINGS

- Small, red, vesicular skin lesions spread unilaterally around the thorax or vertically over the arms or legs
- Vesicles possibly filled with clear fluid or pus
- Vesicles drying, forming scabs, or even becoming gangrenous (see *A look at herpes zoster*)
- Enlarged regional lymph nodes

Geniculate involvement

- Vesicle formation in the external auditory canal and ipsilateral facial palsy
- Hearing loss, dizziness, and loss of taste

Trigeminal involvement

- Eye pain
- Corneal and scleral damage and impaired vision
- Conjunctivitis, extraocular weakness, ptosis, and paralytic mydriasis
- Secondary glaucoma

LABORATORY

- Vesicular fluid and infected tissue analyses show eosinophilic intranuclear inclusions and varicella virus.
- Staining antibodies from vesicular fluid and identification under fluorescent light aids differentiation of herpes zoster from herpes simplex virus.
- Specific antibody immune globulin measurement of varicella antibodies is elevated.
- Cerebrospinal fluid analysis demonstrates increased protein levels and, possibly, pleocytosis.

DIAGNOSTIC PROCEDURES

- Lumbar puncture may indicate increased pressure.

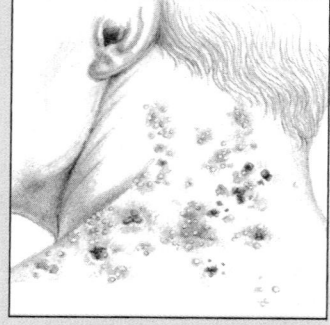

A look at herpes zoster

These characteristic herpes zoster lesions are fluid-filled vesicles that dry and form scabs after about 10 days. Unilateral vesicular lesions in a dermatomal pattern should rapidly lead to a diagnosis of herpes zoster.

TREATMENT

GENERAL
◆ Transcutaneous peripheral nerve stimulation for postherpetic neuralgia
◆ Soothing baths
◆ Cold compresses

MEDICATIONS
◆ Antivirals
◆ Antipruritics
◆ Analgesics
◆ Tricyclic antidepressants
◆ Demulcent and skin protectant
◆ Systemic antibiotic
◆ Corticosteroids
◆ Tranquilizers and sedatives
◆ Patient-controlled analgesia

NURSING CONSIDERATIONS

NURSING DIAGNOSES
◆ Acute pain
◆ Disturbed body image
◆ Impaired skin integrity
◆ Impaired social interaction
◆ Risk for infection

EXPECTED OUTCOMES
The patient will:
◆ express feelings of increased comfort and relief from pain
◆ acknowledge change in body image
◆ exhibit improved or healed lesions or wounds
◆ demonstrate effective social interaction skills in one-on-one and group settings
◆ experience no further signs or symptoms of infection.

NURSING INTERVENTIONS
◆ Give prescribed drugs.
◆ Maintain meticulous hygiene to prevent spreading the infection to other parts of the patient's body.
◆ With open lesions, follow contact isolation precautions to prevent the spread of infection.

MONITORING
◆ Response to treatment
◆ Adverse reaction to medications
◆ Lesions
◆ Signs and symptoms of infection

PATIENT TEACHING

GENERAL
Be sure to cover:
◆ the use of a soft toothbrush, use of a saline- or bicarbonate-based mouthwash and oral anesthetics to decrease discomfort from oral lesions, and the advice to eat soft foods
◆ the need for meticulous hygiene to prevent spreading infection to other body parts
◆ the need to avoid scratching lesions
◆ application of a cold compress if vesicles rupture
◆ local treatment of vesicles.

DISCHARGE PLANNING
◆ Refer the patient to an ophthalmologist for ocular involvement.
◆ Refer the patient to a pain management specialist for postherpetic neuralgia.

RESOURCES
Organizations
Centers for Disease Control and Prevention: *www.cdc.gov*
Harvard University Consumer Health Information: *www.intelihealth.com*
National Health Information Center: *www.health.gov/nhic/*
National Library of Medicine: *www.nlm.nih.gov*

Selected references
Bielan, B. "What's Your Assessment? Herpes Zoster," *Dermatology Nursing* 16(5):431-32, October 2004.
Crider, E.F. "Herpes Zoster," *New England Journal of Medicine* 348(20):2044-2045, May 2003.
Kasper, D.L., et al., eds. *Harrison's Principles of Internal Medicine,* 16th ed. New York: McGraw-Hill Book Co., 2005.
Sandy, M.C. "Herpes Zoster: Medical and Nursing Management," *Clinical Journal of Oncology Nursing* 9(4):443-46, August 2005.
Wung, P.K., et al. "Herpes Zoster in Immunocompromised Patients: Incidence, Timing, and Risk Factors," *American Journal of Medicine* 118(12):1416, December 2005.

Hip fracture LIFE-THREATENING DISORDER

OVERVIEW

- Break in the head or neck of the femur (usually the head)
- Most common fall-related injury resulting in hospitalization
- Leading cause of disability among older adults
- May permanently change level of functioning and independence
- Fatal in almost 25% of patients within 1 year following fracture

PATHOPHYSIOLOGY

- With bone fracture, the periosteum and blood vessels in the marrow, cortex, and surrounding soft tissues are disrupted.
- This results in bleeding from the damaged ends of the bone and from the neighboring soft tissue.
- Clot formation occurs within the medullary canal, between the fractured bone ends, and beneath the periosteum.
- Bone tissue immediately adjacent to the fracture dies, and the necrotic tissue causes an intense inflammatory response.
- Vascular tissue invades the fracture area from surrounding soft tissue and marrow cavity within 48 hours, increasing blood flow to the entire bone.
- Bone-forming cells in the periosteum, endosteum, and marrow are activated to produce subperiosteal procallus along the outer surface of the shaft and over the broken ends of the bone.
- Collagen and matrix, which become mineralized to form callus, are synthesized by osteoblasts within the procallus.
- During the repair process, remodeling occurs; unnecessary callus is resorbed, and trabeculae are formed along stress lines.
- New bone, not scar tissue, is formed over the healed fracture.

CAUSES

- Cancer metastasis
- Falls
- Osteoporosis
- Skeletal disease
- Trauma

INCIDENCE

- Hip fracture affects more than 200,000 people each year.
- This disorder occurs in one of five women by age 80.
- This disorder is more common in females than in males.
- This disorder is more common in white females than in non-white females.

COMPLICATIONS

- Pneumonia
- Venous thrombosis
- Pressure ulcers
- Social isolation
- Depression
- Bladder dysfunction
- Deep vein thrombosis
- Pulmonary embolus
- Hip dislocation
- Death

ASSESSMENT

HISTORY

- Falls or trauma to the bones
- Pain in the affected hip and leg
- Pain worsened by movement

PHYSICAL FINDINGS

- Outward rotation of affected extremity
- Affected extremity possibly appearing shorter
- Limited or abnormal range of motion (ROM)
- Edema and discoloration of the surrounding tissue
- In an open fracture, bone protruding through the skin

DIAGNOSTIC TEST RESULTS

IMAGING

- X-rays show the location of the fracture.
- Computed tomography scan shows abnormalities in complicated fractures.

TREATMENT

GENERAL

- Depends on age, comorbidities, cognitive functioning, support systems, and functional ability
- Possible skin traction
- Non-weight-bearing transfers

DIET

- Well-balanced
- Foods rich in vitamins C and A, calcium, and protein
- Adequate vitamin D

ACTIVITY

- Bed rest, initially
- Ambulation as soon as possible after surgery
- Physical therapy

MEDICATIONS

- Analgesics

SURGERY

- Total hip arthroplasty
- Hemiarthroplasty
- Percutaneous pinning
- Internal fixation using a compression screw and plate

NURSING DIAGNOSES
- Acute pain
- Anxiety
- Dressing or grooming self-care deficit
- Fear
- Impaired physical mobility
- Impaired skin integrity
- Ineffective coping
- Ineffective role performance
- Ineffective tissue perfusion: Peripheral
- Risk for infection
- Risk for injury

EXPECTED OUTCOMES
The patient will:
- verbalize feelings of increased comfort
- express feelings of decreased anxiety
- perform self-care activities to the fullest extent possible
- verbalize fears and concerns
- attain the highest degree of mobility possible within the confines of the injury
- maintain skin integrity
- demonstrate effective coping mechanisms
- carry out previous roles within the limitations of the condition
- exhibit signs of adequate peripheral perfusion
- exhibit no signs or symptoms of infection
- identify factors that increase the potential for injury.

NURSING INTERVENTIONS
- Give prescribed drugs.
- Give prescribed prophylactic anticoagulation after surgery.
- Maintain traction.
- Maintain proper body alignment and posturing.
- Use logrolling techniques to turn the patient in bed.
- Maintain non-weight-bearing status.
- Increase the patient's activity level, as prescribed.
- Consult physical therapy as early as possible.
- Assist with active ROM exercises to unaffected limbs.
- Encourage coughing and deep-breathing exercises.
- Keep the patient's skin clean and dry.
- Prevent skin breakdown.
- Encourage good nutrition; offer high-protein, high-calorie snacks.
- Perform daily wound care.

⚡ **WARNING** *Don't massage the patient's legs and feet to promote circulation because this could increase the risk of thromboembolism.*

MONITORING
- Vital signs
- Intake and output
- Pain
- Mobility and ROM
- Incision and dressings
- Complications
- Coagulation study results
- Signs of bleeding
- Neurovascular status
- Skin integrity
- Signs and symptoms of infection

⚡ **WARNING** *Following surgery, assess the patient for complications, such as deep vein thrombosis, pulmonary embolus, and hip dislocation.*

GENERAL
Be sure to cover:
- the disorder, diagnosis, and treatment
- prescribed drugs and potential adverse effects
- ROM exercises
- meticulous skin care
- proper body alignment
- wound care
- signs of infection
- coughing and deep-breathing exercises and incentive spirometry
- assistive devices
- activity restrictions and lifestyle changes
- safe ambulation practices
- nutritious diet and adequate fluid intake.

DISCHARGE PLANNING
- Refer the patient to physical and occupational therapy programs, as indicated.
- Refer the patient to home health or intermediate care.

RESOURCES
Organizations
American Academy of Orthopaedic Surgeons: *www.aaos.org*
Mayo Clinic: *www.mayoclinic.com*
The Merck Manuals Online Medical Library: *www.merck.com/mmhe*

Selected references
Cole, A. "Nurse-administered Femoral Nerve Block After Hip Fracture," *Nursing Times* 101(37):34-36, September 2005.

Latham, N.K., et al. "Pattern of Functional Change During Rehabilitation of Patients with Hip Fracture," *Archives of Physical Medicine and Rehabilitation* 87(1):111-16, January 2006.

Wald, H., et al. "Extended Use of Indwelling Urinary Catheters in Postoperative Hip Fracture Patients," *Medical Care* 43(10):1009-1017, October 2005.

Williams, A., and Jester, R. "Delayed Surgical Fixation of Fractured Hips in Older People: Impact on Mortality," *Journal of Advanced Nursing* 52(1):63-69, October 2005.

Hirschsprung's disease

- Congenital disorder of the large intestine characterized by the absence or marked reduction of parasympathetic ganglion cells in the colorectal wall
- Usually coexists with other congenital anomalies, particularly trisomy 21 and anomalies of the urinary tract such as megaloureter
- Also called *congenital megacolon* and *congenital aganglionic megacolon*

PATHOPHYSIOLOGY
- Parasympathetic ganglion cells in the colorectal wall are absent or markedly reduced in number.
- The aganglionic bowel segment contracts without the reciprocal relaxation needed to propel feces forward.
- Impaired intestinal motility causes severe, intractable constipation.
- Colonic obstruction can ensue, causing bowel dilation and subsequent occlusion of surrounding blood and lymphatics.
- Ensuing mucosal edema, ischemia, and infarction draw large amounts of fluid into the bowel, causing copious amounts of liquid stool.
- Continued infarction and destruction of the mucosa can lead to infection and sepsis.

CAUSES
- Familial congenital defect

INCIDENCE
- This disorder occurs in 1 in 2,000 to 1 in 5,000 live births.
- Hirschsprung's disease is up to seven times more common in males than in females (although the aganglionic segment is usually shorter in males).
- Hirschsprung's disease is most prevalent in whites.
- Both sexes are equally affected by total aganglionosis.
- Females with Hirschsprung's disease are at higher risk for having affected children.

COMPLICATIONS
- Bowel perforation
- Electrolyte imbalances
- Nutritional deficiencies
- Enterocolitis
- Hypovolemic shock
- Sepsis

HISTORY
- Familial history of difficult stool passage
- Failure to pass meconium within the first 24 to 48 hours after birth
- Vomiting of bile-stained or fecal contents
- Anorexia
- Nausea
- Lethargy
- Constipation

PHYSICAL FINDINGS
- Distended abdomen
- Tachypnea
- Rectum without stools

IMAGING
- Barium enema reveals a narrowed segment of distal colon with a saw-toothed appearance and a funnel-shaped segment above it.
- Upright plain abdominal X-rays shows marked colonic distention.

DIAGNOSTIC PROCEDURES
- A rectal biopsy may confirm the diagnosis by showing the absence of ganglion cells.
- A rectal manometry may detect failure of the internal anal sphincter to relax and contract.

GENERAL

◆ Daily colonic lavage (to empty the infant's bowel until the time of surgery)

DIET

◆ Oral feeding with breast milk or predigested formula when bowel sounds return (infants)

⚡ **WARNING** *Without prompt treatment, an infant with colonic obstruction may die within 24 hours from enterocolitis that leads to severe diarrhea and hypovolemic shock.*

SURGERY

◆ Corrective surgery to pull the normal ganglionic segment through to the anus (usually delayed until the infant is at least age 10 months)
◆ Temporary colostomy or ileostomy to compress the colon in instances of total bowel obstruction

NURSING DIAGNOSES

◆ Constipation
◆ Deficient fluid volume
◆ Imbalanced nutrition: Less than body requirements
◆ Risk for impaired parenting
◆ Risk for impaired skin integrity
◆ Risk for infection

EXPECTED OUTCOMES

The patient (or parents) will:
◆ have bowel function return to normal patterns
◆ attain and maintain normal fluid and electrolyte balance
◆ maintain adequate caloric intake
◆ participate in the infant's care as much as possible (parents)
◆ maintain skin integrity
◆ exhibit no signs or symptoms of infection.

NURSING INTERVENTIONS

◆ Maintain fluid and electrolyte balance and prevent shock.
◆ Provide adequate nutrition and hydrate with I.V. fluids, as needed.
◆ Relieve respiratory distress by keeping the patient in an upright position.

After colostomy or ileostomy

◆ Place the infant in a heated incubator, with the temperature set at 98° to 99° F (36.7° to 37.2° C), or in a radiant warmer.

MONITORING

◆ Vital signs
◆ Signs of sepsis and enterocolitis
◆ Intake and output
◆ Laboratory values

GENERAL

Be sure to cover:
◆ recognizing the signs of fluid loss, dehydration, and enterocolitis
◆ withholding foods that have increased the number of stools previously
◆ that complete continence may take several years to develop and that constipation may recur at times
◆ participating in the child's care as much as possible, if appropriate.

DISCHARGE PLANNING

◆ Refer the parents to an enterostomal therapist for information on ostomy care.

RESOURCES

Organizations

Mayo Clinic: *www.mayoclinic.com*
National Digestive Diseases Information Clearinghouse: *www.niddk.nih.gov/health/digest/nddic.htm*
National Organization for Rare Disorders: *www.rarediseases.org*

Selected references

Brooks, A.S., et al. "Studying the Genetics of Hirschsprung's Disease: Unraveling an Oligogenic Disorder," *Clinical Genetics* 67(1):6-14, January 2005.
Hyman, P.E. "Defecation Disorders after Surgery for Hirschsprung's Disease," *Journal of Pediatric Gastroenterology & Nutrition* 41 (Suppl 1):S62-63, September 2005.
Murphy, F., and Puri, P. "New Insights into the Pathogenesis of Hirschsprung's Associated Enterocolitis," *Pediatric Surgery International* 21(10):773-79, October 2005.

Histoplasmosis

- Fungal infection
- Three forms in the United States
- Primary acute histoplasmosis
- Progressive disseminated histoplasmosis (acute disseminated or chronic disseminated disease)
- Chronic pulmonary (cavitary) histoplasmosis
- Also known as *Ohio Valley disease, Central Mississippi Valley disease, Appalachian Mountain disease*, and *Darling's disease*

PATHOPHYSIOLOGY

- Spores reach alveoli and are transformed into budding forms, carried to regional lymphatics, and then disseminated throughout the body.
- Intense granulomatous reaction occurs and caseation necrosis or calcification (resembling tuberculosis) occurs.
- Transient dissemination can leave granulomas in the spleen.

CAUSES

- *Histoplasma capsulatum*, which is found in the stool of birds and bats and in soil contaminated by their stool (near roosts, chicken coops, barns, caves, and underneath bridges)
- Transmitted to humans by inhalation of *H. capsulatum* or *H. capsulatum var. duboisii* spores or invasion of spores after minor skin trauma

INCIDENCE

- This disease occurs worldwide but most commonly in temperate areas of Asia, Africa, Europe, and North and South America.
- In the United States, it's most prevalent in southeastern, mid-Atlantic, and central states.
- Primary acute histoplasmosis is most common in infants, young children, and immunocompromised patients.

COMPLICATIONS

- Vascular or bronchial obstruction
- Acute pericarditis
- Pleural effusion
- Mediastinal fibrosis or granuloma
- Intestinal ulceration
- Addison's disease
- Endocarditis
- Meningitis

ASSESSMENT

HISTORY

- Possible history of an immunocompromised condition
- Exposure to contaminated soil in an endemic area

PHYSICAL FINDINGS

- Fever, which may rise as high as 105° F (40.6° C)

Primary acute histoplasmosis

- Usually no characteristic signs
- Mild respiratory illness, cough
- Malaise, headache, myalgia, anorexia
- Chest pain

Progressive disseminated histoplasmosis

- Anorexia and weight loss
- Pain
- Hoarseness, tachypnea in later stages
- Ulceration of the oropharynx, dysphagia
- Pallor from anemia
- Jaundice and ascites
- Hepatosplenomegaly
- Lymphadenopathy

Chronic pulmonary histoplasmosis

- Productive cough, dyspnea, hemoptysis
- Shortness of breath, cyanosis
- Extreme weakness, weight loss
- Upper lobe fibrocavitary pneumonia

DIAGNOSTIC TEST RESULTS

LABORATORY

- Blood cultures done by lysis-centrifugation technique reveal organism causing the infection.
- In disseminated histoplasmosis, culture of bone marrow, mucosal lesions, liver, and bronchoalveolar lavage may show organism causing the infection.
- Sputum cultures are preferred in chronic pulmonary histoplasmosis; they may take 2 to 4 weeks to show growth of the organism.
- Radioactive assay for histoplasma antigen in blood or urine shows presence of histoplasma antigen.

IMAGING

- Chest X-rays show lung damage.

TREATMENT

GENERAL
- Oxygen for respiratory distress
- Parenteral fluids for dysphagia caused by oral or laryngeal ulcerations
- Smoking cessation
- Cool mist humidifier

DIET
- Soft, bland foods (with oropharyngeal ulceration)
- Small, frequent meals

ACTIVITY
- Frequent rest periods

MEDICATIONS
- Antifungals
- Glucocorticoids

SURGERY
- Lung resection to remove pulmonary nodules
- Shunt for increased intracranial pressure
- Cardiac repair for constrictive pericarditis

NURSING CONSIDERATIONS

NURSING DIAGNOSES
- Activity intolerance
- Acute pain
- Decreased cardiac output
- Imbalanced nutrition: Less than body requirements
- Impaired gas exchange
- Ineffective airway clearance
- Ineffective breathing pattern
- Risk for injury

EXPECTED OUTCOMES
The patient will:
- demonstrate skill in conserving energy while carrying out daily activities to tolerance level
- be free from pain
- maintain adequate cardiac output
- experience no further weight loss
- maintain adequate ventilation and oxygenation
- maintain a patent airway
- express feelings of comfort in maintaining air exchange
- remain free from complications.

NURSING INTERVENTIONS
- Give prescribed drugs.
- Provide oxygen therapy, if needed.
- Plan rest periods.
- Consult with the dietitian and patient concerning food preferences.

MONITORING
- Hypoglycemia and hyperglycemia, which indicate adrenal dysfunction
- Respiratory status
- Neurologic status

PATIENT TEACHING

GENERAL
Be sure to cover:
- the disorder, diagnosis, and treatment
- medication administration, dosage, and possible adverse effects
- cardiac and pulmonary signs that could indicate effusions
- the need to watch for early signs of this infection and to seek treatment promptly to help prevent histoplasmosis for people in endemic areas
- the need for people who risk occupational exposure to contaminated soil to wear face masks.

DISCHARGE PLANNING
- Stress the need for follow-up care on a regular basis for at least 1 year.
- Refer the patient with chronic pulmonary or disseminated histoplasmosis for psychological support to cope with long-term treatment.
- Refer the patient to a social worker or an occupational therapist, as needed.
- Help the parents of a child with this disease arrange for a visiting teacher.

RESOURCES
Organizations
Centers for Disease Control and Prevention: *www.cdc.gov*
Harvard University Consumer Health Information: *www.intelihealth.com*
National Health Information Center: *www.health.gov/nhic/*
National Library of Medicine: *www.nlm.nih.gov*

Selected references
Adderson, E. "Histoplasmosis," *Pediatric Infectious Disease Journal* 25(1):73-74, January 2006.
Adderson, E. "Histoplasmosis in a Pediatric Oncology Center," *Journal of Pediatrics* 144(1):100-106, January 2004.
Kasper, D.L., et al., eds. *Harrison's Principles of Internal Medicine*, 16th ed. New York: McGraw-Hill Book Co., 2005.
Topin, J., and Mutlu, G.M. "Images in Clinical Medicine. Splenic and Mediastinal Calcifications in Histoplasmosis," *New England Journal of Medicine* 354(2):179, January 2006.

Hodgkin's disease

OVERVIEW

- Neoplastic disorder characterized by painless, progressive enlargement of lymph nodes, spleen, and other lymphoid tissue
- With appropriate treatment, 5-year survival rate about 90%

PATHOPHYSIOLOGY

- Enlarged lymphoid tissue results from proliferation of lymphocytes, histiocytes, eosinophils, and Reed-Sternberg cells. (See *Recognizing Reed-Sternberg cells.*)
- Untreated Hodgkin's disease follows a variable but relentlessly progressive and ultimately fatal course.

CAUSES

- Exact cause unknown

RISK FACTORS

- Genetic factors
- Viral factors
- Environmental factors

INCIDENCE

- Hodgkin's disease occurs in all races, but is slightly more common in whites.
- This disease is most common in people age 15 to 38, except in Japan where it occurs exclusively in people older than age 50.
- The incidence rate is higher in men than in women.

COMPLICATIONS

- Multiple organ failure

ASSESSMENT

HISTORY

- Painless swelling of one of the cervical, axillary, or inguinal lymph nodes
- Persistent fever and night sweats
- Weight loss despite an adequate diet, with resulting fatigue and malaise
- Increasing susceptibility to infection

PHYSICAL FINDINGS

- Edema of the face and neck and jaundice
- Enlarged, rubbery lymph nodes in the neck (these nodes enlarge during periods of fever and then revert to normal size)

DIAGNOSTIC TEST RESULTS

LABORATORY

- Hematologic tests show mild to severe normocytic, normochromic anemia in 50% of patients; elevated, normal, or reduced white blood cell count and differential; and any combination of neutrophilia, lymphocytopenia, monocytosis, and eosinophilia.
- Serum alkaline phosphatase levels are elevated, indicating liver or bone involvement.

DIAGNOSTIC PROCEDURES

- Tests must first rule out other disorders that enlarge the lymph nodes.
- A lymph node biopsy confirms the presence of Reed-Sternberg cells, abnormal histiocyte proliferation, and nodular fibrosis and necrosis. A lymph node biopsy is also used to determine lymph node and organ involvement.
- A staging laparotomy is necessary for patients younger than age 55 and for those without obvious stage III or IV disease, lymphocyte predominance subtype histology, or medical contraindications.

Recognizing Reed-Sternberg cells

The illustration below shows Reed-Sternberg cells. Note the large, distinct nucleoli.

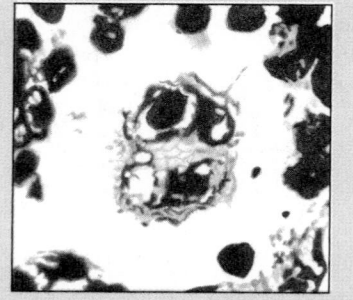

TREATMENT

GENERAL
- For patient with stage I or II disease, radiation therapy alone
- For patient with stage III disease, radiation therapy and chemotherapy
- For patient with stage IV disease, chemotherapy alone (or chemotherapy and radiation therapy to involved sites), sometimes inducing complete remission
- Autologous bone marrow transplantation or autologous peripheral blood sternal transfusions and immunotherapy

DIET
- Well-balanced, high-calorie, high-protein

ACTIVITY
- Frequent rest periods

MEDICATIONS
- Chemotherapy
- Antiemetics
- Sedatives
- Antidiarrheals

NURSING CONSIDERATIONS

NURSING DIAGNOSES
- Acute pain
- Anxiety
- Fatigue
- Fear
- Imbalanced nutrition: Less than body requirements
- Impaired oral mucous membranes
- Impaired skin integrity
- Ineffective coping
- Risk for infection

EXPECTED OUTCOMES
The patient will:
- express feelings of increased comfort and decreased pain
- verbalize feelings of decreased anxiety
- express feelings of increased energy
- express fears and concerns relating to his diagnosis and condition
- maintain weight within an acceptable range
- exhibit intact mucous membranes
- demonstrate adequate skin integrity
- demonstrate effective coping mechanisms
- remain free from all signs and symptoms of infection.

NURSING INTERVENTIONS
- Provide a well-balanced, high-calorie, high-protein diet.
- Provide frequent rest periods.
- Give prescribed drugs.
- Provide emotional support.

MONITORING
- Complications of treatment
- Pain control
- Lymph node enlargement
- Body temperature
- Fatigue
- Daily weight
- Signs and symptoms of infection
- Response to treatment
- Signs and symptoms of dehydration

PATIENT TEACHING

GENERAL
Be sure to cover:
- the disorder, diagnosis, and treatment
- signs and symptoms of infection
- the importance of maintaining good nutrition
- the pacing of activities to counteract therapy-induced fatigue
- the importance of good oral hygiene
- the avoidance of crowds and people with known infection
- the importance of checking the lymph nodes
- medication administration, dosage, and possible adverse effects.

DISCHARGE PLANNING
- Refer the patient to resource and support services.

RESOURCES
Organizations
American Cancer Society:
www.cancer.org
Guide to Internet Resources for Cancer:
www.cancerindex.org
National Cancer Institute:
www.cancer.gov

Selected references
Atlas of Pathophysiology, 2nd ed. Philadelphia: Lippincott Williams & Wilkins, 2005.

Casciato, D.A. *Manual of Clinical Oncology*, 5th ed. Philadelphia: Lippincott Williams & Wilkins, 2004.

Cole, S., and Dunne, K. "Hodgkin's Lymphoma," *Nursing Standard* 18(19):46-52, January 2004.

Krasin, M.J., et al. "Patterns of Treatment Failure in Pediatric and Young Adult Patients with Hodgkin's Disease: Local Disease Control with Combined-Modality Therapy," *Journal of Clinical Oncology* 23(33):8406-413, November 2005.

Kuppers, R., et al. "Advances in Biology, Diagnostics, and Treatment of Hodgkin's Disease," *Biology of Blood and Marrow Transplantation* 12(1 Suppl 1):66-76, January 2006.

Hookworm disease

- Infection of the upper intestine caused by *Ancylostoma duodenale* (in the Eastern Hemisphere) or *Necator americanus* (in the Western Hemisphere)
- Occurs mostly in tropical and subtropical climates
- Also called *uncinariasis* or *ground itch*

PATHOPHYSIOLOGY

- This disease is transmitted to humans through direct skin penetration (usually in the foot) by hookworm larvae in soil contaminated with feces containing hookworm ova.
- These ova develop into infectious larvae in 1 to 3 days.
- The larvae travel through the lymphatics to the pulmonary capillaries, where they penetrate alveoli and move up the bronchial tree to the trachea and epiglottis. There they are swallowed and enter the GI tract.
- When they reach the small intestine, they mature, attach to the jejunal mucosa, and suck blood, oxygen, and glucose from the intestinal wall.
- These mature worms then deposit ova, which are excreted in the stool, starting the cycle anew. Hookworm larvae mature in about 5 to 6 weeks.

CAUSES

- Transmission of *Ancylostoma duodenale* (in the Eastern Hemisphere) or *Necator americanus* (in the Western Hemisphere)

INCIDENCE

- This disorder may produce no symptoms.
- This disorder affects one billion people worldwide.
- This disorder is more common in whites.
- Children are more at risk because of playing or walking barefoot in contaminated soil.

COMPLICATIONS

- Anemia
- Cardiomegaly
- Heart failure
- Generalized massive edema

ASSESSMENT

HISTORY

- Recent walking (barefoot) in an area with contaminated soil
- Irritation and pruritus at entry site
- Fatigue
- Cough, hoarseness
- Abdominal pain
- Fever
- Nausea
- Weight loss
- Dizziness
- Diarrhea

PHYSICAL FINDINGS

- Papulovesicular rash
- Crackles (with lung involvement)
- Irregular respirations
- Bloody sputum
- Black, tarry stools
- Edema

DIAGNOSTIC TEST RESULTS

LABORATORY

- Stool specimen reveals larvae.
- Hemoglobin level is decreased to as low as 5 to 9 g/dl (in severe cases).
- Leukocyte count is increased to as high as 47,000/μl.
- Eosinophil count is increased to as high as 500 to 700/μl.

GENERAL
◆ Blood transfusions (if anemia is severe)

DIET
◆ Nutritious, high-protein, high-iron

ACTIVITY
◆ As tolerated, with frequent rest periods

MEDICATIONS
◆ Mebendazole
◆ Pyrantel pamoate
◆ Albendazole (Albenza)
◆ Iron supplements
◆ Topical thiabendazole (cutaneous larva migrans)

NURSING DIAGNOSES
◆ Delayed growth and development
◆ Diarrhea
◆ Fatigue
◆ Imbalanced nutrition: Less than body requirements
◆ Impaired gas exchange
◆ Ineffective breathing pattern
◆ Risk for infection

EXPECTED OUTCOMES
The patient will:
◆ demonstrate appropriate skills and behaviors to the extent possible
◆ avoid episodes of diarrhea
◆ report having increased energy levels
◆ experience no further weight loss
◆ maintain adequate ventilation
◆ maintain effective breathing pattern
◆ experience no further signs or symptoms of infection.

NURSING INTERVENTIONS
◆ Follow standard precautions.
◆ Isolate the incontinent patient.
◆ Teach proper hand-washing technique.
◆ For severe anemia, administer oxygen, if ordered, at low to moderate flow.
◆ Encourage coughing and deep breathing.
◆ Allow frequent rest periods.
◆ Reposition frequently.
◆ Assess family members for symptoms.

MONITORING
◆ Intake and output
◆ Nutritional status
◆ Quantity and frequency of stools
◆ Daily weight
◆ Skin integrity

GENERAL
Be sure to cover:
◆ proper hand-washing technique
◆ the need to wear shoes when outdoors
◆ nutritious diet
◆ proper hygiene after toileting
◆ use of prescribed iron supplements and how this treatment affects stools
◆ the need to start another course of treatment if stool examination remains positive for larvae.

RESOURCES
Organizations
Centers for Disease Control and Prevention: Division of Parasitic Diseases: *www.cdc.gov/ncidod/dpd/*
National Institute of Allergy and Infectious Diseases: *www.niaid.nih.gov*
World Health Organization: *www.who.int*

Selected references
Brooker, S., et al. "Human Hookworm Infection in the 21st Century," *Advances in Parasitology* 58:197-288, 2004.
Hotez, P.J, et al. "Hookworm Infection," *New England Journal of Medicine* 351(8):799-807, August 2004.
Quinnell, R.J., et al. "The Immunoepidemiology of Human Hookworm Infection," *Parasite Immunology* 26(11-12):443-54, November-December 2004.

Huntington's disease

- Degenerative disease of the brain that causes dementia
- Death usually 10 to 15 years after onset
- Also called *Huntington's chorea, hereditary chorea, chronic progressive chorea,* and *adult chorea*

PATHOPHYSIOLOGY

- Degeneration in the cerebral cortex and basal ganglia leads to chronic progressive chorea (dancelike movements).
- The final stage is mental deterioration, which ends in dementia.

CAUSES

- Genetic link
- Transmitted as autosomal dominant trait (either sex can transmit and inherit it)

INCIDENCE

- Huntington's disease is most common between ages 30 and 50.
- 2% of cases occur in children.
- 5% of cases occur as late as age 60.
- Each child of a parent with this disease has 50% chance of inheritance.
- A child who doesn't inherit it can't pass it on.
- Huntington's disease affects men and women equally.

COMPLICATIONS

- Choking and aspiration
- Pneumonia
- Heart failure
- Infections
- Suicide

HISTORY

- Familial history
- Emotional and mental changes
- Insidious onset
- Total dependency through:
- Intellectual decline
- Emotional disturbances
- Loss of musculoskeletal control
- Described as clumsy, irritable, or impatient
- Subject to fits of anger
- Periods of suicidal depression, apathy, or elation
- Ravenous appetite, especially for sweets
- Loss of bladder and bowel control in later stages

PHYSICAL FINDINGS

- Choreic movements
- Rapid, often violent, and purposeless movements
- Cognitive decline

Early stages

- Mild fidgeting
- Grimacing, tongue smacking
- Dysarthria
- Athetoid movements related to emotional state
- Torticollis
- Deficits in short-term memory

Later stages

- Constant writhing and twitching
- Unintelligible speech
- Difficulty chewing and swallowing
- Ambulation impossible
- Appears emaciated and exhausted

LABORATORY

- DNA analysis may confirm diagnosis.

IMAGING

- Positron emission tomography may confirm diagnosis.
- Magnetic resonance imaging shows characteristic butterfly dilation of the brain's lateral ventricles.
- Computed tomography scan shows brain atrophy.

TREATMENT

GENERAL
- No known cure
- Supportive and symptomatic treatment
- Psychotherapy
- Safety measures
- Electroconvulsive therapy

DIET
- Soft, as needed

MEDICATIONS
- Tranquilizers
- Dopamine agonists
- Neuroleptics
- Selective serotonin reuptake inhibitors
- Antidepressants

NURSING CONSIDERATIONS

NURSING DIAGNOSES
- Anxiety
- Bathing or hygiene self-care deficit
- Chronic low self-esteem
- Disabled family coping
- Impaired physical mobility
- Impaired verbal communication
- Ineffective health maintenance
- Risk for aspiration
- Risk for infection
- Risk for injury
- Total urinary incontinence

EXPECTED OUTCOMES
The patient will:
- identify strategies to reduce anxiety
- perform activities of daily living within the confines of the disorder
- express positive feelings about self
- demonstrate effective coping behaviors, along with family members
- maintain joint mobility and range of motion
- develop alternative means of communication
- identify measures to maintain good health
- show no signs of aspiration
- remain free from signs and symptoms of infection
- remain free from injury
- identify strategies to reduce incontinence episodes.

NURSING INTERVENTIONS
- Provide psychological support.
- Identify self-care deficits.
- Encourage the patient to be independent.
- Provide communication aids.
- Help the patient with difficulty walking.
- Maintain a turning schedule.
- Elevate the head of the bed during eating.
- Give prescribed drugs.
- Protect the patient from infections.

MONITORING
- Response to prescribed drugs
- Possible suicide ideation
- Temperature
- White blood cell count

PATIENT TEACHING

GENERAL
Be sure to cover:
- the disorder, diagnosis, and treatment
- prescribed drugs and possible adverse effects
- aspiration precautions
- signs and symptoms of infection
- communication strategies.

DISCHARGE PLANNING
- Refer the patient to the Huntington's Disease Society of America.
- Refer the patient to appropriate community organizations.
- Refer the family for genetic counseling.
- Refer the patient for psychotherapy, as appropriate.

RESOURCES
Organizations
Huntington's Disease Society of America: *www.hdsa.org*
National Institutes of Health: *www.nih.gov*

Selected references
Diseases, 4th ed. Philadelphia: Lippincott Williams & Wilkins, 2006.
Handbook of Pathophysiology, 2nd ed. Philadelphia: Lippincott Williams & Wilkins, 2005.
King, N. "Palliative Care Management of a Child with Juvenile Onset Huntington's Disease," *International Journal of Palliative Nursing* 11(6):278-83, June 2005.
Skirton, H. "Huntington's Disease: A Nursing Perspective," *Medsurg Nursing* 14(3):167-72, June 2005.

Hydrocele

- A collection of fluid between the visceral and parietal layers of the testicle's tunica vaginalis or along the spermatic cord
- The most common cause of scrotal swelling
- Described as communicating or noncommunicating

PATHOPHYSIOLOGY
Communicating
- A patency between the scrotal sac and the peritoneal cavity allows peritoneal fluids to collect in the scrotum.

Noncommunicating
- Fluid accumulation may be caused by infection, trauma, tumor, an imbalance between the secreting and absorptive capacities of scrotal tissue, or an obstruction of lymphatic or venous drainage in the spermatic cord.
- This leads to a displacement of fluid in the scrotum, outside the testes.
- Subsequent swelling results, leading to reduced blood flow to the testes.

CAUSES
- Congenital malformation (infants)
- Infection of the testes or epididymis
- Testicular tumor
- Trauma to the testes or epididymis

INCIDENCE
- Hydrocele is apparent in 6% of full-term male neonates.
- The incidence rate in adult males is unknown.

COMPLICATIONS
- Epididymitis
- Testicular atrophy
- Infertility

HISTORY
- Scrotal tenderness
- Inguinal hernia

PHYSICAL FINDINGS
- Soft, nontender fullness within the hemiscrotum
- Transillumination of the scrotum revealing a homogenous glow without internal shadows

LABORATORY
- Urinalysis may reveal proteinuria or pyuria.

IMAGING
- Abdominal X-rays distinguish acute hydrocele from an incarcerated hernia.
- Ultrasonography distinguishes spermatoceles from hydroceles and identifies torsion or tumor.

OTHER
- Transillumination distinguishes fluid-filled from solid mass (a tumor doesn't transilluminate).

TREATMENT

GENERAL
◆ Frequently resolves spontaneously
◆ Scrotal elevation

DIET
◆ No restrictions

ACTIVITY
◆ As tolerated
◆ Postoperatively, avoidance of vigorous activity for short time

MEDICATIONS
◆ Nonsteroidal anti-inflammatory drugs
◆ Nonopioid analgesics

SURGERY
◆ Operative exploration if underlying pathology is suspected
◆ Surgical repair to avoid strangulation of the bowel (inguinal hernia with bowel present in the sac)
◆ Aspiration of fluid and injection of sclerosing drug into the scrotal sac for a tense hydrocele that impedes blood circulation or causes pain
◆ Excision of the tunica vaginalis for recurrent hydroceles
◆ Suprainguinal excision for testicular tumor detected by ultrasound

NURSING CONSIDERATIONS

NURSING DIAGNOSES
◆ Acute pain
◆ Anxiety
◆ Risk for situational low self-esteem

EXPECTED OUTCOMES
The patient (or his parents) will:
◆ express feelings of comfort and relief from pain
◆ express feelings of decreased anxiety
◆ express positive feelings about self.

NURSING INTERVENTIONS
◆ Place a rolled towel between the patient's legs and elevate the scrotum to help reduce severe swelling.
◆ Apply heat or ice packs to the scrotum.
◆ Provide preoperative teaching.
◆ Provide postoperative wound care, if appropriate.

MONITORING
◆ Swelling
◆ Worsening of condition

PATIENT TEACHING

GENERAL
Be sure to cover:
◆ the need to wear a loose-fitting athletic supporter lined with soft cotton dressings
◆ how to take a sitz bath
◆ the need to avoid tub baths postoperatively for 5 to 7 days
◆ the possibility that the hydrocele may reaccumulate for 1 month postoperatively because of edema.

DISCHARGE PLANNING
◆ Follow-up visits may be required biweekly, monthly, or every 2 to 3 months, depending on recovery rate.

RESOURCES
Organizations
Cleveland Clinic Health Information Center: *www.clevelandclinic.org/health*
Mayo Clinic: *www.mayoclinic.com*
National Library of Medicine: *www.nlm.nih.gov*

Selected references
Matsumoto, A., et al. "Torsion of the Hernia Sac within a Hydrocele of the Scrotum in a Child," *International Journal of Urology* 11(9):789-91, September 2004.
Shiraishi, K., et al. "Torsion of a Communicating Hydrocele in a Child," *International Journal of Urology* 12(1):111-12, January 2005.

Hydrocephalus

OVERVIEW

- A variety of conditions characterized by an excess of fluid within the cranial vault, subarachnoid space, or both
- Occurs because of interference with cerebrospinal fluid (CSF) flow caused by increased fluid production, obstruction within the ventricular system, or defective reabsorption of CSF
- Types:
  - Noncommunicating hydrocephalus: obstruction within the ventricular system
  - Communicating hydrocephalus: impaired absorption of CSF

PATHOPHYSIOLOGY

- The obstruction of CSF flow associated with hydrocephalus produces dilation of the ventricles proximal to the obstruction.
- The obstructed CSF is under pressure, causing atrophy of the cerebral cortex and degeneration of the white matter tracts. Gray matter is preserved selectively.
- When excess CSF fills a defect caused by atrophy, a degenerative disorder, or a surgical excision, the fluid isn't under pressure, and atrophy and degenerative changes aren't induced.

CAUSES
Noncommunicating hydrocephalus
- Aqueduct stenosis
- Arnold-Chiari malformation
- Congenital abnormalities in the ventricular system
- Mass lesions such as a tumor that compresses one of the structures of the ventricular system

Communicating hydrocephalus
- Adhesions from inflammation, such as with meningitis or subarachnoid hemorrhage
- Cerebral atrophy
- Compression of the subarachnoid space by a mass such as a tumor
- Congenital abnormalities of the subarachnoid space
- Head injury
- High venous pressure within the sagittal sinus

INCIDENCE
- Rare cases of congenital hydrocephalus occur.
- Noncommunicating hydrocephalus is more common in children.
- Communicating hydrocephalus is more common in adults.

COMPLICATIONS
- Mental retardation
- Impaired motor function
- Vision loss
- Death (increased intracranial pressure [ICP])
- Infection and malnutrition (more common in infants)

The infant with hydrocephalus

Characteristic changes of hydrocephalus in infants include marked head enlargement; distended scalp veins; thin, shiny, and fragile-looking scalp skin; and underdeveloped neck muscles.

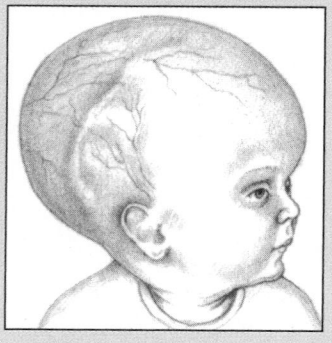

ASSESSMENT

HISTORY
Infants
- History that may disclose cause
- High-pitched, shrill cry; irritability
- Anorexia
- Episodes of projectile vomiting

Adults and older children
- Frontal headaches
- Nausea and vomiting (may be projectile)
- Symptoms causing wakening or occurring on awakening
- Diplopia
- Restlessness

PHYSICAL FINDINGS
Infants
- Enlarged head clearly disproportionate to the infant's growth (see *The infant with hydrocephalus*)
- Head possibly appearing normal in size with bulging fontanels
- Distended scalp veins
- Thin, fragile, and shiny scalp skin
- Underdeveloped neck muscles
- Depression of the roof of the eye orbit
- Displacement of the eyes downward
- Prominent sclera (sunset sign)
- Abnormal leg muscle tone

Adults and older children
- Decreased level of consciousness
- Ataxia
- Impaired intellect
- Incontinence
- Signs of increased ICP

DIAGNOSTIC TEST RESULTS

IMAGING
- Skull X-rays show thinning of the skull with separation of sutures and widening of the fontanels in infants.
- Angiography, computed tomography scan, and magnetic resonance imaging show differentiation between hydrocephalus and intracranial lesions and Arnold-Chiari deformity.

GENERAL
♦ Shunting of CSF directly from the ventricular system to some point beyond the obstruction

DIET
♦ Small, frequent feedings
♦ Slow feeding

ACTIVITY
♦ Decreased movement during and immediately after meals

MEDICATIONS
♦ Possible preoperative and postoperative antibiotics

SURGERY
♦ Surgical correction (the only treatment for hydrocephalus) includes:
– removal of obstruction to CSF flow
– implantation of a ventriculoperitoneal shunt to divert CSF flow from the brain's lateral ventricle into the peritoneal cavity
– with concurrent abdominal problem, ventriculoatrial shunt to divert CSF flow from the brain's lateral ventricle into the right atrium of the heart.

NURSING CONSIDERATIONS

NURSING DIAGNOSES
♦ Acute pain
♦ Anxiety
♦ Decreased intracranial adaptive capacity
♦ Delayed growth and development
♦ Imbalanced nutrition: Less than body requirements
♦ Impaired gas exchange
♦ Impaired skin integrity
♦ Ineffective airway clearance
♦ Ineffective tissue perfusion: Cerebral
♦ Interrupted family processes
♦ Risk for disorganized infant behavior
♦ Risk for infection

EXPECTED OUTCOMES
The patient (or family) will:
♦ exhibit no signs of pain or agitation
♦ identify measures to reduce anxiety
♦ exhibit signs of reduced ICP
♦ achieve age-appropriate growth, behaviors, and skills to the fullest extent possible
♦ show no signs of malnutrition
♦ maintain adequate ventilation and oxygenation
♦ maintain skin integrity without signs of breakdown
♦ maintain a patent airway
♦ maintain and improve current level of consciousness
♦ verbalize the effect of the patient's condition on their daily life
♦ remain free from signs of seizure activity
♦ remain free from signs and symptoms of infection.

NURSING INTERVENTIONS
♦ Elevate the head of the bed 30 degrees or put an infant in an infant seat.
♦ Give prescribed oxygen, as needed.
♦ Provide small, frequent feedings.
♦ Decrease the patient's movement during and immediately after meals.
♦ Provide skin care.

After shunt surgery
♦ Place the patient on the side opposite the operative site.
♦ Give prescribed I.V. fluids.
♦ Give prescribed analgesics.

MONITORING
♦ Fontanels for tension or fullness
♦ Head circumference
♦ Signs and symptoms of increased ICP
♦ Complications
♦ Growth and development
♦ Neurologic status
♦ Intake and output

After surgery
♦ Signs and symptoms of meningitis
♦ Redness, swelling, and other signs and symptoms of local infection
♦ Dressing for drainage
♦ Response to analgesics

⚡ **WARNING** *Monitor the patient for vomiting, which may be an early sign of shunt malfunction.*

GENERAL
Be sure to cover:
♦ the disorder, diagnosis, and treatment
♦ shunt surgery: hair loss and the visibility of a mechanical device
♦ postoperative shunt care
♦ signs and symptoms of increased ICP or shunt malfunction
♦ signs and symptoms of infection
♦ signs and symptoms of paralytic ileus
♦ the need for periodic shunt surgery to lengthen the shunt as the child grows older.

DISCHARGE PLANNING
♦ Refer the patient to special education programs, as appropriate.

RESOURCES
Organizations
The American Academy of Pediatrics: *www.aap.org*
National Institutes of Health: *www.nih.gov*

Selected references
Diseases, 4th ed. Philadelphia: Lippincott Williams & Wilkins, 2006.
Handbook of Pathophysiology, 2nd ed. Philadelphia: Lippincott Williams & Wilkins, 2005.
Mangano, F.T., et al. "Early Programmable Valve Malfunctions in Pediatric Hydrocephalus," *Journal of Neurosurgery* 103(6 Suppl):501-507, December 2005.
McGirt, M.J., et al. "Diagnosis, Treatment, and Analysis of Long-Term Outcomes in Idiopathic Normal-Pressure Hydrocephalus," *Neurosurgery* 57(4):699-705, October 2005.
Rudy, C. "Hydrocephalus," *Journal of Pediatric Health Care* 19(2):111, 127-28, March-April 2005.

Hydronephrosis

OVERVIEW

- Abnormal dilation of the renal pelvis and calyces of one or both kidneys
- Caused by obstruction of urine flow in the genitourinary tract
- May be acute or chronic

PATHOPHYSIOLOGY

- With obstruction in the urethra or bladder, hydronephrosis is usually bilateral.
- With obstruction in a ureter, hydronephrosis is usually unilateral.
- Obstructions distal to the bladder cause the bladder to dilate, acting as a buffer zone, delaying hydronephrosis.
- Total obstruction of urine flow with dilation of the collecting system ultimately causes complete cortical atrophy and glomerular filtration ceases.

CAUSES

- Benign prostatic hyperplasia (BPH)
- Bladder, ureteral, or pelvic tumors
- Blood clots
- Congenital abnormalities
- Gram-negative infection
- Neurogenic bladder
- Renal calculi
- Strictures or stenosis of the ureter or bladder outlet
- Tuberculosis
- Ureterocele
- Urethral strictures

INCIDENCE

- About 1 in 100 people are affected by unilateral hydronephrosis.
- About 1 in 200 people are affected by bilateral hydronephrosis.

COMPLICATIONS

- Renal calculi
- Sepsis
- Renovascular hypertension
- Obstructive nephropathy
- Infection
- Pyelonephritis
- Paralytic ileus
- Renal failure

ASSESSMENT

HISTORY

- Possibly no initial symptoms, but increasing pressure behind the obstruction eventually results in renal dysfunction
- Varies depending on cause of obstruction
- No symptoms or complaint of only mild pain and slightly decreased urine flow
- Severe, colicky renal pain or dull flank pain that radiates to the groin
- Hematuria
- Pyuria
- Dysuria
- Alternating oliguria and polyuria, anuria
- Nausea
- Vomiting
- Abdominal fullness
- Pain on urination
- Dribbling
- Urinary hesitancy
- Change in voiding pattern

PHYSICAL FINDINGS

- Hematuria
- Pyuria
- Urinary tract infection
- Palpable kidney
- Lower extremity edema
- Distended bladder
- Costovertebral angle tenderness

DIAGNOSTIC TEST RESULTS

LABORATORY

- Renal function study results are abnormal.
- Urine studies confirm the inability to concentrate urine.
- Glomerular filtration rate is decreased.
- Pyuria occurs if infection is present.
- Leukocytosis indicates infection.

IMAGING

- Excretory urography, retrograde pyelography, and renal ultrasonography confirm diagnosis.
- I.V. urography shows site of obstruction.
- Nephrography shows delayed appearance time.
- Radionuclide scan shows site of obstruction.
- Computed tomography scan may indicate cause.

TREATMENT

GENERAL
- For inoperable obstructions, decompression and drainage of the kidney, using a nephrostomy tube placed temporarily or permanently in the renal pelvis
- Urinary catheterization

DIET
- If renal function affected, low-protein, low-sodium, and low-potassium

MEDICATIONS
- Antibiotic therapy
- Analgesics
- Oral alkalinization therapy (for uric acid calculi)
- Steroid therapy (for retroperitoneal fibrosis)

SURGERY
- Dilatation for urethral stricture and placement of urethral stents
- Prostatectomy for BPH
- Placement of percutaneous nephrostomy tube

NURSING CONSIDERATIONS

NURSING DIAGNOSES
- Acute pain
- Anxiety
- Deficient fluid volume
- Imbalanced nutrition: Less than body requirements
- Impaired urinary elimination
- Risk for infection
- Risk for injury

EXPECTED OUTCOMES
The patient will:
- report increased comfort
- express feelings of decreased anxiety
- maintain fluid balance
- verbalize appropriate food choices according to the prescribed diet
- maintain adequate urine output
- remain free from signs or symptoms of infection
- avoid or have minimized complications.

NURSING INTERVENTIONS
- Give prescribed drugs.
- Give prescribed I.V. fluids.
- Allow the patient to express his fears and anxieties.

MONITORING
- Renal function studies
- Intake and output
- Vital signs
- Fluid and electrolyte status
- Nephrostomy tube function and drainage, if appropriate
- Wound site (postoperatively)

PATIENT TEACHING

GENERAL
Be sure to cover:
- the disorder, diagnosis, and treatment
- the procedure and postoperative care, if surgery is scheduled
- nephrostomy tube care, if appropriate
- medication administration, dosage, and possible adverse effects
- dietary changes
- hydronephrosis symptom recognition and reporting.

DISCHARGE PLANNING
- Follow-up imaging studies may be required to evaluate recovery.
- Follow-up laboratory studies may be needed to assess renal function.

RESOURCES
Organizations
American Association of Kidney Patients: *www.aakp.org*
National Institute of Diabetes & Digestive & Kidney Diseases: *www.niddk.nih.gov*

Selected references
Diseases, 4th ed. Philadelphia: Lippincott Williams & Wilkins, 2006.
Eskild-Jensen, A., et al. "Interpretation of the Renogram: Problems and Pitfalls in Hydronephrosis in Children," *BJU International* 94(6):887-92, October 2004.
Pates, J.A., and Dashe, J.S. "Prenatal Diagnosis and Management of Hydronephrosis," *Early Human Development* 82(1):3-8, January 2006.
Tsai, J.D., et al. "Intermittent Hydronephrosis Secondary to Ureteropelvic Junction Obstruction: Clinical and Imaging Features," *Pediatrics* 117(1):139-46, January 2006.

Hyperaldosteronism

OVERVIEW

- Hypersecretion of the mineralocorticoid aldosterone by the adrenal cortex
- Causes excessive reabsorption of sodium and water and excessive renal excretion of potassium
- May be primary (uncommon) or secondary

PATHOPHYSIOLOGY

In primary hyperaldosteronism (Conn's syndrome)

- Chronic excessive secretion of aldosterone is independent of the renin-angiotensin system and suppresses plasma renin activity.
- This aldosterone excess enhances sodium and water reabsorption and potassium loss by the kidneys, which leads to mild hypernatremia, hypokalemia, and increased extracellular fluid volume.
- Expansion of intravascular fluid volume also occurs and results in volume-dependent hypertension and increased cardiac output.

⚡ **WARNING** *Excessive ingestion of English black licorice or licorice-like substances can produce a syndrome similar to primary hyperaldosteronism because of the mineralocorticoid action of glycyrrhizic acid.*

In secondary hyperaldosteronism

- An extra-adrenal abnormality stimulates the adrenal gland to increase aldosterone production.

CAUSES

- Bartter's syndrome
- Benign aldosterone-producing adrenal adenoma (in 70% of patients)
- Bilateral adrenocortical hyperplasia (in children) or carcinoma (rarely)
- Conditions that produce a sodium deficit (Wilms' tumor)
- Conditions that reduce renal blood flow and extracellular fluid volume (renal artery stenosis)
- Heart failure
- Hepatic cirrhosis with ascites
- Nephrotic syndrome

INCIDENCE

- Hypoaldosteronism is three times more common in women than in men.
- This disorder is most common between ages 30 and 50.

COMPLICATIONS

- Neuromuscular irritability, tetany, paresthesia
- Seizures
- Left ventricular hypertrophy, heart failure, death
- Metabolic alkalosis, nephropathy, azotemia

ASSESSMENT

HISTORY

- Vision disturbances
- Nocturnal polyuria
- Polydipsia
- Fatigue
- Headaches
- Hypokalemia

PHYSICAL FINDINGS

- Muscle weakness
- Intermittent, flaccid paralysis
- Paresthesia
- High blood pressure
- Abdominal distention

DIAGNOSTIC TEST RESULTS

LABORATORY

- Serum potassium levels are persistenly low.
- Low plasma renin level that fails to increase appropriately during volume depletion (upright posture, sodium depletion) and high plasma aldosterone level during volume expansion by salt loading (confirm primary hyperaldosteronism in a hypertensive patient without edema).
- Serum bicarbonate level is elevated.
- Urine aldosterone levels are markedly increased.
- Plasma aldosterone levels are increased.
- Plasma renin levels (secondary) are increased.
- Suppression test distinguishes between primary and secondary hyperaldosteronism.

IMAGING

- Chest X-rays show left ventricular hypertrophy from chronic hypertension.
- Adrenal angiography or computed tomography scan localize the tumor.

DIAGNOSTIC PROCEDURES

- Electrocardiography may show signs of hypokalemia (ST-segment depression and U waves).

TREATMENT

GENERAL
◆ Treatment of underlying cause (secondary)

DIET
◆ Low-sodium, high-potassium

MEDICATIONS
◆ Potassium-sparing diuretics (primary)

SURGERY
◆ Unilateral adrenalectomy (primary)

NURSING CONSIDERATIONS

NURSING DIAGNOSES
◆ Acute pain
◆ Decreased cardiac output
◆ Excess fluid volume
◆ Impaired physical mobility
◆ Impaired urinary elimination
◆ Ineffective coping
◆ Ineffective tissue perfusion: Cardiopulmonary

EXPECTED OUTCOMES
The patient will:
◆ express feelings of increased comfort
◆ maintain adequate cardiac output
◆ show no signs of circulatory overload
◆ maintain joint range of motion and muscle strength
◆ maintain a normal urine output
◆ demonstrate adaptive coping behaviors
◆ maintain hemodynamic stability.

NURSING INTERVENTIONS
◆ Watch for signs of tetany (muscle twitching, Trousseau's sign, Chvostek's sign).
◆ Give potassium replacement, and keep I.V. calcium gluconate available.
◆ After adrenalectomy, watch for weakness, hyponatremia, rising serum potassium levels, and signs of adrenal hypofunction, especially hypotension.

MONITORING
◆ Intake and output
◆ Vital signs
◆ Weight
◆ Serum electrolyte levels
◆ Cardiac arrhythmias

PATIENT TEACHING

GENERAL
Be sure to cover:
◆ adverse effects of spironolactone, including hyperkalemia, impotence, and gynecomastia, if appropriate
◆ the importance of wearing medical identification jewelry while taking steroid hormone replacement therapy.

RESOURCES
Organizations
Endocrine Society: *www.endo-society.org*
The Merck Manuals Online Medical Library: *www.merck.com/mmhe*
National Adrenal Diseases Foundation: *www.medhelp.org/www/nadf.htm*
National Institute of Diabetes & Digestive & Kidney Diseases: *www.niddk.nih.gov*
National Library of Medicine: *www.nlm.nih.gov*

Selected references

Barzon, L., et al. "Shift from Conn's Syndrome to Cushing's Syndrome in a Recurrent Adrenocortical Carcinoma," *European Journal of Endocrinology* 153(5):629-36, November 2005.

Pizzolo, F., et al. "Primary Hyperaldosteronism: A Frequent Cause of Residual Hypertension After Successful Endovascular Treatment of Renal Artery Disease," *Journal of Hypertension* 23(11):2041-2047, November 2005.

Williams, J.S., et al. "Prevalence of Primary Hyperaldosteronism in Mild to Moderate Hypertension Without Hypokalaemia," *Journal of Human Hypertension* 20(2):129-36, February 2006.

Hyperbilirubinemia, unconjugated

OVERVIEW

- Excessive serum bilirubin levels and mild jaundice
- Caused by hemolytic processes in the neonate
- Can be physiologic (with jaundice the only symptom) or pathologic (resulting from an underlying disease)
- Also called *neonatal jaundice*

PATHOPHYSIOLOGY

- As erythrocytes break down at the end of their neonatal life cycle, hemoglobin separates into globin (protein) and heme (iron) fragments.
- Heme fragments form unconjugated (indirect) bilirubin, which binds with albumin for transport to liver cells to conjugate with glucuronide, forming direct bilirubin.
- Because unconjugated bilirubin is fat-soluble and can't be excreted in the urine or bile, it may escape to extravascular tissue, especially fatty tissue and the brain, resulting in hyperbilirubinemia.
- Hyperbilirubinemia may develop when:
- certain factors disrupt conjugation and usurp albumin-binding sites, including drugs (such as aspirin, tranquilizers, and sulfonamides) and conditions (such as hypothermia, anoxia, hypoglycemia, and hypoalbuminemia)
- decreased hepatic function results in reduced bilirubin conjugation
- increased erythrocyte production or breakdown results from hemolytic disorders or Rh or ABO incompatibility
- biliary obstruction or hepatitis results in blockage of normal bile flow
- maternal enzymes present in breast milk inhibit the infant's glucuronyltransferase conjugating activity.

CAUSES

- Dependent on the age of the infant (see *Causes of hyperbilirubinemia*)

INCIDENCE

- Hyperbilirubinemia is more common in neonates.
- This disease is more common in males than in females.
- This disease is less common in Black infants than in White infants.

COMPLICATIONS

- Kernicterus
- Cerebral palsy
- Epilepsy
- Mental retardation

ASSESSMENT

HISTORY

- Previous sibling with neonatal jaundice
- Familial history of anemia, bile stones, splenectomy, liver disease
- Maternal illness suggestive of viral or other infection
- Maternal drug intake
- Delayed cord clamping
- Birth trauma with bruising

PHYSICAL FINDINGS

- Yellowish skin, particularly in the sclerae

Causes of hyperbilirubinemia

The neonate's age at onset of hyperbilirubinemia may provide clues as to the sources of this jaundice-causing disorder.

DAY 1
- Blood type incompatibility (Rh, ABO, other minor blood groups)
- Intrauterine infection (rubella, cytomegalic inclusion body disease, toxoplasmosis, syphilis and, occasionally, such bacteria as *Escherichia coli, Staphylococcus, Pseudomonas, Klebsiella, Proteus,* and *Streptococcus*)

DAY 2 OR 3
- Infection (usually from gram-negative bacteria)
- Polycythemia
- Enclosed hemorrhage (skin bruises, subdural hematoma)
- Respiratory distress syndrome (hyaline membrane disease)
- Heinz body anemia from drugs and toxins (vitamin K_3, sodium nitrate)
- Transient neonatal hyperbilirubinemia
- Abnormal red blood cell morphology

- Red cell enzyme deficiencies (glucose-6-phosphate dehydrogenase, hexokinase)
- Physiologic jaundice
- Blood group incompatibilities

DAYS 4 AND 5
- Breast-feeding, respiratory distress syndrome, maternal diabetes
- Crigler-Najjar syndrome (congenital nonhemolytic icterus)
- Gilbert syndrome

DAY 6 AND LATER
- Herpes simplex
- Pyloric stenosis
- Hypothyroidism
- Neonatal giant cell hepatitis
- Infection (usually acquired in neonatal period)
- Bile duct atresia
- Galactosemia
- Choledochal cysts

DIAGNOSTIC TEST RESULTS

LABORATORY
◆ Serum bilirubin levels are elevated.

TREATMENT

GENERAL
◆ Phototherapy
◆ Exchange transfusions

MEDICATIONS
◆ Albumin
◆ Phenobarbital (rarely used)
◆ Rh$_o$(D) immune globulin (human) (to Rh-negative mother)

NURSING CONSIDERATIONS

NURSING DIAGNOSES
◆ Anxiety (parents)
◆ Risk for deficient fluid volume
◆ Risk for imbalanced body temperature
◆ Risk for impaired parent/infant/child attachment
◆ Risk for impaired skin integrity

EXPECTED OUTCOMES
The patient (or parents) will:
◆ verbalize reduced anxiety levels
◆ maintain normal fluid balance
◆ exhibit normal body temperature
◆ maintain eye, verbal, and physical contact with the neonate
◆ maintain skin integrity.

NURSING INTERVENTIONS
◆ Reassure parents that most infants experience some degree of jaundice.
◆ Keep emergency equipment available when transfusing blood.
◆ Give Rh$_o$(D) immune globulin (human), to an Rh-negative mother after amniocentesis or — to prevent hemolytic disease in subsequent infants — to an Rh-negative mother in the third trimester of pregnancy, after the birth of an Rh-positive infant, or after spontaneous or elective abortion.

MONITORING
◆ Jaundice
◆ Bilirubin levels
◆ Body temperature
◆ Intake and output
◆ Bleeding and complications

PATIENT TEACHING

GENERAL
Be sure to cover:
◆ the disorder, diagnosis, and treatment
◆ that the infant's stool contains some bile and may be greenish.

RESOURCES
Organizations
The American Academy of Pediatrics: *www.aap.org*
American Liver Foundation: *www.liverfoundation.org*
The Merck Manuals Online Medical Library: *www.merck.com/mmhe*
National Library of Medicine: *www.nlm.nih.gov*

Selected references
Dollberg, G., et al. "Computerized Decision-making Assistance for Managing Neonatal Hyperbilirubinemia," *Pediatrics* 117(1):262-63, January 2006.
Ellis, E., et al. "Successful Treatment of Severe Unconjugated Hyperbilirubinemia via Induction of UGT1A1 by Rifampicin," *Journal of Hepatology* 44(1):243-45, January 2006.
Gourley, G.R. "Another Risk Factor for Neonatal Hyperbilirubinemia," *Journal of Pediatric Gastroenterology and Nutrition* 40(3):388-89, March 2005.
Nettina, S.M. *Lippincott Manual of Nursing Practice,* 8th ed. Philadelphia: Lippincott Williams & Wilkins, 2006.

Hypercalcemia

◆ Excessive levels of serum calcium

PATHOPHYSIOLOGY

◆ Together with phosphorus, calcium is responsible for the formation and structure of bones and teeth.
◆ Calcium helps to maintain cell structure and function.
◆ It plays a role in cell membrane permeability and impulse transmission.
◆ Calcium affects the contraction of cardiac muscle, smooth muscle, and skeletal muscle.
◆ It participates in the blood-clotting process.

CAUSES

◆ Certain cancers
◆ Certain drugs (see *Drugs causing hypercalcemia*)
◆ Hyperparathyroidism
◆ Hypervitaminosis D
◆ Multiple fractures and prolonged immobilization

INCIDENCE

◆ Incidence rate is considerably higher in women than in men.
◆ No gender predominance exists in elevated calcium levels related to cancer.
◆ Incidence rate increases with age.

COMPLICATIONS

◆ Renal calculi
◆ Coma
◆ Cardiac arrest
◆ Osteoporosis

HISTORY

◆ Underlying cause
◆ Lethargy
◆ Weakness
◆ Anorexia
◆ Constipation
◆ Nausea, vomiting
◆ Polyuria
◆ Bone pain
◆ Abdominal upset
◆ Depression

PHYSICAL FINDINGS

◆ Confusion (see *Clinical effects of hypercalcemia*)
◆ Muscle weakness
◆ Hyporeflexia
◆ Decreased muscle tone
◆ Depression

LABORATORY

◆ Serum calcium level is greater than 10.5 mg/dl.
◆ Ionized calcium level is less than 5.3 mg/dl.

DIAGNOSTIC PROCEDURES

◆ Electrocardiography may show shortened QT interval and ventricular arrhythmias.

Drugs causing hypercalcemia

These drugs can cause or contribute to hypercalcemia:
◆ calcium-containing antacids
◆ calcium preparations (oral or I.V.)
◆ lithium
◆ thiazide diuretics
◆ vitamin A
◆ vitamin D.

Clinical effects of hypercalcemia

BODY SYSTEM	EFFECTS
Cardiovascular	◆ Signs of heart block, cardiac arrest, hypertension
Gastrointestinal	◆ Anorexia, nausea, vomiting, constipation, dehydration, polydipsia
Musculoskeletal	◆ Weakness, muscle flaccidity, bone pain, pathologic fractures
Neurologic	◆ Drowsiness, lethargy, headaches, depression or apathy, irritability, confusion
Other	◆ Renal polyuria, flank pain and, eventually, azotemia

TREATMENT

GENERAL
◆ Treatment of the underlying cause

ACTIVITY
◆ As tolerated

MEDICATIONS
◆ Normal saline solution
◆ Loop diuretics

SURGERY
◆ Parathyroidectomy

NURSING CONSIDERATIONS

NURSING DIAGNOSES
◆ Anxiety
◆ Decreased cardiac output
◆ Fear
◆ Impaired gas exchange
◆ Ineffective tissue perfusion: Cardio-pulmonary
◆ Risk for injury

EXPECTED OUTCOMES
The patient will:
◆ identify strategies to reduce anxiety
◆ maintain adequate cardiac output
◆ discuss fears and concerns
◆ maintain adequate ventilation and oxygenation
◆ exhibit signs of adequate cardiopulmonary perfusion
◆ avoid complications.

NURSING INTERVENTIONS
◆ Provide safety measures and institute seizure precautions, if appropriate.
◆ Give prescribed I.V. solutions.
◆ Watch for signs of heart failure.

After parathyroidectomy
◆ Keep a tracheotomy tray and endotracheal tube setup at the patient's bedside.
◆ Maintain seizure precautions.
◆ Place the patient in semi-Fowler's position.
◆ Support the patient's head and neck with sandbags.
◆ Have the patient ambulate as soon as possible.

⚡ **WARNING** *Watch for complaints of tingling in the hands and around the mouth. If these symptoms don't subside quickly, they may be prodromal signs of tetany, so keep I.V. calcium gluconate or calcium chloride available for emergency administration.*

MONITORING
◆ Cardiac rhythm
◆ Seizures
◆ Calcium levels

After parathyroidectomy
◆ Increased neuromuscular activity
◆ Neck edema
◆ Chvostek's sign
◆ Trousseau's sign

PATIENT TEACHING

GENERAL
Be sure to cover:
◆ avoiding over-the-counter drugs that are high in calcium
◆ increasing fluid intake
◆ following a low-calcium diet.

DISCHARGE PLANNING
◆ Refer the patient to a dietitian and social services, if indicated.

RESOURCES
Organizations
Mayo Clinic: *www.mayoclinic.com*
National Cancer Institute: *www.cancer.gov*
National Library of Medicine: *www.nlm.nih.gov*

Selected references
Delaney, M.F., and Carey, J.J. "Hypercalcemia," *Cleveland Clinic Journal of Medicine* 72(12):1075, December 2005.
Guardiano, S.A., and Mason, E. "A Unique Case of Peripartum Hypercalcemia and Joint Pain," *Endocrinologist* 14(1):19-24, January-February 2004.
Shuey, K.M., and Brant, J.M. "Hypercalcemia of Malignancy: Part II," *Clinical Journal of Oncology Nursing* 8(3):321-23, June 2004.

Hyperchloremia

- Excessive serum levels of the chloride anion
- Usually accompanied by sodium and water retention

PATHOPHYSIOLOGY

- Chloride accounts for two-thirds of all serum anions.
- Chloride is secreted by stomach mucosa as hydrochloric acid; it provides an acid medium that aids digestion and activation of enzymes.
- Chloride helps to maintain acid-base and body water balances, influences the osmolality or tonicity of extracellular fluid, plays a role in the exchange of oxygen and carbon dioxide in red blood cells, and helps activate salivary amylase (which, in turn, activates the digestive process).
- An inverse relationship exists between chloride and bicarbonate. When the level of one goes up, the level of the other goes down. (See *Anion gap and metabolic acidosis.*)

CAUSES

- Certain drugs (see *Drugs causing hyperchloremia*)
- Hypernatremia
- Hyperparathyroidism
- Loss of pancreatic secretion
- Metabolic acidosis
- Prolonged diarrhea
- Renal tubular acidosis

COMPLICATIONS

- Coma

HISTORY

- Risk factors for high chloride level
- Altered level of consciousness

PHYSICAL FINDINGS

- Agitation
- Pitting edema
- Dyspnea
- Rapid deep breathing (Kussmaul's respirations)
- Weakness
- Tachypnea
- Hypertension

LABORATORY

- Serum chloride level is greater than 108 mEq/L.
- With metabolic acidosis, serum pH is less than 7.35, serum carbon dioxide level is less than 22 mEq/L, and the anion gap is normal.
- Serum sodium level is greater than 145 mEq/L.

Anion gap and metabolic acidosis

Hyperchloremia increases the likelihood that a patient will develop hyperchloremic metabolic acidosis.

HOW IT HAPPENS

If a patient with metabolic acidosis has a normal anion gap, the acidosis is probably caused by a loss of bicarbonate ions by the kidneys or the GI tract. In such cases, a corresponding increase in chloride ions also occurs.

Acidosis can also result from an accumulation of chloride ions in the form of acidifying salts. A corresponding decrease in bicarbonate ions occurs at the same time.

TREATMENT

GENERAL
◆ Treatment of underlying cause
◆ Restoring fluid, electrolyte, and acid-base balance

DIET
◆ Restricted sodium and chloride intake

ACTIVITY
◆ As tolerated

MEDICATIONS
◆ Sodium bicarbonate I.V.
◆ Lactated Ringer's solution
◆ Diuretics

NURSING CONSIDERATIONS

NURSING DIAGNOSES
◆ Anxiety
◆ Excess fluid volume
◆ Ineffective breathing pattern
◆ Ineffective tissue perfusion: Cardiopulmonary
◆ Risk for injury

EXPECTED OUTCOMES
The patient will:
◆ express feelings of decreased anxiety
◆ attain and maintain normal fluid and electrolyte balance
◆ maintain effective breathing pattern
◆ maintain adequate cardiac output
◆ avoid complications.

NURSING INTERVENTIONS
◆ Provide a safe environment.
◆ Give prescribed I.V. fluids.
◆ Evaluate muscle strength and adjust activity level.
◆ Reorient the confused patient when necessary.

MONITORING
◆ Serum electrolyte levels
◆ Respiratory status
◆ Signs of metabolic alkalosis
◆ Intake and output
◆ Neurologic status
◆ Cardiac rhythm
◆ Arterial blood gas levels

PATIENT TEACHING

GENERAL
Be sure to cover:
◆ the disorder, diagnosis, and treatment
◆ dietary or fluid restrictions, as indicated
◆ medication administration, dosage, and possible adverse effects.

RESOURCES
Organizations
National Digestive Diseases Information Clearinghouse: *www.niddk.nih.gov/health/digest/nddic.htm*
National Library of Medicine: *www.nlm.nih.gov*

Selected references
Diseases, 4th ed. Philadelphia: Lippincott Williams & Wilkins, 2006.
Martin, M., et al. "Diagnosis of Acid-Base Derangements and Mortality Prediction in the Trauma Intensive Care Unit: The Physiochemical Approach," *Journal of Trauma* 58(2):238-43, February 2005.
Strategies for Managing Multisystem Disorders. Philadelphia: Lippincott Williams & Wilkins, 2005.

Drugs causing hyperchloremia

These drugs can cause or contribute to hyperchloremia:
◆ acetazolamide (Diamox)
◆ ammonium chloride
◆ sodium polystyrene sulfonate (Kayexalate)
◆ salicylates (overdose)
◆ triamterene (Dyrenium).

Hyperkalemia LIFE-THREATENING DISORDER

OVERVIEW

- Excessive serum levels of the potassium anion
- Commonly induced by treatments for other disorders

PATHOPHYSIOLOGY

- Potassium facilitates contraction of both skeletal and smooth muscles, including myocardial contraction.
- Potassium figures prominently in nerve impulse conduction, acid-base balance, enzyme action, and cell membrane function.
- Hyperkalemia is often induced by other treatments.
- Slight deviation in serum levels can produce profound clinical consequences.
- Potassium imbalance can lead to muscle weakness and flaccid paralysis because of an ionic imbalance in neuromuscular tissue excitability.

CAUSES

- Adrenal gland insufficiency
- Burns
- Certain drugs (see *Drugs causing hyperkalemia*)
- Crushing injuries
- Decreased urinary excretion of potassium
- Dehydration
- Diabetic acidosis
- Increased intake of potassium
- Large quantities of blood transfusions
- Renal dysfunction or failure
- Severe infection
- Use of potassium-sparing diuretics such as triamterene by patients with renal disease

INCIDENCE

- Hyperkalemia affects males and females equally.
- Up to 8% of hospitalized patients in the United States are diagnosed with this disorder.

COMPLICATIONS

- Cardiac arrhythmia
- Metabolic acidosis
- Cardiac arrest

ASSESSMENT

HISTORY

- Irritability
- Paresthesia
- Muscle weakness
- Nausea
- Abdominal cramps
- Diarrhea

PHYSICAL FINDINGS

- Hypotension
- Irregular heart rate
- Irregular heart rhythm

DIAGNOSTIC TEST RESULTS

LABORATORY

- Serum potassium level is greater than 5 mEq/L.
- Arterial pH is decreased.

DIAGNOSTIC PROCEDURES

- Electrocardiography may show a tall, tented T wave. (See *Clinical effects of hyperkalemia.*)

Drugs causing hyperkalemia

These drugs may increase potassium levels:
- angiotensin-converting enzyme inhibitors
- antibiotics
- beta-adrenergic blockers
- chemotherapeutic drugs
- nonsteroidal anti-inflammatory drugs
- potassium (in excessive amounts)
- spironolactone (Aldactone).

Clinical effects of hyperkalemia

BODY SYSTEM	EFFECTS
Cardiovascular	◆ Tachycardia and later bradycardia, ECG changes (tented and elevated T waves, widened QRS complex, prolonged PR interval, flattened or absent P waves, depressed ST segment), cardiac arrest (with levels > 7 mEq/L)
Gastrointestinal	◆ Nausea, diarrhea, abdominal cramps
Genitourinary	◆ Oliguria, anuria
Musculoskeletal	◆ Muscle weakness, flaccid paralysis
Neurologic	◆ Hyperreflexia progressing to weakness, numbness, tingling, flaccid paralysis
Other	◆ Metabolic acidosis

TREATMENT

GENERAL
- Treatment of the underlying cause
- Hemodialysis or peritoneal dialysis

ACTIVITY
- As tolerated

MEDICATIONS
- Rapid infusion of 10% calcium gluconate (decreases myocardial irritability)
- Insulin and 10% to 50% glucose I.V.
- Sodium polystyrene sulfonate with 70% sorbitol

NURSING CONSIDERATIONS

NURSING DIAGNOSES
- Decreased cardiac output
- Diarrhea
- Risk for injury

EXPECTED OUTCOMES
The patient will:
- maintain adequate cardiac output and hemodynamic stability
- regain normal bowel elimination pattern
- avoid complications.

NURSING INTERVENTIONS
- Check the serum sample. (See *Avoiding false results.*)
- Give prescribed drugs.
- Insert an indwelling urinary catheter.
- Implement safety measures.
- Be alert for signs of hypokalemia after treatment.

MONITORING
- Serum potassium levels
- Cardiac rhythm
- Intake and output

PATIENT TEACHING

GENERAL
Be sure to cover:
- prescribed drugs and potential adverse effects
- monitoring intake and output
- preventing future episodes of hyperkalemia
- need for potassium-restricted diet.

RESOURCES
Organizations
Mayo Clinic: *www.mayoclinic.com*
The Merck Manuals Online Medical Library: *www.merck.com/mmhe*
National Library of Medicine: *www.nlm.nih.gov*

Selected references
Burger, C.M. "Hyperkalemia," *AJN* 104(10):66-70, October 2004.
Tran, H.A. "Extreme Hyperkalemia," *Southern Medical Journal* 98(7):729-32, July 2005.
Vuckovic, K., and Richlin, D. "Bradycardia Induced by Hyperkalemia," *AAOHN Journal* 52(5):186-87, May 2004.

Avoiding false results

When your patient gets a laboratory test result indicating a high potassium level, and the result doesn't make sense, make sure it's a true result. If the sample was drawn using poor technique, the results may be falsely high. These are some of the causes of falsely high potassium levels:
- drawing the sample above an I.V. infusion containing potassium
- using a recently exercised arm or leg for the venipuncture site
- causing hemolysis (cell damage) as the specimen is obtained.

Hyperlipoproteinemia

OVERVIEW

- Increased plasma concentrations of one or more lipoproteins
- Primary form includes at least five distinct and inherited metabolic disorders
- May occur secondary to other conditions such as diabetes mellitus
- Clinical changes range from relatively mild symptoms, managed by diet, to potentially fatal pancreatitis

PATHOPHYSIOLOGY

- Increased low-density lipoprotein (LDL) and decreased high-density lipoprotein (HDL) levels
- Accelerated development of atherosclerosis

CAUSES

- Primary hyperlipoproteinemia
- Types I and III transmitted as autosomal recessive traits
- Types II, IV, and V transmitted as autosomal dominant traits
- Secondary hyperlipoproteinemia
- Diabetes mellitus
- Hypothyroidism
- Pancreatitis
- Renal disease

INCIDENCE

Type I
- This type is relatively rare and is present at birth.

Type II
- The onset of type II is between ages 10 and 30.

Type III
- This type is uncommon and usually occurs after age 20.

Type IV
- This type is relatively common, especially in middle-age men.

Type V
- This type is uncommon and usually occurs in late adolescence or early adulthood.

COMPLICATIONS

- Coronary artery disease (CAD)
- Pancreatitis

ASSESSMENT

HISTORY

Type I
- Recurrent attacks of severe abdominal pain
- Abdominal pain usually preceded by fat intake
- Malaise and anorexia

Type II
- History of premature and accelerated coronary atherosclerosis
- Symptoms typically develop in 20s or 30s

Type III
- No clinical symptoms until after age 20
- Aggravating factors, such as obesity, hypothyroidism, and diabetes mellitus

Type IV
- Atherosclerosis
- Early CAD
- Excessive alcohol consumption
- Poorly controlled diabetes mellitus
- Hormonal contraceptive pills containing estrogen (can precipitate severe hypertriglyceridemia)
- Hypertension
- Hyperuricemia

Type V
- Abdominal pain associated with pancreatitis
- Complaints related to peripheral neuropathy

PHYSICAL FINDINGS

Type I
- Papular or eruptive xanthomas over pressure points and extensor surfaces
- Ophthalmoscopic examination: lipemia retinalis (reddish-white retinal vessels)
- Abdominal spasm, rigidity, or rebound tenderness
- Hepatosplenomegaly, with liver or spleen tenderness
- Possible fever

Type II
- Tendinous xanthomas on the Achilles tendons and tendons of the hands and feet
- Tuberous xanthomas, xanthelasma
- Juvenile corneal arcus

Type III
- Tuberoeruptive xanthomas over elbows and knees
- Palmar xanthomas on the hands, particularly the fingertips

Type IV
- Obesity
- Xanthomas possible during exacerbations

Type V
- Eruptive xanthomas on extensor surface of arms and legs
- Ophthalmoscopic examination: lipemia retinalis
- Hepatosplenomegaly

DIAGNOSTIC TEST RESULTS

LABORATORY

- Serum lipid profile shows elevated levels of total cholesterol, triglycerides, or very-low-density lipoproteins, or decreased HDL levels.

TREATMENT

GENERAL

- Weight reduction
- Elimination or treatment of aggravating factors, such as diabetes mellitus, alcoholism, and hypothyroidism
- Reduction of risk factors for atherosclerosis
- Smoking cessation
- Treatment of hypertension
- Avoidance of hormonal drugs and contraceptives that contain estrogen

DIET
◆ Avoidance of alcohol to decrease plasma triglyceride levels

Type I
◆ Restricted fat intake (less than 20 g/day); 20 to 40 g/day, medium-chain triglyceride diet to supplement calorie intake

Type II
◆ Restricted cholesterol intake (less than 300 mg/day for adults and less than 150 mg/day for children); restricted triglyceride intake (less than 100 mg/day for children and adults); increased polyunsaturated fats

Type III
◆ Restricted cholesterol intake (less than 300 mg/day) and carbohydrates; increased polyunsaturated fats

Type IV
◆ Restricted cholesterol intake; increased polyunsaturated fats

Type V
◆ Long-term maintenance of a low-fat diet; 20 to 40 g/day medium-chain triglyceride diet

ACTIVITY
◆ Maintenance of exercise and physical fitness program

MEDICATIONS
◆ Nicotinic acid
◆ Clofibrate and niacin
◆ Niacin, clofibrate, gemfibrozil (Lopid)
◆ HMG-CoA reductase inhibitors (such as atorvastatin [Lipitor], simvastatin [Zocor], and lovastatin [Mevacor])

SURGERY
◆ If unable to tolerate drug therapy, surgical creation of an ileal bypass
◆ For severely affected homozygote children, portacaval shunt as a last resort to reduce plasma cholesterol levels

NURSING CONSIDERATIONS

NURSING DIAGNOSES
◆ Anxiety
◆ Fear
◆ Ineffective tissue perfusion: Cardiopulmonary
◆ Risk for injury

EXPECTED OUTCOMES
The patient will:
◆ identify strategies to reduce anxiety
◆ verbalize fears and concerns
◆ exhibit signs of adequate cardiopulmonary perfusion
◆ avoid complications.

NURSING INTERVENTIONS
◆ Give prescribed antilipemics.
◆ Prevent or minimize adverse reactions.
◆ Urge the patient to adhere to the prescribed diet.
◆ Assist the patient with additional lifestyle changes.
◆ Encourage verbalization of fears related to premature CAD.

MONITORING
◆ Vital signs
◆ Adverse reactions
◆ Serum lipoproteins
◆ Response to treatment
◆ Signs and symptoms related to CAD or its sequelae

PATIENT TEACHING

GENERAL
Be sure to cover:
◆ the disorder, diagnosis, and treatment
◆ the need to maintain a steady weight and strictly adhere to the prescribed diet (for the 2 weeks preceding serum cholesterol and serum triglyceride tests), and to fast for 12 hours before the test
◆ the need to avoid excessive sugar intake and alcoholic beverages
◆ minimized intake of saturated fats (higher in meats and coconut oil)
◆ increased intake of polyunsaturated fats (vegetable oils)
◆ the need to avoid hormonal contraceptives or drugs that contain estrogen
◆ the need to avoid foods high in cholesterol and saturated fats
◆ the prescribed drug regimen and potential adverse effects
◆ signs and symptoms requiring medical evaluation.

DISCHARGE PLANNING
◆ Refer the patient for a medically supervised exercise program.
◆ Refer the patient to a smoking-cessation program, if indicated.
◆ Refer the patient to a dietitian, if necessary.

RESOURCES
Organizations
American Heart Association: *www.americanheart.org*
Food and Nutritional Information Center: *www.nal.usda.gov/fnic*

Selected references
Burnside, N.J., et al. "Type III Hyperlipoproteinemia with Xanthomas and Multiple Myeloma," *Journal of the American Academy of Dermatology* 53(5 Suppl 1):S281-84, November 2005.
Carroll, M.D., et al. "Trends in Serum Lipids and Lipoproteins of Adults, 1960-2002," *JAMA* 294(14):1773-781, October 2005.
Diseases, 4th ed. Philadelphia: Lippincott Williams & Wilkins, 2006.
Hollman, G., et al. "Meaning of Quality of Life among Patients with Familial Hypercholesterolemia," *Journal of Cardiovascular Nursing* 19(4):243-50, July-August 2004.
Thompson, G.R. "Additive Effects of Plant Sterol and Stanol Esters to Statin Therapy," *American Journal of Cardiology* 96(1A):37D-39D, July 2005.

Hypermagnesemia

OVERVIEW

◆ Excessive serum levels of the magnesium cation

PATHOPHYSIOLOGY

◆ Magnesium enhances neuromuscular integration and stimulates parathyroid hormone secretion, thus regulating intracellular fluid calcium levels.
◆ Magnesium may also regulate skeletal muscles through its influence on calcium utilization by depressing acetylcholine release at synaptic junctions.
◆ Magnesium activates many enzymes for proper carbohydrate and protein metabolism, aids in cell metabolism and the transport of sodium and potassium across cell membranes, and influences sodium, potassium, calcium, and protein levels.
◆ About one-third of magnesium taken into the body is absorbed through the small intestine and is eventually excreted in the urine; remaining unabsorbed magnesium is excreted in the stool.

CAUSES

◆ Addison's disease
◆ Adrenocortical insufficiency
◆ Chronic renal insufficiency
◆ Overcorrection of hypomagnesemia
◆ Overuse of magnesium-containing antacids
◆ Severe dehydration (resulting oliguria can cause magnesium retention)
◆ Untreated diabetic ketoacidosis
◆ Use of laxatives (magnesium sulfate, milk of magnesia, and magnesium citrate solutions), especially with renal insufficiency (see *Drugs and supplements causing hypermagnesemia*)

RISK FACTORS

◆ Advanced age
◆ Pregnancy
◆ Neonates whose mothers received magnesium sulfate during labor
◆ Patients receiving magnesium sulfate to control seizures

INCIDENCE

◆ This disorder rarely occurs in the United States.

COMPLICATIONS

◆ Respiratory depression
◆ Cardiac arrhythmia
◆ Cardiac arrest

ASSESSMENT

HISTORY

◆ Nausea
◆ Vomiting
◆ Drowsiness
◆ Confusion

PHYSICAL FINDINGS

◆ Flushed appearance
◆ Hypotension (see *Clinical effects of hypermagnesemia*)
◆ Weak pulse
◆ Muscle weakness
◆ Hyporeflexia (see *Testing the patellar reflex*)

DIAGNOSTIC TEST RESULTS

LABORATORY

◆ Serum magnesium level is greater than 2.5 mEq/L.

DIAGNOSTIC PROCEDURES

◆ Electrocardiography may show a prolonged PR interval, widened QRS complex, and tall T waves.

TREATMENT

GENERAL

◆ Identification and correction of the underlying cause
◆ Peritoneal dialysis or hemodialysis

DIET

◆ Increased fluid intake

MEDICATIONS

◆ Loop diuretics such as furosemide with impaired renal function
◆ Calcium gluconate (10%)

Drugs and supplements causing hypermagnesemia

Monitor your patient's magnesium level closely if he's receiving any of these drugs that can cause hypermagnesemia:
◆ an antacid (Di-Gel, Gaviscon, Maalox)
◆ a laxative (Milk of Magnesia, Haley's M-O, magnesium citrate)
◆ a magnesium supplement (magnesium oxide, magnesium sulfate).

Clinical effects of hypermagnesemia

BODY SYSTEM	EFFECTS
Cardiovascular	◆ Bradycardia, weak pulse, hypotension, heart block, cardiac arrest
Neurologic	◆ Drowsiness, flushing, lethargy, confusion, diminished sensorium
Neuromuscular	◆ Diminished reflexes, muscle weakness, flaccid paralysis, respiratory muscle paralysis that may cause respiratory embarrassment

NURSING DIAGNOSES
- Anxiety
- Decreased cardiac output
- Impaired gas exchange
- Ineffective tissue perfusion: Renal
- Risk for injury

EXPECTED OUTCOMES
The patient will:
- identify strategies to reduce anxiety
- maintain adequate cardiac output and hemodynamic stability
- maintain adequate ventilation and oxygenation
- exhibit signs of adequate renal perfusion
- avoid complications.

NURSING INTERVENTIONS
- Provide sufficient fluids for adequate hydration and maintenance of renal function.
- Give prescribed drugs.
- Report abnormal serum electrolyte levels immediately.
- Watch patients receiving a cardiac glycoside and calcium gluconate simultaneously because calcium excess enhances the cardiac glycoside.

MONITORING
- Vital signs
- Magnesium levels
- Electrolyte levels
- Intake and output
- Cardiac rhythm
- Neuromuscular system
- Level of consciousness
- Respiratory status

GENERAL
Be sure to cover:
- avoidance of abusing laxatives and antacids containing magnesium, particularly in the elderly or those patients with compromised renal function
- hydration requirements
- prescribed drugs.

RESOURCES
Organizations
The Merck Manuals Online Medical Library: *www.merck.com/mmhe*
National Institute of Diabetes & Digestive & Kidney Diseases: *www.niddk.nih.gov*
National Library of Medicine: *www.nlm.nih.gov*

Selected references
Kraft, M.D., et al. "Treatment of Electrolyte Disorders in Adult Patients in the Intensive Care Unit," *American Journal of Health-System Pharmacy* 62(16):1663-682, August 2005.
Strategies for Managing Multisystem Disorders. Philadelphia: Lippincott Williams & Wilkins, 2006.

Testing the patellar reflex

One way to gauge your patient's magnesium status is to test his patellar reflex, one of the deep tendon reflexes that the magnesium level affects. To test the reflex, strike the patellar tendon just below the patella with the patient sitting or lying in a supine position, as shown. Look for leg extension or contraction of the quadriceps muscle in the front of the thigh.

If the patellar reflex is absent, notify the physician immediately. This finding may mean your patient's magnesium level is 7 mEq/L or higher.

SITTING

Have the patient sit on the side of the bed with his legs dangling freely, as shown here. Then test the reflex.

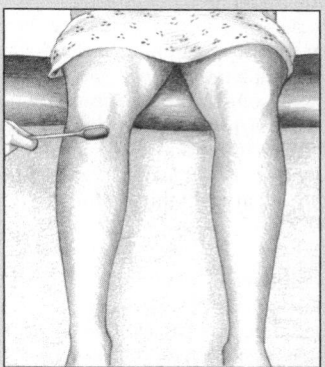

SUPINE POSITION

Flex the patient's knee at a 45-degree angle, and place your nondominant hand behind it for support. Then test the reflex.

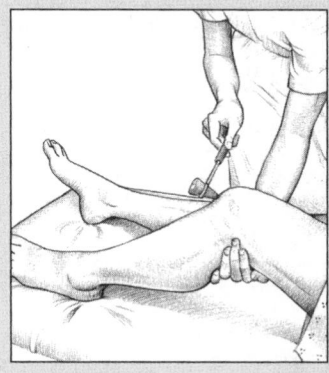

Hypernatremia

- Excessive serum levels of the sodium cation relative to body water

PATHOPHYSIOLOGY

- Sodium is the major cation (90%) in extracellular fluid, and potassium is the major cation in intracellular fluid.
- During repolarization, the sodium-potassium pump continually shifts sodium into the cells and potassium out of the cells; during depolarization, it does the reverse.
- Sodium cation functions include maintaining tonicity and concentration of extracellular fluid, acid-base balance (reabsorption of sodium ion and excretion of hydrogen ion), nerve conduction and neuromuscular function, glandular secretion, and water balance.
- Increased sodium causes high serum osmolality (increased solute concentrations in the body), which stimulates the hypothalamus and initiates the sensation of thirst.

CAUSES

- Antidiuretic hormone deficiency (diabetes insipidus)
- Certain drugs (see *Drugs causing hypernatremia*)
- Decreased water intake
- Excess adrenocortical hormones, as in Cushing's syndrome
- Excessive I.V. administration of sodium solutions
- Salt intoxication (less common), which may be produced by excessive table salt ingestion

RISK FACTORS

- People who can't drink voluntarily

INCIDENCE

- This disorder occurs in about 1% of hospitalized patients (usually elderly patients).
- This disorder affects males and females equally.

COMPLICATIONS

- Seizures
- Coma
- Permanent neurologic damage.

ASSESSMENT

HISTORY

- Fatigue
- Restlessness, agitation
- Weakness
- Disorientation
- Lethargy

PHYSICAL FINDINGS

- Flushed skin (see *Clinical effects of hypernatremia*)
- Dry, swollen tongue
- Sticky mucous membranes
- Low-grade fever
- Twitching
- Hypertension, dyspnea (with hypervolemia)
- Orthostatic hypotension and oliguria (with hypovolemia)

Drugs causing hypernatremia

Ask your patient if he's taking any of these drugs that can elevate his sodium level:
- antacids with sodium bicarbonate
- antibiotics such as ticarcillin disodium-clavulanate potassium (Timentin)
- salt tablets
- sodium bicarbonate injections (such as those given during cardiac arrest)
- I.V. sodium chloride preparations
- sodium polystyrene sulfonate (Kayexalate).

Clinical effects of hypernatremia

BODY SYSTEM	EFFECTS
Cardiovascular	◆ Hypertension, tachycardia, pitting edema, excessive weight gain
Gastrointestinal	◆ Rough, dry tongue; intense thirst
Genitourinary	◆ Oliguria
Integumentary	◆ Flushed skin; dry, sticky membranes
Neurologic	◆ Fever, agitation, restlessness, seizures
Respiratory	◆ Dyspnea, respiratory arrest, death (from dramatic rise in osmotic pressure)

DIAGNOSTIC TEST RESULTS

LABORATORY
◆ Serum sodium level is greater than 145 mEq/L.
◆ Urine sodium level is less than 40 mEq/24 hours, with high serum osmolality.

TREATMENT

GENERAL
◆ Treatment of underlying cause
◆ Administration of salt-free solutions (such as dextrose in water) followed by infusion of half-normal saline solution to prevent hyponatremia
◆ Discontinuation of drugs that promote sodium retention

DIET
◆ Sodium restriction

ACTIVITY
◆ As tolerated

NURSING CONSIDERATIONS

NURSING DIAGNOSES
◆ Anxiety
◆ Deficient fluid volume
◆ Fear
◆ Ineffective tissue perfusion: Cardiopulmonary
◆ Risk for injury

EXPECTED OUTCOMES
The patient will:
◆ identify strategies to reduce anxiety
◆ maintain adequate fluid volume
◆ discuss fears and concerns
◆ exhibit signs of adequate cardiopulmonary perfusion
◆ avoid complications.

NURSING INTERVENTIONS
◆ Obtain a drug history to check for drugs that promote sodium retention.
◆ Assist with oral hygiene.
◆ Observe for signs of cerebral edema during fluid replacement therapy.

MONITORING
◆ Serum sodium levels
◆ Intake and output
◆ Neurologic status

PATIENT TEACHING

GENERAL
Be sure to cover:
◆ the disorder and treatment
◆ the importance of sodium restriction
◆ low-sodium diet
◆ prescribed drugs
◆ signs and symptoms of hypernatremia
◆ avoiding over-the-counter medications that contain sodium.

RESOURCES
Organizations
The Merck Manuals Online Medical Library: *www.merck.com/mmhe*
National Institute of Diabetes & Digestive & Kidney Diseases: *www.niddk.nih.gov*

Selected references
Dickerson, R.N., and Brown, R.O. "Long-term Enteral Nutrition Support and the Risk of Dehydration," *Nutrition in Clinical Practice* 20(6):646-53, December 2005.
Ellison, D.H. "Disorders of Sodium and Water," *American Journal of Kidney Disease* 46(2):356-61, August 2005.
Moritz, M.L., et al. "Breastfeeding-associated Hypernatremia: Are We Missing the Diagnosis?" *Pediatrics* 116(3):e343-47, September 2005.
Strategies for Managing Multisystem Disorders. Philadelphia: Lippincott Williams & Wilkins, 2006.

Hyperparathyroidism

OVERVIEW

- Characterized by a greater than normal secretion of parathyroid hormone (PTH)
- Classified as either primary or secondary

PATHOPHYSIOLOGY

- In primary hyperparathyroidism, one or more of the parathyroid glands enlarges, increasing PTH secretion and elevating serum calcium levels, or an adenoma secretes PTH, unresponsive to negative feedback of serum calcium.
- In secondary hyperparathyroidism, excessive compensatory production of PTH stems from a hypocalcemia-producing abnormality outside the parathyroid gland, which isn't responsive to PTH such as decreased intestinal absorption of calcium or vitamin D.
- Increased PTH levels act directly on the bone and the kidney tubules, resulting in an increase in extracellular calcium.
- Renal excretion and uptake into the soft tissues or skeleton can't compensate for increased calcium.

CAUSES

- Adenoma
- Chronic renal failure
- Decreased intestinal absorption of vitamin D or calcium
- Dietary vitamin D or calcium deficiency
- Genetic disorders
- Idiopathic
- Ingestion of drugs such as phenytoin
- Laxative ingestion
- Multiple endocrine neoplasia
- Osteomalacia

INCIDENCE

- This disorder is more common in women than in men.
- The incidence rate is higher in postmenopausal women.
- Onset of this disorder is usually between ages 35 and 65.

COMPLICATIONS

- Osteoporosis
- Subchondral fractures
- Traumatic synovitis
- Renal calculi and colic
- Renal insufficiency and failure
- Peptic ulcers
- Cholelithiasis
- Cardiac arrhythmias
- Vascular damage
- Heart failure
- Muscle atrophy
- Depression

ASSESSMENT

HISTORY

- Recurring nephrolithiasis
- Polyuria
- Hematuria
- Chronic lower back pain
- Easy fracturing
- Osteoporosis
- Constant, severe epigastric pain that radiates to the back
- Abdominal pain
- Anorexia, nausea, and vomiting
- Constipation
- Polydipsia
- Muscle weakness, particularly in the legs
- Lethargy
- Personality disturbances
- Depression
- Overt psychosis
- Cataracts
- Anemia

PHYSICAL FINDINGS

- Muscle weakness and atrophy
- Psychomotor disturbances
- Stupor and, possibly, coma
- Skin necrosis
- Subcutaneous calcification

DIAGNOSTIC TEST RESULTS

LABORATORY

In primary disease

- Alkaline phosphatase level increases.
- Osteocalcin level increases.
- Tartrate-resistant acid phosphatase level increases.
- Serum PTH level increases.
- Serum calcium level increases.
- Serum phosphorus level decreases.
- Urine and serum calcium and serum chloride levels increase.
- Creatinine level may increase.
- Basal acid secretion may increase.
- Serum amylase level may increase.

In secondary disease

- Serum calcium level is normal or slightly decreased.
- Serum phosphorus level is variable.
- Serum PTH level increases.

IMAGING

- X-rays show diffuse bone demineralization, bone cysts, outer cortical bone absorption, and subperiosteal erosion of the phalanges and distal clavicles in primary disease.
- X-ray spectrophotometry shows increased bone turnover in primary disease.
- Esophagography, thyroid scan, parathyroid thermography, ultrasonography, thyroid angiography, computed tomography scan, and magnetic resonance imaging may show location of parathyroid lesions.

TREATMENT

GENERAL

- In primary disease, treatment to decrease calcium levels
- In renal failure, dialysis
- In secondary disease, treatment to correct underlying cause of parathyroid hypertrophy

DIET

- Increased oral fluid intake

ACTIVITY
◆ As tolerated

MEDICATIONS
Primary disease
◆ Bisphosphonates
◆ Oral sodium or potassium phosphate
◆ Calcitonin (Miacalcin)
◆ Plicamycin (Mithracin), if primary disease is metastatic

Secondary disease
◆ Vitamin D therapy
◆ Aluminum hydroxide
◆ Glucocorticoids

Postoperatively
◆ I.V. magnesium and phosphate
◆ Sodium phosphate
◆ Supplemental calcium
◆ Vitamin D or calcitriol (Calcijex)

SURGERY
◆ With primary hyperparathyroidism, removal of adenoma or all but one-half of one gland

NURSING CONSIDERATIONS

NURSING DIAGNOSES
◆ Activity intolerance
◆ Acute pain
◆ Anxiety
◆ Decreased cardiac output
◆ Disturbed body image
◆ Excess fluid volume
◆ Fear
◆ Imbalanced nutrition: Less than body requirements
◆ Ineffective coping

EXPECTED OUTCOMES
The patient will:
◆ perform activities of daily living without excessive fatigue
◆ express feelings of increased comfort and decreased pain
◆ verbalize strategies to reduce anxiety
◆ maintain adequate cardiac output
◆ express positive feelings about self
◆ maintain normal fluid volume
◆ express fears and concerns

◆ maintain adequate nutrition and hydration
◆ demonstrate adaptive coping behaviors.

NURSING INTERVENTIONS
◆ Obtain baseline serum potassium, calcium, phosphate, and magnesium levels before treatment.
◆ Provide at least 3 qt (3 L) of fluid per day.
◆ Institute safety precautions.
◆ Schedule frequent rest periods.
◆ Provide comfort measures.
◆ Give prescribed drugs.
◆ Help the patient turn and reposition every 2 hours.
◆ Support affected extremities with pillows.
◆ Offer emotional support.
◆ Help the patient develop effective coping strategies.

After parathyroidectomy
◆ Keep a tracheotomy tray and endotracheal tube setup at the bedside.
◆ Maintain seizure precautions.
◆ Place the patient in semi-Fowler's position.
◆ Support the patient's head and neck with sandbags.
◆ Have the patient ambulate as soon as possible.

WARNING *Watch for complaints of tingling in the hands and around the mouth. If these symptoms don't subside quickly, they may be prodromal signs of tetany, so keep I.V. calcium gluconate or calcium chloride available for emergency administration.*

MONITORING
◆ Vital signs
◆ Intake and output
◆ Serum calcium levels
◆ Respiratory status
◆ Cardiovascular status

After parathyroidectomy
◆ Increased neuromuscular irritability
◆ Complications
◆ Neck edema
◆ Chvostek's sign
◆ Trousseau's sign

PATIENT TEACHING

GENERAL
Be sure to cover:
◆ the disorder, diagnosis, and treatment
◆ prescribed drugs and possible adverse effects
◆ when to notify the practitioner
◆ the signs and symptoms of tetany, respiratory distress, and renal dysfunction
◆ the need for periodic blood tests
◆ avoidance of calcium-containing antacids and thiazide diuretics
◆ the need to wear medical identification jewelry.

RESOURCES
Organizations
American Association of Clinical Endocrinologists: *www.aace.com*
Endocrine Society: *www.endo-society.org*

Selected references
Donovan, P.I. "Outpatient Parathyroidectomy: A New Paradigm from a Nursing Perspective," *Current Opinion in Oncology* 17(1):28-32, January 2005.
Levine, M.A. "Primary Hyperparathyroidism: 7,000 Years of Progress," *Cleveland Clinic Journal of Medicine* 72(12):1084-1085, 1088, 1091-1092 passim., December 2005.
Peregrin, T. "Early Assessment of Secondary Hyperparathyroidism," *Journal of the American Dietetic Association* 106(1):22-23, January 2006.
Strategies for Managing Multisystem Disorders. Philadelphia: Lippincott Williams & Wilkins, 2006.

Hyperphosphatemia

OVERVIEW

- Excessive serum levels of phosphate
- Reflects the kidney's inability to excrete excess phosphorus

PATHOPHYSIOLOGY

- Phosphorus exists in combination with calcium in teeth and bones.
- In extracellular fluid, the phosphate ion supports many metabolic functions: B vitamin use, acid-base homeostasis, bone formation, nerve and muscle activity, cell division, transmission of hereditary traits, and metabolism of carbohydrates, proteins, and fats.
- Renal tubular reabsorption of phosphate is inversely regulated by calcium levels — an increase in phosphorus causes a decrease in calcium. An imbalance causes hypophosphatemia or hyperphosphatemia.

CAUSES

- Acid-base imbalance
- Certain drugs (see *Drugs and supplements causing hyperphosphatemia*)
- Hypervitaminosis D
- Hypocalcemia
- Hypoparathyroidism
- Overuse of laxatives with phosphates or phosphate enemas
- Renal failure

RISK FACTORS

- Muscle necrosis
- Infection
- Heat stroke
- Trauma
- Chemotherapy

INCIDENCE

- This disorder occurs most commonly in children, who tend to consume more phosphorus-rich foods and beverages than adults.
- The incidence is higher in children and adults with renal insufficiency.

COMPLICATIONS

- Soft tissue calcifications
- Hypocalcemia
- Bone fractures

ASSESSMENT

HISTORY

- Anorexia
- Decreased mental status
- Nausea and vomiting

PHYSICAL FINDINGS

- Hyperreflexia
- Hypocalcemic electrocardiogram changes
- Muscle weakness and cramps
- Papular eruptions
- Paresthesia
- Presence of Chvostek's or Trousseau's sign
- Abdominal spasm
- Tetany
- Visual impairment
- Conjunctivitis

DIAGNOSTIC TEST RESULTS

LABORATORY

- Serum phosphorus level is greater than 4.5 mg/dl.
- Serum calcium level is less than 8.9 mg/dl.
- Blood urea nitrogen and creatinine levels are increased.

IMAGING

- X-ray studies reveal skeletal changes caused by osteodystrophy in chronic hyperphosphatemia.

DIAGNOSTIC PROCEDURES

- Electrocardiography may show changes characteristic of hypercalcemia.

Drugs and supplements causing hyperphosphatemia

These drugs may cause hyperphosphatemia:

- enemas such as Fleet enemas
- laxatives containing phosphorus or phosphate
- oral phosphorus supplements
- parenteral phosphorus supplements (sodium phosphate, potassium phosphate)
- vitamin D supplements.

TREATMENT

GENERAL
- Treatment of the underlying cause
- Peritoneal dialysis or hemodialysis (if severe)
- Discontinuation of drugs associated with hyperphosphatemia
- I.V. saline solution

DIET
- Low-phosphorus

ACTIVITY
- As tolerated

MEDICATIONS
- Aluminum
- Magnesium
- Calcium gel
- Phosphate-binding antacids

NURSING CONSIDERATIONS

NURSING DIAGNOSES
- Acute pain
- Anxiety
- Risk for injury

EXPECTED OUTCOMES
The patient will:
- express feelings of comfort and decreased pain
- express feelings of decreased anxiety
- avoid injury.

NURSING INTERVENTIONS
- Provide safety measures.
- Be alert for signs of hypocalcemia.
- Give prescribed drugs.
- Give antacids with meals to increase their effectiveness.
- Prepare the patient for dialysis, if appropriate.
- Assist with selecting a low-phosphorus diet.

MONITORING
- Vital signs
- Phosphorus and calcium levels
- Intake and output
- Renal studies

PATIENT TEACHING

GENERAL
Be sure to cover:
- the disorder and treatment
- prescribed drugs
- the need to avoid preparations that contain phosphorus
- the need to avoid high-phosphorus foods. (See *Foods high in phosphorus.*)

DISCHARGE PLANNING
- Refer the patient to a dietitian and social services, if indicated.

RESOURCES
Organizations
American Association of Kidney Patients: *www.aakp.org*
National Institute of Diabetes & Digestive & Kidney Diseases: *www.niddk.nih.gov*

Selected references
Hayes, D.D. "Phosphorus: Here, There, Everywhere," *Nursing Made Incredible Easy!* 2(6):36-41, November-December 2004.
Schucker, J.J., and Ward, K.E. "Hyperphosphatemia and Phosphate Binders," *American Journal of Health-System Pharmacy* 62(22):2355-361, November 2005.
Strategies for Managing Multisystem Disorders. Philadelphia: Lippincott Williams & Wilkins, 2006.

Foods high in phosphorus

These foods have a high phosphorus content:
- beans
- bran
- cheese
- chocolate
- dark-colored sodas
- ice cream
- lentils
- milk
- nuts
- peanut butter
- seeds
- yogurt.

Hyperpituitarism

- Chronic, progressive disease marked by hormonal dysfunction and startling skeletal overgrowth
- Prognosis dependent on cause
- Life expectancy usually reduced
- Appears in two forms: acromegaly and gigantism
- Also referred to as *growth hormone (GH) excess*

PATHOPHYSIOLOGY

- Progressive excessive secretion of pituitary GH occurs.
- Acromegaly occurs after epiphyseal closure, causing bone thickening and transverse growth and visceromegaly.
- Gigantism occurs before epiphyseal closure with excess GH, causing proportional overgrowth of all body tissues.
- A large tumor may cause loss of other trophic hormones, such as thyroid-stimulating hormone, luteinizing hormone, follicle-stimulating hormone, and corticotropin, which may cause dysfunction of target organs.

CAUSES

- Excessive GH-releasing hormone
- Excessive GH secretion
- GH-producing adenoma of the anterior pituitary gland
- Possible genetic cause

INCIDENCE

Acromegaly

- Acromegaly occurs equally in men and women.
- Acromegaly usually occurs between ages 30 and 50.

Gigantism

- Gigantism affects infants and children.

COMPLICATIONS

- Arthritis
- Carpal tunnel syndrome
- Osteoporosis
- Kyphosis
- Hypertension
- Arteriosclerosis
- Cardiomegaly and heart failure
- Blindness
- Severe neurologic disturbances
- Glucose intolerance
- Diabetes mellitus
- Severe psychological stress

ASSESSMENT

HISTORY

- Gradual onset of acromegaly
- Relatively abrupt onset of gigantism
- Soft tissue swelling
- Hypertrophy of the face and extremities
- Diaphoresis, oily skin
- Fatigue, sleep disturbances
- Weight gain
- Headaches, decreased vision
- Decreased libido, impotence
- Oligomenorrhea, infertility
- Joint pain
- Hypertrichosis
- Irritability, hostility, and other psychological disturbances

PHYSICAL FINDINGS

- Enlarged jaw, thickened tongue
- Enlarged and weakened hands
- Coarsened facial features
- Oily or leathery skin
- Prominent supraorbital ridge
- Deep, hollow-sounding voice
- Cartilaginous and connective tissue overgrowth
- Skeletal abnormalities

AGE FACTOR *In infants, inspection reveals a highly arched palate, muscular hypotonia, slanting eyes, and exophthalmos.*

DIAGNOSTIC TEST RESULTS

LABORATORY

- GH radioimmunoassay shows increased plasma GH levels and levels of insulin-like growth factor I.
- Glucose suppression test failing to suppress the hormone level to below the accepted norm of 2 ng/ml.

IMAGING

- Skull X-rays, computed tomography scan, or magnetic resonance imaging show location of pituitary tumor.
- Bone X-rays show a thickening of the cranium and long bones and osteoarthritis in the spine.

TREATMENT

GENERAL

- Treatment to curb overproduction of GH
- Pituitary radiation therapy

MEDICATIONS

- Replacement of thyroid, cortisone, and gonadal hormones postoperatively if entire pituitary removed
- GH synthesis inhibitor
- Long-acting analogue of somatostatin

SURGERY

- Transsphenoidal hypophysectomy

NURSING CONSIDERATIONS

NURSING DIAGNOSES
- Activity intolerance
- Acute pain
- Chronic low self-esteem
- Disturbed body image
- Disturbed sensory perception (visual)
- Impaired oral mucous membrane
- Impaired physical mobility
- Ineffective coping
- Sexual dysfunction

EXPECTED OUTCOMES
The patient will:
- perform activities of daily living within the confines of the disorder
- express feelings of increased comfort
- voice positive feelings related to self-esteem
- express positive feelings related to body image
- maintain optimal functioning within the limits of his visual disturbance
- maintain intact oral mucous membranes
- maintain joint mobility and range of motion (ROM)
- demonstrate effective coping skills
- verbalize feelings regarding actual or perceived sexual impairment.

NURSING INTERVENTIONS
- Provide emotional support.
- Provide reassurance that mood changes result from hormonal imbalances and can be reduced with treatment.
- Give prescribed drugs.
- Provide comfort measures.
- Perform or assist with ROM exercises.
- Evaluate muscle weakness.
- Institute safety precautions.
- Provide meticulous skin care.
- Assist with early postoperative ambulation.

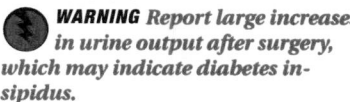 **WARNING** *Report large increases in urine output after surgery, which may indicate diabetes insipidus.*

MONITORING
- Vital signs
- Intake and output
- Serum glucose levels
- Signs and symptoms of hyperglycemia

After surgery
- Signs and symptoms of increased intracranial pressure (ICP) and intracranial bleeding
- Respiratory status
- Surgical incisions and dressings
- Complications
- Signs and symptoms of infection
- Signs and symptoms of hormonal deficiency

PATIENT TEACHING

GENERAL
Be sure to cover:
- the disorder, diagnosis, and treatment
- prescribed drugs and potential adverse effects
- when to notify the practitioner
- avoidance of activities that increase ICP
- deep breathing through the mouth if nasal packing is in place postoperatively
- hormone replacement therapy, if ordered
- the importance of wearing a medical identification bracelet
- follow-up examinations
- possible tumor recurrence.

DISCHARGE PLANNING
- Refer the patient for psychological counseling to help deal with body image changes and sexual dysfunction as needed.
- Refer the patient to an acromegaly center.

RESOURCES
Organizations
Endocrine Society: *www.endo-society.org*
Pituitary Network Association: *www.pituitary.com*

Selected references

Ezzat, S. "Pharmacological Options in the Treatment of Acromegaly," *Current Opinion in Investigational Drugs* 6(10):1023-1027, October 2005.

Hanberg, A. "Common Disorders of the Pituitary Gland: Hyposecretion versus Hypersecretion," *Journal of Infusion Nursing* 28(1); 36-44, January-February 2005.

Strategies for Managing Multisystem Disorders. Philadelphia: Lippincott Williams & Wilkins, 2006.

Hypersplenism

OVERVIEW

- Exaggerated splenic activity and, possibly, splenomegaly
- Results in peripheral blood cell deficiency as the spleen traps and destroys peripheral blood cells
- May be primary or secondary

PATHOPHYSIOLOGY

- The spleen's normal filtering and phagocytic functions accelerate indiscriminately, automatically removing antibody-coated, aging, and abnormal cells, even though some cells may be functionally normal.
- The spleen may also temporarily sequester normal platelets and red blood cells (RBCs), withholding them from circulation. In this manner, the enlarged spleen may trap as many as 90% of the body's platelets and up to 45% of its RBC mass.

CAUSES

- Idiopathic (see *Causes of splenomegaly*)
- An extrasplenic disorder, such as chronic malaria, polycythemia vera, or rheumatoid arthritis

INCIDENCE

- Hypersplenism affects all ages.
- Hypersplenism affects males and females equally.

COMPLICATIONS

- Bleeding
- Postsplenectomy infection and thromboembolic disease

ASSESSMENT

HISTORY

- Frequent bacterial infection
- Frequent bruising
- Spontaneous hemorrhaging from the mucous membranes and GI or genitourinary tract
- Fever
- Weakness
- Palpitations
- Weight loss

PHYSICAL FINDINGS

- Ulcerations of the mouth, legs, and feet
- Bruising
- Splenomegaly
- Jaundice
- Pallor

DIAGNOSTIC TEST RESULTS

LABORATORY

- A high spleen-liver ratio of radioactivity indicates splenic destruction or sequestration.
- Hemoglobin level falls to as low as 4 g/dl.
- White blood cell count is less than 4,000/µl.
- Platelet count is less than 125,000/µl.
- Reticulocyte count is greater than 75,000/µl.

IMAGING

- Ultrasonography or splenic scan may show enlarged spleen or underlying cause such as a tumor.

Causes of splenomegaly

CONGESTIVE

- Cirrhosis, thrombosis

CYSTIC OR NEOPLASTIC

- Cysts, leukemia, lymphoma, myelofibrosis

HYPERPLASTIC

- Hemolytic anemia, polycythemia

INFECTIOUS

- Acute (abscesses, subacute infective endocarditis), chronic (tuberculosis, malaria, Felty's syndrome)

INFILTRATIVE

- Gaucher's disease, Niemann-Pick disease

TREATMENT

GENERAL
◆ Treatment of underlying disease (secondary)

DIET
◆ Nothing by mouth if surgery is indicated

ACTIVITY
◆ Limited, noncontact

MEDICATIONS
◆ Antibiotics if infection present
◆ Pneumococcal vaccine (after splenectomy)

SURGERY
◆ Splenectomy indicated only in transfusion-dependent patients who are refractory to medical therapy

NURSING CONSIDERATIONS

NURSING DIAGNOSES
◆ Anxiety
◆ Disturbed body image
◆ Fear
◆ Impaired skin integrity
◆ Risk for infection
◆ Risk for injury

EXPECTED OUTCOMES
The patient will:
◆ use support systems to assist with anxiety and fear
◆ verbalize feelings about changed body image
◆ verbalize feelings of anxiety and fear
◆ maintain skin integrity
◆ avoid infection and other complications
◆ sustain no harm or injury.

NURSING INTERVENTIONS
◆ If splenectomy is scheduled, administer preoperative transfusions of blood or blood products (fresh frozen plasma and platelets) to replace deficient blood elements.
◆ Treat symptoms or complications of any underlying disorder.
◆ Provide emotional support.

MONITORING
◆ Vital signs
◆ Signs of bleeding
◆ Complete blood cell count
◆ Signs of infection

After surgery
◆ Pain control
◆ Wound site

PATIENT TEACHING

GENERAL
Be sure to cover:
◆ the disorder, diagnosis, and treatment
◆ signs and symptoms of infection
◆ activity restrictions.

RESOURCES
Organizations
National Heart, Lung, and Blood Institute: *www.nhlbi.nih.gov*
National Library of Medicine: *www.nlm.nih.gov*

Selected references
Arya, L.S., et al. "Significance of Splenomegaly in Childhood Hodgkin's Disease," *Journal of Pediatric Hematology/Oncology* 26(12):807-12, December 2004.

Diseases, 4th ed. Philadelphia: Lippincott Williams & Wilkins, 2006.

Iso, Y., et al. "Hepatobiliary and Pancreatic: Massive Splenomegaly," *Journal of Gastroenterology & Hepatology* 20(12):1942, December 2005.

Mohan, A., et al. "Sarcoidosis Manifesting as Massive Splenomegaly: A Rare Occurrence," *American Journal of Medical Sciences* 328(3):170-72, September 2004.

Hypertension

- Intermittent or sustained elevation of diastolic or systolic blood pressure
- Usually begins as benign disease, slowly progressing to accelerated or malignant state
- Two major types: essential (also called primary or idiopathic) hypertension and secondary hypertension, which results from renal disease or another identifiable cause
- Malignant hypertension, a medical emergency, is a severe, fulminant form commonly arising from both types

PATHOPHYSIOLOGY
Several theories
- Changes in arteriolar bed cause increased peripheral vascular resistance.
- Abnormally increased tone in the sympathetic nervous system originates in the vasomotor system centers, causing increased peripheral vascular resistance.
- Increased blood volume results from renal or hormonal dysfunction.
- Increase in arteriolar thickening is caused by genetic factors, leading to increased peripheral vascular resistance.
- Abnormal renin release results in the formation of angiotensin II, which constricts the arterioles and increases blood volume.

CAUSES
- Unknown

RISK FACTORS
- Family history
- Blacks in the United States
- Stress
- Obesity
- High-sodium, high-saturated fat diet
- Use of tobacco
- Use of hormonal contraceptives
- Excessive alcohol intake
- Sedentary lifestyle
- Aging

INCIDENCE
- This disorder affects 15% to 20% of adults in the United States.
- Essential hypertension accounts for 90% to 95% of cases.

COMPLICATIONS
- Cardiac disease
- Renal failure
- Blindness
- Stroke

ASSESSMENT

HISTORY
- In many cases, no symptoms, and disorder revealed incidentally during evaluation for another disorder or during a routine blood pressure screening program
- Symptoms that reflect the effect of hypertension on the organ systems
- Awakening with a headache in the occipital region, which subsides spontaneously after a few hours
- Dizziness, fatigue, and confusion
- Palpitations, chest pain, dyspnea
- Epistaxis
- Hematuria
- Blurred vision

PHYSICAL FINDINGS
- Bounding pulse
- S_4
- Peripheral edema in late stages
- Hemorrhages, exudates, and papilledema of the eye in late stages if hypertensive retinopathy present
- Pulsating abdominal mass, suggesting an abdominal aneurysm
- Elevated blood pressure on at least two consecutive occasions after initial screenings
- Bruits over the abdominal aorta and femoral arteries or the carotids

DIAGNOSTIC TEST RESULTS

LABORATORY
- Urinalysis may show protein, red blood cells, or white blood cells, suggesting renal disease, or glucose, suggesting diabetes mellitus.
- Serum potassium levels less than 3.5 mEq/L may indicate adrenal dysfunction (primary hyperaldosteronism).
- Blood urea nitrogen levels normal or elevated to more than 20 mg/dl and serum creatinine levels normal or elevated to more than 1.5 mg/dl suggest renal disease.

IMAGING
- Excretory urography reveals renal atrophy, indicating chronic renal disease; one kidney more than $5/8''$ (1.6 cm) shorter than the other suggests unilateral renal disease.
- Chest X-rays demonstrate cardiomegaly.
- Renal arteriography shows renal artery stenosis.

DIAGNOSTIC PROCEDURES
- Electrocardiography may show left ventricular hypertrophy or ischemia.
- An oral captopril challenge may be done to test for renovascular hypertension.
- Ophthalmoscopy reveals arteriovenous nicking and, in hypertensive encephalopathy, edema.

TREATMENT

GENERAL
- Lifestyle modification, such as weight control, limiting alcohol, regular exercise, and smoking cessation
- For a patient with secondary hypertension, correction of the underlying cause and control of hypertensive effects

DIET
◆ Low–saturated fat and low-sodium
◆ Adequate calcium, magnesium, and potassium

ACTIVITY
◆ Regular exercise

MEDICATIONS
◆ Diuretics
◆ Beta-adrenergic blockers
◆ Calcium channel blockers
◆ Angiotensin-converting enzyme inhibitors
◆ Alpha-receptor antagonists
◆ Vasodilators
◆ Angiotensin-receptor blockers
◆ Aldosterone antagonist

NURSING CONSIDERATIONS

NURSING DIAGNOSES
◆ Fatigue
◆ Ineffective coping
◆ Ineffective tissue perfusion: Cardiopulmonary
◆ Noncompliance (therapeutic regimen)
◆ Risk for injury

EXPECTED OUTCOMES
The patient will:
◆ express feelings of increased energy
◆ demonstrate adaptive coping behaviors
◆ maintain adequate cardiac output and hemodynamic stability
◆ comply with the therapy regimen
◆ remain free from complications.

NURSING INTERVENTIONS
◆ Give prescribed drugs.
◆ Encourage dietary changes, as appropriate.
◆ Help the patient identify risk factors and modify his lifestyle, as appropriate.

MONITORING
◆ Vital signs, especially blood pressure
◆ Signs and symptoms of target end-organ damage
◆ Complications
◆ Response to treatment
◆ Risk factor modification
◆ Adverse effects of antihypertensive agents

PATIENT TEACHING

GENERAL
Be sure to cover:
◆ the disorder, diagnosis, and treatment
◆ how to use a self-monitoring blood pressure cuff and to record the reading in a journal for review by the practitioner
◆ the importance of compliance with antihypertensive therapy and establishing a daily routine for taking prescribed drugs
◆ the need to report adverse effects of drugs
◆ the need to avoid high sodium antacids and over-the-counter cold and sinus medications containing harmful vasoconstrictors
◆ examining and modifying lifestyle, including diet
◆ the need for a routine exercise program, particularly aerobic walking
◆ dietary restrictions
◆ the importance of follow-up care.

DISCHARGE PLANNING
◆ Refer the patient to stress-reduction therapies or support groups, as needed.
◆ Refer the patient to weight-reduction or smoking-cessation groups, as needed.

RESOURCES
Organizations
American Heart Association:
www.americanheart.org
American Medical Association:
www.ama-assn.org

Selected references
Cheng, S.L. "Treating HTN Crisis. How Low? How Fast?" *RN* 68(6):37-41, June 2005.
Coy, V. "Genetics of Essential Hypertension," *Journal of the American Academy of Nurse Practitioners* 17(6):219-24, June 2005.
Jacobs, T.F., and Ramsey, L.A. "Angiotensin Receptor Blockers. Applications Beyond Hypertension," *Advanced Nurse Practitioner* 13(1):27-30, January 2005.
Lloyd-Jones, D.M., et al. "Hypertension in Adults Across the Age Spectrum: Current Outcomes and Control in the Community," *JAMA* 294(4):466-72, July 2005.
Nettina, S.M. *Lippincott Manual of Nursing Practice*, 8th ed. Philadelphia: Lippincott Williams & Wilkins, 2006.

Hypertension, gestational — LIFE-THREATENING DISORDER

OVERVIEW

- High blood pressure, most often occurring after the 20th week of gestation in a nulliparous woman
- Carries a high risk for fetal mortality because of the increased incidence of premature delivery
- Among the most common causes of maternal death in developed countries (especially when complications occur)
- Nonconvulsive form (also called *preeclampsia*) occurring after the 20th week of gestation; may be mild or severe
- Convulsive form (also called *eclampsia*) occurring between the 24th week of gestation and the end of the first postpartum week

PATHOPHYSIOLOGY

- Generalized arteriolar vasoconstriction is thought to cause decreased blood flow through the placenta and maternal organs.
- This leads to intrauterine growth retardation or restriction, placental infarcts, and abruptio placentae.

CAUSES

- Unknown
- Contributing factors:
  - Autointoxication
  - Autolysis of placental infarcts
  - Diabetes
  - Geographic, ethnic, racial, nutritional, immunologic, and familial factors
  - Maternal age
  - Maternal sensitization to total proteins
  - Preexisting vascular disease
  - Pyelonephritis
  - Uremia

AGE FACTOR *Adolescents and primiparas older than age 35 are at higher risk for preeclampsia.*

RISK FACTORS

- First-time pregnancy
- Multiple fetuses
- History of vascular disease

INCIDENCE

- This condition occurs in about 7% of pregnancies and is more common in women from lower socioeconomic groups.
- There is roughly a 5% incidence of preeclampsia progressing to eclampsia.

COMPLICATIONS

- Abruptio placentae
- HELLP syndrome: hemolysis, elevated liver enzyme levels, low platelet count
- Coagulopathy
- Stillbirth
- Seizures
- Coma
- Premature labor
- Renal failure
- Maternal hepatic damage

ASSESSMENT

HISTORY

- Sudden weight gain
- Irritability
- Emotional tension
- Severe frontal headache
- Blurred vision
- Epigastric pain or heartburn

PHYSICAL FINDINGS

- Preeclampsia: blood pressure of 160/110 mm Hg or higher
- Eclampsia: systolic blood pressure of 180 or 200 mm Hg or higher
- Generalized edema, especially of the face
- Pitting edema of the legs and feet
- Hyperreflexia
- Oliguria
- Vascular spasm, papilledema, retinal edema or detachment, and arteriovenous nicking or hemorrhage (seen on ophthalmoscopy)
- Seizures

DIAGNOSTIC TEST RESULTS

LABORATORY

- In preeclampsia, proteinuria exceeds 300 mg/24 hours [1+].
- In severe eclampsia, proteinuria is 5 g/24 hours [5+] or more.
- In HELLP syndrome, hemolysis, elevated liver enzymes, and decreased platelet count are present.

IMAGING

- Ultrasonography aids evaluation of fetal well-being.

DIAGNOSTIC PROCEDURES

- Stress and nonstress tests and biophysical profiles help evaluate fetal well-being.

TREATMENT

GENERAL

- Measures to halt progression of the disorder and ensure fetal survival
- Prompt labor induction, especially if the patient is near term (advocated by some clinicians)
- Adequate nutrition

DIET

- Low-sodium, if indicated
- Limited caffeine

ACTIVITY

- Complete bed rest
- Left lateral lying position

MEDICATIONS

- Antihypertensives
- Magnesium sulfate
- Oxytocin
- Oxygen

SURGERY

- Possible cesarean delivery

NURSING DIAGNOSES
- Activity intolerance
- Anxiety
- Disturbed sensory perception (visual)
- Excess fluid volume
- Fear
- Impaired urinary elimination
- Ineffective coping
- Ineffective tissue perfusion: Cerebral, peripheral
- Risk for injury

EXPECTED OUTCOMES
The patient will:
- perform activities of daily living without excessive fatigue
- identify strategies to reduce anxiety
- maintain optimal functioning within the confines of the visual impairment
- maintain normal fluid volume
- verbalize fears and concerns
- maintain urine output within normal limits
- demonstrate adaptive coping behaviors
- exhibit signs of adequate cerebral and peripheral perfusion
- avoid complications.

NURSING INTERVENTIONS
- Give prescribed drugs.
- Elevate edematous arms or legs.
- Eliminate constricting hose, slippers, and bed linens.
- Assist with or insert an indwelling urinary catheter, if necessary.
- Provide a quiet, darkened room.
- Enforce absolute bed rest.
- Provide emotional support.
- Encourage the patient to express feelings.
- Help the patient develop effective coping strategies. (See *Emergency interventions for gestational hypertension.*)

MONITORING
- Vital signs
- Fetal heart rate
- Vision
- Edema
- Daily weight
- Intake and output
- Level of consciousness
- Deep tendon reflexes
- Headache unrelieved by medication
- Complications

Emergency interventions for gestational hypertension

When caring for a patient with gestational hypertension, be prepared to perform the following interventions:
- Observe for signs of fetal distress by closely monitoring results of stress and nonstress tests.
- Keep emergency resuscitative equipment and anticonvulsants at hand in case of seizures and cardiac or respiratory arrest.
- Carefully monitor magnesium sulfate administration. Signs of drug toxicity include absence of patellar reflexes, flushing, muscle flaccidity, decreased urinary output, significant blood pressure drop (> 15 mm Hg), and a respiratory rate less than 12 per minute. Keep calcium gluconate at the bedside to counteract the toxic effects of magnesium sulfate.
- Prepare for emergency cesarean delivery, if indicated. Alert the anesthesiologist and pediatrician.
- To protect the patient from injury, maintain seizure precautions. Don't leave an unstable patient unattended. Maintain a patent airway, and have supplemental oxygen readily available.

GENERAL
Be sure to cover:
- the disorder, diagnosis, and treatment
- signs and symptoms of preeclampsia and eclampsia
- importance of bed rest in the left lateral position, as ordered
- adequate nutrition and a low-sodium diet
- good prenatal care
- control of preexisting hypertension
- early recognition and prompt treatment of preeclampsia
- likelihood that the neonate will be small for gestational age, with the probability that he'll do better than other premature neonates of the same weight.

DISCHARGE PLANNING
- Refer the patient for professional counseling, as indicated.

RESOURCES
Organizations
American College of Obstetricians and Gynecologists: *www.acog.org*
American Heart Association: *www.americanheart.org*
American Society for Reproductive Medicine: *www.asrm.org*

Selected references
Kisters, K., et al. "Preventing Pregnancy-induced Hypertension: The Role of Calcium and Magnesium," *Journal of Hypertension* 24(1):201, January 2006.
Nettina, S.M. *Lippincott Manual of Nursing Practice,* 8th ed. Philadelphia: Lippincott Williams & Wilkins, 2006.
Roberts, J.M., and Gammill, H.S. "Preeclampsia: Recent Insights," *Hypertension* 46(6):1243-249, December 2005.
Sibai, B.M. "Diagnosis and Management of Gestational Hypertension and Preeclampsia," *Obstetrics & Gynecology* 102(1):181-92, July 2003.

Hyperthyroidism

OVERVIEW

- An alteration in thyroid function in which thyroid hormones (TH) exert greater than normal responses
- Management determined by cause
- Hyperthyroidism: a form of thyrotoxicosis in which excess thyroid hormones are secreted by the thyroid gland
- Thyrotoxicoses not associated with hyperthyroidism: subacute thyroiditis, ectopic thyroid tissue, and ingestion of excessive TH
- Graves' disease (also known as *toxic diffuse goiter*): an autoimmune disease, the most common form of hyperthyroidism
- Also known as *thyrotoxicosis*

PATHOPHYSIOLOGY

- In Graves' disease, thyroid-stimulating antibodies bind to and stimulate the thyroid-stimulating hormone (TSH) receptors of the thyroid gland.
- The trigger for this autoimmune disease is unclear.
- It's associated with the production of autoantibodies possibly caused by a defect in suppressor T-lymphocyte function that allows the formation of these autoantibodies.

CAUSES

- Diseases that can cause hyperthyroidism:
- Genetic and immunologic factors
- Graves' disease
- Increased TSH secretion
- Thyroid cancer
- Toxic multinodular goiter
- Precipitating factors:
- Diabetic ketoacidosis
- Excessive iodine intake
- Infection
- Stress
- Surgery
- Toxemia of pregnancy

INCIDENCE

- Graves' disease is most common between ages 30 and 60, and is more common in women than in men.
- Graves' disease has an increased incidence rate among monozygotic twins.
- This disease is more common in those with a family history of thyroid abnormalities.
- Only 5% of hyperthyroid patients younger than age 15 develop Graves' disease.

COMPLICATIONS

- Arrhythmias
- Left ventricular hypertrophy
- Heart failure
- Muscle weakness and atrophy
- Paralysis
- Osteoporosis
- Vitiligo
- Skin hyperpigmentation
- Corneal ulcers
- Myasthenia gravis
- Impaired fertility
- Decreased libido
- Gynecomastia
- Thyrotoxic crisis or thyroid storm
- Hepatic or renal failure

ASSESSMENT

HISTORY
Graves' disease
- Nervousness, tremor
- Heat intolerance
- Weight loss despite increased appetite
- Sweating
- Frequent bowel movements
- Palpitations
- Poor concentration
- Shaky handwriting
- Clumsiness
- Emotional instability and mood swings
- Thin, brittle nails
- Hair loss
- Nausea and vomiting
- Weakness and fatigue
- Oligomenorrhea or amenorrhea
- Fertility problems
- Diminished libido
- Diplopia

PHYSICAL FINDINGS
Graves' disease
- Enlarged thyroid (goiter)
- Exophthalmos
- Tremor
- Smooth, warm, flushed skin
- Fine, soft hair
- Premature graying and increased hair loss
- Friable nails and onycholysis
- Pretibial myxedema
- Thickened skin
- Accentuated hair follicles
- Tachycardia at rest
- Full, bounding pulses
- Arrhythmias, especially atrial fibrillation
- Wide pulse pressure
- Possible systolic murmur
- Dyspnea
- Hepatomegaly
- Hyperactive bowel sounds
- Weakness, especially in proximal muscles, and atrophy
- Possible generalized or localized paralysis
- Gynecomastia in males
- Increased tearing

DIAGNOSTIC TEST RESULTS

LABORATORY
- Radioimmunoassay shows increased serum triiodothyronine and thyroxine concentrations.
- Serum protein-bound iodine level increases.
- Serum cholesterol and total lipid levels decrease.
- TSH level decreases.

IMAGING
- Thyroid scan shows increased uptake of radioactive iodine (^{131}I).
- Ultrasonography shows subclinical ophthalmopathy.

DIET
◆ Adequate caloric intake

ACTIVITY
◆ As tolerated

MEDICATIONS
◆ Treatment with ^{131}I: a single oral dose; treatment of choice for women past reproductive age or men and women not planning to have children
◆ Thyroid hormone antagonists
◆ Beta-adrenergic antagonists
◆ Corticosteroids
◆ Sedatives

SURGERY
◆ Subtotal (partial) thyroidectomy
◆ Surgical decompression

NURSING CONSIDERATIONS

NURSING DIAGNOSES
◆ Decreased cardiac output
◆ Diarrhea
◆ Disturbed body image
◆ Imbalanced nutrition: Less than body requirements
◆ Ineffective coping
◆ Risk for deficient fluid volume
◆ Risk for imbalanced body temperature

EXPECTED OUTCOMES
The patient will:
◆ maintain normal cardiac output
◆ have normal bowel movements
◆ express positive feelings about body
◆ maintain adequate nutrition and hydration with no further weight loss
◆ demonstrate adaptive coping behaviors
◆ maintain an adequate fluid balance
◆ remain normothermic.

NURSING INTERVENTIONS
◆ Minimize physical and emotional stress.
◆ Balance rest and activity periods.

◆ Keep the patient's room cool and quiet and the lights dim.
◆ Encourage the patient to dress in loose-fitting, cotton clothing.
◆ Consult a dietitian to ensure a nutritious diet with adequate calories and fluids.
◆ Offer small, frequent meals.
◆ Provide meticulous skin care.
◆ Reassure the patient and his family that mood swings and nervousness usually subside with treatment.
◆ Encourage verbalization of feelings.
◆ Help the patient identify and develop coping strategies.
◆ Offer emotional support.
◆ Give prescribed drugs.
◆ Avoid excessive palpation of the thyroid.

After thyroidectomy
◆ Change dressings and perform wound care, as ordered.
◆ Keep the patient in semi-Fowler's position.
◆ Support the patient's head and neck with sandbags.

MONITORING
◆ Vital signs
◆ Daily weight
◆ Intake and output
◆ Daily neck circumference
◆ Serum electrolyte results
◆ Hyperglycemia and glycosuria
◆ Electrocardiogram for arrhythmias and ST-segment changes
◆ Complete blood count results
◆ Signs and symptoms of heart failure
◆ Frequency and characteristics of stools

After thyroidectomy
◆ Dressings
◆ Signs and symptoms of hemorrhage into the neck
◆ Surgical incision
◆ Dysphagia or hoarseness
◆ Signs and symptoms of hypocalcemia

PATIENT TEACHING

GENERAL
Be sure to cover:
◆ the disorder, diagnosis, and treatment
◆ prescribed drugs and potential adverse effects
◆ when to notify the practitioner
◆ the need for regular medical follow-up visits
◆ the need for lifelong thyroid hormone replacement
◆ the importance of wearing medical identification jewelry
◆ precautions with ^{131}I therapy
◆ signs and symptoms of hypothyroidism and hyperthyroidism
◆ eye care for ophthalmopathy.

RESOURCES
Organizations
American Association of Clinical Endocrinologists: *www.aace.com*
Endocrine and Metabolic Diseases Information Service: *www.endocrine.niddk.nih.gov*
Endocrine Society: *www.endo-society.org*

Selected references
Amer, K.S. "Advances in Assessment, Diagnosis, and Treatment of Hyperthyroidism in Children," *Journal of Pediatric Nursing* 20(2):119-26, April 2005.
Franklyn, J.A., et al. "Thyroid Function and Mortality in Patients Treated for Hyperthyroidism," *JAMA* 294(1):71-80, July 2005.
Holcomb, S.S. "Detecting Thyroid Disease," *Nursing* 35(10 Suppl):4-8, October 2005.
Strategies for Managing Multisystem Disorders. Philadelphia: Lippincott Williams & Wilkins, 2006.
Waltman, P.A., et al. "Thyroid Storm During Pregnancy: A Medical Emergency," *Critical Care Nurse* 24(2):74-79, April 2004.

Hypocalcemia

◆ Deficient serum levels of calcium

PATHOPHYSIOLOGY
◆ Together with phosphorous, calcium is responsible for the formation and structure of bones and teeth.
◆ Calcium helps maintain cell structure and function.
◆ It plays a role in cell membrane permeability and impulse transmission.
◆ It affects the contraction of cardiac muscle, smooth muscle, and skeletal muscle.
◆ It also participates in the blood-clotting process.

CAUSES
◆ Hypomagnesemia
◆ Hypoparathyroidism
◆ Inadequate dietary intake of calcium and vitamin D
◆ Malabsorption or loss of calcium from the GI tract
◆ Overcorrection of acidosis
◆ Pancreatic insufficiency
◆ Renal failure
◆ Severe infections or burns

INCIDENCE
◆ Hypocalcemia occurs equally in males and females.
◆ This disorder affects persons of all ages.

COMPLICATIONS
◆ Laryngeal spasm
◆ Seizures
◆ Cardiac arrhythmia
◆ Respiratory arrest

ASSESSMENT

HISTORY
◆ Underlying cause
◆ Anxiety
◆ Irritability
◆ Seizures
◆ Muscle cramps
◆ Diarrhea

PHYSICAL FINDINGS
◆ Twitching (see *Clinical effects of hypocalcemia*)
◆ Carpopedal spasm
◆ Tetany
◆ Hypotension
◆ Confusion
◆ Positive Chvostek's and Trousseau's signs (see *Eliciting signs of hypocalcemia*)

DIAGNOSTIC TEST RESULTS

LABORATORY
◆ Serum calcium level is less than 8.5 mg/dl.
◆ Ionized calcium level is less than 4.5 mg/dl.

DIAGNOSTIC PROCEDURES
◆ Electrocardiography shows lengthened QT interval, prolonged ST segment, and arrhythmias.

TREATMENT

GENERAL
◆ Treatment of the underlying cause

DIET
◆ High in calcium and vitamin D

ACTIVITY
◆ As tolerated

MEDICATIONS
◆ Oral calcium and vitamin D supplements
◆ Calcium gluconate I.V.

Clinical effects of hypocalcemia

BODY SYSTEM	EFFECTS
Cardiovascular	◆ Arrhythmias, hypotension
Gastrointestinal	◆ Increased GI motility, diarrhea
Musculoskeletal	◆ Paresthesia, tetany or painful tonic muscle spasms, facial spasms, abdominal cramps, muscle cramps, spasmodic contractions
Neurologic	◆ Anxiety, irritability, twitching around mouth, laryngospasm, seizures, Chvostek's sign, Trousseau's sign
Other	◆ Blood-clotting abnormalities

NURSING DIAGNOSES
- Anxiety
- Decreased cardiac output
- Fear
- Impaired gas exchange
- Ineffective tissue perfusion: Cardiopulmonary
- Risk for injury

EXPECTED OUTCOMES
The patient will:
- identify strategies to reduce anxiety
- maintain adequate cardiac output
- discuss fears and concerns
- maintain adequate ventilation and oxygenation
- exhibit signs of adequate cardiopulmonary perfusion
- avoid complications.

NURSING INTERVENTIONS
- Provide safety measures; institute seizure precautions, if appropriate.
- Give prescribed calcium replacement.
- Assess I.V. sites if administering calcium I.V. (infiltration causes sloughing).

MONITORING
- Cardiac rhythm
- Seizures
- Calcium levels

GENERAL
Be sure to cover:
- proper administration of calcium supplements
- importance of following a high-calcium diet.

DISCHARGE PLANNING
- Refer the patient to a dietitian and social services, if indicated.

RESOURCES
Organizations
Endocrine and Metabolic Diseases Information Service:
www.endocrine.niddk.nih.gov
Mayo Clinic: *www.mayoclinic.com*
National Library of Medicine:
www.nlm.nih.gov

Selected references
Bellazzini, M.A., and Howes, D.S. "Pediatric Hypocalcemia Seizures: A Case of Rickets," *Journal of Emergency Medicine* 28(2):161-64, February 2005.
Krueger, D., and Tasota, F.J. "Keeping an Eye on Calcium Levels," *Nursing* 3(6):68, 70, June 2003.
Strategies for Managing Multisystem Disorders. Philadelphia: Lippincott Williams & Wilkins, 2006.
Vivien, B., et al. "Early Hypocalcemia in Severe Trauma," *Critical Care Medicine* 33(9):1946-952, September 2005.

Eliciting signs of hypocalcemia

When the patient complains of muscle spasms and paresthesia in his limbs, try eliciting Chvostek's and Trousseau's signs — indications of tetany associated with calcium deficiency.

Follow the procedures described here, keeping in mind the discomfort they typically cause. If you detect these signs, notify the practitioner immediately. During these tests, watch the patient for laryngospasm, monitor his cardiac status, and have resuscitation equipment nearby.

CHVOSTEK'S SIGN
To elicit this sign, tap the patient's facial nerve just in front of the earlobe and below the zygomatic arch or between the zygomatic arch and the corner of the mouth, as shown at right.

A positive response (indicating latent tetany) ranges from simple mouth-corner twitching to twitching of all facial muscles on the side tested. Simple twitching may be normal in some patients. However, a more pronounced response usually confirms Chvostek's sign.

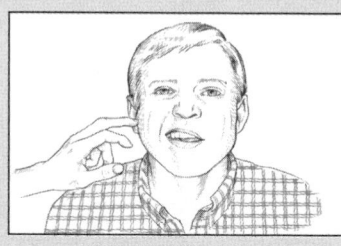

TROUSSEAU'S SIGN
In this test, occlude the brachial artery by inflating a blood pressure cuff on the patient's upper arm to a level between diastolic and systolic blood pressure. Maintain this inflation for 3 minutes while observing the patient for carpal spasm (shown at right), which is Trousseau's sign.

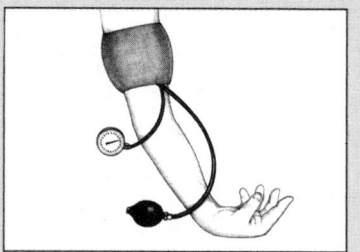

Hypochloremia

OVERVIEW

- Deficient serum levels of the chloride anion
- When serum chloride levels drop, levels of sodium, potassium, calcium, and other electrolytes may be affected
- When chloride levels decrease, bicarbonate levels rise to compensate

PATHOPHYSIOLOGY

- Chloride accounts for two-thirds of all serum anions.
- Chloride is secreted by the stomach's mucosa as hydrochloric acid; it provides an acid medium that aids digestion and activation of enzymes.
- It participates in maintaining acid-base and body water balances, influences the osmolality or tonicity of extracellular fluid, plays a role in the exchange of oxygen and carbon dioxide in red blood cells, and helps activate salivary amylase (which, in turn, activates the digestive process).

CAUSES

- Addison's disease
- Administration of dextrose I.V. without electrolytes
- Certain drugs (see *Drugs causing hypochloremia*)
- Chloride-deficient formula (for infants)
- Loss of hydrochloric acid in gastric secretions due to vomiting, gastric suctioning, or gastric surgery
- Prolonged diarrhea or diaphoresis
- Prolonged use of mercurial diuretics
- Salt-restricted diets
- Untreated diabetic ketoacidosis

RISK FACTORS

- Cystic fibrosis
- Pyloric obstruction
- Draining fistula
- Ileostomy
- Heart failure

COMPLICATIONS

- Respiratory arrest
- Seizures
- Coma

ASSESSMENT

HISTORY

- Risk factors for low chloride levels
- Agitation
- Irritability

PHYSICAL FINDINGS

- Muscle weakness
- Twitching
- Tetany
- Shallow, depressed breathing
- Hyperactive deep tendon reflexes
- Muscle cramps
- Cardiac arrhythmias

DIAGNOSTIC TEST RESULTS

LABORATORY

- Serum chloride level is less than 98 mEq/L.
- Serum sodium level is less than 135 mEq/L.
- Supportive values in metabolic alkalosis:
- – Serum pH is greater than 7.45.
- – Serum carbon dioxide level is greater than 32 mEq/L.

Drugs causing hypochloremia

These kinds of diuretics may cause hypochloremia:
- loop (such as furosemide [Lasix])
- osmotic (such as mannitol [Osmitrol])
- thiazide (such as hydrochlorothiazide [Esidrix]).

TREATMENT

GENERAL
◆ Treatment of underlying condition
◆ Treatment of associated metabolic acidosis or electrolyte imbalances

DIET
◆ High-sodium

ACTIVITY
◆ As tolerated

MEDICATIONS
◆ Normal saline I.V. solution
◆ Ammonium chloride
◆ Potassium chloride (for metabolic acidosis)

NURSING CONSIDERATIONS

NURSING DIAGNOSES
◆ Anxiety
◆ Ineffective breathing pattern
◆ Ineffective tissue perfusion: Cardiopulmonary
◆ Risk for injury

EXPECTED OUTCOMES
The patient will:
◆ express feelings of decreased anxiety
◆ maintain effective breathing pattern
◆ maintain adequate cardiac output
◆ avoid complications.

NURSING INTERVENTIONS
◆ Offer foods high in chloride. (See *Dietary sources of chloride.*)
◆ Provide environmental safety.
◆ Give prescribed I.V. fluids and drugs.

MONITORING
◆ Level of consciousness
◆ Muscle strength and movement
◆ Cardiac rhythm
◆ Arterial blood gas levels
◆ Serum electrolyte levels
◆ Respiratory status
◆ Signs of metabolic alkalosis

PATIENT TEACHING

GENERAL
Be sure to cover:
◆ the disorder, diagnosis, and treatment
◆ signs and symptoms of electrolyte imbalance
◆ dietary supplements
◆ prescribed drugs.

RESOURCES
Organizations
Endocrine and Metabolic Diseases Information Service: *www.endocrine.niddk.nih.gov*
National Institute of Diabetes & Digestive & Kidney Diseases: *www.niddk.nih.gov*

Selected references
Elgart, H.N. "Assessment of Fluids and Electrolytes," *AACN Clinical Issues: Advanced Practice in Acute & Critical Care* 15(4):607-21, October-December 2004.
Strategies for Managing Multisystem Disorders. Philadelphia: Lippincott Williams & Wilkins, 2006.

Dietary sources of chloride

These foods provide chloride:
◆ fruits
◆ vegetables
◆ table salt
◆ salty foods
◆ processed meats
◆ canned vegetables.

Hypokalemia ^{LIFE-THREATENING DISORDER}

OVERVIEW

- Deficient serum levels of the potassium anion
- Normal range for a serum potassium level narrow (3.5 to 5 mEq/L); a slight decrease can have a profound consequence

PATHOPHYSIOLOGY

- Potassium facilitates contraction of both skeletal and smooth muscles, including myocardial contraction.
- Potassium figures prominently in nerve impulse conduction, acid-base balance, enzyme action, and cell membrane function.
- A slight deviation in serum levels can produce profound clinical consequences.
- Potassium imbalance can lead to muscle weakness and flaccid paralysis because of an ionic imbalance in neuromuscular tissue excitability.

CAUSES

- Acid-base imbalances
- Certain drugs, especially potassium-wasting diuretics, steroids, and certain sodium-containing antibiotics (carbenicillin) (see *Drugs causing hypokalemia*)
- Chronic renal disease, with tubular potassium wasting
- Cushing's syndrome
- Excessive GI or urinary losses, such as vomiting, gastric suction, diarrhea, dehydration, anorexia, or chronic laxative abuse
- Excessive ingestion of licorice
- Hyperglycemia
- Low-potassium diet
- Primary hyperaldosteronism
- Prolonged potassium-free I.V. therapy
- Severe serum magnesium deficiency
- Trauma (injury, burns, or surgery)

INCIDENCE

- Hypokalemia affects up to 20% of hospitalized patients, but is significant in only about 4% to 5% of these patients.
- Up to 14% of all outpatients are affected mildly.

- About 80% of patients who receive diuretics become hypokalemic.
- Males and females are affected equally.

COMPLICATIONS

- Cardiac arrhythmia
- Cardiac arrest
- Rhabdomyolysis

ASSESSMENT

HISTORY

- Muscle weakness
- Paresthesia
- Abdominal cramps
- Anorexia
- Nausea, vomiting
- Constipation
- Polyuria

PHYSICAL FINDINGS

- Hyporeflexia (see *Clinical effects of hypokalemia*)
- Weak, irregular pulse
- Orthostatic hypotension
- Decreased bowel sounds

Drugs causing hypokalemia

These drugs can deplete potassium and cause hypokalemia:
- adrenergics, such as albuterol (Proventil) and epinephrine
- antibiotics, such as amphotericin B, carbenicillin (Geocillin), and gentamicin
- cisplatin
- corticosteroids
- diuretics, such as furosemide and thiazide
- insulin
- laxatives (when used excessively).

Clinical effects of hypokalemia

BODY SYSTEM	EFFECTS
Cardiovascular	Dizziness, hypotension, arrhythmias, electrocardiogram changes (flattened T waves, elevated U waves, decreased ST segments), cardiac arrest (with levels < 2.5 mEq/L)
Gastrointestinal	Nausea, vomiting, anorexia, diarrhea, abdominal distention, paralytic ileus or decreased peristalsis
Genitourinary	Polyuria
Musculoskeletal	Muscle weakness and fatigue, leg cramps
Neurologic	Malaise, irritability, confusion, mental depression, speech changes, decreased reflexes, respiratory paralysis
Other	Metabolic alkalosis

DIAGNOSTIC TEST RESULTS

LABORATORY
◆ Serum potassium level is less than 3.5 mEq/L.
◆ Bicarbonate and pH levels are elevated.
◆ Serum glucose level is slightly elevated.

DIAGNOSTIC PROCEDURES
◆ Characteristic electrocardiogram changes may be seen, including flattened T wave and depressed ST segment and U wave.

TREATMENT

GENERAL
◆ Treatment of the underlying cause
◆ High-potassium diet
◆ Activity, as tolerated

MEDICATIONS
◆ Potassium chloride (I.V. or orally)
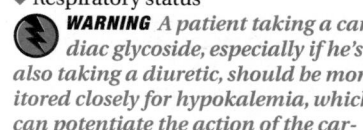 **WARNING** *A patient taking a diuretic may be switched to a potassium-sparing diuretic to prevent excessive urinary loss of potassium.*

NURSING CONSIDERATIONS

NURSING DIAGNOSES
◆ Decreased cardiac output
◆ Diarrhea
◆ Fatigue
◆ Risk for injury

EXPECTED OUTCOMES
The patient will:
◆ maintain adequate cardiac output and hemodynamic stability
◆ regain normal bowel elimination pattern
◆ express feelings of increased energy
◆ avoid complications.

NURSING INTERVENTIONS
◆ Give prescribed drugs.
◆ Insert an indwelling urinary catheter.
◆ Implement safety measures.
◆ Be alert for signs of hyperkalemia after treatment.
◆ Administer I.V. fluids.

MONITORING
◆ Serum potassium levels
◆ Cardiac rhythm
◆ Intake and output
◆ Vital signs
◆ Respiratory status
WARNING *A patient taking a cardiac glycoside, especially if he's also taking a diuretic, should be monitored closely for hypokalemia, which can potentiate the action of the cardiac glycoside and cause toxicity.*

PATIENT TEACHING

GENERAL
Be sure to cover:
◆ the disorder and treatment
◆ prescribed drugs and potential adverse effects
◆ monitoring intake and output
◆ preventing future episodes of hypokalemia
◆ need for a high-potassium diet
◆ warning signs and symptoms to report to the practitioner.

RESOURCES
Organizations
American Heart Association: *www.americanheart.org*
The Merck Manuals Online Medical Library: *www.merck.com/mmhe*
National Institute of Diabetes & Digestive & Kidney Diseases: *www.niddk.nih.gov*
National Library of Medicine: *www.nlm.nih.gov*

Selected references
Lewin, H. "A Close Call with Hypokalemia: For One Woman, Diarrhea Signaled a Dangerous Potassium Loss," *AJN* 104(11):65, November 2004.
Stern, E. "Hypokalemia," *AJN* 105(4):15, April 2005.
Strategies for Managing Multisystem Disorders. Philadelphia: Lippincott Williams & Wilkins, 2006.
Sweeney, J. "What Causes Sudden Hypokalemia?" *Nursing* 35(4):12, April 2005.

⚡ Hypomagnesemia LIFE-THREATENING DISORDER

OVERVIEW

- Deficient serum levels of the magnesium cation
- Relatively common imbalance

PATHOPHYSIOLOGY

- Magnesium enhances neuromuscular integration and stimulates parathyroid hormone secretion, thus regulating intracellular fluid calcium levels.
- Magnesium may also regulate skeletal muscles through its influence on calcium utilization by depressing acetylcholine release at synaptic junctions.
- It activates many enzymes for proper carbohydrate and protein metabolism, aids in cell metabolism and the transport of sodium and potassium across cell membranes, and influences sodium, potassium, calcium, and protein levels.
- About one-third of magnesium taken into the body is absorbed through the small intestine and is eventually excreted in the urine; the remaining unabsorbed magnesium is excreted in the stool.

CAUSES

- Administration of parenteral fluids without magnesium salts
- Certain drugs (see *Drugs causing hypomagnesemia*)
- Chronic alcoholism
- Chronic diarrhea
- Diabetic acidosis
- Excessive release of adrenocortical hormones
- Hyperaldosteronism
- Hypercalcemia
- Hyperparathyroidism
- Hypoparathyroidism
- Malabsorption syndrome
- Nasogastric suctioning
- Postoperative complications after bowel resection
- Prolonged diuretic therapy
- Severe dehydration
- Starvation or malnutrition

RISK FACTORS

- Sepsis
- Serious burns
- Wounds requiring debridement

INCIDENCE

- Hypomagnesemia occurs in 10% to 20% of hospitalized patients, and in 50% to 60% of patients in the intensive care unit.
- Hypomagnesemia occurs in 25% of outpatients with diabetes.
- Hypomagnesemia occurs in 30% to 80% of alcoholics.
- Hypomagnesemia affects males and females equally.

COMPLICATIONS

- Laryngeal stridor
- Seizures
- Respiratory depression
- Cardiac arrhythmia
- Cardiac arrest

ASSESSMENT

HISTORY

- Dysphagia
- Nausea
- Vomiting
- Drowsiness
- Confusion
- Leg and foot cramps

PHYSICAL FINDINGS

- Tachycardia
- Hypertension (see *Clinical effects of hypomagnesemia*)
- Muscle weakness, tremors, twitching
- Hyperactive deep tendon reflexes
- Chvostek's and Trousseau's signs
- Cardiac arrhythmia

Drugs causing hypomagnesemia

Monitor your patient's magnesium level if he's taking any of these drugs that can cause or contribute to hypomagnesemia:
- aminoglycoside antibiotic, such as amikacin, gentamicin, streptomycin, or tobramycin
- amphotericin B
- cisplatin
- cyclosporine
- insulin
- laxative
- loop or thiazide diuretic, such as bumetanide, furosemide, or torsemide
- pentamidine isethionate.

LABORATORY
◆ Serum magnesium level is less than 1.5 mEq/L.
◆ Serum potassium or calcium level is below normal.

DIAGNOSTIC PROCEDURES
◆ Electrocardiography may show abnormalities, such as prolonged QT interval and atrioventricular block.

TREATMENT

GENERAL
◆ Treatment of the underlying cause

DIET
◆ Replacement of magnesium

ACTIVITY
◆ As tolerated

MEDICATIONS
◆ Magnesium oxide
◆ Magnesium sulfate (I.M. or I.V.)

NURSING CONSIDERATIONS

NURSING DIAGNOSES
◆ Anxiety
◆ Decreased cardiac output
◆ Imbalanced nutrition: Less than body requirements
◆ Risk for injury

EXPECTED OUTCOMES
The patient will:
◆ identify strategies to reduce anxiety
◆ maintain adequate cardiac output and hemodynamic stability
◆ maintain daily calorie requirements
◆ avoid complications.

NURSING INTERVENTIONS
◆ Institute seizure precautions.
◆ Give prescribed drugs.
◆ Report abnormal serum electrolyte levels immediately.

⚡ **WARNING** *A low magnesium level may increase the body's retention of a cardiac glycoside. Be alert for signs of digoxin toxicity if your patient is taking digoxin.*

◆ Ensure patient safety.
◆ Reorient the patient as needed.

MONITORING
◆ Vital signs
◆ Magnesium levels
◆ Electrolyte levels
◆ Intake and output
◆ Cardiac rhythm
◆ Level of consciousness
◆ Respiratory status

PATIENT TEACHING

GENERAL
Be sure to cover:
◆ the disorder and treatment
◆ prescribed drugs
◆ avoidance of drugs that deplete magnesium, such as diuretics and laxatives
◆ the need to adhere to a high-magnesium diet
◆ danger signs and when to report them.

DISCHARGE PLANNING
◆ Refer the patient to Alcoholics Anonymous, if appropriate.

RESOURCES
Organizations
Endocrine and Metabolic Diseases Information Service: *www.endocrine.niddk.nih.gov*
The Merck Manuals Online Medical Library: *www.merck.com/mmhe*
National Institute of Diabetes & Digestive & Kidney Diseases: *www.niddk.nih.gov*
National Library of Medicine: *www.nlm.nih.gov*

Selected references
Richette, P., et al. "Hypomagnesemia and Chondrocalcinosis in Short Bowel Syndrome," *Journal of Rheumatology* 32(12):2434-436, December 2005.
Shechter, M., and Shechter, A. "Magnesium and Myocardial Infarction," *Clinical Calcium* 15(11):111-15, November 2005.
Strategies for Managing Multisystem Disorders. Philadelphia: Lippincott Williams & Wilkins, 2006.
Tong, G.M., and Rude, R.K. "Magnesium Deficiency in Critical Illness," *Journal of Intensive Care Medicine* 20(1):3-17, January-February 2005.

Clinical effects of hypomagnesemia

BODY SYSTEM	EFFECTS
Cardiovascular	◆ Arrhythmias, vasomotor changes (vasodilation and hypotension) and, occasionally, hypertension
Neurologic	◆ Confusion, delusions, hallucinations, seizures
Neuromuscular	◆ Hyperirritability, tetany, leg and foot cramps, Chvostek's sign (facial muscle spasms induced by tapping the branches of the facial nerve)

Hyponatremia

- Deficient serum levels of the sodium cation in relation to body water

PATHOPHYSIOLOGY

- Sodium is the major cation (90%) in extracellular fluid; potassium, the major cation in intracellular fluid.
- During repolarization, the sodium-potassium pump continually shifts sodium into the cells and potassium out of the cells; during depolarization, it does the reverse.
- Sodium cation functions include maintaining tonicity and concentration of extracellular fluid, acid-base balance (reabsorption of sodium ion and excretion of hydrogen ion), nerve conduction and neuromuscular function, glandular secretion, and water balance.

CAUSES

- Adrenal gland insufficiency (Addison's disease) or hypoaldosteronism
- Certain drugs, such as chlorpropamide and clofibrate (see *Drugs causing hyponatremia*)
- Cirrhosis of the liver with ascites
- Diarrhea
- Excessive perspiration or fever
- Excessive water intake
- Infusion of I.V. dextrose in water without other solutes
- Low-sodium diet, usually in combination with one of the other causes
- Malnutrition or starvation
- Suctioning
- Syndrome of inappropriate antidiuretic hormone, resulting from brain tumor, stroke, pulmonary disease, or neoplasm with ectopic antidiuretic hormone production
- Tap water enemas
- Trauma, surgery (wound drainage), or burns
- Use of potent diuretics
- Vomiting

INCIDENCE

- Hyponatremia occurs in about 1% of hospitalized patients.
- This disorder is more common in the very young and very old.
- This disorder affects males and females equally.

COMPLICATIONS

- Seizures
- Coma
- Permanent neurologic damage

HISTORY

- Altered level of consciousness
- Nausea
- Headache
- Muscle weakness
- Abdominal cramps

PHYSICAL FINDINGS

- Orthostatic hypotension (see *Clinical effects of hyponatremia*)
- Dry mucous membranes
- Poor skin turgor
- Rapid, bounding pulse
- Muscle twitching

Drugs causing hyponatremia

Drugs can contribute to the development of hyponatremia by potentiating the action of antidiuretic hormone, by causing syndrome of inappropriate antidiuretic hormone secretion, or by inhibiting sodium reabsorption in the kidney (diuretics).

ANTICONVULSANTS
- carbamazepine (Tegretol)

ANTIDIABETICS
- chlorpropamide (Diabinese)
- tolbutamide (rarely)

ANTINEOPLASTICS
- cyclophosphamide (Cytoxan)
- vincristine

ANTIPSYCHOTICS
- fluphenazine (Prolixin)
- thioridazine
- thiothixene (Navane)

DIURETICS
- bumetanide (Bumex)
- ethacrynic acid (Edecrin)
- furosemide (Lasix)
- thiazides

SEDATIVES
- barbiturates
- morphine

Clinical effects of hyponatremia

BODY SYSTEM	EFFECTS
Cardiovascular	◆ Hypotension; tachycardia; with severe deficit, vasomotor collapse, thready pulse
Gastrointestinal	◆ Nausea, vomiting, abdominal cramps
Genitourinary	◆ Oliguria or anuria
Integumentary	◆ Cold, clammy skin; decreasing skin turgor
Neurologic	◆ Anxiety, headaches, muscle twitching and weakness, seizures
Respiratory	◆ Cyanosis with severe deficiency

DIAGNOSTIC TEST RESULTS

LABORATORY
- Serum sodium level is less than 135 mEq/L.
- Urine specific gravity is less than 1.010.
- Serum osmolality is less than 280 mOsm/kg (dilute blood).
- Urine specific gravity is increased and urine sodium is elevated (0.2 mEq/L).

TREATMENT

GENERAL
- Treatment of the underlying cause

DIET
- Restricted fluid intake
- High-sodium

ACTIVITY
- As tolerated

MEDICATIONS
- Oral sodium supplements
- Demeclocycline or lithium (Eskalith)
- Administration of normal saline solution
- Hypertonic (3% or 5%) saline solutions (with serum sodium levels below 110 mEq/L)

NURSING CONSIDERATIONS

NURSING DIAGNOSES
- Anxiety
- Fear
- Ineffective tissue perfusion: Cardiopulmonary
- Risk for imbalanced fluid volume
- Risk for injury

EXPECTED OUTCOMES
The patient will:
- identify strategies to reduce anxiety
- discuss fears and concerns
- exhibit signs of adequate cardiopulmonary perfusion
- attain and maintain normal fluid volume and electrolyte balance
- avoid complications.

NURSING INTERVENTIONS
- Restrict fluid intake.
- Give prescribed I.V. fluids.
- Provide a safe environment.

MONITORING
- Vital signs
- Serum sodium levels
- Urine specific gravity
- Intake and output
- Neurologic status

PATIENT TEACHING

GENERAL
Be sure to cover:
- the disorder and treatment
- drug therapy and possible adverse effects
- dietary changes and fluid restrictions
- monitoring daily weight
- signs and symptoms to report to the practitioner.

RESOURCES
Organizations
Endocrine and Metabolic Diseases Information Service: *www.endocrine.niddk.nih.gov*
Mayo Clinic: *www.mayoclinic.com*
National Institute of Diabetes & Digestive & Kidney Diseases: *www.niddk.nih.gov*
National Library of Medicine: *www.nlm.nih.gov*

Selected references
Allison, S.P., and Lobo, D.N. "Fluid and Electrolytes in the Elderly," *Current Opinion in Clinical Nutrition and Metabolic Care* 7(1):27-33, January 2004.
Bhananker, S.M., et al. "Water Intoxication and Symptomatic Hyponatremia after Outpatient Surgery," *Anesthesia & Analgesia* 98(5):1294-296, May 2004.
Strategies for Managing Multisystem Disorders. Philadelphia: Lippincott Williams & Wilkins, 2006.

Hypoparathyroidism

OVERVIEW

- Deficiency in parathyroid hormone (PTH) secretion by the parathyroid glands or the decreased action of PTH in the periphery
- Because parathyroid glands primarily regulate calcium balance, neuromuscular symptoms range from paresthesia to tetany
- May be acute or chronic
- Classified as idiopathic, acquired, or reversible

PATHOPHYSIOLOGY

- PTH normally maintains serum calcium levels by increasing bone resorption and by stimulating renal conversion of vitamin D to its active form, which enhances GI absorption of calcium and bone resorption.
- PTH also maintains the inverse relationship between serum calcium and phosphate levels by inhibiting phosphate reabsorption in the renal tubules and enhancing calcium reabsorption.
- Abnormal PTH production in hypoparathyroidism disrupts this delicate balance.

CAUSES

- Abnormalities of the calcium-sensor receptor
- Accidental removal of or injury to one or more parathyroid glands during surgery
- Amyloidosis
- Autoimmune genetic disorder
- Congenital absence or malformation of the parathyroid glands
- Delayed maturation of parathyroid function
- Hemochromatosis
- Hypomagnesemia-induced impairment of hormone secretion
- Ischemia or infarction of the parathyroid glands during surgery
- Massive thyroid irradiation
- Neoplasms
- Sarcoidosis
- Suppression of normal gland function due to hypercalcemia
- Trauma
- Tuberculosis

INCIDENCE

- Idiopathic and reversible forms of this disorder are most common in children.
- The acquired form of this disorder is most common in older patients who have undergone thyroid gland surgery.

COMPLICATIONS

- Heart failure
- Cataracts
- Tetany
- Increased intracranial pressure
- Irreversible calcification of basal ganglia
- Bone deformities
- Laryngospasm, respiratory stridor, anoxia
- Vocal cord paralysis
- Seizures
- Death

 AGE FACTOR *Hypoparathyroidism that develops during childhood results in malformed teeth.*

ASSESSMENT

HISTORY

- Neck surgery or irradiation
- Malabsorption disorders
- Alcoholism
- Tingling in the fingertips, around the mouth and, occasionally, in the feet
- Muscle tension and spasms
- Feeling like throat is constricted
- Dysphagia
- Difficulty walking and a tendency to fall
- Nausea, vomiting, abdominal pain
- Constipation or diarrhea
- Personality changes
- Fatigue

PHYSICAL FINDINGS

- Brittle nails
- Dry skin
- Coarse hair, alopecia
- Transverse and longitudinal ridges in the fingernails
- Loss of eyelashes and fingernails
- Stained, cracked, and decayed teeth
- Tetany
- Positive Chvostek's and Trousseau's signs
- Increased deep tendon reflexes
- Irregular, slow or rapid pulse

DIAGNOSTIC TEST RESULTS

LABORATORY
- Radioimmunoassay for PTH is decreased.
- Serum and urine calcium levels are decreased.
- Serum phosphate level is increased.
- Urine creatinine level is decreased.

IMAGING
- Computed tomography scan shows frontal lobe and basal ganglia calcifications.
- X-rays show increased bone density and bone malformation.

DIAGNOSTIC PROCEDURES
- Electrocardiography shows a prolonged QT interval.

TREATMENT

GENERAL
- To restore the calcium and associated mineral balance within the body
- Supportive care necessary for an acute, life-threatening attack or hypoparathyroid tetany

DIET
- High-calcium, low-phosphorus

ACTIVITY
- As tolerated

MEDICATIONS
- Vitamin D
- Supplemental calcium
- Calcitriol (Rocaltrol)

Acute, life-threatening tetany
- I.V. administration of 10% calcium gluconate, 10% calcium gluceptate, or 10% calcium chloride
- Sedatives
- Anticonvulsants

SURGERY
- To treat underlying cause such as a tumor

NURSING CONSIDERATIONS

NURSING DIAGNOSES
- Anxiety
- Decreased cardiac output
- Disturbed body image
- Impaired skin integrity
- Ineffective breathing pattern
- Ineffective coping
- Risk for injury
- Risk for peripheral neurovascular dysfunction

EXPECTED OUTCOMES
The patient will:
- identify strategies to reduce anxiety
- maintain normal cardiac output
- express positive feelings about body
- maintain skin integrity
- maintain adequate ventilation
- demonstrate adaptive coping behaviors
- be able to recognize signs and symptoms of neurovascular impairment
- avoid injury and complications.

NURSING INTERVENTIONS
- Give prescribed drugs.
- Maintain a patent I.V. line.
- Keep emergency equipment readily available.
- Maintain seizure precautions.
- Provide meticulous skin care.
- Institute safety precautions.
- Encourage the patient to express his feelings.
- Offer emotional support.
- Help the patient develop effective coping strategies.

MONITORING
- Vital signs
- Intake and output
- Serum calcium and phosphorus levels
- Electrocardiogram for QT-interval changes and arrhythmias
- Signs and symptoms of decreased cardiac output
- Chvostek's sign
- Trousseau's sign

⚡ **WARNING** *Closely monitor the patient receiving digoxin and calcium because calcium potentiates the effect of digoxin. Stay alert for signs of digoxin toxicity.*

PATIENT TEACHING

GENERAL
Be sure to cover:
- the disorder, diagnosis, and treatment
- prescribed drugs and potential adverse effects
- when to notify the practitioner
- follow-up care
- complications
- periodic checks of serum calcium levels.

DISCHARGE PLANNING
- Refer the patient to a mental health professional for additional counseling, if necessary.

RESOURCES
Organizations
American Association of Clinical Endocrinologists: *www.aace.com*
Endocrine Society: *www.endo-society.org*

Selected references
Adorni, A., et al. "Extensive Brain Calcification and Dementia in Postsurgical Hypoparathyroidism," *Neurology* 65(9):1501, November 2005.
Diseases, 4th ed. Philadelphia: Lippincott Williams & Wilkins, 2006.
Heymann, R.S., et al. "Anaplastic Thyroid Carcinoma with Thyrotoxicosis and Hypoparathyroidism," *Endocrine Practice* 11(4):281-84, July-August 2005.

Hypophosphatemia

◆ Deficient serum phosphate levels

PATHOPHYSIOLOGY

◆ Phosphorus exists primarily in inorganic combinations with calcium in teeth and bones.
◆ In extracellular fluid, the phosphate ion supports several metabolic functions: Utilization of B vitamins, acid-base homeostasis, bone formation, nerve and muscle activity, cell division, transmission of hereditary traits, and metabolism of carbohydrates, proteins, and fats.
◆ Renal tubular reabsorption of phosphate is inversely regulated by calcium levels — an increase in phosphorus causes a decrease in calcium. An imbalance causes hypophosphatemia or hyperphosphatemia.

CAUSES

◆ Chronic diarrhea
◆ Chronic use of antacids containing aluminum hydroxide
◆ Diabetic acidosis
◆ Hyperparathyroidism with resultant hypercalcemia
◆ Hypomagnesemia
◆ Inadequate dietary intake
◆ Intestinal malabsorption
◆ Commonly related to malnutrition resulting from a prolonged catabolic state or chronic alcoholism
◆ Renal tubular defects
◆ Tissue damage in which phosphorus is released by injured cells
◆ Use of parenteral nutrition solution with inadequate phosphate content
◆ Vitamin D deficiency

INCIDENCE

◆ Incidence rates for this disorder vary according to the underlying cause.

COMPLICATIONS

◆ Heart failure
◆ Shock
◆ Arrhythmias
◆ Rhabdomyolysis
◆ Seizures
◆ Coma

ASSESSMENT

HISTORY

◆ Anorexia
◆ Memory loss
◆ Muscle and bone pain
◆ Fractures
◆ Chest pain

PHYSICAL FINDINGS

◆ Tremor and weakness in speaking voice
◆ Confusion
◆ Bruising and bleeding

DIAGNOSTIC TEST RESULTS

LABORATORY

◆ Serum phosphorus level is less than 2.5 mg/dl.

TREATMENT

GENERAL
- Treatment of the underlying cause
- Discontinuation of drugs that may cause hypophosphatemia (see *Drugs that may cause hypophosphatemia*)

DIET
- High-phosphorus

ACTIVITY
- As tolerated

MEDICATIONS
- Phosphate salt tablets or capsules
- Potassium phosphate I.V.

NURSING CONSIDERATIONS

NURSING DIAGNOSES
- Acute pain
- Anxiety
- Impaired gas exchange
- Risk for injury

EXPECTED OUTCOMES
The patient will:
- express feelings of comfort
- identify strategies to reduce anxiety
- maintain adequate ventilation
- avoid injury and complications.

NURSING INTERVENTIONS
- Provide safety measures.
- Give prescribed phosphorus replacement.
- Assist with ambulation and activities of daily living.

MONITORING
- Respiratory status
- Neurologic status
- Phosphorus and calcium levels
- Intake and output

PATIENT TEACHING

GENERAL
Be sure to cover:
- proper administration of phosphorus supplements
- importance of adhering to a high-phosphorus diet. (See *Foods high in phosphorus*, page 397.)

DISCHARGE PLANNING
- Refer the patient to a dietitian and social services, if indicated.

RESOURCES
Organizations
Alcoholics Anonymous: *www.alcoholicsanonymous.org*
Endocrine and Metabolic Diseases Information Service: *www.endocrine.niddk.nih.gov*
National Institute of Diabetes & Digestive & Kidney Diseases: *www.niddk.nih.gov*
National Library of Medicine: *www.nlm.nih.gov*

Selected references
Gaasbeek, A., and Meinders, A.E. "Hypophosphatemia: An Update on Its Etiology and Treatment," *American Journal of Medicine* 118(10):1094-101, October 2005.
Marinella, M.A. "Refeeding Syndrome and Hypophosphatemia," *Journal of Intensive Care Medicine* 20(3):155-59, May-June 2005.
Strategies for Managing Multisystem Disorders. Philadelphia: Lippincott Williams & Wilkins, 2006.

Drugs that may cause hypophosphatemia

These drugs may cause hypophosphatemia:
- acetazolamide (Diamox), thiazide diuretics (chlorothiazide [Diuril] and hydrochlorothiazide [Esidrix]), loop diuretics (bumetanide [Bumex] and furosemide [Lasix]), and other diuretics
- antacids, such as aluminum carbonate, aluminum hydroxide, calcium carbonate, and magnesium oxide
- insulin
- laxatives.

Hypopituitarism

- Partial or complete failure of the anterior pituitary gland to produce its vital hormones: corticotropin, thyroid-stimulating hormone (TSH), luteinizing hormone (LH), follicle-stimulating hormone (FSH), growth hormone (GH), and prolactin
- May be primary or secondary, resulting from dysfunction of the hypothalamus
- Development of clinical features typically slow and not apparent until 75% of the pituitary gland is destroyed
- Total loss of all hormones fatal without treatment
- Prognosis good with adequate replacement therapy and correction of the underlying causes
- Panhypopituitarism: absence of all hormones

PATHOPHYSIOLOGY
- The pituitary gland is extremely vulnerable to ischemia and infarction because it's highly vascular.
- Any event that leads to circulatory collapse and compensatory vasospasm may result in gland ischemia, tissue necrosis, or edema.
- Expansion of the pituitary within the fixed compartment of the sella turcica further impedes blood supply to the pituitary.

CAUSES
- Congenital defects
- Deficiency of hypothalamus-releasing hormones
- Granulomatous disease
- Idiopathic
- Infection
- Partial or total hypophysectomy by surgery, irradiation, or chemical agents
- Pituitary gland hypoplasia or aplasia
- Pituitary infarction
- Trauma
- Tumor

INCIDENCE
- Hypopituitarism is relatively rare.

- Hypopituitarism occurs in adults and children.
- Males and females are equally affected by this disorder.

COMPLICATIONS
- Any combination of deficits in the production of the six major hormones
- GH deficiency
- TSH deficiency
- Corticotropin deficiency
- Gonadotropin and prolactin deficiency
- Pituitary apoplexy (a medical emergency)
- High fever, shock, coma, and death
- Diabetes insipidus

  AGE FACTOR *In children, hypopituitarism can cause dwarfism and pubertal delay.*

HISTORY
- Signs and symptoms depend on which pituitary hormones are deficient, patient's age, and severity of disorder.

Gonadotropin (FSH and LH) deficiency in women
- Amenorrhea
- Dyspareunia
- Infertility
- Reduced libido

Gonadotropin (FSH and LH) deficiency in men
- Impotence
- Reduced libido

TSH deficiency
- Cold intolerance
- Constipation
- Menstrual irregularity
- Lethargy
- Severe growth retardation in children despite treatment

Corticotropin deficiency
- Fatigue
- Nausea, vomiting, anorexia
- Weight loss

Prolactin deficiency
- Absent postpartum lactation
- Amenorrhea

PHYSICAL FINDINGS
GH deficiency
- Physical signs possibly not apparent in neonate
- Growth retardation usually apparent at age 6 months

In children
- Chubbiness from fat deposits in the lower trunk
- Short stature
- Delayed secondary tooth eruption
- Delayed puberty
- Average height of 4' (1.2 m), with normal proportions
- More subtle signs in adults (fine wrinkles near the mouth and eyes)

Gonadotropin (FSH and LH) deficiency in women
- Breast atrophy
- Sparse or absent axillary and pubic hair
- Dry skin

Gonadotropin (FSH and LH) deficiency in men
- Decreased muscle strength
- Testicular softening and shrinkage
- Retarded secondary sexual hair growth

TSH deficiency
- Dry, pale, puffy skin
- Slow thought processes
- Bradycardia

Corticotropin deficiency
- Depigmentation of skin and nipples
- Hypothermia and hypotension during periods of stress

Prolactin deficiency
- Sparse or absent growth of pubic and axillary hair

Panhypopituitarism
- Mental abnormalities, including lethargy and psychosis
- Physical abnormalities, including orthostatic hypotension and bradycardia

DIAGNOSTIC TEST RESULTS

LABORATORY

- Serum thyroxin level is decreased in diminished thyroid gland function due to lack of TSH.
- Radioimmunoassay shows decreased plasma levels of some or all of the pituitary hormones.
- Increased prolactin levels may indicate a lesion in the hypothalamus or pituitary stalk.

IMAGING

- Computed tomography scans, magnetic resonance imaging, or cerebral angiography show intrasellar or extrasellar tumors.

OTHER

- Oral administration of metyrapone shows the source of low hydroxycorticosteroid levels.
- Insulin administration shows low levels of corticotropin, indicating pituitary or hypothalamic failure.
- Dopamine antagonist administration evaluates prolactin secretory reserve.
- I.V. administration of gonadotropin-releasing hormone distinguishes pituitary and hypothalamic causes of gonadotropin deficiency.
- Provocative testing shows persistently low GH and insulin-like growth factor-1 levels, confirming GH deficiency.

TREATMENT

GENERAL

- If caused by a lesion or tumor, removal, radiation, or both, followed by possible lifelong hormone replacement therapy
- Endocrine substitution therapy for affected organs

DIET

- High-calorie, high-protein

ACTIVITY

- Regular exercise
- Rest periods for fatigue

MEDICATIONS

- Hormone replacement

AGE FACTOR *Children with hypopituitarism may also need adrenal and thyroid hormone replacement and, as they approach puberty, sex hormones.*

SURGERY

- For pituitary tumor

NURSING CONSIDERATIONS

NURSING DIAGNOSES

- Chronic low self-esteem
- Delayed growth and development
- Disturbed body image
- Disturbed sensory perception (visual)
- Hypothermia
- Imbalanced nutrition: Less than body requirements
- Ineffective coping
- Risk for infection
- Sexual dysfunction

EXPECTED OUTCOMES

The patient will:

- verbalize feelings of positive self-esteem
- demonstrate age-appropriate skills and behavior to the extent possible
- express positive feelings about self
- maintain optimal functioning within the limits of the visual impairment
- maintain normal body temperature
- maintain body weight
- agree, along with family members, to seek help from peer support groups or professional counselors to increase adaptive coping behaviors
- remain free from signs and symptoms of infection
- verbalize feelings regarding impaired sexual function.

NURSING INTERVENTIONS

- Give prescribed drugs.
- Encourage maintenance of adequate calorie intake.
- Offer small, frequent meals.
- Keep the patient warm.
- Institute safety precautions.
- Provide emotional support.
- Encourage the patient to express his feelings.

MONITORING

- Laboratory tests for hormonal deficiencies
- Calorie intake
- Daily weight
- Vital signs
- Neurologic status
- Signs and symptoms of pituitary apoplexy, a medical emergency
- Signs and symptoms of hypoglycemia

PATIENT TEACHING

GENERAL

Be sure to cover:

- the disorder, diagnosis, and treatment
- long-term hormonal replacement therapy and adverse reactions
- when to notify the practitioner
- regular follow-up appointments
- energy-conservation techniques
- the need for adequate rest
- the need for a balanced diet.

DISCHARGE PLANNING

- Refer the parents for psychological counseling or to community resources.

RESOURCES

Organizations

American Association of Clinical Endocrinologists: *www.aace.com*
National Organization for Rare Diseases: *www.rarediseases.org*

Selected references

Agha, A., et al. "The Natural History of Post-Traumatic Hypopituitarism: Implications for Assessment and Treatment," *American Journal of Medicine* 118(12):1416, December 2005.

Hanberg, A. "Common Disorders of the Pituitary Gland: Hyposecretion versus Hypersecretion," *Journal of Infusion Nursing* 28(1):36-44, January-February 2005.

Mondok, A., et al. "Treatment of Pituitary Tumors: Radiation," *Endocrine* 28(1):77-85, October 2005.

Morton, A., and Kannan, S. "Peripartum Cardiomyopathy in a Woman with Hypopituitarism," *BJOG* 113(1):123-24, January 2006.

Hypothyroidism

- Clinical condition characterized by either decreased circulating levels of or resistance to free TH
- Classified as primary or secondary
- Severe hypothyroidism known as *myxedema*

PATHOPHYSIOLOGY

- In primary hypothyroidism, a decrease in TH production is a result of the loss of thyroid tissue.
- This results in an increased secretion of TSH that leads to a goiter.
- In secondary hypothyroidism, the pituitary typically fails to synthesize or secrete adequate amounts of TSH, or target tissues fail to respond to normal blood levels of TH.
- Either type may progress to myxedema, which is clinically more severe and considered a medical emergency. (See *Managing myxedema coma*.)

CAUSES

- Amyloidosis
- Antithyroid drugs
- Autoimmune thyroiditis (Hashimoto's) (most common cause)
- Congenital defects
- Drugs, such as iodides and lithium
- Endemic iodine deficiency
- External radiation to the neck
- Hypothalamic failure to produce thyrotropin-releasing hormone
- Idiopathic
- Inflammatory conditions
- Pituitary failure to produce TSH
- Pituitary tumor
- Postpartum pituitary necrosis
- Radioactive iodine therapy
- Sarcoidosis
- Thyroid gland surgery

INCIDENCE

- This disorder is most prevalent in women.
- In the United States, incidence increases in people older than age 40.

COMPLICATIONS

Cardiovascular complications

- Hypercholesterolemia
- Arteriosclerosis
- Ischemic heart disease
- Peripheral vascular disease
- Cardiomegaly
- Heart failure
- Pleural and pericardial effusion

GI complications

- Achlorhydria
- Anemia
- Dynamic colon
- Megacolon
- Intestinal obstruction
- Bleeding tendencies

Other complications

- Conductive or sensorineural deafness
- Psychiatric disturbances
- Carpal tunnel syndrome
- Benign intracranial hypertension
- Impaired fertility
- Myxedema coma

HISTORY

- Vague and varied symptoms that developed slowly over time
- Energy loss, fatigue
- Forgetfulness
- Sensitivity to cold
- Unexplained weight gain
- Constipation
- Anorexia
- Decreased libido
- Menorrhagia
- Paresthesia
- Joint stiffness
- Muscle cramping

PHYSICAL FINDINGS

- Slight mental slowing to severe obtundation
- Thick, dry tongue
- Hoarseness; slow, slurred speech
- Dry, flaky, inelastic skin
- Puffy face, hands, and feet
- Periorbital edema; drooping upper eyelids
- Dry, sparse hair with patchy hair loss
- Loss of outer third of eyebrow

Managing myxedema coma

Myxedema coma is a medical emergency that is commonly fatal. Progression is usually gradual, but when stress aggravates severe or prolonged hypothyroidism, coma may develop abruptly. Examples of severe stress are infection, exposure to cold, and trauma. Other precipitating factors include thyroid medication withdrawal and the use of a sedative, an opioid, or an anesthetic.

Patients in myxedema coma have significantly depressed respirations, so their partial pressure of carbon dioxide in arterial blood may increase. Decreased cardiac output and worsening cerebral hypoxia may also occur. The patient is stuporous and hypothermic, and her vital signs reflect bradycardia and hypotension.

LIFESAVING INTERVENTIONS

If your patient becomes comatose, begin these interventions as soon as possible:
- Maintain airway patency with ventilatory support if necessary.
- Maintain circulation through I.V. fluid replacement.
- Provide continuous electrocardiogram monitoring.
- Monitor arterial blood gas levels to detect hypoxia and metabolic acidosis.
- Warm the patient by wrapping her in blankets. Don't use a warming blanket because it might increase peripheral vasodilation, causing shock.
- Monitor body temperature until stable with a low-reading thermometer.
- Replace thyroid hormone by administering large doses of I.V. levothyroxine, as ordered. Monitor vital signs because rapid correction of hypothyroidism can cause adverse cardiac reactions.
- Monitor intake and output and daily weight. With treatment, urine output should increase and body weight should decrease; if not, report this to the practitioner.
- Replace fluids and other substances such as glucose. Monitor serum electrolyte levels.
- Administer a corticosteroid, as ordered.
- Check for possible sources of infection, such as blood, sputum, or urine, which may have precipitated coma. Treat infections or any other underlying illness.

- Thick, brittle nails with transverse and longitudinal grooves
- Ataxia, intention tremor; nystagmus
- Doughy skin that feels cool
- Weak pulse and bradycardia
- Muscle weakness
- Sacral or peripheral edema
- Delayed reflex relaxation time
- Possible goiter
- Absent or decreased bowel sounds
- Hypotension
- A gallop or distant heart sounds
- Adventitious breath sounds
- Abdominal distention or ascites

DIAGNOSTIC TEST RESULTS

LABORATORY
- Radioimmunoassay show decreased serum levels of triiodothyronine and thyroxine.
- Serum TSH level increases with thyroid insufficiency and decreases with hypothalamic or pituitary insufficiency.
- Serum cholesterol, alkaline phosphatase, and triglycerides levels are elevated.
- Serum electrolyte levels show low serum sodium levels in myxedema coma.
- Arterial blood gas results show decreased pH and increased partial pressure of carbon dioxide in myxedema coma.

IMAGING
- Skull X-rays, computed tomography scan, and magnetic resonance imaging show pituitary or hypothalamic lesions.

TREATMENT

GENERAL
- To restore and maintain a normal thyroid state
- Need for long-term thyroid replacement

DIET
- Low-fat, low-cholesterol, high-fiber, low-sodium
- Possibly fluid restriction

ACTIVITY
- As tolerated

MEDICATIONS
- Synthetic hormone levothyroxine
- Synthetic liothyronine

SURGERY
- For underlying cause such as pituitary tumor

NURSING CONSIDERATIONS

NURSING DIAGNOSES
- Chronic low self-esteem
- Constipation
- Decreased cardiac output
- Disturbed body image
- Excess fluid volume
- Ineffective coping
- Ineffective tissue perfusion: Cardiopulmonary
- Risk for impaired skin integrity

EXPECTED OUTCOMES
The patient will:
- express feelings about self-esteem
- resume a normal bowel elimination pattern
- maintain adequate cardiac output
- express positive feelings about self
- maintain balanced fluid volume
- demonstrate adaptive coping behaviors
- remain hemodynamically stable
- maintain skin integrity.

NURSING INTERVENTIONS
- Give prescribed drugs.
- Provide adequate rest periods.
- Apply antiembolism stockings.
- Encourage coughing and deep-breathing exercises.
- Maintain fluid restrictions and a low-salt diet.
- Provide a high-bulk, low-calorie diet.
- Reorient the patient, as needed.
- Offer support and encouragement.
- Provide meticulous skin care.
- Keep the patient warm, as needed.
- Encourage the patient to express his feelings.
- Help the patient develop effective coping strategies.

MONITORING
- Vital signs
- Intake and output
- Daily weight
- Cardiovascular status
- Pulmonary status
- Edema
- Bowel sounds, abdominal distention, frequency of bowel movements
- Mental and neurologic status
- Signs and symptoms of hyperthyroidism

PATIENT TEACHING

GENERAL
Be sure to cover:
- disorder, diagnosis, and treatment
- drugs and possible adverse effects
- when to notify the practitioner
- physical and mental changes
- signs and symptoms of myxedema
- the need for lifelong hormone replacement therapy
- the need to wear a medical identification bracelet
- the importance of keeping accurate records of daily weight
- the need for a well-balanced, high-fiber, low-sodium diet
- energy-conservation techniques.

DISCHARGE PLANNING
- Refer the patient and family members to a mental health professional for additional counseling, if needed.

RESOURCES
Organizations
American Foundation of Thyroid Patients: *www.thyroidfoundation.org*
American Thyroid Association: *www.thyroid.org*
Thyroid Foundation of America, Inc.: *www.tsh.org*

Selected references
Col, N.F., et al. "Subclinical Thyroid Disease: Clinical Applications," *JAMA* 291(2):239-43, January 2004.
Holcomb, S.S. "Detecting Thyroid Disease," *Nursing* 35(10 Suppl):4-8, October 2005.
Strategies for Managing Multisystem Disorders. Philadelphia: Lippincott Williams & Wilkins, 2006.

Idiopathic thrombocytopenic purpura

OVERVIEW

- A deficiency of platelets that occurs when the immune system destroys the body's own platelets
- May be acute, as in postviral thrombocytopenia, or chronic, as in essential thrombocytopenia or autoimmune thrombocytopenia
- Excellent prognosis for acute form; nearly four out of five patients recover without treatment
- Good prognosis for chronic form; remissions commonly lasting weeks or years, especially among women

PATHOPHYSIOLOGY

- Circulating immunoglobulin (Ig) G molecules react with host platelets, which are then destroyed in the spleen and, to a lesser degree, in the liver.
- Normally, the life span of platelets in circulation is 7 to 10 days. In idiopathic thrombocytopenic purpura (ITP), platelets survive 1 to 3 days or less.

CAUSES

- Drug reactions
- Immunization with a live virus vaccine
- Immunologic disorders
- Viral infection

INCIDENCE

AGE FACTOR *Acute ITP usually affects children between ages 2 and 6; chronic ITP mainly affects adults younger than age 50, especially women between ages 20 and 40.*

COMPLICATIONS

- Hemorrhage
- Cerebral hemorrhage
- Purpuric lesions of vital organs (such as the brain and kidney)

ASSESSMENT

HISTORY

- Epistaxis
- Bleeding gums
- Menorrhagia
- Recent viral illness

PHYSICAL FINDINGS

- Petechiae or ecchymosis
- Bleeding into mucous membranes
- Splenomegaly

DIAGNOSTIC TEST RESULTS

LABORATORY

- Platelet count is less than $20,000/\mu l$.
- Bleeding time is prolonged.
- Platelets size and appearance are abnormal.
- Hemoglobin level is decreased (if bleeding occurred).
- Bone marrow studies show abundant megakaryocytes (platelet precursor cells) and a circulating platelet survival time of only several hours to a few days.
- Humoral tests measure platelet-associated IgG (50% of all patients with ITP display elevated IgG levels).

Living with ITP

When teaching a patient how to live safely at home with idiopathic thrombocytopenic purpura (ITP), include the following points:
- Caution the patient to avoid aspirin and other drugs that impair coagulation. Teach him how to recognize aspirin compounds and nonsteroidal anti-inflammatory drugs listed on labels of over-the-counter drugs.
- Instruct the patient to use a humidifier at night if he frequently experiences nosebleeds. Suggest that he moisten his inner nares twice a day with an anti-infective ointment.
- Teach the patient how to examine his skin for ecchymoses and petechiae and how to test his stools for occult blood.
- Explain the importance of reporting signs of bleeding, such as tarry stools, coffeeground vomitus, and gum or urinary tract bleeding.

TREATMENT

GENERAL
◆ Platelet replacement

DIET
◆ Well-balanced

ACTIVITY
◆ Rest periods between activities
◆ Complete bed rest during active bleeding

MEDICATIONS
Acute
◆ Glucocorticoids to prevent further platelet destruction
◆ Ig to prevent platelet destruction
◆ Plasmapheresis
◆ Platelet pheresis

Chronic
◆ Vitamin K
◆ Corticosteroids

SURGERY
◆ Splenectomy (when splenomegaly accompanies the initial thrombocytopenia)

OTHER
◆ Immunosuppressants to help stop platelet destruction
◆ High-dose I.V. Ig
◆ Immunoabsorption apheresis using staphylococcal protein A columns

NURSING CONSIDERATIONS

NURSING DIAGNOSES
◆ Activity intolerance
◆ Anxiety
◆ Disturbed body image
◆ Fatigue
◆ Impaired skin integrity
◆ Ineffective coping
◆ Ineffective protection
◆ Risk for deficient fluid volume
◆ Risk for infection
◆ Risk for injury

EXPECTED OUTCOMES
The patient will:
◆ verbalize the importance of balancing activity, as tolerated, with rest
◆ verbalize strategies to reduce anxiety
◆ express positive feelings about body
◆ express feelings of increased energy
◆ experience healing of wounds and lesions without complications
◆ demonstrate effective coping mechanisms
◆ demonstrate the use of protective measures, including conserving energy, maintaining a balanced diet, and getting plenty of rest
◆ maintain balanced fluid volume
◆ remain free from all signs and symptoms of infection
◆ verbalize appropriate safety and preventive measures.

NURSING INTERVENTIONS
◆ Give prescribed platelets.
◆ Provide emotional support.
◆ Protect all areas of petechiae and ecchymoses from further injury.

MONITORING
◆ Signs of bleeding
◆ Platelet count
◆ Intake and output
◆ Vital signs

When receiving immunosuppressants
◆ Bone marrow depression
◆ Infection
◆ Mucositis
◆ GI ulcers
◆ Severe diarrhea or vomiting

PATIENT TEACHING

GENERAL
Be sure to cover:
◆ how to observe for petechiae, ecchymoses, and other signs of recurrence (see *Living with ITP*)
◆ avoiding aspirin and ibuprofen
◆ avoiding straining during defecation and coughing.

DISCHARGE PLANNING
◆ Advise the patient to carry medical identification to alert others about the condition.

RESOURCES
Organizations
Mayo Clinic: *www.mayoclinic.com*
National Heart, Lung, and Blood Institute: *www.nhlbi.nih.gov*
National Organization for Rare Disorders: *www.rarediseases.org*

Selected references
Blackwell, J., and Goolsby, M.J. "Diagnosis and Treatment of Idiopathic Thrombocytopenic Purpura," *Journal of the American Academy of Nurse Practitioners* 15(6):244-45, June 2003.
Ferrara, M., et al. "Side Effects of Corticosteroid Therapy in Children with Chronic Idiopathic Thrombocytopenic Purpura," *Hematology* 10(5);401-403, October 2005.
Panepinto, J.A., and Brousseau, D.C. "Acute Idiopathic Thrombocytopenic Purpura of Childhood-Diagnosis and Treatment," *Pediatric Emergency Care* 21(10):691-95, October 2005.

Impetigo

- Highly contagious, superficial, gram-positive bacterial infection of the superficial skin layers
- Nonbullous and bullous forms
- May complicate chickenpox, eczema, and other skin disorders marked by open lesions
- Most commonly appears on face, arms, and legs

PATHOPHYSIOLOGY
Nonbullous impetigo
- Eruption occurs when bacteria inoculate traumatized skin cells.
- Lesions begin as small vesicles, which rapidly erode.
- Honey-colored crusts surrounded by erythema are formed.

Bullous impetigo
- Eruption occurs in nontraumatized skin via bacterial toxin or exotoxin.
- Lesions begin as thin-walled bullae and vesicles.
- Lesions contain clear to turbid yellow fluid; some crusting exists. (See *Recognizing impetigo.*)

CAUSES
Nonbullous impetigo
- Beta-hemolytic streptococci

Bullous impetigo
- Coagulase-positive *Staphylococcus aureus*

RISK FACTORS
- Poor hygiene
- Untreated minor trauma
- Overcrowded living conditions
- Lesions of preexisting eczema, chickenpox, scabies
- Other skin rashes
- Anemia
- Malnutrition

INCIDENCE
- Impetigo is most common among infants, children, and young adults.
- This disorder occurs more commonly in warm ambient temperatures.
- This disorder occurs predominantly during late summer and early fall.

COMPLICATIONS
- Acute glomerulonephritis (streptococcal impetigo)
- Ecthyma (see *Comparing ecthyma and impetigo*)
- Exfoliative eruption (staphylococcal scalded skin syndrome)

HISTORY
- Presence of risk factors
- Absence of pain
- Possible pruritus

PHYSICAL FINDINGS
Nonbullous impetigo
- Small, red macule or vesicle that becomes pustular within a few hours
- Characteristic thick, honey-colored crust formed from the exudate
- Satellite lesions caused by autoinoculation

Bullous impetigo
- Thin-walled vesicle
- Thin, clear crust formed from exudate
- Lesion that appears as a central clearing circumscribed by an outer rim

Recognizing impetigo

In impetigo, when the vesicles break, crust forms from the exudate. This infection is especially contagious among young children.

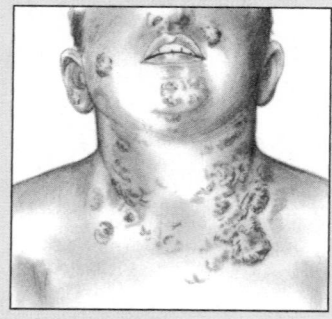

DIAGNOSTIC TEST RESULTS

LABORATORY
- Gram stain of vesicular fluid shows infecting organism.
- Culture and sensitivity testing of exudate or denuded crust shows infecting organism.
- White blood cell count is elevated.

TREATMENT

GENERAL
- Removal of exudate by washing lesions two to three times per day with soap and water
- Warm soaks or compresses of normal saline solution or a diluted soap solution for stubborn crusts
- Prevention by benzoyl peroxide soap

MEDICATIONS
- Antibiotics
- Antihistamines

Comparing ecthyma and impetigo

Ecthyma is a superficial skin infection that usually causes scarring. It generally results from infection by group A beta-hemolytic streptococci.

Ecthyma differs from impetigo in that its characteristic ulcer results from deeper penetration of the skin by the infecting organism (involving the lower epidermis and dermis), and the overlying crust tends to be raised (⅜″ to 1¼″) [1 to 3 cm]).

These lesions are usually found on the legs after a scratch or an insect bite. Autoinoculation can transmit ecthyma to other parts of the body, especially to sites that have been scratched open.

Therapy for ecthyma is basically the same as for impetigo, beginning with removal of the crust, but the patient's response may be slower. Parenteral antibiotics are also used.

NURSING CONSIDERATIONS

NURSING DIAGNOSES
- Acute pain
- Disturbed body image
- Impaired skin integrity
- Impaired tissue integrity
- Risk for infection

EXPECTED OUTCOMES
The patient will:
- report feelings of increased comfort
- verbalize feelings about changed body image
- exhibit improved or healed wounds or lesions
- experience decreased redness, swelling, and pain at the site of impaired tissue
- avoid or minimize the risk of secondary skin infection.

NURSING INTERVENTIONS
- Use meticulous hand-washing technique.
- Follow standard precautions.
- Remove crusts by gently washing with bactericidal soap and water.
- Soften stubborn crusts with cool compresses.
- Give prescribed drugs.
- Encourage verbalization of feelings about body image.
- Comply with local public health standards and guidelines.

MONITORING
- Response to treatment
- Adverse drug reactions
- Complications

PATIENT TEACHING

GENERAL
Be sure to cover:
- the disorder, diagnosis, and treatment
- meticulous hand-washing technique
- trimming fingernails short
- regular bathing with bactericidal soap
- avoiding sharing clothes and linens
- identification of characteristic lesions
- completion of prescribed medications
- potential adverse reactions
- lesion care.

DISCHARGE PLANNING
- Encourage the patient to schedule follow-up appointments as recommended by his practitioner.

RESOURCES
Organizations
American Academy of Dermatology: *www.aad.org*
Dermatology Foundation: *www.dermfnd.org*

Selected references
Kuniyuki, S., et al. "Topical Antibiotic Treatment of Impetigo with Tetracycline," *Journal of Dermatology* 32(10):788-92, October 2005.
Sandhu, K., and Kanwar, A.J. "Generalized Bullous Impetigo in a Neonate," *Pediatric Dermatology* 21(6):667-69, November-December 2004.
Watkins, P. "Impetigo: Aetiology, Complications and Treatment Options," *Nursing Standard* 19(36):50-54, May 2005.

Infectious mononucleosis

- An acute infectious disease that causes fever, sore throat, and cervical lymphadenopathy (see *Differentiating mononucleosis*)

PATHOPHYSIOLOGY

- Virus enters and replicates in epithelial cells of the oropharynx and B cells of tonsillar tissue, causing alteration of shape and function of the infected cells.
- Infected B cells cause activation of cell-mediated immunity with proliferation of abnormal cytotoxic T cells in lymphoid tissues.
- Lymphoproliferation stops when cytotoxic T cells are able to destroy infected B cells.

CAUSES

- Epstein-Barr virus (EBV), a member of the herpes group
- Spread by contact with oral secretions (kissing)
- Transmitted during bone marrow transplantation and blood transfusion

INCIDENCE

- This disease primarily affects young adults and children.
- This disease is common and widespread in early childhood in developing countries and socioeconomically depressed populations.

COMPLICATIONS

- Splenic rupture
- Aseptic meningitis
- Encephalitis
- Hemolytic anemia
- Pericarditis
- Guillain-Barré syndrome

HISTORY

- Contact with a person who has infectious mononucleosis
- Headache
- Malaise
- Fatigue
- Sore throat
- Fever

PHYSICAL FINDINGS

- Exudative tonsillitis, pharyngitis
- Palatal petechiae
- Periorbital edema
- Maculopapular rash that resembles rubella
- Cervical adenopathy; possible inguinal and axillary adenopathy
- Splenomegaly, hepatomegaly, jaundice

LABORATORY

- White blood cell (WBC) count is increased to 10,000 to 20,000/µl during the second and third weeks of illness; lymphocytes and monocytes account for 50% to 70% of the total WBC count; and 10% of the lymphocytes are atypical.
- A fourfold increase in heterophil antibodies (agglutinins for sheep red blood cells) occurs during the acute phase and at 3- to 4-week intervals.
- Antibodies to EBV and cellular antigens are shown by indirect immunofluorescence.
- Liver function study results are abnormal.

Differentiating mononucleosis

Mononucleosis needs to be differentiated from acute infection with cytomegalovirus (CMV), toxoplasma, human immunodeficiency virus, human herpesvirus 6, and hepatitis virus as well as drug hypersensitivity reactions. CMV commonly affects older patients, causing less severe sore throat, splenomegaly, and lymphadenopathy. In addition, rubella, acute infectious lymphocytosis in children, and lymphoma or leukemia share some of the same features as infectious mononucleosis.

TREATMENT

GENERAL
◆ Essentially supportive

DIET
◆ Well-balanced
◆ Soft food (with throat soreness)

ACTIVITY
◆ Frequent rest periods
◆ Avoidance of strenuous activity or contact sports until fully recovered

MEDICATIONS
◆ Aspirin or other salicylate
◆ Steroids
◆ Antibiotics

SURGERY
◆ Splenectomy for splenic rupture

NURSING CONSIDERATIONS

NURSING DIAGNOSES
◆ Activity intolerance
◆ Acute pain
◆ Fatigue
◆ Hyperthermia
◆ Imbalanced nutrition: Less than body requirements
◆ Impaired skin integrity
◆ Impaired social interaction
◆ Impaired swallowing
◆ Risk for deficient fluid volume

EXPECTED OUTCOMES
The patient will:
◆ demonstrate skill in conserving energy while performing daily activities to tolerance level
◆ articulate factors that intensify pain and change behavior accordingly
◆ report an increased energy level
◆ maintain temperature within normal limits
◆ achieve adequate nutritional intake
◆ experience healed lesions or wounds without complications
◆ engage in appropriate social interaction with others
◆ report relief from sore throat to allow for appropriate swallowing
◆ maintain balanced fluid volume.

NURSING INTERVENTIONS
◆ Give prescribed drugs.
◆ Provide warm saline gargles for symptomatic relief of sore throat.
◆ Provide adequate fluids and nutrition.
◆ Plan care to provide frequent rest periods.

MONITORING
◆ Response to treatment
◆ Fatigue
◆ Nutritional status
◆ Liver function tests
◆ Complications

PATIENT TEACHING

GENERAL
Be sure to cover:
◆ the disorder, diagnosis, and treatment
◆ expectation that convalescence may take several weeks
◆ importance of bed rest during the acute illness
◆ explanation that there's a period of prolonged communicability (stress good hand washing and avoidance of salivary contamination)
◆ benefits of bland foods, milk shakes, fruit juices, and broths to minimize throat discomfort.

DISCHARGE PLANNING
◆ Refer the patient to an otolaryngologist for marked tonsillar swelling or a neurologist for a central nervous system complication.

RESOURCES
Organizations
Centers for Disease Control and Prevention: *www.cdc.gov*
Harvard University Consumer Health Information: *www.intelihealth.com*
National Health Information Center: *www.health.gov/nhic*
National Institute of Allergy and Infectious Diseases: *www.niaid.nih.gov*
National Library of Medicine: *www.nlm.nih.gov*

Selected references
Diseases, 4th ed. Philadelphia: Lippincott Williams & Wilkins, 2006.
Foreman, B.H., et al. "Clinical Inquiries. Can We Prevent Splenic Rupture for Patients with Infectious Mononucleosis?" *Journal of Family Practice* 54(6):547-48, June 2005.
Kasper, D.L., et al., eds. *Harrison's Principles of Internal Medicine,* 16th ed. New York: McGraw-Hill Book Co., 2005.
Statter, M.B., and Liu, D.C. "Nonoperative Management of Blunt Splenic Injury in Infectious Mononucleosis," *The American Surgeon* 71(5):376-78, May 2005.

Influenza

- An acute, highly contagious infection of the respiratory tract
- Has capacity for antigenic variation (ability to mutate into different strains so that no immunologic resistance is present in those at risk)
- Antigenic variation characterized as antigenic drift (minor changes that occur yearly or every few years) and antigenic shift (major changes that lead to pandemics)
- Also called the *grippe* or *flu*

PATHOPHYSIOLOGY

- The virus invades the epithelium of the respiratory tract, causing inflammation and desquamation.
- After attaching to the host cell, viral ribonucleic acid enters the cell and uses host components to replicate its genetic material and protein, which are then assembled into new virus particles.
- Newly produced viruses burst forth to invade other healthy cells.
- Viral invasion destroys host cells, impairing respiratory defenses (especially mucociliary transport system) and predisposing the patient to secondary bacterial infection.

CAUSES

- Infection transmitted by inhaling a respiratory droplet from an infected person or by indirect contact (drinking from a contaminated glass)
- Type A most prevalent, strikes annually with new serotypes, causes epidemics every 3 years
- Type B strikes annually, causes epidemics every 4 to 6 years
- Type C endemic, causes only sporadic cases

INCIDENCE

- Influenzae affects all age-groups, but the highest incidence is among school-age children.
- Influenza occurs most severely (may lead to death) in young children, elderly people, and those with chronic diseases

- Influenza occurs sporadically or in epidemics (usually during colder months), and its incidence peaks within 2 to 3 weeks after initial cases and lasts 2 to 3 months.

COMPLICATIONS

- Pneumonia
- Myositis
- Exacerbation of chronic obstructive pulmonary disease
- Reye's syndrome
- Myocarditis
- Pericarditis
- Transverse myelitis
- Encephalitis

HISTORY

- Usually, recent exposure (typically within 48 hours) to a person with influenza
- No influenza vaccine received during the past season
- Headache
- Malaise
- Myalgia
- Fatigue, listlessness, weakness

PHYSICAL FINDINGS

- Fever (usually higher in children)
- Signs of croup, dry cough
- Red, watery eyes; clear nasal discharge
- Erythema of the nose and throat without exudate
- Tachypnea, shortness of breath, cyanosis
- With bacterial pneumonia, purulent or bloody sputum
- Cervical adenopathy and tenderness
- Breath sounds may be diminished in areas of consolidation

DIAGNOSTIC TEST RESULTS

GENERAL
- After an epidemic is confirmed, diagnosis requires only observation of clinical signs and symptoms.

LABORATORY
- Inoculation of chicken embryos with nasal secretions from infected patients shows influenza virus.
- Throat swabs, nasopharyngeal washes, or sputum culture isolate the influenza virus.
- Immunodiagnostic techniques show viral antigens in tissue culture or in exfoliated nasopharyngeal cells obtained by washings.
- White blood cell (WBC) count is elevated in secondary bacterial infection.
- WBC count is decreased in overwhelming viral or bacterial infection.

TREATMENT

GENERAL
- Fluid and electrolyte replacements
- Oxygen and assisted ventilation, if indicated

DIET
- Increased fluid intake

ACTIVITY
- Rest periods, as needed

MEDICATIONS
- Acetaminophen (Tylenol) or aspirin
- Guaifenesin (Mucinex) or expectorant
- Amantadine (Symmetrel)
- Antibiotics

NURSING CONSIDERATIONS

NURSING DIAGNOSES
- Acute pain
- Fatigue
- Hyperthermia
- Ineffective breathing pattern
- Ineffective health maintenance
- Risk for deficient fluid volume
- Risk for infection

EXPECTED OUTCOMES
The patient will:
- express feelings of increased comfort and relief from pain
- report increased energy level
- maintain a normal temperature
- maintain respiratory rate within 5 breaths/minute of baseline
- maintain current health status
- maintain adequate fluid volume
- experience no further signs or symptoms of infection

NURSING INTERVENTIONS
- Give prescribed drugs.
- Follow standard precautions.
- Administer oxygen therapy, if warranted.

MONITORING
- Temperature
- Signs and symptoms of dehydration
- Respiratory status
- Response to treatment
- Complications

PATIENT TEACHING

GENERAL
Be sure to cover:
- the disorder, diagnosis, and treatment
- mouthwash or warm saline gargles to ease sore throat
- importance of increased fluids to prevent dehydration
- warm bath or a heating pad to relieve myalgia
- proper hand-washing technique and tissue disposal to prevent the virus from spreading
- influenza immunization.

RESOURCES
Organizations
Centers for Disease Control and Prevention: *www.cdc.gov*
Harvard University Consumer Health Information: *www.intelihealth.com*
National Health Information Center: *www.health.gov/nhic*
National Institute of Allergy and Infectious Diseases: *www.niaid.nih.gov*
National Library of Medicine: *www.nlm.nih.gov*

Selected references
Hara, M., et al. "Immune Response to Influenza Vaccine in Healthy Adults and the Elderly: Association with Nutritional Status," *Vaccine* 23(12):1457-463, February 2005.
Kasper, D.L., et al., eds. *Harrison's Principles of Internal Medicine,* 16th ed. New York: McGraw-Hill Book Co., 2005.
Munoz, F.M., et al. "Safety of Influenza Vaccination during Pregnancy," *American Journal of Obstetrics & Gynecology* 192(4):1098-106, April 2005.
Nelson, R. "Health Care Workers: Few Feel the Flu Shot," *AJN* 104(10):24-25, October 2004.

Inguinal hernia

OVERVIEW

- Part of an internal organ that protrudes through an abnormal opening in the wall of the cavity that surrounds it
- The most common type of hernia (see *Common sites of hernia*)
- May be direct or indirect
- Also called *ruptures*

PATHOPHYSIOLOGY

- In an inguinal hernia, the large or small intestine, omentum, or bladder protrudes into the inguinal canal.
- In an indirect hernia, abdominal viscera leave the abdomen through the inguinal ring and follow the spermatic cord (in males) or round ligament (in females); they emerge at the external ring and extend down into the inguinal canal, often into the scrotum or labia.
- In a direct inguinal hernia, instead of entering the canal through the internal ring, the hernia passes through the posterior inguinal wall, protrudes directly through the transverse fascia of the canal (in an area known as Hesselbach's triangle), and comes out at the external ring.

CAUSES

- Direct — weakness in fascial floor of inguinal canal
- Either — weak abdominal muscles (caused by congenital malformation, trauma, or aging) or increased intra-abdominal pressure (caused by heavy lifting, pregnancy, obesity, or straining)
- Indirect — weakness in fascial margin of internal inguinal ring

INCIDENCE

- Indirect hernias are more common; they may develop at any age, are three times more common in males, and are especially prevalent in infants.
- Direct hernias occur more often in middle-age and older people.

COMPLICATIONS

- Strangulation
- Intestinal obstruction
- Infection (after surgery)

ASSESSMENT

HISTORY

- Sharp or "catching" pain when lifting or straining

PHYSICAL FINDINGS

- Obvious swelling or lump in the inguinal area (large hernia) (see *Identifying a hernia*)

DIAGNOSTIC TEST RESULTS

LABORATORY

- White blood cell count is elevated, with intestinal obstruction.

OTHER

- Physical examination helps to confirm the diagnosis.

Common sites of hernia

There are four common sites of hernia: umbilical, incisional, inguinal, and femoral. Here are descriptions of each type with an illustration demonstrating where each type is located.

UMBILICAL

Umbilical hernia results from abnormal muscular structures around the umbilical cord. This hernia is quite common in neonates but also occurs in women who are obese or who have had several pregnancies. Because most umbilical hernias in infants close spontaneously, surgery is warranted only if the hernia persists for more than 4 or 5 years. Taping or binding the affected area or supporting it with a truss may relieve symptoms until the hernia closes. A severe congenital umbilical hernia, which allows the abdominal viscera to protrude outside the body, must be repaired immediately.

INCISIONAL

Incisional (ventral) hernia develops at the site of previous surgery, usually along vertical incisions. This hernia may result from a weakness in the abdominal wall, caused by an infection, impaired wound healing, inadequate nutrition, extreme abdominal distention, or obesity. Palpation of an incisional hernia may reveal several defects in the surgical scar. Effective repair requires pulling the layers of the abdominal wall together without creating tension or, if this isn't possible, the use of Teflon, Marlex mesh, or tantalum mesh to close the opening.

INGUINAL

Inguinal hernia can be direct or indirect. An indirect inguinal hernia causes the abdominal

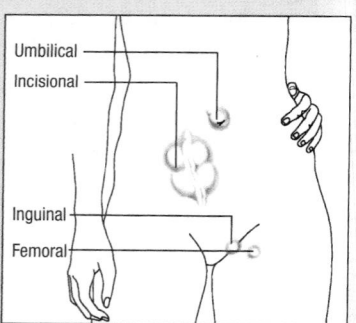

viscera to protrude through the inguinal ring and follow the spermatic cord (in males) or round ligament (in females). A direct inguinal hernia results from a weakness in the fascial floor of the inguinal canal.

FEMORAL

Femoral hernia occurs where the femoral artery passes into the femoral canal. Typically, a fatty deposit within the femoral canal enlarges and eventually creates a hole big enough to accommodate part of the peritoneum and bladder. A femoral hernia appears as a swelling or bulge at the pulse point of the large femoral artery. It's usually a soft, pliable, reducible, nontender mass but commonly becomes incarcerated or strangulated.

TREATMENT

GENERAL
◆ Manual reduction
◆ Truss

DIET
◆ Nothing by mouth (if surgery necessary)

ACTIVITY
◆ As tolerated

MEDICATIONS
◆ Analgesics
◆ Antibiotics
◆ Electrolyte replacement

SURGERY
◆ Herniorrhaphy
◆ Hernioplasty
◆ Bowel resection (with strangulation or necrosis)

NURSING CONSIDERATIONS

NURSING DIAGNOSES
◆ Activity intolerance
◆ Acute pain
◆ Ineffective tissue perfusion: GI
◆ Risk for infection
◆ Risk for injury

EXPECTED OUTCOMES
The patient will:
◆ perform activities of daily living within the confines of the disease process
◆ express feelings of increased comfort
◆ have normal GI function
◆ remain free from signs or symptoms of infection
◆ avoid complications.

NURSING INTERVENTIONS
◆ Apply a truss after a hernia has been reduced.
◆ Give prescribed drugs for pain.
◆ Encourage coughing and deep breathing.

MONITORING
◆ Vital signs
◆ Pain control
◆ Signs of strangulation or incarceration

PATIENT TEACHING

GENERAL
Be sure to cover:
◆ avoiding lifting heavy objects or straining during bowel movements
◆ signs and symptoms of infection (oozing, tenderness, warmth, and redness) at the incision site
◆ wound care
◆ after surgery, not resuming normal activity or returning to work without the surgeon's permission.

DISCHARGE PLANNING
◆ Encourage the patient to schedule follow-up appointments as recommended by the surgeon.

RESOURCES
Organizations
Mayo Clinic: *www.mayoclinic.com*
The Merck Manuals Online Medical Library: *www.merck.com/mmhe*
National Digestive Diseases Information Clearinghouse: *www.niddk.nih.gov/health/digest/nddic.htm*

Selected references
Twu, C.M., et al. "Predicting Risk Factors for Inguinal Hernia after Radical Retropubic Prostatectomy," *Urology* 66(4):814-18, October 2005.
Zisholtz, B. "Laparoscopic Inguinal Hernia Repair," *Journal of the American College of Surgeons* 201(3):488-89, September 2005.

Identifying a hernia

Palpation of the inguinal area while the patient is performing Valsalva's maneuver confirms the diagnosis of inguinal hernia. To detect a hernia in a male patient, ask the patient to stand with his ipsilateral leg slightly flexed and his weight resting on the other leg. Insert an index finger into the lower part of the scrotum and invaginate the scrotal skin so the finger advances through the external inguinal ring to the internal ring (about $1/2$″ to 2″ [1 to 5 cm] through the inguinal canal). Tell the patient to cough. If pressure is felt against the fingertip, an indirect hernia exists; if pressure is felt against the side of the finger, a direct hernia exists.

Insect bites and stings

OVERVIEW

- Bite or sting from an insect or other arthropod, such as a tick, brown recluse spider, black widow spider, scorpion, bee, wasp, yellow jacket, or fire ant, that causes pain or a local systemic reaction

PATHOPHYSIOLOGY

- A bite or sting can injure the skin, and secretions released from a bite or sting can cause a physiologic response specific to the insect or arthropod.
- Reactions to secretion exposure range from barely noticeable to life-threatening.
- Transmission of disease may result from a bite or sting.
- Mouth parts of insect or arthropod are classified as piercing-sucking, sponging, or biting-chewing.

CAUSES

- Hypersensitivity response
- Toxic effects of venom

INCIDENCE

- The incidence of this disorder is unknown.

COMPLICATIONS

- Anaphylaxis
- Hemolytic anemia
- Rarely, thrombocytopenia (brown recluse spider only)

ASSESSMENT

HISTORY
Tick bite
- Itching at the affected site
- Tick exposure lesion

Brown recluse spider bite
- Minimal initial pain that increases over time
- Fever, chills, malaise, weakness
- Nausea, vomiting
- Joint pain, arthralgias

Black widow spider bite
- Pinprick sensation, followed by dull, numbing pain
- Leg bite: severe pain and large muscle cramping
- Vertigo
- Chills and sweats

Bee, wasp, or yellow jacket sting
- Pain and pruritus
- Generalized weakness
- Chest tightness
- Dizziness
- Nausea and vomiting
- Abdominal cramps
- Throat constriction

Fire ant sting
- Immediate pain, itching, and burning

PHYSICAL FINDINGS
Tick bite
- Tick paralysis
- Expanding skin lesion, erythema migrans

Brown recluse spider bite
- Bleb (blister)
- Bluish ring around bite
- Joint pain
- Seizures
- Petechiae

Black widow spider bite
- Rigid, painful abdomen
- Rigidity and pain in the chest, shoulders, and back (if arm bite)
- Extreme restlessness (systemic)
- Pallor
- Seizures, especially in children
- Hyperactive reflexes
- Hypertension
- Tachycardia with thready pulse
- Circulatory collapse and shock
- Tiny red fang marks

Bee, wasp, or yellow jacket sting
- Raised, reddened wheal, possibly with a protruding stinger from the bee, wasp, or yellow jacket
- Wheezing
- Hypotension

Fire ant sting
- Clear vesicles with surrounding erythema
- Pustule

DIAGNOSTIC TEST RESULTS

LABORATORY
- Urinalysis shows hematuria (black widow spider bite).
- White blood cell count is increased (black widow spider bite).
- Anemia panel shows hemolytic anemia (brown recluse spider bite).
- Platelet count shows thrombocytopenia (brown recluse spider bite).

OTHER
- Identification of the insect is difficult unless the patient is stung by a honeybee or bumblebee, which commonly leaves a stinger with a venom sac in the lesion.

TREATMENT

GENERAL
Tick bite
- Tick removal
- Symptomatic therapy for severe symptoms

Brown recluse spider bite
- Cool compresses and elevation of extremity
- I.V. fluids

Black widow spider bite
- Ice packs

Bee, wasp, yellow jacket, or fire ant sting
- Ice application
- Elevation of affected extremity
- Supportive treatment

DIET
- No restrictions
- Nothing by mouth if severe, systemic reaction

ACTIVITY
- Rest to limit toxic effects of venom

MEDICATIONS

Tick bite
- Antipruritics
- Antibiotics (Lyme disease treatment or Rocky Mountain spotted fever treatment)

Brown recluse spider bite
- Corticosteroids
- Antibiotics
- Antihistamines
- Tranquilizers
- Tetanus prophylaxis

Black widow spider bite
- Antivenin I.V.
- Calcium gluconate I.V.
- Muscle relaxants
- Adrenaline or antihistamines
- Tetanus immunization
- Benzodiazepines
- Antibiotics
- Oxygen for respiratory difficulty

Bee, wasp, yellow jacket, or fire ant sting
- Antihistamines
- Steroids for severe reactions

SURGERY
- Lesion excision for brown recluse spider bite

NURSING CONSIDERATIONS

NURSING DIAGNOSES
- Acute pain
- Deficient fluid volume
- Impaired skin integrity
- Ineffective airway clearance
- Ineffective breathing pattern
- Ineffective tissue perfusion: Cardiopulmonary
- Risk for poisoning

EXPECTED OUTCOMES
The patient will:
- express feelings of increased comfort and relief of pain
- maintain normal fluid volume
- regain skin integrity
- maintain a patent airway
- maintain adequate ventilation
- exhibit signs of adequate cardiopulmonary perfusion
- verbalize methods to prevent insect bites and stings.

NURSING INTERVENTIONS
- Keep the affected part immobile.
- Clean the bite or sting site with antiseptic.
- Apply ice.
- Give prescribed drugs.
- Provide emergency resuscitation.

Tick bite
- Remove the tick promptly and carefully.
- Use tweezers to grasp the tick near its head or mouth, and gently pull to remove the whole tick without crushing it.
- If possible, seal the tick in a plastic bag and keep it in case the patient needs to see a practitioner. Otherwise, flush the tick down the toilet or burn it.

Brown recluse spider bite
- Clean the lesion with a 1:20 Burow's aluminum acetate solution.
- Apply antibiotic ointment, as ordered.

Black widow spider bite
- Remove all jewelry.
- Apply cool compresses.
- Avoid cutting into the wound or applying suction.

Scorpion sting
- Wash the bite area thoroughly.
- Remove all jewelry.
- Apply cool compresses.
- Avoid cutting into the wound or applying suction.
- Provide analgesia for pain relief.

Bee, wasp, or yellow jacket sting
- Scrape stinger off; don't pull or squeeze it, which releases more toxin.

Fire ant sting
- Apply cool compresses.
- Gently wash the bite area, leaving the blister intact.
- Be prepared to intervene for an acute severe allergic reaction (rare).

MONITORING
- Vital signs
- Respiratory status
- General appearance
- Changes at the bite or sting site

PATIENT TEACHING

GENERAL
Be sure to cover:
- avoidance of insect bites and stings
- examination of the body for ticks after being outdoors
- removal of ticks
- medical identification jewelry or card
- anaphylaxis kit use
- insect repellent use.

RESOURCES

Organizations
American Academy of Allergy, Asthma, and Immunology: *www.aaaai.org*
National Center for Injury Prevention and Control: *www.cdc.gov/ncipc*
National Institutes of Health: *ww.nih.gov*

Selected references
McIntyre, C.L., et al. "Administration of Epinephrine for Life-Threatening Allergic Reactions in School Settings," *Pediatrics* 116(5):1134-140, November 2005.
Nunnelee, J.D. "Summer Injuries. Bites & Stings," *RN* 68(4):56-58, 60-61, April 2005.
Rash, E.M. "Arthropod Bites and Stings. Recognition and Treatment," *Advance for Nurse Practitioners* 11(9):87-90, 92, 102, September 2003.
Wolfson, A.B., et al. *Harwood-Nuss' Clinical Practice of Emergency Medicine*, 4th ed. Philadelphia: Lippincott Williams & Wilkins, 2005.

Intestinal obstruction LIFE-THREATENING DISORDER

OVERVIEW

- Partial or complete blockage of the lumen of the small or large bowel
- Commonly a medical emergency
- Most likely after abdominal surgery or with congenital bowel deformities
- Without treatment, complete obstruction in any part of bowel can cause death within hours from shock and vascular collapse

PATHOPHYSIOLOGY

- Mechanical or nonmechanical (neurogenic) blockage of the lumen occurs.
- Fluid, air, or gas collects near the site.
- Peristalsis increases temporarily in an attempt to break through the blockage.
- Intestinal mucosa is injured, and distention at and above the site of obstruction occurs.
- Venous blood flow is impaired, and normal absorptive processes cease.
- Water, sodium, and potassium are secreted by the bowel into the fluid pooled in the lumen.

CAUSES
Mechanical obstruction
- Adhesions
- Carcinomas
- Compression of the bowel wall from stenosis, intussusception, volvulus of the sigmoid or cecum, tumors, and atresia
- Foreign bodies
- Strangulated hernias

Nonmechanical obstruction
- Electrolyte imbalances
- Neurogenic abnormalities
- Paralytic ileus
- Thrombosis or embolism of mesenteric vessels
- Toxicity, such as that associated with uremia or generalized infection

RISK FACTORS
- Abdominal surgery
- Radiation therapy
- Gallstones
- Inflammatory bowel disease

INCIDENCE
- Intestinal obstruction is diagnosed in approximately 20% of hospital admissions for abdominal illness.
- This disorder occurs equally in men and women.

COMPLICATIONS
- Perforation
- Peritonitis
- Septicemia
- Secondary infection
- Metabolic alkalosis or acidosis
- Death

ASSESSMENT

HISTORY
- Recent change in bowel habits
- Hiccups

Mechanical obstruction
- Colicky pain
- Nausea, vomiting
- Constipation

Nonmechanical obstruction
- Diffuse abdominal discomfort
- Frequent vomiting
- Severe abdominal pain (if obstruction results from vascular insufficiency or infarction)

PHYSICAL FINDINGS
Mechanical obstruction
- Distended abdomen
- Borborygmi and rushes (occasionally loud enough to be heard without a stethoscope)
- Abdominal tenderness
- Rebound tenderness

Nonmechanical obstruction
- Abdominal distention
- Decreased bowel sounds (early), then absent bowel sounds

DIAGNOSTIC TEST RESULTS

LABORATORY
- Serum sodium, chloride, and potassium levels are decreased.
- White blood cell count is elevated.
- Serum amylase level is increased (if pancreas is irritated by a bowel loop).
- Blood urea nitrogen is increased (with dehydration).

IMAGING
- Abdominal X-rays reveal the presence and location of intestinal gas or fluid; in small bowel obstruction, typical "stepladder" pattern emerges, with alternating fluid and gas levels apparent in 3 to 4 hours.
- Barium enema reveals a distended, air-filled colon or a closed loop of sigmoid with extreme distention (in sigmoid volvulus).

TREATMENT

GENERAL
- Correction of fluid and electrolyte imbalances
- Decompression of the bowel to relieve vomiting and distention
- Treatment of shock and peritonitis

DIET
- Nothing by mouth if surgery is planned
- Parenteral nutrition until bowel is functioning
- High-fiber, when obstruction is relieved

ACTIVITY
- Bed rest during acute phase
- Postoperatively, avoidance of lifting and contact sports

MEDICATIONS
- Broad-spectrum antibiotics
- Analgesics
- Blood replacement

SURGERY
- Usually the treatment of choice (exception is paralytic ileus in which nonoperative therapy is usually attempted first)
- Type of surgery depends on cause of blockage

NURSING CONSIDERATIONS

NURSING DIAGNOSES
- Acute pain
- Constipation
- Deficient fluid volume
- Imbalanced nutrition: Less than body requirements
- Ineffective tissue perfusion: GI

EXPECTED OUTCOMES
The patient will:
- express feelings of increased comfort
- return to normal bowel function
- maintain normal fluid volume
- maintain caloric requirement
- exhibit signs of adequate GI perfusion.

NURSING INTERVENTIONS
- Insert a nasogastric (NG) tube and attach to low-pressure, intermittent suction.
- Maintain the patient in semi-Fowler's position.
- Provide mouth and nose care.
- Begin and maintain I.V. therapy as ordered.
- Give prescribed drugs.

MONITORING
- Vital signs
- Signs and symptoms of shock
- Bowel sounds and signs of returning peristalsis
- NG tube function and drainage
- Pain control
- Abdominal girth measurement to detect progressive distention
- Hydration and nutritional status
- Electrolytes and signs and symptoms of metabolic derangements
- Wound site (postoperatively)

PATIENT TEACHING

GENERAL
Be sure to cover:
- the disorder (focusing on the patient's type of intestinal obstruction), diagnosis, and treatment
- techniques for coughing and deep breathing, and use of incentive spirometry
- colostomy or ileostomy care, if appropriate
- incision care
- postoperative activity limitations and why these restrictions are necessary
- proper use of prescribed medications, focusing on their correct administration, desired effects, and possible adverse reactions
- importance of following a structured bowel regimen, particularly if the patient had a mechanical obstruction from fecal impaction.

DISCHARGE PLANNING
- Refer the patient to an enterostomal therapist if indicated.

RESOURCES
Organizations
Digestive Disease National Coalition: *www.ddnc.org*
National Digestive Diseases Information Clearinghouse: *www.niddk.nih.gov/health/digest/nddic.htm*

Selected references
Ben-Sassi, A., et al. "Distal Intestinal Obstruction Syndrome: A Childhood Illness Now Seen in Adults," *Colorectal Disease Supplement* 6 (Suppl 1):83, July 2004.
Handbook of Diseases, 3rd ed. Philadelphia: Lippincott Williams & Wilkins, 2004.
Hughes, E. "Caring for a Patient with an Intestinal Obstruction," *Nursing Standard* 19(47):56-64, August 2005.
Saddler, D. "A Literature Review of Fecal Impaction," *Gastroenterology Nursing* 28(1):49-50, January-February 2005.

Intussusception

OVERVIEW

- Condition in which a portion of the bowel telescopes or invaginates into an adjacent bowel portion (see *Understanding intussusception*)
- Can be fatal if treatment delayed more than 24 hours
- Pediatric emergency

PATHOPHYSIOLOGY

- A bowel section invaginates and is propelled by peristalsis.
- More bowel is pulled in, causing edema, obstruction, and pain.

CAUSES

- May be linked to viral infections due to seasonal peaks

In infants

- Unknown

In older children

- Alterations in intestinal motility
- Hemangioma
- Lymphoid hyperplasia
- Lymphosarcoma
- Meckel's diverticulum
- Polyps

In adults

- Appendiceal stump
- Benign or malignant tumors (65% of patients)
- Gastroenterostomy with herniation
- Meckel's diverticulum
- Polyps

INCIDENCE

- Intussusception is most common in infants.
- Males are affected three times more commonly than females.
- About 87% of children with intussusception are younger than age 2 and about 70% of these children are between ages 4 and 11 months.
- Seasonal incidence peaks in late spring and early summer.

COMPLICATIONS

- Strangulation of the intestine
- Gangrene of the bowel
- Shock
- Bowel perforation
- Peritonitis
- Death

ASSESSMENT

HISTORY

- Intermittent attacks of colicky pain
- Pain that causes the child to scream, draw his legs up to his abdomen, turn pale and diaphoretic and, possibly, grunt
- Vomiting, initially stomach contents; later, bile-stained or fecal material
- "Currant jelly" stools, which contain mixture of blood and mucus

PHYSICAL FINDINGS

- Distended, tender abdomen
- Guarding over the intussusception site
- Palpable, sausage-shaped abdominal mass in the right upper quadrant or in the midepigastric area if transverse colon is involved
- Bloody mucus found on rectal examination
- In adults, abdominal pain localized in right lower quadrant, radiating to the back, and increasing with eating

---

Understanding intussusception

In intussusception, a bowel section invaginates and is propelled along by peristalsis, pulling in more bowel. This illustration shows intussusception of a portion of the transverse colon. Intussusception typically produces edema, hemorrhage from venous engorgement, incarceration, and obstruction.

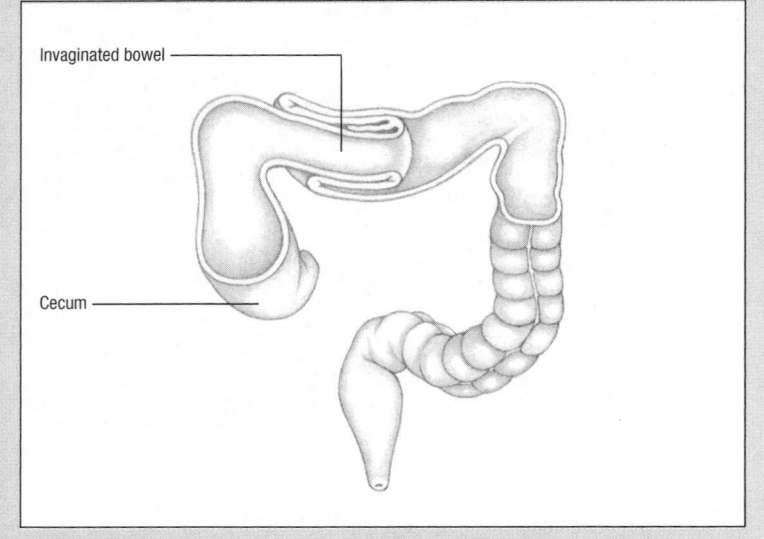

Invaginated bowel

Cecum

DIAGNOSTIC TEST RESULTS

LABORATORY
◆ White blood cell count up to 15,000/μl indicates obstruction; greater than 15,000/μl, strangulation; and more than 20,000/μl, bowel infarction.

IMAGING
◆ Barium enema confirms colonic intussusception by showing the characteristic coiled spring sign; it also delineates the extent of intussusception.
◆ Upright abdominal X-rays show a soft tissue mass and signs of complete or partial obstruction, with dilated loops of bowel.

TREATMENT

GENERAL
◆ Hydrostatic reduction
◆ Bowel decompression

DIET
◆ Nothing by mouth until bowel functions properly

ACTIVITY
◆ Bed rest until condition is resolved

MEDICATIONS
◆ Analgesics
◆ Antibiotics

SURGERY
◆ Indicated for children with recurrent intussusception, those who show signs of shock or peritonitis, and those in whom symptoms present longer than 24 hours
◆ In adults, always the treatment of choice

NURSING CONSIDERATIONS

NURSING DIAGNOSES
◆ Acute pain
◆ Anxiety
◆ Deficient fluid volume
◆ Fear
◆ Ineffective tissue perfusion: GI
◆ Risk for infection

EXPECTED OUTCOMES
The patient will:
◆ express feelings of increased comfort
◆ identify strategies to reduce anxiety
◆ maintain normal fluid volume
◆ discuss fears and concerns
◆ exhibit signs of adequate GI perfusion
◆ remain free from signs and symptoms of infection.

NURSING INTERVENTIONS
◆ Offer reassurance and emotional support to the patient and, if the patient is a child, to his parents.
◆ Give prescribed I.V. fluids.
◆ Encourage coughing and deep breathing.
◆ Give prescribed antibiotics.

MONITORING
◆ Vital signs
◆ Intake and output
◆ Hydration status
◆ Nasogastric tube function and drainage
◆ Bowel sounds, stools, abdominal distention
◆ Wound site (after surgery)
◆ For recurrence in the first 36 to 48 hours after reduction

PATIENT TEACHING

GENERAL
Be sure to cover:
◆ the disorder, diagnosis, and treatment
◆ medication administration, dosage, and possible adverse effects
◆ wound care
◆ signs and symptoms of infection
◆ parental participation in their child's care to minimize the stress of hospitalization (visiting hours should be flexible).

DISCHARGE PLANNING
◆ Encourage the patient's family to make follow-up appointments as recommended by his practitioner.

RESOURCES
Organizations
Digestive Disease National Coalition: *www.nddc.org*
National Digestive Diseases Information Clearinghouse: *www.niddk.nih.gov/health/digest/nddic.htm*

Selected references
Grosfeld, J.L. "Intussusception Then and Now: A Historical Vignette," *Journal of the American College of Surgeons* 201(6):830-33, December 2005.
Handbook of Diseases, 3rd ed. Philadelphia: Lippincott Williams & Wilkins, 2004.
Kim, K.H., et al. "Intussusception after Gastric Surgery," *Endoscopy* 37(12): 1237-243, December 2005.
McNally, P. *GI/Liver Secrets*, 3rd ed. Philadelphia: Hanley & Belfus, Inc., 2006.

Irritable bowel syndrome

- Common condition marked by chronic or periodic diarrhea alternating with constipation
- Accompanied by straining and abdominal cramps
- Initial episodes early in life and late teens to 20s
- Prognosis good
- Also known as *spastic colon, spastic colitis, mucous colitis*

PATHOPHYSIOLOGY

- Precise etiology is unclear.
- A change occurs in bowel motility, reflecting an abnormality in the neuromuscular control of intestinal smooth muscle.

CAUSES

- Anxiety and stress
- Dietary factors, such as fiber, raw fruits, coffee, alcohol, and foods that are cold, highly seasoned, or laxative in nature

Other possible triggers

- Allergy to certain foods or drugs
- Hormones
- Lactose intolerance
- Laxative abuse

INCIDENCE

- Irritable bowel syndrome occurs mostly in women, with symptoms first emerging before age 40.

COMPLICATIONS

- Diverticulitis and colon cancer
- Chronic inflammatory bowel disease

HISTORY

- Chronic constipation, diarrhea, or both
- Lower abdominal pain (typically in the left lower quadrant) usually relieved by defecation or passage of gas
- Small stools with visible mucus or pasty, pencil-like stools instead of diarrhea
- Dyspepsia
- Abdominal bloating
- Heartburn
- Faintness and weakness
- Contributing psychological factors, such as a recent stressful life change, that may have triggered or aggravated symptoms
- Anxiety and fatigue

PHYSICAL FINDINGS

- Normal bowel sounds
- Tympany over a gas-filled bowel

GENERAL

- Assessment involves studies to rule out other, more serious disorders.

LABORATORY

- Stool examination is negative for occult blood, parasites, and pathogenic bacteria.
- Complete blood count, serologic tests, serum albumin, and erythrocyte sedimentation rate are normal.

IMAGING

- Barium enema reveals colonic spasm and a tubular appearance of the descending colon; also used to rule out certain other disorders, such as diverticula, tumors, and polyps.

DIAGNOSTIC PROCEDURES

- Sigmoidoscopy may disclose spastic contractions.

TREATMENT

GENERAL
- Stress management
- Lifestyle modifications

DIET
- Based on the patient's symptoms
- Initially, elimination diet
- Avoidance of sorbitol, nonabsorbable carbohydrates, and foods that contain lactose
- Increased bulk
- Increased fluids

ACTIVITY
- Regular exercise

MEDICATIONS
- Anticholinergic, antispasmodic drugs
- Antidiarrheals
- Laxatives
- Antiemetics
- Simethicone
- Mild tranquilizers
- Tricyclic antidepressants

NURSING CONSIDERATIONS

NURSING DIAGNOSES
- Acute pain
- Constipation
- Diarrhea
- Disturbed body image
- Ineffective coping

EXPECTED OUTCOMES
The patient will:
- express feelings of increased comfort
- have stool that's soft and passes easily
- have normal bowel function
- express positive feelings about body
- demonstrate adaptive coping behaviors.

NURSING INTERVENTIONS
- Because the patient with irritable bowel syndrome isn't hospitalized, nursing interventions almost always focus on patient teaching.

MONITORING
- Weight
- Diet
- Bowel movements

PATIENT TEACHING

GENERAL
Be sure to cover:
- the disorder, diagnosis, and treatment
- dietary plans and implementation
- importance of drinking 8 to 10 glasses of water or other compatible fluids daily
- proper use of prescribed medication, reviewing desired effects and possible adverse reactions
- importance of implementing lifestyle changes that reduce stress
- smoking cessation
- importance of regular physical examinations. (For patients older than age 40, emphasize the need for colorectal cancer screening, including annual proctosigmoidoscopy and rectal examinations.)

RESOURCES
Organizations
Digestive Disease National Coalition: *www.nddc.org*
National Digestive Diseases Information Clearinghouse: *www.niddk.nih.gov/health/digest/nddic.htm*

Selected references
Bruno, M. "Irritable Bowel Syndrome and Inflammatory Bowel Disease in Pregnancy," *Journal of Perinatal & Neonatal Nursing* 18(4):341-50, October-December 2004.
Handbook of Diseases, 3rd ed. Philadelphia: Lippincott Williams & Wilkins, 2004.
McNally, P. *GI/Liver Secrets*, 3rd ed. Philadelphia: Hanley & Belfus, Inc., 2006.
Tierney, L., et al. *Current Medical Diagnosis & Treatment 2006*. New York: McGraw-Hill Book Co., 2006.
Watson, A.R., and Bowling, T.E. "Irritable Bowel Syndrome: Diagnosis and Symptom Management," *British Journal of Community Nursing* 10(3):118-22, March 2005.

Juvenile rheumatoid arthritis

OVERVIEW

- Several inflammatory conditions characterized by chronic synovitis and joint swelling, pain, and tenderness
- Major types: systemic (Still's disease or acute febrile type), polyarticular, and pauciarticular

PATHOPHYSIOLOGY

- If juvenile rheumatoid arthritis (JRA) isn't arrested, the inflammatory process in the joints occurs in four stages:
- Synovitis develops from congestion and edema of the synovial membrane and joint capsule.
- Pannus covers and invades cartilage and eventually destroys the joint capsule and bone.
- Fibrous tissue and ankylosis occludes the joint space.
- Fibrous tissue calcifies, resulting in bony ankylosis and total immobility.

CAUSES

- Suggested link to genetic factors or an abnormal immune response
- Viral or bacterial (streptococcal) infection, trauma, and emotional stress

INCIDENCE

- JRA may occur as early as age 6 weeks but seldom before age 6 months; peak onset is between ages 1 and 3, and ages 8 and 12.
- JRA occurs in an estimated 150,000 to 250,000 children in the United States; it affects twice as many girls as boys.

COMPLICATIONS

- Flexion contractures
- Ocular damage and loss of vision
- Retarded growth and development

ASSESSMENT

HISTORY

- Common complaint of joint stiffness in the morning or after periods of inactivity
- In young children, typically irritability and listlessness

PHYSICAL FINDINGS

Systemic JRA

- Mild, transient arthritis or frank polyarthritis with fever and rash
- Behavior that clearly suggests joint pain and fatigue
- Painful breathing and nonspecific abdominal pain
- Fatigue, shortness of breath, palpitations, and fever
- Resting or exertional tachycardia, arrhythmias, jugular vein distention, and heart murmurs
- Hepatic, splenic, and lymph node enlargement
- Friction rub associated with pericarditis

Polyarticular JRA

- Pain in the wrists, elbows, knees, ankles, and small joints of the hands and feet
- Pain in larger joints, including the temporomandibular, cervical spine, hips, and shoulders
- Tenderness, stiffness, and swelling of joints
- Possible low-grade fever with daily peaks
- Weight loss
- Noticeable developmental retardation
- Hepatic, splenic, and lymph node enlargement
- Subcutaneous nodules on the elbows or heels

Pauciarticular JRA

- Pain in the hips, knees, heels, feet, ankles, and elbows
- Eye redness, blurred vision, and photophobia
- Lower back pain

DIAGNOSTIC TEST RESULTS

LABORATORY

- Blood tests show decreased hemoglobin levels, increased neutrophil (neutrophilia) and platelet (thrombocytosis) counts, an elevated erythrocyte sedimentation rate, and elevated C-reactive protein, haptoglobin, immunoglobulin, and C3 complement levels.
- Antinuclear antibody test result is positive in patients with polyarticular JRA and in those with pauciarticular JRA with chronic iridocyclitis.
- Rheumatoid factor (RF) appears in about 15% of patients with JRA. (In contrast, about 85% of patients with rheumatoid arthritis [RA] test positive for RF.) Patients with polyarticular JRA may test positive for RF.
- The presence of human leukocyte antigen-B27 forecasts the later development of ankylosing spondylitis.

IMAGING

- X-ray studies show early structural changes associated with JRA, including soft tissue swelling, effusion, and periostitis in affected joints, and later evidence, including osteoporosis and accelerated bone growth followed by subchondral erosions, joint-space narrowing, bone destruction, and fusion.

TREATMENT

GENERAL

- Physical therapy
- Splints
- Heat application during passive exercise

DIET

- Adequate iron, protein, calcium, and caloric intake

ACTIVITY

- As tolerated

MEDICATIONS

- Aspirin

- Nonsteroidal anti-inflammatory drugs (NSAIDs)
- Gold salts
- Hydroxychloroquine (Plaquenil)
- Penicillamine (Cuprimine)
- Low-dose cytotoxics
- Monoclonal antibodies

SURGERY
- Soft-tissue releases to improve mobility
- Joint replacement (delayed until child matures physically and can tolerate vigorous rehabilitation)

NURSING CONSIDERATIONS

NURSING DIAGNOSES
- Activity intolerance
- Acute pain
- Compromised family coping
- Delayed growth and development
- Disturbed sensory perception: Visual
- Fatigue
- Impaired physical mobility
- Ineffective coping
- Ineffective role performance
- Powerlessness
- Risk for injury

EXPECTED OUTCOMES
The patient (and family) will:
- verbalize the importance of balancing activity, as tolerated, with rest
- express feelings of increased comfort and decreased pain
- assist the child in all physical and emotional areas
- demonstrate age-appropriate skills and behaviors to the extent possible
- maintain optimal functioning within the limits of the visual impairment
- express feelings of increased energy
- maintain optimal mobility within the confines of the disease
- demonstrate effective coping behaviors
- recognize and express feelings about limitations due to illness
- express feelings of control over his well-being
- identify factors that increase potential for injury.

NURSING INTERVENTIONS
- Focus nursing care on reducing pain and promoting mobility.
- During inflammatory exacerbations, administer NSAIDs or prescribed medication on a regular schedule.
- Allow the patient to rest frequently throughout the day to conserve energy for times when he must be mobile.
- Arrange the patient's environment for participation in activities of daily living so that he feels capable of accomplishing tasks.

MONITORING
- Pain level
- Response to treatment
- Signs and symptoms of bleeding
- Nutritional status
- Joint mobility
- Adverse drug reactions

PATIENT TEACHING

GENERAL
Be sure to cover:
- the disorder, diagnosis, and treatment
- the need to encourage the child to be as independent as possible
- the need for regular slit-lamp examinations to enable early diagnosis and treatment of iridocyclitis
- signs and symptoms of bleeding caused by aspirin or NSAID therapy (instructing the patient to take these medications with meals or milk to reduce adverse GI reactions)
- signs and symptoms of exacerbation, and the need to notify the practitioner about these symptoms
- the need for proper nutrition and caloric consumption
- child's special needs (tell teachers and the school principal).

DISCHARGE PLANNING
- Consult an occupational therapist to assess the patient's home care needs.

RESOURCES
Organizations
American Academy of Pediatrics: *www.aap.org*
Arthritis Foundation: *www.arthritis.org*

Selected references
Kasper, D.L., et al., eds. *Harrison's Principles of Internal Medicine,* 16th ed. New York: McGraw-Hill Book Co., 2005.
Mason, T.G., and Reed, A.M. "Update in Juvenile Rheumatoid Arthritis," *Arthritis and Rheumatism* 53(5):796-99, October 2005.
The Merck Manual of Diagnosis & Therapy, 18th ed. Whitehouse Station, N.J.: Merck & Co., Inc., 2006.
Phelan, J.D., et al. "Susceptibility to JRA/JIA: Complementing General Autoimmune and Arthritis Traits," *Genes and Immunity* 7(1):1-10, January 2006.
Schikler, K.N. "Growth Hormone Therapy in Juvenile Arthritis: Importance of Classification," *Journal of Pediatrics* 145(3):423-24, September 2004.

Kaposi's sarcoma

- Most common acquired immunodeficiency syndrome (AIDS)–related cancer
- External lesions characterized by obvious, colorful lesions
- Most common internal sites: lungs and GI tract (esophagus, oropharynx, and epiglottis)

PATHOPHYSIOLOGY

- Kaposi's sarcoma causes structural and functional damage.
- When associated with AIDS, it progresses aggressively, involving the lymph nodes, the viscera and, possibly, GI structures.

CAUSES

- Exact cause unknown

RISK FACTORS

- Immunosuppression
- Genetic or hereditary predisposition

INCIDENCE

- Kaposi's sarcoma originally affected 35% of AIDS patients; incidence is now declining with the earlier detection of AIDS.
- It may be more common in middle-age and older Mediterranean, Eastern European, and Jewish men.

COMPLICATIONS

- Severe pulmonary involvement, resulting in respiratory distress
- GI involvement, leading to digestive problems

HISTORY

- Possible history of AIDS
- Pain (in advanced cases)

PHYSICAL FINDINGS

- Several lesions of various shapes, sizes, and colors (ranging from red-brown to dark purple) on the skin, buccal mucosa, hard and soft palates, lips, gums, tongue, tonsils, conjunctiva, and sclera (the most common sites)
- Lesions that may merge, becoming one large plaque, in advanced disease
- Untreated lesions that may appear as large, ulcerative masses
- Dyspnea
- Edema from lymphatic obstruction
- Wheezing and hypoventilation

DIAGNOSTIC PROCEDURES

- Tissue biopsy shows the type and stage of the lesion. (See *Laubenstein's stages in Kaposi's sarcoma.*)

Laubenstein's stages in Kaposi's sarcoma

L.J. Laubenstein proposed this staging system to evaluate and treat patients with acquired immunodeficiency syndrome and Kaposi's sarcoma:

- Stage I — locally indolent cutaneous lesions
- Stage II — locally aggressive cutaneous lesions
- Stage III — mucocutaneous lesions and lymph node involvement
- Stage IV — visceral involvement.

Within each stage, a patient may have different symptoms further classified as stage subtype A or B, which are:

- Subtype A — no systemic signs or symptoms
- Subtype B — one or more systemic signs and symptoms, including 10% weight loss, fever of unknown origin that exceeds 100° F (37.8° C) for longer than 2 weeks, chills, lethargy, night sweats, anorexia, and diarrhea.

TREATMENT

GENERAL
◆ Radiation therapy for palliation of symptoms (pain from obstructing lesions in the oral cavity or extremities and edema caused by lymphatic blockage); also for cosmetic improvement

DIET
◆ High-calorie, high-protein
◆ Small meals

ACTIVITY
◆ Limited
◆ Frequent rest periods

MEDICATIONS
◆ Chemotherapy
◆ Biologic response modifier

SURGERY
◆ Removal of lesion from skin (especially if lesion is small) using local excision, electrodesiccation and curettage, or cryotherapy

NURSING CONSIDERATIONS

NURSING DIAGNOSES
◆ Acute pain
◆ Anticipatory grieving
◆ Anxiety
◆ Disturbed body image
◆ Fatigue
◆ Fear
◆ Imbalanced nutrition: Less than body requirements
◆ Impaired gas exchange
◆ Impaired skin integrity
◆ Ineffective breathing pattern
◆ Ineffective coping
◆ Risk for infection

EXPECTED OUTCOMES
The patient will:
◆ report feelings of comfort and reduced pain
◆ express feelings about potential loss
◆ verbalize feelings of reduced anxiety
◆ express positive feelings about body
◆ express feelings of increased energy
◆ verbalize fears and concerns
◆ maintain weight within an acceptable range
◆ maintain adequate ventilation
◆ exhibit improved or healed lesions or wounds
◆ maintain an effective breathing pattern
◆ demonstrate effective coping mechanisms
◆ remain free from signs and symptoms of infection.

NURSING INTERVENTIONS
◆ Encourage verbalization and offer support.
◆ Inspect the skin for new lesions and skin breakdown.
◆ Give prescribed drugs.
◆ Provide rest periods.

MONITORING
◆ Adverse effects of treatment
◆ Vital signs
◆ Pain control
◆ Nutritional status
◆ Respiratory status

PATIENT TEACHING

GENERAL
Be sure to cover:
◆ the disorder, diagnosis, and treatment
◆ medication administration, dosage, and possible adverse effects
◆ infection-prevention techniques and, if necessary, basic hygiene measures to prevent infection (especially if the patient also has AIDS)
◆ the need for ongoing treatment and care.

DISCHARGE PLANNING
◆ Refer the patient to available resources and support services.

RESOURCES
Organizations
American Cancer Society: *www.cancer.org*
Guide to Internet Resources for Cancer: *www.cancerindex.org*
National Cancer Institute: *www.cancer.gov*

Selected references
Casciato, D.A. *Manual of Clinical Oncology,* 5th ed. Philadelphia: Lippincott Williams & Wilkins, 2004.
Guttman-Yassky, E., et al. "Classic Kaposi Sarcoma," *Cancer* 106(2):413-19, January 2006.

Kawasaki syndrome

OVERVIEW

- A noncontagious, febrile, self-limited disorder of unknown origin
- Affects the mucous membranes, lymph nodes, blood vessels, and heart
- Occurs in stages: acute, subacute, and convalescent
- Cardiac complications most serious sequelae (2% of patients die from coronary vasculitis)
- Full recovery expected
- Also known as *mucocutaneous lymph node syndrome* and *infantile polyarteritis*

PATHOPHYSIOLOGY

- An infection results in altered immune function.
- Antibodies increase because of the infection and cause inflammation of blood vessels.
- Blood vessel inflammation increases platelet accumulation and results in thrombus formation.
- Thrombi result in obstruction of the heart and blood vessels.

CAUSES

- Possible genetic role after exposure to an unknown virus, bacteria, or other pathogen

RISK FACTORS

- None known
- No known preventive measures

INCIDENCE

- Incidence peaks in boys younger than age 4, but the disease can occur up to puberty.
- Kawasaki disease affects boys 1½ times more commonly than girls.
- It occurs more commonly in late winter and in spring.
- It's most common in Japan or in Japanese or Korean children living elsewhere.
- It commonly occurs in clusters within a geographic location.
- The disease rarely occurs twice in the same household.

COMPLICATIONS

- Vasculitis leading to aneurysm and myocardial infarction
- Future coronary bypass surgery, if coronary artery disease develops
- Myocarditis
- Pericarditis
- Cardiac arrhythmias
- Abnormal valve functioning
- Death

ASSESSMENT

HISTORY

- Fever for 5 days or more that's unresponsive to antipyretics
- Occurrence of characteristic symptoms

PHYSICAL FINDINGS

- Reddened, swollen hands and feet
- Inflamed mucous membranes of the eyes
- "Strawberry" tongue with red, cracked lips
- Rash in trunk area
- Enlarged cervical lymph nodes
- Reddened, swollen joints
- Possible enlarged gallbladder

DIAGNOSTIC TEST RESULTS

LABORATORY

- White blood cell count and erythrocyte sedimentation rate are elevated in the acute phase.
- Platelet count is elevated in the subacute phase.
- Lumbar puncture results reveal aseptic meningitis.
- Liver function test levels are elevated.
- Hemoglobin levels are decreased, indicating anemia.
- Urinalysis may show pyuria or proteinuria.

IMAGING

- Sequential echocardiograms detect artery disease.
- Chest X-ray rules out cardiomegaly and subclinical pneumonitis.

TREATMENT

GENERAL

- Hospitalization
- Symptomatic treatment
- Prevention of complications

DIET

- Soft, nonirritating foods
- Avoidance of citrus fruits and juices (mouth sores)

ACTIVITY

- As tolerated

MEDICATIONS

- I.V. gamma globulin
- Aspirin
- Dipyridamole (Persantine)

NURSING DIAGNOSES

◆ Activity intolerance
◆ Acute pain
◆ Decreased cardiac output
◆ Fatigue
◆ Hyperthermia
◆ Imbalanced nutrition: Less than body requirements
◆ Impaired oral mucous membrane
◆ Impaired skin integrity
◆ Ineffective tissue perfusion: Cardiopulmonary, peripheral
◆ Risk for infection

EXPECTED OUTCOMES

The patient will:
◆ verbalize the importance of balancing activity, as tolerated, with rest
◆ experience increased comfort and decreased pain
◆ maintain adequate cardiac output and hemodynamic stability
◆ express feelings of increased energy
◆ maintain temperature within normal limits
◆ maintain adequate nutrition
◆ maintain intact oral mucous membranes
◆ maintain skin integrity
◆ exhibit signs of adequate cardiopulmonary and peripheral perfusion
◆ remain free from all signs and symptoms of infection.

NURSING INTERVENTIONS

◆ Observe for signs of heart failure: tachycardia, dyspnea, crackles, edema.
◆ Inspect the extremities for color, temperature, and capillary refill.
◆ Observe and report joint swelling and redness.
◆ Observe and report nature of rash.
◆ Keep clothing from constricting or irritating rash.
◆ Moisten lips with lip balm to prevent cracking.
◆ Offer frequent fluids.
◆ Observe for signs of GI upset, such as nausea and vomiting.
◆ Avoid pressure on the extremities with edema.
◆ Give prescribed drugs.

MONITORING

◆ Complications, such as chest pain, arrhythmias, and electrocardiogram changes
◆ Edema changes
◆ Intake and output
◆ Nutritional status
◆ Response to treatment
◆ Adverse effects of I.V. immunoglobulin: allergic reactions, fever, chills, headache, transfusion reactions, and pulmonary edema

GENERAL

Be sure to cover:
◆ aspirin therapy during and after hospitalization
◆ the need to report exposure to viral illnesses, such as influenza or chickenpox, while taking aspirin, in order to prevent Reye's syndrome
◆ the possibility of long-term management if cardiac complications exist
◆ the need to delay immunizations (especially the measles-mumps-rubella and chickenpox vaccines) when immunoglobulin is given.

DISCHARGE PLANNING

◆ Encourage the patient to schedule a follow-up examination in 2 to 3 weeks.

RESOURCES

Organizations

American Heart Association: *www.americanheart.org*
Harvard University Consumer Health Information: *www.intelihealth.com*
Mayo Foundation for Medical Education and Research: *www.mayoclinic.com*
National Center for Infectious Diseases: *www.cdc.gov/ncidod*

Selected references

Bastian, J.F., and Kushner, H.I. "Diagnosing Kawasaki Syndrome," *Rheumatology (Oxford)* 45(2):240-41, February 2006.
Benseler, S.M., et al. "Infections and Kawasaki Disease: Implications for Coronary Artery Outcome," *Pediatrics* 116(6):e760-66, December 2005.
Wang, C.L., et al. "Kawasaki Disease: Infection, Immunity and Genetics," *Pediatric Infectious Disease Journal* 24(11):998-1004, November 2005.

Keratitis

- Infection of the cornea
- Usually affects only one eye
- May be acute or chronic

PATHOPHYSIOLOGY

- Inflammation of the cornea results from corneal infection.
- Inflammation may be deep or superficial.

CAUSES

- Congenital syphilis
- Denervation
- Immune reactions
- Ischemia
- Tear deficiency
- Trauma
- Viral, bacterial, or fungal infection

INCIDENCE

- Keratitis is fairly common.
- It may develop at any age.

COMPLICATIONS

- Blindness
- Corneal scarring or perforation

HISTORY

- Recent upper respiratory tract infection accompanied by cold sores
- Eye pain
- Central vision loss
- Sensitivity to light
- Sensation of a foreign body in the eye
- Blurred vision

PHYSICAL FINDINGS

- Cornea lacking normal luster
- Characteristic branched lesion of the cornea with herpes simplex virus type 1

DIAGNOSTIC PROCEDURES

- Slit-lamp examination with sodium fluorescein staining may show corneal inflammation or abrasion; small branchlike (dendritic) lesions indicate possible herpes simplex virus infection. (See *Examining the eye with a slit lamp.*)

Examining the eye with a slit lamp

An ophthalmologist uses the slit lamp, an instrument equipped with a special lighting system and a binocular microscope, to view the eyelids, eyelashes, conjunctiva, sclera, cornea, tear film, anterior chamber, iris, crystalline lens, and vitreous face. The examiner may adjust the size, shape, intensity, and depth of the light source as well as the magnification of the microscope to evaluate normally transparent or near-transparent ocular fluids and tissues. If he notes abnormalities, he can attach special devices to the slit lamp to allow more detailed investigation.

PREPARING THE PATIENT

- Tell the patient that the slit-lamp examination evaluates the front portion of the eyes and that it requires that he remain still. Reassure him that the examination is painless.
- If the patient wears contact lenses, tell him to remove them for the test, unless the test is being performed to evaluate the fit of the lens.
- If the test calls for dilating eyedrops, check the patient's history for adverse reactions to mydriatics and for the presence of angle-closure glaucoma before giving the drops. Dilating eyedrops aren't used in routine eye examinations, but some diseases require pupillary dilation before slit-lamp examination.

TREATMENT

GENERAL
◆ Eye shield or patch

MEDICATIONS
Acute keratitis
◆ Trifluridine eyedrops
◆ Vidarabine ophthalmic ointment
◆ Broad-spectrum antibiotic

Chronic keratitis
◆ Vidarabine therapy
◆ Long-term topical therapy, if necessary

Fungal keratitis
◆ Natamycin (Natacyn)

SURGERY
◆ Corneal transplantation for severe ulcerations with residual scarring

NURSING CONSIDERATIONS

NURSING DIAGNOSES
◆ Acute pain
◆ Disturbed sensory perception: Visual
◆ Ineffective health maintenance
◆ Risk for infection
◆ Risk for injury

EXPECTED OUTCOMES
The patient will:
◆ express increased feelings of comfort
◆ regain normal visual functioning
◆ maintain current health status
◆ show no further signs or symptoms of infection
◆ avoid injury.

NURSING INTERVENTIONS
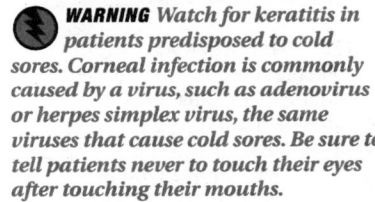 **WARNING** *Watch for keratitis in patients predisposed to cold sores. Corneal infection is commonly caused by a virus, such as adenovirus or herpes simplex virus, the same viruses that cause cold sores. Be sure to tell patients never to touch their eyes after touching their mouths.*
◆ Wear gloves when in contact with the eyes or ocular drainage of patients with herpes simplex virus.
◆ Apply warm compresses.
◆ Dim the lights in case of photophobia.
◆ Give prescribed drugs.

MONITORING
◆ Response to treatment
◆ Visual acuity

PATIENT TEACHING

GENERAL
Be sure to cover:
◆ the disorder, diagnosis, and treatment
◆ medication and possible adverse effects
◆ how stress, traumatic injury, fever, colds, and sun overexposure can trigger a flare-up
◆ the need to wear sunglasses for photophobia
◆ the importance of meticulous hand washing
◆ preventing spread of infection.

RESOURCES
Organizations
American Academy of Ophthalmology: *www.aao.org*
National Eye Institute: *www.nei.nih.gov*

Selected references
Gagnon, M.R., and Walter, K.A. "A Case of Acanthamoeba Keratitis as a Result of a Cosmetic Contact Lens," *Eye & Contact Lens* 32(1):37-38, January 2006.
Parmar, P., et al. "Microbial Keratitis at Extremes of Age," *Cornea* 25(2):153-58, February 2006.
Sun, X., et al. "Acanthamoeba Keratitis Clinical Characteristics and Management," *Ophthalmology* 113(3):412-16, March 2006.

Kidney cancer

- Proliferation of cancer cells in the kidney
- 85% originating in the kidneys; 15% metastasizing from various primary site carcinomas
- Also called *nephrocarcinoma, renal carcinoma, hypernephroma,* and *Grawitz' tumor*

PATHOPHYSIOLOGY

- Most kidney tumors are large, firm, nodular, encapsulated, unilateral, and solitary.
- Kidney cancer may affect either kidney; occasionally tumors are bilateral or multifocal. (See *Unilateral kidney tumor.*)
- Renal cancers arise from the tubular epithelium.
- Tumor margins are usually clearly defined.
- Tumors can include areas of ischemia, necrosis, and focal hemorrhage.
- Tumor cell characteristics may range from well differentiated to anaplastic.
- Kidney cancer can be separated histologically into clear cell, granular cell, and spindle cell types.
- The prognosis is better for patients with the clear cell type than for those with the other types; in general, however, the prognosis depends more on the cancer's stage than on its type. The overall prognosis has improved considerably, with the current 5-year survival rate being about 50%.

CAUSES

- Unknown

RISK FACTORS

- Heavy cigarette smoking
- Regular hemodialysis treatments
- Obesity
- Occupational exposure to petroleum products, asbestosis, or heavy metals

INCIDENCE

- Kidney cancer is twice as common in men as in women.
- It's more common after age 40.
- Renal pelvic tumors and Wilms' tumor are most common in children.

COMPLICATIONS

- Hemorrhage
- Metastasis

HISTORY

- Hematuria
- Dull, aching flank pain
- Weight loss (rare)
- Fever
- Night sweats

PHYSICAL FINDINGS

- Palpable smooth, firm, nontender abdominal or flank mass
- Gross hematuria
- Hypertension
- Supraclavicular adenopathy

LABORATORY

- Alkaline phosphatase, bilirubin, and transaminase levels are increased.
- Prothrombin time is prolonged.

IMAGING

- Renal ultrasonography and computed tomography can be used to verify renal cancer.
- Excretory urography, nephrotomography, and kidney-ureter-bladder radiography are used to aid diagnosis and help in staging.

Unilateral kidney tumor

In kidney cancer, tumors such as this one in the upper kidney pole, usually occur unilaterally.

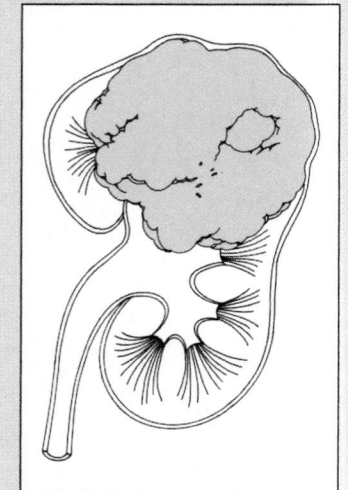

TREATMENT

GENERAL
◆ Because of radiation resistance, radiotherapy limited to cases in which cancer has spread into the perinephric region or lymph nodes, or when primary tumor or metastatic sites can't be completely excised

DIET
◆ Low-protein diet

ACTIVITY
◆ No heavy lifting or contact sports for 6 to 8 weeks postoperatively

MEDICATIONS
◆ Chemotherapy
◆ Biotherapy with lymphokine-activated killer cells plus recombinant interleukin-2
◆ Interferon

SURGERY
◆ Radical nephrectomy, with or without regional lymph node dissection

NURSING CONSIDERATIONS

NURSING DIAGNOSES
◆ Acute pain
◆ Anxiety
◆ Fear
◆ Impaired physical mobility
◆ Ineffective breathing pattern
◆ Ineffective tissue perfusion: Renal
◆ Readiness for enhanced management of therapeutic regimen
◆ Risk for imbalanced fluid volume

EXPECTED OUTCOMES
The patient will:
◆ report increased comfort
◆ identify strategies to reduce anxiety
◆ express fears and concerns relating to his condition and prognosis
◆ maintain joint mobility and range of motion
◆ maintain effective breathing pattern
◆ exhibit signs of adequate renal perfusion
◆ communicate understanding of medical regimen, medications, diet, and activity restrictions
◆ maintain fluid balance.

NURSING INTERVENTIONS
◆ Give prescribed drugs.
◆ Encourage verbalization and provide support.

MONITORING
◆ Wound site
◆ Intake and output
◆ Complete blood count; serum chemistry results
◆ Pain control

PATIENT TEACHING

GENERAL
Be sure to cover:
◆ the disorder, diagnosis, and treatment
◆ medication administration, dosage, and possible adverse effects
◆ the need for a healthy, well-balanced diet and regular exercise
◆ the importance of checking with the practitioner before taking vitamins or other dietary supplements
◆ the importance of follow-up care.

DISCHARGE PLANNING
◆ Refer the patient to support services.
◆ Refer the patient to a program for weight reduction, if indicated.
◆ Refer the patient to a program for smoking cessation, if indicated.

RESOURCES
Organizations
American Cancer Society: *www.cancer.org*
Guide to Internet Resources for Cancer: *www.cancerindex.org*
National Cancer Institute: *www.cancer.gov*
National Institute of Diabetes & Digestive & Kidney Diseases: *www.niddk.nih.gov*

Selected references
Atlas of Pathophysiology, 2nd ed. Philadelphia: Lippincott Williams & Wilkins, 2005.
Galli, B., et al. "Laparoscopic Radical Nephrectomy in Renal Cell Carcinoma," *Urologic Nursing* 25(2):83-86, April 2005.
Weiss, R.H., and Lin, P.Y. "Kidney Cancer: Identification of Novel Targets for Therapy," *Kidney International* 69(2):224-32, January 2006.
Weizer, A.Z., et al. "Complications after Percutaneous Radiofrequency Ablation of Renal Tumors," *Urology* 66(6):1176-80, December 2005.

Klinefelter's syndrome

- Relatively common genetic abnormality that results from an extra X chromosome, creating an XXY sex chromosome constitution
- Affects only males and usually becomes apparent at puberty, when secondary sex characteristics develop
- Involves failure of the testicles to mature and degenerative testicular changes that eventually result in irreversible infertility

PATHOPHYSIOLOGY

- The extra chromosome responsible for Klinefelter syndrome probably results from either meiotic nondisjunction during parental gametogenesis or mitotic nondisjunction in the zygote.
- The incidence of meiotic nondisjunction increases with maternal age.

CAUSES

- A 47,XXY complement, instead of the normal 46,XY complement, created by an extra X chromosome
- In the rare mosaic form: some cells containing extra X chromosomes and others containing the normal XY complement

INCIDENCE

- In the United States, about 1 in 500 to 1,000 males is born with an extra X chromosome.
- Over 3,000 affected males are born annually.

COMPLICATIONS

- Aspermatogenesis and infertility
- Learning disabilities and behavioral problems
- Osteoporosis
- Breast cancer (because of the extra X chromosome)

HISTORY

- Delayed puberty
- Sexual dysfunction (infertility, lack of libido)
- Behavioral problems beginning in adolescence, in some individuals
- Increased incidence of pulmonary disease and varicose veins

PHYSICAL FINDINGS

- Small testicles in adolescence
- Sparse facial and abdominal hair
- Feminine distribution of pubic hair (triangular shape)
- Gynecomastia in fewer than 50% of patients
- Delay of pathologic changes and resulting infertility in the mosaic form
- Abnormal body build (long legs with short, obese trunk)
- Tall stature

LABORATORY

- A karyotype (chromosome analysis) is determined by culturing lymphocytes from the patient's peripheral blood.
- Excretion of follicle-stimulating hormone is increased.
- Plasma testosterone levels are decreased after puberty.

TREATMENT

GENERAL
◆ Psychological counseling

DIET
◆ As tolerated

ACTIVITY
◆ As tolerated

MEDICATIONS
◆ Supplemental testosterone to induce secondary sexual characteristics of puberty for body image problems or emotional maladjustment due to sexual dysfunction

SURGERY
◆ Mastectomy in patients with persistent gynecomastia

NURSING CONSIDERATIONS

NURSING CONSIDERATIONS
◆ Chronic low self-esteem
◆ Delayed growth and development
◆ Disturbed body image
◆ Disturbed personal identity
◆ Ineffective coping
◆ Ineffective sexuality patterns
◆ Risk for disproportionate growth
◆ Sexual dysfunction
◆ Social isolation

EXPECTED OUTCOMES
The patient will:
◆ express positive feelings about self
◆ achieve age-appropriate growth, behaviors, and skills to the fullest extent possible
◆ verbalize feelings about changed body image
◆ express feelings related to personal identity
◆ demonstrate effective coping mechanisms
◆ express feelings about potential or actual changes in sexual activity
◆ express understanding of norms for growth and development
◆ identify measures to maintain sexual function as tolerated
◆ interact with family or friends.

NURSING INTERVENTIONS
◆ Encourage the patient to discuss feelings of confusion and rejection that may arise, and try to reinforce his male identity.
◆ Give prescribed drugs.

MONITORING
◆ Response to treatment

PATIENT TEACHING

GENERAL
Be sure to cover:
◆ the potential benefits and adverse effects of testosterone administration.

DISCHARGE PLANNING
◆ Send the fertile patient with the mosaic form of the syndrome for genetic counseling.

RESOURCES
Organizations
Klinefelter Syndrome Support Group: *www.klinefeltersyndrome.org*
National Institute of Child Health & Human Development: *www.nichd.nih.gov*
National Organization for Rare Disorders: *www.rarediseases.org*

Selected references
Schulman, G.S., et al. "Taurodontism and Learning Disabilities in Patients with Klinefelter Syndrome," *Pediatric Dentistry* 27(5):389-94, September-October 2005.

Swerdlow, A.J., et al. "Cancer Incidence and Mortality in Men with Klinefelter Syndrome: A Cohort Study," *Journal of the National Cancer Institute* 97(16):1204-210, August 2005.

Wattendorf, D.J., and Muenke, M. "Klinefelter Syndrome," *American Family Physician* 72(11):2259-262, December 2005.

Labyrinthitis

- Inflammation of the labyrinth of the inner ear
- Typically produces severe vertigo with head movement and sensorineural hearing loss
- Viral labyrinthitis most prevalent form

PATHOPHYSIOLOGY

- Lesion within vestibular pathways (inner ear to cerebral cortex) results in an imbalance in the vestibular system.

CAUSES

- Cholesteatoma
- Drug toxicity
- Head injury
- Tumor
- Vasculitis
- Viral or bacterial infections

INCIDENCE

- Labyrinthitis affects individuals of all ages beyond infancy.
- It affects men and women equally.

COMPLICATIONS

- Meningitis
- Permanent balance disability
- Permanent hearing loss

HISTORY

- Severe vertigo from any movement of the head
- Nausea and vomiting
- Unilateral or bilateral hearing loss
- Recent upper respiratory tract infection
- Loss of balance and falling in the direction of the affected ear

PHYSICAL FINDINGS

- Spontaneous nystagmus
- Jerking movements of eyes toward the unaffected ear
- Purulent drainage

LABORATORY

- Culture and sensitivity tests show the infecting organism.

IMAGING

- Computed tomography scan results rule out brain lesion.

DIAGNOSTIC PROCEDURES

- Audiometric testing reveals sensorineural hearing loss.
- A flat tympanogram may suggest fluid in the middle ear, a perforated tympanic membrane, or impacted cerumen. Fluctuations on the tympanogram, synchronous with the patient's pulse, suggest a glomangioma in the middle ear.
- Electronystagmography may show decreased velocity from one side that indicates hypofunction or canal paresis. An inability to induce nystagmus with ice water denotes a dead labyrinth.

TREATMENT

GENERAL
◆ Based on relieving symptoms

DIET
◆ Increased oral fluids

ACTIVITY
◆ Bed rest in darkened room with head immobilized between pillows during acute attacks

MEDICATIONS
◆ Meclizine (Antivert) to relieve vertigo
◆ Antiemetics
◆ Antibiotics
◆ I.V. fluids for severe dehydration

SURGERY
◆ Surgical excision of cholesteatoma
◆ Drainage of middle and inner ear infected areas
◆ Labyrinthectomy

Managing labyrinthitis

◆ Tell the patient to avoid sudden position changes.
◆ Help the patient assess how much this disability will affect his daily life.
◆ Work with the patient to identify hazards in the home, such as throw rugs and dark stairways.
◆ Discuss the patient's anxieties and concerns about vertigo attacks and decreased hearing.
◆ Stress the importance of maintaining and resuming normal diversions or social activities when balance disturbance is absent.

NURSING CONSIDERATIONS

NURSING DIAGNOSES
◆ Activity intolerance
◆ Anxiety
◆ Disturbed sensory perception: Auditory
◆ Fear
◆ Risk for deficient fluid volume
◆ Risk for falls
◆ Risk for infection
◆ Risk for injury

EXPECTED OUTCOMES
The patient will:
◆ perform activities of daily living to the fullest extent possible
◆ identify strategies to reduce anxiety
◆ regain hearing or develop other means of communication
◆ express fears and concerns
◆ maintain normal fluid volumes
◆ identify measures to safeguard the home environment to prevent falls
◆ remain free from signs and symptoms of infection
◆ avoid injury.

NURSING INTERVENTIONS
◆ Offer the patient reassurance when appropriate.
◆ Maintain bed rest in a darkened room with the patient's head immobilized during acute attacks.
◆ Give prescribed drugs.
◆ Encourage oral fluid intake.

For patient with hearing loss
◆ Encourage expression of concerns about hearing loss.
◆ Give clear, concise explanations.
◆ Face patient when speaking.
◆ Enunciate words clearly, slowly, and in a normal tone.
◆ Provide a pencil and paper to aid communication.
◆ Alert staff to communication needs.

MONITORING
◆ Response to medication
◆ Vital signs
◆ Signs of dehydration
◆ Intake and output
◆ Auditory acuity
◆ Complications

PATIENT TEACHING

GENERAL
Be sure to cover:
◆ the disorder, diagnosis, and treatment
◆ limitation of activities to avoid danger from vertigo
◆ recovery time (up to 6 weeks)
◆ the need for prompt treatment of upper respiratory tract and systemic infections
◆ the need to control use of salicylates and other potentially toxic substances
◆ completion of the prescribed medication regimen
◆ adverse drug reactions
◆ preoperative and postoperative instructions as indicated
◆ management of labyrinthitis. (See *Managing labyrinthitis.*)

RESOURCES
Organizations
American Academy of Otolaryngology — Head and Neck Surgery: *www.entnet.org*
The Vestibular Disorders Association: *www.vestibular.org*

Selected references
Barreire, S.O. "Spin Cycle: Evaluation and Management of Dizziness and Vertigo," *Advance for Nurse Practitioners* 13(3):22-27, March 2005.
Trinidad, A., et al. "Labyrinthitis Secondary to Experimental Otitis Media," *American Journal of Otolaryngology* 26(4):226-29, July-August 2005.
Westerlaan, H.E., et al. "Labyrinthitis Ossificans Associated with Sensorineural Deafness," *Ear, Nose, & Throat Journal* 84(1):14-15, January 2005.

Lactose intolerance

- Inability to digest and absorb lactose, the main carbohydrate in milk
- Stems from an insufficiency of the enzyme lactase
- May be congenital (rare) or acquired
- Deficiency continues for life

PATHOPHYSIOLOGY
- Lactose intolerance stems from deficient supplies of the enzyme lactase. (See *Understanding lactase insufficiency*.)

CAUSES
- Genetic basis
- Ionizing radiation to the abdomen and abdominal surgery
- Medical conditions that disrupt the intestinal mucosa (secondary)
- Medications that cause GI disturbances

INCIDENCE
- There is a high incidence of lactose intolerance among certain ethnic groups, including Blacks, Asians, Native Americans, Greek Cypriots, and some Ashkenazic Jews.

COMPLICATIONS
- Dehydration

HISTORY
- GI signs and symptoms, such as diarrhea, abdominal cramping, discomfort, distention, flatulence, and borborygmus (intestinal rumbling), following ingestion of milk products
- History of a medical disorder or treatment that disrupts the GI mucosa

PHYSICAL FINDINGS
- Abdominal distention
- Nonverbal signs of patient distress, such as doubling over or holding of the abdomen
- Rectal tissue irritation and excoriation related to diarrhea
- Hyperactive bowel sounds

Understanding lactase insufficiency

Normally, the enzyme lactase hydrolyzes dietary lactose in the jejunum and proximal ileus. The hydrolysis splits lactose into glucose and galactose, which bind to glucose carriers and eventually pass into the portal vein. If lactase levels are insufficient to split the lactose, a chain of effects is triggered.

> Available lactase is insufficient to hydrolyze dietary lactose.

↓

> Unsplit lactose remains as unabsorbed glucose in the small intestine.

↓

> Unabsorbed glucose acts osmotically to draw in and retain intraluminal fluid, leading to diarrhea.

↓

> Intestinal bacteria ferment the lactose, breaking it down into hydrogen, carbon dioxide, water, and organic acids.

↓

> Accumulation of gases causes discomfort, flatulence, and distention.

LABORATORY
- Lactose tolerance test: A blood sample is taken after the patient has fasted overnight. The patient then ingests a specified oral lactose load. Glucose levels are measured from blood samples drawn at specified intervals following lactose ingestion and from the fasting blood sample. A minimal increase (less than 20 mg/dl) in the serum glucose level and GI symptoms (cramping, flatulence, and perhaps, diarrhea) confirm lactase deficiency.
- Breath hydrogen analysis measures excess hydrogen exhalation resulting from bacterial fermentation of lactose in the colon. (Hydrogen from the colon passes to the blood and then to the lungs.) Increased hydrogen content of expired air confirms lactose intolerance.

OTHER
- Lactose challenge test produces diarrhea and bloating within minutes to hours.
- Lactose-free diet test eliminates lactose from the patient's diet for a period of time, such as 5 days. If he becomes asymptomatic, the diagnosis is upheld.
- Small-bowel biopsy (rarely used) determines whether lactose intolerance is primary or secondary. Only the secondary form shows abnormal epithelium.

TREATMENT

DIET
- Lactose-free

MEDICATIONS
- Lactase enzyme products (LactAid, Lactrase)
- Antidiarrheal

NURSING CONSIDERATIONS

NURSING DIAGNOSES
- Acute pain
- Diarrhea
- Imbalanced nutrition: Less than body requirements
- Impaired skin integrity
- Risk for deficient fluid volume

EXPECTED OUTCOMES
The patient will:
- express feelings of increased comfort
- have normal bowel function
- maintain adequate caloric intake
- maintain skin integrity
- have fluid volume within normal parameters.

NURSING INTERVENTIONS
- Give prescribed antidiarrheal agents.
- Give prescribed lactase enzyme products.
- Assess the patient for abdominal discomfort.
- Encourage relaxation and diversion techniques to relieve discomfort.
- Initiate patient care measures to protect the rectal skin and mucous membranes.
- Assess the patient for signs of dehydration.
- Offer emotional support.
- Provide patient privacy.

MONITORING
- Elimination pattern
- Diet
- Skin integrity

PATIENT TEACHING

GENERAL
Be sure to cover:
- lactose intolerance and its associated signs and symptoms, risks, and treatment, especially dietary management
- the need to avoid foods that contain lactose, such as milk (whole, low-fat, skim, evaporated, condensed, buttermilk, cream), ice cream, cheese, sour cream, custards, milk-based puddings, butter, drinks prepared with chocolate or malted milk powder, cream sauces and gravies, cream-based soups, chocolate candy, instant potatoes, baked products made with milk, and frozen or canned fruits and vegetables containing lactose
- the importance of checking product labels carefully for lactose content and avoiding products that list milk solids, milk sugars, whey, or casein
- the need to eliminate all sources of lactose from the patient's diet until he's symptom-free
- how to use lactase enzyme products
- the need to avoid deficiencies of vitamin D and calcium.

RESOURCES
Organizations
American Gastroenterological Association: *www.gastro.org*
National Digestive Diseases Information Clearinghouse: *www.digestive.niddk.nih.gov*

Selected references
Byers, K.G., and Savaiano, D.A. "The Myth of Increased Lactose Intolerance in African-Americans," *Journal of the American College of Nutrition* 24(6 Suppl):569S-73S, December 2005.
He, T., et al. "Colonic Fermentation May Play a Role in Lactose Intolerance in Humans," *Journal of Nutrition* 136(1):58-63, January 2006.
Ojetti, V., et al. "High Prevalence of Celiac Disease in Patients with Lactose Intolerance," *Digestion* 71(2):106-10, March 2005.
Roberson, C.M. "Lactose Intolerance," *The Alabama Nurse* 31(4):23-24, December 2004-February 2005.

Laryngeal cancer

OVERVIEW

- Malignant cells in the tissues of the larynx or voice box
- Squamous cell carcinoma — most common form (95% of cases)
- Adenocarcinoma and sarcoma — rare (5% of cases)
- Intrinsic tumor (located on the true vocal cords; tends not to spread because underlying connective tissues lack lymph nodes) or extrinsic tumor (located on another part of the larynx; tends to spread easily)

PATHOPHYSIOLOGY

- Laryngeal cancer is classified by its location:
- supraglottic (on the false vocal cords)
- glottic (on the true vocal cords)
- subglottic (rare downward extension from the vocal cords).
- Malignant cells that proliferate can cause swallowing and breathing impairment.
- A tumor can decrease mobility of the vocal cords.

CAUSES

- Unknown

RISK FACTORS

- Smoking
- Alcoholism
- Chronic inhalation of noxious fumes
- Familial disposition
- History of gastroesophageal reflux disease

INCIDENCE

- Laryngeal cancer is about nine times more common in men than in women.
- Most patients are between ages 50 and 65.

COMPLICATIONS

- Increased swallowing difficulty and pain
- Metastasis

ASSESSMENT

HISTORY

Stage I
- Complaints of local throat irritation
- 2-week history of hoarseness

Stages II and III
- Hoarseness
- Sore throat
- Voice volume reduced to a whisper

Stage IV
- Pain radiating to ears
- Dysphagia
- Dyspnea

PHYSICAL FINDINGS

Stage I
- None

Stage II
- Possible abnormal movement of vocal cords

Stage III
- Abnormal movement of vocal cords
- Possible lymphadenopathy

Stage IV
- Neck mass or enlarged cervical lymph nodes

DIAGNOSTIC TEST RESULTS

IMAGING

- Xeroradiography, laryngeal tomography, computed tomography, and laryngography confirm the presence of a mass.
- Chest X-ray rules out metastasis.

DIAGNOSTIC PROCEDURES

- Results of the biopsy of multiple specimens obtained during laryngoscopy establish a primary diagnosis, determine the extent of the disease, and identify additional premalignant specimens or second primary tumors.

OTHER

- Biopsy results identify cancer cells.

TREATMENT

GENERAL

- Precancerous lesions — laser surgery
- Early lesions — laser surgery or radiation therapy
- Tumors limited to true vocal cords — radiation
- Subglottic tumors — laryngectomy with or without neck dissection
- Speech preservation
- Speech rehabilitation (when speech preservation is impossible) — esophageal speech, prosthetic devices, or experimental surgical reconstruction of the voice box

DIET

- Based on treatment options
- Enteral feeding possibly required

ACTIVITY

- Frequent rest periods

MEDICATIONS

- Chemotherapeutic agents
- Analgesics

SURGERY

- Cordectomy
- Partial or total laryngectomy
- Supraglottic laryngectomy or total laryngectomy with laryngoplasty

NURSING CONSIDERATIONS

NURSING DIAGNOSES

- Acute pain
- Anxiety
- Disturbed body image
- Energy field disturbance
- Impaired gas exchange
- Impaired skin integrity
- Impaired swallowing
- Impaired verbal communication
- Ineffective airway clearance
- Ineffective breathing pattern
- Ineffective coping
- Ineffective role performance
- Risk for infection

EXPECTED OUTCOMES

The patient will:

- express feelings of increased comfort
- verbalize feelings of decreased anxiety
- express positive feelings about body image
- express an increased sense of well-being
- maintain adequate ventilation
- experience no complications with surgical wounds
- swallow without coughing or choking
- use language or an alternative speech method to effectively communicate needs
- maintain a patent airway
- maintain an effective breathing pattern
- demonstrate positive coping mechanisms
- continue to function in usual roles as much as possible
- not exhibit signs or symptoms of infection.

NURSING INTERVENTIONS

- Provide supportive psychological, preoperative, and postoperative care.
- Encourage verbalization and provide support.

- Assist with establishing a method of communication.
- Prepare the patient for functional losses (inability to smell, blow his nose, whistle, gargle, sip, or suck on a straw).
- Provide frequent mouth care.
- Suction when needed.
- After total laryngectomy, elevate the head of the bed 30 to 45 degrees, and support the back of the neck to prevent tension on sutures and, possibly, wound dehiscence.

MONITORING

(See *Recognizing and managing complications of laryngeal surgery.*)

After partial laryngectomy

- Hydration and nutritional status
- Tracheostomy tube care
- Use of voice

After total laryngectomy

- Laryngectomy tube care
- Vital signs
- Postoperative complications (airway obstruction, hemorrhage, carotid artery rupture, and fistula formation)
- Pain control
- Nasogastric (NG) tube placement and function

GENERAL

Be sure to cover:

- the disorder, diagnosis, and treatment
- appropriate oral hygiene practices (before partial or total laryngectomy)
- postoperative procedures, such as suctioning, NG tube feeding, and laryngectomy tube care
- preparation for any functional losses.

DISCHARGE PLANNING

- Arrange for rehabilitation measures (including laryngeal speech, esophageal speech, an artificial larynx, and various mechanical devices).
- Refer the patient to local resources and support services.

RESOURCES

Organizations

American Cancer Society:
www.cancer.org
International Association of Laryngectomees: *www.larynxlink.com*
National Cancer Institute:
www.cancer.gov

Selected references

Atlas of Pathophysiology, 2nd ed. Philadelphia: Lippincott Williams & Wilkins, 2005.

Blanco, A.I., and Chao, C. "Management of Radiation-induced Head and Neck Injury," *Cancer Treatment and Research* 128:23-41, 2006.

Dias, F.L. "Therapeutic Options in Advanced Laryngeal Cancer: An Overview," *ORL Journal* 67(6):311-18, December 2005.

Garavello, W., et al. "Type of Alcoholic Beverage and the Risk for Laryngeal Cancer," *European Journal of Cancer Prevention* 15(1);69-73, February 2006.

Nishiike, S., et al. "Laryngeal Tuberculosis Following Laryngeal Carcinoma," *Journal of Laryngology and Otology* 120(2):151-53, February 2006.

Recognizing and managing complications of laryngeal surgery

Once the patient returns from surgery, you'll need to monitor his recovery, watching carefully for complications, such as fistula formation, a ruptured carotid artery, and stenosis of the tracheostomy site.

FISTULA FORMATION

Warning signs of fistula formation include redness, swelling, and secretions on the suture line. The fistula may form between the reconstructed hypopharynx and the skin. This eventually heals spontaneously, although the process may take weeks or months.

Feed the patient who has a fistula through a nasogastric tube. Otherwise, food will leak through the fistula and delay healing.

RUPTURED CAROTID ARTERY

Bleeding, a cardinal sign of a ruptured carotid artery, may occur in a patient who received

preoperative radiation therapy or in a patient with a fistula that constantly bathes the carotid artery with oral secretions.

If rupture occurs, apply pressure to the site. Call for help immediately, and take the patient to the operating room for carotid ligation.

TRACHEOSTOMY STENOSIS

Constant shortness of breath alerts you to tracheostomy stenosis, which may occur weeks to months after laryngectomy.

Management includes fitting the patient with successively larger tracheostomy tubes until he can tolerate insertion of a full-sized one.

Laryngitis

- Acute or chronic inflammation of the vocal cords
- Isolated infection or part of a generalized bacterial or viral upper respiratory tract infection
- Viral infection typically mild and of limited duration
- Inflammatory changes caused by repeated attacks (associated with chronic laryngitis)

PATHOPHYSIOLOGY

- Inflammatory response to cell damage caused by viruses results in hyperemia and fluid exudation.
- Irritant receptors are triggered.
- Kinins and other inflammatory mediators may induce spasm of upper airway smooth muscle.

AGE FACTOR Developmental differences in the upper airway structures of young children may result in severe narrowing of the upper airways with inflammation, to the degree that respiratory failure may result from hypoventilation.

CAUSES

- Alcohol abuse
- Aspiration of caustic chemicals
- Chronic laryngitis
- Chronic upper respiratory tract disorders
- Constant exposure to dust or other irritants
- Gastroesophageal reflux
- Infection
- Inhalation of smoke or fumes
- Mouth breathing
- Overuse of the voice
- Reflux esophagitis
- Smoking

INCIDENCE

- Laryngitis is a common disorder.
- It affects all ages.
- It affects men and women equally.

COMPLICATIONS

- Chronic hoarseness
- Permanent laryngeal tissue changes
- Airway obstruction

HISTORY

- Hoarseness ranging from mild to complete loss of voice
- Feeling of throat rawness
- Throat pain
- Dry cough
- Malaise
- Difficulty swallowing

PHYSICAL FINDINGS

- Cough
- Fever
- Regional lymphadenopathy
- Stridor (in children)

LABORATORY

- White blood cell count is elevated in bacterial infections.

DIAGNOSTIC PROCEDURES

- Indirect laryngoscopy reveals red, inflamed, and occasionally, hemorrhagic vocal cord exudate.

TREATMENT

GENERAL
- Based on symptoms
- Elimination of underlying cause
- Resting the voice (primary treatment)
- Humidification
- Avoidance of smoking
- Avoidance of whispering

DIET
- Cold fluids

ACTIVITY
- Rest during febrile period, with head of bed elevated

MEDICATIONS
- Analgesics
- Throat lozenges
- Antibiotics (bacterial infection)
- Systemic corticosteroids

SURGERY
- Tracheotomy in chronic laryngitis

NURSING CONSIDERATIONS

NURSING DIAGNOSES
- Acute pain
- Anxiety
- Fatigue
- Fear
- Impaired verbal communication
- Ineffective airway clearance
- Ineffective breathing pattern
- Risk for aspiration

EXPECTED OUTCOMES
The patient will:
- express feelings of increased comfort
- identify strategies to reduce anxiety
- report feeling well rested
- express fears and concerns
- develop other means of communication
- maintain a patent airway
- exhibit an effective breathing pattern
- show no signs or symptoms of aspiration.

NURSING INTERVENTIONS
- Encourage communication of concerns.
- Keep tracheotomy tray at bedside.
- Encourage modification of predisposing factors.
- Restrict verbal communication.
- Provide alternative communication means.
- Anticipate patient needs.
- Give prescribed drugs.

MONITORING
- Response to treatment
- Respiratory status

⚡ **WARNING** *In severe, acute laryngitis, monitor the patient for signs and symptoms of airway obstruction.*

PATIENT TEACHING

GENERAL
Be sure to cover:
- the disorder, diagnosis, and treatment
- why the patient shouldn't talk
- alternate methods of communication
- the importance of speaking softly rather than whispering
- the need to maintain adequate humidification
- smoking cessation
- medication and potential adverse reactions
- the importance of completing prescribed antibiotic treatment
- avoidance of occupational hazards.

DISCHARGE PLANNING
- Refer the patient to a smoking-cessation program, if indicated.
- Refer the patient to voice retraining, as needed.

RESOURCES
Organizations
Johns Hopkins Center for Laryngeal and Voice Disorders — Laryngitis: *www.hopkinsmedicine.org/voice/disorders.html*
National Institute of Allergy and Infectious Diseases: *www3.niaid.nih.gov*

Selected references
Beaver, M.E., et al. "Acute Ulcerative Laryngitis," *Ear, Nose, & Throat Journal* 84(5):268, May 2005.
Ebell, M.H. "Antibiotics for Acute Laryngitis in Adults," *American Family Physician* 72(1):76-77, July 2005.
Savoy, N.B. "Differentiating Stridor in Children at Triage: It's Not Always Croup," *Journal of Emergency Nursing* 31(5):503-5, October 2005.

Latex allergy LIFE-THREATENING DISORDER

OVERVIEW

- An immunoglobulin (Ig) E-mediated immediate hypersensitivity reaction to products that contain natural latex
- Can range from local dermatitis to life-threatening anaphylactic reaction

PATHOPHYSIOLOGY

- Mast cells release histamine and other secretory products in response to contact with latex-containing products.
- Vascular permeability increases, and vasodilation and bronchoconstriction occur.
- Chemical sensitivity dermatitis is a type IV delayed hypersensitivity reaction to the chemicals used in the processing rather than to the latex itself.
- In a cell-mediated allergic reaction, sensitized T lymphocytes are triggered, stimulating the proliferation of other lymphocytes and mononuclear cells, resulting in tissue inflammation and contact dermatitis.

CAUSES

- Frequent contact with latex-containing products (see *Products that contain latex*)

RISK FACTORS

- Medical and dental professionals
- Workers in latex manufacturing or supply companies
- Patients with spina bifida or other conditions that require multiple surgeries involving latex material
- History of:
- asthma or other allergies, especially to bananas, avocados, tropical fruits, or chestnuts
- multiple intra-abdominal or genitourinary surgeries
- frequent intermittent urinary catheterization

INCIDENCE

- Latex allergy is present in 1% to 5% of the U.S. population.
- It affects 10% to 30% of health care workers.

- It's most prevalent (20% to 68%) in patients with spina bifida and urogenital abnormalities.
- It affects men and women equally.

COMPLICATIONS

- Respiratory obstruction
- Systemic vascular collapse
- Death

ASSESSMENT

HISTORY

- Exposure to latex

PHYSICAL FINDINGS

- Signs of anaphylaxis
- Rash
- Angioedema
- Conjunctivitis
- Wheezing, stridor

DIAGNOSTIC TEST RESULTS

LABORATORY

- Radioallergosorbent test results show specific IgE antibodies to latex (safest for use in patients with a history of type I hypersensitivity).

OTHER

- Diagnosis of latex allergy is based mainly on history and physical assessment.
- Patch test reaction is positive, as indicated by hives with itching or redness.

Products that contain latex

MEDICAL PRODUCTS

- Adhesive bandages
- Airways, Levin tube
- Handheld resuscitation bags
- Blood pressure cuff, tubing, and bladder
- Catheters
- Catheter leg straps
- Dental dams
- Elastic bandages
- Electrode pads
- Fluid-circulating hypothermia blankets
- Hemodialysis equipment
- I.V. catheters
- Latex or rubber gloves
- Medication vials
- Pads for crutches
- Protective sheets
- Reservoir breathing bags
- Rubber airways and endotracheal tubes
- Tape
- Tourniquets

NONMEDICAL PRODUCTS

- Adhesive tape
- Balloons (excluding Mylar)
- Cervical diaphragms
- Condoms
- Disposable diapers
- Elastic stockings
- Glue
- Latex paint
- Nipples and pacifiers
- Rubber bands
- Tires

GENERAL
◆ Prevention of exposure, including use of latex-free products, to decrease possible exacerbation of hypersensitivity
◆ Maintenance of patent airway

MEDICATIONS
Before and after possible exposure to latex:
◆ Corticosteroids
◆ Antihistamines
◆ Histamine-2 receptor blockers

Acute treatment
◆ Epinephrine (1:1,000)
◆ Oxygen therapy
◆ Volume expanders
◆ I.V. vasopressors
◆ Aminophylline and albuterol

NURSING DIAGNOSES
◆ Impaired gas exchange
◆ Impaired skin integrity
◆ Ineffective airway clearance
◆ Ineffective breathing pattern
◆ Latex allergy response
◆ Risk for injury

EXPECTED OUTCOMES
The patient will:
◆ maintain adequate ventilation and oxygenation
◆ maintain skin integrity
◆ maintain a patent airway
◆ maintain effective breathing pattern
◆ exhibit no signs or symptoms of latex allergy response
◆ exhibit no signs of complications.

NURSING INTERVENTIONS
◆ Maintain airway, breathing, and circulation.
◆ Give prescribed drugs.

⚡ **WARNING** *When adding medication to an I.V. bag, inject the drug through the spike port, not the rubber latex port.*

◆ Monitor the patient for sensitivity to tropical nuts or bananas.
◆ Keep the patient's environment latex-free.

MONITORING
◆ Vital signs
◆ Respiratory status

GENERAL
Be sure to cover:
◆ the disorder, diagnosis, and treatment
◆ the potential for life-threatening reaction
◆ the importance of wearing medical identification jewelry that identifies allergy
◆ how to use an epinephrine autoinjector.

RESOURCES
Organizations
American Academy of Allergy Asthma & Immunology: *www.aaaai.org*
American Latex Allergy Association: *www.latexallergyresources.org*
U.S. Department of Labor Occupational Safety & Health Administration: *www.osha-slc.gov*

Selected references
Filon, F.L., and Radman, G. "Latex Allergy: A Follow-up Study of 1,040 Healthcare Workers," *Occupational and Environmental Medicine* 63(2):121-25, February 2006.
Reines, H.D., and Seifert, P.C. "Patient Safety: Latex Allergy," *Surgical Clinics of North America* 85(6):1329-340, December 2005.
Rolland, J.M., et al. "Advances in Development of Hypoallergenic Latex Immunotherapy," *Current Opinion in Allergy and Clinical Immunology* 5(6):544-51, December 2005.

Legg-Calvé-Perthes disease

OVERVIEW

- Ischemic necrosis leading to eventual flattening of the head of the femur due to vascular interruption
- Typically unilateral (bilateral in 20% of patients)
- Usually runs its course in 3 to 4 years
- May lead to premature osteoarthritis later in life from misalignment of the acetabulum and flattening of the femoral head
- Also called *coxa plana*

PATHOPHYSIOLOGY

- The first of four stages, synovitis, is characterized by synovial inflammation and increased joint fluid and typically lasts 1 to 3 weeks.
- In the second (avascular) stage, vascular interruption causes necrosis of the ossification center of the femoral head (usually in several months to 1 year).
- In the third stage, revascularization, a new blood supply causes bone resorption and deposition of immature bone cells. New bone replaces necrotic bone, and the femoral head gradually reforms.
- The final, or residual stage, involves healing and regeneration. Immature bone cells are replaced by normal bone cells, thereby fixing the joint's shape. There may or may not be residual deformity, based on the degree of necrosis that occurs in stage 2.

CAUSES

- Cause of vascular obstructive changes that initiate disease unknown
- Current theories include:
- increased blood viscosity, resulting in stasis and decreased blood flow
- trauma to retinacular vessels
- vascular irregularities (congenital or developmental)
- vascular occlusion secondary to increased intracapsular pressure from acute transient synovitis
- venous obstruction with secondary intraepiphyseal thrombosis.

INCIDENCE

- Legg-Calvé-Perthes disease occurs most frequently in boys ages 4 to 10.
- Higher incidence occurs within families.

COMPLICATIONS

- Permanent disability
- Premature osteoarthritis

ASSESSMENT

HISTORY

- Family history of the disease
- Limp that becomes progressively worse
- Persistent pain in the groin, anterior thigh, or knee that's aggravated by activity and relieved by rest

PHYSICAL FINDINGS

- Muscle atrophy
- Slight shortening of the affected leg
- Restricted hip abduction and internal rotation
- Adductor muscle spasm in the affected hip

DIAGNOSTIC TEST RESULTS

IMAGING

- Hip X-rays taken every 3 to 4 months confirm the diagnosis, with findings that vary according to the stage of the disease.
- Anterior-posterior X-rays and magnetic resonance imaging enhance early diagnosis of necrosis and visualization of articular surface.

OTHER

- Physical examination and clinical history aid in diagnosis.

GENERAL
♦ Protection of the femoral head from further stress and damage by containing it within the acetabulum

DIET
♦ Well-balanced

ACTIVITY
♦ Reduced weight bearing by means of bed rest in bilateral split counterpoised traction; then application of hip abduction splint or cast, or weight bearing while a splint, cast, or brace holds the leg in abduction (braces may remain in place for 6 to 18 months)
♦ Physical therapy with passive and active range-of-motion exercises after cast removal

MEDICATIONS
♦ Analgesics

SURGERY
♦ Osteotomy and subtrochanteric derotation for a young child in the early stages of the disease (requires a postoperative spica cast for about 2 months)

NURSING DIAGNOSES
♦ Acute pain
♦ Anxiety
♦ Deficient diversional activity
♦ Dressing or grooming self-care deficit
♦ Imbalanced nutrition: More than body requirements
♦ Risk for impaired skin integrity

EXPECTED OUTCOMES
The patient will:
♦ express feelings of increased comfort and decreased pain
♦ identify strategies to reduce anxiety
♦ perform meaningful activities in spare time
♦ perform activities of daily living within the confines of the disease
♦ consume a nutritious diet with specified calorie intake
♦ maintain adequate skin integrity.

NURSING INTERVENTIONS
♦ Provide cast care.
♦ Give prescribed analgesics.
♦ Provide emotional support.

MONITORING
♦ Intake and output
♦ Neurovascular status of affected extremity
♦ Skin integrity

GENERAL
Be sure to cover:
♦ the disorder, diagnosis, and treatment
♦ proper cast care and monitoring of skin integrity.

RESOURCES
Organizations
American Academy of Orthopaedic Surgeons: *www.aaos.org*
American Orthopaedic Association: *www.aoassn.org*

Selected references
Dezateux, C., and Roposch, A. "The Puzzles of Perthes' Disease: Definitive Studies of Causal Factors are Needed," *Journal of Bone and Joint Surgery (British volume)* 87(11):1463-464, November 2005.

Grzegorzewski, A., et al. "Leg Length Discrepancy in Legg-Calvé-Perthes Disease," *Journal of Pediatric Orthopedics* 25(2):206-209, March-April 2005.

Rab, G.T. "Theoretical Study of Subluxation in Early Legg-Calvé-Perthes Disease," *Journal of Pediatric Orthopedics* 25(6):728-33, November-December 2005.

Legionnaires' disease

- An acute bronchopneumonia produced by a gram-negative bacteria
- Illness ranging from mild (with or without pneumonitis) to serious multilobed pneumonia, with mortality as high as 15%
- Epidemic outbreaks (usually in late summer and early fall) or outbreaks confined to a few cases

PATHOPHYSIOLOGY

- The *Legionella* organisms enter the lungs after aspiration or inhalation.
- Although alveolar macrophages phagocytize *Legionella*, the organisms aren't killed and proliferate intracellularly.
- The cells rupture, releasing *Legionella*, and the cycle starts again.
- Lesions develop a nodular appearance, and alveoli become filled with fibrin, neutrophils, and alveolar macrophages.

CAUSES

- *Legionella pneumophila*, an aerobic, gram-negative bacillus that's most likely transmitted by air
- Water distribution systems (such as whirlpool spas and decorative fountains) and air-conditioning vents, which are reservoirs for the organism

INCIDENCE

- Legionnaires' disease is most likely to affect men more than women.
- Others at increased risk include:
- elderly patients
- immunocompromised patients
- patients with chronic underlying disease such as diabetes
- alcoholics
- cigarette smokers.

COMPLICATIONS

- Hypoxia and acute respiratory failure
- Hypotension
- Delirium
- Seizures
- Heart failure
- Arrhythmias
- Renal failure
- Shock

HISTORY

- Presence at a suspected source of infection
- Prodromal symptoms, including anorexia, malaise, myalgia, and headache

PHYSICAL FINDINGS

- Rapidly rising fever with chills
- Grayish or rust-colored, nonpurulent, occasionally blood-streaked sputum
- Chest pain
- Tachypnea
- Bradycardia (in about 50% of patients)
- Neurologic signs (altered level of consciousness [LOC])
- Dullness over areas of secretions and consolidation or pleural effusions
- Fine crackles that develop into coarse crackles as the disease progresses

LABORATORY

- Gram staining reveals numerous neutrophils but no organism.
- Definitive method of diagnosis involves isolation of the organisms from respiratory secretions or bronchial washings or through thoracentesis.
- Definitive tests include direct immunofluorescence of *L. pneumophila* and indirect fluorescent serum antibody testing.
- Complete blood count results show leukocytosis and an increased erythrocyte sedimentation rate.
- Partial pressure of arterial oxygen is decreased, and partial pressure of arterial carbon dioxide is initially decreased.
- Blood tests reveal hyponatremia (serum sodium level less than 131 mg/L).

IMAGING

- Chest X-ray typically shows patchy, localized infiltration, which progresses to multilobed consolidation (usually involving the lower lobes) and pleural effusion.
- In fulminant disease, chest X-ray reveals opacification of the entire lung.

TREATMENT

GENERAL
- Fluid replacement
- Oxygen administration
- Mechanical ventilation as needed

MEDICATIONS
- Antibiotics
- Antipyretics
- Pressor drugs

NURSING CONSIDERATIONS

NURSING DIAGNOSES
- Acute pain
- Deficient fluid volume
- Hyperthermia
- Impaired gas exchange
- Ineffective airway clearance
- Ineffective breathing pattern
- Ineffective tissue perfusion: Cardiopulmonary

EXPECTED OUTCOMES
The patient will:
- report decreased or absence of pain
- regain and maintain normal fluid and electrolyte balance
- remain afebrile
- express feelings of increased comfort in maintaining gas exchange
- cough effectively
- expectorate sputum effectively
- maintain cardiopulmonary tissue perfusion and cellular oxygenation.

NURSING INTERVENTIONS
- Give tepid sponge baths or use hypothermia blankets to lower fever.
- Provide frequent mouth care. If necessary, apply soothing cream to irritated nostrils.
- Replace fluids and electrolytes as needed.
- Institute seizure precautions.
- Give prescribed drugs.

MONITORING
- Vital signs
- Respiratory status and arterial blood gases
- LOC

PATIENT TEACHING

GENERAL
Be sure to cover:
- the disorder, diagnosis, and treatment
- prevention of infection
- the importance of disinfection of water supply
- purpose of postural drainage and how to perform coughing and deep-breathing exercises
- proper hand washing and disposal of soiled tissues to prevent disease transmission.

DISCHARGE PLANNING
- Refer the patient to a pulmonologist, if necessary.

RESOURCES

Organizations
Centers for Disease Control and Prevention: *www.cdc.gov*
Harvard University Consumer Health Information: *www.intelihealth.com*
National Health Information Center: *www.health.gov/nhic*
National Institute of Allergy and Infectious Diseases: *www3.niaid.nih.gov*
National Library of Medicine: *www.nlm.nih.gov*

Selected references
Kasper, D.L., et al., eds. *Harrison's Principles of Internal Medicine*, 16th ed. New York: McGraw-Hill Book Co., 2005.
Makin, T. "Legionella Bacteria and Water Systems in Health Care Premises," *Nursing Times* 101(39):48-49, September-October 2005.
Murray, S. "Legionella Infection," *Canadian Medical Association Journal* 173(11):1322, November 2005.
Todd, B. "Legionella Pneumonia: Many Cases of Legionnaire Disease Go Unreported or Unrecognized," *AJN* 105(11);35-36, 38, November 2005.

Leprosy

- A chronic, systemic infection characterized by progressive cutaneous lesions
- Three distinct forms:
- Lepromatous leprosy: The most serious form, causes damage to the upper respiratory tract, eyes, testes, nerves, and skin
- Tuberculoid leprosy: Affects peripheral nerves and, occasionally, the surrounding skin, especially on the face, arms, legs, and buttocks
- Borderline (dimorphous) leprosy: Characteristics of both lepromatous and tuberculoid leprosy, with skin lesions appearing diffuse and poorly defined
- Incubation time frequently 3 to 5 years but has been reported 6 months to several decades
- Good prognosis with timely and correct treatment
- Also called *Hansen's disease*

PATHOPHYSIOLOGY

- *Mycobacterium leprae*, an acid-fast bacillus, attacks cutaneous tissue and peripheral nerves, especially the ulnar, radial, posteropopliteal, anterotibial, and facial nerves.
- The central nervous system appears highly resistant.

CAUSES

- Airborne respiratory droplets that contain *M. leprae*
- Inoculation through skin breaks (from a contaminated hypodermic or tattoo needle, for instance)
- Transmitted by humans most commonly, though a few cases transmitted by animals (armadillos and primates)

RISK FACTORS

- Close contact with individuals who have the disease
- Travel into countries where the disease is endemic

INCIDENCE

- Highest susceptibility to the disease is during childhood; susceptibility seems to decrease with age (although leprosy is rarely seen in children younger than age 3).
- In the United States, 90% of patients with leprosy are immigrants from leprosy-endemic regions (Mexico, India, and Southeast Asia).

COMPLICATIONS

- Erythema nodosum leprosum: seen in lepromatous leprosy, may produce fever, malaise, lymphadenopathy, and painful, red skin nodules, usually but not always during antimicrobial treatment
- Lucio's phenomenon: generalized reddened lesions with necrotic centers, which may extend into muscle and fascia; seen in patients in Mexico and other Central American countries
- Amyloidosis, deformity contractures, ocular disorders that can result in blindness, secondary bacterial infection of skin ulcers, and rarely, hepatitis and exfoliative dermatitis

HISTORY

- Anesthesia, anhidrosis, and dryness when the bacilli damage the skin's fine nerves
- Motor nerve damage, weakness, and pain followed by peripheral anesthesia, muscle paralysis, or atrophy, if a large nerve trunk is attacked
- Treatment for clawhand, footdrop, or visual disturbances, such as photophobia and blindness, in the later stages of the disease

PHYSICAL FINDINGS

- Hepatosplenomegaly revealed upon palpation in a patient with lepromatous leprosy; lesions all superficial and easily palpable

In lepromatous leprosy

- Early multiple lesions appearing symmetrical and erythematous
- Lesions possibly erupting as macules or papules with smooth surfaces
- Later enlarging and forming plaques or nodules, called lepromas, appearing on the earlobes, nose, eyebrows, and forehead, giving the patient a characteristic leonine appearance
- *M. leprae* possibly infiltrating the entire skin surface in advanced stages
- Loss of eyebrows and eyelashes
- Loss of sebaceous and sweat gland function
- Conjunctival and scleral nodules
- Epistaxis, ulcerated uvula and tonsils, septal perforation, and nasal collapse
- Orchitis and resultant testicular atrophy
- Scars and contractures

In tuberculoid leprosy affecting the skin

- Large, raised, erythematous plaques or macules with clearly defined borders
- Progressing lesions that become rough, hairless, and hypopigmented
- Numbness in the resultant scars

In borderline leprosy

- Numerous skin lesions that are smaller and less sharply defined than those of tuberculoid leprosy
- Possible patient reports of feeling in the lesions

LABORATORY

- Identification of acid-fast bacilli in skin and nasal mucosal scrapings confirms diagnosis.
- Evaluation of skin biopsy specimen and scrapings determines the percentage of fully intact cells (morphologic index) and measures the amount of bacteria present (bacterial index).

DIAGNOSTIC PROCEDURES

- Skin biopsy results show the typical histologic pattern of nerve changes.

TREATMENT

GENERAL
- Rigid-soled footwear or walking plaster casts to prevent plantar ulcers
- Ophthalmologic examinations

ACTIVITY
- Physical therapy to prevent contractures of the hand

MEDICATIONS
- Antimicrobial with a sulfone, primarily oral dapsone
- Rifampin (Rifadin)
- Clofazimine
- Multidrug regimens (combined dapsone, rifampin, and clofazimine therapies)

SURGERY
- Reconstructive surgery
- Nerve and tendon transplants
- Plastic surgery for facial deformities

NURSING CONSIDERATIONS

NURSING DIAGNOSES
- Acute pain
- Disturbed body image
- Impaired physical mobility
- Impaired skin integrity
- Risk for infection
- Risk for injury
- Social isolation

EXPECTED OUTCOMES
The patient will:
- state relief from pain
- communicate his feelings about his changed body image
- maintain full range of motion in his joints
- exhibit improved or healed lesions or wounds
- experience no further signs or symptoms of infection
- remain free from complications
- interact with family or friends.

NURSING INTERVENTIONS
- Provide supportive patient care, taking steps to control acute infection, prevent complications, speed recovery and rehabilitation, and provide emotional encouragement.
- Give antipyretics, analgesics, and sedatives as needed. Watch for and report erythema nodosum leprosum, Lucio's phenomenon, and other complications.
- Take precautions against the possible spread of infection, even though leprosy isn't highly contagious.
  - Instruct patients to cover coughs or sneezes with a paper tissue and to dispose of used tissues properly.
  - Use infection precautions when handling clothing or articles that touch open skin lesions.
  - The patient is no longer infectious soon after beginning multidrug antibiotic therapy.
- Plan care to promote adequate rest and optimal nutrition.
- Give the patient and his family opportunities to express their feelings.
- Initiate or participate in consultations with other health team members, especially for the patient with deformities. An interdisciplinary rehabilitation program, including physiotherapy and plastic surgery, may be necessary.
- Inspect the patient's skin and report observed changes. Assist with general hygiene and comfort measures, and provide a skin care program.

MONITORING
- The patient's response to medications
- Signs and symptoms of possible complications
- Skin integrity

PATIENT TEACHING

GENERAL
Be sure to cover:
- the disorder, diagnosis, and treatment
- the need to avoid injuring an anesthetized leg by putting too much weight on it
- the need to carefully test bath water to avoid scalding
- suggestions to wear sturdy footwear and to soak feet in warm water after any kind of exercise, even a short walk, to prevent ulcerations
- the need to rub the feet with petrolatum, oil, or lanolin
- the need to use a tear substitute two times per day and to protect the eyes, especially if experiencing decreased corneal sensation and lacrimation
- avoiding rubbing the eyes and wearing sunglasses (to help prevent the corneal irritation and ulceration that lead to blindness)
- the need to take antimicrobial medications exactly as prescribed for the entire length of time prescribed — in some cases, for life.

DISCHARGE PLANNING
- Refer the patient to a regional treatment center, such as the National Hansen's Disease Programs in Baton Rouge, Louisiana, if appropriate.

RESOURCES
Organizations
American Leprosy Missions: *www.leprosy.org*
Centers for Disease Control and Prevention: *www.cdc.gov*
World Health Organization: *www.who.int/en*

Selected references
Araoz, R., et al. "Antigen Discovery: A Postgenomic Approach to Leprosy Diagnosis," *Infection and Immunity* 74(1):175-82, January 2006.
Ellertsen, L.K., et al. "Allergic Sensitisation in Tuberculosis and Leprosy Patients," *International Archives of Allergy and Immunology* 138(3):217-24, November 2005.
Gupta, R., et al. "Genital Involvement and Type I Reaction in Childhood Leprosy," *Leprosy Review* 76(3)253-57, September 2005.

Leukemia, acute
LIFE-THREATENING DISORDER

OVERVIEW

- Malignant proliferation of white blood cell (WBC) precursors, or blasts, in bone marrow or lymph tissue; blasts accumulate in peripheral blood, bone marrow, and body tissues
- Most common form of cancer among children
- Common forms:
- Acute lymphoblastic (lymphocytic) leukemia (ALL) — characterized by abnormal growth of lymphocyte precursors (lymphoblasts)
- Acute myeloblastic (myelogenous) leukemia (AML) — causes rapid accumulation of myeloid precursors (myeloblasts)
- Acute monoblastic (monocytic) leukemia, or Schilling's type — results in a marked increase in monocyte precursors (monoblasts)
- ALL: Treatment induces remissions in 90% of children (average survival: 5 years) and in 65% of adults (average survival: 1 to 2 years); children ages 2 to 8 have the best survival rate (about 50%) with intensive therapy
- AML: Average survival is only 1 year after diagnosis, even with aggressive treatment (remissions lasting 2 to 10 months in 50% of children; adult survival only about 1 year after diagnosis, even with treatment)
- Invariably fatal without treatment

PATHOPHYSIOLOGY

- Immature, nonfunctioning WBCs appear to accumulate first in the tissue where they originate (lymphocytes in lymphatic tissue and granulocytes in bone marrow).
- The immature, nonfunctioning WBCs spill into the bloodstream and overwhelm red blood cells (RBCs) and platelets; from there, they infiltrate other tissues.

CAUSES

- Unknown

RISK FACTORS

- Radiation (especially prolonged exposure)

- Certain chemicals and drugs
- Viruses
- Genetic abnormalities
- Chronic exposure to benzene

In children

- Down syndrome
- Ataxia
- Telangiectasia
- Congenital disorders, such as albinism and congenital immunodeficiency syndrome

INCIDENCE

- Acute leukemia is more common in men and boys than in women and girls.
- It's more common in whites (especially of Jewish ancestry).
- It's more common in children between ages 2 and 5 (80% of leukemias in this age group are ALL) and in those who live in urban and industrialized areas.

COMPLICATIONS

- Infection
- Organ malfunction through encroachment or hemorrhage

ASSESSMENT

HISTORY

- Sudden onset of high fever
- Abnormal bleeding
- Fatigue and night sweats
- Weakness, lassitude, recurrent infections, and chills
- Abdominal or bone pain in patients with ALL, AML, or acute monoblastic leukemia

PHYSICAL FINDINGS

- Tachycardia, palpitations, and a systolic ejection murmur
- Decreased ventilation
- Pallor
- Lymph node enlargement
- Liver or spleen enlargement

DIAGNOSTIC TEST RESULTS

LABORATORY

- Blood counts show thrombocytopenia and neutropenia, and a WBC differential shows the cell type.

IMAGING

- Computed tomography scan shows the affected organs, and cerebrospinal fluid analysis shows abnormal WBC invasion of the central nervous system.

DIAGNOSTIC PROCEDURES

- Bone marrow aspiration results showing a proliferation of immature WBCs confirm acute leukemia. If the aspirate is dry or free from leukemic cells, but the patient has other typical signs of leukemia, biopsy of the bone marrow, usually of the posterior superior iliac spine, must be performed.
- Lumbar puncture is used to detect meningeal involvement.

TREATMENT

GENERAL

- Transfusions of platelets to prevent bleeding
- Transfusions of RBCs to prevent anemia
- Bone marrow transplantation in some patients
- Radiation treatment in the case of brain or testicular infiltration
- Chemotherapy and radiation treatment, depending on diagnosis

DIET

- Well-balanced

ACTIVITY

- Frequent rest periods

MEDICATIONS
For meningeal infiltration

- Intrathecal instillation of methotrexate or cytarabine with cranial irradiation

For ALL

- Vincristine, prednisone, high-dose cytarabine, and daunorubicin
- Intrathecal methotrexate or cytarabine, because ALL carries a 40% risk of meningeal infiltration

For AML

- Combination of I.V. daunorubicin and cytarabine (If these fail to induce remission, treatment involves some or all of the following drugs: a combination of cyclophosphamide, vincristine, prednisone, or methotrexate; high-dose cytarabine alone or with other drugs; amsacrine; etoposide; and 5-azacytidine and mitoxantrone.)

For acute monoblastic leukemia

- Cytarabine and thioguanine with daunorubicin or doxorubicin
- Anti-infective agents, such as antibiotics, antifungals, and antiviral drugs, and granulocyte colony-stimulating factor injections

NURSING CONSIDERATIONS

NURSING DIAGNOSES

- Acute pain
- Anticipatory grieving
- Anxiety
- Fatigue
- Fear
- Imbalanced nutrition: Less than body requirements
- Impaired oral mucous membrane
- Impaired tissue integrity
- Ineffective coping
- Ineffective protection
- Risk for imbalanced body temperature
- Risk for infection
- Risk for injury

EXPECTED OUTCOMES

The patient (or family) will:

- express feelings of increased comfort and reduced pain
- express feelings about potential loss
- verbalize feelings of reduced anxiety
- express feelings of increased energy
- express fears regarding the patient's diagnosis and condition

- maintain weight within an acceptable range
- exhibit intact mucous membranes
- exhibit improved or healed lesions or wounds
- demonstrate positive coping behaviors
- demonstrate use of protective measures, including conserving energy, maintaining a balanced diet, and getting adequate rest
- maintain a normal body temperature
- experience no chills, fever, or other signs and symptoms of illness
- remain free from injury and complications.

NURSING INTERVENTIONS

- Encourage verbalization and provide comfort.
- Provide adequate hydration.
- After bone marrow transplantation, keep the patient in a sterile room, administer antibiotics, and transfuse packed RBCs as necessary.
- Give prescribed drugs.
- Control mouth ulceration by checking often for obvious ulcers and gum swelling and by providing frequent mouth care and saline rinses.

MONITORING

- Complications from treatment
- Hydration and nutritional status
- Urine pH (should be above 7.5)
- Vital signs
- Signs and symptoms of bleeding

PATIENT TEACHING

GENERAL

Be sure to cover:

- the disorder, diagnosis, and treatment
- medication, including administration, dosage, and possible adverse effects
- the need to use a soft toothbrush and to avoid hot, spicy foods and commercial mouthwashes
- signs and symptoms of infection
- signs and symptoms of abnormal bleeding
- the importance of planned rest periods during the day.

DISCHARGE PLANNING

- Refer the patient to available resources and support services.

RESOURCES
Organizations

American Cancer Society:
www.cancer.org
Guide to Internet Resources for Cancer:
www.cancerindex.org
The Leukemia and Lymphoma Society:
www.leukemia.org
National Cancer Institute:
www.cancer.gov

Selected references

Atlas of Pathophysiology, 2nd ed. Philadelphia: Lippincott Williams & Wilkins, 2005.

Dick, J.E. and Lapidot, T. "Biology of Normal and Acute Myeloid Leukemia Stem Cells," *International Journal of Hematology* 82(5):389-96, December 2005.

Mohren, M., et al. "Increased Risk for Thromboembolism in Patients with Acute Leukaemia," *British Journal of Cancer* 94(2):200-202, January 2006.

Leukemia, chronic granulocytic

- Type of leukemia characterized by abnormal overgrowth of granulocytic precursors (myeloblasts, promyelocytes, metamyelocytes, and myelocytes) in bone marrow, peripheral blood, and body tissues
- Always fatal (average survival is 3 to 4 years after onset of chronic phase and 3 to 6 months after onset of acute phase)
- Clinical course proceeds in two distinct phases:
- Insidious chronic phase (characterized by anemia and bleeding abnormalities)
- Acute phase (blast crisis, or myeloblasts, the most primitive granulocytic precursors, proliferate rapidly)
- May involve development of either lymphoblastic or myeloblastic disease during acute phase (rapid advancement after acute phase, despite vigorous treatment)
- Also called *chronic myelogenous (or myelocytic) leukemia (CML)*

PATHOPHYSIOLOGY
- CML is a myeloproliferative disorder originating in a progenitor stem cell.
- Malignant transformation is identified in erythroid, megakaryocytic, and macrophage cell lines.
- Malignant transformation arises from pluripotential or lymphoid stem cells.

CAUSES
- Exact cause unknown

RISK FACTORS
- Presence of the Philadelphia chromosome (found in almost 90% of patients)
- Myeloproliferative diseases

INCIDENCE
- CML is most common in young and middle-age adults.
- It's slightly more common in men than in women, and it's rare in children.

- In the United States, there are 3,000 to 4,000 cases annually (accounting for about 20% of all leukemias).

COMPLICATIONS
- Infection
- Hemorrhage
- Pain

ASSESSMENT

HISTORY
- Renal calculi or gouty arthritis
- Fatigue, weakness, dyspnea, decreased exercise tolerance, and headache
- Recent weight loss and anorexia

PHYSICAL FINDINGS
- Evidence of bleeding and clotting disorders
- Low-grade fever and tachycardia
- Pallor
- Difficulty breathing
- Retinal hemorrhage
- Hepatosplenomegaly with abdominal discomfort and pain
- Sternal and rib tenderness

DIAGNOSTIC TEST RESULTS

LABORATORY
- Chromosomal studies of peripheral blood or bone marrow show the Philadelphia chromosome.
- Low serum leukocyte alkaline phosphatase levels confirm CML.
- Complete blood count (CBC) shows white blood cell (WBC) abnormalities, including:
- Leukocytosis (WBC count greater than 50,000/µl, rising as high as 250,000/µl)
- Leukopenia (WBC count less than 5,000/µl) occasionally
- Neutropenia (neutrophil count less than 1,500/µl) despite high WBC count
- Bone marrow aspiration results show increased circulating myeloblasts.
- Blood tests show decreased hemoglobin levels (less than 10 g/dl) and low hematocrit (less than 30%).

- CBC shows thrombocytosis (greater than 1 million thrombocytes/µl).
- Serum uric acid level may exceed 8 mg/dl.

IMAGING
- Computed tomography scan may show the affected organs.

DIAGNOSTIC PROCEDURES
- Results of bone marrow aspirate or biopsy (performed only if the aspirate is dry) may show hypercellular marrow, with characteristic infiltration shown by a significantly increased number of myeloid elements; in the acute phase, myeloblasts predominate.

TREATMENT

GENERAL
- Bone marrow transplantation (more than 60% of patients who receive transplant during chronic phase achieve remission)
- Local splenic irradiation
- Leukapheresis (selective leukocyte removal) to reduce WBC count

DIET
- Well-balanced

ACTIVITY
- Frequent rest periods

MEDICATIONS
- Busulfan (Busulfex) and hydroxyurea (Droxia)
- Aspirin
- Allopurinol
- Antibiotic treatment

SURGERY
- Splenectomy

NURSING DIAGNOSES

- Acute pain
- Anticipatory grieving
- Anxiety
- Constipation
- Fatigue
- Fear
- Imbalanced nutrition: Less than body requirements
- Impaired oral mucous membrane
- Impaired tissue integrity
- Ineffective coping
- Ineffective protection
- Risk for imbalanced body temperature
- Risk for infection
- Risk for injury

EXPECTED OUTCOMES

The patient (or family) will:
- express feelings of increased comfort and reduced pain
- express feelings about potential loss
- verbalize feelings of reduced anxiety
- regain normal bowel elimination pattern
- express feelings of increased energy
- express fears about the patient's diagnosis and condition
- maintain weight within an acceptable range
- exhibit intact mucous membranes
- exhibit improved or healed lesions or wounds
- demonstrate positive coping behaviors
- demonstrate use of protective measures, including conserving energy, maintaining a balanced diet, and getting adequate rest
- maintain a normal body temperature
- experience no chills, fever, or other signs and symptoms of illness
- remain free from injury and complications.

NURSING INTERVENTIONS

- Plan care to minimize fatigue.
- Regularly check skin and mucous membranes for pallor, petechiae, and bruising.
- Encourage deep-breathing and coughing exercises.
- Encourage verbalization and provide comfort.
- Give prescribed drugs.
- After bone marrow transplantation, keep the patient in a sterile room and give prescribed antibiotics and packed red blood cells.

MONITORING

- Adverse effects of treatment
- Signs and symptoms of bleeding
- Signs and symptoms of infection
- Complete blood count
- Vital signs
- Hydration and nutritional status

GENERAL

Be sure to cover:
- the disorder, diagnosis, and treatment
- how to minimize bleeding and infection risks (such as by using a soft-bristled toothbrush, an electric razor, and other safety devices)
- the need for a high-calorie, high-protein diet
- reinforcement of the practitioner's explanation of bone marrow transplantation, possible outcome, and potential adverse effects, if appropriate
- medication, including administration, dosage, and possible adverse effects
- signs and symptoms of infection and thrombocytopenia.

DISCHARGE PLANNING

- Refer the patient to available resources and support services.

RESOURCES

Organizations

American Cancer Society: *www.cancer.org*
Guide to Internet Resources for Cancer: *www.cancerindex.org*
The Leukemia and Lymphoma Society: *www.leukemia.org*
National Cancer Institute: *www.cancer.gov*

Selected references

Atlas of Pathophysiology, 2nd ed. Philadelphia: Lippincott Williams & Wilkins, 2005.

D'Antonio, J. "Chronic Myelogenous Leukemia," *Clinical Journal of Oncology Nursing* 9(5):535-38, October 2005.

Goldman, J. "Is Imatinib a Cost-Effective Treatment for Newly Diagnosed Chronic Myeloid Leukemia Patients?" *Nature Clinical Practice Oncology* 2(3):126-27, March 2005.

Morris, E.L., and Dutcher, J.P. "Blastic Phase of Chronic Myelogenous Leukemia," *Clinical Advances in Hematology and Oncology* 3(7):547-52, July 2005.

Leukemia, chronic lymphocytic

OVERVIEW

- The most benign and slowly progressive form of leukemia
- Poor prognosis if anemia, thrombocytopenia, neutropenia, bulky lymphadenopathy, and severe lymphocytosis develop

PATHOPHYSIOLOGY

- Chronic lymphocytic leukemia is a generalized, progressive disease marked by an uncontrollable spread of abnormal, small lymphocytes in lymphoid tissue, blood, and bone marrow.
- Once these cells infiltrate bone marrow, lymphoid tissue, and organ systems, clinical signs begin to appear.
- Gross bone marrow replacement by abnormal lymphocytes is the most common cause of death, usually within 5 years of diagnosis.

CAUSES

- Exact cause unknown

RISK FACTORS

- Hereditary factors
- Undefined chromosomal abnormalities
- Certain immunologic defects, such as acquired agammaglobulinemia or ataxia telangiectasia

INCIDENCE

- Chronic lymphocytic leukemia is most common in elderly people; nearly all afflicted are men older than age 50.
- It accounts for almost one-third of new leukemia cases annually.
- Higher incidence is recorded within families.

COMPLICATIONS

- Infection
- Anemia, progressive splenomegaly, leukemic cell replacement of the bone marrow, and profound hypogammaglobulinemia, usually terminating with fatal septicemia, in end-stage disease

ASSESSMENT

HISTORY

- Fatigue, malaise, fever, weight loss, and frequent infections
- Weakness, palpitations

PHYSICAL FINDINGS

- Macular or nodular eruptions and evidence of skin infiltration
- Enlarged lymph nodes, liver, and spleen
- Bone tenderness and edema from lymph node obstruction
- Pallor, dyspnea, tachycardia, bleeding, and infection from bone marrow involvement
- Signs of opportunistic fungal, viral, or bacterial infections

DIAGNOSTIC TEST RESULTS

LABORATORY

- Miscellaneous blood tests reveal the disease. (Typically, chronic lymphocytic leukemia is an incidental finding during a routine complete blood count that reveals numerous abnormal lymphocytes.)
- In the early stages, the white blood cell (WBC) count is mildly but persistently elevated; granulocytopenia is the rule, although the WBC count climbs as the disease progresses.
- Hemoglobin level is less than 11g/dl.
- WBC differential shows neutropenia (less than 1,500/µl) and lymphocytosis (greater than 10,000/µl).
- Platelet count shows thrombocytopenia (less than 150,000/µl).
- Serum protein electrophoresis shows hypogammaglobulinemia.

IMAGING

- Computed tomography scan shows affected organs.

DIAGNOSTIC PROCEDURES

- Results of bone marrow aspiration and biopsy show lymphocytic invasion.

TREATMENT

GENERAL

- Radiation therapy to relieve symptoms (generally for patient with enlarged lymph nodes, painful bony lesions, or massive splenomegaly)

DIET

- High-calorie, high-protein
- Avoidance of hot and spicy foods for patient with impaired oral membranes

ACTIVITY

- Frequent rest periods

MEDICATIONS

- Systemic chemotherapy

NURSING DIAGNOSES

- Acute pain
- Anticipatory grieving
- Anxiety
- Fatigue
- Fear
- Imbalanced nutrition: Less than body requirements
- Impaired oral mucous membrane
- Impaired tissue integrity
- Ineffective coping
- Ineffective protection
- Risk for infection
- Risk for injury

EXPECTED OUTCOMES

The patient (or family) will:
- express feelings of increased comfort and reduced pain
- express feelings about potential loss
- verbalize feelings of reduced anxiety
- express feelings of increased energy
- express fears regarding the patient's diagnosis and condition
- maintain weight within an acceptable range
- exhibit intact mucous membranes
- exhibit improved or healed lesions or wounds
- demonstrate positive coping behaviors
- demonstrate use of protective measures, including conserving energy, maintaining a balanced diet, and getting adequate rest
- experience no chills, fever, or other signs and symptoms of illness
- remain free from injury and complications.

NURSING INTERVENTIONS

- Help establish an appropriate rehabilitation program during remission.
- Place in reverse isolation, if necessary.
- Give prescribed drugs.
- Encourage verbalization and provide support.
- Administer blood component therapy as necessary.

MONITORING

- Signs and symptoms of bleeding and thrombocytopenia
- Adverse effects of treatment
- Induration, swelling, erythema, skin discoloration, and drainage in rectal area
- Pain control
- Vital signs

GENERAL

Be sure to cover:
- the disorder, diagnosis, and treatment
- the use of a soft toothbrush and avoidance of commercial mouthwashes to prevent irritating the mouth ulcers that result from chemotherapy
- medication, including administration, dosage, and possible adverse effects
- signs and symptoms of infection, bleeding, and recurrence
- the need to stay away from anyone with an infection
- the importance of follow-up care
- signs and symptoms of recurrence.

DISCHARGE PLANNING

- Refer the patient to available resources and support services.

RESOURCES

Organizations

American Cancer Society:
www.cancer.org
Guide to Internet Resources for Cancer:
www.cancerindex.org
The Leukemia and Lymphoma Society:
www.leukemia.org
National Cancer Institute:
www.cancer.gov

Selected references

Abbott, B.L. "Chronic Lymphocytic Leukemia: Recent Advances in Diagnosis and Treatment," *Oncologist* 11(1):21-30, January 2006.
Atlas of Pathophysiology, 2nd ed. Philadelphia: Lippincott Williams & Wilkins, 2005.
Hamblin, T.J. "Autoimmune Complications of Chronic Lymphocytic Leukemia," *Seminars in Oncology* 33(2):230-39, April 2006.

Listeriosis

OVERVIEW

- An infection caused by the weakly hemolytic, gram-positive bacillus *Listeria monocytogenes* (a nonspore-producing, motile organism with aerobic and anaerobic characteristics)
- Occurs most commonly in fetuses, in neonates (during the first 3 weeks of life), and in older or immunosuppressed adults; infected fetus usually stillborn or born prematurely, almost always with lethal listeriosis
- Produces milder illness in pregnant women and varying degrees of illness in older and immunosuppressed patients; prognosis depends on the severity of underlying illness

PATHOPHYSIOLOGY

- *L. monocytogenes* grows best at neutral to slightly alkaline pH.
- Transmission occurs:
- – in utero (through the placenta) or during passage through an infected birth canal
- – by inhalation of contaminated dust
- – by drinking of contaminated, unpasteurized milk
- – by contact with infected animals, contaminated sewage or mud, or soil contaminated with feces organism. (See *Avoiding listeriosis.*)

CAUSES

- Contamination with *L. monocytogenes*

INCIDENCE

- There are 7.4 cases of listeriosis per million population annually.
- It affects women of childbearing age.

COMPLICATIONS

- Stillbirth
- Meningitis
- Septic arthritis
- Endocarditis

ASSESSMENT

HISTORY

- Ingestion of infected food
- Eye or skin exposure to laboratory animals or animals seen in veterinary practice
- Back pain and malaise
- Fever

PHYSICAL FINDINGS

- Skin lesions on trunk and extremities
- Signs of sepsis

DIAGNOSTIC TEST RESULTS

LABORATORY

- Culture of blood, spinal fluid, drainage from cervical or vaginal lesions, or lochia from a mother with an infected infant produces positive result (isolation of the organism from these specimens is usually difficult).
- A wet mount of the culture identifies *L. monocytogenes* by its diagnostic tumbling motility.

Avoiding listeriosis

Follow these general guidelines to avoid listeriosis:
- Thoroughly cook raw food from animal sources, such as beef, pork, or poultry.
- Wash raw vegetables thoroughly before eating.
- Keep uncooked meats separate from vegetables and from cooked foods and ready-to-eat foods.
- Avoid unpasteurized (raw) milk or foods made from unpasteurized milk.
- Wash hands, knives, and cutting boards after handling uncooked foods.

Patients at high risk, such as those with weakened immune systems and pregnant women, should follow the general guidelines, plus the following:
- Avoid hot dogs, luncheon meats, and delicatessen meats, unless they are reheated until steaming hot.
- Avoid cross-contaminating other foods, utensils, and food preparation surfaces with fluid from hot dog packages, and wash hands after handling hot dogs, luncheon meats, and delicatessen meats.
- Don't eat soft cheeses, such as feta, Brie, Camembert, blue-veined cheeses, and Mexican-style cheeses such as queso blanco fresco.
- Don't eat refrigerated pâtés or meat spreads. Canned or shelf-stable pâtés and meat spreads may be eaten.
- Don't eat refrigerated smoked seafood, such as salmon, trout, whitefish, cod, tuna, or mackerel, unless it's in a cooked dish such as a casserole.

TREATMENT

GENERAL
◆ Treatment of symptoms

DIET
◆ As tolerated

ACTIVITY
◆ As tolerated

MEDICATIONS
◆ Antibiotics

NURSING CONSIDERATIONS

NURSING DIAGNOSES
◆ Acute pain
◆ Disabled family coping
◆ Impaired skin integrity
◆ Ineffective tissue perfusion: Cardiopulmonary, cerebral, renal
◆ Risk for deficient fluid volume
◆ Risk for disorganized infant behavior
◆ Risk for infection
◆ Risk for injury

EXPECTED OUTCOMES
The patient will:
◆ express feelings of comfort or absence of pain at rest
◆ contact appropriate sources of support outside the family
◆ maintain skin integrity
◆ maintain tissue perfusion and cellular oxygenation
◆ maintain fluid balance
◆ not exhibit signs of seizure activity or meningitis (infant)
◆ experience no further signs or symptoms of infection
◆ remain free from complications.

NURSING INTERVENTIONS
◆ Follow standard precautions.
◆ Provide adequate nutrition by total parenteral nutrition, nasogastric tube feedings, or a soft diet, as ordered.

MONITORING
◆ Neurologic status
◆ Fontanels (in neonates)
◆ Vital signs
◆ Intake and output

PATIENT TEACHING

GENERAL
Be sure to cover:
◆ the disorder, diagnosis, and treatment
◆ how to avoid infective materials on farms where listeriosis is endemic among livestock.

RESOURCES
Organizations
Centers for Disease Control and Prevention Division of Bacterial and Mycotic Diseases: *www.cdc.gov/ncidod/dbmd/diseaseinfo*
U.S. Department of Agriculture Food Safety and Inspection Service: *www.fsis.usda.gov*

Selected references
Cito, G., et al. "Listeriosis in Pregnancy: A Case Report," *Journal of Maternal-Fetal & Neonatal Medicine* 18(6):367-68, December 2005.
Ivanek, R., et al. "The Cost and Benefit of *Listeria monocytogenes* Food Safety Measures," *Critical Reviews in Food Science and Nutrition* 44(7-8):513-23, 2004.
Ogunmodede, F., et al. "Listeriosis Prevention Knowledge among Pregnant Women in the USA," *Obstetrical & Gynecological Survey* 60(11):704-705, November 2005.

Liver cancer

- Malignant cells growing in the tissues of the liver
- Rapidly fatal, usually within 6 months
- Second leading cause of fatal hepatic disease (after cirrhosis)
- Liver metastasis occurring as a solitary lesion (the first sign of recurrence after a remission)

PATHOPHYSIOLOGY

- Most primary liver tumors (90%) are hepatomas originating in the parenchymal cells. Others originate in the intrahepatic bile ducts (cholangiomas).
- About 30% to 70% of patients with hepatomas also have cirrhosis.
- Rare tumors include a mixed cell type, Kupffer cell sarcoma, and hepatoblastoma.
- The liver is one of the most common sites of metastasis from other primary cancers. Cells metastasize to the gallbladder, mesentery, peritoneum, and diaphragm by direct extension.

CAUSES

- Immediate cause unknown
- Androgens and oral estrogens, possibly
- Environmental exposure to carcinogens
- Hepatitis B virus
- Hepatitis C virus
- Hepatitis D virus

RISK FACTORS

- Cirrhosis
- Excessive alcohol intake
- Malnutrition

INCIDENCE

- Liver cancer is most prevalent in men older than age 60.
- Primary liver cancer accounts for roughly 2% of all cancers in North America and for 10% to 50% of cancers in Africa and parts of Asia.

COMPLICATIONS

- GI hemorrhage
- Progressive cachexia
- Liver failure

ASSESSMENT

HISTORY

- Dull aching abdominal pain initially
- Weight loss
- Weakness, fatigue, and fever
- Severe pain in the epigastrium or right upper quadrant

PHYSICAL FINDINGS

- Jaundice
- Dependent edema
- Abdominal bruit, hum, or rubbing sound
- Tender, nodular, enlarged liver
- Ascites
- Palpable mass in the right upper quadrant

DIAGNOSTIC TEST RESULTS

LABORATORY

- Liver function study results are abnormal.
- Alpha-fetoprotein levels are greater than 500 mcg/ml.
- Electrolyte study results are abnormal.

IMAGING

- Liver scan may show filling defects and lesions in the liver.
- Arteriography may define large tumors.
- Ultrasonography and computed tomography scans may reveal lesions in the liver.

DIAGNOSTIC PROCEDURES

- Biopsy of the liver reveals cancerous cells.

TREATMENT

GENERAL
◆ Radiation therapy (alone or with chemotherapy)

DIET
◆ High-calorie, low-protein

ACTIVITY
◆ Frequent rest periods
◆ Postoperative avoidance of heavy lifting and contact sports

MEDICATIONS
◆ Chemotherapeutic drugs
◆ Analgesics

SURGERY
◆ Resection (lobectomy or partial hepatectomy)
◆ Liver transplantation

NURSING CONSIDERATIONS

NURSING DIAGNOSES
◆ Acute pain
◆ Anxiety
◆ Excess fluid volume
◆ Fatigue
◆ Fear
◆ Hyperthermia
◆ Imbalanced nutrition: Less than body requirements
◆ Impaired gas exchange
◆ Impaired skin integrity
◆ Ineffective coping
◆ Ineffective tissue perfusion: Cardiopulmonary

EXPECTED OUTCOMES
The patient will:
◆ express feelings of increased comfort
◆ express feelings of decreased anxiety
◆ maintain normal fluid volume
◆ express feelings of increased energy
◆ verbalize fears and concerns about his diagnosis and condition
◆ maintain a normal body temperature
◆ achieve adequate nutritional intake through oral foods or I.V. fluids
◆ maintain adequate ventilation
◆ maintain skin integrity
◆ exhibit adequate coping behaviors
◆ exhibit signs of adequate cardiopulmonary perfusion.

NURSING INTERVENTIONS
◆ Give prescribed drugs.
◆ Provide meticulous skin care.
◆ Encourage verbalization and provide support.

MONITORING
◆ Vital signs
◆ Hydration and nutritional status
◆ Weight
◆ Pain control
◆ Neurologic status
◆ Complete blood count; liver function tests
◆ Postoperative complications
◆ Wound site

PATIENT TEACHING

GENERAL
Be sure to cover:
◆ the disorder, diagnosis, and treatment
◆ dietary restrictions
◆ relaxation techniques
◆ medication, including administration, dosage, and possible adverse effects.

DISCHARGE PLANNING
◆ Refer the patient and family members to support services.

RESOURCES
Organizations
American Cancer Society:
www.cancer.org
Guide to Internet Resources for Cancer:
www.cancerindex.org
National Cancer Institute:
www.cancer.gov

Selected references
Atlas of Pathophysiology, 2nd ed. Philadelphia: Lippincott Williams & Wilkins, 2005.

Weber, S.M., and Lee, F.T. Jr. "Expanded Treatment of Hepatic Tumors with Radiofrequency Ablation and Cryoablation," *Oncology* (Williston Park) 19(11 Suppl 4):27-32, October 2005.

Yoshida, H., et al. "Early Liver Cancer: Concepts, Diagnosis, and Management," *International Journal of Clinical Oncology* 10(6):384-90, December 2005.

Zavaglia, C., et al. "Predictors of Long-term Survival after Liver Transplantation for Hepatocellular Carcinoma," *American Journal of Gastroenterology* 100(12):2708-716, December 2005.

Liver failure

- Inability of the liver to function properly, usually as the end result of any liver disease
- Causes a complex syndrome involving the impairment of many different organs and body functions (see *Understanding liver functions*)
- Two conditions occurring in liver failure — hepatic encephalopathy and hepatorenal syndrome
- Liver transplantation only cure
- Poor prognosis in patients younger than age 10 and older than age 40

PATHOPHYSIOLOGY

- Manifestations of liver failure include hepatic encephalopathy and hepatorenal syndrome.

Hepatic encephalopathy

- The liver can no longer detoxify the blood.
- Liver dysfunction and collateral vessels that shunt blood around the liver to the systemic circulation permit toxins absorbed from the GI tract to circulate freely to the brain.
- The normal liver converts ammonia (a by-product of protein metabolism) to urea, which the kidneys excrete.
- When the liver is no longer able to convert ammonia to urea, ammonia blood levels rise and the ammonia is delivered to the brain.
- Short-chain fatty acids, serotonin, tryptophan, and false neurotransmitters may also accumulate in the blood.

Hepatorenal syndrome

- Renal failure is concurrent with liver disease; the kidneys appear to be normal but abruptly cease functioning.
- Blood volume expands, hydrogen ions accumulate, and electrolyte disturbances occur.
- The cause may be the accumulation of vasoactive substances that cause inappropriate constriction of renal arterioles, leading to decreased glomerular filtration and oliguria.

- The vasoconstriction may also be a compensatory response to portal hypertension and the pooling of blood in the splenic circulation.

CAUSES

- Acetaminophen toxicity
- Cirrhosis
- Liver cancer
- Nonviral hepatitis
- Viral hepatitis

INCIDENCE

- More than 60,000 United States residents die each year from liver failure.

COMPLICATIONS

- Variceal bleeding
- GI hemorrhage
- Coma
- Death

Understanding liver functions

To understand how liver disease affects the body, you need to understand its main functions. The liver:

- detoxifies poisonous chemicals, including alcohol and drugs (prescribed and over-the-counter as well as illegal substances)
- makes bile to help digest food
- stores energy by stockpiling sugar (carbohydrates, glucose, and fat) until needed
- stores iron reserves as well as vitamins and minerals
- manufactures new proteins
- produces important plasma proteins necessary for blood coagulation, including prothrombin and fibrinogen
- serves as a site for hematopoiesis during fetal development.

HISTORY

- Liver disorder
- Fatigue
- Weight loss
- Nausea
- Anorexia
- Pruritus

PHYSICAL FINDINGS

- Jaundice
- Abdominal tenderness
- Splenomegaly
- Ascites
- Peripheral edema
- Decreased level of consciousness

LABORATORY

- Liver function test results reveal elevated levels of aspartate aminotransferase, alanine aminotransferase, alkaline phosphatase, and bilirubin.
- Blood studies reveal anemia, impaired red blood cell production, prolonged bleeding and clotting times, low blood glucose levels, and increased serum ammonia levels.
- Urine osmolarity is increased.

TREATMENT

GENERAL
- Paracentesis to remove ascitic fluid
- Balloon tamponade to control bleeding varices

DIET
- Low-protein, high-carbohydrate

ACTIVITY
- As tolerated

MEDICATIONS
- Lactulose
- Potassium-sparing diuretics (for ascites)
- Potassium supplements
- Vasoconstrictor drugs (for variceal bleeding)
- Vitamin K

SURGERY
- Sclerosis to stop bleeding varices
- Shunt placement
- Liver transplantation

NURSING CONSIDERATIONS

NURSING DIAGNOSES
- Acute pain
- Anxiety
- Diarrhea
- Fear
- Imbalanced nutrition: Less than body requirements
- Ineffective tissue perfusion: GI, cerebral
- Risk for injury

EXPECTED OUTCOMES
The patient will:
- express feelings of increased comfort
- identify strategies to reduce anxiety
- have normal bowel movements
- discuss fears and concerns
- achieve adequate caloric and nutritional intake
- maintain adequate GI and cerebral perfusion
- avoid or minimize complications.

NURSING INTERVENTIONS
- Reorient patient as needed.
- Provide a safe environment.
- Provide emotional support.

MONITORING
- Level of consciousness
- Vital signs
- Laboratory values
- Intake and output
- Weight and abdominal girth

PATIENT TEACHING

GENERAL
Be sure to cover:
- the disorder, diagnosis, and treatment
- signs of complications and when to notify the practitioner
- the importance of following a low-protein diet
- the importance of avoiding alcohol.

DISCHARGE PLANNING
- Refer the patient to available support services, as appropriate.

RESOURCES
Organizations
American Liver Foundation: *www.liverfoundation.org*
Cleveland Clinic Health Information Center: *www.clevelandclinic.org/health*

Selected references
Day, H.L., and Taylor, R.M. "The Liver. Part 5: Acute Liver Failure," *Nursing Times* 102(2):26-27, January 2006.
Koroneos, A., et al. "Acute Liver Failure as the First Manifestation of Severe Traumatic Tricuspid Valve Insufficiency," *Intensive Care Medicine* 32(2): 336-37, February 2006.
Su, D.H., et al. "Liver Failure in a Patient Receiving Rosiglitazone Therapy," *Diabetic Medicine* 23(1):105-106, January 2006.
Wolf, D.C., et al. "Emergent Stent Occlusion for TIPS-induced Liver Failure," *Digestive Diseases and Sciences* 50(12):2356-358, December 2005.

Lung cancer

- Malignant tumors arising from the respiratory epithelium
- Most common types are epidermoid (squamous cell), adenocarcinoma, small-cell (oat cell), and large-cell (anaplastic)
- Most common site is wall or epithelium of bronchial tree
- Poor prognosis for most patients, depending on the extent of the cancer, when it was diagnosed, and the cell growth rate (5-year survival after diagnosis only in about 13% of patients with lung cancer)

PATHOPHYSIOLOGY

- Individuals with lung cancer demonstrate bronchial epithelial changes progressing from squamous cell alteration or metaplasia to carcinoma in situ.
- Tumors originating in the bronchi are thought to be more mucus producing.
- Partial or complete obstruction of the airway occurs with tumor growth, resulting in lobar collapse distal to the tumor.
- There is early metastasis to other thoracic structures, such as hilar lymph nodes or the mediastinum.
- Distant metastasis to the brain, liver, bone, and adrenal glands occurs.

CAUSES

- Exact cause unknown

RISK FACTORS

- Smoking: increases the risk 13-fold
- Exposure to carcinogenic and industrial air pollutants (asbestos, arsenic, chromium, coal dust, iron oxides, nickel, radioactive dust, and uranium)
- Genetic predisposition

INCIDENCE

- There is a family susceptibility to lung cancer.
- **AGE FACTOR** *Lung cancer is the most common cause of death from cancer for men and women ages 50 to 75.*

COMPLICATIONS

- Spread of primary tumor to intrathoracic structures
- Tracheal obstruction
- Esophageal compression with dysphagia
- Phrenic nerve paralysis with hemidiaphragm elevation and dyspnea
- Sympathetic nerve paralysis with Horner's syndrome
- Spinal cord compression
- Lymphatic obstruction with pleural effusion
- Hypoxemia
- Anorexia and weight loss, sometimes leading to cachexia, digital clubbing, and hypertrophic osteoarthropathy
- Neoplastic and paraneoplastic syndromes, including Pancoast's syndrome and syndrome of inappropriate secretion of antidiuretic hormone

HISTORY

- Possibly no symptoms
- Exposure to carcinogens
- Coughing
- Hemoptysis
- Shortness of breath
- Hoarseness
- Fatigue

PHYSICAL FINDINGS

- Dyspnea on exertion
- Digital clubbing
- Edema of the face, neck, and upper torso
- Dilated chest and abdominal veins (superior vena cava syndrome)
- Weight loss
- Enlarged lymph nodes
- Enlarged liver
- Decreased breath sounds
- Wheezing
- Pleural friction rub

LABORATORY

- Cytologic sputum analysis shows diagnostic evidence of pulmonary malignancy.
- Liver function test results are abnormal, especially with metastasis.

IMAGING

- Chest X-rays show advanced lesions and can show a lesion up to 2 years before signs and symptoms appear; findings may indicate tumor size and location.
- Contrast studies of the bronchial tree (chest computed tomography [CT], bronchography) demonstrate size and location as well as spread of lesion.
- Bone scan is used to detect metastasis.
- CT of the chest is used to detect malignant pleural effusion.
- CT of the brain is used to detect metastasis.
- Positron emission tomography aids in the diagnosis of primary and metastatic sites.
- MRI may reveal tumor invasion.
- Gallium scans of the liver and spleen help to detect metastasis.

DIAGNOSTIC PROCEDURES

- Bronchoscopy can be used to identify the tumor site. Bronchoscopic washings provide material for cytologic and histologic study.
- Needle biopsy of the lungs (relies on biplanar fluoroscopic visual control to locate peripheral tumors before withdrawing a tissue specimen for analysis) allows firm diagnosis in 80% of patients.
- Tissue biopsy of metastatic sites (including supraclavicular and mediastinal lymph nodes and pleura) is used to assess disease extent. Based on histologic findings, staging describes the disease extent and prognosis, and is used to direct treatment.
- Thoracentesis allows chemical and cytologic examination of pleural fluid.
- Exploratory thoracotomy is performed to obtain biopsy specimen.

GENERAL

- Various combinations of surgery, radiation therapy, and chemotherapy to improve prognosis
- Palliative (most treatments)
- Preoperative and postoperative radiation therapy
- Laser therapy (experimental)

DIET

- Well-balanced

ACTIVITY

- As tolerated, according to breathing capacity

MEDICATIONS

- Chemotherapy drug combinations
- Immunotherapy (investigational)

SURGERY

- Partial removal of lung (wedge resection, segmental resection, lobectomy, radical lobectomy)
- Total removal of lung (pneumonectomy, radical pneumonectomy)

NURSING DIAGNOSES

- Acute pain
- Anxiety
- Deficient fluid volume
- Fatigue
- Imbalanced nutrition: Less than body requirements
- Impaired gas exchange
- Impaired physical mobility
- Impaired skin integrity
- Ineffective airway clearance
- Ineffective breathing pattern
- Risk for infection
- Risk for injury

EXPECTED OUTCOMES

The patient will:
- express feelings of increased comfort and decreased pain
- identify strategies to reduce anxiety
- maintain normal fluid volume
- carry out activities of daily living without weakness or fatigue
- maintain daily calorie requirements
- maintain adequate ventilation
- maintain muscle strength and joint range of motion
- have surgical wounds that remain pink and free from complications
- maintain a patent airway
- maintain an effective breathing pattern
- remain free from signs or symptoms of infection
- remain free from injury or complications.

NURSING INTERVENTIONS

- Provide supportive care.
- Encourage verbalization.
- Give prescribed drugs.

MONITORING

- Chest tube function and drainage
- Postoperative complications
- Wound site
- Vital signs
- Sputum production
- Hydration and nutrition
- Oxygenation
- Pain control

GENERAL

Be sure to cover:
- the disorder, diagnosis, and treatment
- postoperative procedures and equipment
- chest physiotherapy
- exercises to prevent shoulder stiffness
- medications, including dosage, administration, and possible adverse effects
- risk factors for recurrent cancer.

DISCHARGE PLANNING

- Refer smokers to local branches of the American Cancer Society or SmokEnders.
- Provide information about group therapy, individual counseling, and hypnosis.
- Refer the patient to available resources and support services.

RESOURCES

Organizations

American Cancer Society: *www.cancer.org*
Guide to Internet Resources for Cancer: *www.cancerindex.org*
National Cancer Institute: *www.cancer.gov*
SmokEnders: *www.smokenders.com*

Selected references

Godtfredsen, N.S., et al. "Effect of Smoking Reduction on Lung Cancer Risk," *JAMA* 294(12):1505-510, September 2005.

Haiman, C.A., et al. "Ethnic and Racial Differences in the Smoking-related Risk for Lung Cancer," *New England Journal of Medicine* 354(4):333-42, January 2006.

Thompson, E., et al. "Non-invasive Interventions for Improving Well-being and Quality of Life in Patients with Lung Cancer — a Systematic Review of the Evidence," *Lung Cancer* 50(2):163-76, November 2005.

Tishelman, C., et al. "Symptoms in Patients with Lung Carcinoma: Distinguishing Distress from Intensity," *Cancer* 104(9):2013-2021, November 2005.

Lupus erythematosus

- A chronic inflammatory disorder of the connective tissues appearing in two forms: discoid lupus erythematosus, which affects only the skin, and systemic lupus erythematosus (SLE), which affects multiple organ systems as well as the skin and can be fatal
- Recurring remissions and exacerbations with SLE, especially common during the spring and summer
- Prognosis improved with early detection and treatment; remains poor for patients who develop cardiovascular, renal, or neurologic complications, or severe bacterial infections

PATHOPHYSIOLOGY

- Autoimmunity is believed to be the prime mechanism involved in SLE.
- The body produces antibodies against components of its own cells, such as the antinuclear antibody (ANA), and immune complex disease follows.
- Patients with SLE may produce antibodies against many different tissue components, such as red blood cells (RBCs), neutrophils, platelets, lymphocytes, or almost any organ or tissue in the body.

CAUSES

- Exact cause unknown

RISK FACTORS

- Physical or mental stress
- Streptococcal or viral infections
- Exposure to sunlight or ultraviolet light
- Immunization
- Pregnancy
- Abnormal estrogen metabolism
- Treatment with certain drugs, such as procainamide (Pronestyl), hydralazine (Apresoline), and anticonvulsants

INCIDENCE

- SLE affects 14 to 50 people per 100,000 population in the United States.
- It affects women more than men.

- It affects all ages, but peak incidence occurs in young adulthood.

COMPLICATIONS

- Concomitant infections
- Urinary tract infections
- Renal failure
- Osteonecrosis of the hip from long-term steroid use

HISTORY

- History of a contributing factor
- Fever
- Weight loss
- Malaise
- Fatigue
- Polyarthralgia
- Abdominal pain
- Headaches, irritability, and depression (common)
- Nausea, vomiting, diarrhea, or constipation
- Irregular menstrual periods or amenorrhea during the active phase of SLE

PHYSICAL FINDINGS

- Rashes (see *Signs of systemic lupus erythematosus*)
- Joint involvement, similar to rheumatoid arthritis (although the arthritis of lupus is usually nonerosive)
- Skin lesions, most commonly an erythematous rash in areas exposed to light (classic butterfly rash over the nose and cheeks in less than 50% of patients) or a scaly, papular rash (mimics psoriasis), especially in sun-exposed areas
- Vasculitis (especially in the digits), possibly leading to infarctive lesions, necrotic leg ulcers, or digital gangrene
- Patchy alopecia and painless ulcers of the mucous membranes
- Lymph node enlargement (diffuse or local, and nontender)

LABORATORY

- Results of anti-double-stranded deoxyribonucleic acid antibody (anti-dsDNA) test (most specific test for SLE) correlate with disease activity, especially renal involvement, and help monitor response to therapy (anti-dsDNA may be low or absent in remission).
- Complete blood count (CBC) with differential possibly shows anemia and a decreased white blood cell (WBC) count.
- CBC shows a decreased platelet count.
- Erythrocyte sedimentation rate is elevated.
- CBC reveals hypergammaglobulinemia.

Signs of systemic lupus erythematosus

Systemic lupus erythematosus (SLE) often mimics other diseases, making it difficult to diagnose. Symptoms may be vague and vary greatly among patients.

For these reasons, the American Rheumatism Association issued a list of criteria for classifying SLE, to be used primarily for consistency in epidemiologic surveys. Usually, four or more of these signs are present at some time during the course of the disease:

- malar or discoid rash
- photosensitivity
- oral or nasopharyngeal ulcerations
- nonerosive arthritis (of two or more peripheral joints)
- pleuritis or pericarditis
- profuse proteinuria (greater than 0.5 g/day) or excessive cellular casts in the urine
- seizures or psychoses
- hemolytic anemia, leukopenia, lymphopenia, or thrombocytopenia
- anti-double-stranded deoxyribonucleic acid or positive findings of antiphospholipid antibodies (elevated immunoglobulin [Ig] G or IgM anticardiolipin antibodies, positive test result for lupus anticoagulant, or false-positive serologic test results for syphilis)
- abnormal antinuclear antibody titer

- ANA and lupus erythematosus cell test results are positive in active SLE.
- Urine study results possibly show RBCs and WBCs, urine casts and sediment, and significant protein loss (greater than 0.5 g/24 hours).
- Blood study results show decreased serum complement (C3 and C4) levels, indicating active disease.
- Lupus anticoagulant and anticardiolipin test results are positive in some patients (usually in patients prone to antiphospholipid syndrome of thrombosis, abortion, and thrombocytopenia).

IMAGING
- Chest X-ray possibly shows pleurisy or lupus pneumonitis.

DIAGNOSTIC PROCEDURES
- Electrocardiography possibly shows a conduction defect with cardiac involvement or pericarditis.
- Results of a biopsy of the kidney determine disease stage and extent of renal involvement.

TREATMENT

GENERAL
- Symptomatic
- Dialysis or kidney transplantation for renal failure

DIET
- Restrictions based on extent of disorder

ACTIVITY
- As tolerated
- Frequent rest periods

MEDICATIONS
- Nonsteroidal anti-inflammatory drugs, including aspirin
- Topical corticosteroid creams, such as hydrocortisone buteprate (Pandel) or triamcinolone (Aristocort)
- Intralesional corticosteroids or antimalarials such as hydroxychloroquine sulfate (Plaquenil)
- Systemic corticosteroids
- Methotrexate (Trexall)

NURSING CONSIDERATIONS

NURSING DIAGNOSES
- Acute pain
- Constipation
- Decreased cardiac output
- Diarrhea
- Disturbed body image
- Fatigue
- Imbalanced nutrition: Less than body requirements
- Impaired oral mucous membrane
- Impaired physical mobility
- Impaired skin integrity
- Impaired tissue integrity
- Impaired urinary elimination
- Ineffective breathing pattern
- Risk for infection
- Risk for peripheral neurovascular dysfunction

EXPECTED OUTCOMES
The patient will:
- express feelings of comfort and decreased pain
- pass soft, regular stool without straining
- maintain adequate cardiac output
- resume a normal bowel elimination pattern
- verbalize feelings about a changed body image
- express feelings of increased energy
- show no signs of malnutrition
- maintain intact oral mucous membranes
- maintain joint mobility and range of motion
- maintain skin integrity
- have reduced pain, redness, and swelling at the site of impaired tissue
- maintain fluid balance; intake will equal output
- maintain an effective breathing pattern
- remain free from infection
- report alterations in sensation or pain in the extremities
- recognize steps and warning signs and symptoms to prevent worsening.

NURSING INTERVENTIONS
- Provide a balanced diet. For renal involvement, provide a low-sodium, low-protein diet.

- Urge the patient to get plenty of rest. Schedule diagnostic tests and procedures to allow adequate rest.
- Explain all tests and procedures.
- Apply heat packs to relieve joint pain and stiffness.
- Encourage regular exercise to maintain full range of motion (ROM) and prevent contractures.

MONITORING
- Signs and symptoms
- Vital signs
- Intake and output
- Laboratory reports

PATIENT TEACHING

GENERAL
Be sure to cover:
- ROM exercises as well as body alignment and postural techniques
- expected benefit of prescribed medications, as well as adverse effects
- cosmetic tips, such as suggesting the use of hypoallergenic makeup and referral to a hairdresser who specializes in scalp disorders.

DISCHARGE PLANNING
- Arrange for physical therapy and occupational counseling, if needed.
- Refer the patient to the Lupus Foundation of America and the Arthritis Foundation as necessary.

RESOURCES
Organizations
Arthritis Foundation: *www.arthritis.org*
Lupus Foundation of America: *www.lupus.org*

Selected references
Chu, Y.T., and Chiou, S.S. "Painless Massive Ascites and Hypoalbuminemia as the Major Manifestations of Systemic Lupus Erythematosus," *Journal of Microbiology, Immunology, and Infection* 39(1):78-81, February 2006.
Rooney, J. "Systemic Lupus Erythematosus: Unmasking a Great Imitator," *Nursing* 35(11):54-60, November 2005.
Shirato, S. "How CAM Helps Systemic Lupus Erythematosus," *Holistic Nursing Practice* 19(1):36-39, January-February 2005.

Lyme disease

OVERVIEW

- A multisystem disorder caused by a spirochete

PATHOPHYSIOLOGY

- A tick injects spirochete-laden saliva into the bloodstream or deposits fecal matter on the skin.
- After incubating for 3 to 32 days, the spirochetes migrate outward on the skin, causing a rash, and disseminate to other skin sites or organs through the bloodstream or lymphatic system.
- Spirochetes may survive for years in the joints or die after triggering an inflammatory response in the host.

CAUSES

- The spirochete *Borrelia burgdorferi*, carried by the minute tick *Ixodes dammini* (also called *I. scapularis*) or another tick in the Ixodidae family

INCIDENCE

- Lyme disease affects all ages and both sexes.
- Disease onset occurs during the summer months.
- Lyme disease occurs primarily in three geographic regions of the United States.

COMPLICATIONS

- Myocarditis
- Pericarditis
- Arrhythmias
- Meningitis
- Encephalitis
- Cranial or peripheral neuropathies
- Arthritis

ASSESSMENT

HISTORY

- Recent exposure to ticks
- Onset of symptoms in warmer months
- Severe headache and stiff neck with rash eruption
- Fever (up to 104° F [40° C]) and chills

PHYSICAL FINDINGS

- Regional lymphadenopathy
- Tenderness in the skin lesion site or the posterior cervical area

Early stage

- Tachycardia or irregular heartbeat
- Mild dyspnea
- Erythema migrans
- Headache
- Myalgia
- Arthralgia

Later stage

- Neurologic signs such as memory impairment
- Bell's palsy
- Intermittent arthritis (see *Differentiating Lyme disease*)
- Cardiac symptoms, such as heart failure, pericarditis, and dyspnea
- Neurologic symptoms, such as memory impairment and myelitis
- Fibromyalgia
- Ocular signs such as conjunctivitis

DIAGNOSTIC TEST RESULTS

LABORATORY

- Results of assays for anti-*B. burgdorferi* (anti-B) show evidence of previous or current infection.
- Enzyme-linked immunosorbent assay technology or indirect fluorescence assay show immunoglobulin (Ig) M levels that peak 3 to 6 weeks after infection; IgG antibodies detected several weeks after infection may continue to develop for several months and generally persist for years.
- Results of Western blot assay show serologic evidence of past or current infection with *B. burgdorferi*.
- Polymerase chain reaction test is used when joint and cerebrospinal fluid involvement are present and detects the genetic material found in the Lyme disease bacteria.

    WARNING *Serologic testing isn't useful early in the course of Lyme disease because of its low sensitivity. However, it may be more useful in later disease stages, when sensitivity and specificity of the test are improved.*

DIAGNOSTIC PROCEDURES

- Analysis of cerebrospinal fluid obtained by lumbar puncture may show antibodies to *B. burgdorferi*.
- Biopsy of skin specimen may be performed to detect *B. burgdorferi*.

TREATMENT

GENERAL
◆ Prompt tick removal using proper technique

ACTIVITY
◆ Rest periods when needed

MEDICATIONS
◆ I.V. or oral antibiotics (initiated as soon as possible after infection)

NURSING CONSIDERATIONS

NURSING DIAGNOSES
◆ Acute pain
◆ Fatigue
◆ Hyperthermia
◆ Impaired physical mobility
◆ Impaired skin integrity
◆ Risk for infection

EXPECTED OUTCOMES
The patient will:
◆ express relief from pain
◆ return to a normal energy level during recovery
◆ remain afebrile
◆ attain the highest degree of mobility possible
◆ experience a decrease in the size of the rash
◆ experience no further signs or symptoms of infection.

NURSING INTERVENTIONS
◆ Plan care to provide adequate rest.
◆ Give prescribed drugs.
◆ Assist with range-of-motion and strengthening exercises (with arthritis).
◆ Encourage verbalization and provide support.

MONITORING
◆ Skin lesions
◆ Response to treatment
◆ Adverse drug reactions
◆ Complications

PATIENT TEACHING

GENERAL
Be sure to cover:
◆ the disorder, diagnosis, and treatment
◆ medication administration, dosage, and possible adverse effects
◆ the importance of follow-up care and reporting recurrent or new symptoms to the practitioner
◆ methods for preventing Lyme disease, such as avoiding tick-infested areas, covering the skin with clothing, using insect repellants, inspecting exposed skin for attached ticks at least every 4 hours, and removing ticks
◆ information about the vaccine for persons at risk for contracting Lyme disease.

DISCHARGE PLANNING
◆ If the patient is in the late stages of the disease, refer him to a dermatologist, neurologist, cardiologist, or infectious disease specialist, as indicated.

RESOURCES
Organizations
Centers for Disease Control and Prevention: *www.cdc.gov*
Harvard University Consumer Health Information: *www.intelihealth.com*
National Health Information Center: *www.health.gov/nhic*
National Institute of Allergy and Infectious Diseases: *www.niaid.nih.gov*
National Library of Medicine: *www.nlm.nih.gov*

Selected references
Bratton, R.L., and Corey, R. "Tick-borne Disease," *American Family Physician* 71(12):2323-330, June 2005.
Kasper, D.L., et al., eds. *Harrison's Principles of Internal Medicine,* 16th ed. New York: McGraw-Hill Book Co., 2005.
Phillips, S.E., et al. "Rash Decisions about Southern Tick-associated Rash Illness and Lyme Disease," *Clinical Infectious Diseases* 42(2):306-307, January 2006.
Rudd-Arieta, M.P. "Lyme Disease in Children. An Overview," *Advance for Nurse Practitioners* 11(6):77-78, June 2003.

Differentiating Lyme disease

Lyme disease, or chronic neuroborreliosis, needs to be differentiated from chronic fatigue syndrome and fibromyalgia, which is difficult late in the disease because of chronic pain and fatigue. The other diseases produce more generalized and disabling symptoms; also, patients lack evidence of joint inflammation, have normal neurologic test results, and have a greater degree of anxiety and depression than patients with Lyme disease have.

Lymphocytic choriomeningitis

OVERVIEW

- A mild, biphasic, febrile illness lasting about 2 weeks
- Asymptomatic in one-third of individuals and resolving without serious sequelae in most cases
- Rarely fatal (less than 1% mortality)
- Also known as *LCM* or *lymphocytic meningitis*

PATHOPHYSIOLOGY

- Infected mice or other hosts excrete lymphocytic choriomeningitis virus (LCMV) in saliva, urine, and feces.
- Human infection is through inhalation of infectious aerosolized particles of host urine, feces, or saliva; ingestion of food contaminated with virus; or contamination of mucous membranes, skin lesions, or cuts with infected body fluids.
- The incubation period is 8 to13 days and is followed by a biphasic, febrile illness.
- The initial viremia extensively seeds extra-central nervous system tissue and sometimes cortical tissue.
- The leptomeninges are infiltrated mainly by lymphocytes and histiocytes, and only by a few neutrophils.
- The host's immune response to the infected cells produces various symptoms.
- Natural killer cells are first to respond, then cytotoxic T cells respond by producing interferon.
- Meningeal symptoms appear in 15 to 21 days.

CAUSES

- Arenavirus
- LCMV

RISK FACTORS

- Handling infected animals or their excreta

INCIDENCE

- The prevalence of LCM in humans is 2% to 10%, but it's important to note that LCM has historically been underreported.
- Individuals of all ages are susceptible, but young adults are infected more commonly.
- Cases have been reported in Europe, North America, South America, Australia, and Japan, but most cases occur in the northeast and eastern seaboard areas of the United States.
- LCM is more common during fall and winter.
- Infection occurs equally in men and women.

COMPLICATIONS

- Temporary or permanent neurologic damage possible (meningitis, paralysis, coma)
- Possible maternal transmission (Pregnancy-related infection is associated with abortion, congenital hydrocephalus, chorioretinitis, and mental retardation.)
- Myelitis presenting with muscle weakness, paralysis, or changes in body sensation
- Guillain-Barré–type syndrome
- Orchitis (usually unilateral) or parotitis
- Cardiac involvement such as myocarditis
- Psychosis
- Joint pain and arthritis during convalescence, especially in the metacarpophalangeal and proximal interphalangeal joints
- Prolonged convalescence, with continuing dizziness, somnolence, and fatigue

ASSESSMENT

HISTORY

- Exposure to rodents, hamsters, or their excreta 1 to 3 weeks before symptom onset

PHYSICAL FINDINGS

- Lymphadenopathy
- Maculopapular rash
- Fever
- Cough
- Possible bradycardia

DIAGNOSTIC TEST RESULTS

LABORATORY
Phase I

- White blood cell (WBC) count is decreased (leukopenia).
- Platelet count is decreased (thrombocytopenia).
- Liver enzymes are mildly elevated.

Phase II

- Protein levels are increased.
- WBC count is increased.
- Glucose levels in cerebrospinal fluid (CSF) are decreased.

DIAGNOSTIC PROCEDURES

- Results of enzyme-linked immunosorbent assay of serum or CSF (the preferred diagnostic test) detect immunoglobulin M antibodies.
- CSF obtained by lumbar puncture in patients with meningeal signs was typically abnormal (increased opening pressure, increased protein levels, and a lymphocytic pleocytosis, usually in the range of several hundred WBCs).

TREATMENT

GENERAL
◆ Hospitalization and supportive treatment based on severity

ACTIVITY
◆ As tolerated

MEDICATIONS
◆ No specific treatment
◆ Anti-inflammatory drugs possibly useful
◆ Ribavirin (effective against LCMV in vitro)
◆ Analgesics (for symptom relief)

SURGERY
◆ Surgical shunting possibly required to relieve increased intracranial pressure in acute hydrocephalus

NURSING CONSIDERATIONS

NURSING DIAGNOSES
◆ Anxiety
◆ Decreased cardiac output
◆ Hyperthermia
◆ Impaired gas exchange
◆ Impaired skin integrity

EXPECTED OUTCOMES
The patient will:
◆ express feelings of decreased anxiety
◆ maintain hemodynamic stability
◆ maintain a normal body temperature
◆ maintain adequate ventilation and oxygenation
◆ maintain skin integrity.

NURSING INTERVENTIONS
◆ Encourage rest and fluids postlumbar puncture.
◆ Give prescribed drugs.
◆ Administer total parental care, if the patient is paralyzed or in a coma.
◆ Encourage diet and activity as tolerated.

MONITORING
◆ Vital signs
◆ Signs of acute hydrocephalus
◆ Cardiac signs and symptoms
◆ Skin integrity
◆ Complications of lumbar puncture

PATIENT TEACHING

GENERAL
Be sure to cover:
◆ rodent control measures
◆ basic hygiene practices
◆ the use of a personal respirator
◆ the importance of adequate ventilation
◆ the use of a liquid disinfectant such as a diluted household bleach solution to clean up rodent droppings.

DISCHARGE PLANNING
◆ Refer pregnant patients to an obstetrician for monitoring.
◆ Refer paralyzed or comatose patients to physical therapy or occupational therapy as needed.
◆ Refer psychotic patients for follow-up with a psychiatrist.

RESOURCES
Organizations
Centers for Disease Control and Prevention: *www.cdc.gov*

Selected references
Banarer, M., et al. "Chronic Lymphocytic Meningitis in an Adolescent," *Journal of Pediatrics* 147(5):686-90, November 2005.

Hoey, J. "Lymphocytic Choriomeningitis Virus," *Canadian Medical Association Journal* 173(9):1033, October 2005.

Storm, P., et al. "Perforin-deficient CD8+ T cells Mediate Fatal Lymphocytic Choriomeningitis Despite Impaired Cytokine Production," *Journal of Virology* 80(3):1222-230, February 2006.

Lymphoma, non-Hodgkin's

- Heterogeneous group of malignant diseases that originate in lymph glands and other lymphoid tissue
- Usually classified according to histologic, anatomic, and immunomorphic characteristics developed by the National Cancer Institute (Rappaport histologic and Lukes and Collins classifications also used in some facilities)
- New categories of non-Hodgkin's lymphoma (mantle zone lymphoma and marginal zone lymphoma) identified recently
- Also called *malignant lymphoma* and *lymphosarcoma*

PATHOPHYSIOLOGY

- Non-Hodgkin's lymphoma seems to be similar to Hodgkin's disease, but Reed-Sternberg cells aren't present, and the lymph node destruction is different.
- Lymphoid tissue is characterized by a pattern of either diffuse or nodular infiltration. Nodular lymphomas yield a better prognosis than the diffuse form, but in both the prognosis is less hopeful than in Hodgkin's disease.

CAUSES

- Exact cause unknown

RISK FACTORS

- History of autoimmune disease

INCIDENCE

- Non-Hodgkin's lymphoma is three times more common than Hodgkin's disease.
- Incidence of the disease is increasing, especially in patients with autoimmune disorders and those receiving immunosuppressant treatments or in those with acquired immunodeficiency syndrome (AIDS).

  AGE FACTOR *Men older than age 60 have the highest incidence of non-Hodgkin's lymphoma.*

COMPLICATIONS

- Hypercalcemia
- Hyperuricemia
- Lymphomatosis
- Meningitis
- Anemia
- Liver, kidney, and lung problems (with tumor growth)
- Increased intracranial pressure (with central nervous system involvement)

ASSESSMENT

HISTORY

- Symptoms mimic those of Hodgkin's disease
- Painless, swollen lymph glands (swelling may have appeared and disappeared over several months)
- Complaints of fatigue, malaise, weight loss, fever, and night sweats
- Trouble breathing, cough (usually children)

PHYSICAL FINDINGS

- Enlarged tonsils and adenoids
- Rubbery nodes in the cervical and supraclavicular areas

DIAGNOSTIC TEST RESULTS

LABORATORY

- Complete blood count shows anemia.
- Uric acid levels are normal or elevated.
- Calcium levels are elevated, resulting from bone lesions.

IMAGING

- Miscellaneous scans (chest X-rays; lymphangiography; liver, bone, and spleen scans; computed tomography of the abdomen; and excretory urography) show disease progression.

DIAGNOSTIC PROCEDURES

- Results of biopsies of lymph nodes, tonsils, bone marrow, liver, bowel, skin, or, as needed, of tissue removed during exploratory laparotomy help to differentiate non-Hodgkin's lymphoma from Hodgkin's disease.
- The same staging system used for Hodgkin's disease is used for non-Hodgkin's lymphoma.

TREATMENT

GENERAL
- Radiation therapy mainly during the localized stage of the disease
- Total nodal irradiation usually effective in nodular and diffuse lymphomas

DIET
- Well-balanced, high-calorie, high-protein
- Increased fluid intake
- Small, frequent meals

ACTIVITY
- Limited
- Frequent rest periods

MEDICATIONS
- Combination chemotherapy regimens

SURGERY
- Debulking procedure (subtotal or, in some cases, total gastrectomy) required before chemotherapy for perforation (common in patients with gastric lymphomas)

NURSING CONSIDERATIONS

NURSING DIAGNOSES
- Acute pain
- Anxiety
- Fatigue
- Fear
- Imbalanced nutrition: Less than body requirements
- Ineffective coping
- Ineffective protection
- Risk for infection

EXPECTED OUTCOMES
The patient will:
- express feelings of increased comfort and decreased pain
- verbalize feelings of reduced anxiety
- express feelings of increased energy
- discuss fears and concerns
- maintain weight within an acceptable range
- demonstrate effective coping mechanisms
- demonstrate the use of protective measures, including conserving energy, maintaining a balanced diet, and getting adequate rest
- not exhibit signs or symptoms of infection.

NURSING INTERVENTIONS
- Give prescribed drugs.
- Provide time for rest periods.
- Encourage verbalization and provide support.

MONITORING
- Adverse effects of treatment
- Vital signs
- Pain control
- Hydration and nutritional status

PATIENT TEACHING

GENERAL
Be sure to cover:
- the disorder, diagnosis, and treatment
- preoperative and postoperative procedures
- dietary plan
- mouth care using a soft-bristled toothbrush and avoidance of commercial mouthwashes
- relaxation and comfort measures
- medication, including administration, dosage, and possible adverse effects
- symptoms that require immediate attention.

DISCHARGE PLANNING
- Refer the patient to available resources and support services.

RESOURCES
Organizations
American Cancer Society:
www.cancer.org
Guide to Internet Resources for Cancer:
www.cancerindex.org
The Leukemia and Lymphoma Society:
www.leukemia.org
National Cancer Institute:
www.cancer.gov

Selected references
Atlas of Pathophysiology, 2nd ed. Philadelphia: Lippincott Williams & Wilkins, 2005.

Casciato, D.A. *Manual of Clinical Oncology,* 5th ed. Philadelphia: Lippincott Williams & Wilkins, 2004.

Grulich, A.E., and Vajdic, C.M. "The Epidemiology of non-Hodgkin's Lymphoma," *Pathology* 37(6):409-19, December 2005.

Hohenstein, M., et al. "Patient-specific Vaccine Therapy for non-Hodgkin's Lymphoma," *Clinical Journal of Oncology Nursing* 9(1):85-90, February 2005.

Lee, W.J., et al. "Asthma History, Occupational Exposure to Pesticides and the Risk for non-Hodgkin's Lymphoma," *International Journal of Cancer* 118(12):3174-76, June 2006.

Major depression LIFE-THREATENING DISORDER

OVERVIEW

- Persistent sad, dysphoric mood
- Unipolar depressive disorder with onset in early adulthood and recurrences throughout life (at least two more episodes in 50% to 60% of patients)
- May occur in clusters or sporadically (with increasing frequency); may recur after symptom-free period

PATHOPHYSIOLOGY

- Changes occur in the receptor-neurotransmitter relationships in the limbic system.
- Changes in the hypothalamic-pituitary-adrenal regulation system may be an adaptive deregulation of the stress response.
- Chromosome II or X may be defective.

CAUSES

- Genetic, familial, biochemical, physical, psychological, and social causes
- Many physical causes result in secondary depression
- Psychological stress
- Seasonal depression

RISK FACTORS

- Female sex
- Family history of major depression or bipolar disorder
- Chronic illness
- Chronic pain
- Substance abuse
- Adverse reaction to medication such as beta-adrenergic blockers

INCIDENCE

- Major depression affects about 17.6 million people in the United States each year.
- It affects 5% to 20% of the general population at some time in their lives.
- The diagnostic criteria for major depression are met in 6% to 8% of patients in health care settings.
- Incidence increases with age.
- It's twice as common in women as in men, regardless of age.

COMPLICATIONS

- Profound alteration in social, family, and occupational functioning
- Suicide

ASSESSMENT

HISTORY

- Profound loss of pleasure in all enjoyable activities for a full month to 1 or more years
- Life problems or losses
- Physical disorder
- Use of prescription, nonprescription, or illegal drugs
- Change in eating and sleeping patterns
- Lack of interest in sex
- Constipation or diarrhea

PHYSICAL FINDINGS

- Difficulty concentrating or thinking clearly
- Easily distracted
- Indecisiveness
- Delusions of persecution or guilt
- Agitation
- Psychomotor retardation
- Somatic delusions

DSM-IV-TR *criteria*

A diagnosis is confirmed when five or more of these symptoms occur in the same 2-week period and represent a change from previous functioning:

- Depressed mood (irritable mood in children and adolescents) most of the day, nearly every day, as indicated by either subjective account or observation by others
- Markedly diminished interest or pleasure in all, or almost all, activities most of the day, nearly every day
- Significant weight loss or weight gain (greater than 5% of the patient's body weight in a month) when not dieting, or a change in appetite
- Insomnia or hypersomnia
- Psychomotor agitation or retardation
- Fatigue or loss of energy
- Feelings of worthlessness and excessive or inappropriate guilt

---

Suicide prevention guidelines

To help deter potential suicide attempt in the patient with major depression, keep in mind these guidelines.

ASSESS FOR CLUES TO SUICIDE

Watch for such clues as communicating suicidal thoughts, threats, and messages; hoarding medication; talking about death and feelings of futility; giving away prized possessions; describing a suicide plan; and changing behavior, *most* especially as depression begins to lift.

PROVIDE A SAFE ENVIRONMENT

Check patient areas and correct dangerous conditions, such as exposed pipes, windows without safety glass, and access to the roof or open balconies.

REMOVE DANGEROUS OBJECTS

Remove such objects as belts, razors, suspenders, light cords, glass, knives, nail files, and clippers from the patient's environment.

CONSULT WITH STAFF

Recognize and document verbal and nonverbal suicidal behaviors, keep the practitioner informed, share data with all staff, clarify the patient's specific restrictions, assess risk and plan for observation, and clarify day and night staff responsibilities and frequency of consultation.

OBSERVE THE SUICIDAL PATIENT

Place the patient on constant (one-on-one) supervision. Be alert when the patient's using a sharp object (shaving), taking medication, or using the bathroom (to prevent hanging or other injury). Assign the patient to a room near the nurses' station. Continuously observe the acutely suicidal patient.

MAINTAIN PERSONAL CONTACT

Help the suicidal patient feel that he isn't alone or without resources or hope. Encourage continuity of care and consistency of primary nurses. Building emotional ties to others is the ultimate technique for preventing suicide.

- Diminished ability to think or concentrate, or indecisiveness
- Recurrent thoughts of death, recurrent suicidal ideation without a specific plan, or suicide attempt or a specific plan for committing suicide (see *Suicide prevention guidelines*)
- Symptoms not due to a mixed episode (mania, depression), a medical condition, the effects of a medication or other substance, or bereavement

DIAGNOSTIC TEST RESULTS

LABORATORY
- Toxicology screening suggests a drug-induced depression.

DIAGNOSTIC PROCEDURES
- Dexamethasone suppression test results may show a failure to suppress cortisol secretion.

OTHER
- Beck Depression Inventory results show the onset, severity, duration, and progression of depressive symptoms.

TREATMENT

GENERAL
- Electroconvulsive therapy
- Short-term psychotherapy (a combination of individual, family, or group psychotherapy)

DIET
- Well-balanced

ACTIVITY
- Scheduled activities of daily living

MEDICATIONS
- Selective serotonin-reuptake inhibitors
- Maprotiline
- Tricyclic antidepressants
- Monoamine oxidase inhibitors (MAOIs)

NURSING CONSIDERATIONS

NURSING DIAGNOSES
- Anxiety
- Chronic low self-esteem
- Disturbed sleep pattern
- Dysfunctional grieving
- Fatigue
- Impaired home maintenance
- Impaired social interaction
- Ineffective coping
- Ineffective role performance
- Risk for other-directed violence
- Risk for self-directed violence
- Social isolation
- Spiritual distress

EXPECTED OUTCOMES
The patient will:
- verbalize strategies to reduce anxiety
- verbally and behaviorally demonstrate a positive self-evaluation
- resume normal sleep patterns
- use support groups to work through the grieving process
- verbalize the importance of adequate rest periods
- comply with the medication regimen
- engage in social interactions
- develop effective coping behaviors
- maintain roles and responsibilities to the fullest extent possible
- not harm others
- make a verbal contract not to harm self while in the facility
- maintain family and peer relationships
- verbalize the importance of inner resources.

NURSING INTERVENTIONS
- Encourage participation in individual and group therapy.
- Encourage expression of feelings.
- Listen attentively and respectfully.
- Provide a structured routine.
- Encourage interaction with others.
- Document observations and significant conversations.
- Assume an active role in starting communication.
- Plan activities for when the patient's energy levels are highest.
- Provide distraction from self-absorption.

MONITORING
- Adverse effects of medication
- Suicidal ideation
- Self-care
- Social interaction
- Functioning level
- Response to treatment

PATIENT TEACHING

GENERAL
Be sure to cover:
- disorder, diagnosis, and treatment
- depression and effects on daily living
- prescribed medications
- the need to adhere to drug regimen
- medication administration, dosage, and possible adverse reactions and interactions with other substances
- dietary restrictions if taking MAOIs.

DISCHARGE PLANNING
- Refer the patient to available support services and community assistance.

RESOURCES
Organizations
American Association of Suicidology: *www.suicidology.org*
American Psychiatric Association: *www.psych.org*
American Psychological Association: *www.apa.org*

Selected references
Diagnostic and Statistical Manual of Mental Disorders, Fourth Edition, Text Revision. Washington, D.C.: American Psychiatric Association, 2000.
Ebmeier, K.P., et al. "Recent Developments and Current Controversies in Depression," *Lancet* 367(9505):153-67, January 2006.
Gunderson, A., and Tomkowiak, J. "Major Depression in Rehabilitation Care," *Rehabilitation Nursing* 30(6):219-20, November-December 2005.
Kendler, K.S., et al. "Toward a Comprehensive Developmental Model for Major Depression in Men," *American Journal of Psychiatry* 163(1):115-24, January 2006.
Montgomery, S.A. "Why Do We Need New and Better Antidepressants?" *International Clinical Psychopharmacology* 21(Suppl 1):S1-10, February 2006.

Malabsorption

- A defect in the GI tract in which the intestinal mucosa fails to absorb single or multiple nutrients efficiently
- May impair absorption of amino acids, fat, sugar, or vitamins
- Results in inadequate movement of nutrients from the small intestine to the bloodstream or lymphatic system
- Manifestations dependent on the specific nutrients not being absorbed

PATHOPHYSIOLOGY

- The mechanism of malabsorption depends on the cause.
- In celiac sprue, dietary gluten — a product of wheat, barley, rye, and oats — is toxic to the patient, causing injury to the mucosal villi. The mucosa appears flat and has lost absorptive surface. Symptoms generally disappear when gluten is removed from the diet.
- Lactase deficiency is a disaccharide deficiency syndrome. Lactase is an intestinal enzyme that splits nonabsorbable lactose (a disaccharide) into the absorbable monosaccharides glucose and galactose. Production may be deficient, or another intestinal disease may inhibit the enzyme.
- After gastrectomy, poor mixing of chyme with gastric secretions is the cause of postsurgical malabsorption.
- In Zollinger-Ellison syndrome, increased acidity in the duodenum inhibits release of cholecystokinin, which stimulates pancreatic enzyme secretion. Pancreatic enzyme deficiency leads to decreased breakdown of nutrients and malabsorption.
- Bacterial overgrowth in the duodenal stump (loop created in the Billroth II gastrectomy) causes malabsorption of vitamin B_{12}.

CAUSES

- Disease of the small intestine such as celiac disease
- Drug toxicity
- Hepatobiliary disease
- Hereditary disorders
- Pancreatic disorders
- Prior gastric surgery (see *Causes of malabsorption*)

INCIDENCE

- Incidence depends on the cause of the malabsorption.

COMPLICATIONS

- Fractures
- Anemias
- Bleeding disorders
- Tetany
- Malnutrition

HISTORY

- Fatigue
- Diarrhea
- Steatorrhea

PHYSICAL FINDINGS

- Orthostatic hypotension
- Signs of weight loss or muscle wasting
- Abdominal distention
- Hyperactive bowel sounds
- Pallor
- Ecchymosis
- Peripheral edema

Causes of malabsorption

Many disorders — from systemic to organ-specific diseases — may lead to malabsorption.

DISEASES OF THE SMALL INTESTINE

Primary small-bowel disease
- Bacterial overgrowth from stasis in afferent loop after Billroth II gastrectomy
- Massive bowel resection
- Nontropical sprue (celiac disease)
- Regional enteritis
- Tropical sprue

Ischemic small-bowel disease
- Chronic heart failure
- Mesenteric atherosclerosis

Systemic disease involving small bowel
- Acute enteritis
- Giardiasis

DRUG-INDUCED MALABSORPTION
- Calcium carbonate
- Neomycin

HEPATOBILIARY DISEASE
- Biliary fistula
- Biliary tract obstruction
- Cirrhosis and hepatitis

HEREDITARY DISORDER
- Primary lactase deficiency

PANCREATIC DISORDERS
- Chronic pancreatitis
- Cystic fibrosis
- Pancreatic cancer
- Pancreatic resection
- Zollinger-Ellison syndrome

PREVIOUS GASTRIC SURGERY
- Billroth II gastrectomy
- Pyloroplasty
- Total gastrectomy
- Vagotomy

DIAGNOSTIC TEST RESULTS

LABORATORY
- Analysis of stool specimen for fat content reveals the excretion of greater than 6 g of fat per day.
- D-xylose absorption test results shows less than 20% of 25 g of D-xylose in the urine after 5 hours (reflects disorders of proximal bowel).
- Results of Schilling test reveal a deficiency of vitamin B_{12} absorption.
- Culture of duodenal and jejunal contents confirms a bacterial overgrowth in the proximal bowel.

IMAGING
- GI barium studies show the characteristic features of malabsorption in the small intestine.

DIAGNOSTIC PROCEDURES
- Results of biopsy of the small intestine reveal the atrophy of mucosal villi.

TREATMENT

GENERAL
- Identification of cause and appropriate correction

DIET
- Gluten-free to stop progression of celiac disease and malabsorption
- Lactose-free to treat lactase deficiency

MEDICATIONS
- Dietary supplementation
- Vitamin B_{12} injections

NURSING CONSIDERATIONS

NURSING DIAGNOSES
- Diarrhea
- Fatigue
- Imbalanced nutrition: Less than body requirements
- Risk for imbalanced fluid volume
- Risk for injury

EXPECTED OUTCOMES
The patient will:
- have normal bowel movements
- express feelings of increased energy
- have improved absorption of nutrients and maintain or improve weight
- maintain balanced fluid volume status
- avoid injury and complications.

NURSING INTERVENTIONS
- Watch for signs of dehydration, such as dry skin and mucous membranes and poor skin turgor.
- Protect patients with osteomalacia from injury by keeping the side rails up and assisting with ambulation as necessary.

MONITORING
- Nutritional status
- Calorie intake
- Weight
- Intake and output
- Laboratory values

PATIENT TEACHING

GENERAL
Be sure to cover:
- the disorder, diagnosis, and treatment
- following a gluten-free diet.

DISCHARGE PLANNING
- Encourage follow-up visits as ordered.

RESOURCES
Organizations
Celiac Sprue Association: *www.csaceliacs.org*
National Institute of Diabetes & Digestive & Kidney Diseases: *www.niddk.nih.gov*

Selected references
Lee, S.K., and Green, P.H. "Celiac Sprue (the Great Modern-Day Imposter)," *Current Opinion in Rheumatology* 18(1):101-107, January 2006.
Littlewood, J.M., et al. "Diagnosis and Treatment of Intestinal Malabsorption in Cystic Fibrosis," *Pediatric Pulmonology* 41(1):35-49, January 2006.
Schiller, L.R. "Nutrition Management of Chronic Diarrhea and Malabsorption," *Nutrition in Clinical Practice* 21(1):34-39, February 2006.

Malaria

- An acute infectious disease caused by protozoa of the genus *Plasmodium*: *P. falciparum, P. vivax, P. malariae,* and *P. ovale*
- Transmitted to humans by mosquito vectors
- *P. falciparum* malaria the most severe form of the disease
- Untreated primary attacks lasting from a week to a month or longer
- Relapses occurring commonly, with sporadic disease recurrence for several years
- Hepatic parasites (*P. vivax, P. ovale,* and *P. malariae*) possibly persisting for years in the liver (responsible for the chronic carrier state)

PATHOPHYSIOLOGY

- *Plasmodium* sporozoites are injected by the bite of a mosquito vector.
- The infective sporozoites migrate by blood circulation to parenchymal cells of the liver; there they form cyst-like structures containing thousands of merozoites.
- Upon release, each merozoite invades an erythrocyte and feeds on hemoglobin.
- Eventually, the erythrocyte ruptures, releasing heme (malaria pigment), cell debris, and more merozoites, which, unless destroyed by phagocytes, enter other erythrocytes.

CAUSES

- Bite of female *Anopheles* mosquitoes

INCIDENCE

- There are 300 to 500 million cases annually (internationally).
- Since 1940, few cases of malaria have been contracted in the United States; most of these were transmitted through blood transfusions or the use of contaminated needles by drug addicts.

COMPLICATIONS

- Renal failure
- Liver failure
- Heart failure
- Pulmonary edema
- Disseminated intravascular coagulation
- Circulatory collapse
- Severe normocytic anemia
- Seizures
- Hypoglycemia
- Splenic rupture
- Cerebral dysfunction
- Death

ASSESSMENT

HISTORY

- Travel to endemic area
- Recent blood transfusion
- I.V. drug abuse
- Chills, fever
- Headache, backache

PHYSICAL FINDINGS

- Pale skin
- Urticaria
- Jaundice
- Petechial rash
- Hepatosplenomegaly (*P. vivax* and *P. ovale*)

DIAGNOSTIC TEST RESULTS

LABORATORY

- Peripheral blood smears identify the parasites in red blood cells.
- Complete blood count (CBC) shows decreased hemoglobin levels.
- CBC shows possible decreased leukocyte count (as low as 3,000/µl).
- Urinalysis results are positive for protein and leukocytes.

P. falciparum *malaria*

- CBC shows a reduced number of platelets (20,000 to 50,000/µl).
- Prothrombin time is prolonged (18 to 20 seconds).
- Partial thromboplastin time is prolonged (60 to 100 seconds).
- Plasma fibrinogen levels are reduced.

Special considerations for antimalarial drugs

CHLOROQUINE

- Perform baseline and periodic ophthalmologic examinations, and report blurred vision, increased sensitivity to light, and muscle weakness to the practitioner.
- Consult with the practitioner about altering therapy if muscle weakness appears in a patient on long-term therapy.
- Monitor the patient for tinnitus and other signs of ototoxicity, such as nerve deafness and vertigo.
- Caution the patient to avoid excessive exposure to the sun to prevent exacerbating drug-induced dermatoses.

PRIMAQUINE

- Give with meals or antacids.
- Discontinue administration if you observe a sudden fall in hemoglobin concentration or in erythrocyte or leukocyte count, or a marked darkening of the urine, suggesting impending hemolytic reaction.

PYRIMETHAMINE

- Give with meals to minimize GI distress.
- Check blood counts (including platelets) twice a week. If signs of folic or folinic acid deficiency develop, reduce or discontinue dosage while patient receives parenteral folinic acid until blood counts become normal.

QUININE

- Use with caution in patients with cardiovascular conditions, asthma, hemolytic anemia, and granulocytosis.
- Monitor blood pressure frequently while administering quinine I.V. infusion. Rapid administration causes marked hypotension.

TREATMENT

GENERAL
◆ Symptomatic

DIET
◆ Increased fluid intake

ACTIVITY
◆ As tolerated (bed rest during acute phase)

MEDICATIONS
◆ Oral chloroquine (for all forms except those caused by chloroquine-resistant *P. falciparum*)
◆ Oral quinine (for malaria caused by *P. falciparum*) given concurrently with pyrimethamine and a sulfonamide such as sulfadiazine
◆ Primaquine phosphate (for hepatic phase) (see *Special considerations for antimalarial drugs*)
◆ Antipyretics

NURSING CONSIDERATIONS

NURSING DIAGNOSES
◆ Activity intolerance
◆ Acute pain
◆ Anxiety
◆ Decreased cardiac output
◆ Deficient fluid volume
◆ Fatigue
◆ Hyperthermia
◆ Impaired gas exchange
◆ Impaired physical mobility
◆ Impaired skin integrity
◆ Risk for infection
◆ Risk for injury

EXPECTED OUTCOMES
The patient will:
◆ participate in self-care activities as tolerated
◆ report decreased levels or absence of pain
◆ acknowledge fears, feelings, and concerns about the current situation
◆ maintain adequate cardiac output
◆ have adequate fluid volume
◆ report an increased energy level
◆ remain afebrile
◆ maintain adequate ventilation and oxygenation
◆ maintain joint mobility and range of motion
◆ maintain skin integrity
◆ experience no further signs or symptoms of infection
◆ avoid injury and complications.

NURSING INTERVENTIONS
◆ Obtain a detailed patient history.
◆ Follow proper hand-washing and aseptic techniques.
◆ Follow standard precautions.
◆ Record symptom pattern, fever, type of malaria, and systemic signs.
◆ Report all cases of malaria to local public health authorities.

MONITORING
◆ Vital signs
◆ Response to treatment
◆ Intake and output

PATIENT TEACHING

GENERAL
Be sure to cover:
◆ the disorder, diagnosis, and potential for relapse
◆ proper administration of medication and possible adverse effects.

RESOURCES
Organizations
Centers for Disease Control and Prevention: *www.cdc.gov*
Malaria Foundation International: *www.malaria.org*
World Health Organization: *www.who.int*

Selected references
Anand, A.C., and Puri, P. "Jaundice in Malaria," *Journal of Gastroenterology & Hepatology* 20(9):1322-332, September 2005.
Butcher, C.A. "Malaria: A Parasitic Disease," *AAOHN Journal* 52(7):302-309, July 2004.
Riley, E.M., et al. "Regulating Immunity to Malaria," *Parasite Immunology* 28(1-2):35-49, January 2006.

Mastitis

- Inflammation of the breast tissue
- Lactating breast infection
- Good prognosis

PATHOPHYSIOLOGY

- A pathogen (typically originating in nursing infant's nose or pharynx) invades the breast tissue, entering through a fissured or abraded nipple.
- The result is parenchymatous inflammation of the mammary glands, which disrupts normal lactation.
- Systemic manifestations of inflammation may result.

CAUSES

- Disseminated tuberculosis (rare)
- Mumps virus (rare)
- *Staphylococcus aureus* most common pathogen; less frequently, *S. epidermidis* or beta-hemolytic streptococci

RISK FACTORS

- Fissure or abrasion of the nipple
- Blocked milk ducts
- Incomplete letdown reflex
- Tight bra
- Prolonged intervals between breast feedings

INCIDENCE

- Mastitis occurs in about 1% of lactating women.
- It's more common in breast-feeding primiparas.
- It occurs occasionally in nonlactating women.
- Mastitis is rare in men.

COMPLICATIONS

- Abscess

HISTORY

- Fever
- Malaise
- Flulike symptoms
- Tenderness

PHYSICAL FINDINGS

- Nipple abrasion or fissure
- Enlarged axillary lymph nodes
- Red, edematous, warm, and hard involved breast

LABORATORY

- Results of cultures of expressed milk confirm generalized mastitis.
- Results of cultures of breast skin confirm localized mastitis.

Preventing mastitis

To help the patient prevent mastitis from recurring, follow these guidelines:
- Stress to the patient the importance of emptying the breasts completely because milk stasis can cause infection and mastitis.
- Teach the patient to alternate feeding positions and to rotate pressure areas on the nipples.
- Remind the patient to position the infant properly on the breast with the entire areola in his mouth.
- Advise the patient to expose sore nipples to the air as often as possible.
- Teach the patient proper hand-washing technique and personal hygiene.
- Instruct the patient to get plenty of rest and consume sufficient fluids and a balanced diet to enhance breast-feeding.
- Suggest that the patient apply a warm, wet towel to the affected breast or take a warm shower to relax and improve breast-feeding.

TREATMENT

GENERAL
◆ Warm soaks
◆ Avoidance of tight bras and clothing
◆ Continuation of breast-feeding on both breasts to prevent engorgement, with proper infant sucking and changing of feeding positions to drain the milk

MEDICATIONS
◆ Broad-spectrum antibiotics
◆ Analgesics

SURGERY
◆ Breast abscess incision and drainage

NURSING CONSIDERATIONS

NURSING DIAGNOSES
◆ Acute pain
◆ Ineffective breast-feeding
◆ Risk for impaired skin integrity
◆ Risk for infection

EXPECTED OUTCOMES
The patient will:
◆ express feelings of increased comfort
◆ resume breast-feeding without further complications
◆ maintain skin integrity
◆ remain free from signs and symptoms of infection.

NURSING INTERVENTIONS
◆ Give prescribed drugs.
◆ Provide warm soaks.
◆ Use meticulous hand-washing technique.
◆ Provide meticulous skin care.

MONITORING
◆ Signs and symptoms of infection
◆ Abscess development
◆ Breast engorgement
◆ Skin integrity
◆ Breast-feeding process

PATIENT TEACHING

GENERAL
Be sure to cover:
◆ the disorder, diagnosis, and treatment
◆ prescribed antibiotic therapy and potential adverse reactions
◆ reassurance that breast-feeding won't harm the infant because he's the source of the infection
◆ the need to offer the infant the unaffected breast first to promote complete emptying and prevent clogged ducts
◆ the need to stop breast-feeding with abscessed breast
◆ the need to use a breast pump until abscess heals
◆ continuation of breast-feeding on the unaffected side
◆ prevention of mastitis (see *Preventing mastitis*).

DISCHARGE PLANNING
◆ Refer the patient to a lactation specialist, if indicated.

RESOURCES
Organizations
American College of Obstetricians and Gynecologists: *www.acog.org*
La Leche League International: *www.lalecheleague.org*

Selected references
Mass, S. "Breast Pain: Engorgement, Nipple Pain and Mastitis," *Clinical Obstetrics and Gynecology* 47(3):676-82, September 2004.
Potter, B. "A Multi-method Approach to Measuring Mastitis Incidence," *Community Practitioner* 78(5):169-73, May 2005.
Potter, B. "Women's Experiences of Managing Mastitis," *Community Practitioner* 78(6):209-12, June 2005.

Melanoma, malignant

OVERVIEW

- Neoplasm that arises from melanocytes
- Potentially the most lethal of the skin cancers
- Common sites in those exposed to excessive sunlight: head and neck in men, legs in women, and backs in men and women
- Four types:
- Superficial spreading melanoma: Most common type; usually develops between ages 40 and 50
- Nodular melanoma: Grows vertically, invades the dermis, and metastasizes early; usually develops between ages 40 and 50
- Acral lentiginous melanoma: Occurs on the palms and soles and under the tongue; most common among Hispanics, Asians, and Blacks
- Lentigo maligna melanoma: Relatively rare; most benign, slowest growing, and least aggressive of the four types; most commonly occurs in areas heavily exposed to the sun; arises from a lentigo maligna on an exposed skin surface; usually occurs between ages 60 and 70

PATHOPHYSIOLOGY

- Melanomas arise because of malignant degeneration of melanocytes located either along the basal layer of the epidermis or in a benign melanocytic nevus.
- Up to 70% of malignant melanomas arise from a preexisting nevus.
- Malignant melanoma spreads through the lymphatic and vascular systems and metastasizes to the regional lymph nodes, skin, liver, lungs, and central nervous system.
- Malignant melanoma follows an unpredictable course; recurrence and metastasis may not appear for more than 5 years after resection of the primary lesion.

CAUSES

- Skin damage associated with exposure to ultraviolet rays from the sun

RISK FACTORS

- Excessive exposure to sunlight
- Skin type (blond or red hair, fair skin, and blue eyes; prone to sunburn; and Celtic or Scandinavian ancestry)
- Hormonal factors (pregnancy)
- Family history
- Past history of melanoma
- Preexisting pigmented mole or nevus

INCIDENCE

- Malignant melanoma accounts for 1% to 2% of all malignant tumors.
- It's slightly more common in women than in men.
- It's unusual in children.
- Peak incidence occurs between ages 50 and 70, but incidence in younger age groups is increasing.

COMPLICATIONS

- Metastasis to the lungs, liver, or brain

ASSESSMENT

HISTORY

- A sore that doesn't heal, a persistent lump or swelling, or changes in preexisting skin markings, such as moles, birthmarks, scars, freckles, or warts
- Preexisting skin lesion or nevus that enlarges, changes color, becomes inflamed or sore, itches, ulcerates, bleeds, changes texture, or shows signs of surrounding pigment regression

PHYSICAL FINDINGS

- Lesions on the ankles or the inside surfaces of the knees
- Uniformly discolored nodule on knee or ankle
- Small, elevated tumor nodules that may ulcerate and bleed
- Palpable polypoid nodules that resemble the surface of a blackberry
- Pigmented lesions on the palms and soles or under the nails
- Long-standing lesion that has ulcerated
- Flat nodule with smaller nodules scattered over the surface

DIAGNOSTIC TEST RESULTS

LABORATORY

- Complete blood count (CBC) with differential shows anemia.
- Erythrocyte sedimentation rate is elevated.
- Platelet count is abnormal if metastasis has occurred.
- Liver function study results are abnormal, if metastasis has occurred.

IMAGING

- Chest X-rays assist in disease staging.

DIAGNOSTIC PROCEDURES

- The results of excisional biopsy and full-depth punch biopsy with histologic examination can show tumor thickness and disease stage.

GENERAL
- Close long-term follow-up care to detect metastases and recurrences
- Radiation therapy (usually for metastatic disease)
- Avoidance of sun exposure

DIET
- Well-balanced

MEDICATIONS
- Chemotherapy
- Biotherapy
- Immunotherapy
- Immunostimulants

SURGERY
- Surgical resection to remove tumor and 3-cm to 5-cm margin
- Regional lymphadenectomy

NURSING CONSIDERATIONS

NURSING DIAGNOSES
- Acute pain
- Anticipatory grieving
- Anxiety
- Disturbed body image
- Fear
- Imbalanced nutrition: Less than body requirements
- Impaired skin integrity
- Ineffective coping
- Risk for infection

EXPECTED OUTCOMES
The patient will:
- express feelings of increased comfort
- verbalize problems associated with grief
- express feelings of decreased anxiety
- express positive feelings about self-image
- verbalize fears and concerns associated with the diagnosis and condition
- maintain weight within an acceptable range
- experience healing of wound without signs of infection

- demonstrate effective coping mechanisms
- remain free from signs and symptoms of infection.

NURSING INTERVENTIONS
- Encourage verbalization and provide support.
- Provide appropriate wound care.
- Give prescribed drugs.
- Provide a high-protein, high-calorie diet.

MONITORING
- Complications of treatment
- Pain control
- Wound site
- Postoperative complications

PATIENT TEACHING

GENERAL
Be sure to cover:
- the disorder, diagnosis, and treatment
- preoperative and postoperative care
- the need for close follow-up care to detect recurrences early
- signs and symptoms of recurrence
- detrimental effects of overexposure to solar radiation and benefits of regular use of a sunblock or a sunscreen and protective clothing.

DISCHARGE PLANNING
- Refer the patient to available resources and support services.

RESOURCES
Organizations
American Cancer Society:
www.cancer.org
Guide to Internet Resources for Cancer:
www.cancerindex.org
National Cancer Institute:
www.cancer.gov
The Melanoma Research Foundation:
www.melanoma.org

Selected references
Atlas of Pathophysiology, 2nd ed. Philadelphia: Lippincott Williams & Wilkins, 2005.

Casciato, D.A. *Manual of Clinical Oncology,* 5th ed. Philadelphia: Lippincott Williams & Wilkins, 2004.

Christopoulou, A., et al. "Integration of Gamma Knife Surgery in the Management of Cerebral Metastases from Melanoma," *Melanoma Research* 16(1):51-57, February 2006.

Demierre, M.F., et al. "New Treatments for Melanoma," *Dermatology Nursing* 17(4):287-95, August 2005.

Lee, D.A., et al. "Are All Melanomas the Same? Spitzoid Melanoma is a Distinct Subtype of Melanoma," *Cancer* 106(4):907-13, February 2006.

Niendorf, K.B., and Tsao, H. "Cutaneous Melanoma: Family Screening and Genetic Testing," *Dermatologic Therapy* 19(1):1-8, January-February 2006.

Ménière's disease

OVERVIEW

- Inner ear disease that results from a labyrinthine dysfunction
- Causes severe vertigo, sensorineural hearing loss, and tinnitus
- Usually involves only one ear
- Possible incapacitating residual tinnitus and hearing loss after multiple attacks over several years
- Also known as *endolymphatic hydrops*

PATHOPHYSIOLOGY

- Ménière's disease may result from overproduction or decreased absorption of endolymph — the fluid contained in the labyrinth of the ear.
- Accumulated endolymph dilates the semicircular canals, utricle, and saccule and causes degeneration of the vestibular and cochlear hair cells.
- Overstimulation of the vestibular branch of cranial nerve VIII impairs postural reflexes and stimulates the vomiting reflex. (See *Normal vestibular function.*)
- Perception of sound is impaired as a result of this excessive cranial nerve stimulation, and injury to sensory receptors for hearing may affect auditory acuity.

CAUSES

- Unknown

RISK FACTORS

- Autonomic nervous system dysfunction
- Family history
- Head trauma
- Immune disorder
- Middle ear infection
- Migraine headaches
- Premenstrual edema

  WARNING *In some women, premenstrual edema may precipitate outbreaks of Ménière's disease.*

INCIDENCE

- Ménière's disease usually affects adults between ages 30 and 60; it's rare in children.
- It's slightly more common in men than in women.

COMPLICATIONS

- Continued tinnitus
- Hearing loss
- Injury

ASSESSMENT

HISTORY

- Vertigo
- Nausea
- Tinnitus
- Falls

PHYSICAL FINDINGS

- Inability to maintain upright posture
- Unsteady gait
- Diplopia
- Hypotension

DIAGNOSTIC TEST RESULTS

IMAGING

- Computed tomography and magnetic resonance imaging are used to rule out acoustic neuroma as a cause of symptoms.

DIAGNOSTIC PROCEDURES

- Audiometric test results show a sensorineural hearing loss and a loss of discrimination and recruitment.
- Electronystagmography results show normal or reduced vestibular response on the affected side.
- Cold caloric test results show impairment of the oculovestibular reflex.
- Electrocochleography results show an increased ratio of summating potential to action potential.
- Brain stem evoked response audiometry test is used to rule out acoustic neuroma, brain tumor, and vascular lesions in the brain stem.

OTHER

- Patient history may reveal a family history of the disorder.

Normal vestibular function

The three semicircular canals and the vestibule of the inner ear are responsible for equilibrium and balance. Each of the semicircular canals lies at a 90-degree angle to the others. Head movement in one direction causes the endolymph inside each semicircular canal to move in the opposite direction and causes vestibular otoliths (crystals of calcium salts) to shift in their gel medium. This movement stimulates hair cells, sending electrical impulses to the brain through the vestibular portion of cranial nerve VIII. Together, these organs help detect the body's present position as well as any change in its direction or motion.

TREATMENT

ACTIVITY
- Lying down to minimize head movement, and avoiding sudden movements and glaring lights to reduce dizziness (during an attack)

MEDICATIONS
For short-term management
- Promethazine (Phenergan) or prochlorperazine (Compazine)
- Atropine
- Dimenhydrinate (Dramamine)
- Central nervous system depressants, such as lorazepam (Ativan) or diazepam (Valium)
- Antihistamines, such as meclizine (Antivert) or diphenhydramine (Benadryl)

For long-term management
- Diuretics
- Betahistine dihydrochloride
- Vasodilators
- Sodium restriction
- Antihistamines or mild sedatives
- Systemic streptomycin (chemical ablation)

SURGERY
- Endolymphatic drainage and shunt procedures
- Vestibular nerve resection
- Labyrinthectomy
- Cochlear implantation

NURSING CONSIDERATIONS

NURSING DIAGNOSES
- Acute pain
- Anxiety
- Deficient fluid volume
- Disturbed sensory perception: Auditory
- Fear
- Hopelessness
- Imbalanced nutrition: More than body requirements
- Ineffective coping
- Powerlessness
- Risk for falls
- Risk for injury

EXPECTED OUTCOMES
The patient will:
- express feelings of increased comfort
- identify strategies to reduce anxiety
- maintain adequate fluid balance
- regain hearing or develop other means of communication
- express fears and concerns
- participate in decisions about care
- identify appropriate food choices according to a prescribed diet
- seek appropriate support to assist with coping
- express feelings of control over well-being
- identify strategies to safeguard home environment to prevent falls
- avoid injury.

NURSING INTERVENTIONS
- Maintain a safe environment; provide assistance when necessary.
- Give prescribed drugs.

MONITORING
- Intake and output
- Frequency of attacks
- Response to treatment

PATIENT TEACHING

GENERAL
Be sure to cover:
- the need to avoid reading and exposure to glaring lights, to reduce dizziness
- the need to avoid sudden position changes and any tasks that vertigo makes hazardous.

RESOURCES
Organizations
Ménière's Disease Information Center: *www.menieresinfo.com*
Menieres.org: *www.menieres.org*
National Institute on Deafness and Other Communication Disorders: *www.nidcd.nih.gov*

Selected references
Ervin, S.E. "Ménière's Disease: Identifying Classic Symptoms and Current Treatments," *AAOHN Journal* 52(4):156-58, April 2004.
Gottshall, K.R., et al. "The Role of Vestibular Rehabilitation in the Treatment of Ménière's Disease," *Otolaryngology — Head and Neck Surgery* 133(3):326-28, September 2005.
Strupp, M, and Brandt, T. "Pharmacological Advances in the Treatment of Neuro-otological and Eye Movement Disorders," *Current Opinion in Neurology* 19(1):33-40, February 2006.

Meningitis LIFE-THREATENING DISORDER

OVERVIEW

- Inflammation of brain and spinal cord meninges
- May affect all three meningeal membranes (dura mater, arachnoid membrane, and pia mater)
- Usually follows onset of respiratory symptoms
- Sudden onset, causing serious illness within 24 hours
- Prognosis good; complications rare
- Bacterial meningitis: acute infection in the subarachnoid space

 AGE FACTOR *Prognosis is poor for infants and elderly people.*

PATHOPHYSIOLOGY

- Inflammation of pia-arachnoid and subarachnoid space progresses to congestion of adjacent tissues.
- Nerve cells are destroyed.
- Intracranial pressure (ICP) increases because of exudates.
- Results can include:
- – engorged blood vessels
- – disrupted blood supply
- – edema of the brain tissue
- – thrombosis
- – rupture
- – acute hydrocephalus.

CAUSES

- Bacterial infection, usually with *Neisseria meningitidis* and *Streptococcus pneumoniae* (Before the 1990s, *Haemophilus influenzae* type b [Hib] was the leading cause of bacterial meningitis. However, new vaccines have reduced its occurrence in children.)
- Fungal infection
- Protozoal infection
- Secondary to another bacterial infection such as pneumonia
- Skull fracture, penetrating head wound, lumbar puncture, or ventricular shunting procedures
- Viral infection

INCIDENCE

- Infants, children, and elderly people are at highest risk for meningitis.
- It's an increasing threat to college students.

COMPLICATIONS

- Visual impairment, optic neuritis
- Cranial nerve palsies
- Deafness
- Paresis or paralysis
- Endocarditis
- Coma
- Vasculitis
- Cerebral infarction
- Seizures

ASSESSMENT

HISTORY

- Headache
- Fever
- Nausea, vomiting
- Weakness
- Myalgia
- Photophobia
- Confusion, delirium
- Seizures

PHYSICAL FINDINGS

- Meningismus
- Rigors
- Profuse sweating
- Kernig's and Brudzinski's signs (elicited in only 50% of adults)
- Declining level of consciousness (LOC)
- Cranial nerve palsies
- Rash (with meningococcemia)
- Focal neurologic deficits such as visual field defects
- Signs of increased ICP (in later stages)

AGE FACTOR *Meningismus and fever are commonly absent in neonates, and the only clinical clues may be nonspecific, such as refusal to feed, high-pitched cry, and irritability.*

AGE FACTOR *Elderly patients may experience an insidious onset, exhibiting lethargy and variable signs of meningismus and no fever.*

DIAGNOSTIC TEST RESULTS

LABORATORY

- White blood cell count shows leukocytosis.
- Blood cultures are positive in bacterial meningitis, depending on the pathogen.
- Coagglutination test results reveal the causative agent.

IMAGING

- Chest X-rays may reveal a coexisting pneumonia.
- Neuroimaging techniques, such as computed tomography and magnetic resonance imaging, may detect complications and a parameningeal source of infection.

DIAGNOSTIC PROCEDURES

- Lumbar puncture and cerebrospinal fluid (CSF) analysis show:
- – increased opening pressure (due to inflammation)
- – neutrophilic pleocytosis
- – elevated protein level
- – hypoglycorrhachia
- – positive Gram stain
- – positive culture
- – decreased glucose level (CSF is milky or cloudy).

TREATMENT

GENERAL
- Fever reduction
- Fluid therapy
- Pain control

ACTIVITY
- Bed rest (in acute phase)

MEDICATIONS
- I.V. antibiotics
- Oral antibiotics
- Antiarrhythmics
- Osmotic diuretics
- Anticonvulsants
- Aspirin or acetaminophen

NURSING CONSIDERATIONS

NURSING DIAGNOSES
- Acute pain
- Anxiety
- Hyperthermia
- Impaired gas exchange
- Risk for deficient fluid volume
- Risk for impaired skin integrity

EXPECTED OUTCOMES
The patient will:
- express feelings of increased comfort and pain relief
- identify strategies to reduce anxiety
- have a normal body temperature
- maintain adequate ventilation
- maintain normal fluid volume
- maintain skin integrity.

NURSING INTERVENTIONS
- Follow standard precautions.
- Maintain respiratory isolation for the first 24 hours (with meningococcal meningitis).
- Give prescribed oxygen.
- Position the patient in proper body alignment.
- Encourage active range-of-motion (ROM) exercises when appropriate.
- Provide passive ROM exercises when appropriate.
- Maintain adequate nutrition.
- Give prescribed laxatives or stool softeners.
- Provide meticulous skin and mouth care.
- Give prescribed drugs.

MONITORING
- Neurologic status
- Vital signs
- Signs and symptoms of cranial nerve involvement
- Signs and symptoms of increased ICP
- LOC
- Seizures
- Respiratory status
- Arterial blood gas results
- Fluid balance
- Response to medications
- Complications

PATIENT TEACHING

GENERAL
Be sure to cover:
- the disorder, diagnosis, and treatment
- contagion risks for close contacts
- medication regimen
- adverse drug effects
- signs and symptoms of meningitis
- exercise to promote muscle strength and mobility
- polysaccharide meningococcal vaccine, pneumococcal vaccine, and Hib vaccine.

DISCHARGE PLANNING
- Refer the patient to community resources.

RESOURCES
Organizations
Mayo Foundation for Medical Education and Research: *www.mayoclinic.com*
Meningitis Research Foundation: *www.meningitis.org*
National Institutes of Health: *www.nih.gov*
WebMD: *www.webmd.com*

Selected references
Diseases, 4th ed. Philadelphia: Lippincott Williams & Wilkins, 2006.
Estep, M. "Meningococcal Meningitis in Critical Care: An Overview, New Treatments/Preventions, and a Case Study," *Critical Care Nursing Quarterly* 28(2):111-21, April-June 2005.
Handbook of Pathophysiology, 2nd ed. Philadelphia: Lippincott Williams & Wilkins, 2005.
Harrison, L.H. "Prospects for Vaccine Prevention of Meningococcal Infection," *Clinical Microbiology Reviews* 19(1):142-64, January 2006.
Snyder, C.H. "Coccidioidal Meningitis Presenting as Memory Loss," *Journal of the American Academy of Nurse Practitioners* 17(5):181-16, May 2005.

Mesotheliomas

- Originate in the serosal lining of the pleural cavity
- Account for less than 10% of all cancer-related deaths
- Latency period ranging from 20 to 45 years from environmental exposure to tumor discovery
- Typically, less than a 2-year period between the onset of symptoms and death
- Invariably fatal

PATHOPHYSIOLOGY

- It's unknown whether mesotheliomas begin in the visceral or parietal pleura; in animals, tumor-causing asbestos fibers migrate to mesothelial cells, penetrating the pleura.
- From there, the pleural lymphatics carry the mesothelial cells to the pleural surface.
- Signs and symptoms result from pleural effusion, restricted lung function, tumor mass, infection, and advanced disease.

CAUSES

- Asbestos exposure link well established
- Predisposition, chronic inflammation, radiation, and recurrent lung infection seldom involved

RISK FACTORS

- Asbestos exposure
- Smoking coupled with asbestos exposure (about a 50% increased risk)

INCIDENCE

- The incidence of mesotheliomas is high in asbestos workers and their immediate families.
- Incidence is high among people who live along major routes used for transporting large quantities of asbestos.
- The disease usually occurs in people older than age 50.

COMPLICATIONS

- Severe dyspnea
- Infection
- Complications of immobility such as skin breakdown

ASSESSMENT

HISTORY

- Asbestos exposure at some time in the patient's life
- Chief complaints possibly chest pain and dyspnea
- Other complaints of cough, hoarseness, anorexia, weight loss, weakness, and fatigue

PHYSICAL FINDINGS

- Elevated temperature
- Shortness of breath
- Finger clubbing
- Dullness over lung fields on chest percussion
- Diminished chest sounds on auscultation

DIAGNOSTIC TEST RESULTS

LABORATORY

- Histologic study of pleural biopsy specimen confirms the diagnosis.

IMAGING

- Chest X-rays exhibit nodular, irregular, unilateral pleural thickening and varying degrees of unilateral pleural effusion.
- Results of a computed tomography scan of the chest define the extent of the tumor.

DIAGNOSTIC PROCEDURES

- Open pleural biopsy is necessary to obtain a specimen for histologic analysis.

TREATMENT

GENERAL

- No standard treatment
- Surgery, radiation therapy, chemotherapy, and a combination of treatments (usually tried but seldom control the disease in most patients)

MEDICATIONS

- Chemotherapeutic drugs (cisplatin-mitomycin combinations most successful)
- Doxorubicin and methotrexate (less successful)

SURGERY

- Pleuropneumonectomy

NURSING DIAGNOSES

- Acute pain
- Anxiety
- Excess fluid volume
- Fatigue
- Hopelessness
- Impaired gas exchange
- Impaired physical mobility
- Impaired skin integrity
- Ineffective airway clearance
- Ineffective breathing pattern
- Risk for infection

EXPECTED OUTCOMES

The patient will:

- express feelings of comfort and decreased pain
- express that he feels less anxious
- maintain normal fluid volume
- carry out activities of daily living without weakness or fatigue
- begin to make decisions on his own behalf
- maintain adequate ventilation
- maintain muscle strength and joint range of motion
- maintain skin integrity
- maintain a patent airway
- maintain an effective breathing pattern
- remain free from signs or symptoms of infection.

NURSING INTERVENTIONS

- Listen to the patient's fears and concerns. Give clear, concise explanations of all procedures and actions, and remain with him during periods of severe anxiety.
- Encourage the patient to identify actions that promote comfort. Then be sure to perform them and to encourage the patient and family to help.
- Include the patient in decisions related to his care whenever possible.
- Give ordered pain medication as required. Monitor and document the medication's effectiveness.
- Perform comfort measures, such as repositioning and assisting with relaxation techniques.
- Monitor respiratory status. Provide oxygen as ordered, and assist the patient to a comfortable position (Fowler's position, for example) that allows for maximal chest expansion to relieve respiratory distress.
- If mobility decreases, turn the patient frequently. Provide skin care, particularly over bony prominences. Encourage him to be as active as possible.
- Prevent infection. Adhere to strict aseptic technique when suctioning the patient, changing dressings or I.V. tubing, and performing any type of invasive procedure.

MONITORING

- Body temperature
- White blood cell count
- I.V. fluid intake
- Treatment complications
- Laboratory studies
- Vital signs

GENERAL

Be sure to cover:

- how to perform relaxation techniques
- breathing and positioning variations to ease the dyspnea associated with progressive disease
- all procedures and treatments
- measures (such as increasing fluid intake) to minimize adverse effects of treatment
- procedures to maximize breathing and prevent the complications of immobility
- how to practice meticulous hand washing and aseptic techniques to avoid infection.

DISCHARGE PLANNING

- Refer the patient to the social services department, support groups, and community or professional mental health resources to help him and his family cope with terminal illness.

RESOURCES

Organizations

Lung Cancer & Mesothelioma: *www.mesothelioma-lung-cancer.org*
Memorial Sloan-Kettering Cancer Center: *www.mskcc.org*
Mesothelioma Web: *www.mesotheliomaweb.org*

Selected references

Dunleavey, R. "Malignant Mesothelioma: Risk Factors and Current Management," *Nursing Times* 100(16):40-43, April 2004.

Munoz, A., et al. "Malignant Mesothelioma," *New England Journal of Medicine* 354(3):305-307, January 2006.

Orbaugh, K.K. "Nursing Considerations for Administering Pemetrexed (Alimta) in Combination with Cisplatin for Malignant Pleural Mesothelioma," *Clinical Journal of Oncology Nursing* 8(3):242-47, June 2004.

Metabolic syndrome

OVERVIEW

- A cluster of symptoms triggered by insulin resistance: abdominal fat; obesity; high blood pressure; and high levels of blood glucose, triglycerides, and cholesterol
- Associated with increased risk of diabetes, heart disease, and stroke
- Often unrecognized
- Also known as *syndrome X, insulin resistance syndrome, dysmetabolic syndrome*, and *multiple metabolic syndrome*

PATHOPHYSIOLOGY

- The body breaks food down into basic components, one of which is glucose.
- Glucose provides energy for cellular activity.
- Excess glucose is stored in cells for future use. It's guided into storage cells by insulin, which is secreted by the pancreas.
- In those with metabolic syndrome, glucose doesn't respond to insulin's attempt to guide it into storage cells. This is called insulin resistance.
- To overcome this resistance, the pancreas produces excess insulin, which causes damage to arterial lining.
- Excessive insulin secretion also promotes fat storage deposits and prevents fat breakdown.
- This series of events can lead to diabetes, blood clots, and coronary events.

CAUSES

- Acquired factors (see "Risk factors")
- Genetic predisposition

RISK FACTORS

- Obesity
- High fat, high-carbohydrate diet
- Insufficient physical activity
- Aging
- Hyperinsulinemia/impaired glucose tolerance
- Previous heart attack

INCIDENCE

- Metabolic syndrome affects an estimated 47 million people in the United States.
- It's most common in Mexican Americans (highest rate at 32%).
- In Black and Mexican-American individuals, women are more susceptible than men; otherwise, men and women are equally affected.

COMPLICATIONS

- Coronary artery disease
- Diabetes
- Hyperlipidemia
- Premature death

ASSESSMENT

HISTORY

- Familial history
- Hypertension
- High low-density lipoprotein (LDL) and triglyceride levels
- Low high-density lipoprotein (HDL) levels
- Abdominal obesity
- Sedentary lifestyle
- Poor diet

PHYSICAL FINDINGS

- Abdominal obesity (see *Why abdominal obesity is dangerous*)

DIAGNOSTIC TEST RESULTS

LABORATORY

- Glucose level is elevated.
- LDL and triglyceride levels are increased.
- HDL level is decreased.
- Blood tests show hyperinsulinemia.
- Serum uric acid level is elevated.

OTHER

- Blood pressure is greater than 130/85 mm Hg.

Why abdominal obesity is dangerous

People with excess weight around the waist have a greater risk of developing metabolic syndrome than people with excess weight around the hips. That's because intra-abdominal fat tends to be more resistant to insulin than fat in other areas of the body. Insulin resistance increases the release of free fatty acid into the portal system, leading to increased apolipoprotein B, increased low-density lipoprotein, decreased high-density lipoprotein, and increased triglyceride levels. As a result, the risk of cardiovascular disease increases.

TREATMENT

GENERAL
◆ Weight-reduction program

DIET
◆ Low alcohol intake
◆ Low-cholesterol
◆ High in complex carbohydrates (grains, beans, vegetables, fruit) and low in refined carbohydrates (soda, table sugar, high-fructose corn syrup)

ACTIVITY
◆ Daily physical activity of at least 20 minutes

MEDICATIONS
◆ Oral antidiabetic agents
◆ Antihypertensives
◆ Statins

NURSING CONSIDERATIONS

NURSING DIAGNOSES
◆ Fatigue
◆ Imbalanced nutrition: More than body requirements
◆ Risk for injury

EXPECTED OUTCOMES
The patient will:
◆ express feelings of increased energy
◆ identify appropriate food choices according to a prescribed diet and maintain a healthy weight
◆ avoid complications associated with the disorder.

NURSING INTERVENTIONS
◆ Promote lifestyle changes and give appropriate support.

MONITORING
◆ Blood pressure
◆ Ordered laboratory tests

PATIENT TEACHING

GENERAL
Be sure to cover:
◆ the disorder, diagnosis, and treatment
◆ principles of a healthy diet
◆ relationship of diet, inactivity, and obesity to metabolic syndrome
◆ benefits of increased physical activity
◆ prescribed medication, administration, and possible adverse reactions.

RESOURCES
Organizations
American Diabetes Association: *www.diabetes.org*
American Heart Association: *www.americanheart.org*
Cleveland Clinic Health Information Center: *www.clevelandclinic.org/health*

Selected references
Appel, S.J. "Sizing Up Patients for Metabolic Syndrome," *Nursing* 35(12):20-21, December 2005.
Bell-Anderson, K., and Samman, S. "Nutrition and Metabolism: Race, Sex and the Metabolic Syndrome," *Current Opinion in Lipidology* 17(1):82-84, February 2006.
Fowler, S.B., et al. "Metabolic Syndrome: Contributing Factors and Treatment Strategies," *Journal of Neuroscience Nursing* 37(4):220-23, August 2003.
Venkatapuram, S., and Shannon, R.P. "Managing Atherosclerosis in Patients with Type 2 Diabetes and Metabolic Syndrome," *American Journal of Therapeutics* 13(1):64-71, January-February 2006.

Methicillin-resistant *Staphylococcus aureus*

OVERVIEW

- A mutation of a very common bacterium easily spread by direct person-to-person contact
- Also known as *MRSA*

PATHOPHYSIOLOGY

- 90% of *Staphylococcus aureus* isolates or strains are penicillin-resistant, and about 27% of all *S. aureus* isolates are resistant to methicillin, a penicillin derivative. These strains may also resist cephalosporins, aminoglycosides, erythromycin, tetracycline, and clindamycin.
- When natural defense systems break down (after invasive procedures, trauma, or chemotherapy), the usually benign bacteria can invade tissue, proliferate, and cause infection.
- The most frequent colonization site is the anterior nares (40% of adults and most children become transient nasal carriers). The groin, armpits, and intestines are less common colonization sites.

CAUSES

- MRSA that enters a health care facility through an infected or colonized patient (symptom-free carrier of the bacteria) or colonized health care worker
- Transmission of bacteria mainly by health care workers' hands

RISK FACTORS

- Immunosuppression
- Prolonged facility stays
- Extended therapy with multiple or broad-spectrum antibiotics
- Proximity to others colonized or infected with MRSA

INCIDENCE

- MRSA is endemic in nursing homes, long-term care facilities, and community facilities.

COMPLICATIONS

- Sepsis
- Death

ASSESSMENT

HISTORY

- Possible risk factors for MRSA
- Carrier patient commonly asymptomatic

PHYSICAL FINDINGS

- Signs and symptoms related to the primary diagnosis (respiratory, cardiac, or other major system symptoms) in symptomatic patients

DIAGNOSTIC TEST RESULTS

LABORATORY

- Results of cultures from suspicious wounds, skin, urine, or blood show MRSA.

TREATMENT

GENERAL
- Transmission precautions: Contact isolation for wound, skin, and urine infection; respiratory isolation for sputum infection
- No treatment needed for patients with colonization only

DIET
- High-protein

ACTIVITY
- Rest periods as needed

MEDICATIONS
- Linezolid (Zyvox)

NURSING CONSIDERATIONS

NURSING DIAGNOSES
- Acute pain
- Decreased cardiac output
- Deficient fluid volume
- Hyperthermia
- Impaired gas exchange
- Impaired tissue integrity
- Ineffective tissue perfusion: Cardiopulmonary

EXPECTED OUTCOMES
The patient will:
- express feelings of comfort and decreased pain
- maintain adequate cardiac output
- have an adequate fluid volume
- remain afebrile
- maintain adequate ventilation and oxygenation
- have wounds that remain free from infection
- attain hemodynamic stability and maintain collateral circulation.

NURSING INTERVENTIONS
- Provide emotional support to the patient and family members.
- Consider grouping infected patients together and having the same nursing staff care for them.
- Use proper hand-washing technique.
- Use contact precautions and standard precautions.

MONITORING
- Vital signs
- Culture results
- Response to treatment
- Adverse drug reactions
- Complications

PATIENT TEACHING

GENERAL
Be sure to cover:
- the disorder, diagnosis, and treatment
- the difference between MRSA infection and colonization
- prevention of MRSA spread
- proper hand-washing technique
- the need for family and friends to wear protective garb (and to dispose of it properly) when they visit the patient
- medication administration, dosage, and possible adverse effects
- the need to take antibiotics for the full prescription period, even if the patient begins to feel better.

DISCHARGE PLANNING
- Refer the patient to an infectious disease specialist, if indicated.

RESOURCES
Organizations
Centers for Disease Control and Prevention: *www.cdc.gov*
Harvard University Consumer Health Information: *www.intelihealth.com*
National Health Information Center: *www.health.gov/nhic*
National Library of Medicine: *www.nlm.nih.gov*

Selected references
Cowan, T. "A Victory Against MRSA," *Journal of Wound Care* 14(8):372, September 2005.
Kasper, D.L., et al., eds. *Harrison's Principles of Internal Medicine*, 16th ed. New York: McGraw-Hill Book Co., 2005.
Mylotte, J.M. "Nursing Home-acquired Bloodstream Infection," *Infection Control and Hospital Epidemiology* 26(10):833-37, October 2005.
Ott, M., et al. "Evidence-based Practice for Control of Methicillin-resistant Staphylococcus aureus," *AORN Journal* 81(2):361-64, 367-72, February 2005.

Mitral stenosis

OVERVIEW

- Narrowing of the mitral valve orifice, which is normally 3 to 6 cm
- Mild mitral stenosis: Valve orifice of 2 cm
- Moderate mitral stenosis: Valve orifice between 1 and 2 cm
- Severe mitral stenosis: Valve orifice of 1 cm

PATHOPHYSIOLOGY

- Valve leaflets become diffusely thickened by fibrosis and calcification.
- The mitral commissures and the chordae tendineae fuse and shorten, the valvular cusps become rigid, and the valve's apex becomes narrowed.
- This obstructs blood flow from the left atrium to the left ventricle, resulting in incomplete emptying.
- Left atrial volume and pressure increase, and the atrial chamber dilates.
- Increased resistance to blood flow causes pulmonary hypertension, right ventricular hypertrophy, and eventually, right-sided heart failure and reduced cardiac output.

CAUSES

- Atrial myxoma
- Congenital anomalies
- Endocarditis
- Fenfluramine and phentermine combination (Fen-phen diet drug) adverse effects
- Rheumatic fever

INCIDENCE

- Two-thirds of all patients with mitral stenosis are female.
- It occurs in approximately 40% of patients with rheumatic heart disease.

COMPLICATIONS

- Cardiac arrhythmias, especially atrial fibrillation
- Thromboembolism

ASSESSMENT

HISTORY
Mild mitral stenosis
- Asymptomatic

Moderate to severe mitral stenosis
- Gradual decline in exercise tolerance
- Dyspnea on exertion, shortness of breath
- Paroxysmal nocturnal dyspnea
- Orthopnea
- Weakness
- Fatigue
- Palpitations
- Cough

PHYSICAL FINDINGS

- Hemoptysis
- Peripheral and facial cyanosis
- Malar rash
- Jugular vein distention
- Ascites
- Peripheral edema
- Hepatomegaly
- A loud S_1 or opening snap
- A diastolic murmur at the apex (see *Identifying the murmur of mitral stenosis*)
- Crackles over lung fields
- Right ventricular lift
- Resting tachycardia; irregularly irregular heart rhythm

Identifying the murmur of mitral stenosis

A low, rumbling crescendo-decrescendo murmur in the mitral valve area characterizes mitral stenosis.

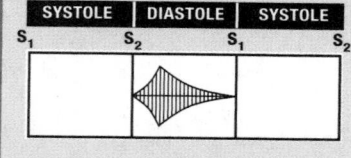

DIAGNOSTIC TEST RESULTS

IMAGING

- Chest X-rays show left atrial and ventricular enlargement (in severe mitral stenosis), straightening of the left border of the cardiac silhouette, enlarged pulmonary arteries, dilation of the upper lobe pulmonary veins, and mitral valve calcification.
- Echocardiography results disclose thickened mitral valve leaflets and left atrial enlargement.

DIAGNOSTIC PROCEDURES

- Cardiac catheterization results show a diastolic pressure gradient across the valve, elevated pulmonary artery wedge pressure (greater than 15 mm Hg), and pulmonary artery pressure in the left atrium with severe pulmonary hypertension.
- Electrocardiography results reveal left atrial enlargement, right ventricular hypertrophy, right axis deviation, and (in 40% to 50% of cases) atrial fibrillation.

TREATMENT

GENERAL

- Synchronized electrical cardioversion to correct atrial fibrillation

DIET

- Sodium-restricted

ACTIVITY

- As tolerated

MEDICATIONS

- Digoxin (Lanoxin)
- Diuretics
- Oxygen
- Beta-adrenergic blockers
- Calcium channel blockers
- Anticoagulants
- Infective endocarditis antibiotic prophylaxis
- Nitrates

SURGERY

- Commissurotomy or valve replacement
- Percutaneous balloon valvuloplasty

NURSING CONSIDERATIONS

NURSING DIAGNOSES

- Activity intolerance
- Decreased cardiac output
- Excess fluid volume
- Fatigue
- Impaired gas exchange
- Impaired physical mobility
- Ineffective coping
- Ineffective role performance
- Ineffective tissue perfusion: Cardiopulmonary
- Risk for infection

EXPECTED OUTCOMES

The patient will:
- carry out activities of daily living without weakness or fatigue
- maintain hemodynamic stability and adequate cardiac output, and have no arrhythmias
- experience no complications from fluid excess
- verbalize the importance of balancing activity with adequate rest periods
- maintain adequate ventilation and oxygenation
- maintain joint mobility and muscle strength
- exhibit adequate coping mechanisms
- express feelings about diminished capacity to perform usual roles
- maintain adequate cardiopulmonary perfusion
- remain free from signs and symptoms of infection.

NURSING INTERVENTIONS

- Check for hypersensitivity reaction to antibiotics.
- Stress the importance of bed rest, if needed.
- Provide a bedside commode.
- Allow the patient to express concerns over his inability to meet responsibilities because of activity restrictions.

- Place the patient in an upright position to relieve dyspnea, if needed.
- Provide a low-sodium diet.

MONITORING

- Vital signs and hemodynamics
- Intake and output
- Signs and symptoms of heart failure and pulmonary edema
- Signs and symptoms of thromboembolism
- Adverse drug reactions
- Cardiac arrhythmias
- Hypotension, arrhythmias, and thrombus formation postoperatively

PATIENT TEACHING

GENERAL

Be sure to cover:
- the disorder, diagnosis, and treatment
- the need to plan for periodic rest in daily routine
- how to take the pulse
- dietary restrictions
- prescribed medications and potential adverse effects
- signs and symptoms to report
- the importance of consistent follow-up care
- when to notify the practitioner
- the need to use prophylactic antibiotics for invasive procedures such as dental work.

RESOURCES
Organizations

American Heart Association: *www.americanheart.org*
Cleveland Clinic Health Information Center: *www.clevelandclinic.org/health*
HeartCenterOnline: *www.heart.healthcentersonline.com*
Mayo Foundation for Medical Education and Research: *www.mayoclinic.com*
National Institutes of Health: *www.nih.gov*

Selected references

Kasper, D.L., et al., eds. *Harrison's Principles of Internal Medicine*, 16th ed. New York: McGraw-Hill Book Co., 2005.
The Merck Manual of Diagnosis & Therapy, 18th ed. Whitehouse Station N.J.: Merck & Co., Inc., 2006.
Sebag, I.A., et al. "Usefulness of Three-dimensionally Guided Assessment of Mitral Stenosis Using Matrix-Array Ultrasound," *American Journal of Cardiology* 96(8):1151-156, October 2005.
Todd, B.A., and Higgins, K. "Recognizing Aortic and Mitral Valve Disease," *Nursing* 35(6):58-63, June 2005.

Mitral valve insufficiency

OVERVIEW

- Valvular disease of the mitral valve that allows the backflow of blood from the left ventricle to the left atrium
- May be acute (sudden volume overload of the left ventricle), chronic compensated (left ventricle compensates and left ventricular enlargement occurs), or chronic decompensated (left ventricle unable to sustain forward cardiac output)
- Also known as *mitral regurgitation*

PATHOPHYSIOLOGY

- Blood from the left ventricle flows back into the left atrium during systole, causing the atrium to enlarge to accommodate the backflow.
- As a result, the left ventricle dilates to accommodate the increased volume of blood from the atrium and to compensate for diminishing cardiac output.
- Ventricular hypertrophy and increased end-diastolic pressure result in increased pulmonary artery pressure, eventually leading to left- and right-sided heart failure.

CAUSES

- Hypertrophic cardiomyopathy
- Infective endocarditis
- Mitral valve prolapse
- Myocardial infarction
- Rheumatic fever
- Ruptured chordae tendineae
- Scleroderma
- Severe left-sided heart failure
- Systemic lupus erythematosus
- Trauma

RISK FACTORS

- Congenital anomalies such as transposition of the great arteries

INCIDENCE

- Mitral valve insufficiency can occur at any age.
- It affects both sexes equally.

COMPLICATIONS

- Heart failure
- Pulmonary edema
- Thromboembolism
- Endocarditis
- Arrhythmias

ASSESSMENT

HISTORY

- Causal occurrence
- Orthopnea
- Dyspnea
- Fatigue
- Angina
- Palpitations

PHYSICAL FINDINGS

- Tachycardia
- Crackles in the lungs
- Hepatomegaly (right-sided failure)
- Holosystolic murmur at the apex (see *Identifying the murmur of mitral valve insufficiency*)
- Possible split S_2
- S_3

DIAGNOSTIC TEST RESULTS

IMAGING

- Chest X-ray reveals left atrial and ventricular enlargement and pulmonary congestion.
- Echocardiogram shows abnormal valve leaflet motion and left atrial enlargement.

DIAGNOSTIC PROCEDURES

- Results of cardiac catheterization reveal mitral valve insufficiency with increased left ventricular end-diastolic volume and pressure, increased atrial pressure and pulmonary artery wedge pressure, and decreased cardiac output.
- Electrocardiography may show left atrial and ventricular hypertrophy, sinus tachycardia, or atrial fibrillation.

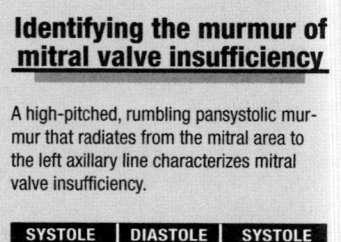

Identifying the murmur of mitral valve insufficiency

A high-pitched, rumbling pansystolic murmur that radiates from the mitral area to the left axillary line characterizes mitral valve insufficiency.

SYSTOLE	DIASTOLE	SYSTOLE
S_1	S_2	S_1 S_2

TREATMENT

GENERAL
◆ Appropriate treatment of underlying cause

DIET
◆ Low-sodium

ACTIVITY
◆ As tolerated

MEDICATIONS
◆ Diuretics
◆ Inotropic agents
◆ Angiotensin-converting enzyme inhibitors
◆ Oxygen
◆ Anticoagulants
◆ Prophylactic antibiotics before and after surgery or dental care to prevent endocarditis
◆ Beta-adrenergic blockers or digoxin to slow the ventricular rate in atrial fibrillation or atrial flutter

SURGERY
◆ Annuloplasty or valvuloplasty to reconstruct or repair the valve
◆ Valve replacement with a prosthetic valve

NURSING CONSIDERATIONS

NURSING DIAGNOSES
◆ Activity intolerance
◆ Decreased cardiac output
◆ Excess fluid volume
◆ Fatigue
◆ Impaired gas exchange
◆ Impaired physical mobility
◆ Ineffective coping
◆ Ineffective tissue perfusion: Cardiopulmonary
◆ Risk for infection

EXPECTED OUTCOMES
The patient will:
◆ carry out activities of daily living without weakness or fatigue
◆ maintain hemodynamic stability and adequate cardiac output, and have no arrhythmias
◆ experience no complications from fluid excess
◆ verbalize the importance of balancing activity with adequate rest periods
◆ maintain adequate ventilation and oxygenation
◆ maintain joint mobility and muscle strength
◆ exhibit adequate coping mechanisms
◆ maintain adequate cardiopulmonary perfusion
◆ remain free from signs and symptoms of infection.

NURSING INTERVENTIONS
◆ Give prescribed oxygen.
◆ Watch for signs of heart failure or pulmonary edema.

MONITORING
◆ Vital signs and pulse oximetry
◆ Cardiac rhythm
◆ Pulmonary artery catheter readings
◆ Intake and output
◆ Adverse effects of drug therapy

PATIENT TEACHING

GENERAL
Be sure to cover:
◆ the disorder, diagnosis, and treatment
◆ dietary restrictions
◆ medication.

RESOURCES
Organizations
American Heart Association: *www.americanheart.org*
Cleveland Clinic Health Information Center: *www.clevelandclinic.org/health*
HeartCenterOnline: *www.heart.healthcentersonline.com*
Mayo Foundation for Medical Education and Research: *www.mayoclinic.com*
National Institutes of Health: *www.nih.gov*

Selected references
Sanchez, P.L., et al. "The Impact of Age in the Immediate and Long-term Outcomes of Percutaneous Mitral Balloon Valvuloplasty," *Journal of Interventional Cardiology* 18(4):217-25, August 2005.
Todd, B.A., and Higgins, K. "Recognizing Aortic and Mitral Valve Disease," *Nursing* 35(6):58-63, June 2005.
Ziegler, K., and Quillen, T.F. "Mitral Valve Regurgitation after Myocardial Infarction," *Nursing* 35(11):88, November 2005.

Mitral valve prolapse

- A condition involving the prolapse of a portion of the mitral valve (MV) into the left atrium during ventricular contraction (systole)
- Also known as *MVP*

PATHOPHYSIOLOGY

- Myxomatous degeneration of MV leaflets with redundant tissue leads to prolapse of the MV into the left atrium during systole.
- In some patients, this results in leakage of blood into the left atrium from the left ventricle.

CAUSES

- Acquired heart disease, such as coronary artery disease and rheumatic heart disease
- Congenital heart disease
- Connective tissue disorders, such as systemic lupus erythematosus and Marfan syndrome

INCIDENCE

- MVP is more prevalent in women than in men.
- It's usually detected in young adulthood.
- It affects 2.5% to 5% of the general population.

 AGE FACTOR *Mitral valve prolapse is most common in women ages 20 to 40.*

COMPLICATIONS

- Arrhythmias
- Infective endocarditis
- Mitral insufficiency from chordal rupture
- Mitral regurgitation

HISTORY

- Usually asymptomatic
- Possible fatigue, syncope, palpitations, chest pain, or dyspnea on exertion

PHYSICAL FINDINGS

- Orthostatic hypotension
- Mid-to-late systolic click and late systolic murmur

IMAGING

- Echocardiogram may reveal MVP with or without mitral insufficiency.

DIAGNOSTIC PROCEDURES

- Electrocardiogram (ECG) is usually normal but may reveal atrial or ventricular arrhythmia.
- Signal-averaged ECG may show ventricular and supraventricular arrhythmias.
- Holter monitor worn for 24 hours may show an arrhythmia.

TREATMENT

GENERAL
- Usually requires no treatment; regular monitoring only

DIET
- Decreased caffeine intake
- Fluid intake to maintain hydration

MEDICATIONS
- Antibiotic prophylaxis
- Beta-adrenergic blockers
- Anticoagulants
- Antiarrhythmics

NURSING CONSIDERATIONS

NURSING DIAGNOSES
- Activity intolerance
- Anxiety
- Decreased cardiac output
- Fatigue
- Impaired gas exchange
- Ineffective tissue perfusion: Cardiopulmonary
- Risk for infection

EXPECTED OUTCOMES
The patient will:
- carry out activities of daily living without weakness or fatigue
- express feelings of decreased anxiety
- maintain adequate cardiac output, without arrhythmias
- verbalize the importance of balancing activity with adequate rest periods
- maintain adequate ventilation and oxygenation
- maintain adequate cardiopulmonary perfusion
- remain free from signs or symptoms of infection.

NURSING INTERVENTIONS
- Provide reassurance and comfort if the patient experiences anxiety.
- If fatigue is a concern, plan rest periods.

MONITORING
- Vital signs
- Blood pressure while lying, sitting, and standing
- Heart sounds
- Signs and symptoms of mitral valve insufficiency
- Serial echocardiograms
- ECG for arrhythmias

PATIENT TEACHING

GENERAL
Be sure to cover:
- disorder, diagnosis, and treatment
- the need to perform the most important activities of the day when energy levels are highest
- the patient's drug therapy including dosage, adverse reactions, and when to notify the practitioner if a problem arises
- the importance of hydration
- the need for antibiotic prophylaxis before dental or surgical procedures as indicated (not all patients with MVP require antibiotic prophylaxis)
- the need to avoid foods and beverages high in caffeine.

DISCHARGE PLANNING
- If the patient is being discharged with a Holter monitor, make sure he understands the importance of documenting his activities throughout the monitoring process.
- Refer him to an MVP support group.

RESOURCES
Organizations
American Heart Association: *www.americanheart.org*
Cleveland Clinic Health Information Center: *www.clevelandclinic.org/health*
Mayo Foundation for Medical Education and Research: *www.mayoclinic.com*
National Heart, Lung, and Blood Institute: *www.nhlbi.nih.gov*
National Institutes of Health: *www.nih.gov*

Selected references
Kasper, D.L., et al., eds. *Harrison's Principles of Internal Medicine*, 16th ed. New York: McGraw-Hill Book Co., 2005.
The Merck Manual of Diagnosis & Therapy, 18th ed. Whitehouse Station N.J.: Merck & Co., Inc., 2006.
Scordo, K.A. "Mitral Valve Prolapse Syndrome Health Concerns, Symptoms, and Treatments," *Western Journal of Nursing Research* 27(4):390-405, June 2005.
Weyman, A.E., and Scherrer-Crosbie, M. "Marfan Syndrome and Mitral Valve Prolapse," *Journal of Clinical Investigation* 114(11):1543-546, December 2004.

Monkeypox

- A rare, viral disease that occurs primarily in the rainforest countries of central and west Africa
- Virus originally discovered in laboratory monkeys in 1958, then later recovered from an African squirrel (thought to be the natural host)
- May also infect other rodents (rats and mice) and rabbits
- First human cases of monkeypox reported in remote African locations in 1970

PATHOPHYSIOLOGY

- The monkeypox virus (related to variola virus [smallpox] and cowpox), belonging to the *Orthopoxvirus* group of viruses, causes monkeypox.
- The virus is less infectious than smallpox.

CAUSES

- Direct contact with an infected person's body fluids or with virus-contaminated objects, such as bedding or clothing
- Person-to-person spread via respiratory droplets during direct and prolonged face-to-face contact
- Transmission to humans by an infected animal through a bite or direct contact with the animal's blood, body fluids, or lesions

INCIDENCE

- In June 2003, an outbreak occurred in the United States involving individuals who became ill following contact with infected prairie dogs.

COMPLICATIONS

- May include encephalitis and death (rare)
- Fatal in 10% of those who contract the disease in Africa

HISTORY

- Signs and symptoms similar to those of smallpox but milder
- Fever, headache, myalgia, backache, swollen lymph nodes, and a general feeling of discomfort and exhaustion possibly reported after a 12-day incubation period
- Duration of 2 to 4 weeks

PHYSICAL FINDINGS

- A papular rash begins on the face or other area of the body within 1 to 3 days of the onset of the fever.
- Lesions go through several stages before crusting and falling off.

LABORATORY

- The virus may be isolated from vesicular fluid to aid in diagnosis and differentiation from other rash-producing viruses.

OTHER

- Diagnosis is based on the patient's history and his presenting signs and symptoms.

GENERAL
◆ No specific treatment

MEDICATIONS
◆ Smallpox vaccine (recommended by the CDC for people who are investigating monkeypox outbreaks, people caring for infected individuals or animals, and those exposed to individuals or animals confirmed to have monkeypox [up to 14 days after exposure])
◆ Immune globulin vaccination for severely immunocompromised patients
◆ Cidofovir (Vistide) for human monkeypox cases (no effectiveness data available)

NURSING DIAGNOSES
◆ Acute pain
◆ Fatigue
◆ Impaired skin integrity

EXPECTED OUTCOMES
The patient will:
◆ express feelings of comfort and relief from pain
◆ report increased levels of energy
◆ maintain warm, dry, and intact skin with healed or improved lesions or wounds.

NURSING INTERVENTIONS
◆ Notify the local health department immediately if you suspect monkeypox in a patient.
◆ A combination of standard, contact, and droplet precautions should be applied in all health care settings. Because of the risk of airborne transmission, droplet precautions should be applied whenever possible using a NIOSH-certified N95 (or comparable) filtering disposable respirator that has been fit-tested. Surgical masks may be worn if a respirator is not available. Isolation should continue until all lesions are crusted over or until the local or state health department advises that isolation is no longer necessary.
◆ Perform strict hand washing after contact with an infected patient or contaminated objects.
◆ Eye protection should be used if splash or spray of body fluids is possible.
◆ Place the patient in a private room. Use a negative pressure room, if available.
◆ When transporting the patient, place a mask over his nose and mouth, and cover the exposed skin lesions with a sheet or gown. If the patient is to remain at home, he should maintain the same precautions.

GENERAL
Be sure to cover:
◆ the disorder, diagnosis, and treatment
◆ the need to wear a mask over his nose and mouth and to cover exposed lesions with a sheet or gown when he's in contact with others
◆ proper hand-washing practices.

RESOURCES
Organizations
Centers for Disease Control and Prevention: *www.cdc.gov*
U.S. Food and Drug Administration: *www.fda.gov*
World Health Organization: *www.who.int*

Selected references
Fishman, M., et al. "Patient Safety Tools: SARS, Smallpox, Monkeypox, and Avian Flu," *Disaster Management & Response* 3(3):86-90, July-September 2005.
Nalca, A., et al. "Reemergence of Monkeypox: Prevalence, Diagnostics, and Countermeasures," *Clinical Infectious Diseases* 41(12):1765-771, December 2005.
Seguin, D., and Stoner Halpern, J. "Triage of a Febrile Patient with a Rash: A Comparison of Chickenpox, Monkeypox, and Smallpox," *Disaster Management & Response* 2(3):81-86, July-September 2004.

Multiple myeloma

OVERVIEW

- Disseminated neoplasm of marrow plasma cells
- Prognosis usually poor (by the time it's diagnosed, it has already infiltrated the vertebrae, pelvis, skull, ribs, clavicles, and sternum); leads to vertebral collapse without treatment (within 3 months of diagnosis, 52% of patients die; within 2 years, 90% die)
- Life often prolonged by 3 to 5 years with early diagnosis and treatment
- Also called *malignant plasmacytoma, plasma cell myeloma,* and *myelomatosis*

PATHOPHYSIOLOGY

- Infiltration of the bone produces osteolytic lesions throughout the skeleton.
- In late stages, the malignant plasma cells infiltrate into the lymph nodes, liver, spleen, and kidneys.

CAUSES

- Exact cause unknown

RISK FACTORS

- Genetic factors
- Occupational exposure to radiation

INCIDENCE

- Multiple myeloma is most common in men older than age 40.

COMPLICATIONS

- Infections (such as pneumonia)
- Pyelonephritis, renal calculi, and renal failure
- Hematologic imbalance
- Fractures
- Hypercalcemia
- Hyperuricemia
- Dehydration

ASSESSMENT

HISTORY

- History of neoplastic fractures
- Severe, constant back pain that may increase with exercise
- Arthritic symptoms
- Peripheral paresthesia
- Progressive weakness
- History of pneumonia
- Pain on movement or weight bearing, especially in the thoracic and lumbar vertebrae

PHYSICAL FINDINGS

- Noticeable thoracic deformities and reduction in body height of 5" (12.7 cm)

Bence Jones protein

The Bence Jones protein is the hallmark of multiple myeloma. This protein — a light chain of gamma globulin — was named for Henry Bence Jones, an English physician. In 1848 he noticed that patients with a certain bone disease excreted a unique protein, unique in that it coagulated at 113° to 131° F (45° to 55° C), then redissolved when heated to boiling.

Otto Kahler, an Austrian, demonstrated in 1889 that Bence Jones protein was related to myeloma. Bence Jones protein isn't found in the urine of all multiple myeloma patients, but it's almost never found in patients without the disease.

DIAGNOSTIC TEST RESULTS

LABORATORY

- Complete blood count shows moderate or severe anemia; the differential may show 40% to 50% lymphocytes but seldom more than 3% plasma cells; the differential smear shows rouleau formation (often the first clue); and the erythrocyte sedimentation rate is elevated.
- Urinalysis results may show proteinuria, Bence Jones protein, and hypercalciuria; the absence of Bence Jones protein doesn't rule out multiple myeloma, but its presence almost invariably confirms the disease. (See *Bence Jones protein.*)
- Serum electrophoresis results show a globulin spike that's electrophoretically and immunologically abnormal.

IMAGING

- X-rays may reveal only diffuse osteoporosis during the early stages of the disease. Eventually, they show the characteristic lesions of multiple myeloma — multiple, sharply circumscribed osteolytic, or punched out lesions, particularly on the skull, pelvis, and spine.

DIAGNOSTIC PROCEDURES

- Bone marrow aspiration results reveal myelomatous cells and an abnormal number of immature plasma cells (10% to 95% instead of the normal 3% to 5%).

TREATMENT

GENERAL
- Adjuvant local radiation
- Dialysis (if renal complications develop)
- Plasmapheresis to remove the M protein from the blood and return the cells to the patient (temporary effect)
- Peripheral blood stem cell transplantation

DIET
- Well-balanced

ACTIVITY
- As tolerated

MEDICATIONS
- Bisphosphonates
- Analgesics
- Chemotherapeutic agents
- Possible use of thalidomide
- Immunotherapy

SURGERY
- Laminectomy, if the patient develops vertebral compression

NURSING CONSIDERATIONS

NURSING DIAGNOSES
- Acute pain
- Anxiety
- Energy field disturbance
- Fear
- Hopelessness
- Imbalanced nutrition: Less than body requirements
- Impaired physical mobility
- Ineffective breathing pattern
- Ineffective coping
- Ineffective protection

EXPECTED OUTCOMES
The patient will:
- express feelings of increased comfort and decreased pain
- identify strategies to reduce anxiety
- express feelings of increased energy
- verbalize fears and concerns relating to the diagnosis and condition
- maintain optimal nutrition
- demonstrate the use of protective measures, including conserving energy, maintaining a balanced diet, and getting adequate rest
- make decisions on his own behalf
- maintain muscle strength and joint range of motion
- maintain adequate ventilation
- demonstrate effective coping skills.

NURSING INTERVENTIONS
- Encourage fluid intake (3 to 4 qt [3 to 4 L] daily).
- Give prescribed drugs.

After surgery
- Encourage mobilization.

MONITORING
- Complications of treatment
- Signs and symptoms of severe anemia and fractures
- Proper positioning (alignment)
- Pain control

PATIENT TEACHING

GENERAL
Be sure to cover:
- the disorder, diagnosis, and treatment
- the importance of deep breathing and changing position every 2 hours after surgery
- the importance of appropriate dress for weather conditions (because the patient may be sensitive to cold)
- the need to avoid crowds and people with infections
- medication administration, dosage, and possible adverse effects.

DISCHARGE PLANNING
- Refer the patient to available resources and support services.

RESOURCES
Organizations
American Cancer Society: *www.cancer.org*
Guide to Internet Resources for Cancer: *www.cancerindex.org*
International Myeloma Foundation: *www.myeloma.org*
National Cancer Institute: *www.cancer.gov*

Selected references
Atlas of Pathophysiology, 2nd ed. Philadelphia: Lippincott Williams & Wilkins, 2005.
Casciato, D.A. *Manual of Clinical Oncology*, 5th ed. Philadelphia: Lippincott Williams & Wilkins, 2004.
Collins, C.D. "Problems Monitoring Response in Multiple Myeloma," *Cancer Imaging* 5(Suppl):S119-126, November 2005.
Hideshima, T., et al. "Current Therapeutic Uses of Lenalidomide in Multiple Myeloma," *Expert Opinion on Investigational Drugs* 15(2):171-79, February 2006.
Richardson, P., and Anderson, K. "Thalidomide and Dexamethasone: A New Standard of Care for Initial Therapy in Multiple Myeloma," *Journal of Clinical Oncology* 24(3):334-36, January 2006.

Multiple sclerosis

OVERVIEW

- Progressive demyelination of white matter of brain and spinal cord
- Characterized by exacerbations and remissions
- May progress rapidly, causing death within months
- Prognosis varies (70% of patients with multiple sclerosis lead active lives with prolonged remissions)
- Also known as *MS*

PATHOPHYSIOLOGY

- Sporadic patches of demyelination occur in the central nervous system, resulting in widespread and varied neurologic dysfunction. (See *Describing multiple sclerosis.*)

CAUSES

- Exact cause unknown
- Allergic response
- Autoimmune response of the nervous system
- Events that precede the onset:
- – emotional stress
- – overwork
- – fatigue
- – pregnancy
- – acute respiratory tract infections
- Genetic factors possibly also involved
- Slow-acting viral infection

RISK FACTORS

- Trauma
- Anoxia
- Toxins
- Nutritional deficiencies
- Vascular lesions
- Anorexia nervosa

INCIDENCE

- The incidence of multiple sclerosis is higher in women than in men.
- It's higher among people in northern urban areas.
- Incidence is increased among those in higher socioeconomic groups.
- There is a low incidence in Japan.
- Family history increases incidence.
- Increased incidence is associated with living in a cold, damp climate.

- Multiple sclerosis is a major cause of chronic disability in young adults ages 20 to 40.

COMPLICATIONS

- Injuries from falls
- Urinary tract infections
- Constipation
- Contractures
- Pressure ulcers
- Pneumonia
- Depression

ASSESSMENT

HISTORY

- Symptoms related to the extent and site of myelin destruction, extent of remyelination, and adequacy of subsequently restored synaptic transmission
- Symptoms possibly transient or lasting for hours or weeks
- Symptoms unpredictable and difficult to describe
- Visual problems and sensory impairment (the first signs)
- Blurred vision or diplopia
- Urinary problems
- Emotional lability
- Dysphagia
- Bowel disturbances (involuntary evacuation or constipation)
- Fatigue and weakness (typically the most disabling symptom)

PHYSICAL FINDINGS

- Poor articulation
- Muscle weakness of the involved area
- Spasticity; hyperreflexia
- Intention tremor
- Gait ataxia
- Paralysis, ranging from monoplegia to quadriplegia
- Nystagmus; scotoma
- Optic neuritis
- Ophthalmoplegia

DIAGNOSTIC TEST RESULTS

LABORATORY

- Cerebrospinal fluid analysis results show mononuclear cell pleocytosis, an elevation in total immunoglobulin (Ig) G levels, and the presence of oligoclonal IgG.

IMAGING

- Magnetic resonance imaging is the most sensitive method of detecting multiple sclerosis focal lesions.

OTHER

- Electroencephalography abnormalities occur in one-third of patients with multiple sclerosis.
- Evoked potential study results show slowed conduction of nerve impulses.
- Years of testing and observation may be required for diagnosis.

Describing multiple sclerosis

Various types (or stages) of multiple sclerosis (MS) can be identified:

- *Relapsing-remitting:* Clear relapses (or acute attacks or exacerbations) with full recovery and lasting disability (Between attacks, the disease doesn't worsen.)
- *Primary progressive:* Steadily progressing or worsening with minor recovery or plateaus (This form is uncommon and may involve different brain and spinal cord damage from other forms.)
- *Secondary progressive:* Beginning as a pattern of clear-cut relapses and recovery but becoming steadily progressive and worsening between acute attacks
- *Progressive-relapsing:* Steadily progressing from the onset but also involving clear, acute attacks. (This form is rare.)

In addition, differential diagnosis must rule out spinal cord compression, foramen magnum tumor (which may mimic the exacerbations and remissions of MS), multiple small strokes, syphilis or another infection, thyroid disease, and chronic fatigue syndrome.

TREATMENT

GENERAL
◆ Symptomatic treatment for acute exacerbations and related signs and symptoms

DIET
◆ High-fluid and high-fiber (for constipation)

ACTIVITY
◆ Frequent rest periods

MEDICATIONS
◆ I.V. steroids followed by oral steroids
◆ Immunosuppressants
◆ Antimetabolites
◆ Alkylating agents
◆ Biological response modifiers
◆ Antidepressants
◆ Glatiramer acetate (Copaxone)

NURSING CONSIDERATIONS

NURSING DIAGNOSES
◆ Activity intolerance
◆ Acute pain
◆ Chronic low self-esteem
◆ Constipation
◆ Disabled family coping
◆ Fatigue
◆ Imbalanced nutrition: Less than body requirements
◆ Impaired physical mobility
◆ Impaired urinary elimination
◆ Ineffective coping
◆ Ineffective role performance
◆ Interrupted family processes
◆ Risk for infection
◆ Risk for injury

EXPECTED OUTCOMES
The patient (or family) will:
◆ perform activities of daily living within the confines of the disorder
◆ express feeling of comfort and relief from pain
◆ voice feelings of increased self-esteem
◆ maintain a normal bowel elimination pattern
◆ use available support systems and coping mechanisms
◆ express feelings of increased energy and decreased fatigue
◆ show no signs of malnutrition
◆ maintain joint mobility and range of motion
◆ develop regular bowel and bladder habits
◆ demonstrate effective coping skills
◆ resume regular roles and responsibilities to the fullest extent possible
◆ discuss the impact of the patient's condition on the family unit
◆ remain free from signs and symptoms of infection
◆ remain free from injury.

NURSING INTERVENTIONS
◆ Provide emotional and psychological support.
◆ Assist with physical therapy program.
◆ Provide adequate rest periods.
◆ Promote emotional stability.
◆ Keep the bedpan or urinal readily available because the need to void is immediate.
◆ Provide bowel and bladder training, if indicated.
◆ Give prescribed drugs.
◆ Schedule activities of daily living in the morning to conserve the patient's energy.

MONITORING
◆ Response to medications
◆ Adverse drug reactions
◆ Sensory impairment
◆ Muscle dysfunction
◆ Energy level
◆ Signs and symptoms of infection
◆ Speech
◆ Elimination patterns
◆ Vision changes
◆ Laboratory results

PATIENT TEACHING

GENERAL
Be sure to cover:
◆ the disease process
◆ medication and adverse effects
◆ the need to avoid stress, infections, and fatigue
◆ the importance of maintaining independence
◆ the need to avoid exposure to bacterial and viral infections
◆ nutritional management
◆ the importance of adequate fluid intake and regular urination.

DISCHARGE PLANNING
◆ Refer the patient to the National Multiple Sclerosis Society.
◆ Refer the patient to physical and occupational rehabilitation programs, as indicated.

RESOURCES
Organizations
Multiple Sclerosis Association of America: *www.msaa.com*
National Institutes of Health: *www.nih.gov*
National Multiple Sclerosis Society: *www.nmss.org*

Selected references
Coyle, P.K., et al. "Multiple Sclerosis Gender Issues: Clinical Practices of Women Neurologists," *Multiple Sclerosis* 10(5):582-88, October 2004.
Diseases, 4th ed. Philadelphia: Lippincott Williams & Wilkins, 2006.
Handbook of Pathophysiology, 2nd ed. Philadelphia: Lippincott Williams & Wilkins, 2005.
Rieckmann, P. "Improving MS Patient Care," *Journal of Neurology* 251(Suppl 5):v69-v73, September 2004.
Traboulsee, A.L., and Li, D.K. "The Role of MRI in the Diagnosis of Multiple Sclerosis," *Advances in Neurology* 98:125-46, 2006.

Mumps

- An acute viral infection of one or both parotid glands and sometimes the sublingual or submaxillary glands
- Also called *infectious* or *epidemic parotitis*

PATHOPHYSIOLOGY

- Virus replication occurs in the epithelium of the upper respiratory tract, leading to viremia.
- Infection of the central nervous system (CNS) or glandular tissues (or both) occurs, resulting in perivascular and interstitial mononuclear cell infiltrates with edema.
- Necrosis of acinar and epithelial duct cells occurs in the salivary glands and germinal epithelium of the seminiferous tubules.

CAUSES

- A paramyxovirus found in the saliva of an infected person
- Transmission by droplets or by direct contact with the saliva of an infected person

INCIDENCE

- Mumps seldom occur in infants younger than age 1 because of passive immunity from maternal antibodies.
- About 50% of cases occur in young adults; the remainder occur in young children or immunocompromised adults.
- Peak incidence is during late winter and early spring.

COMPLICATIONS

- Epididymo-orchitis
- Meningoencephalitis
- Sterility
- Pancreatitis
- Transient sensorineural hearing loss
- Arthritis
- Nephritis
- Spontaneous abortion (with contact during the first trimester)

ASSESSMENT

HISTORY

- Inadequate immunization and exposure to someone with mumps within the preceding 2 to 3 weeks
- Myalgia
- Headache
- Malaise
- Fever
- Earache aggravated by chewing

PHYSICAL FINDINGS

- Swelling and tenderness of the parotid glands
- Simultaneous or subsequent swelling of one or more other salivary glands (see *Parotid inflammation in mumps*)

DIAGNOSTIC TEST RESULTS

LABORATORY

- Serologic test results show mumps antibodies.

OTHER

- Glandular swelling confirms the diagnosis.

Parotid inflammation in mumps

The mumps virus (paramyxovirus) attacks the parotid glands — the main salivary glands. Inflammation causes characteristic swelling and discomfort with eating, drinking, swallowing, and talking.

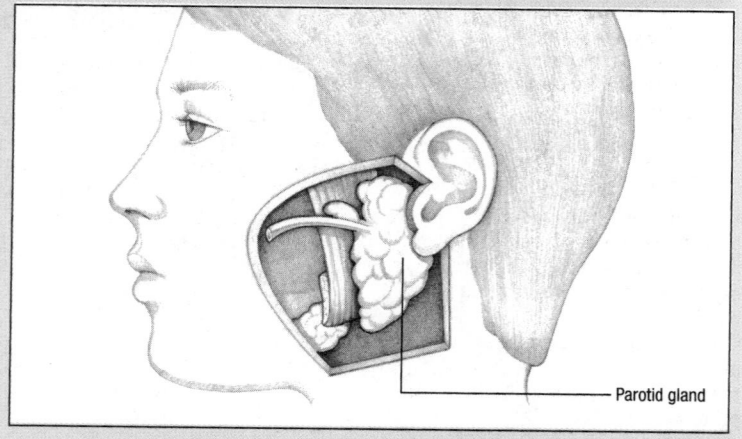

Parotid gland

TREATMENT

GENERAL
◆ Rest
◆ Cold compresses for swollen glands
◆ Use of athletic supporter, if testicles are tender

DIET
◆ Clear liquid to mechanical soft diet until able to swallow
◆ Increased fluid intake

ACTIVITY
◆ Bed rest until fever resolves
◆ Rest periods when fatigued

MEDICATIONS
◆ Analgesics
◆ Antipyretics

NURSING CONSIDERATIONS

NURSING DIAGNOSES
◆ Acute pain
◆ Deficient fluid volume
◆ Disturbed body image
◆ Hyperthermia
◆ Imbalanced nutrition: Less than body requirements
◆ Impaired swallowing
◆ Risk for infection

EXPECTED OUTCOMES
The patient will:
◆ express feelings of increased comfort and decreased pain
◆ maintain adequate fluid volume
◆ verbalize feelings about changed body image
◆ remain afebrile
◆ achieve adequate nutritional intake
◆ swallow without pain or aspiration
◆ remain free from signs and symptoms of infection.

NURSING INTERVENTIONS
◆ Apply cool compresses to the neck area to relieve pain.
◆ Give prescribed drugs.
◆ Provide scrotal support, if needed.
◆ Report all cases of mumps to local public health authorities.
◆ Disinfect articles soiled with nose and throat secretions.

MONITORING
◆ Response to treatment
◆ Signs of CNS involvement
◆ Auditory acuity
◆ Complications

PATIENT TEACHING

GENERAL
Be sure to cover:
◆ the disorder, diagnosis, and treatment
◆ the need to stay away from school or work from days 12 through 25 after exposure
◆ the importance of having children immunized with live attenuated mumps vaccine at age 15 months or older, if applicable
◆ reassurance that epididymo-orchitis, if it occurs, won't cause impotence or sterility (occurs only with bilateral orchitis)
◆ the need for bed rest during febrile period
◆ the need to avoid spicy, irritating foods and those that require much chewing (advise a soft, bland diet)
◆ the need for family members to follow respiratory isolation precautions until symptoms subside.

DISCHARGE PLANNING
◆ Refer the patient to a urologist for orchitis, if indicated.

RESOURCES
Organizations
Centers for Disease Control and Prevention: *www.cdc.gov*
Harvard University Consumer Health Information: *www.intelihealth.com*
National Health Information Center: *www.health.gov/nhic*
National Institute of Allergy and Infectious Diseases: *www3.niaid.nih.gov*
National Library of Medicine: *www.nlm.nih.gov*

Selected references
Bedford, H. "Mumps: Current Outbreaks and Vaccination Recommendations," *Nursing Times* 101(39):53-54, 56, September-October 2005.
Francois, G., et al. "Vaccine Safety Controversies and the Future of Vaccination Programs," *Pediatric Infectious Disease Journal* 24(11):953-61, November 2005.
Hviid, A., et al. "Childhood Vaccination and Nontargeted Infectious Disease Hospitalization," *JAMA* 294(6):699-705, August 2005.

Muscular dystrophy

- Hereditary disorder characterized by progressive symmetrical wasting of skeletal muscles
- No neural or sensory defects
- Four main types: Duchenne's (pseudohypertrophic), Becker's (benign pseudohypertrophic), Landouzy-Dejerine (facioscapulohumeral), and Erb's (limb-girdle)
- Duchenne's muscular dystrophy (most common) beginning in early childhood with death occurring in 10 to 15 years

PATHOPHYSIOLOGY

- Muscle fibers necrotize and regenerate in various states.
- Regeneration slows and degeneration dominates.
- Connective tissue replaces muscle fibers.
- Weakness and wasting result.

CAUSES

- Autosomal dominant (Landouzy-Dejerine type)
- Autosomal recessive, usually (Erb's type)
- Genetic mechanisms of various types (band Xp21)
- X-linked recessive (Duchenne's and Becker's types)

INCIDENCE

- Duchenne's and Becker's muscular dystrophy types affect males almost exclusively.
- Landouzy-Dejerine and Erb's types affect both sexes about equally.

COMPLICATIONS

- Crippling disability
- Contractures
- Pneumonia
- Arrhythmias
- Cardiac hypertrophy
- Dysphagia
- Spinal deformity
- Fractures
- Speech impairment

ASSESSMENT

HISTORY

- Evidence of genetic transmission
- Progressive muscle weakness

Duchenne's muscular dystrophy

- Onset insidious
- Onset between ages 3 and 5
- Pelvic muscle weakness
- Interferes with child's ability to run, climb, and walk

Becker's muscular dystrophy

- Onset after age 5
- Same symptoms as with Duchenne's muscular dystrophy but slower progression

Landouzy-Dejerine muscular dystrophy

- Onset before age 10
- Weakness of eye, face, and shoulder muscles
- Inability to raise arms over head
- Inability to close eyes
- Inability to pucker lips or whistle
- Abnormal facial movements
- Absence of facial movements when laughing or crying
- Weakening of pelvic muscles as disease progresses

Erb's muscular dystrophy

- Same symptoms as with Landouzy-Dejerine muscular dystrophy but slower progression
- Less of a disability than with Landouzy-Dejerine muscular dystrophy
- Onset between ages 6 and 10
- Muscle weakness of upper arm and pelvic muscles

PHYSICAL FINDINGS

Duchenne's and Becker's types

- Wide stance and waddling gait
- Gowers' sign when rising from a sitting or supine position
- Muscle hypertrophy and atrophy
- Calves enlarged because of fat infiltration into the muscle
- Posture changes
- Lordosis and a protuberant abdomen
- Scapular "winging" or flaring when raising arms (see Detecting muscular dystrophy)
- Contractures
- Tachypnea and shortness of breath

Landouzy-Dejerine type

- Pendulous lower lip
- Possible disappearance of nasolabial fold
- Diffuse facial flattening leading to a masklike expression
- Inability to suckle (infants)
- Scapulae with a winglike appearance; inability to raise arms above head

---

Detecting muscular dystrophy

In muscular dystrophy, the trapezius muscle typically rises, creating a stepped appearance at the shoulder's point.

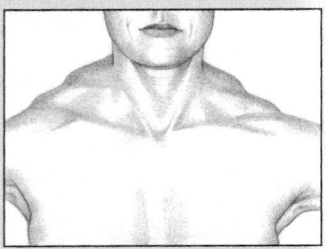

From the posterior view, the scapulae ride over the lateral thoracic region, giving them a winged appearance. In Duchenne's and Becker's dystrophies, this winglike sign appears when the patient raises his arms. In other dystrophies, the sign is obvious without arm raising (in fact, the patient can't raise his arms).

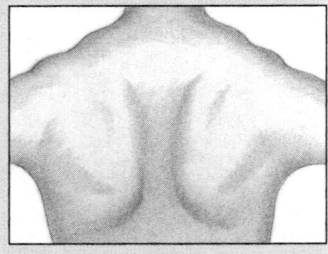

Erb's type
- Muscle weakness effects apparent
- Muscle wasting
- Winging of the scapulae
- Lordosis with abdominal protrusion
- Waddling gait
- Poor balance
- Inability to raise the arms

DIAGNOSTIC TEST RESULTS

LABORATORY
- Urine creatinine, serum creatine kinase, lactate dehydrogenase, alanine aminotransferase, and aspartate aminotransferase levels are elevated.

DIAGNOSTIC PROCEDURES
- Results of biopsy of the muscle confirm the diagnosis.
- Immunologic and biologic test results facilitate prenatal and postnatal diagnosis.
- Electromyogram shows abnormal muscle movements.
- Amniocentesis results detect the sex of a fetus in a high-risk family.

OTHER
- Genetic testing may be used to detect the gene defect that leads to muscular dystrophy in some families.

TREATMENT

GENERAL
- No known treatment to stop progression
- Orthopedic appliances to help the patient achieve mobility

DIET
- Low-calorie, high-protein, high-fiber
- Tube feedings as needed

ACTIVITY
- Exercise as tolerated
- Physical therapy

MEDICATIONS
- Stool softeners
- Possible steroids

SURGERY
- Surgery to correct contractures
- Spinal fusion

NURSING CONSIDERATIONS

NURSING DIAGNOSES
- Activity intolerance
- Bathing or hygiene self-care deficit
- Disabled family coping
- Disturbed body image
- Impaired physical mobility
- Ineffective breathing pattern
- Ineffective coping
- Risk for disuse syndrome
- Risk for injury

EXPECTED OUTCOMES
The patient (or family) will:
- perform activities of daily living without muscle fatigue or intolerance
- participate in self-care activities to the fullest extent possible
- demonstrate adaptive coping behaviors
- express positive feelings about body image
- achieve the highest degree of mobility possible within the confines of the disease
- maintain respiratory rate within 5 breaths/minute of baseline
- use support measures and exhibit adaptive coping behaviors
- maintain muscle strength, joint mobility, and range of motion
- show no evidence of complications of the disorder.

NURSING INTERVENTIONS
- Encourage coughing and deep-breathing exercises.
- Take steps to prevent muscle atrophy.
- Use splints, braces, grab bars, and overhead slings.
- Use a footboard or high-topped shoes and a foot cradle.
- Provide a low-calorie, high-protein, high-fiber diet.

MONITORING
- Intake and output
- Respiratory status
- Joint mobility

- Muscle weakness
- Complications

PATIENT TEACHING

GENERAL
Be sure to cover:
- the disorder, diagnosis, and treatment
- the importance of maintaining peer relationships
- how to maintain mobility and independence
- possible complications and prevention
- signs and symptoms of respiratory tract infections
- the need for a low-calorie, high-protein, high-fiber diet
- the need to avoid long periods of bed rest and inactivity.

DISCHARGE PLANNING
- Refer the patient for sexual counseling, if indicated.
- Refer the patient for physical therapy, vocational rehabilitation, social services, and financial assistance.
- Refer the patient to the Muscular Dystrophy Association.
- Refer the patient for genetic counseling.

RESOURCES
Organizations
The American Academy of Pediatrics: *www.aap.org*
Muscular Dystrophy Association: *www.mda.org*
National Institutes of Health: *www.nih.gov*

Selected references
Bostrom, K., and Ahlstrom, G. "Quality of Life in Patients with Muscular Dystrophy and Their Next of Kin," *Internal Journal of Rehabilitation Research* 28(2):103-109, June 2005.

Hoogerwaard, E.M., et al. "Dystrophin Analysis in Carriers of Duchenne and Becker Muscular Dystrophy," *Neurology* 65(12):1984-986, December 2005.

Parker, A.E., et al. "Analysis of an Adult Duchenne Muscular Dystrophy Population," *QJM* 98(10):729-36, October 2005.

Myasthenia gravis LIFE-THREATENING DISORDER

OVERVIEW

- An acquired autoimmune disorder characterized by abnormal fatigability of striated (skeletal) muscles
- Sporadic but progressive weakness
- Muscle weakness exacerbated by exercise and repetitive movement
- Initial symptoms related to cranial nerves
- Possibly life-threatening if there's respiratory system involvement
- Spontaneous remissions occurring in about 25% of patients

PATHOPHYSIOLOGY

- Blood cells and thymus gland produce antibodies that block, destroy, or weaken neuroreceptors (which transmit nerve impulses).
- The result is failure in transmission of nerve impulses at the neuromuscular junction.

CAUSES

- Autoimmune disorder associated with the thymus gland
- Other immune and thyroid disorders causing secondary symptoms
- Rheumatoid arthritis
- Systemic lupus erythematosus
- Thyrotoxicosis

INCIDENCE

- Myasthenia gravis occurs at any age.
- It's three times more common in women than in men.
- Highest incidence in women is from ages 18 to 25.
- Highest incidence in men is from ages 50 to 60.
- Transient myasthenia occurs in about 20% of infants born to myasthenic mothers.

COMPLICATIONS

- Respiratory distress
- Pneumonia
- Aspiration

ASSESSMENT

HISTORY

- Varying assessment findings
- Progressive muscle weakness
- Extreme muscle weakness and fatigue (cardinal symptoms)
- Ptosis and diplopia (the most common sign and symptom)
- Difficulty chewing and swallowing
- Jaw hanging open (especially when tired)
- Head bobbing
- Symptoms that are milder on awakening and worsen as the day progresses
- Short rest periods that temporarily restore muscle function
- Symptoms that intensify before the menstrual period, during pregnancy, after emotional stress, after prolonged exposure to sunlight or cold, and with infections

PHYSICAL FINDINGS

- Sleepy, masklike expression
- Drooping jaw
- Ptosis
- Decreased breath sounds
- Decreased tidal volume
- Respiratory distress and myasthenic crisis
- Diplopia
- Difficulty swallowing or chewing
- Limb weakness

DIAGNOSTIC TEST RESULTS

IMAGING

- Chest X-rays or computed tomography scan results show thymoma.

OTHER

- Results of Tensilon test are positive, showing temporary improved muscle function and confirming the diagnosis.
- Electrodiagnostic test results show a rapid reduction of more than 10% in the amplitude of evoked responses.

TREATMENT

GENERAL
- Plasmapheresis
- Emergency airway and ventilation management

DIET
- As tolerated

ACTIVITY
- As tolerated (exercise possibly worsening symptoms; planned rest periods possibly slowing symptoms)

MEDICATIONS
- Anticholinesterase agents
- Corticosteroids
- I.V. immune globulin

SURGERY
- Thymectomy

NURSING CONSIDERATIONS

NURSING DIAGNOSES
- Activity intolerance
- Anxiety
- Bathing or hygiene self-care deficit
- Chronic low self-esteem
- Disturbed body image
- Dressing or grooming self-care deficit
- Fatigue
- Feeding self-care deficit
- Impaired gas exchange
- Impaired physical mobility
- Ineffective airway clearance

EXPECTED OUTCOMES
The patient will:
- perform activities of daily living within the confines of the disease process
- identify strategies to reduce anxiety
- perform bathing and hygiene activities to the fullest extent possible
- voice feelings related to increased self-esteem
- express positive feelings about body image
- perform dressing and grooming activities to the fullest extent possible
- verbalize the importance of balancing activity with adequate rest periods
- perform self-care needs related to feeding to the fullest extent possible
- maintain adequate ventilation and oxygenation
- maintain range of motion and joint mobility
- maintain a patent airway.

NURSING INTERVENTIONS
- Provide psychological support.
- Provide frequent rest periods.
- Maintain nutritional management program.
- Maintain social activity.
- Give prescribed drugs.

MONITORING
- Neurologic and respiratory function
- Response to medications

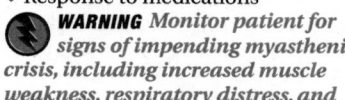 **WARNING** *Monitor patient for signs of impending myasthenic crisis, including increased muscle weakness, respiratory distress, and difficulty talking or chewing.*

PATIENT TEACHING

GENERAL
Be sure to cover:
- the disorder, diagnosis, and treatment
- surgery (preoperative and postoperative teaching)
- energy-conservation techniques
- medication and adverse effects
- the need to avoid strenuous exercise, stress, infection, and unnecessary exposure to the sun or cold weather
- nutritional management program
- swallowing therapy program.

DISCHARGE PLANNING
- Refer the patient to the Myasthenia Gravis Foundation.

RESOURCES
Organizations
Myasthenia Gravis Foundation of America: *www.myasthenia.org*
National Institutes of Health: *www.nih.gov*

Selected references
Burch, J., et al. "Myasthenia Gravis — A Rare Presentation with Tongue Atrophy and Fasciculation," *Age and Aging* 35(1):87-88, January 2006.
Diseases, 4th ed. Philadelphia: Lippincott Williams & Wilkins, 2006.
Handbook of Pathophysiology, 2nd ed. Philadelphia: Lippincott Williams & Wilkins, 2005.
Hughes, T. "The Early History of Myasthenia Gravis," *Neuromuscular Disorders* 15(12):878-86, December 2005.
Wagner, A.J., et al. "Long-term Follow-up after Thymectomy for Myasthenia Gravis: Thoracoscopic vs. Open," *Journal of Pediatric Surgery* 41(1):50-54, January 2006.

Myocardial infarction LIFE-THREATENING DISORDER

OVERVIEW

- Reduced blood flow through one or more coronary arteries causing myocardial ischemia and necrosis
- Infarction site depending on the vessels involved
- Also called *MI* and *heart attack*

PATHOPHYSIOLOGY

- One or more coronary arteries become occluded.
- If coronary occlusion causes ischemia lasting longer than 30 to 45 minutes, irreversible myocardial cell damage and muscle death occur.
- Every MI has a central area of necrosis surrounded by an area of hypoxic injury. This injured tissue is potentially viable and may be salvaged if circulation is restored, or it may progress to necrosis.

CAUSES

- Atherosclerosis
- Coronary artery stenosis or spasm
- Platelet aggregation
- Thrombosis

RISK FACTORS

- Increased age (40 to 70)
- Diabetes mellitus
- Elevated serum triglyceride, low-density lipoprotein, and cholesterol levels, and decreased serum high-density lipoprotein levels
- Excessive intake of saturated fats, carbohydrates, or salt
- Hypertension
- Obesity
- Family history of coronary artery disease (CAD)
- Sedentary lifestyle
- Smoking
- Stress or a type A personality
- Use of drugs, such as amphetamines or cocaine

INCIDENCE

- Men are more susceptible than premenopausal women.
- Incidence is increasing among women who smoke and take hormonal contraceptives.
- Incidence in postmenopausal women is similar to that in men.

COMPLICATIONS

- Arrhythmias
- Cardiogenic shock
- Heart failure causing pulmonary edema
- Pericarditis
- Rupture of the atrial or ventricular septum or of the ventricular wall
- Ventricular aneurysm
- Cerebral or pulmonary emboli
- Extension of the original infarction
- Mitral insufficiency

ASSESSMENT

HISTORY

- Possible CAD with increasing anginal frequency, severity, or duration
- Persistent, crushing substernal pain or pressure possibly radiating to the left arm, jaw, neck, and shoulder blades, and possibly persisting for 12 or more hours (cardinal symptom of MI)
- Pain possibly absent in elderly patients or those with diabetes; pain possibly mild and with confusion and indigestion in others
- A feeling of impending doom, fatigue, nausea, vomiting, and shortness of breath
- Sudden death (may be the first and only indication of MI)

PHYSICAL FINDINGS

- Extreme anxiety and restlessness
- Dyspnea
- Diaphoresis
- Tachycardia
- Hypertension
- Bradycardia and hypotension in inferior MI
- An S_4, an S_3, and paradoxical splitting of S_2 in ventricular dysfunction
- Systolic murmur of mitral insufficiency
- Pericardial friction rub in transmural MI or pericarditis
- Low-grade fever during the next few days

DIAGNOSTIC TEST RESULTS

LABORATORY

- Levels of serum creatine kinase (CK), especially the CK-myocardial bound (CK-MB) isoenzyme (the cardiac muscle fraction of CK), are elevated.
- Serum lactate dehydrogenase (LD) levels are elevated; there are higher levels of LD1 isoenzyme (found in cardiac tissue) than LD2 (in serum).
- White blood cell count usually appears elevated on the second day and through 1 week.
- Myoglobin (the hemoprotein found in cardiac and skeletal muscle that's released with muscle damage) is detected as soon as 2 hours after MI.
- Levels of troponin I , a structural protein found in cardiac muscle, are elevated only when there's cardiac muscle damage (more specific than the CK-MB level, because troponin levels increase within 4 to 6 hours of myocardial injury and may remain elevated for 5 to 11 days).

IMAGING

- Nuclear medicine scans, using I.V. technetium Tc 99m pertechnetate, can identify acutely damaged muscle by picking up accumulations of radioactive nucleotide, which appear as "hot spots" on the film. Myocardial perfusion imaging with thallium Tl 201 reveals a "cold spot" in most patients during the first few hours after a transmural MI.
- Echocardiography shows ventricular wall dyskinesia in transmural MI and helps to evaluate the ejection fraction.

DIAGNOSTIC PROCEDURES

- Serial 12-lead electrocardiography (ECG) readings may be normal or inconclusive during the first few hours after an MI. Characteristic abnormalities include serial ST-segment depression in subendocardial MI, and ST-segment elevation and Q waves (representing scarring and necrosis) in transmural MI.
- Pulmonary artery catheterization may be performed to detect left- or

right-sided heart failure and to monitor response to treatment.

TREATMENT

GENERAL
- Pacemaker implantation or electrical cardioversion for arrhythmias
- Intra-aortic balloon pump for cardiogenic shock

DIET
- Low-fat, low-cholesterol
- Calorie restriction, if indicated

ACTIVITY
- Bed rest with bedside commode
- Gradual increase in activity as tolerated

MEDICATIONS
- I.V. thrombolytic therapy started within 3 hours of onset of symptoms
- Aspirin
- Antiarrhythmics, antianginals
- Calcium channel blockers
- I.V. heparin
- I.V. morphine
- Inotropic agents
- Beta-adrenergic blockers
- Angiotensin-converting enzyme inhibitors
- Stool softeners
- Oxygen

SURGERY
- Surgical revascularization (coronary artery bypass graft)
- Percutaneous revascularization (percutaneous transluminal coronary angioplasty and stenting)

NURSING CONSIDERATIONS

NURSING DIAGNOSES
- Activity intolerance
- Acute pain
- Anxiety
- Decreased cardiac output
- Excess fluid volume
- Fatigue
- Imbalanced nutrition: Less than body requirements
- Ineffective coping
- Ineffective denial
- Ineffective sexuality patterns
- Ineffective tissue perfusion: Cardiopulmonary

EXPECTED OUTCOMES
The patient will:
- perform activities of daily living without excessive fatigue or exhaustion
- express feelings of increased comfort and decreased pain
- verbalize strategies to reduce anxiety and stress
- maintain adequate cardiac output
- develop no complications of fluid volume excess
- verbalize the importance of balancing activity, as tolerated, with rest
- achieve ideal weight
- exhibit adequate coping skills
- recognize his acute condition and accept the lifestyle changes he needs to make
- voice feelings about changes in sexual patterns
- maintain hemodynamic stability and develop no arrhythmias.

NURSING INTERVENTIONS
- Assess pain and give prescribed analgesics. Record the severity, location, type, and duration of pain. Avoid I.M. injections.
- Check the patient's blood pressure before and after giving nitroglycerin.
- During chest pain, obtain ECG.
- Organize patient care and activities to provide uninterrupted rest.
- Provide a low-cholesterol, low-sodium diet with caffeine-free beverages.
- Allow the patient to use a commode.
- Help with range-of-motion exercises.
- Provide emotional support, and help to reduce stress and anxiety.
- If the patient has undergone percutaneous transluminal coronary angioplasty, sheath care is necessary. Watch for bleeding. Keep the leg with the sheath insertion site immobile. Maintain strict bed rest. Check peripheral pulses in affected leg often.

MONITORING
- Serial ECGs
- Vital signs, heart and breath sounds

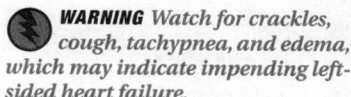 **WARNING** *Watch for crackles, cough, tachypnea, and edema, which may indicate impending left-sided heart failure.*
- Daily weight
- Intake and output
- Cardiac enzyme levels
- Coagulation study results
- Cardiac rhythm for reperfusion arrhythmias (treat according to facility protocol)

PATIENT TEACHING

GENERAL
Be sure to cover:
- procedures
- drug dosages, adverse reactions, and signs of toxicity to watch for
- dietary restrictions
- progressive resumption of sexual activity
- appropriate responses to symptoms
- types of chest pain to report.

DISCHARGE PLANNING
- Refer the patient to a cardiac rehabilitation program.
- Refer the patient to a smoking-cessation program, if needed.
- Refer the patient to a weight-reduction program, if needed.

RESOURCES
Organizations
American Heart Association: *www.americanheart.org*

Selected references
DeVon, H.A., and Ryan, C.J. "Chest Pain and Associated Symptoms of Acute Coronary Syndrome," *Journal of Cardiovascular Nursing* 20(4):232-38, July-August 2005.
Gershlick, A.H., et al. "Rescue Angioplasty after Failed Thrombolytic Therapy for Acute Myocardial Infarction," *New England Journal of Medicine* 353(26):2758-68, December 2005.
Quinn, T. "The Role of Nurses in Improving Emergency Cardiac Care," *Nursing Standard* 19(48):41-48, August 2005.
Vorchheimer, D.A., and Becker, R. "Platelets in Atherothrombosis," *Mayo Clinic Proceedings* 81(1):59-68, January 2006.

Myocarditis

- Focal or diffuse inflammation of the myocardium that's typically uncomplicated and self-limiting
- May be acute or chronic
- Recovery usually spontaneous and without residual defects

PATHOPHYSIOLOGY

- An infectious organism triggers an autoimmune, cellular, and humoral reaction.
- Inflammation may lead to hypertrophy, fibrosis, and inflammatory changes of the myocardium and conduction system.
- Heart muscle weakens, and contractility is reduced.

CAUSES

- Bacteria
- Chronic alcoholism
- Helminthic infections such as trichinosis
- Hypersensitive immune reactions such as acute rheumatic fever
- Parasitic infections
- Radiation therapy
- Viruses

INCIDENCE

- Myocarditis can occur at any age.

COMPLICATIONS

- Left-sided heart failure
- Cardiomyopathy
- Chronic valvulitis (when it results from rheumatic fever)
- Arrhythmias
- Thromboembolism

HISTORY

- Possible recent upper respiratory tract infection with fever, viral pharyngitis, or tonsillitis
- Nonspecific symptoms, such as fatigue, dyspnea, palpitations, persistent tachycardia, and persistent fever
- Mild, continuous pressure or soreness in the chest

PHYSICAL FINDINGS

- S_3 and S_4 gallops, muffled S_1
- Pericardial friction rub

LABORATORY

- Levels of cardiac enzymes, including creatine kinase (CK), CK-myocardial bound (CK-MB), aspartate aminotransferase, and lactate dehydrogenase are elevated.
- White blood cell count and erythrocyte sedimentation rate are elevated.
- Antibody titers, such as antistreptolysin-O titer in rheumatic fever, are elevated.
- Results of cultures of stools, throat or pharyngeal washings, or other body fluids show the causative bacteria or virus.

DIAGNOSTIC PROCEDURES

- Biopsy of the endomyocardium can be used to confirm a myocarditis diagnosis.
- Electrocardiogram typically shows diffuse ST-segment and T-wave abnormalities (as in pericarditis), conduction defects (prolonged PR interval), and ventricular and supraventricular ectopic arrhythmias.

TREATMENT

GENERAL
- Hospitalization until stabilized, for patient with signs and symptoms of heart failure
- Oxygen therapy, if indicated

DIET
- Avoidance of alcohol
- Low-sodium

ACTIVITY
- Modified bed rest
- As tolerated

MEDICATIONS
- Anti-infectives
- Antiarrhythmics
- Anticoagulants
- Anti-inflammatory agents
- Angiotensin-converting enzyme inhibitors
- Diuretics
- Inotropic agents

SURGERY
- Pacemaker implantation
- Ventricular assist device implantation
- Heart transplantation

NURSING CONSIDERATIONS

NURSING DIAGNOSES
- Activity intolerance
- Anxiety
- Decreased cardiac output
- Deficient diversional activity
- Impaired gas exchange
- Ineffective role performance

EXPECTED OUTCOMES
The patient will:
- carry out activities of daily living without weakness or fatigue
- cope with current medical condition without demonstrating severe signs of anxiety
- maintain hemodynamic stability and adequate cardiac output without arrhythmia
- express interest in using leisure time meaningfully
- maintain adequate ventilation and oxygenation
- express feelings about diminished capacity to perform usual roles.

NURSING INTERVENTIONS
- Stress the importance of bed rest. Provide a bedside commode.
- Allow the patient to express his concerns about the effects of activity restrictions on his responsibilities and routines.
- Give prescribed oxygen.
- Give prescribed parenteral anti-infectives and other drugs.

MONITORING
- Vital signs
- Cardiovascular status
- Intake and output
- Signs and symptoms of heart failure
- Signs of digoxin toxicity
- Cardiac rhythm
- Arterial blood gas levels
- Daily weight
- Response to treatment

PATIENT TEACHING

GENERAL
Be sure to cover:
- the disorder, diagnosis, and treatment
- prescribed medications and potential adverse reactions
- prevention of myocarditis
- signs and symptoms of heart failure
- for a patient taking cardiac glycosides at home, how to check the pulse for 1 full minute before taking the dose, and the need to withhold the dose and notify the practitioner if the heart rate falls below the predetermined rate (usually 60 beats/minute)
- when to notify the practitioner.

RESOURCES
Organizations
American Heart Association: *www.americanheart.org*
Mayo Foundation for Medical Education and Research: *www.mayoclinic.com*
National Heart, Lung, and Blood Institute: *www.nhlbi.nih.gov*

Selected references
Kasper, D.L., et al., eds. *Harrison's Principles of Internal Medicine*, 16th ed. New York: McGraw-Hill Book Co., 2005.
The Merck Manual of Diagnosis & Therapy, 18th ed. Whitehouse Station N.J.: Merck & Co., Inc., 2006.
Pulerwitz, T.C., et al. "Mortality in Primary and Secondary Myocarditis," *American Heart Journal* 147(4):746-50, April 2004.
Takkenberg, J., et al. "Eosinophilic Myocarditis in Patients Awaiting Heart Transplantation," *Critical Care Medicine* 32(3):714-21, March 2004.
Williams, P., and Lainchbury, J. "Enteritis-associated Myocarditis," *Heart, Lung & Circulation* 13(1):106-109, March 2004.

◼ Near drowning LIFE-THREATENING DISORDER

OVERVIEW

- Victim surviving physiologic effects of submersion
- Primary problems include hypoxemia and acidosis
- "Dry" near drowning: Fluid not aspirated; respiratory obstruction or asphyxia
- "Wet" near drowning: Fluid aspirated; asphyxia or secondary changes from fluid aspiration
- "Secondary" near drowning: Recurrence of respiratory distress

PATHOPHYSIOLOGY

- Submersion stimulates hyperventilation.
- Voluntary apnea occurs.
- Laryngospasm develops.
- Hypoxemia develops and can lead to brain damage and cardiac arrest.

CAUSES

- Blow to the head while in the water
- Boating accident
- Dangerous water conditions
- Decompression sickness from deep-water diving
- Excessive alcohol consumption before swimming
- Inability to swim
- Panic
- Sudden acute illness
- Suicide attempt
- Venomous stings from aquatic animals

INCIDENCE

- Near drowning is the most common cause of injury and death in children ages 1 month to 14 years.
- The incidence is greater in males.

COMPLICATIONS

- Neurologic impairment
- Seizure disorder
- Pulmonary edema
- Renal damage
- Bacterial aspiration
- Pulmonary complications
- Cardiac complications

ASSESSMENT

HISTORY

- Victim found in water

PHYSICAL FINDINGS

- Fever or hypothermia
- Rapid, slow, or absent pulse
- Shallow, gasping, or absent respirations
- Altered level of consciousness
- Seizures
- Cyanosis or pink, frothy sputum, or both
- Abdominal distention
- Crackles, rhonchi, wheezing, or apnea
- Tachycardia
- Irregular heartbeat

DIAGNOSTIC TEST RESULTS

LABORATORY

- Arterial blood gas (ABG) levels show degree of hypoxia, intrapulmonary shunt, and acid-base balance.
- Electrolyte levels are imbalanced.
- Complete blood count shows hemolysis.
- Blood urea nitrogen and creatinine levels reveal impaired renal function.
- Urinalysis results show signs of impaired renal function.

IMAGING

- Cervical spine X-ray may show evidence of fracture.
- Serial chest X-rays may show pulmonary edema.

DIAGNOSTIC PROCEDURES

- Electrocardiography may show myocardial ischemia, infarct, or cardiac arrhythmias.

TREATMENT

GENERAL
◆ Stabilizing neck with cervical collar
◆ Establishing airway and providing ventilation
◆ Correcting abnormal laboratory values
◆ Warming measures, if hypothermic

DIET
◆ Nothing by mouth until swallowing ability has returned

ACTIVITY
◆ Based on extent of injury and success of resuscitation

MEDICATIONS
◆ Bronchodilators
◆ Cardiac drug therapy, if appropriate
◆ Prophylactic antibiotics

NURSING CONSIDERATIONS

NURSING DIAGNOSES
◆ Anxiety
◆ Decreased cardiac output
◆ Hypothermia
◆ Impaired gas exchange
◆ Ineffective airway clearance
◆ Ineffective breathing pattern
◆ Ineffective coping
◆ Risk for aspiration
◆ Risk for infection

EXPECTED OUTCOMES
The patient will:
◆ express feelings of decreased anxiety
◆ maintain adequate cardiac output
◆ maintain a normal body temperature
◆ maintain adequate ventilation
◆ have a patent airway
◆ maintain effective breathing pattern
◆ develop effective coping mechanisms
◆ show no signs of aspiration
◆ remain free from signs and symptoms of infection.

NURSING INTERVENTIONS
◆ Perform cardiopulmonary resuscitation as indicated.
◆ Perform active external rewarming and passive rewarming measures for mild hypothermia (93.2° to 96.8° F [34° to 36° C]), active external rewarming of truncal areas only and passive rewarming measures for moderate hypothermia (86° to 93.2° F [30° to 34° C], and active internal rewarming measures for severe hypothermia (less than 86° F [30° C]).
◆ Protect the cervical spine.
◆ Give prescribed drugs.
◆ Provide emotional support.

MONITORING
◆ Electrolyte and ABG measurement results
◆ Cardiac rhythm
◆ Vital signs
◆ Neurologic status
◆ Respiratory status
◆ Core body temperature
◆ Psychological state

PATIENT TEACHING

GENERAL
Be sure to cover:
◆ the injury, diagnosis, and treatment
◆ the need to avoid using alcohol or drugs before swimming
◆ water safety measures (such as the "buddy system").

DISCHARGE PLANNING
◆ Recommend a water safety course given by the Red Cross, YMCA, or YWCA.
◆ Refer the patient or family for psychological counseling if appropriate.
◆ Refer the patient or family to resource and support services.

RESOURCES
Organizations
American Academy of Neurology: *www.aan.com*
Brain Injury Association of America: *www.biausa.org*
Harborview Injury Prevention and Research Center: *www.depts.washington.edu/hiprc*
National Center for Injury Prevention and Control: *www.cdc.gov/ncipc*

Selected references
Burford, A.E., et al. "Drowning and Near-drowning in Children and Adolescents: A Succinct Review for Emergency Physicians and Nurses," *Pediatric Emergency Care* 21(9):610-16, September 2005.

Pierro, M.M., et al. "Anoxic Brain Injury Following Near-drowning in Children. Rehabilitation Outcome: Three Case Reports," *Brain Injury* 19(13):1147-155, December 2005.

Robles, L.A., and Curiel, A. "Posttraumatic Cervical Disc Herniation: An Unusual Cause of Near Drowning," *American Journal of Emergency Medicine* 23(7):905-907, November 2005.

Ross, J.L. "Summer Injuries: Near Drowning," *RN* 68(7):36-38, July 2005.

◪ Necrotizing fasciitis LIFE-THREATENING DISORDER

OVERVIEW

- A progressive, rapidly spreading inflammatory infection of the deep fascia
- Mortality rate of 70% to 80%
- Most commonly called *flesh-eating bacteria*
- Also called *hemolytic streptococcal gangrene, acute dermal gangrene, suppurative fasciitis,* and *synergistic necrotizing cellulitis*

PATHOPHYSIOLOGY

- Infecting bacteria enter the host through a local tissue injury or a breach in a mucous membrane barrier.
- Organisms proliferate in an environment of tissue hypoxia caused by trauma, recent surgery, or a medical condition that compromises the patient.
- Necrosis of the surrounding tissue results, accelerating the disease process by creating a favorable environment for organisms to proliferate.
- The fascia and fat tissues are destroyed, resulting in secondary necrosis of subcutaneous tissue.

CAUSES

- Group A beta-hemolytic streptococci (GAS) and *Staphylococcus aureus,* alone or together, as the most common primary infecting bacteria (epidemiology of GAS infections complex because of the more than 80 types of the causative bacteria, *Streptococcus pyogenes*)

INCIDENCE

- Necrotizing fasciitis is three times more likely to occur in men than in women.
- It rarely occurs in children, except in countries with poor hygiene practices.
- The mean age of individuals diagnosed is 38 to 44.
- Elderly or immunocompromised patients and those with chronic illnesses or using steroids are at increased risk for the disease.

COMPLICATIONS

- Renal failure
- Septic shock
- Scarring with cosmetic deformities
- Myositis
- Myonecrosis
- Amputation

ASSESSMENT

HISTORY

- Associated risk factors
- Pain
- Tissue injury

PHYSICAL FINDINGS

- Rapidly progressing erythema at the site of insult
- Fluid-filled blisters and bullae (indicate rapid progression of the necrotizing process)
- Large areas of gangrenous skin by days 4 and 5
- Extensive necrosis of the subcutaneous tissue by days 7 to 10
- Fever
- Sepsis
- Hypovolemia
- Hypotension
- Respiratory insufficiency
- Deterioration in level of consciousness
- Signs of sepsis

DIAGNOSTIC TEST RESULTS

LABORATORY

- Results of biopsy of tissue show infiltration of the deep dermis, fascia, and muscular planes with bacteria and polymorphonuclear cells, and necrosis of fatty and muscular tissue.
- Results of cultures of microorganisms from the periphery of the spreading infection or from deeper tissues during surgical debridement identify the causative organism.
- Results of Gram stain and culture of biopsied tissue identify the causative organism.

IMAGING

- Radiographic study results may pinpoint the presence of subcutaneous gases.
- Computed tomography scan results may show the anatomic site of involvement by locating the area of necrosis.
- Magnetic resonance imaging results show areas of necrosis and areas that require surgical debridement.

TREATMENT

GENERAL
- Wound care
- Hyperbaric oxygen therapy

DIET
- High-protein, high-calorie
- Increased fluid intake

ACTIVITY
- Bed rest until treatment is effective

MEDICATIONS
- Antimicrobials
- Analgesics

SURGERY
- Immediate surgical debridement, fasciectomy, or amputation

NURSING CONSIDERATIONS

NURSING DIAGNOSES
- Acute pain
- Decreased cardiac output
- Deficient fluid volume
- Hyperthermia
- Impaired tissue integrity
- Ineffective tissue perfusion: Cardiopulmonary, peripheral

EXPECTED OUTCOMES
The patient will:
- express feeling of comfort and relief from pain
- maintain adequate cardiac output
- maintain adequate fluid volume
- remain afebrile
- receive adequate blood supply to the wound
- maintain collateral circulation and hemodynamic stability.

NURSING INTERVENTIONS
- Give prescribed drugs.
- Provide supportive care and supplemental oxygen as appropriate.
- Provide emotional support.

MONITORING
- Signs and symptoms of complications
- Vital signs
- Mental status
- Wound status
- Pain control

PATIENT TEACHING

GENERAL
Be sure to cover:
- the disorder, diagnosis, and treatment
- the importance of strict sterile technique and proper hand-washing technique for wound care
- drug administration, dosage, and possible adverse effects
- the importance of recognizing and reporting signs and symptoms of complications.

DISCHARGE PLANNING
- Refer the patient for follow-up with an infectious disease specialist and surgeon as indicated.
- Refer the patient for physical rehabilitation, if indicated.
- For education and support, refer the patient to organizations such as the National Necrotizing Fasciitis Foundation.

RESOURCES
Organizations
Centers for Disease Control and Prevention: *www.cdc.gov*
Harvard University Consumer Health Information: *www.intelihealth.com*
National Institute of Allergy and Infectious Diseases: *www3.niaid.nih.gov*
National Necrotizing Fasciitis Foundation: *www.nnff.org*

Selected references
Kasper, D.L., et al., eds. *Harrison's Principles of Internal Medicine*, 16th ed. New York: McGraw-Hill Book Co., 2005.

McGee, E.J. "Necrotizing Fasciitis: Review of Pathophysiology, Diagnosis, and Treatment," *Critical Care Nursing Quarterly* 28(1):80-84, January-March 2005.

Rodreguez, R.M., et al. "A Pilot Study of Cytokine Levels and White Blood Cell Counts in the Diagnosis of Necrotizing Fasciitis," *American Journal of Emergency Medicine* 24(1):58-61, January 2006.

Young, M.H., et al. "Therapies for Necrotising Fasciitis," *Expert Opinion on Biological Therapy* 6(2):155-65, February 2006.

Nephrotic syndrome

- Kidney disorder characterized by marked proteinuria, hypoalbuminemia, hyperlipidemia, increased coagulation, and edema
- Results from a glomerular defect that affects permeability, indicating renal damage
- Prognosis highly variable, depending on underlying cause
- Some forms possibly progressing to end-stage renal failure
- Classified as primary or secondary

PATHOPHYSIOLOGY

- Glomerular protein permeability increases.
- Urinary excretion of protein, especially albumin, increases.
- Hypoalbuminemia develops and causes decreased colloidal oncotic pressure.
- Leakage of fluid into interstitial spaces leads to acute, generalized edema.
- Vascular volume loss leads to increased blood viscosity and coagulation disorders.
- The renin-angiotensin system is triggered, causing tubular reabsorption of sodium and water and contributing to edema.

CAUSES

- Certain neoplastic diseases such as multiple myeloma
- Circulatory diseases
- Collagen vascular disorders
- Focal glomerulosclerosis (can develop spontaneously at any age, occur after kidney transplantation, or result from heroin injection; develops in about 10% of childhood cases and up to 20% of adult cases)
- Lipid nephrosis (main cause in children younger than age 8)
- Membranoproliferative glomerulonephritis (may follow infection, particularly streptococcal infection; occurs primarily in children and young adults)
- Membranous glomerulonephritis (most common lesion in adult idiopathic nephrotic syndrome)
- Metabolic diseases
- Primary (idiopathic) glomerulonephritis (about 75% of cases)

RISK FACTORS

- Nephrotoxins
- Infection
- Allergic reactions
- Pregnancy
- Hereditary nephritis
- Chronic analgesic abuse

INCIDENCE

- The incidence in children is 1 in 50,000 population per year.
- The incidence in adults is 1 or 2 in 50,000 population per year.
- Peak incidence in children is between ages 2 and 3.
- It's slightly more common in men than in women.
- Incidence is higher in Native American, Hispanic, and Black populations.

COMPLICATIONS

- Malnutrition
- Infection
- Coagulation disorders
- Thromboembolic vascular occlusion
- Accelerated atherosclerosis
- Acute renal failure

HISTORY

- Lethargy
- Depression
- Anorexia
- Underlying cause
- Presence of risk factor
- Decreased urination
- Frothy urine

PHYSICAL FINDINGS

- Periorbital edema
- Mild to severe dependent edema
- Orthostatic hypotension
- Ascites
- Swollen external genitalia
- Signs of pleural effusion
- Pallor

LABORATORY

- Urinalysis results reveal an increased number of hyaline, granular, waxy, fatty casts, oval fat bodies, and consistent, heavy proteinuria (levels greater than 3.5 mg/dl for 24 hours).
- Serum cholesterol, phospholipid, and triglyceride levels are elevated, and serum albumin level is decreased.

DIAGNOSTIC PROCEDURES

- Renal biopsy results allow histologic identification of the lesion.

GENERAL
◆ Correction of the underlying cause, if possible
◆ Diet consisting of 0.6 g of protein per kilogram of body weight
◆ Restricted sodium intake
◆ Frequent rest periods

MEDICATIONS
◆ Diuretics
◆ Antibiotics for infection
◆ Glucocorticoids
◆ Possible alkylating agents
◆ Possible cytotoxics
◆ I.V. albumin
◆ Angiotensin-converting enzyme inhibitors (cornerstone of treatment in adults)

NURSING DIAGNOSES
◆ Disturbed body image
◆ Excess fluid volume
◆ Imbalanced nutrition: Less than body requirements
◆ Ineffective tissue perfusion: Renal
◆ Risk for infection
◆ Risk for injury

EXPECTED OUTCOMES
The patient will:
◆ express positive feelings about body image
◆ maintain fluid balance
◆ show no signs of malnutrition
◆ maintain adequate urine output
◆ remain free from signs and symptoms of infection
◆ avoid or have minimal complications of the disorder.

NURSING INTERVENTIONS
◆ Offer the patient reassurance and support, especially during the acute phase, when severe edema changes body image.
◆ Provide information regarding dietary restrictions and fluid restriction.

MONITORING
◆ Urine for protein
◆ Intake and output
◆ Daily weight
◆ Plasma albumin and transferrin levels
◆ Edema

GENERAL
Be sure to cover:
◆ the disorder, diagnosis, and treatment
◆ signs of infection that should be reported
◆ the importance of adherence to diet
◆ drug administration, dosage, and possible adverse effects.

DISCHARGE PLANNING
◆ Refer the patient to resource and support services.

RESOURCES
Organizations
American Association of Kidney Patients: *www.aakp.org*
National Institute of Diabetes & Digestive & Kidney Diseases: *www.niddk.nih.gov*

Selected references
Broome, L.F. "Treating Pediatric Nephrotic Syndrome: A Clinical Challenge," *Nephrology Nursing Journal* 30(6):662-63, 667, December 2003.
Diseases, 4th ed. Philadelphia: Lippincott Williams & Wilkins, 2006.
Papez, K.E., and Smoyer, W.E. "Recent Advances in Congenital Nephrotic Syndrome," *Current Opinion in Pediatrics* 16(2):165-70, April 2004.
Yakupoglu, U., et al. "Post-transplant Nephrotic Syndrome: A Comprehensive Clinicopathologic Study," *Kidney International* 65(6):2360-370, June 2004.

Neural tube defects

OVERVIEW

- Birth defects that involve the spine or skull
- Result from neural tube's failure to close about 28 days after conception
- Different forms include spina bifida (50% of cases), anencephaly (40%), and encephalocele (10%)

PATHOPHYSIOLOGY

- Spina bifida occulta, the least severe neural tube defect (NTD), is characterized by incomplete closure of one or more vertebrae without protrusion of the spinal cord or meninges. When defects of neural tube closure occur, such as meningocele and myelomeningocele, an accompanying vertebral defect allows the protrusion of the neural tube contents. (See *Types of spinal cord defects.*)
- In encephalocele, a saclike portion of the meninges and brain protrudes through a defective opening in the skull. Usually it occurs in the occipital area, but it may also occur in the parietal, nasopharyngeal, or frontal area.
- In anencephaly, the closure defect occurs at the cranial end of the neuraxis and, as a result, part or the entire top of the skull is missing, severely damaging the brain. Portions of the brain stem and spinal cord may also be missing. This condition is fatal.

CAUSES

- A combination of genetic and environmental factors (possibly a lack of folic acid in the mother's diet)
- Exposure to a teratogen
- Trisomy 18 or trisomy 13 syndrome, or another multiple malformation syndrome

INCIDENCE

- Spina bifida occulta is the most common NTD.
- The incidence of NTD in North Carolina and South Carolina is at least twice that in the rest of the United States.
- NTD is more common in Whites than in Blacks.

COMPLICATIONS

- Paralysis below the level of the defect
- Infection such as meningitis
- Hydrocephalus
- Death

ASSESSMENT

HISTORY

- Maternal history revealing factors that cause defect

PHYSICAL FINDINGS

Spina bifida occulta
- Possibly a depression or dimple, tuft of hair, soft fatty deposit, port wine nevi, or a combination of these abnormalities on the skin over the spinal area
- Saclike protrusion over the spinal cord
- Flaccid or spastic paralysis

Encephalocele
- Saclike protrusion through a defective opening in the skull
- Paralysis

Anencephaly
- Part or entire top of skull missing

DIAGNOSTIC TEST RESULTS

LABORATORY

- Levels of maternal alpha-fetoprotein (AFP), amniotic fluid AFP, and amniotic fluid acetylcholinesterase are elevated, indicating the need for further testing.
- Results of fetal karyotype analysis detect chromosomal abnormalities (present in 5% to 7% of NTDs).
- Results of maternal serum AFP screening, combined with screening for other serum markers, such as human chorionic gonadotropin (hCG), free beta-hCG, and unconjugated estriol (for patients with a lower risk of NTDs and those who will be younger than age 34½ at the time of delivery), estimate the risk of fetal NTD and possible perinatal complications (premature rupture of the membranes, abruptio placentae, and fetal death).

IMAGING

- Ultrasonography (used when family history or abnormal serum screening results indicate an increased risk of open NTD) isn't conclusive for open NTDs or ventral wall defects.
- Spinal X-rays reveal spina bifida occulta.
- Myelography results differentiate spina bifida occulta from other spinal abnormalities, especially spinal cord tumors.
- Skull X-rays, cephalic measurements, and computed tomography (CT) scan demonstrate associated hydrocephalus.
- X-rays show a basilar, bony skull defect (CT scan and ultrasonography results further define the defect [for encephalocele]).

OTHER

- Transillumination of the protruding sac distinguishes between myelomeningocele (typically doesn't transilluminate) and meningocele (typically transilluminates).

TREATMENT

GENERAL

- Symptomatic treatment according to neurologic effects of defect
- Assessment of growth and development throughout lifetime

DIET

- As tolerated

ACTIVITY

- Physical therapy

MEDICATIONS

- Antibiotics as indicated

SURGERY

- Surgical closure of the protruding sac
- Shunt placement to relieve associated hydrocephalus
- Surgery during infancy to place protruding tissues back in the skull, ex-

cise the sac, and correct associated craniofacial abnormalities (for encephalocele)

NURSING DIAGNOSES
- Decreased intracranial adaptive capacity
- Delayed growth and development
- Impaired parenting
- Impaired physical mobility
- Impaired skin integrity
- Impaired urinary elimination
- Ineffective tissue perfusion: Peripheral
- Risk for impaired parent/infant/child attachment
- Risk for infection
- Risk for injury

EXPECTED OUTCOMES
The patient (or family) will:
- maintain a stable head circumference and soft, flat fontanels
- achieve age-appropriate growth, skills, and behaviors to the fullest extent possible
- identify realistic goals for their child
- maintain joint mobility and range of motion
- maintain adequate skin integrity
- maintain balance in intake and output

- exhibit signs of adequate peripheral perfusion
- show signs of bonding with their infant and participate in his care
- remain free from signs and symptoms of infection
- show no signs of complications of the disorder.

NURSING INTERVENTIONS
- Provide psychological support.

Before surgery
- Clean the defect gently with sterile saline solution or other solutions as ordered.
- Handle the infant carefully, and don't apply pressure to the defect.
- Provide adequate time for parent-child bonding, if possible.

After surgery
- Change the dressing regularly, as ordered, and check and report any signs of drainage, wound rupture, and infection.
- Place the infant prone to protect and assess the site.
- If leg casts have been applied, watch for signs that the child is outgrowing the cast. Regularly check distal pulses to ensure adequate circulation.

MONITORING
Before surgery
- Neurologic status
- Feeding ability
- Nutritional status

After surgery
- Signs of infection
- Signs of increased intracranial pressure
- Intake and output
- Vital signs

PATIENT TEACHING

GENERAL
Be sure to cover:
- the disorder, diagnosis, and treatment
- how to prevent contractures, pressure ulcers, and urinary tract infections.

DISCHARGE PLANNING
- Refer the prospective parents to a genetic counselor when an NTD has been diagnosed prenatally.
- Refer the family for psychological and support services.

RESOURCES
Organizations
American Academy of Neurology: *www.aan.com*
Centers for Disease Control and Prevention: *www.cdc.gov*
The Merck Manual of Medical Information — Second Home Edition, Online Version: *www.merck.com/mmhe*

Selected references
Mowatt, D.J., et al. "Tissue Expansion for the Delayed Closure of Large Myelomeningoceles," *Journal of Neurosurgery* 103(6 Suppl):544-48, December 2005.
Neville-Jan, A. "The Problem with Prevention: The Case of Spina Bifida," *American Journal of Occupational Therapy* 59(5):527-39, September-October 2005.
Ryan, M. "Folic Acid to Prevent Neural Tube Defects: A Potential Pharmacy Initiative with Public Health Implications," *Hospital Pharmacy* 39(10):962-69, October 2004.

Types of spinal cord defects

There are three major types of spinal cord defects. *Spina bifida occulta* is characterized by a depression or raised area and a tuft of hair over the defect. In *myelomeningocele*, an external sac contains meninges, cerebrospinal fluid, and a portion of the spinal cord or nerve roots. *Meningocele* is characterized by an external sac containing only meninges and cerebrospinal fluid.

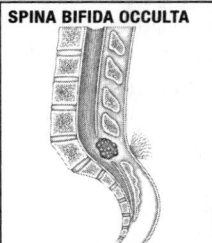

SPINA BIFIDA OCCULTA

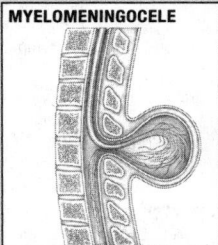

MYELOMENINGOCELE

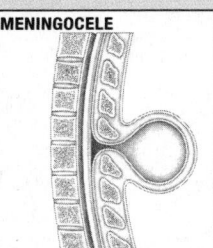

MENINGOCELE

Neurogenic bladder

OVERVIEW

- All types of bladder dysfunction caused by an interruption of normal bladder innervation by the nervous system
- Can be hyperreflexic (hypertonic, spastic, or automatic) or flaccid (hypotonic, atonic, or autonomous)
- Also known as *neuromuscular dysfunction of the lower urinary tract, neurologic bladder dysfunction,* and *neuropathic bladder*

PATHOPHYSIOLOGY

- An upper motor neuron lesion (at or above T12) causes spastic neurogenic bladder, with spontaneous contractions of detrusor muscles, increased intravesical voiding pressure, bladder wall hypertrophy with trabeculation, and urinary sphincter spasms.
- A lower motor neuron lesion (at or below S2 to S4) affects the spinal reflex that controls micturition. The result is a flaccid neurogenic bladder, with decreased intravesical pressure, increased bladder capacity, residual urine retention, and poor detrusor contraction. The bladder may not empty spontaneously.
- Interruption of the efferent nerves at the cortical level results in loss of voluntary control. Higher centers also control micturition, and voiding may be incomplete. Sensory neuron interruption leads to dribbling and overflow incontinence. (See *Types of neurogenic bladder.*)

CAUSES

- Acute infectious diseases
- Cerebral disorders
- Chronic alcoholism
- Collagen diseases
- Heavy metal toxicity
- Herpes zoster
- Metabolic disturbances
- Sacral agenesis (absence of a completely formed sacrum)
- Spinal cord disease
- Trauma
- Vascular diseases

INCIDENCE

- Incidence is based on the type of neurogenic bladder disorder.

COMPLICATIONS

- Incontinence
- Residual urine retention
- Urinary tract infections (UTIs)
- Calculus formation
- Renal failure

ASSESSMENT

HISTORY

- Frequent UTIs
- Hyperactive autonomic reflexes (autonomic dysreflexia) when the bladder is distended and the lesion is at upper thoracic or cervical level
- Involuntary or frequent, scant urination without a feeling of bladder fullness
- Overflow incontinence and diminished anal sphincter tone, due to flaccid neurogenic bladder

PHYSICAL FINDINGS

- Severe hypertension, bradycardia, and vasodilation (blotchy skin) above the level of the lesion
- Piloerection and profuse sweating above the level of the lesion
- Spontaneous spasms (caused by voiding) of the arms and legs
- Increased anal sphincter tone
- Greatly distended bladder without feeling of bladder fullness due to sensory impairment

DIAGNOSTIC TEST RESULTS

IMAGING

- Retrograde urethrography results show strictures and diverticula.

DIAGNOSTIC PROCEDURES

- Voiding cystourethrography results evaluate bladder neck function, vesicoureteral reflux, and continence.
- Results of urodynamic studies evaluate how urine is stored in the bladder, how well the bladder empties urine, and the movement of urine out of the bladder during voiding.
- Urine flow study (uroflow) results show diminished or impaired urine flow.

Types of neurogenic bladder

NEURAL LESION	TYPE	CAUSE
Upper motor	Uninhibited	- Lack of voluntary control in infancy - Multiple sclerosis
	Reflex or automatic	- Spinal cord transection - Cord tumors - Multiple sclerosis
Lower motor	Autonomous	- Sacral cord trauma - Tumors - Herniated disk - Abdominal surgery with transection of pelvic parasympathetic nerves
	Motor paralysis	- Lesions at levels S2, S3, S4 - Poliomyelitis - Trauma - Tumors
	Sensory paralysis	- Posterior lumbar nerve roots - Diabetes mellitus - Tabes dorsalis

- Cystometry results evaluate bladder nerve supply, detrusor muscle tone, and intravesical pressures during bladder filling and contraction.
- Results of urethral pressure profile determine urethral function with respect to the urethra's length and outlet pressure resistance.
- Results of sphincter electromyelography correlate neuromuscular function of the external sphincter with bladder muscle function during bladder filling and contraction; they also evaluate how well the bladder and urinary sphincter muscles work together.
- Videourodynamic study results correlate visual documentation of bladder function with pressure studies.

TREATMENT

GENERAL
- Use of incontinence products
- Insertion of urethral occlusive devices
- Catheterization of the bladder
- Bladder training program

DIET
- Avoidance of dietary stimulants, such as spicy foods, citrus fruits, and chocolate
- Avoidance of excessive fluid intake
- Avoidance of caffeinated and carbonated products

ACTIVITY
- Pelvic muscle exercises

MEDICATIONS
- Anticholinergics
- Alpha-adrenergic stimulators
- Antispasmodics

SURGERY
- External sphincterotomy, urethral dilation, urinary diversion, or transurethral resection of the bladder neck to correct structural impairment
- Possible implantation of an artificial urinary sphincter, if permanent incontinence follows surgery

NURSING CONSIDERATIONS

NURSING DIAGNOSES
- Acute pain
- Deficient fluid volume
- Disturbed body image
- Impaired skin integrity
- Impaired urinary elimination
- Risk for infection
- Risk for injury
- Sexual dysfunction
- Urinary retention

EXPECTED OUTCOMES
The patient will:
- report increased comfort and decreased pain
- maintain fluid balance
- express positive feelings about body image
- maintain skin integrity
- regain normal voiding habits
- remain free from signs and symptoms of infection
- avoid or minimize complications of the disorder
- reestablish sexual activity to the fullest extent possible
- completely evacuate the bladder with voiding or through alternative methods.

NURSING INTERVENTIONS
- Catheterize the patient as appropriate.
- Provide emotional support as appropriate.

MONITORING
- Intake and output
- Signs of infection

PATIENT TEACHING

GENERAL
Be sure to cover:
- the disorder, diagnosis, and treatment
- dietary adjustments
- pelvic exercises
- bladder evacuation techniques.

RESOURCES
Organizations
American Urological Association: *www.auanet.org*
National Institute of Diabetes & Digestive & Kidney Diseases: *www.niddk.nih.gov*

Selected references
Lemke, J.R., et al. "Intermittent Catheterization for Patients with Neurogenic Bladder: Sterile Versus Clean: Using Evidence-based Practice at the Staff Nurse Level," *Journal of Nursing Care Quality* 20(4):302-306, October-December 2005.
Misawa, T., et al. "Neurogenic Bladder in Patients with Cervical Compressive Myelopathy," *Journal of Spinal Disorders & Techniques* 18(4):315-20, August 2005.
Zickler, C.F., and Richardson, V. "Achieving Continence in Children with Neurogenic Bowel and Bladder," *Journal of Pediatric Health Care* 18(6):276-83, November-December 2004.

Nocardiosis

- Acute, subacute, or chronic bacterial infection caused by a weakly gram-positive species of the genus *Nocardia* — usually *Nocardia asteroides*

PATHOPHYSIOLOGY

- *Nocardia* are aerobic gram-positive bacteria with branching filaments resembling fungi.
- Normally found in soil, these organisms cause occasional sporadic disease in humans and animals throughout the world.
- Their incubation period is unknown but probably lasts several weeks.
- The usual mode of transmission is inhalation of organisms suspended in dust. Transmission by direct inoculation through puncture wounds or abrasions is less common.

CAUSES

- Inhalation or inoculation of *Nocardia* bacteria

RISK FACTORS

- Immunocompromised state
- Alcoholism
- Pulmonary alveolar proteinosis
- Male sex

INCIDENCE

- About 500 to 1,000 cases occur annually in the United States.
- It's more common in men (3:1), especially those with a compromised immune system.
- Mortality exceeds 80% in patients with brain infection; mortality is 50% in other forms.

COMPLICATIONS

- Pleurisy
- Intrapleural effusions
- Empyema
- Tracheitis
- Bronchitis
- Pericarditis
- Endocarditis
- Peritonitis
- Mediastinitis
- Septic arthritis
- Keratoconjunctivitis
- Purulent meningitis
- Seizures

ASSESSMENT

HISTORY

- Immunocompromising condition
- Chills
- Night sweats
- Anorexia
- Malaise
- Weight loss
- Dyspnea
- Pleural pain
- Puncture wound or abrasion

PHYSICAL FINDINGS

- Fever
- Cellulitis
- Productive cough
- Subcutaneous abscesses that lack induration
- Crackles

DIAGNOSTIC TEST RESULTS

LABORATORY

- Results of culture from site of infection identify causative organism.

IMAGING

- Chest X-rays vary and may show fluffy or interstitial infiltrates, nodules, or abscesses.

DIAGNOSTIC PROCEDURES

- Biopsy of lung or other tissue shows the causative organism.
- In brain infection with meningitis, lumbar puncture results show nonspecific changes such as increased opening pressure; analysis of cerebrospinal fluid shows increased white blood cell count and protein levels, and decreased glucose levels compared with serum glucose analysis.

TREATMENT

GENERAL
- Safety measures

DIET
- As tolerated

ACTIVITY
- As tolerated (bed rest during acute phase)

MEDICATIONS
- Antimicrobial therapy for at least 6 months
- Combination drug therapy (sulfonamide, ceftriaxone) and amikacin
- Antipyretics

SURGERY
- Drainage of abscesses and excision of necrotic tissue

NURSING CONSIDERATIONS

NURSING DIAGNOSES
- Acute pain
- Hyperthermia
- Imbalanced nutrition: Less than body requirements
- Impaired gas exchange
- Impaired physical mobility
- Ineffective airway clearance
- Ineffective tissue perfusion: Cerebral, cardiopulmonary
- Risk for injury

EXPECTED OUTCOMES
The patient will:
- report pain relief with analgesia or other measures
- remain afebrile
- experience no further weight loss
- maintain adequate ventilation
- resume normal physical mobility during recovery
- cough effectively and maintain a patent airway
- maintain tissue perfusion and cellular oxygenation
- remain free from complications of the disorder.

NURSING INTERVENTIONS
- Encourage coughing and deep-breathing exercises.
- Provide psychological support.
- Give prescribed antibiotics.
- Provide adequate nourishment.
- Give tepid sponge baths to reduce fever.
- Perform chest physiotherapy.
- Assist with range-of-motion exercises.

MONITORING
- Vital signs
- Respiratory status
- Sputum production and character
- Compliance with treatment
- Allergic reaction to antibiotics

PATIENT TEACHING

GENERAL
Be sure to cover:
- the disorder, diagnosis, and treatment
- the need for long-term antibiotic therapy
- signs of worsening infection
- signs of allergic reaction to antibiotics.

DISCHARGE PLANNING
- Encourage follow-up care as indicated.

RESOURCES
Organizations
Centers for Disease Control and Prevention: *www.cdc.gov*
National Library of Medicine: *www.nlm.nih.gov*
WebMD: *www.webmd.com*

Selected references
Cheng, H.M., et al. "Disseminated Nocardiosis with Initial Manifestation Mimicking Disease Flare-up of Systemic Lupus Erythematosus in an SLE Patient," *American Journal of Medicine* 118(11):1297-298, November 2005.
Diseases, 4th ed. Philadelphia: Lippincott Williams & Wilkins, 2006.
Lederman, E.R., and Crum, N.F. "A Case Series and Focused Review of Nocardiosis: Clinical and Microbiologic Aspects," *Medicine* 83(5):300-313, September 2004.
Soy, M., et al. "Nocardiosis in a Patient with Primary Anti-phospholipid Syndrome," *Rheumatology International* 26(5):461-64, March 2006.

Obesity

OVERVIEW

- An excess of body fat, generally 20% above ideal body weight
- Body mass index (BMI) of 30 or greater (see *BMI measurements*)
- Second-leading cause of preventable deaths

PATHOPHYSIOLOGY

- Fat cells increase in size in response to dietary intake.
- When the cells can no longer expand, they increase in number.
- With weight loss, the size of the fat cells decreases, but the number of cells doesn't.

CAUSES

- Excessive caloric intake combined with inadequate energy expenditure
- Theories to explain obesity include:
- abnormal absorption of nutrients
- environmental factors
- genetic predisposition
- hypothalamic dysfunction of hunger and satiety centers
- impaired action of GI and growth hormones and of hormonal regulators such as insulin
- psychological factors
- socioeconomic status

INCIDENCE

- More than 50% of people in the United States are overweight.
- Obesity affects one in five children.

COMPLICATIONS

- Respiratory difficulties
- Hypertension
- Cardiovascular disease
- Diabetes mellitus
- Renal disease
- Gallbladder disease
- Psychosocial difficulties
- Premature death

ASSESSMENT

HISTORY

- Increasing weight
- Complications of obesity

PHYSICAL FINDINGS

- BMI of 30 or greater

DIAGNOSTIC TEST RESULTS

GENERAL

- Comparison of height and weight with a standard table helps determine obesity.
- Measurement of the thickness of subcutaneous fat folds with calipers approximates total body fat. (See *Taking anthropometric arm measurements.*)
- BMI calculation helps to confirm obesity.

TREATMENT

GENERAL

- Hypnosis and behavior modification techniques
- Psychological counseling

DIET

- Reduction in daily caloric intake

ACTIVITY

- Increase in daily activity level

SURGERY

- Vertical banded gastroplasty
- Gastric bypass

NURSING CONSIDERATIONS

NURSING DIAGNOSES

- Chronic low self-esteem
- Disturbed body image
- Imbalanced nutrition: More than body requirements
- Ineffective coping
- Sedentary lifestyle

EXPECTED OUTCOMES

The patient will:
- voice feelings related to self-esteem
- express positive feelings about self
- safely reduce weight and reduce BMI to a normal level
- demonstrate effective coping mechanisms to deal with long-term compliance
- state the need to increase activity level.

NURSING INTERVENTIONS

- Obtain an accurate diet history to identify the patient's eating patterns and the importance of food to his lifestyle.
- Promote increased physical activity as appropriate.

MONITORING

- Diet
- Intake and output
- Vital signs
- Weight and BMI

BMI measurements

Use these steps to calculate body mass index (BMI):
- Multiply weight in pounds by 705.
- Divide this number by height in inches.
- Then divide this by height in inches again.
- Compare results to these standards:
- 18.5 to 24.9: normal
- 25 to 29.9: overweight
- 30 to 39.9: obese
- 40 or greater: morbidly obese.

Taking anthropometric arm measurements

Follow these steps to determine triceps skin-fold thickness, midarm circumference, and midarm muscle circumference.

TRICEPS SKIN-FOLD THICKNESS

◆ Find the midpoint circumference of the arm by placing the tape measure halfway between the axilla and the elbow. Grasp the patient's skin with your thumb and forefinger, about ⅜" (1 cm) above the midpoint, as shown below.
◆ Place calipers at the midpoint, and squeeze for 3 seconds.
◆ Record the measurement to the nearest millimeter.
◆ Take two more readings, and use the average.

MIDARM CIRCUMFERENCE AND MIDARM MUSCLE CIRCUMFERENCE

◆ At the midpoint, measure the midarm circumference, as shown below. Record the measurement in centimeters.

◆ Calculate the midarm muscle circumference by multiplying the triceps skin-fold thickness — measured in millimeters — by 3.14.
◆ Subtract this number from the midarm circumference.

RECORDING THE MEASUREMENTS

Record all three measurements as a percentage of the standard measurements (see table below), using this formula:

$$\frac{\text{Actual measurement}}{\text{Standard measurement}} \times 100\%$$

Remember, a measurement less than 90% of the standard indicates caloric deprivation. A measurement over 90% indicates adequate or more-than-adequate energy reserves.

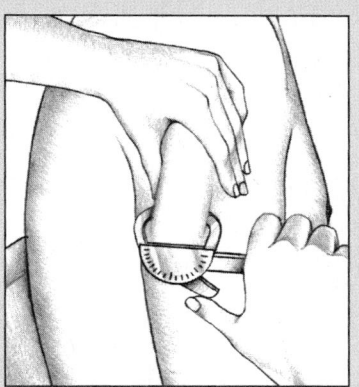 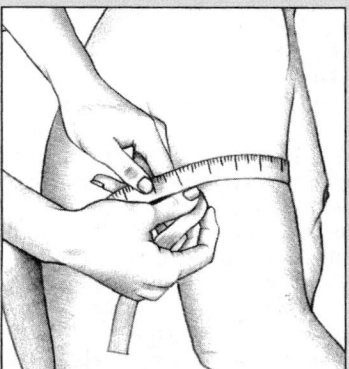

MEASUREMENT	STANDARD	90%
Triceps skin-fold thickness	Men: 12.5 mm Women: 16.5 mm	Men: 11.3 mm Women: 14.9 mm
Midarm circumference	Men: 29.3 cm Women: 28.5 cm	Men: 26.4 cm Women: 25.7 cm
Midarm muscle circumference	Men: 25.3 cm Women: 23.3 cm	Men: 22.8 cm Women: 20.9 cm

GENERAL

Be sure to cover:
◆ need for long-term maintenance after desired weight is achieved
◆ dietary guidelines
◆ safe weight-loss practices.

DISCHARGE PLANNING

◆ Refer the patient to a weight-reduction program.

RESOURCES

Organizations

American Obesity Association: *www.obesity.org*
Obesity Help, Inc.: *www.obesityhelp.com*
The Obesity Society: *www.naaso.org*

Selected references

Brown, I. "Nurses' Attitudes Towards Adult Patients Who Are Obese: Literature Review," *Journal of Advanced Nursing* 53(2):221-32, January 2006.

Dietz, W.H., and Robinson, T.N. "Clinical Practice. Overweight Children and Adolescents," *New England Journal of Medicine* 352(20):2100-09, May 2005.

Lapane, K.L., and Resnik, L. "Obesity in Nursing Homes: An Escalating Problem," *Journal of the American Geriatrics Society* 53(8):1386-91, August 2005.

Yensel, C.S., et al. "Childhood Obesity and Insulin-Resistant Syndrome," *Journal of Pediatric Nursing* 19(4):238-46, August 2004.

Obsessive-compulsive disorder

- Obsessive thoughts and compulsive behaviors that impair everyday functioning
- May be simple or complex and ritualized
- Also known as *OCD*

PATHOPHYSIOLOGY

- This anatomic-physiologic disturbance is thought to involve an alteration in the frontal-subcortical neural circuitry of the brain.

CAUSES

- Decrease in caudate nucleus volume

RISK FACTORS

- Coexisting mental disorder
- Tic disorders

INCIDENCE

- OCD affects 1 in 50 people in the United States.
- The disorder may develop at any age.
- It's more common in males and in first-born children.

COMPLICATIONS

- Impairment of occupational and social functioning
- Endangerment of health and safety

HISTORY

- Presence of obsessive thoughts, words, or mental images that persistently and involuntarily invade the consciousness
- Moderate to severe impairment of social and occupational functioning
- Patient usually rigid and conscientious, with great aspirations
- Patient serious about responsibility, having difficulty making decisions
- Patient lacking creativity and the ability to find alternate solutions to problems

PHYSICAL FINDINGS

- Formal, reserved manner
- Patient accurate and precise, carefully qualifying statements and anticipating moves and gestures of person to whom he speaks
- Flat, unemotional affect, except for controlled anxiety
- Intellectual self-awareness, without accompanying emotion or feeling

DSM-IV-TR *criteria*

Diagnosis is confirmed when the patient meets these criteria:

- For obsessions
- Patient experiences recurrent and persistent ideas, thoughts, impulses, or images as intrusive and senseless.
- Patient attempts to ignore or suppress such thoughts or impulses or to neutralize them with some other thought or action.
- Patient recognizes that the obsessions are products of his mind, not externally imposed.
- Patient's obsession is unrelated to another Axis I disorder.
- For compulsions
- Patient performs repetitive, purposeful, and intentional behaviors in response to an obsession or according to certain rules or in a stereotypical manner.
- Behavior is intended to neutralize or prevent discomfort or some dreaded event or situation, but the behavior isn't connected in a realistic way with intended outcome, or is clearly excessive.
- Patient recognizes that the behavior is excessive or unreasonable.

GENERAL

- No specific diagnostic test exists for this disorder.
- Diagnosis depends on confirmation by *DSM-IV-TR* criteria.

TREATMENT

GENERAL
- Behavioral therapy
- Increasing exposure to stressful situations
- Keeping a diary of daily stressors
- Substituting new activities for compulsive behavior

MEDICATIONS
- Selective serotonin-reuptake inhibitors

NURSING CONSIDERATIONS

NURSING DIAGNOSES
- Anxiety
- Chronic low self-esteem
- Fear
- Impaired social interaction
- Ineffective coping
- Ineffective role performance
- Risk for injury
- Social isolation

EXPECTED OUTCOMES
The patient will:
- express feelings of anxiety as they occur
- express positive feelings about self
- express fears and concerns
- cope with stress without excessive obsessive-compulsive behavior
- reduce the amount of time spent each day on obsessing and ritualizing
- demonstrate effective social interaction skills
- produce no harmful effects from ritualistic behavior
- maintain family and peer relationships.

NURSING INTERVENTIONS
- Provide an accepting, patient atmosphere.
- Allow time for ritualistic behavior (unless it's dangerous) until distraction occurs.
- Provide for basic needs.
- Make reasonable demands and set reasonable limits; make the patient's purpose clear.
- Explore patterns leading to the behavior or recurring problems.
- Encourage active diversional resources.
- Assist with individualized problem solving.
- Identify insight and improved behavior.

MONITORING
- Behavioral changes
- Disturbing topics of conversation
- Effective interventions
- Effects of pharmacologic therapy

PATIENT TEACHING

GENERAL
Be sure to cover:
- the disorder, diagnosis, and treatment
- how to identify progress
- importance of realistic expectations of self and others
- stress relief by channeling emotional energy
- relaxation and breathing techniques.

DISCHARGE PLANNING
- Refer the patient to social services and support services.

RESOURCES
Organizations
American Psychiatric Association: *www.psych.org*
American Psychological Association: *www.apa.org*
Anxiety Disorders Association of America: *www.adaa.org*
Obsessive Compulsive Foundation: *www.ocfoundation.org*

Selected references
Diagnostic and Statistical Manual of Mental Disorders, Fourth Edition, Text Revision. Washington, D.C.: American Psychiatric Association, 2000.

Grover, S., and Gupta, N. "Shared Obsessive-Compulsive Disorder," *Psychopathology* 39(2):99-101, January 2006.

Hohenhaus, S.M. "Caring for OCD Patients in the Emergency Department," *Journal of Emergency Nursing* 30(3):249, June 2004.

Mancebo, M.C., et al. "Obsessive Compulsive Personality Disorder and Obsessive Compulsive Disorder: Clinical Characteristics, Diagnostic Difficulties, and Treatment," *Annals of Clinical Psychiatry* 17(4):197-204, October-December 2005.

Moritz, S., et al. "Quality of Life in Obsessive-Compulsive Disorder Before and After Treatment," *Comprehensive Psychiatry* 46(6):453-59, November-December 2005.

Shoval, G., et al. "Clinical Characteristics of Inpatient Adolescents with Severe Obsessive-Compulsive Disorder," *Depression and Anxiety* 23(2):62-70, 2006.

Osgood-Schlatter disease

OVERVIEW

- Partial separation of the epiphysis of the tibial tubercle from the tibial shaft, leading to tendinitis
- Affects one or both knees
- Also known as *osteochondrosis*

PATHOPHYSIOLOGY

- Bone growth is faster than soft-tissue growth.
- Muscle tendon tightness occurs across the joint.
- Flexibility is decreased.
- Mechanical inefficiency of the extensor mechanism follows incomplete separation of the epiphysis from the shaft.
- Tendinitis of the knee results.

CAUSES

- Exercise
- Genetic factors
- Locally deficient blood supply
- Traumatic avulsion of the proximal tibial tuberosity at the patellar tendon insertion

RISK FACTORS

- Male gender
- Age 11 to 18
- Rapid skeletal growth
- Repetitive jumping sports

INCIDENCE

- Osgood-Schlatter disease is most common in active adolescent boys after undergoing a rapid growth spurt.

COMPLICATIONS

- Irregular growth of the proximal tibial epiphysis
- Partial avascular necrosis of the proximal tibial epiphysis
- Chronic pain
- Patellar tendon avulsion

ASSESSMENT

HISTORY

- Intermittent aching, pain, swelling, and tenderness below the kneecap
- Pain that worsens from running, jumping, squatting, and ascending or descending stairs
- Symptoms relieved with rest
- Precipitating trauma

PHYSICAL FINDINGS

- Soft-tissue swelling
- Localized heat and tenderness
- Decreased flexibility and restriction in the hamstrings, triceps surae, and quadriceps muscle
- Pain at 30-degree flexion with tibia starting at 90 degrees in internal rotation
- Palpable firm mass

DIAGNOSTIC TEST RESULTS

IMAGING

- X-rays show epiphyseal closings, soft-tissue swelling, and bone fragmentation.
- Bone scan may reveal increased uptake in the area of the tibial tuberosity.

TREATMENT

GENERAL
- Ice application for 20 minutes every 2 to 4 hours
- Reinforced elastic knee support, plaster cast, or splint

ACTIVITY
- Reduction of sports activities or exercise
- Avoidance of exercises that demand quadriceps contraction
- In severe cases, immobilization for 6 to 8 weeks
- Rehabilitation exercises

MEDICATIONS
- Nonsteroidal anti-inflammatory drugs
- Analgesics

SURGERY
- Removal or fixation of the epiphysis

NURSING CONSIDERATIONS

NURSING DIAGNOSES
- Acute pain
- Delayed growth and development
- Disturbed body image
- Dressing or grooming self-care deficit
- Fear
- Impaired physical mobility

EXPECTED OUTCOMES
The patient will:
- express feelings of increased comfort and decreased pain
- exhibit developmental milestones within the confines of the disease process
- express positive feelings about self
- perform activities of daily living within the confines of the disease
- discuss fears and concerns
- maintain joint mobility and range of motion.

NURSING INTERVENTIONS
- Give prescribed analgesics and assess response.
- Ensure proper application of knee support or splint.
- Provide the patient with crutches if needed.
- Promote and allow adequate time for self-care.
- Encourage verbalization and provide support.

MONITORING
- Limitation of movement
- Muscle atrophy
- After surgery: circulation, sensation, and pain
- Excessive bleeding

PATIENT TEACHING

GENERAL
Be sure to cover:
- the disorder, diagnosis, and treatment
- prescribed exercise program
- use of crutches if needed
- protection of the injured knee
- avoidance of activities that require deep knee bending for 2 to 4 months.

DISCHARGE PLANNING
- Refer the patient for occupational and physical therapy, as appropriate.

RESOURCES
Organizations
American Orthopaedic Association: *www.aoassn.org*
National Institutes of Health: *www.nih.gov*

Selected references
Diseases, 4th ed. Philadelphia: Lippincott Williams & Wilkins, 2006.
Handbook of Pathophysiology, 2nd ed. Philadelphia: Lippincott Williams & Wilkins, 2005.
Ishida, K., et al. "Infrapatellar Bursal Osteochondromatosis Associated with Unresolved Osgood-Schlatter Disease. A Case Report," *Journal of Bone and Joint Surgery* 87(12):2780-83, December 2005.

Osteoarthritis

- Chronic degeneration of joint cartilage
- Most common form of arthritis
- Disability from minor limitation to near immobility
- Most commonly affects the hips and knees
- Varying progression rates

PATHOPHYSIOLOGY

- Deterioration of the joint cartilage occurs.
- Reactive new bone forms at the margins and subchondral areas.
- Breakdown of chondrocytes occurs.
- Cartilage flakes irritate synovial lining.
- The cartilage lining becomes fibrotic.
- Joint movement is limited.
- Synovial fluid leaks into bone defects, causing cysts.

CAUSES

- Advancing age
- Congenital abnormality
- Endocrine disorders such as diabetes mellitus
- Hereditary, possibly
- Metabolic disorders such as chondrocalcinosis
- Secondary osteoarthritis
- Traumatic injury

INCIDENCE

- Osteoarthritis occurs equally in both sexes.
- The disease typically develops after age 40.

COMPLICATIONS

- Flexion contractures
- Subluxation
- Deformity
- Ankylosis
- Bony cysts
- Gross bony overgrowth
- Central cord syndrome
- Nerve root compression
- Cauda equina syndrome

HISTORY

- Predisposing traumatic injury
- Deep, aching joint pain
- Pain after exercise or weight bearing
- Pain possibly relieved by rest
- Stiffness in morning and after exercise
- Aching during changes in weather
- "Grating" feeling when the joint moves
- Limited movement

PHYSICAL FINDINGS

- Contractures
- Joint swelling
- Muscle atrophy
- Deformity of the involved areas
- Gait abnormalities
- Hard nodes that may be red, swollen, and tender on the distal and proximal interphalangeal joints (see *Signs of osteoarthritis*)
- Loss of finger dexterity
- Muscle spasms, limited movement, and joint instability

LABORATORY

- Synovial fluid analysis rules out inflammatory arthritis.

IMAGING

- X-rays of the affected joint may show a narrowing of the joint space or margin, cystlike bony deposits in the joint space and margins, sclerosis of the subchondral space, joint deformity or articular damage, bony growths at weight-bearing areas, and possible joint fusion.
- Radionuclide bone scan may be used to rule out inflammatory arthritis by showing normal uptake of the radionuclide.
- Magnetic resonance imaging shows affected joint, adjacent bones, and disease progression.

DIAGNOSTIC PROCEDURES

- Neuromuscular tests may show reduced muscle strength.
- Arthroscopy shows internal joint structures and identifies soft-tissue swelling.

TREATMENT

GENERAL
◆ Relieve pain
◆ Improve mobility
◆ Minimize disability

ACTIVITY
◆ As tolerated
◆ Physical therapy
◆ Assistive mobility devices

MEDICATIONS
◆ Analgesics

SURGERY
◆ Arthroplasty (partial or total)
◆ Arthrodesis
◆ Osteoplasty
◆ Osteotomy

Signs of osteoarthritis

Heberden's nodes appear on the dorsolateral aspect of the distal interphalangeal joints. These bony and cartilaginous enlargements are usually hard and painless. They typically occur in middle-aged and elderly patients with osteoarthritis. Bouchard's nodes are similar to Heberden's nodes but are less common and appear on the proximal interphalangeal joints.

HEBERDEN'S NODES	BOUCHARD'S NODES
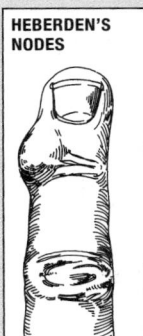	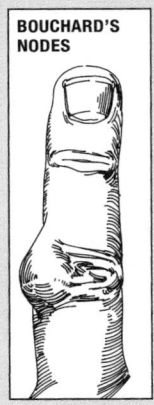

NURSING CONSIDERATIONS

NURSING DIAGNOSES
◆ Acute pain
◆ Anxiety
◆ Disturbed body image
◆ Disturbed sleep pattern
◆ Dressing or grooming self-care deficit
◆ Impaired physical mobility
◆ Ineffective coping

EXPECTED OUTCOMES
The patient will:
◆ express feelings of increased comfort and decreased pain
◆ identify strategies to reduce anxiety
◆ express positive feelings about self
◆ report feeling well-rested
◆ perform activities of daily living within confines of the disease
◆ achieve the highest level of mobility
◆ exhibit adequate coping behaviors.

NURSING INTERVENTIONS
◆ Allow adequate time for self-care.
◆ Adjust pain medications to allow maximum rest.
◆ Identify techniques that promote rest and relaxation.
◆ Give prescribed anti-inflammatories.
◆ For affected hand joints, use hot soaks and paraffin dips.
◆ For affected lumbosacral spinal joints, provide a firm mattress.
◆ For affected cervical spinal joints, apply a cervical collar.
◆ For an affected hip, apply moist heat pads and give antispasmodics.
◆ For an affected knee, help with range-of-motion (ROM) exercises.
◆ Apply elastic supports or braces.
◆ Check crutches, cane, braces, or walker for proper fit.

MONITORING
◆ Pain pattern
◆ Response to analgesics
◆ ROM

PATIENT TEACHING

GENERAL
Be sure to cover:
◆ the disorder, diagnosis, and treatment
◆ need for adequate rest during the day, after exertion, and at night
◆ energy conservation methods
◆ need to take medications exactly as prescribed
◆ adverse reactions to drugs
◆ wearing support shoes that fit well and repairing worn heels
◆ installation of safety devices at home
◆ ROM exercises, performing them as gently as possible
◆ need to maintain proper body weight
◆ use of crutches or other orthopedic devices.

DISCHARGE PLANNING
◆ Refer the patient to occupational or physical therapist as indicated.

RESOURCES
Organizations
Arthritis Foundation: *www.arthritis.org*
National Institutes of Health: *www.nih.gov*

Selected references
Cuddy, M.L. "Geriatric Pharmacology: Osteoarthritis," *Journal of Practical Nursing* 55(1):6-15, Spring 2005.
Diseases, 4th ed. Philadelphia: Lippincott Williams & Wilkins, 2006.
Handbook of Pathophysiology, 2nd ed. Philadelphia: Lippincott Williams & Wilkins, 2005.
Sharma, L., et al. "Epidemiology of Osteoarthritis: An Update," *Current Opinion in Rheumatology* 18(2):147-56, March 2006.
Wang, T.J. "A Theoretical Model for Preventing Osteoarthritis-related Disability," *Rehabilitation Nursing* 30(2):62-67, March-April 2005.

Osteogenesis imperfecta

OVERVIEW

- Genetic disease in which bones are thin, poorly developed, and fracture easily
- Expression varies, depending on whether the defect is carried as a trait or is clinically obvious
- Also called *little bone disease*

PATHOPHYSIOLOGY

- The pathogenesis begins when mutations in the genes change the structure of collagen.
- Possible mutations in other genes may cause variations in the assembly and maintenance of bone and other connective tissues.
- Collectively or alone, these mutated genes lead to pathologic fractures and impaired healing.

CAUSES

- Autosomal recessive carriage of gene defects producing osteogenesis imperfecta in homozygotes (osteoporosis in some)
- Genetic disease, typically autosomal dominant (characterized by a defect in the synthesis of connective tissue)

RISK FACTORS

- One parent with disorder (child has 50% chance of having disorder)

INCIDENCE

- This autosomal dominant disorder occurs in about 1 in 30,000 people.
- Osteogenesis imperfecta affects males and females equally.

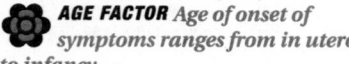 **AGE FACTOR** *Age of onset of symptoms ranges from in utero to infancy.*

COMPLICATIONS

- Deafness
- Stillbirth or death within the first year of life (autosomal-recessive disorder)
- Hyperplastic callus formation
- Repeated respiratory infections
- Cord compression
- Cerebral hemorrhage caused by birth trauma

ASSESSMENT

HISTORY

- Fractures early in life
- Hearing loss
- Easy bruising

PHYSICAL FINDINGS

- Blue sclerae, showing that mutation is expressed in more than one connective tissue
- Short trunk
- Hearing loss
- Fractures
- Kyphoscoliosis

DIAGNOSTIC TEST RESULTS

LABORATORY

- Serum alkaline phosphatase levels are elevated during periods of rapid bone formation and cellular injury.
- Skin culture shows reduced quantity of fibroblasts.

IMAGING

- Echocardiography may show mitral insufficiency or floppy mitral valves.
- Prenatal ultrasonography (during second trimester) reveals bowing of long bones, fractures, limb shortening, and decreased skull echogenicity.
- Skull, long-bone, and pelvic X-rays reveal thin bones, fractures with deformities, beaded ribs, and osteopenia.

TREATMENT

GENERAL
◆ Prevention of fractures

DIET
◆ Nutritious, well-balanced

ACTIVITY
◆ Safety during periods of activity
◆ Physical therapy

MEDICATIONS
◆ Antibiotics (when infection occurs)

SURGERY
◆ Internal fixation of fractures to ensure stabilization and prevent deformities
◆ Spinal fusion for scoliosis

NURSING CONSIDERATIONS

NURSING DIAGNOSES
◆ Acute pain
◆ Delayed growth and development
◆ Impaired physical mobility
◆ Risk for infection
◆ Risk for injury

EXPECTED OUTCOMES
The patient (or family) will:
◆ express feelings of comfort and decreased pain
◆ demonstrate appropriate skills and behaviors to the fullest extent possible
◆ maintain joint mobility, range of motion, and muscle strength
◆ remain free from signs and symptoms of infection
◆ follow safety measures to prevent fractures or injuries.

NURSING INTERVENTIONS
◆ Ensure a safe environment.
◆ Encourage activities based on ability.
◆ Provide psychological support.

MONITORING
◆ Environment
◆ Bone condition

PATIENT TEACHING

GENERAL
Be sure to cover:
◆ safe handling of infant
◆ how to recognize fractures and correctly splint them
◆ how to protect the child during diapering, dressing, and other activities of daily living
◆ encouraging interests that don't require strenuous physical activity
◆ the importance of good nutrition to heal bones and promote growth
◆ use of shock-absorbing footwear
◆ importance of not letting infants younger than age 1 year sit upright.

DISCHARGE PLANNING
◆ Refer the child and his parents for genetic counseling to assess the recurrence risk.
◆ Instruct the parents to provide their child with medical identification jewelry.

RESOURCES
Organizations
National Institutes of Health — Osteoporosis and Related Bone Diseases National Resource Center: *www.osteo.org*
The Osteogenesis Imperfecta Clinic: *www.osteogenesisimperfecta.org*
Osteogenesis Imperfecta Foundation: *www.oif.org*

Selected references
Cho, T.J., et al. "Efficacy of Oral Alendronate in Children with Osteogenesis Imperfecta," *Journal of Pediatric Orthopedics* 25(5):607-12, September-October 2005.
Millington-Ward, S., et al. "Emerging Therapeutic Approaches for Osteogenesis Imperfecta," *Trends in Molecular Medicine* 11(6):299-305, June 2005.
Plotkin, H. "Two Questions about Osteogenesis Imperfecta," *Journal of Pediatric Orthopedics* 26(1):148-49, January-February 2006.

Osteomalacia and rickets

OVERVIEW

- Vitamin D deficiency that doesn't allow bone to calcify normally
- Prognosis good with treatment
- Possible disappearance of bone deformities in adults; usually persist in children
- Called *rickets* in infants and young children; *osteomalacia* in adults

PATHOPHYSIOLOGY

- Vitamin D regulates the absorption of calcium ions from the intestine.
- When vitamin D is lacking, falling serum calcium concentration stimulates synthesis and secretion of parathyroid hormone.
- This causes the release of calcium from bone, decreasing renal calcium excretion and increasing renal phosphate excretion.
- When the concentration of phosphate in the bone decreases, osteoid may be produced but mineralization can't proceed normally.
- This causes large quantities of osteoid to accumulate, coating the trabeculae and linings of the haversian canals and areas beneath the periosteum.
- When bone matrix mineralization is delayed or inadequate, bone is disorganized in structure and lacks density. The result is gross deformity of both spongy and compact bone.

CAUSES

- Conditions reducing the absorption of fat-soluble vitamin D
- Hepatic or renal disease
- Inadequate dietary intake of vitamin D
- Inadequate exposure to sunlight
- Inherited impairment of renal tubular reabsorption of phosphate (from vitamin D insensitivity) in vitamin D–resistant rickets (refractory rickets, familial hypophosphatemia)
- Malabsorption of vitamin D
- Malfunctioning parathyroid gland contributing to calcium deficiency and interfering with vitamin D activation in the kidneys

RISK FACTORS

- Older age
- Malnourishment
- Sun-deprived geographic location

INCIDENCE

- The disorder is rare in the United States.
- It appears occasionally in breast-fed infants who don't receive a vitamin D supplement or in infants fed a formula with a nonfortified milk base.
- The disorder typically occurs in overcrowded, urban areas where smog limits sunlight penetration.

⚡ **WARNING** *Incidence of rickets is highest in children with darkly pigmented skin who, because of their pigmentation, absorb less sunlight.*

COMPLICATIONS

- Spontaneous multiple fractures
- Tetany in infants
- Bone deformities

ASSESSMENT

HISTORY

- Poor diet
- Leg and lower back pain

PHYSICAL FINDINGS

- Bowed legs
- Knock knees
- Rachitic rosary (beading of ends of ribs)
- Enlarged wrists and ankles
- Pigeon breast (protruding ribs and sternum)
- Bulging forehead
- Poorly developed muscles (pot belly)
- Kyphoscoliosis

DIAGNOSTIC TEST RESULTS

LABORATORY

- Serum calcium concentration less than 7.5 mg/dl
- Serum inorganic phosphorus concentration less than 3 mg/dl
- Serum citrate level less than 2.5 mg/dl
- Alkaline phosphatase level less than 4 Bodansky units/dl

IMAGING

- X-rays showing characteristic bone deformities and abnormalities such as Looser transformation zones (radiolucent bands perpendicular to the surface of the bones indicating reduced bone ossification confirm the diagnosis)

TREATMENT

GENERAL
- Sufficient sun exposure
- Treatment of bone deformities or fractures

DIET
- High in vitamin D (fortified milk, fish-liver oils, herring, liver, and egg yolks)

MEDICATIONS
- Massive oral doses of vitamin D or cod-liver oil
- For rickets refractory to vitamin D, or in rickets accompanied by hepatic or renal disease, 25-hydroxycholecalciferol, 1,25-dihydroxycholecalciferol, or a synthetic analogue of active vitamin D

SURGERY
- Possible surgical intervention for intestinal disease
- Appropriate repair of bone fractures

NURSING CONSIDERATIONS

NURSING DIAGNOSES
- Acute pain
- Delayed growth and development
- Disturbed body image
- Imbalanced nutrition: Less than body requirements
- Impaired physical mobility
- Risk for infection
- Risk for injury

EXPECTED OUTCOMES
The patient (or family) will:
- express feelings of comfort and decreased pain
- demonstrate appropriate skills and behaviors to the fullest extent possible
- express positive feelings about self
- have increased vitamin D intake
- maintain joint mobility, range of motion, and muscle strength
- remain free from signs and symptoms of infection
- follow safety measures to prevent fractures or injuries.

NURSING INTERVENTIONS
- Obtain a dietary history to assess the patient's vitamin D intake.

MONITORING
- Dietary intake
- Bone integrity

PATIENT TEACHING

GENERAL
Be sure to cover:
- symptoms of vitamin D toxicity (headache, nausea, constipation and, after prolonged use, renal calculi).

DISCHARGE PLANNING
- If the patient's vitamin D deficiency appears to be linked to adverse socioeconomic conditions, refer him to an appropriate community agency.

RESOURCES
Organizations
Mayo Clinic: *www.mayoclinic.com*
National Library of Medicine: *www.nlm.nih.gov*

Selected references
Holick, M.F. "The Vitamin D Epidemic and its Health Consequences," *Journal of Nutrition* 135(11):2739S-48S, November 2005.
Jan de Beur, S.M. "Tumor-induced Osteomalacia," *JAMA* 294(10):1260-67, September 2005.
Levy, Y., and Davidovits, M. "Nutritional Rickets in Children with Cows' Milk Allergy: Calcium Deficiency or Vitamin D Deficiency?" *Pediatric Allergy and Immunology* 16(6):553, September 2005.
Lyman, D. "Undiagnosed Vitamin D Deficiency in the Hospitalized Patient," *American Family Physician* 71(2):299-304, January 2005.

Osteomyelitis

OVERVIEW

- Chronic or acute pyogenic bone infection
- Good prognosis for acute form (with prompt treatment)
- Poor prognosis for chronic form

PATHOPHYSIOLOGY

- Organisms settle in a hematoma or weakened area and spread directly to bone.
- Pus is produced and pressure builds within the rigid medullary cavity.
- Pus is forced through the haversian canals.
- Subperiosteal abscess forms.
- Bone is deprived of its blood supply.
- Necrosis results and new bone formation is stimulated.
- Dead bone detaches and exits through an abscess or the sinuses.
- Osteomyelitis becomes chronic.

CAUSES

- Acute infection originating elsewhere in the body
- *Escherichia coli*
- Fungi or viruses
- Minor traumatic injury
- *Proteus vulgaris*
- *Pseudomonas aeruginosa*
- *Staphylococcus aureus*
- *Streptococcus pyogenes*

RISK FACTORS

- Older age
- Obesity
- Immunosuppression
- Diabetes
- Rheumatoid arthritis
- Long-term steroid therapy

INCIDENCE

- The incidence of both types of osteomyelitis is declining, except in drug abusers.

AGE FACTOR *The acute form affects rapidly growing children, especially boys.*

COMPLICATIONS

- Chronic infection
- Skeletal deformities
- Joint deformities
- Disturbed bone growth in children
- Differing leg lengths
- Impaired mobility

ASSESSMENT

HISTORY

- Previous injury, surgery, or primary infection
- Sudden, severe pain in the affected bone
- Pain unrelieved by rest and worse with motion
- Related chills, nausea, and malaise
- Refusal to use the affected area

PHYSICAL FINDINGS

- Tachycardia and fever
- Swelling and restricted movement over the infection site
- Tenderness and warmth over the infection site
- Persistent pus drainage from an old pocket in a sinus tract

DIAGNOSTIC TEST RESULTS

LABORATORY

- White blood cell count shows leukocytosis.
- Erythrocyte sedimentation rate is increased.
- Blood culture identifies pathogen.

IMAGING

- X-rays may show bone involvement.
- Bone scans may detect early infection.
- Computed tomography scan and magnetic resonance imaging can show extent of infection.

TREATMENT

GENERAL
- Decrease internal bone pressure
- Prevent bone necrosis
- Hyperbaric oxygen therapy
- Free tissue transfers
- I.V. fluids as needed

DIET
- High-protein, rich in vitamin C

ACTIVITY
- Bed rest
- Immobilization of involved bone and joint with a cast or traction

MEDICATIONS
- I.V. antibiotics
- Analgesics
- Intracavitary instillation of antibiotics for open wounds

SURGERY
- Surgical drainage
- Local muscle flaps
- Sequestrectomy
- Amputation for chronic and unrelieved symptoms

NURSING CONSIDERATIONS

NURSING DIAGNOSES
- Activity intolerance
- Acute pain
- Anxiety
- Excess fluid volume
- Fear
- Impaired physical mobility
- Impaired tissue integrity

EXPECTED OUTCOMES
The patient will:
- perform activities of daily living without excessive pain or fatigue
- experience increased comfort and decreased pain
- identify strategies to reduce anxiety
- exhibit adequate fluid volume
- express fears and concerns
- maintain joint mobility and range of motion
- exhibit adequate tissue perfusion and pulses distally.

NURSING INTERVENTIONS
- Control infection.
- Protect the bone from injury.
- Provide emotional support.
- Promote and allow adequate time for self-care.
- Promote activities that promote rest and relaxation.
- Use strict sterile technique.
- With skeletal traction, cover the pin insertion points with small, dry dressings.
- Provide firm pillows.
- Provide thorough skin care.
- Provide complete cast care.
- Give prescribed analgesics.

MONITORING
- Vital signs
- Wound appearance and healing
- Pain control
- Drainage and suctioning equipment
- Sudden malpositioning of the limb

PATIENT TEACHING

GENERAL
Be sure to cover:
- the disorder, diagnosis, and treatment
- drug administration, dosage, and possible adverse effects
- techniques for promoting rest and relaxation
- wound site care
- signs of recurring infection
- importance of follow-up examinations.

DISCHARGE PLANNING
- Refer the patient for occupational therapy as appropriate.

RESOURCES
Organizations
American Orthopaedic Association: *www.aoassn.org*
Cleveland Clinic Health Information Center: *www.clevelandclinic.org/health*
The Merck Manuals Online Medical Library: *www.merck.com/mmhe*

Selected references
Diseases, 4th ed. Philadelphia: Lippincott Williams & Wilkins, 2006.
Embil, J.M., and Trepman, E. "Microbiological Evaluation of Diabetic Foot Osteomyelitis," *Clinical Infectious Diseases* 42(1):63-65, January 2006.
Gamble, K., et al. "Osteomyelitis of the Pubic Symphysis in Pregnancy," *Obstetrics and Gynecology* 107(2):477-81, February 2006.
Handbook of Pathophysiology, 2nd ed. Philadelphia: Lippincott Williams & Wilkins, 2005.
Singh, G., et al. "Cervical Osteomyelitis Associated With Intravenous Drug Use," *Emergency Medicine Journal* 23(2):e16, February 2006.

Osteoporosis

- Loss of calcium and phosphate from bones causing increased vulnerability to fractures
- Primary or secondary to underlying disease
- Types of primary osteoporosis: post-menopausal osteoporosis (type I) and age-associated osteoporosis (type II)
- Secondary osteoporosis: caused by an identifiable agent or disease

PATHOPHYSIOLOGY

- The rate of bone resorption accelerates as the rate of bone formation decelerates.
- Decreased bone mass results and bones become porous and brittle.

CAUSES

- Exact cause unknown
- Alcoholism
- Bone immobilization
- Hyperthyroidism
- Lactose intolerance
- Liver disease
- Malabsorption
- Malnutrition
- Osteogenesis imperfecta
- Prolonged therapy with steroids or heparin
- Rheumatoid arthritis
- Scurvy
- Sudeck's atrophy (localized in hands and feet, with recurring attacks)

RISK FACTORS

- Mild, prolonged negative calcium balance
- Declining gonadal adrenal function
- Faulty protein metabolism (caused by estrogen deficiency)
- Sedentary lifestyle

INCIDENCE

- Idiopathic osteoporosis affects children and adults and appears to affect both sexes equally.
- Type I (or postmenopausal) osteoporosis typically affects women ages 51 to 75.
- Type II (or senile) osteoporosis is most common between ages 70 and 85.

COMPLICATIONS

- Bone fractures (vertebrae, femoral neck, and distal radius)

ASSESSMENT

HISTORY

- Postmenopausal patient
- Condition known to cause secondary osteoporosis
- Snapping sound or sudden pain in lower back when bending down to lift something
- Possible slow development of pain (over several years)
- With vertebral collapse, backache and pain radiating around the trunk
- Pain aggravated by movement or jarring

PHYSICAL FINDINGS

- Humped back
- Markedly aged appearance
- Loss of height
- Muscle spasm
- Decreased spinal movement with flexion more limited than extension

DIAGNOSTIC TEST RESULTS

LABORATORY

- Serum calcium, phosphorus, and alkaline levels are normal.
- Parathyroid hormone level is elevated.

IMAGING

- X-ray studies show characteristic degeneration in the lower thoracolumbar vertebrae.
- Computed tomography scan assesses spinal bone loss.
- Bone scans show injured or diseased areas.

DIAGNOSTIC PROCEDURES

- Bone biopsy shows thin, porous, but otherwise normal bone.

OTHER

- Dual- or single-photon absorptiometry (measurement of bone mass) shows loss of bone mass.

TREATMENT

GENERAL
- Control of bone loss
- Prevention of additional fractures
- Control of pain
- Reduction and immobilization of fractures
- Supportive devices

DIET
- Rich in vitamin D, calcium, and protein

ACTIVITY
- Physical therapy program of gentle exercise and activity

MEDICATIONS
- Estrogen
- Sodium fluoride (Fluoritab)
- Calcium and vitamin D supplements
- Calcitonin (Miacalcin)

SURGERY
- Open reduction and internal fixation for femur fractures

NURSING CONSIDERATIONS

NURSING DIAGNOSES
- Chronic pain
- Disturbed body image
- Dressing or grooming self-care deficit
- Imbalanced nutrition: Less than body requirements
- Impaired physical mobility
- Risk for impaired skin integrity
- Risk for injury

EXPECTED OUTCOMES
The patient will:
- experience increased comfort and decreased pain
- express positive feelings about self
- perform activities of daily living within the confines of the disease
- maintain adequate dietary intake
- maintain joint mobility and range of motion (ROM)
- maintain skin integrity
- demonstrate measures to prevent injury.

NURSING INTERVENTIONS
- Encourage careful positioning, ambulation, and prescribed exercises.
- Promote self-care while allowing adequate time.
- Encourage mild exercise.
- Assist with walking.
- Perform passive ROM exercises.
- Promote physical therapy sessions.
- Use safety precautions.
- Give prescribed analgesics.
- Apply heat.

MONITORING
- Skin for redness, warmth, and new pain sites
- Response to analgesia
- Nutritional status
- Height
- Exercise tolerance
- Joint mobility

PATIENT TEACHING

GENERAL
Be sure to cover:
- the disorder, diagnosis, and treatment
- drug administration, dosage, and possible adverse effects
- performing monthly breast self-examination while on estrogen therapy
- need to report vaginal bleeding promptly
- need to report new pain sites immediately
- sleeping on a firm mattress
- avoiding excessive bed rest
- use of back brace if appropriate
- proper body mechanics
- home safety devices
- diet rich in calcium.

DISCHARGE PLANNING
- Refer the patient for physical and occupational therapy, as appropriate.

RESOURCES
Organizations
National Institutes of Health — Osteoporosis and Related Bone Diseases National Resource Center: *www.osteo.org*
National Osteoporosis Foundation: *www.nof.org*

Selected references
Chang, S. "A Cross-sectional Survey of Calcium Intake in Relation to Knowledge of Osteoporosis and Beliefs in Young Adult Women," *International Journal of Nursing Practice* 12(1):21-27, February 2006.
Diseases, 4th ed. Philadelphia: Lippincott Williams & Wilkins, 2006.
Handbook of Pathophysiology, 2nd ed. Philadelphia: Lippincott Williams & Wilkins, 2005.
Kessenich, C.R. "Osteoporosis: New Options for Pain Relief," *Nurse Practitioner* 31(2):44-47, February 2006.
Reginster, J., and Sarlet, N. "The Treatment of Severe Postmenopausal Osteoporosis: A Review of Current and Emerging Therapeutic Options," *Treatments in Endocrinology* 5(1):15-23, 2006.

Otitis externa

- Acute or chronic inflammation of the external ear canal
- With treatment, usually subsides within 7 days
- May become chronic; tends to recur
- If severe and chronic, may reflect underlying diabetes mellitus, hypothyroidism, or nephritis
- Also known as *external otitis* and *swimmer's ear*

PATHOPHYSIOLOGY

- External ear canal inflammation results from invasion by infecting organisms.

CAUSES

- Bacteria (common) and fungi (less common)
- Occasionally, dermatologic conditions, such as seborrhea or psoriasis
- Trauma or excessive moisture that predisposes canal to infection

RISK FACTORS

- Swimming in contaminated water
- Cleaning ear canal with cotton-tipped applicator, bobby pin, finger, or other object
- Exposure to dust, hair care products, or other irritants
- Regular use of earphones, earplugs, or earmuffs
- Chronic drainage from a perforated tympanic membrane

INCIDENCE

- Otitis externa is most common in the summer but can occur any time of the year.

COMPLICATIONS

- Complete closure of the ear canal
- Significant hearing loss
- Otitis media
- Cellulitis
- Abscesses
- Disfigurement of the pinna
- Lymphadenopathy
- Osteitis
- Septicemia
- Stenosis

HISTORY

- Repeated exposure to ear trauma, water, use of earphones, or allergic response to hair spray, dye, or other hair care products
- Mild to severe ear itching or pain aggravated by jaw motion, clenching the teeth, opening the mouth, or chewing
- Fungal otitis externa possibly not producing symptoms

PHYSICAL FINDINGS

- Swollen, inflamed ear canal
- Ear discharge that may be foul-smelling and yellow to green
- Thick red epithelium in canal with chronic otitis externa
- Increased pain or itching on palpation or manipulation

LABORATORY

- Microscopic examination shows the causative organism.

DIAGNOSTIC PROCEDURES

- Audiometric testing may reveal a partial hearing loss.
- Otoscopy reveals a swollen external ear canal, periauricular lymphadenopathy and, occasionally, regional cellulitis.

TREATMENT

GENERAL
- Cleaning of debris from canal under direct visualization
- With mild, chronic otitis externa, use of specially fitted earplugs for showering or swimming

MEDICATIONS
- Analgesics
- Antibiotic drops
- Oral antibiotics if lymphadenopathy is present, or if external ear is swollen

SURGERY
- Excision and abscess drainage

Preventing otitis externa

- To prevent recurrence, tell the patient to avoid potential irritants, such as hair care products and earrings.
- Advise the patient to use lamb's wool earplugs coated with petroleum jelly to keep water out of the ears when showering or shampooing.
- Inform the parents of a young child that modeling clay makes a tight seal and can be used to prevent water from getting into the external canal.
- Tell the patient to wear earplugs or to keep his head above water when swimming and to instill two or three drops of 3% boric acid solution in 70% alcohol into the ear before and after swimming to toughen the skin of the external ear canal.
- Warn against cleaning the ears with cotton-tipped applicators or other objects.

NURSING CONSIDERATIONS

NURSING DIAGNOSES
- Acute pain
- Disturbed sensory perception: Auditory
- Fear
- Impaired skin integrity
- Impaired verbal communication
- Risk for infection

EXPECTED OUTCOMES
The patient will:
- express feelings of increased comfort
- regain hearing function or develop other ways to communicate
- express feelings and concerns
- experience wound or lesion healing without complications
- communicate needs
- show no signs or symptoms of infection.

NURSING INTERVENTIONS
- Clean and dry the ear gently and thoroughly.
- Use wet soaks on infected skin.
- Give prescribed drugs.

With hearing loss
- Encourage discussion of concerns.
- Reassure the patient that hearing loss from an external ear infection is temporary.
- Face the patient when speaking.
- Enunciate words clearly, slowly, and in a normal tone.
- Allow adequate time to grasp what was said.
- Provide a pencil and paper to aid communication.
- Alert staff to the communication problem.

MONITORING
- Vital signs, especially temperature
- Auditory acuity
- Type and amount of aural drainage
- Response to treatment
- Complications

PATIENT TEACHING

GENERAL
Be sure to cover:
- the disorder, diagnosis, and treatment
- proper hand washing and daily ear cleaning
- administration of eardrops, ointment, and ear wash
- antibiotics, as prescribed
- recognizing and reporting adverse reactions
- preventing recurrence. (See *Preventing otitis externa*.)

RESOURCES
Organizations
American Academy of Allergy, Asthma and Immunology: *www.aaaai.org*
American Academy of Audiology: *www.audiology.org*

Selected references
Antonelli, P.J., et al. "Inflammatory Proteases in Chronic Otitis Externa," *Laryngoscope* 115(4):651-54, April 2005.

Block, S.L. "Otitis Externa: Providing Relief while Avoiding Complications," *Journal of Family Practice* 54(8):669-76, August 2005.

Emgard, P., and Hellstom, S. "A Group III Steroid Solution without Antibiotic Components: An Effective Cure for External Otitis," *Journal of Laryngology and Otology* 119(5):342-47, May 2005.

Tierney, L., et al. *Current Medical Diagnosis & Treatment 2006.* New York: McGraw-Hill Book Co., 2006.

Otitis media

OVERVIEW

- Inflammation of the middle ear associated with fluid accumulation
- Acute, chronic, suppurative, or secretory

PATHOPHYSIOLOGY

- The disease process differs according to type of otitis media.

Suppurative form

- Nasopharyngeal flora reflux through the eustachian tube and colonize the middle ear.
- Respiratory tract infections, allergic reactions, and position changes allow reflux of nasopharyngeal flora through the eustachian tube and colonization in the middle ear.

Secretory form

- Obstruction of the eustachian tube promotes transudation of sterile serous fluid from blood vessels in the middle ear membrane.

CAUSES

- Acute otitis media: disruption of eustachian tube patency
- Secretory otitis media: viral infection, allergy, or barotrauma
- Suppurative otitis media: bacterial infection with pneumococci, group A beta-hemolytic streptococci, staphylococci, and gram-negative bacteria
- Chronic secretory otitis media: adenoidal tissue overgrowth, edema, chronic sinus infection, or inadequate treatment of acute suppurative otitis media
- Chronic suppurative otitis media: inadequate treatment of acute otitis episodes or infection by resistant strains of bacteria

INCIDENCE

- Otitis media occurs most commonly in infants and children.
  - **AGE FACTOR** *Acute otitis media is an emergency in an immunocompromised child.*
- Otitis media peaks between ages 6 and 24 months.

- The incidence of otitis media subsides after age 3.
- The disease is most common during the winter months, paralleling the seasonal increase in nonbacterial respiratory tract infections.

COMPLICATIONS

- Spontaneous rupture of the tympanic membrane
- Persistent perforation
- Chronic otitis media
- Mastoiditis
- Meningitis
- Cholesteatomas
- Abscesses, septicemia
- Lymphadenopathy, leukocytosis
- Permanent hearing loss and tympanosclerosis
- Vertigo

ASSESSMENT

HISTORY

- Upper respiratory tract infection
- Allergies
- Severe, deep, throbbing ear pain
- Dizziness
- Nausea, vomiting

Acute secretory otitis media

- Sensation of fullness in the ear
- Popping, crackling, or clicking sounds on swallowing or moving the jaw
- Describes hearing an echo when speaking

Tympanic membrane rupture

- Pain that suddenly stops
- Recent air travel or scuba diving

PHYSICAL FINDINGS

- Sneezing and coughing with upper respiratory tract infection
- Mild to high fever
- Painless, purulent discharge in chronic suppurative otitis media
- Obscured or distorted bony landmarks of the tympanic membrane in acute suppurative otitis media
- Tympanic membrane retraction in acute secretory otitis media
- Clear or amber fluid behind the tympanic membrane

- Blue-black tympanic membrane with hemorrhage into the middle ear
- Pulsating discharge with tympanic perforation
- Conductive hearing loss (varies with the size and type of tympanic membrane perforation and ossicular destruction)

Chronic otitis media

- Thickening and scarring of tympanic membrane
- Decreased or absent tympanic membrane mobility
- Cholesteatoma

DIAGNOSTIC TEST RESULTS

LABORATORY

- Culture and sensitivity tests of exudate show the causative organism.
- Complete blood count shows leukocytosis.

IMAGING

- Radiographic studies demonstrate mastoid involvement.

DIAGNOSTIC PROCEDURES

- Tympanometry detects hearing loss and evaluates the condition of the middle ear.
- Audiometry shows degree of hearing loss.
- Pneumatic otoscopy may show decreased tympanic membrane mobility.
  - **WARNING** *In adults, unilateral serous otitis media should always be evaluated for a nasopharyngeal-obstructing lesion such as carcinoma.*

TREATMENT

GENERAL

- In acute secretory otitis media, Valsalva's maneuver several times per day (may be the only treatment required)
- Concomitant treatment of the underlying cause

- Elimination of eustachian tube obstruction

MEDICATIONS
- Antibiotic therapy
- Aspirin or acetaminophen (Tylenol)
- Analgesics
- Sedatives (small children)
- Nasopharyngeal decongestant therapy

SURGERY
- Myringotomy and aspiration of middle ear fluid, followed by insertion of a polyethylene tube into the tympanic membrane
- Myringoplasty
- Tympanoplasty
- Mastoidectomy
- Cholesteatoma excision
- Stapedectomy for otosclerosis

NURSING CONSIDERATIONS

NURSING DIAGNOSES
- Acute pain
- Disturbed sensory perception (auditory)
- Disturbed sleep pattern
- Impaired verbal communication
- Risk for infection
- Risk for injury

EXPECTED OUTCOMES
The patient will:
- express feelings of increased comfort
- regain hearing or develop compensatory mechanisms
- resume normal sleep patterns

- communicate feelings and needs
- remain free from signs and symptoms of infection
- avoid injury.

NURSING INTERVENTIONS
- Answer all questions.
- Encourage discussion of concerns about hearing loss.

With hearing loss
- Offer reassurance, when appropriate, that hearing loss caused by serious otitis media is temporary.
- Provide clear, concise explanations.
- Face the patient when speaking and enunciate clearly and slowly.
- Allow time for the patient to grasp what was said.
- Provide a pencil and paper.
- Alert the staff to the patient's communication problem.

After myringotomy
- Wash hands before and after ear care.
- Maintain drainage flow.
- Place sterile cotton loosely in the external ear to absorb drainage and prevent infection. Change the cotton when damp. Avoid placing cotton or plugs deep in ear canal.
- Give prescribed analgesics.
- Give antiemetics after tympanoplasty and reinforce dressings.

MONITORING
- Pain level
- Excessive bleeding or discharge
- Auditory acuity
- Response to treatment

- Complications

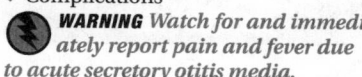 **WARNING** *Watch for and immediately report pain and fever due to acute secretory otitis media.*

PATIENT TEACHING

GENERAL
Be sure to cover:
- proper instillation of ointment, drops, and ear wash, as ordered
- drug administration, dosage, and possible adverse effects
- importance of taking antibiotics
- adequate fluid intake
- correct instillation of nasopharyngeal decongestants
- use of fitted earplugs for swimming after myringotomy and tympanostomy tube insertion
- notification of the practitioner if tube falls out and for ear pain, fever, or pus-filled discharge
- preventing recurrence. (See *Preventing otitis media.*)

RESOURCES
Organizations
American Academy of Allergy, Asthma and Immunology: *www.aaaai.org*
American Academy of Audiology: *www.audiology.org*

Selected references
Carlson, L., and Scudder, L. "Controversies in the Management of Pediatric Otitis Media. Are More Definitive Answers on the Horizon?" *Advance for Nurse Practitioners* 12(2):73-77, February 2004.
Friedman, N.R., et al. "Development of a Practical Tool for Assessing the Severity of Acute Otitis Media," *Pediatric Infectious Disease Journal* 25(2):101-07, February 2006.
Leskinen, K., and Jero, J. "Acute Complications of Otitis Media in Adults," *Clinical Otolaryngology* 30(6):511-16, December 2005.
Montgomery, D. "A New Approach to Treating Acute Otitis Media," *Journal of Pediatric Health Care* 19(1):505-02, January-February 2005.

Preventing otitis media

For a patient recovering from otitis media at home, instruct the patient or his family to follow these guidelines to help prevent a recurrence:
- Teach the patient how to recognize upper respiratory tract infections, and encourage early treatment of them.
- Instruct parents not to feed an infant in a supine position and not to put him to bed with a bottle. Explain that doing so could cause reflux of nasopharyngeal flora.

- If appropriate, teach the patient to promote eustachian tube patency by performing Valsalva's maneuver several times per day, especially during airplane travel.
- After tympanoplasty, advise the patient not to blow his nose or get his ear wet when bathing.
- Explain adverse reactions to the prescribed medication, emphasizing those that require immediate medical attention.

Otosclerosis

OVERVIEW

- Bone disease that occurs only in the middle ear and results in an overgrowth of abnormal bone, usually involving the stapes bone
- Most common cause of conductive hearing loss
- With surgery, prognosis good
- Also known as *hardening of the ear* and *otospongiosis*

PATHOPHYSIOLOGY

- Normal bone of otic capsule is gradually replaced with highly vascular spongy bone.
- Spongy bone immobilizes the footplate of the normally mobile stapes.
- Conduction of vibrations from the tympanic membrane to the cochlea is disrupted, and conductive hearing loss results.
- If the inner ear is involved, sensorineural hearing loss may develop.

CAUSES

- Genetic factor transmitted as an autosomal dominant trait
- Pregnancy (may trigger the onset)

RISK FACTORS

- Pregnancy
- Family history

INCIDENCE

- Otosclerosis occurs in at least 10% of whites.
- It's twice as common in women as in men.
- The disease usually occurs between ages 15 and 50.

COMPLICATIONS

- Bilateral conductive hearing loss
- Taste disturbance

ASSESSMENT

HISTORY

- Family history of hearing loss (excluding presbycusis)
- Tinnitus
- Ability to hear a conversation better in a noisy environment than in a quiet one (paracusis of Willis)
- Vertigo, especially after bending over

PHYSICAL FINDINGS

- Tympanic membrane appears normal
- Schwartze's sign (faint pink blush throughout the tympanic membrane from vascularity of active otosclerotic bone)

DIAGNOSTIC TEST RESULTS

DIAGNOSTIC PROCEDURES

- Rinne test result shows bone-conducted tone is heard longer than air-conducted tone.
- Weber's test result shows that sound lateralizes to the more damaged ear.
- Audiometric testing reveals hearing loss.

TREATMENT

GENERAL

- Hearing aids

ACTIVITY

- Avoidance of activities that provoke dizziness

MEDICATIONS

- Antibiotics
- Sodium fluoride (may prevent further worsening of hearing)

SURGERY

- Stapedectomy
- Prosthesis insertion to restore partial or total hearing
- Fenestration
- Stapes mobilization

NURSING CONSIDERATIONS

NURSING DIAGNOSES
- Anxiety
- Fear
- Disturbed sensory perception: Auditory
- Impaired verbal communication
- Ineffective coping
- Risk for infection
- Risk for injury

EXPECTED OUTCOMES
The patient will:
- identify strategies to reduce anxiety
- verbalize fears and concerns
- regain hearing function or develop other ways to communicate
- express needs and feelings
- demonstrate adaptive coping mechanisms
- remain free from signs and symptoms of infection
- avoid injury.

NURSING INTERVENTIONS
- Encourage discussion of concerns about hearing loss.
- Offer reassurance with hearing loss, when appropriate.
- Give clear, concise explanations.
- Face the patient when speaking.
- Enunciate clearly and slowly, in a normal tone.
- Allow adequate time to grasp what was said.
- Provide a pencil and paper to aid communication.
- Alert the staff to communication problem.

After surgery
- Position as ordered.
- Assist with ambulation when indicated.
- Give prescribed drugs for pain.
- Reassure the patient that taste disturbance is common and usually subsides in a few weeks.

MONITORING
- For vertigo
- Response to medication
- Hearing loss

 WARNING *Watch for and report postoperative facial drooping, which may indicate swelling of or around the facial nerve.*

PATIENT TEACHING

GENERAL
Be sure to cover:
- the disorder, diagnosis, and treatment
- preoperative and postoperative teaching, if indicated
- slow movement to prevent vertigo
- drug administration, dosage, and possible adverse effects
- importance of protecting ears against the cold
- need to avoid activities that provoke dizziness
- avoidance of anyone with upper respiratory tract infection
- changing external ear dressing and incision care
- completion of prescribed drug regimen
- need for follow-up care
- how hearing may be masked by packing, dressing, and postoperative edema
- why hearing may not be noticeably improved for 1 to 4 weeks after surgery
- avoidance of loud noises and sudden pressure changes until healing is complete
- avoidance of blowing nose for at least 1 week to prevent contaminated air and bacteria from entering the eustachian tube
- avoidance of sudden movements
- avoidance of wetting head in shower or swimming for about 6 weeks
- avoidance of getting water in the ear for an additional 4 weeks
- prevention of constipation and avoidance of straining while defecating.

RESOURCES
Organizations
Alexander Graham Bell Association for the Deaf and Hard of Hearing: *www.agbell.org*
Hearing Loss Association of America: *www.shhh.org*

Selected references
Karosi, T., et al. "Two Subgroups of Stapes Fixation: Otosclerosis and Pseudo-Otosclerosis," *Laryngoscope* 115(11): 1968-73, November 2005.

Knox, G.W., and Reitan, H. "Shape-Memory Stapes Prosthesis for Otosclerosis Surgery," *Laryngoscope* 115(8):1340-46, August 2005.

Menger, D.J., et al. "The Genetics of Otosclerosis," *Clinical Otolaryngology & Allied Sciences* 29(4):435, August 2004.

Rama-Lopez, J., et al. "Cochlear Implantation of Patients with Far-Advanced Otosclerosis," *Otology & Neurotology* 27(2):153-58, February 2006.

Ovarian cancer

- Malignancy arising from the ovary; a rapidly progressing cancer that's difficult to diagnose
- Prognosis varying with histologic type and stage
- 90% primary epithelial tumors
- Stromal and germ cell tumors also important tumor types

PATHOPHYSIOLOGY

- Ovarian cancer spreads rapidly intraperitoneally by local extension or surface seeding and, occasionally, through the lymphatics and the bloodstream.
- Metastasis to the ovary can occur from breast, colon, gastric, and pancreatic cancers.

CAUSES

- Exact cause unknown

RISK FACTORS

- Infertility problems or nulliparity
- Celibacy
- Exposure to asbestos and talc
- History of breast or uterine cancer
- Family history of ovarian cancer
- Diet high in saturated fat

INCIDENCE

- After lung, breast, and colon cancer, primary ovarian cancer is the most common cause of cancer death among women in the United States (about 40% survive for 5 years).
- Ovarian cancer is more common after age 50.
- Women in industrialized nations are at greater risk for this disease.
- Metastatic ovarian cancer is more common than cancer at any other site in women with previously treated breast cancer.

COMPLICATIONS

- Depression
- Fluid and electrolyte imbalance
- Leg edema
- Ascites
- Intestinal obstruction
- Profound cachexia
- Recurrent malignant effusions

ASSESSMENT

HISTORY

- Lack of obvious signs, or signs and symptoms that vary with tumor size and extent of metastasis (disease usually metastasized before diagnosis is made)
- In later stages: urinary frequency, constipation, pelvic discomfort, distention, weight loss, abdominal pain

PHYSICAL FINDINGS

- Gaunt appearance
- Grossly distended abdomen accompanied by ascites
- Palpable abdominal mass with rocky hardness or rubbery or cystlike quality

DIAGNOSTIC TEST RESULTS

LABORATORY

- Laboratory tumor marker studies (such as ovarian carcinoma antigen, carcinoembryonic antigen, and human chorionic gonadotropin) show abnormalities that may indicate complications.

IMAGING

- Abdominal ultrasonography, computed tomography scan, or X-rays delineate tumor size.

DIAGNOSTIC PROCEDURES

- Aspiration of ascitic fluid can reveal atypical cells.

OTHER

- Exploratory laparotomy, including lymph node evaluation and tumor resection, is required for accurate diagnosis and staging.

TREATMENT

GENERAL
- Radiation therapy (not commonly used because it causes myelosuppression, which limits effectiveness of chemotherapy)
- Radioisotopes as adjuvant therapy

DIET
- High-protein
- Small, frequent meals

MEDICATIONS
- Chemotherapy after surgery
- Immunotherapy (under investigation)
- Hormone replacement therapy in prepubertal girls who had bilateral salpingo-oophorectomy

SURGERY
- Total abdominal hysterectomy and bilateral salpingo-oophorectomy with tumor resection
- Omentectomy, appendectomy, lymph node palpation with probable lymphadenectomy, tissue biopsies, and peritoneal washings
- Resection of involved ovary
- Biopsies of omentum and uninvolved ovary
- Peritoneal washings for cytologic examination of pelvic fluid

NURSING CONSIDERATIONS

NURSING DIAGNOSES
- Acute pain
- Anticipatory grieving
- Anxiety
- Excess fluid volume
- Fear
- Hopelessness
- Imbalanced nutrition: Less than body requirements
- Impaired skin integrity
- Ineffective coping
- Risk for infection
- Sexual dysfunction

EXPECTED OUTCOMES
The patient will:
- express feelings of increased comfort and decreased pain
- express feelings about the potential loss
- express feelings of decreased anxiety
- maintain appropriate fluid balance
- verbalize fears and concerns related to the diagnosis and treatment
- begin to make decisions on own behalf
- maintain weight within an acceptable range
- maintain skin integrity
- demonstrate positive coping behaviors
- exhibit no signs of infection
- verbalize concerns about actual or potential impairment in sexual function.

NURSING INTERVENTIONS
- Encourage verbalization and provide support.
- Give prescribed drugs.
- Provide abdominal support, and be alert for abdominal distention.
- Encourage coughing and deep breathing.

MONITORING
- Vital signs
- Intake and output
- Wound site
- Pain control
- Effects of medication
- Hydration and nutrition status

PATIENT TEACHING

GENERAL
Be sure to cover:
- the disorder, diagnosis, and treatment
- dietary needs
- relaxation techniques
- importance of preventing infection, emphasizing proper hand-washing technique
- drug administration, dosage, and possible adverse effects.

DISCHARGE PLANNING
- Refer the patient to resource and support services.

RESOURCES
Organizations
American Cancer Society: *www.cancer.org*
Guide to Internet Resources for Cancer: *www.cancerindex.org*
National Cancer Institute: *www.cancer.gov*

Selected references
Atlas of Pathophysiology, 2nd ed. Philadelphia: Lippincott Williams & Wilkins, 2005.

Brooks, S.E., et al. "Ovarian Cancer: A Clinician's Perspective," *Pathology Case Reviews* 11(1):3-8, January-February 2006.

Ferrell, B., et al. "Perspectives on the Impact of Ovarian Cancer: Women's Views of Quality of Life," *Oncology Nursing Forum* 32(6):1143-49, November 2005.

Lecuru, F., et al. "Impact of Initial Surgical Access on Staging and Survival of Patients with Stage I Ovarian Cancer," *International Journal of Gynecological Cancer* 16(1):87-94, January-February 2006.

Schildkraut, J.M., et al. "Analgesic Drug Use and Risk of Ovarian Cancer," *Epidemiology* 17(1):104-07, January 2006.

Ovarian cysts

- Nonneoplastic sacs on an ovary that contain fluid or semisolid material
- Usually small and not producing symptoms
- May be single or multiple (polycystic ovarian disease)
- Include follicular cysts, theca-lutein cysts, and corpus luteum cysts
- Can develop any time between puberty and menopause, including during pregnancy
- Excellent prognosis for nonneoplastic ovarian cysts (The risk of ovarian malignancy isn't increased with a functional [physiologic] ovarian cyst.)

PATHOPHYSIOLOGY

- Follicular cysts are generally very small and arise from follicles that overdistend, either because they haven't ruptured or have ruptured and resealed before their fluid was reabsorbed. (See *Follicular cyst.*)
- Luteal cysts develop if a mature corpus luteum persists abnormally and continues to secrete progesterone. They consist of blood or fluid that accumulates in the cavity of the corpus luteum and typically produce more symptoms than follicular cysts.
- When luteal cysts persist into menopause, they secrete excessive amounts of estrogen in response to the hypersecretion of follicle-stimulating hormone and luteinizing hormone that normally occurs during menopause.

CAUSES

- Choriocarcinoma
- Granulosa-lutein cysts (excessive accumulation of blood during menstruation)
- Hormone therapy
- Hydatidiform mole
- Theca-lutein cysts

INCIDENCE

- Ovarian cysts can develop at any age but are more common in women of reproductive age.

COMPLICATIONS

- Torsion or rupture of cyst
- Infertility
- Amenorrhea
- Secondary dysmenorrhea
- Oligomenorrhea

HISTORY

- Mild pelvic discomfort
- Lower back pain
- Dyspareunia
- Irregular bleeding

PHYSICAL FINDINGS

- Abdominal tenderness
- Abdominal distention
- Rigid abdomen
- Enlarged ovaries

LABORATORY

- Human chorionic gonadotropin (hCG) titer is elevated (theca-lutein cyst).
- Urine 17-ketosteroids are slightly elevated (polycystic ovarian disease).

IMAGING

- Ultrasound reveals cyst.

OTHER

- Laparoscopy (usually for another condition) reveals cyst.

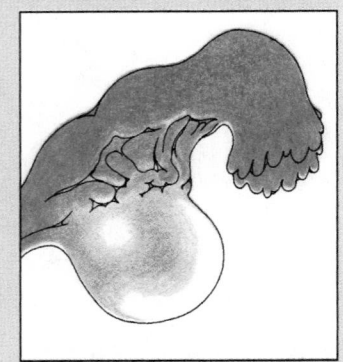

Follicular cyst

A common type of ovarian cyst, a follicular cyst is usually semitransparent and overdistended, with watery fluid visible through its thin walls.

TREATMENT

GENERAL
- Follicular cysts: no treatment because cysts commonly disappear spontaneously within one to two menstrual cycles (excision of persistent cysts to rule out malignancy)
- Theca-lutein cysts: discontinuation of hCG or clomiphene citrate therapy
- Ruptured cysts: culdocentesis to drain intraperitoneal fluid

ACTIVITY
- As tolerated

MEDICATIONS
- Hormonal contraceptives
- Gonadotropin-releasing hormonal agonists
- Analgesics

SURGERY
- Laparoscopy or exploratory laparotomy with possible ovarian cystectomy or oophorectomy for persistent or suspicious ovarian cyst

NURSING CONSIDERATIONS

NURSING DIAGNOSES
- Acute pain
- Anxiety
- Deficient fluid volume
- Ineffective coping
- Ineffective sexuality patterns
- Risk for infection

EXPECTED OUTCOMES
The patient will:
- express feelings of comfort and relief from pain
- identify strategies to reduce anxiety
- maintain normal fluid volume
- demonstrate adaptive coping behaviors
- express with partner feelings about the condition and its effect on their sexual relationship
- remain free from signs and symptoms of infection.

NURSING INTERVENTIONS
- Provide emotional support.

After surgery
- Encourage early ambulation.

MONITORING
- Signs of rupture
- Vital signs
- Vaginal bleeding

PATIENT TEACHING

GENERAL
Be sure to cover:
- the disorder, diagnosis, and treatment
- importance of follow-up care
- need to report increased menstrual bleeding
- need to report abdominal mass.

RESOURCES
Organizations
American College of Obstetricians and Gynecologists: *www.acog.org*
American Society for Reproductive Medicine: *www.asrm.org*
Mayo Clinic: *www.mayoclinic.com*

Selected references
McCook, J.G., et al. "Health-related Quality of Life Issues in Women with Polycystic Ovary Syndrome," *Journal of Obstetric, Gynecologic, and Neonatal Nursing* 34(1):12-20, January-February 2005.
Patel, S.M., and Nestler, J.E. "Fertility in Polycystic Ovary Syndrome," *Endocrinology and Metabolism Clinics of North America* 35(1):137-55, vii, March 2006.
Snyder, B.S. "Polycystic Ovary Syndrome (PCOS) in the Adolescent Patient: Recommendations for Practice," *Pediatric Nursing* 31(5):416-21, September-October 2005.

Paget's disease

- Bone disorder that causes an irregular bone formation
- Affects one or several skeletal areas (spine, pelvis, femur, and skull)
- Slow and progressive
- Causes malignant bone changes in about 5% of patients
- Can be fatal, particularly when associated with heart failure, bone sarcoma, or giant cell tumors
- Also known as *osteitis deformans*

  ⚡ WARNING *Paget's disease of the breast, a form of breast cancer, is a different disorder from Paget's disease. (See* Paget's disease of the breast.*)*

PATHOPHYSIOLOGY
- In the initial phase (osteoclastic phase) excessive bone resorption occurs.
- The second phase (osteoblastic phase) involves excessive abnormal bone formation.
- Affected bones enlarge and soften.
- New bone structure is chaotic, fragile, and weak.

CAUSES
- Exact cause unknown
- Thought to be caused by a slow or dormant viral infection (possibly mumps)

INCIDENCE
- Paget's disease is more common after age 40.
- Men and women are affected equally.

COMPLICATIONS
- Fractures
- Paraplegia
- Blindness and hearing loss with tinnitus and vertigo
- Osteoarthritis
- Sarcoma
- Hypertension
- Renal calculi
- Hypercalcemia
- Gout
- Heart failure

ASSESSMENT

HISTORY
- Severe, persistent pain
- Impaired mobility
- Pain that worsens with weight bearing
- Increased hat size
- Headaches

PHYSICAL FINDINGS
- Cranial enlargement over frontal and occipital areas
- Kyphosis
- Barrel-shaped chest
- Asymmetrical bowing of the tibia and femur
- Warmth and tenderness over affected sites

Paget's disease of the breast

Commonly misdiagnosed as a dermatologic problem, this rare type of breast cancer appears as a red, scaly crust on the nipple, causing itchiness and burning. Biopsy confirms the diagnosis. Treatment should be started to prevent spread of malignancy to the lymph nodes and other parts of the body.

DIAGNOSTIC TEST RESULTS

LABORATORY
- Red blood cell count shows anemia.
- Serum alkaline phosphatase level is elevated.
- Level of 24-hour urine hydroxyproline is elevated.

IMAGING
- X-ray studies show bone expansion and increased bone density.
- Bone scans clearly show early pagetic lesions.

DIAGNOSTIC PROCEDURES
- Bone biopsy shows a characteristic mosaic pattern of bone tissue.

TREATMENT

GENERAL
- Heat therapy
- Massage
- Weight management

DIET
- Adequate levels of calcium and vitamin D

ACTIVITY
- As tolerated
- Regular exercise
- Pacing of activities
- Use of assistive devices such as cane or walker, if needed, to prevent falls

MEDICATIONS
- Calcitonin
- Nonsteroidal anti-inflammatory drugs
- Bisphosphonates
- Calcium supplements
- Vitamin D

SURGERY
- Reduction of pathologic fractures
- Correction of secondary deformities
- Relief of neurologic impairment

NURSING CONSIDERATIONS

NURSING DIAGNOSES
- Chronic pain
- Dressing or grooming self-care deficit
- Impaired physical mobility
- Risk for impaired skin integrity
- Risk for injury

EXPECTED OUTCOMES
The patient will:
- express feelings of increased comfort and decreased pain
- perform activities of daily living to the extent possible
- maintain joint mobility and range of motion
- maintain adequate skin integrity
- demonstrate measures to prevent self-injury.

NURSING INTERVENTIONS
- Take measures to prevent pressure ulcers.
- Instruct the patient with footdrop to wear high-topped sneakers or use a footboard.

MONITORING
- Pain level, response to analgesic therapy
- New areas of pain
- New movement restrictions
- Sensory and motor disturbances
- Serum calcium and alkaline phosphatase levels
- Intake and output

PATIENT TEACHING

GENERAL
Be sure to cover:
- the disorder, diagnosis, and treatment
- pacing of activities
- use of assistive devices
- exercise program
- use of a firm mattress or a bed board
- home safety measures
- how to take prescribed drugs
- adverse reactions to report.

DISCHARGE PLANNING
- Refer the patient to community resource and support sources, as appropriate.
- Refer the patient to physical and occupational therapy.

RESOURCES
Organizations
Arthritis Foundation: *www.arthritis.org*
National Institutes of Health: *www.nih.gov*
Paget Foundation for Paget's Disease of Bone and Related Disorders: *www.paget.org*

Selected references
Handbook of Pathophysiology, 2nd ed. Philadelphia: Lippincott Williams & Wilkins, 2005.
Hosking, D. "Pharmacological Therapy of Paget's and Other Metabolic Bone Disease," *Bone* 38(2 Suppl 2):3-7, February 2006.
Lee, G.C., et al. "Total Knee Arthroplasty in Patients with Paget's Disease of Bone at the Knee," *Journal of Arthroplasty* 20(6):689-93, September 2005.
Professional Guide to Diseases, 8th ed. Philadelphia: Lippincott Williams & Wilkins, 2005.
Rendina, D., et al. "Paget's Disease and Bisphosphonates," *New England Journal of Medicine* 353(24):2616-18, December 2005.

Pancreatic cancer

◆ Proliferation of cancer cells in the pancreas
◆ Fifth most lethal type of carcinoma
◆ Poor prognosis (most patients die within 1 year of diagnosis)

PATHOPHYSIOLOGY

◆ Pancreatic cancer is almost always adenocarcinoma.
◆ Nearly two-thirds of tumors appear in the head of the pancreas; islet cell tumors are rare.
◆ Two main tissue types form fibrotic nodes. Cylinder cells arise in ducts and degenerate into cysts; large, fatty, granular cells arise in parenchyma.
◆ A high-fat or excessive protein diet induces chronic hyperplasia of the pancreas, with increased cell turnover.

CAUSES

◆ Possible link to inhalation or absorption of carcinogens (such as cigarette smoke, excessive fat and protein, food additives, and industrial chemicals), which the pancreas then excretes

RISK FACTORS

◆ Chronic pancreatitis
◆ Diabetes
◆ Chronic alcohol abuse
◆ Smoking
◆ Occupational exposure to chemicals
◆ High-fat diet

INCIDENCE

◆ Pancreatic cancer is three to four times more common in smokers than nonsmokers.
◆ Pancreatic cancer incidence is highest in black men ages 35 to 70.
◆ Incidence is highest in Israel, United States, Sweden, and Canada; it's lowest in Switzerland, Belgium, and Italy.

COMPLICATIONS

◆ Depression
◆ Nutrient malabsorption
◆ Type 1 diabetes
◆ Liver and GI problems

◆ Mental status changes
◆ Hemorrhage
◆ Pulmonary congestion

ASSESSMENT

HISTORY

◆ Colicky, dull, or vague intermittent epigastric pain, which may radiate to the right upper quadrant or dorsolumbar area; unrelated to posture or activity and aggravated by meals
◆ Anorexia, nausea, and vomiting
◆ Rapid, profound weight loss

PHYSICAL FINDINGS

◆ Jaundice
◆ Large, palpable, well-defined mass in the subumbilical or left hypochondrial region
◆ Abdominal bruit or pulsation

DIAGNOSTIC TEST RESULTS

LABORATORY

◆ The secretin test reveals an absence of pancreatic enzymes.
◆ Serum bilirubin is increased.
◆ Serum lipase and amylase levels may be increased.
◆ Thrombin time is prolonged.
◆ Aspartate aminotransferase and alanine aminotransferase levels are elevated (if liver cell necrosis is present).
◆ Alkaline phosphatase level is markedly elevated (in biliary obstruction).
◆ Insulin level is measurable in serum (if islet cell tumor is present).
◆ Hypoglycemia or hyperglycemia may be present.
◆ Specific tumor markers for pancreatic cancer are elevated, including carcinoembryonic antigen, pancreatic oncofetal antigen, alpha-fetoprotein, and serum immunoreactive elastase I.

IMAGING

◆ Barium swallow, retroperitoneal insufflation, cholangiography, and scintigraphy locate the neoplasm and detect changes in the duodenum or stomach.
◆ Ultrasonography and computed tomography scans identify masses.
◆ Magnetic resonance imaging scan discloses tumor location and size.
◆ Angiography reveals tumor vascularity.
◆ Endoscopic retrograde cholangiopancreatography allows tumor visualization and specimen biopsy.

DIAGNOSTIC PROCEDURES

◆ Percutaneous fine-needle aspiration biopsy may detect tumor cells.
◆ Laparotomy with biopsy allows definitive diagnosis.

TREATMENT

GENERAL
◆ Mainly palliative
◆ May involve radiation therapy as adjunct to fluorouracil chemotherapy

DIET
◆ Well-balanced, as tolerated
◆ Small, frequent meals

ACTIVITY
◆ Postoperative avoidance of lifting and contact sports
◆ After recovery, no activity restrictions

MEDICATIONS
◆ Chemotherapy
◆ Antibiotics
◆ Anticholinergics
◆ Antacids
◆ Diuretics
◆ Insulin
◆ Analgesics
◆ Pancreatic enzymes

SURGERY
◆ Total pancreatectomy
◆ Cholecystojejunostomy, choledochoduodenostomy, and choledochojejunostomy
◆ Gastrojejunostomy
◆ Whipple's operation or radical pancreatoduodenectomy

NURSING CONSIDERATIONS

NURSING DIAGNOSES
◆ Acute pain
◆ Anxiety
◆ Constipation
◆ Deficient fluid volume
◆ Imbalanced nutrition: Less than body requirements
◆ Impaired skin integrity
◆ Ineffective coping
◆ Risk for injury

EXPECTED OUTCOMES
The patient will:
◆ verbalize increased comfort and pain relief
◆ express feelings of reduced anxiety
◆ experience return to normal bowel movements
◆ maintain normal fluid volume status
◆ maintain an adequate weight
◆ maintain skin integrity
◆ demonstrate positive coping behaviors
◆ avoid injury.

NURSING INTERVENTIONS
◆ Give prescribed drugs and blood transfusions.
◆ Provide small, frequent meals.
◆ Ensure adequate rest and sleep.
◆ Assist with range-of-motion and isometric exercises, as appropriate.
◆ Perform scrupulous skin care.
◆ Apply antiembolism stockings.
◆ Encourage verbalization and provide emotional support.

MONITORING
◆ Fluid balance and nutrition
◆ Abdominal girth, metabolic state, and daily weight
◆ Blood glucose levels
◆ Complete blood count
◆ Pain control
◆ Bleeding

PATIENT TEACHING

GENERAL
Be sure to cover:
◆ the disorder, diagnosis, and treatment
◆ end-of-life issues
◆ drug administration, dosage, and possible adverse effects
◆ expected postoperative care
◆ information about diabetes, including signs and symptoms of hypoglycemia and hyperglycemia
◆ adverse effects of radiation therapy and chemotherapy.

DISCHARGE PLANNING
◆ Refer the patient to community resource and support services.
◆ Refer the patient to hospice care if indicated.
◆ Refer the patient to the American Cancer Society.

RESOURCES
Organizations
American Cancer Society:
www.cancer.org
American Diabetes Association:
www.diabetes.org
Guide to Internet Resources for Cancer:
www.cancerindex.org
National Cancer Institute:
www.cancer.gov
National Institute of Diabetes & Digestive & Kidney Diseases: *www.niddk.nih.gov*

Selected references
Atlas of Pathophysiology, 2nd ed. Philadelphia: Lippincott Williams & Wilkins, 2005.
Leonard, G.D., et al. "Metastases to the Breast from Primary Pancreatic Cancer," *Breast Journal* 11(6):503, November-December 2005.
Lerch, M.M. "Anticipating Disaster: The Genetics of Familial Pancreatic Cancer," *Gut* 55(2):150-51, February 2006.
Wasan, S.M., and Ross, W.A. "Use of Expandable Metallic Biliary Stents in Resectable Pancreatic Cancer," *Journal of Vascular & Interventional Radiology* 17(1):192, January 2006.

Pancreatitis

OVERVIEW

- Inflammation of the pancreas
- Occurs in acute and chronic forms; acute form has 10% mortality
- Irreversible tissue damage with chronic form, which tends to progress to significant pancreatic function loss
- Can be idiopathic but sometimes associated with biliary tract disease, alcoholism, trauma, and certain drugs

PATHOPHYSIOLOGY

- Enzymes normally excreted into the duodenum by the pancreas are activated in the pancreas or its ducts and start to autodigest pancreatic tissue.
- Consequent inflammation causes intense pain, third spacing of large fluid volumes, pancreatic fat necrosis with consumption of serum calcium and, occasionally, hemorrhage.

CAUSES

- Abnormal organ structure
- Alcoholism
- Biliary tract disease
- Metabolic or endocrine disorders
- Pancreatic cysts or tumors
- Penetrating peptic ulcers
- Penetrating trauma
- Viral or bacterial infection

RISK FACTORS

- Use of glucocorticoids, sulfonamides, thiazides, and hormonal contraceptives
- Renal failure and kidney transplantation
- Endoscopic retrograde cholangiopancreatography (ERCP)
- Heredity
- Emotional or neurogenic factors

INCIDENCE

- Acute pancreatitis occurs in 2 out of every 10,000 people.
- Chronic pancreatitis occurs in 2 out of every 25,000 people.
- The disorder affects more men than women.
- It's four times more common in Blacks than in Whites.

COMPLICATIONS

- Diabetes mellitus
- Massive hemorrhage
- Diabetic acidosis
- Shock and coma
- Acute respiratory distress syndrome
- Atelectasis and pleural effusion
- Pneumonia
- Paralytic ileus
- GI bleeding
- Pancreatic abscess and cancer
- Pseudocysts
- Renal failure

ASSESSMENT

HISTORY

- Intense epigastric pain centered close to the umbilicus and radiating to the back, between the 10th thoracic and 6th lumbar vertebrae
- Pain aggravated by fatty foods, alcohol consumption, or recumbent position
- Weight loss with nausea and vomiting
- Predisposing factor

PHYSICAL FINDINGS

- Hypotension
- Tachycardia
- Fever
- Dyspnea, orthopnea
- Generalized jaundice
- Cullen's sign (bluish periumbilical discoloration)
- Turner's sign (bluish flank discoloration)
- Steatorrhea (with chronic pancreatitis)
- Abdominal tenderness, rigidity, and guarding

DIAGNOSTIC TEST RESULTS

LABORATORY

In acute pancreatitis

- Serum amylase and lipase levels are elevated.
- White blood cell count is elevated.
- Serum bilirubin level is elevated.
- Transient hyperglycemia and glycosuria are present.
- Urine amylase level is increased.

In chronic pancreatitis

- Serum alkaline phosphatase, amylase, and bilirubin levels are elevated.
- Serum glucose level is transiently elevated.
- Lipid and trypsin levels in stools are elevated.

IMAGING

- Abdominal and chest X-rays differentiate pancreatitis from other diseases that cause similar symptoms; they also detect pleural effusions.
- Computed tomography scans and ultrasonography show increased pancreatic diameter, pancreatic cysts, and pseudocysts.

DIAGNOSTIC PROCEDURES

- ERCP shows pancreatic anatomy, identifies ductal system abnormalities, and differentiates pancreatitis from other disorders.

TREATMENT

GENERAL
- Emergency treatment of shock as needed; vigorous I.V. replacement of fluid, electrolytes, and proteins
- Blood transfusions (for hemorrhage)
- Nasogastric suctioning

DIET
- Nothing by mouth
- Once crisis starts to resolve, oral low-fat, low-protein feedings implemented gradually
- Alcohol and caffeine abstention

ACTIVITY
- As tolerated

MEDICATIONS
- Analgesics
- Antacids
- Histamine antagonists
- Antibiotics
- Anticholinergics
- Total parenteral nutrition
- Pancreatic enzymes
- Insulin
- Albumin

SURGERY
- Not indicated in acute pancreatitis unless complications occur
- For chronic pancreatitis: sphincterotomy
- Pancreaticojejunostomy

NURSING CONSIDERATIONS

NURSING DIAGNOSES
- Acute pain
- Deficient fluid volume
- Disturbed body image
- Hopelessness
- Imbalanced nutrition: Less than body requirements
- Ineffective breathing pattern
- Risk for impaired skin integrity
- Risk for injury

EXPECTED OUTCOMES
The patient will:
- verbalize feelings of increased comfort
- maintain normal fluid volume
- express positive feelings about self
- participate in decisions about care
- achieve adequate caloric and nutritional intake
- maintain an effective breathing pattern
- maintain skin integrity
- avoid complications.

NURSING INTERVENTIONS
- Give prescribed drugs and I.V. therapy.
- Encourage the patient to express his feelings.
- Provide emotional support.

MONITORING
- Vital signs
- Nasogastric tube function and drainage
- Respiratory status
- Acid-base balance
- Serum glucose level
- Fluid and electrolyte balance
- Daily weight
- Pain control
- Nutritional status and metabolic requirements

PATIENT TEACHING

GENERAL
Be sure to cover:
- the disorder, diagnosis, and treatment
- identification and avoidance of acute pancreatitis triggers
- dietary needs
- medication administration, dosage, and possible adverse effects.

DISCHARGE PLANNING
- Refer the patient to community resource and support services, as needed.

RESOURCES
Organizations
Alcoholics Anonymous: *www.aa.org*
Digestive Disease National Coalition: *www.ddnc.org*
National Digestive Diseases Information Clearinghouse: *www.niddk.nih.gov/health/digest/nddic.htm*

Selected references
Handbook of Diseases, 3rd ed. Philadelphia: Lippincott Williams & Wilkins, 2004.
Hughes, E. "Understanding the Care of Patients with Acute Pancreatitis," *Nursing Standard* 18(18):45-52, January 2004.
Shrikhande, S.V., et al. "Management of Pain in Small Duct Chronic Pancreatitis," *Journal of Gastrointestinal Surgery* 10(2):227-33, February 2006.
Swaroop, V.S., et al. "Severe Acute Pancreatitis," *JAMA* 291(23):2865-68, June 2004.
Tierney, L., et al. *Current Medical Diagnosis & Treatment 2006.* New York: McGraw-Hill Book Co., 2006.

Panic disorder

OVERVIEW

- Anxiety in its most severe form, characterized by recurrent episodes of intense apprehension, terror, and impending doom
- May be associated with specific situations or tasks
- Commonly exists concurrently with agoraphobia
- May be triggered by severe separation anxiety experienced during early childhood
- Can persist for years without treatment, with alternating exacerbations and remissions

PATHOPHYSIOLOGY

- Sensitivity to adrenergic central nervous system discharges is increased with hypersensitivity of presynaptic alpha-2 receptors.

CAUSES

- Brain biochemistry alterations, especially in norepinephrine, serotonin, and gamma-aminobutyric acid activity
- Combination of physiologic and psychological factors
- Hereditary
- Persistent pattern of maladaptive behavior acquired by learning
- Stressful events or unconscious conflicts from early childhood
- Temporal lobe dysfunction

INCIDENCE

- Men and women are affected equally.
- Panic disorder with agoraphobia is about twice as common in women as in men.
- Typical onset is in late adolescence or early adulthood, commonly in response to a sudden loss.

COMPLICATIONS

- Psychoactive substance use disorder

ASSESSMENT

HISTORY

- Repeated episodes of unexpected apprehension or fear

PHYSICAL FINDINGS

- During a panic attack
- Trembling
- Digestive disturbances
- Hyperventilation
- Tachycardia
- Profuse sweating

DSM-IV-TR *criteria*

Diagnosis of panic disorder confirmed when the patient meets the following criteria:

- Recurrent, unexpected panic attacks with at least one of the attacks having been followed by 1 month (or more) of one (or more) of the following:
- persistent concern about having additional attacks
- worry about the attack's implications or consequences
- significant change in behavior related to the attack
- agoraphobia
- Attacks not due to the direct physiologic effects of a substance or a general medical condition
- Attacks not better accounted for by another mental disorder, such as social phobia, specific phobia, obsessive-compulsive disorder, posttraumatic stress disorder, or separation anxiety.

DIAGNOSTIC TEST RESULTS

LABORATORY

- Urine and serum toxicology tests may reveal the presence of psychoactive substances that can precipitate panic attacks, including barbiturates, caffeine, and amphetamines.

OTHER

- Various tests may be ordered to rule out an organic basis for the symptoms.

TREATMENT

GENERAL
- Behavioral therapy
- Supportive psychotherapy

MEDICATIONS
- Anxiolytics
- Antidepressants

NURSING CONSIDERATIONS

NURSING DIAGNOSES
- Anxiety
- Chronic low self-esteem
- Impaired social interaction
- Impaired verbal communication
- Ineffective coping

EXPECTED OUTCOMES
The patient will:
- experience reduced anxiety by identifying internal precipitating situation
- verbalize feelings related to self-esteem
- exhibit effective social interaction skills
- verbalize his needs
- develop effective coping mechanisms.

NURSING INTERVENTIONS
- Stay with the patient until the attack subsides.
- Speak in short, simple sentences and slowly give one direction at a time. Avoid giving lengthy explanations and asking too many questions.
- Give prescribed drugs.

MONITORING
- Response to therapy
- Vital signs during an attack

PATIENT TEACHING

GENERAL
Be sure to cover:
- relaxation techniques such as focusing on slow, deep breathing
- drug administration, dosage, and possible adverse effects.

DISCHARGE PLANNING
- Encourage the patient and his family to use community resources such as the Anxiety Disorders Association of America.

RESOURCES
Organizations
American Psychiatric Association: *www.psych.org*
American Psychological Association: *www.apa.org*
Anxiety Disorders Association of America: *www.adaa.org*

Selected references
Diagnostic and Statistical Manual of Mental Disorders, Fourth Edition, Text Revision. Washington, D.C.: American Psychiatric Association, 2000.

Fava, G.A., et al. "Sequential Treatment of Mood and Anxiety Disorders," *Journal of Clinical Psychiatry* 66(11):1392-400, November 2005.

Overbeek, T., and Schruers, K. "Cognitive Behavioural Therapy Reduces Nocturnal Panic in People with Panic Disorder," *Evidence-Based Mental Health* 9(1):13, February 2006.

Overbeek, T., et al. "Sleep Complaints in Panic Disorder Patients," *Journal of Nervous & Mental Disease* 193(7):488-93, July 2005.

Parkinson's disease

OVERVIEW

- Brain disorder causing progressive deterioration, with muscle rigidity, akinesia, and involuntary tremors
- Usual cause of death: aspiration pneumonia
- One of the most common crippling diseases in the United States

PATHOPHYSIOLOGY

- Dopaminergic neurons degenerate, causing loss of available dopamine.
- Dopamine deficiency prevents affected brain cells from performing their normal inhibitory function.
- Excess excitatory acetylcholine occurs at synapses.
- Nondopaminergic receptors are also involved.
- Motor neurons are depressed. (See *Understanding Parkinson's disease.*)

CAUSES

- Usually unknown
- Drug-induced (haloperidol [Haldol], methyldopa, reserpine)
- Exposure to such toxins as manganese dust and carbon monoxide
- Possible genetic or viral cause
- Type A encephalitis

INCIDENCE

- Parkinson's disease is more common in men than in women.
- It develops in middle age or later.
- Parkinson's disease is rare in blacks.

COMPLICATIONS

- Injury from falls
- Food aspiration
- Urinary tract infections
- Skin breakdown
- Pneumonia
- Depression
- Dementia
- Constipation
- Sleep problems
- Sexual dysfunction

ASSESSMENT

HISTORY

- Muscle rigidity
- Akinesia
- Insidious (unilateral pill-roll) tremor, which increases during stress or anxiety and decreases with purposeful movement and sleep
- Dysphagia
- Fatigue with activities of daily living
- Muscle cramps of legs, neck, and trunk
- Oily skin
- Increased perspiration
- Insomnia
- Mood changes
- Dysarthria

PHYSICAL FINDINGS

- High-pitched, monotonous voice
- Drooling
- Masklike facial expression
- Difficulty walking
- Lack of parallel motion in gait
- Loss of posture control with walking
- Oculogyric crises (eyes fixed upward, with involuntary tonic movements)
- Muscle rigidity causing resistance to passive muscle stretching
- Difficulty pivoting
- Loss of balance
- Tremors of hands and feet

DIAGNOSTIC TEST RESULTS

IMAGING

- Computed tomography scan or magnetic resonance rules out other disorders such as intracranial tumors.

TREATMENT

GENERAL

- Environmental safety measures
- Assistance with activities of daily living

DIET

- Small, frequent meals
- High-bulk foods

ACTIVITY

- Physical therapy and occupational therapy
- Assistive devices to aid ambulation
- Fall prevention measures

MEDICATIONS

- Dopamine replacement drugs
- Anticholinergics
- Antihistamines
- Antiviral agents
- Enzyme-inhibiting agents
- Tricyclic antidepressants
- Dopamine agonists

SURGERY

- Used when drug therapy fails
- Stereotaxic neurosurgery
- Destruction of ventrolateral nucleus of thalamus
- Deep brain stimulation

Understanding Parkinson's disease

Research on the pathogenesis of Parkinson's disease focuses on damage to the substantia nigra from oxidative stress. Oxidative stress is believed to:

- alter the brain's iron content
- impair mitochondrial function
- alter antioxidant and protective systems
- reduce glutathione
- damage lipids, proteins, and deoxyribonucleic acid.

NURSING DIAGNOSES
- Bathing or hygiene self-care deficit
- Chronic low self-esteem
- Constipation
- Disabled family coping
- Disturbed body image
- Dressing or grooming self-care deficit
- Feeding self-care deficit
- Imbalanced nutrition: Less than body requirements
- Impaired physical mobility
- Impaired social interaction
- Impaired verbal communication
- Ineffective coping
- Interrupted family processes
- Risk for injury

EXPECTED OUTCOMES
The patient (or family) will:
- perform bathing and hygiene activities to the fullest extent possible
- verbalize feelings regarding self-esteem
- resume a normal bowel elimination pattern
- seek support resources and develop adequate coping behaviors
- express positive feelings about self
- perform dressing and grooming activities to the fullest extent possible
- perform self-care needs related to feeding to the fullest extent possible
- consume adequate daily calories as required
- maintain maximal mobility within the confines of the disorder
- maintain family and peer relationships
- develop alternative means of communication
- demonstrate effective coping skills
- discuss the impact of the patient's condition on the family unit
- remain free from injury.

NURSING INTERVENTIONS
- Take measures to prevent aspiration.
- Protect the patient from injury.
- Stress the importance of rest periods between activities.
- Ensure adequate nutrition.
- Provide frequent warm baths and massage.
- Encourage the patient to enroll in a physical therapy program.
- Provide emotional and psychological support.
- Encourage the patient to be independent.
- Assist with ambulation and range-of-motion exercises

MONITORING
- Vital signs
- Intake and output
- Drug therapy
- Adverse reactions to medications
- Postoperatively: signs of hemorrhage and increased intracranial pressure
- Swallowing
- Self-care abilities

GENERAL
Be sure to cover:
- the disorder, diagnosis, and treatment
- drug administration, dosage, and possible adverse effects
- measures to prevent pressure ulcers and contractures
- household safety measures
- importance of daily bathing
- methods to improve communication
- swallowing therapy regimen (aspiration precautions).

DISCHARGE PLANNING
- Refer the patient for occupational and physical rehabilitation, as indicated.

RESOURCES
Organizations
American Parkinson Disease Association: *www.apdaparkinson.org*
National Institutes of Health: *www.nih.gov*
National Parkinson Foundation: *www.parkinson.org*
Parkinson's Disease Foundation: *www.pdf.org*

Selected references
Aarsland, D., et al. "Neuroleptic Sensitivity in Parkinson's Disease and Parkinsonian Dementias," *Journal of Clinical Psychiatry* 66(5):633-37, May 2005.
Diseases, 4th ed. Philadelphia: Lippincott Williams & Wilkins, 2006.
Eriksen, J.L., et al. "Molecular Pathogenesis of Parkinson Disease," *Archives of Neurology* 62(3):353-57, March 2005.
Grosset, K.A., et al. "Measuring Therapy Adherence in Parkinson's Disease: A Comparison of Methods," *Journal of Neurology, Neurosurgery & Psychiatry* 77(2):249-51, February 2006.
Habermann, B., and Davis, L.L. "Caring for Family with Alzheimer's Disease and Parkinson's Disease: Needs, Challenges and Satisfaction," *Journal of Gerontological Nursing* 31(6):49-54, June 2005.
Handbook of Pathophysiology, 2nd ed. Philadelphia: Lippincott Williams & Wilkins, 2005.

Patent ductus arteriosus

- Heart condition in which the lumen of the ductus (fetal blood vessel that connects the pulmonary artery to the descending aorta) remains open after birth
- Initially may produce no clinical effects, but in time can precipitate pulmonary vascular disease, causing symptoms to appear by age 40
- Good prognosis if the shunt is small or surgical repair is effective; otherwise, may advance to intractable heart failure, which may be fatal

PATHOPHYSIOLOGY

- The lumen of the ductus remains open after birth and creates a left-to-right shunt of blood from the aorta to the pulmonary artery, resulting in recirculation of arterial blood through the lungs.
- The condition is prevalent in premature infants, probably as a result of abnormalities in oxygenation or the relaxant action of prostaglandin E, which prevents ductal spasm and contracture necessary for closure.

CAUSES

- Prematurity
- Rubella syndrome

RISK FACTORS

- Other congenital defects, such as coarctation of the aorta, ventricular septal defect, and pulmonary and aortic stenoses

INCIDENCE

- The disorder is twice as common in females as in males.
- It's the most common congenital heart defect found in adults.

COMPLICATIONS

- Chronic pulmonary hypertension
- Intractable left-sided heart failure
- Respiratory distress

HISTORY

- Prematurity
- Rubella
- Difficulty breathing

PHYSICAL FINDINGS

- Gibson murmur during systole and diastole
- Thrill at the left sternal border
- Prominent left ventricular impulse
- Bounding peripheral arterial pulses (Corrigan's pulse)
- Widened pulse pressure

IMAGING

- Chest X-rays may show increased pulmonary vascular markings, prominent pulmonary arteries, and enlargement of the left ventricle and aorta.
- Echocardiography detects and helps estimate the size of a patent ductus arteriosus (PDA). It also reveals an enlarged left atrium and left ventricle or right ventricular hypertrophy from pulmonary vascular disease.

DIAGNOSTIC PROCEDURES

- Electrocardiography may be normal or may indicate left atrial or ventricular hypertrophy and, in pulmonary vascular disease, biventricular hypertrophy.
- Cardiac catheterization shows pulmonary arterial oxygen content higher than right ventricular content because of the influx of aortic blood.

TREATMENT

GENERAL
◆ No immediate treatment (if no symptoms are produced)

DIET
◆ Fluid restriction

ACTIVITY
◆ As tolerated

MEDICATIONS
◆ Diuretics
◆ Cardiac glycosides
◆ Antibiotics (preoperatively)

SURGERY
◆ Ligation of the ductus

⚙ *AGE FACTOR If symptoms are mild, surgical correction is usually delayed until at least age 1. Before surgery, children with PDA require antibiotics to protect against infective endocarditis.*

◆ Cardiac catheterization to deposit a plug in the ductus to stop shunting or for I.V. administration of indomethacin (a prostaglandin inhibitor that's an alternative to surgery in premature infants) to induce ductus spasm and closure

NURSING CONSIDERATIONS

NURSING DIAGNOSES
◆ Activity intolerance
◆ Decreased cardiac output
◆ Delayed growth and development
◆ Fatigue
◆ Impaired gas exchange
◆ Impaired parenting
◆ Ineffective breathing pattern
◆ Ineffective tissue perfusion: Cardiopulmonary
◆ Risk for infection

EXPECTED OUTCOMES
The patient (or parents) will:
◆ carry out activities of daily living without weakness or fatigue
◆ maintain adequate cardiac output and remain free from arrhythmias
◆ demonstrate age-appropriate skills and behaviors to the extent possible
◆ express feelings of increased energy
◆ maintain adequate ventilation and oxygenation
◆ agree to seek help from peer support groups or professional counselors to ensure adaptive coping behaviors
◆ maintain an effective breathing pattern
◆ maintain hemodynamic stability
◆ remain free from signs and symptoms of infection.

NURSING INTERVENTIONS
◆ Give prescribed drugs.
◆ Provide emotional support to the patient and her family.

MONITORING
◆ Respiratory status
◆ Vital signs
◆ Cardiac rhythm
◆ Intake and output

PATIENT TEACHING

GENERAL
Be sure to cover:
◆ activity restrictions based on the child's tolerance and energy levels
◆ importance of informing any practitioner who treats the child about her history of surgery for PDA — even if the child is being treated for an unrelated medical problem.

DISCHARGE PLANNING
◆ Stress the need for regular medical follow-up examinations.

RESOURCES
Organizations
American Heart Association: *www.americanheart.org*
National Heart, Lung, and Blood Institute: *www.nhlbi.nih.gov*

Selected references
Arora, R. "Transcatheter Closure of Patent Ductus Arteriosus," *Expert Review of Cardiovascular Therapy* 3(5):865-74, September 2005.
Bancalari, E., et al. "Patent Ductus Arteriosus and Respiratory Outcome in Premature Infants," *Biology of the Neonate* 88(3):192-201, 2005.
Ozmen, J., et al. "Operation for Adult Patent Ductus Arteriosus Using an Aortic Stent-Graft Technique," *Heart, Lung & Circulation* 14(1):54-57, March 2005.
Tanner, K., et al. "Cardiovascular Malformations among Preterm Infants," *Pediatrics* 116(6):e833-38, December 2005.

Pediculosis

OVERVIEW

- Infestation of human parasitic lice, which feed exclusively on human blood and lay eggs (nits) on body hairs or clothing fibers; after nits hatch, lice must feed within 24 hours or die (see *Types of lice*)
- Pediculosis capitis (head lice): confined to scalp and, occasionally, eyebrows, eyelashes, and beard
- Pediculosis corporis (body lice): found next to skin in clothing seams; move to the host only to feed on blood
- Pediculosis pubis (crab lice): found primarily in pubic hairs; may extend to eyebrows, eyelashes, and axillary or body hair

PATHOPHYSIOLOGY

- Lice crawl and attach superficially to the epidermis and hair. One female louse deposits approximately 60 to 150 nits to hair shafts. Nits survive by ingesting blood from the human host.
- A louse bite injects a toxin into the skin. Mild irritation and a purpuric spot result.
- Repeated bites cause sensitization to the toxin, leading to more serious inflammation. In severe cases, sensitization causes wheals or a rash on the trunk.
- Scratching may result in secondary bacterial infection.

CAUSES

Pediculosis capitis
- *Pediculus humanus var. capitis, P. humanus var. corporis*
- Spreads through shared clothing, hats, combs, and hairbrushes

Pediculosis corporis
- *P. humanus var. corporis*
- Spreads through shared clothing and bedding, especially with environmental overcrowding, prolonged wearing of same clothing, or poor personal hygiene

Pediculosis pubis
- *Phthirus pubis*
- Spreads through sexual intercourse or contact with clothing, bedding, or towels harboring lice

---

Types of lice

HEAD LOUSE

Pediculus humanus var. *capitis* (head louse) resembles *P. humanus* var. *corporis* (body louse).

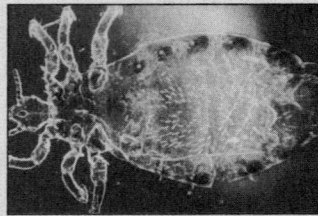

BODY LOUSE

Pediculus humanus var. *corporis* (body louse) has a long abdomen, and its legs are all about the same length.

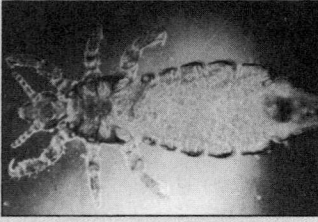

PUBIC LOUSE

Phthirus pubis (pubic, or crab, louse) is slightly translucent. Its first set of legs is shorter than its second and third sets.

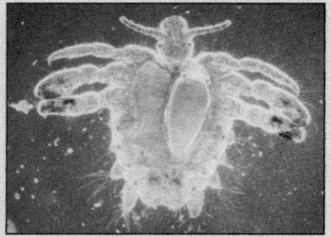

RISK FACTORS
- Poor hygiene
- Overcrowded living conditions

INCIDENCE
- *P. capitis* is more common in children.
- *P. pubis* is more common in adults.

COMPLICATIONS
- Skin excoriation
- Secondary bacterial infections
- Hyperpigmentation or residual scarring

ASSESSMENT

HISTORY
- Exposure to causative organism
- Headache
- Fever
- Malaise
- Pruritus
- Cutaneous changes

PHYSICAL FINDINGS
Pediculosis capitis
- Visible lice
- Skin excoriation on the scalp and neck
- Matted, lusterless hair (in severe cases)
- Occipital and cervical lymphadenopathy
- Oval, gray-white nits visible on hair shafts

Pediculosis corporis
- Red papules or macules, usually on the shoulders, trunk, or buttocks
- Excoriations from scratching
- Nits on clothing seams

Pediculosis pubis
- Visible brownish-gray lice
- Erythematous papules
- Small macules on the thighs, buttocks, or lower abdomen
- Coarse, grainy-feeling, white-gray nits attached to pubic hairs

DIAGNOSTIC TEST RESULTS

DIAGNOSTIC PROCEDURES
- Direct inspection with hand lens shows visible lice or nits.
- Wood's light examination shows fluorescence of live nits (dead nits don't fluoresce).

TREATMENT

GENERAL
- Use of fine-toothed comb dipped in vinegar
- Hair-washing with ordinary shampoo
- Laundering of potentially contaminated clothing and bed linen
- Bathing with soap and water
- Petroleum jelly applied to eyebrows or eyelashes

MEDICATIONS
Pediculosis capitis
- Permethrin or pyrethrins

Pediculosis corporis
- Pediculicide cream (for severe infestation)

Pediculosis pubis
- Pediculicide shampoo

NURSING CONSIDERATIONS

NURSING DIAGNOSES
- Acute pain
- Disturbed body image
- Impaired skin integrity
- Risk for infection

EXPECTED OUTCOMES
The patient (or family) will:
- report feelings of increased comfort
- demonstrate understanding of the appropriate skin care regimen
- verbalize feelings about changed body image
- avoid or minimize the risk of secondary infection.

NURSING INTERVENTIONS
- Give prescribed drugs.
- Use personal protective equipment when administering delousing treatment.
- Notify the school if infestation occurs in a child.
- Encourage the patient to express feelings about the infestation.

MONITORING
- Adverse reactions to insecticide treatment
- Complications
- Response to treatment

PATIENT TEACHING

GENERAL
Be sure to cover:
- how to inspect for lice, eggs, and lesions
- how to decontaminate infestation sources
- how to apply insecticidal agents
- removal of nits and lice
- importance of not sharing personal articles
- adverse reactions to treatment, including when to notify the practitioner
- notification and treatment of sexual contacts within previous 30 days.

RESOURCES
Organizations
American Academy of Dermatology: *www.aad.org*
Dermatology Foundation: *www.dermfnd.org*

Selected references
Elston, D.M. "Drugs Used in the Treatment of Pediculosis," *Journal of Drugs in Dermatology* 4(2):207-11, March-April 2005.
Ko, C.J., and Elston, D.M. "Pediculosis," *Journal of the American Academy of Dermatology* 50(1):1-12, January 2004.
Leung, A.K., et al. "Pediculosis Capitis," *Journal of Pediatric Health Care* 19(6):369-73, November-December 2005.
Schoessler, S.Z. "Treating and Managing Head Lice: The School Nurse Perspective," *American Journal of Managed Care* 10(9 Suppl):S273-76, September 2004.

Pelvic inflammatory disease

OVERVIEW

- General term that refers to any acute, subacute, recurrent, or chronic infection of the oviducts and ovaries, with adjacent tissue involvement
- Includes inflammation of the cervix (cervicitis), uterus (endometritis), fallopian tubes (salpingitis), and ovaries (oophoritis)
- Possible extension of the inflammation to connective tissue lying between the broad ligaments (parametritis)
- Commonly called *PID*

PATHOPHYSIOLOGY

- Various conditions, procedures, or instrumentation can alter or destroy the cervical mucus, which normally serves as a protective barrier.
- As a result, bacteria enter the uterine cavity, causing inflammation of various structures.

CAUSES

- Aerobic or anaerobic organisms (commonly, overgrowth of one or more of the bacterial species found in the cervical mucus)
- Diverticulitis of the sigmoid colon
- Infected drainage from a chronically infected fallopian tube
- Pelvic abscess
- Ruptured appendix
- Septicemia
- Sexually transmitted infections (*Neisseria gonorrhoeae* and *Chlamydia trachomatis*)
- Use of intrauterine device

RISK FACTORS

- Multiple sex partners
- Sexual intercourse at a young age
- Conditions or procedures that alter or destroy cervical mucus
- Procedures that risk transfer of contaminated cervical mucus into the endometrial cavity by an instrument
- Infection during or after pregnancy
- Cigarette smoking
- Multiparity
- Douching
- Intercourse during menses
- Therapeutic abortion

INCIDENCE

- The disorder primarily affects women ages 16 to 40.

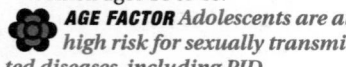 **AGE FACTOR** *Adolescents are at high risk for sexually transmitted diseases, including PID.*

COMPLICATIONS

- Septicemia (potentially fatal)
- Pulmonary embolism
- Infertility
- Peritonitis
- Shock
- Death
- Ectopic pregnancy

ASSESSMENT

HISTORY

- Profuse, purulent vaginal discharge
- Low-grade fever
- Malaise
- Lower abdominal pain
- Vaginal bleeding

PHYSICAL FINDINGS

- Pain with cervical movement or adnexal palpation
- Vaginal discharge
- Unilaterally or bilaterally tender adnexal mass

DIAGNOSTIC TEST RESULTS

LABORATORY

- Culture and sensitivity and Gram stain of endocervix or cul-de-sac secretions show the causative agent.
- Urethral and rectal secretions show the causative agent.
- C-reactive protein level is elevated.

IMAGING

- Transvaginal ultrasonography may show the presence of thickened, fluid-filled fallopian tubes.
- Computed tomography scan may show complex tubo-ovarian abscesses and is useful in diagnosing PID.
- Magnetic resonance imaging provides images of soft tissue; useful not only for establishing the diagnosis of PID but also for detecting other processes responsible for symptoms.

DIAGNOSTIC PROCEDURES

- Culdocentesis obtains peritoneal fluid or pus for culture and sensitivity testing.
- Diagnostic laparoscopy identifies cul-de-sac fluid, tubal distention, and masses in pelvic abscess.

TREATMENT

GENERAL
◆ Frequent perineal care if vaginal discharge occurs

ACTIVITY
◆ Bed rest

MEDICATIONS
◆ Antibiotics
◆ Analgesics
◆ I.V. fluids as needed

SURGERY
◆ Drainage of pelvic abscess

WARNING *A ruptured pelvic abscess is a life-threatening condition. The patient may need a total abdominal hysterectomy with bilateral salpingo-oophorectomy.*

NURSING CONSIDERATIONS

NURSING DIAGNOSES
◆ Acute pain
◆ Anxiety
◆ Deficient fluid volume
◆ Ineffective coping
◆ Ineffective sexuality patterns
◆ Risk for infection

EXPECTED OUTCOMES
The patient will:
◆ express feelings of increased comfort
◆ identify strategies to reduce anxiety
◆ maintain fluid balance
◆ demonstrate adaptive coping behaviors
◆ express feelings about potential or actual changes in sexual activity
◆ remain free from signs or symptoms of infection.

NURSING INTERVENTIONS
◆ Give prescribed antibiotics and analgesics.
◆ Provide frequent perineal care.
◆ Use meticulous hand-washing technique.
◆ Encourage the patient to discuss her feelings, and offer emotional support.
◆ Help the patient develop effective coping strategies.
◆ Assess discharge.

MONITORING
◆ Vital signs
◆ Fluid intake and output
◆ Signs and symptoms of dehydration

WARNING *Watch for and report abdominal rigidity and distention. These signs may indicate development of peritonitis.*

PATIENT TEACHING

GENERAL
Be sure to cover:
◆ disorder, diagnosis, and treatment
◆ ways to prevent a recurrence
◆ avoiding multiple sexual partners
◆ need for patient's sexual partner to be examined and treated for infection
◆ condom use
◆ causes of PID
◆ signs and symptoms of infection after a minor gynecologic procedure

WARNING *Tell the patient to immediately report fever, increased vaginal discharge, or pain, especially after a minor gynecologic procedure.*

◆ avoidance of douching or intercourse for at least 7 days after a minor gynecologic procedure.

DISCHARGE PLANNING
◆ Refer patient to infertility counseling if indicated.
◆ Refer the patient to a smoking-cessation program if indicated.

RESOURCES
Organizations
American College of Obstetricians and Gynecologists: *www.acog.org*
American Fertility Association: *www.theafa.org*
American Society for Reproductive Medicine: *www.asrm.org*

Selected references
Banikarim, C., and Chacko, M.R. "Pelvic Inflammatory Disease in Adolescents," *Seminars in Pediatric Infectious Diseases* 16(3):175-80, July 2005.

Dahlberg, D.L., et al. "Differential Diagnosis of Abdominal Pain in Women of Childbearing Age. Appendicitis or Pelvic Inflammatory Disease?" *Advance for Nurse Practitioners* 12(1):40-45, January 2004.

Mahon, B.E., et al. "Pelvic Inflammatory Disease During the Post-partum Year," *Infectious Diseases in Obstetrics and Gynecology* 13(4):191-96, December 2005.

Ness, R.B., et al. "Effectiveness of Treatment Strategies of Some Women with Pelvic Inflammatory Disease: A Randomized Trial," *Obstetrics and Gynecology* 106(3):573-80, September 2005.

Peptic ulcer

- Circumscribed lesion in the mucosal membrane of the lower esophagus, stomach, duodenum, or jejunum
- Occurs in two major forms: duodenal ulcer and gastric ulcer (both forms chronic)
- Duodenal ulcers: represent about 80% of peptic ulcers; affect the proximal part of the small intestine and follow a chronic course characterized by remissions and exacerbations (about 5% to 10% of patients with duodenal ulcers develop complications that necessitate surgery)

PATHOPHYSIOLOGY

- *Helicobacter pylori* releases a toxin that promotes mucosal inflammation and ulceration.
- In a peptic ulcer resulting from *H. pylori,* acid isn't the dominant cause of bacterial infection but contributes to the consequences.
- Ulceration stems from inhibition of prostaglandin synthesis, increased gastric acid and pepsin secretion, reduced gastric mucosal blood flow, or decreased cytoprotective mucus production.

CAUSES

- *H. pylori*
- Nonsteroidal anti-inflammatory drug (NSAID) or glucocorticoid use
- Pathologic hypersecretory states

RISK FACTORS

- Type A blood (for gastric ulcer)
- Type O blood (for duodenal ulcer)
- Other genetic factors
- Exposure to irritants
- Cigarette smoking
- Trauma
- Psychogenic factors
- Normal aging

INCIDENCE

- Gastric ulcers are most common in middle-aged and elderly men, especially those who are poor and undernourished; incidence is higher in chronic users of aspirin or alcohol.
- Duodenal ulcers are most common in men ages 20 to 50.

COMPLICATIONS

- GI hemorrhage
- Abdominal or intestinal infarction
- Ulcer penetration into attached structures

ASSESSMENT

HISTORY

- Periods of symptom exacerbation and remission, with remissions lasting longer than exacerbations
- History of predisposing factor
- Left epigastric pain described as heartburn or indigestion, accompanied by feeling of fullness or distention

Gastric ulcer
- Recent weight or appetite loss
- Nausea or vomiting
- Pain triggered or worsened by eating

Duodenal ulcer
- Pain relieved by eating; may occur 1½ to 3 hours after food intake
- Pain that awakens the patient from sleep
- Weight gain

PHYSICAL FINDINGS

- Pallor
- Epigastric tenderness
- Hyperactive bowel sounds

DIAGNOSTIC TEST RESULTS

LABORATORY

- Complete blood count shows anemia.
- Occult blood is found in stools.
- Venous blood sample shows *H. pylori* antibodies.
- White blood cell count is elevated.
- Urea breath test reveals low levels of exhaled carbon-13.
- Fasting serum gastrin level rules out Zollinger-Ellison syndrome.

IMAGING

- Barium swallow or upper GI and small-bowel series may reveal the ulcer.
- Upper GI tract X-rays reveal mucosal abnormalities.

DIAGNOSTIC PROCEDURES

- Upper GI endoscopy or esophagogastroduodenoscopy confirm the ulcer and permit cytologic studies and biopsy to rule out *H. pylori* or cancer.
- Gastric secretory studies show hyperchlorhydria.

TREATMENT

GENERAL
- Treatment of symptoms
- Iced saline lavage, possibly containing norepinephrine
- Laser or cautery during endoscopy
- Stress reduction
- Smoking cessation

DIET
- Avoidance of dietary irritants
- Nothing by mouth if GI bleeding evident

MEDICATIONS
For H. pylori
- Amoxicillin, clarithromycin (Biaxin), and omeprazole (Prilosec)

For gastric or duodenal ulcer
- Proton pump inhibitors
- Antacids
- Histamine-receptor antagonists or gastric acid pump inhibitors
- Coating agents (for duodenal ulcer)
- Antisecretory agents if ulcer resulted from NSAID use, when NSAIDs must be continued
- Sedatives and tranquilizers (for gastric ulcer)
- Anticholinergics (for duodenal ulcers; usually contraindicated in gastric ulcers)
- Prostaglandin analogs

SURGERY
- Indicated for perforation, lack of response to conservative treatment, suspected cancer, or other complications
- Type varies with ulcer location and extent; major operations: bilateral vagotomy, pyloroplasty, and gastrectomy

NURSING CONSIDERATIONS

NURSING DIAGNOSES
- Acute pain
- Anxiety
- Deficient fluid volume
- Disturbed sleep pattern
- Imbalanced nutrition: Less than body requirements
- Risk for injury

EXPECTED OUTCOMES
The patient will:
- express feelings of increased comfort
- identify strategies to reduce anxiety
- maintain adequate fluid volume
- resume regular sleep patterns
- achieve adequate caloric and nutritional intake
- avoid or minimize complications.

NURSING INTERVENTIONS
- Give prescribed drugs.
- Provide six small meals or small hourly meals, as ordered.
- Offer emotional support.

MONITORING
- Medication effects
- Vital signs
- Signs and symptoms of bleeding
- Pain control

After surgery
- Nasogastric tube function and drainage
- Bowel function
- Fluid and nutritional status
- Wound site
- Signs and symptoms of metabolic alkalosis or perforation

PATIENT TEACHING

GENERAL
Be sure to cover:
- the disorder, diagnosis, and treatment
- drug administration, dosage, and possible adverse effects
- warnings against over-the-counter medications, especially aspirin, aspirin-containing products, and NSAIDs, unless the practitioner approves
- warnings against caffeine and alcohol intake during exacerbations
- appropriate lifestyle changes
- dietary modifications.

DISCHARGE PLANNING
- Refer the patient to a smoking-cessation program if indicated.

RESOURCES
Organizations
Digestive Disease National Coalition: *www.ddnc.org*
National Digestive Diseases Information Clearinghouse: *www.niddk.nih.gov/health/digest/nddic.htm*

Selected references
Gisbert, J.P., et al. "Risk Assessment and Outpatient Management in Bleeding Peptic Ulcer," *Journal of Clinical Gastroenterology* 40(2):129-34, February 2006.
Goldstein, J.L., et al. "Healing of Gastric Ulcers with Esomeprazole versus Ranitidine in Patients who Continued to Receive NSAID Therapy: A Randomized Trial," *American Journal of Gastroenterology* 100(12):2650-57, December 2005.
Handbook of Diseases, 3rd ed. Philadelphia: Lippincott Williams & Wilkins, 2004.
Krumberger, J.M. "How to Manage an Acute Upper GI Bleed," *RN* 68(3):34-39, March 2005.
Tierney, L., et al. *Current Medical Diagnosis & Treatment 2006.* New York: McGraw-Hill Book Co., 2006.
Yuan, Y., et al. "Peptic Ulcer Disease Today," *Nature Clinical Practice – Gastroenterology & Hepatology* 3(2):80-89, February 2006.

Pericarditis

- Inflammation of the pericardium — the fibroserous sac that envelops, supports, and protects the heart
- Occurs in acute and chronic forms
- Acute form: can be fibrinous or effusive; characterized by serous, purulent, or hemorrhagic exudate
- Chronic form: characterized by dense fibrous pericardial thickening
- Chronic form called *constrictive pericarditis*

PATHOPHYSIOLOGY

- Pericardial tissue is damaged by bacteria or another substance that releases chemical mediators of inflammation into surrounding tissue.
- Friction occurs as the inflamed layers rub against each other.
- Chemical mediators dilate blood vessels and increase vessel permeability.
- Vessel walls leak fluids and proteins, causing extracellular edema.

CAUSES

- Aortic aneurysm with pericardial leakage
- Bacterial, fungal, or viral infection (in infectious pericarditis)
- Chest trauma
- Drugs, such as hydralazine or procainamide
- High-dose chest radiation
- Hypersensitivity or autoimmune disease
- Idiopathic factors
- Myocardial infarction (MI)
- Myxedema with cholesterol deposits in pericardium
- Neoplasms (primary or metastatic)
- Radiation
- Rheumatologic conditions
- Tuberculosis
- Uremia

INCIDENCE

- Pericarditis is more common in males than in females.
- The disorder is most common in men ages 20 to 50.

COMPLICATIONS

- Pericardial effusion
- Cardiac tamponade

HISTORY

- Predisposing factor
- Sharp, sudden pain, usually starting over the sternum and radiating to the neck, shoulders, back, and arms
- Pleuritic pain, increasing with deep inspiration and decreasing when the patient sits up and leans forward
- Dyspnea
- Chest pain (may mimic MI pain)

PHYSICAL FINDINGS

- Pericardial friction rub
- Diminished apical impulse
- Fluid retention, ascites, hepatomegaly (resembling those of chronic right-sided heart failure)
- With pericardial effusion: tachycardia
- With cardiac tamponade: pallor, clammy skin, hypotension, pulsus paradoxus, jugular vein distention, and dyspnea

LABORATORY

- White blood cell count is elevated, especially in infectious pericarditis.
- Erythrocyte sedimentation rate is elevated.
- Serum creatine kinase-MB levels is slightly elevated with associated myocarditis.
- Pericardial fluid culture may identify a causative organism in bacterial or fungal pericarditis.
- Blood urea nitrogen level is elevated in uremia.
- Elevated antistreptolysin-O titers; may indicate rheumatic fever.
- Positive reaction in purified protein derivative skin test indicates tuberculosis.

IMAGING

- Echocardiography shows an echo-free space between the ventricular wall and the pericardium, which indicates pericardial effusion.
- High-resolution computed tomography and magnetic resonance imaging reveal pericardial thickness.

DIAGNOSTIC PROCEDURES

- Electrocardiography shows initial ST-segment elevation across the precordium.

TREATMENT

GENERAL
◆ Management of rheumatic fever, uremia, tuberculosis, or other underlying disorder

DIET
◆ Restrictions based on underlying disorder

ACTIVITY
◆ Bed rest as long as fever and pain persist

MEDICATIONS
◆ Nonsteroidal anti-inflammatory drugs
◆ Corticosteroids
◆ Antibiotics

SURGERY
◆ Surgical drainage
◆ Pericardiocentesis
◆ Partial pericardectomy (for recurrent pericarditis)
◆ Total pericardectomy (for constrictive pericarditis)

NURSING CONSIDERATIONS

NURSING DIAGNOSES
◆ Acute pain
◆ Anxiety
◆ Decreased cardiac output
◆ Deficient diversional activity
◆ Impaired gas exchange
◆ Ineffective breathing pattern
◆ Ineffective role performance

EXPECTED OUTCOMES
The patient will:
◆ verbalize feelings of increased comfort and decreased pain
◆ express feelings of decreased anxiety
◆ maintain hemodynamic stability and adequate cardiac output
◆ express interest in using leisure time meaningfully
◆ maintain adequate ventilation and oxygenation
◆ maintain an effective breathing pattern
◆ express feelings about diminished capacity to perform usual roles.

NURSING INTERVENTIONS
◆ Give prescribed analgesics and oxygen.
◆ Give prescribed antibiotics on time.
◆ Stress the importance of bed rest. Provide a bedside commode.
◆ Place the patient upright to relieve dyspnea and chest pain.
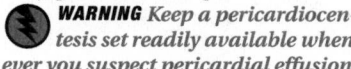 **WARNING** *Keep a pericardiocentesis set readily available whenever you suspect pericardial effusion.*
◆ Encourage the patient to express concerns about the effects of activity restrictions on responsibilities and routines.
◆ Review the patient's allergy history.
◆ Provide appropriate postoperative care.

MONITORING
◆ Vital signs
◆ Heart rhythm
◆ Heart sounds
◆ Hemodynamic values

PATIENT TEACHING

GENERAL
Be sure to cover:
◆ the disorder, diagnosis, and treatment
◆ how to perform deep-breathing and coughing exercises
◆ the need to resume daily activities slowly and to schedule rest periods in daily routine, as instructed by the practitioner.

RESOURCES
Organizations
Mayo Clinic: *www.mayoclinic.org*
National Heart, Lung, and Blood Institute: *www.nhlbi.nih.gov*

Selected references
Demmler, G.J. "Infectious Pericarditis in Children," *Pediatric Infectious Disease Journal* 25(2):165-66, February 2006.

Imazio, M., et al. "Management, Risk Factors, and Outcomes in Recurrent Pericarditis," *American Journal of Cardiology* 96(5):736-69, September 2005.

Kasper, D.L., et al, eds. *Harrison's Principles of Internal Medicine*, 16th ed. New York: McGraw-Hill Book Co., 2005.

Mayosi, B.M., et al. "Tuberculous Pericarditis," *Circulation* 112(23):3608-16, December 2005.

The Merck Manual of Diagnosis & Therapy, 18th ed., Whitehouse Station N.J.: Merck and Co., Inc., 2006.

Rheuban, K.S. "Pericarditis," *Current Treatment Options in Cardiovascular Medicine* 7(5):419-27, October 2005.

Peritonitis

- Inflammation of the peritoneum; may extend throughout the peritoneum or localize as an abscess
- Commonly decreases intestinal motility and causes intestinal distention with gas
- Fatal in 10% of cases, with bowel obstruction the usual cause of death
- Can be acute or chronic

PATHOPHYSIOLOGY

- Bacteria invade the peritoneum after inflammation and perforation of the GI tract.
- Fluid containing protein and electrolytes accumulates in the peritoneal cavity; normally transparent, the peritoneum becomes opaque, red, inflamed, and edematous.
- Infection may localize as an abscess rather than disseminate as a generalized infection.

CAUSES

- Bacterial or chemical inflammation
- GI tract perforation (from appendicitis, diverticulitis, peptic ulcer, or ulcerative colitis)
- Ruptured ectopic pregnancy
- Peritoneal dialysis
- Ascites

INCIDENCE

- Peritonitis is more common in men.

COMPLICATIONS

- Abscess
- Septicemia
- Respiratory compromise
- Bowel obstruction
- Shock

HISTORY
Early phase

- Vague, generalized abdominal pain
- If localized: pain over a specific area (usually the inflammation site)
- If generalized: diffuse pain over the abdomen

With progression

- Increasingly severe and constant abdominal pain that increases with movement and respirations
- Possible referral of pain to shoulder or thoracic area
- Anorexia, nausea, and vomiting
- Inability to pass stools and flatus
- Hiccups

PHYSICAL FINDINGS

- Fever
- Tachycardia
- Hypotension
- Shallow breathing
- Signs of dehydration
- Positive bowel sounds (early); absent bowel sounds (later)
- Abdominal rigidity
- General abdominal tenderness
- Rebound tenderness
- Typical patient positioning: lying very still with knees flexed

LABORATORY

- Complete blood count shows leukocytosis.

IMAGING

- Abdominal X-rays show edematous and gaseous distention of the small and large bowel. With perforation of a visceral organ, X-rays show air in the abdominal cavity.
- Chest X-rays may reveal elevation of the diaphragm.
- Computed tomography reveals fluid and inflammation.

DIAGNOSTIC PROCEDURES

- Paracentesis shows the exudate's nature and permits bacterial culture testing.

GENERAL
- I.V. fluids
- Nasogastric (NG) intubation

DIET
- Nothing by mouth until bowel function returns
- Gradual increase in diet
- Parenteral nutrition if necessary

ACTIVITY
- Bed rest until condition improves
- Semi-Fowler's position
- Avoidance of lifting for at least 6 weeks postoperatively

MEDICATIONS
- Antibiotics, based on infecting organism
- Electrolyte replacement
- Analgesics

SURGERY
- Treatment of choice; procedure varies with the cause of peritonitis

NURSING DIAGNOSES
- Acute pain
- Anxiety
- Deficient fluid volume
- Fear
- Imbalanced nutrition: Less than body requirements
- Ineffective tissue perfusion: GI

EXPECTED OUTCOMES
The patient will:
- express feelings of increased comfort
- identify strategies to reduce anxiety
- maintain normal fluid volume
- discuss fears and concerns
- maintain adequate caloric intake
- exhibit signs of adequate GI perfusion and regain normal bowel function.

NURSING INTERVENTIONS
- Give prescribed drugs.
- Encourage early postoperative ambulation.
- Encourage the patient to express his feelings.
- Provide emotional support.

MONITORING
- Fluid and nutritional status
- Pain control
- Vital signs
- NG tube function and drainage
- Bowel function
- Wound site
- Signs and symptoms of dehiscence

WARNING *Watch for signs and symptoms of abscess formation, including persistent abdominal tenderness and fever.*

GENERAL
Be sure to cover:
- the disorder, diagnosis, and treatment
- preoperatively, coughing and deep-breathing techniques
- postoperative care procedures
- signs and symptoms of infection
- proper wound care
- drug administration, dosage, and possible adverse effects
- dietary and activity limitations (depending on type of surgery).

RESOURCES
Organizations
Digestive Disease National Coalition: *www.ddnc.org*
National Digestive Diseases Information Clearinghouse: *www.niddk.nih.gov/health/digest/nddic.htm*

Selected references
Akman, S., et al. "Value of the Urine Strip Test in the Early Diagnosis of Bacterial Peritonitis," *Pediatrics International* 47(5):523-27, October 2005.

Courtney, A.E., and Doherty, C.C. "Fulminant Sclerosing Peritonitis Immediately Following Acute Bacterial Peritonitis," *Nephrology Dialysis Transplantation* 21(2):532-34, February 2006.

Handbook of Diseases, 3rd ed. Philadelphia: Lippincott Williams & Wilkins, 2004.

McNally, P. *GI/Liver Secrets,* 3rd ed. Philadelphia: Hanley & Belfus, Inc., 2006.

Yamamoto, N., et al. "Gastrointestinal: Sclerosing Encapsulating Peritonitis," *Journal of Gastroenterology & Hepatology* 20(6):952, June 2005.

Pertussis

OVERVIEW

- Highly contagious respiratory infection
- Typically causes an irritating cough that becomes paroxysmal and ends in a high-pitched, inspiratory whoop
- Follows a 6- to 8-week course that includes three 2-week stages with varying symptoms
- Also called *whooping cough*

PATHOPHYSIOLOGY

- The infecting organism adheres to ciliated epithelial cells and multiplies.
- The resulting local mucosal damage induces paroxysmal coughing, which enhances disease transmission.
- Various toxins produced during the infection impair local defenses and cause local tissue damage. Toxins may cause direct central nervous system injury.

CAUSES

- Nonmotile, gram-negative coccobacillus *Bordetella pertussis*; occasionally, *B. parapertussis* or *B. bronchiseptica* (see Bordetella pertussis)
- Spreads indirectly through soiled linen and other articles contaminated by respiratory secretions
- Typically transmitted by direct inhalation of contaminated droplets from someone in the acute disease stage

INCIDENCE

- Fifty percent of cases of pertussis are seen in underimmunized children younger than age 1.
- The disease commonly occurs in schools, nursing homes, and residential facilities.
- Epidemics occur every 3 to 5 years without seasonal variation.

COMPLICATIONS

- Increased venous pressure
- Anterior eye chamber hemorrhage
- Detached retina and blindness
- Rectal prolapse
- Inguinal or umbilical hernia
- Encephalopathy, seizures
- Atelectasis or pneumonitis
- In infants: apnea, anoxia
- Otitis media
- Pneumonia
- Cerebral hemorrhage

ASSESSMENT

HISTORY

- Possible lack of immunization coupled with exposure to pertussis during previous 3 weeks

PHYSICAL FINDINGS

- Low or normal body temperature
- Mild conjunctivitis
- Listlessness
- Engorged neck veins
- Epistaxis during paroxysmal coughing
- Exhaustion and cyanosis after coughing spell
- Diminished breath sounds, upper airway wheezing
- Cough that produces a high-pitched "whooping" sound
- Vomiting from repeated coughing
- Choking spells (in infants)

DIAGNOSTIC TEST RESULTS

LABORATORY

- White blood cell count and differential show lymphocytosis.
- *B. pertussis* is found in nasopharyngeal swabs and sputum culture in early disease stages.
- Direct immunofluorescence shows antigen.

Bordetella pertussis

This microscopic enlargement shows *Bordetella pertussis*, the nonmotile, gram-negative coccobacillus that commonly causes whooping cough. After entering the tracheobronchial tree, pertussis causes mucus to become increasingly tenacious. The classic 6-week course of whooping cough follows.

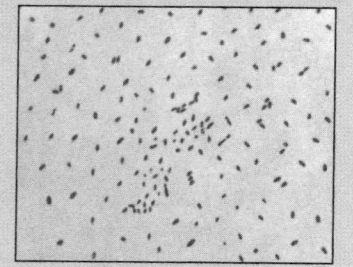

TREATMENT

GENERAL
◆ For infants and elderly patients: hospitalization with vigorous supportive therapy and fluid and electrolyte replacement

DIET
◆ Adequate nutrition with small, frequent meals
◆ Increased fluid intake

ACTIVITY
◆ Rest periods when fatigued

MEDICATIONS
◆ Oxygen
◆ Antibiotics

NURSING CONSIDERATIONS

NURSING DIAGNOSES
◆ Activity intolerance
◆ Acute pain
◆ Anxiety
◆ Deficient fluid volume
◆ Impaired gas exchange
◆ Ineffective airway clearance
◆ Ineffective breathing pattern
◆ Risk for infection
◆ Risk for injury

EXPECTED OUTCOMES
The patient will:
◆ return to a normal activity level as patient recovers
◆ report decreased levels or absence of pain
◆ identify strategies to reduce anxiety
◆ attain and maintain normal fluid and electrolyte balance
◆ maintain adequate ventilation and oxygenation
◆ maintain a patent airway
◆ remain free from adventitious breath sounds
◆ show no evidence of pathogens in cultures
◆ remain free from complications.

NURSING INTERVENTIONS
◆ Maintain respiratory isolation (mask only) for 5 to 7 days after antibiotic therapy begins.
◆ Provide oxygen and moist air as ordered; if needed, assist respiration.
◆ Suction secretions as necessary. Elevate the head of the bed to ease breathing.
◆ Create a quiet environment to decrease coughing stimulation.
◆ Assess for complications caused by excessive coughing.
◆ Provide emotional support to the patient and parents, as appropriate.
◆ Report pertussis cases to local public health authorities.

MONITORING
◆ Respiratory status
◆ Acid-base balance
◆ Fluid and electrolyte balance

PATIENT TEACHING

GENERAL
Be sure to cover:
◆ the disease process and medical procedures
◆ need for the patient's close contacts to get medical care
◆ when to notify the practitioner
◆ importance of immunization and vaccinations and the need to notify the practitioner of adverse reactions to the vaccine.

DISCHARGE PLANNING
◆ Refer the patient to a pulmonologist for follow-up care as indicated.

RESOURCES
Organizations
American Lung Association: *www.lungusa.org*
Centers for Disease Control and Prevention: *www.cdc.gov*
Harvard Medical School's Consumer Health Information: *www.intelihealth.com*
National Health Information Center: *www.health.gov/nhic/*
National Institute of Allergy and Infectious Diseases: *www.niaid.nih.gov*
National Library of Medicine: *www.nlm.nih.gov*

Selected references
Casey, J.R., and Pichichero, M.E. "Acellular Pertussis Vaccine Safety and Efficacy in Children, Adolescents and Adults," *Drugs* 65(10):1367-89, 2005.
Edwards, K., and Freeman, D.M. "Adolescent and Adult Pertussis: Disease Burden and Prevention," *Current Opinion in Pediatrics* 18(1):77-80, February 2006.
Hu, J.J., et al. "Survey of Pertussis in Patients with Prolonged Cough," *Journal of Microbiology, Immunology, and Infection* 39(1):54-58, February 2006.
Kasper, D.L., et al, eds. *Harrison's Principles of Internal Medicine*, 16th ed. New York: McGraw-Hill Book Co., 2005.

Pharyngitis

- Acute or chronic inflammation of the pharynx
- Most common throat disorder
- Usually subsides in 3 to 10 days unless complications occur

PATHOPHYSIOLOGY

- Cellular damage caused by a virus or bacteria causes an inflammatory response.
- Hyperemia and fluid exudation result.

CAUSES

- Beta-hemolytic streptococci (15% to 20% of acute pharyngitis cases)
- Mononucleosis
- Viral, fungal, or bacterial infection

In children

- Streptococcal bacteria infections

Gonococcal pharyngitis

- Release of a toxin produced by *Corynebacterium diphtheriae*

Fungal pharyngitis

- Prolonged antibiotic use (in immunosuppressed patients)

INCIDENCE

- Pharyngitis is widespread among adults who:
- live or work in dusty or dry environments
- use their voices excessively
- use tobacco or alcohol habitually
- suffer from chronic sinusitis, persistent coughs, or allergies.

COMPLICATIONS

- Otitis media
- Sinusitis
- Mastoiditis
- Rheumatic fever
- Nephritis

HISTORY

- Sore throat
- Slight difficulty swallowing (swallowing saliva more painful than swallowing food)
- Sensation of a lump in the throat
- Constant, aggravating urge to swallow
- Headache
- Muscle and joint pain

PHYSICAL FINDINGS

- Mild fever
- Fiery red appearance of the posterior pharyngeal wall
- Swollen, exudate-flecked tonsils
- Lymphoid follicles

Bacterial pharyngitis

- Acutely inflamed throat, with patches of white and yellow follicles
- Strawberry-red tongue
- Enlarged, tender cervical lymph nodes

LABORATORY

- Throat culture identifies the causative organism.
- Rapid strep test shows group A beta-hemolytic streptococcal infection.
- White blood cell count and differential show atypical lymphocytes.

IMAGING

- Computed tomography scans identify abscesses.

TREATMENT

GENERAL
- Warm saline gargles
- Hospitalization for dehydration
- Elimination of the underlying cause
- Adequate humidification

DIET
- Adequate fluid intake
- Avoidance of citrus juices

ACTIVITY
- Bed rest while febrile

MEDICATIONS
- Anesthetic throat lozenges
- Analgesics as needed
- Antibiotics
- Antifungal agents (for fungal pharyngitis)
- Antipyretics
- Equine antitoxins (for diphtherial pharyngitis)

SURGERY
- Abscess drainage

NURSING CONSIDERATIONS

NURSING DIAGNOSES
- Acute pain
- Fatigue
- Imbalanced nutrition: Less than body requirements
- Impaired oral mucous membrane
- Risk for deficient fluid volume

EXPECTED OUTCOMES
The patient will:
- express feelings of increased comfort
- verbalize the importance of adequate rest periods
- achieve adequate daily calorie intake
- maintain intact mucous membranes
- maintain normal fluid volume.

NURSING INTERVENTIONS
- Give prescribed drugs.
- Obtain throat cultures as ordered.
- Instruct the patient to use warm saline gargles.
- Encourage adequate oral fluid intake.
- Perform meticulous mouth care.
- Maintain a restful environment.

MONITORING
- Intake and output
- Signs and symptoms of dehydration

  WARNING *Examine the patient's skin twice per day for rashes caused by drug sensitivity or rashes that could indicate a communicable disease.*

PATIENT TEACHING

GENERAL
Be sure to cover:
- the disorder, diagnosis, and treatment
- importance of completing prescribed antibiotic therapy
- drug administration, dosage, and possible adverse effects
- preventive measures
- avoidance of excessive exposure to air conditioning
- smoking cessation
- ways to minimize environmental sources of throat irritation
- importance of throat cultures for all family members if the patient has a streptococcal infection.

DISCHARGE PLANNING
- Refer the patient to a smoking-cessation program if indicated.

RESOURCES
Organizations
American Academy of Allergy, Asthma and Immunology: *www.aaaai.org*
National Institute of Allergy and Infectious Diseases: *www.niaid.nih.gov*

Selected references
Linder, J.A., et al. "Antibiotic Treatment of Children with Sore Throat," *JAMA* 294(18):2315-22, November 2005.
Moukarel, R.V., et al. "Acute Pharyngitis: An Unusual Presentation of Acute Enemic Typhus," *Otolaryngology – Head and Neck Surgery* 133(4):645, October 2005.
Summers, A. "Sore Throats," *Accident and Emergency Nursing* 13(1):15-17, January 2005.
Woolley, S.L., et al. "Sore Throat in Adults — Does the Introduction of a Clinical Scoring System Improve the Management of these Patients in a Secondary Care Setting?" *Journal of Laryngology and Otology* 119(7):550-55, July 2005.

Pheochromocytoma

OVERVIEW

- Catecholamine-producing tumor, typically benign; usually derived from adrenal medullary cells
- Most common cause of adrenal medullary hypersecretion
- Usually produces norepinephrine; large tumors secrete both epinephrine and norepinephrine
- Potentially fatal, but with treatment carries a good prognosis
- Also known as *chromaffin tumor*

PATHOPHYSIOLOGY

- Pheochromocytoma causes excessive catecholamine production from autonomous tumor functioning.
- The tumor stems from a chromaffin cell tumor of the adrenal medulla or sympathetic ganglia (more commonly in the right adrenal gland than in the left).
- Extra-adrenal pheochromocytomas may occur in the abdomen, thorax, urinary bladder, and neck and in association with the 9th and 10th cranial nerves.

CAUSES

- May be inherited as an autosomal dominant trait

INCIDENCE

- Pheochromocytoma is rare; it's seen in about 0.5% of newly diagnosed hypertensive patients.
- The disease occurs equally among all races.
- It affects both sexes equally.
- Pheochromocytoma is typically familial.
- It occurs most commonly in patients ages 30 to 50.

COMPLICATIONS

- Stroke
- Retinopathy
- Irreversible kidney damage
- Acute pulmonary edema
- Cholelithiasis
- Cardiac arrhythmias
- Heart failure

WARNING *Pheochromocytoma may occur during pregnancy when uterine pressure on the tumor causes more frequent hypertensive crises. These crises carry a high risk for spontaneous abortion and can be fatal for both the mother and fetus.*

ASSESSMENT

HISTORY

- Unpredictable episodes of hypertensive crisis
- Paroxysmal symptoms suggesting a seizure disorder or anxiety attack
- Hypertension that responds poorly to conventional treatment
- Hypotension or shock after surgery or diagnostic procedures

During paroxysms or crises

- Throbbing headache
- Palpitations
- Visual blurring
- Nausea and vomiting
- Severe diaphoresis
- Feelings of impending doom
- Precordial or abdominal pain
- Moderate weight loss
- Dizziness or light-headedness when moving to an upright position

PHYSICAL FINDINGS
During paroxysms or crises

- Hypertension
- Tachypnea
- Pallor or flushing
- Profuse sweating
- Tremor
- Seizures
- Tachycardia

DIAGNOSTIC TEST RESULTS

LABORATORY

- Levels of vanillylmandelic acid and metanephrine are increased in 24-hour urine specimen.
- Total plasma catecholamine levels are 10 to 50 times higher than normal on direct assay.

IMAGING

- Computed tomography (CT) scan or magnetic resonance imaging of adrenal glands may show intra-adrenal lesions.
- CT scan, chest X-rays, or abdominal aortography may reveal extra-adrenal pheochromocytoma.
- Iodine-131–meta-iodobenzyl-guanidine scan locates or confirms pheochromocytoma.

GENERAL
◆ Measures to control blood pressure

DIET
◆ High-protein with adequate calories

ACTIVITY
◆ Rest during acute attacks

MEDICATIONS
◆ Alpha-adrenergic blockers
◆ Catecholamine-synthesis antagonists
◆ Beta-adrenergic blockers
◆ Calcium channel blockers
◆ I.V. phentolamine or nitroprusside during paroxysms or crises

⚡ **WARNING** *Because severe and occasionally fatal paroxysms have been induced by opiates, histamine, and other drugs, all medications should be considered carefully and administered cautiously in patients with known or suspected pheochromocytoma.*

SURGERY
◆ Removal of pheochromocytoma

NURSING CONSIDERATIONS

NURSING DIAGNOSES
◆ Acute pain
◆ Anxiety
◆ Fear
◆ Imbalanced nutrition: Less than body requirements
◆ Ineffective coping
◆ Ineffective tissue perfusion: Cardiopulmonary, renal
◆ Risk for infection

EXPECTED OUTCOMES
The patient will:
◆ express feelings of increased comfort
◆ identify strategies to reduce anxiety
◆ discuss fears and concerns
◆ identify appropriate food choices according to a prescribed diet
◆ demonstrate adaptive coping behaviors

◆ exhibit signs of adequate cardiopulmonary and renal perfusion
◆ remain free from signs and symptoms of infection.

NURSING INTERVENTIONS
◆ Take orthostatic blood pressures.
◆ Give prescribed drugs.
◆ Ensure the reliability of urine catecholamine measurements.
◆ Watch for signs of hypertensive crisis.
◆ Prepare the patient and family for surgery.
◆ Provide comfort measures.
◆ Consult a dietitian as needed.
◆ Tell the patient to report symptoms of an acute attack.
◆ Encourage the patient to express his feelings.
◆ Help the patient develop effective coping strategies.

⚡ **WARNING** *Be aware that postoperative hypertension is common because the stress of surgery and adrenal gland manipulation stimulate catecholamine secretion.*

MONITORING
◆ Vital signs, especially blood pressure
◆ Serum glucose level
◆ Daily weight
◆ Neurologic status
◆ Renal function
◆ Cardiovascular status
◆ Adverse reactions to medications

After adrenalectomy
◆ Vital signs
◆ Bowel sounds
◆ Wound dressings
◆ Incision
◆ Signs and symptoms of hemorrhage
◆ Pain

PATIENT TEACHING

GENERAL
Be sure to cover:
◆ the disorder, diagnosis, and treatment
◆ drug administration, dosage, and possible adverse effects
◆ when to notify the practitioner
◆ ways to prevent paroxysmal attacks
◆ signs and symptoms of adrenal insufficiency
◆ importance of wearing medical identification jewelry
◆ how to monitor his own blood pressure.

DISCHARGE PLANNING
◆ Refer family members for genetic counseling if autosomal dominant transmission of pheochromocytoma is suspected.

RESOURCES
Organizations
American Association of Clinical Endocrinologists: *www.aace.com*
American Society of Human Genetics: *www.faseb.org/genetics*
Endocrine Society: *www.endo-society.org*
Pheochromocytoma Support and Awareness Group: *www.ndrf.org/pheochro.htm*

Selected references
Dahia, P.L. "Evolving Concepts in Pheochromocytoma and Paraganglioma," *Current Opinion in Oncology* 18(1):1-8, January 2006.
Guller, U., et al. "Detecting Pheochromocytoma: Defining the Most Sensitive Test," *Annals of Surgery* 243(1):102-07, January 2006.
Ilias, I., and Pacak, K. "Diagnosis and Management of Tumors of the Adrenal Medulla," *Hormone and Metabolic Research* 37(12):717-21, December 2005.
Nettina, S.M. *Lippincott Manual of Nursing Practice,* 8th ed. Philadelphia: Lippincott Williams & Wilkins, 2006.
Sullivan, J., et al. "Presenting Signs and Symptoms of Pheochromocytoma in Pediatric-aged Patients," *Clinical Pediatrics* 44(8):715-19, October 2005.

Pituitary tumors

OVERVIEW

- Nonmalignant intracranial tumor; accounts for 10% of all intracranial neoplasms
- Most common tumor tissue types: chromophobe adenoma (90%), basophil adenoma, and eosinophil adenoma
- Most common site: anterior pituitary (adenohypophysis)
- Considered a neoplastic condition because of the tumor's invasive growth
- Carries a fair to good prognosis, depending on how far the tumor spreads beyond the sella turcica

PATHOPHYSIOLOGY

- As a pituitary adenoma grows, it replaces normal glandular tissue and enlarges the sella turcica (which houses it).
- Chromophobe adenoma may be associated with production of corticotropin, melanocyte-stimulating hormone, growth hormone, and prolactin.
- Basophil adenoma may be associated with excess corticotropin production and, consequently, Cushing's syndrome.
- Eosinophil adenoma may be associated with excessive growth hormone.

CAUSES

- Unknown

RISK FACTORS

- Autosomal dominant trait

INCIDENCE

- Pituitary tumor affects adults of both sexes between ages 30 and 50.
- It's twice as common in females as in males.

COMPLICATIONS

- Endocrine abnormalities throughout the body, unless lost hormones are replaced
- Diabetes insipidus from tumor compression of the hypothalamus

ASSESSMENT

HISTORY

- Neurologic and endocrine abnormalities
- Personality changes or dementia
- Amenorrhea
- Decreased libido
- Impotence
- Lethargy, weakness, increased fatigability
- Sensitivity to cold
- Constipation
- Seizures
- With cranial nerve involvement: diplopia and dizziness

PHYSICAL FINDINGS

- Rhinorrhea
- Head tilting during physical examination
- Skin changes
- Strabismus

DIAGNOSTIC TEST RESULTS

LABORATORY

- Protein level in cerebrospinal fluid (CSF) is increased.

IMAGING

- Skull X-rays with tomography may show an enlarged sella turcica or erosion of its floor; if growth hormone secretion predominates, X-rays show enlargement of the paranasal sinuses and mandible, thickened cranial bones, and separated teeth.
- Carotid angiography may identify displacement of the anterior cerebral and internal carotid arteries from tumor enlargement and may rule out intracerebral aneurysm.
- Computed tomography scan may confirm an adenoma and accurately depict its size.
- Magnetic resonance imaging scan differentiates healthy, benign, and malignant tissues and blood vessels.

TREATMENT

GENERAL
◆ Radiation therapy used for small, nonsecretory tumors confined to the sella turcica or for patients considered poor surgical risks

DIET
◆ Individualized according to tumor manifestations; possible sodium or caloric restriction

ACTIVITY
◆ In initial postoperative period, avoidance of coughing, sneezing, bending, and other movements that may increase intracranial pressure (ICP) or cause CSF leakage

MEDICATIONS
◆ Corticosteroids or thyroid or sex hormones
◆ Electrolyte replacement
◆ Insulin
◆ Bromocriptine (a dopamine agent)

SURGERY
◆ Transfrontal removal of a large tumor impinging on the optic apparatus
◆ Transsphenoidal resection for a smaller tumor confined to the pituitary fossa
◆ Cryohypophysectomy

NURSING CONSIDERATIONS

NURSING DIAGNOSES
◆ Acute pain
◆ Constipation
◆ Disturbed sensory perception (visual)
◆ Fatigue
◆ Ineffective coping
◆ Risk for injury
◆ Sexual dysfunction

EXPECTED OUTCOMES
The patient will:
◆ express feelings of comfort and decreased pain
◆ report a normal elimination pattern
◆ maintain optimal functioning within the limits of the visual impairment
◆ exhibit increased energy
◆ demonstrate adaptive coping behaviors
◆ remain free from injury
◆ maintain a positive attitude toward his sexuality and sexual performance.

NURSING INTERVENTIONS
◆ Give prescribed drugs.
◆ Maintain patient safety.
◆ Provide rest periods to avoid fatigue.
◆ Establish a supportive, trusting relationship with the patient.

MONITORING
After supratentorial or transsphenoidal hypophysectomy
◆ Proper positioning (head of the bed elevated 30 degrees)
◆ Intake and output
◆ Signs and symptoms of infection
◆ Blood glucose level

After craniotomy
◆ Vital signs
◆ Neurologic status
◆ Signs and symptoms of increased ICP

PATIENT TEACHING

GENERAL
Be sure to cover:
◆ the disorder, diagnosis, and treatment
◆ preoperative instructions on surgery, treatments, and postoperative course
◆ avoidance of coughing, sneezing, and bending
◆ importance of immediately reporting persistent postnasal drip or constant swallowing.

DISCHARGE PLANNING
◆ Encourage the patient to wear medical identification that indicates his medical condition and its proper treatment.

RESOURCES
Organizations
American Brain Tumor Association: *www.abta.org*
American Cancer Society: *www.cancer.org*
Guide to Internet Resources for Cancer: *www.cancerindex.org*
National Cancer Institute: *www.cancer.gov*
Pituitary Network Association: *www.pituitary.org*

Selected references
Akabane, A., et al. "Gamma Knife Radiosurgery for Pituitary Adenomas," *Endocrine* 28(1):87-92, October 2005.
Atlas of Pathophysiology, 2nd ed. Philadelphia: Lippincott Williams & Wilkins, 2005.
Barahona, M.J., et al. "Determinants of Neurosurgical Outcome in Pituitary Tumors," *Journal of Endocrinological Investigation* 28(9):787-94, October 2005.
Kontogeorgos, G. "Classification and Pathology of Pituitary Tumors," *Endocrine* 28(1):27-35, October 2005.
Seilicovich, A., et al. "Gene Therapy for Pituitary Tumors," *Current Gene Therapy* 5(6):559-72, December 2005.

Placenta previa

- Placental implantation in the lower uterine segment, encroaching on the internal cervical os
- Common cause of bleeding during the second half of pregnancy (Among patients who develop placenta previa during the second trimester, less than 15% have persistent previa at term.)
- Carries good maternal prognosis if hemorrhage can be controlled
- Usually necessitates pregnancy termination if bleeding is heavy
- Fetal prognosis dependent on gestational age and amount of blood lost; risk of death greatly reduced by frequent monitoring and prompt management

PATHOPHYSIOLOGY
- The placenta covers all or part of the internal cervical os. (See *Three types of placenta previa*.)

CAUSES
- Unknown
- Factors that may affect the site of placental attachment to the uterine wall:
- Advanced maternal age
- Defective vascularization of the decidua
- Endometriosis
- Multiparity
- Multiple pregnancy
- Previous uterine surgery
- Smoking

INCIDENCE
- Placenta previa occurs in about 1 of 200 pregnancies.
- The disorder is more common in multigravidas than in primigravidas.
- It's more common after age 35.

COMPLICATIONS
- Anemia
- Hemorrhage
- Disseminated intravascular coagulation
- Shock
- Renal damage
- Cerebral ischemia
- Maternal or fetal death

ASSESSMENT

HISTORY
- Onset of painless, bright red, vaginal bleeding after 20th week of pregnancy
- Vaginal bleeding before labor onset, typically episodic and stopping spontaneously
- May not produce symptoms

PHYSICAL FINDINGS
- Soft, nontender uterus
- Fetal malpresentation
- Minimal descent of fetal presenting part
- Good fetal heart tones

DIAGNOSTIC TEST RESULTS

LABORATORY
- Maternal hemoglobin level is decreased.

IMAGING
- Transvaginal ultrasound scanning determines placental position.

DIAGNOSTIC PROCEDURES
- Pelvic examination confirms diagnosis.

  WARNING *Pelvic examination isn't commonly performed because it increases maternal bleeding and can dislodge more of the placenta.*

Three types of placenta previa

The degree of placenta previa depends largely on the extent of cervical dilation at the time of examination because the dilating cervix gradually uncovers the placenta, as shown below.

MARGINAL PLACENTA PREVIA

If the placenta covers just a fraction of the internal cervical os, the patient has marginal, or low-lying, placenta previa.

PARTIAL PLACENTA PREVIA

The patient has the partial, or incomplete, form of the disorder if the placenta caps a larger part of the internal os.

TOTAL PLACENTA PREVIA

If the placenta covers all of the internal os, the patient has total, complete, or central placenta previa.

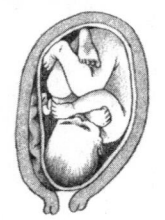
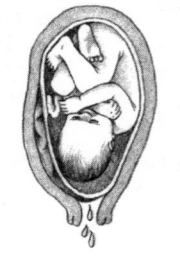
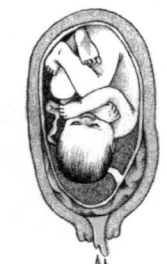

TREATMENT

GENERAL
- Control of blood loss, blood replacement
- Delivery of viable neonate
- Prevention of coagulation disorders
- With premature fetus, careful observation to give fetus more time to mature
- With complete placenta previa, hospitalization
- Possible vaginal delivery if bleeding is minimal and placenta previa is marginal or when labor is rapid

⚡ **WARNING** *Because of possible fetal blood loss through the placenta, a pediatric team should be on hand during delivery to immediately assess and treat neonatal shock, blood loss, and hypoxia.*

DIET
- Nothing by mouth initially, then as guided by clinical status

ACTIVITY
- Bed rest

MEDICATIONS
- I.V. fluids, using large-bore catheter

SURGERY
- Immediate cesarean delivery in case of severe hemorrhage or as soon as fetus is sufficiently mature

NURSING CONSIDERATIONS

NURSING DIAGNOSES
- Acute pain
- Anxiety
- Deficient fluid volume
- Dysfunctional grieving
- Fear
- Ineffective coping
- Risk for injury

EXPECTED OUTCOMES
The patient will:
- express feelings of increased comfort
- express feelings of decreased anxiety
- maintain normal fluid volume
- express feelings about the current condition
- discuss fears and concerns
- use available support systems, such as family and friends, to aid coping
- avoid complications.

NURSING INTERVENTIONS
- Obtain blood samples for complete blood count and blood type and crossmatch.
- Initiate external electronic fetal monitoring.
- Give prescribed I.V. fluids and blood products.
- If the patient is Rh-negative, give $Rh_o(D)$ immune globulin (RhoGAM) after every bleeding episode, as ordered.
- Offer emotional support during labor.
- Provide information about labor progress and the condition of the fetus.
- Encourage the patient to express her feelings.
- Help the patient develop effective coping strategies.

MONITORING
- Vital signs
- Vaginal bleeding, including character of blood loss
- Central venous pressure
- Intake and output
- Fetal heart tones
- Signs and symptoms of hemorrhage and shock

PATIENT TEACHING

GENERAL
Be sure to cover:
- the disorder, diagnosis, and treatment
- signs and symptoms of placenta previa
- possibility of emergency cesarean delivery
- possibility of the birth of a premature neonate
- possibility of neonatal death
- postpartum physical and emotional changes to expect.

DISCHARGE PLANNING
- Refer the patient for professional counseling if necessary.

RESOURCES
Organizations
American College of Obstetricians and Gynecologists: *www.acog.org*
American Society for Reproductive Medicine: *www.asrm.org*

Selected references
Luo, G., et al. "Failure of Conservative Management of Placenta Previa-Percreta," *Journal of Perinatal Medicine* 33(6):564-68, 2005.
MacMullen, N.J., et al. "Red Alert: Perinatal Hemorrhage," *American Journal of Maternal Child Nursing* 30(1):46-51, January-February 2005.
Wu, S., et al. "Abnormal Placentation: Twenty-Year Analysis," *American Journal of Obstetrics and Gynecology* 192(5):1458-61, May 2005.
Zlatnik, M., et al. "Placenta Previa & the Attributable Risk of Preterm Delivery," *American Journal of Obstetrics & Gynecology* 193 Supplement 6:S122, February 2006.

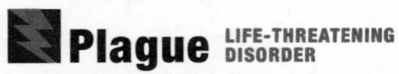

Plague   LIFE-THREATENING DISORDER

OVERVIEW

- Acute, febrile, zoonotic infection caused by the gram-negative, non-sporulating bacillus *Yersinia pestis*
- Usually transmitted to humans through the bite of a flea from an infected rodent host, such as a rat or squirrel; occasional transmission from handling infected animals or their tissues (see *Bubonic plague carrier*)
- Potential bioterrorism and biological warfare agent

FORMS OF PLAGUE

- Bubonic: most common form; causes swollen and sometimes suppurating, lymph glands (buboes)
- Septicemic: rapid, severe systemic form
- Pneumonic: can be primary or secondary to the other two forms; highly contagious, with secondary spread a serious concern (Primary pneumonic plague is an acutely fulminant form causing acute prostration, respiratory distress, and death, possibly within 2 to 3 days after onset. Secondary pneumonic plague is transmitted by contaminated respiratory droplets.)
- Without treatment, 60% mortality in bubonic plague and nearly 100% in septicemic and pneumonic plague; with treatment, 18% mortality

Bubonic plague carrier

Bubonic plague is usually transmitted to humans through the bite of an infected flea (*Xenopsylla cheopis*), shown here.

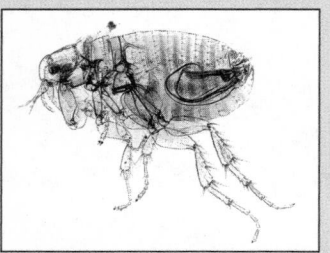

PATHOPHYSIOLOGY

- *Y. pestis* is one of the most invasive bacterium known; mechanisms by which it causes disease aren't fully understood.
- Once inoculated through the skin or mucous membranes, *Y. pestis* usually invades cutaneous lymphatic vessels and regional lymph nodes; direct bloodstream inoculation may also occur.
- Organisms probably are phagocytized by mononuclear phagocytes without being destroyed and are then disseminated to distant sites in the body.
- Plague can involve almost any organ and usually results in massive and widespread tissue destruction, especially if left untreated.

CAUSES

- *Y. pestis* infection

INCIDENCE

- Plague is becoming more prevalent in the United States.
- Plague occurs most commonly between May and September; in hunters who skin wild animals, between October and February.
- It affects both sexes equally.

COMPLICATIONS

- Peritoneal or pleural effusions
- Septicemia
- Fulminant pneumonia
- Pericarditis
- Seizures
- Diffuse interstitial myocarditis
- Multifocal hepatic necrosis
- Diffuse hemorrhagic splenic necrosis
- Respiratory failure
- Cardiovascular collapse
- Disseminated intravascular coagulation
- Meningitis
- Death

ASSESSMENT

HISTORY
Bubonic plague
- Characteristic buboes

- History of exposure to rodents

Milder form of bubonic plague
- History of exposure to rodents
- Malaise
- Fever
- Excruciatingly painful buboes

Severe form of bubonic plague
- Sudden fever of 103° to 106° F (39.4° to 41.1° C)
- Chills, myalgia, and headache
- Restlessness, disorientation
- Abdominal pain, nausea, and vomiting
- Constipation followed by bloody diarrhea

PHYSICAL FINDINGS
Bubonic plague
- Fever
- Prostration
- Restlessness, disorientation, delirium
- Toxemia
- Staggering gait
- Skin mottling, petechiae
- Circulatory collapse
- Coma

Milder form of bubonic plague
- Fever
- Pain or tenderness in regional lymph nodes
- Painful, inflamed, and possibly suppurative buboes (usually in the axillary, cervical, or inguinal areas)
- Necrotization of hemorrhagic areas
- Moribund state within hours after onset

DIAGNOSTIC TEST RESULTS

LABORATORY
- *Y. pestis* is found in capsular antigen testing, Wayson stain, or fluorescent antibody stain.
- White blood cell count is above 20,000/µl, with increased polymorphonuclear leukocytes and hemoagglutination reaction.
- *Y. pestis* is present in culture and Gram stain of skin-lesion needle aspirate or lymph node aspirate, blood, or sputum.

IMAGING

◆ Chest X-rays show fulminating pneumonia in pneumonic plague.

TREATMENT

GENERAL

◆ Supportive management to control fever, shock, and seizures and maintain fluid balance
◆ Warm, moist compresses on buboes

DIET

◆ As tolerated
◆ Tube feedings or total parenteral nutrition, if required
◆ Supplemental I.V. fluids

ACTIVITY

◆ Bed rest during the acute phase

MEDICATIONS

◆ Antibiotics
◆ Oxygen
◆ Corticosteroids
◆ Benzodiazepines
◆ Anticonvulsants
◆ Antipyretics

SURGERY

◆ Incision and drainage of necrotic buboes

NURSING CONSIDERATIONS

NURSING DIAGNOSES

◆ Acute pain
◆ Anxiety
◆ Decreased cardiac output
◆ Fatigue
◆ Fear
◆ Hyperthermia
◆ Imbalanced nutrition: Less than body requirements
◆ Impaired gas exchange
◆ Impaired skin integrity
◆ Ineffective coping
◆ Ineffective tissue perfusion: Cerebral, cardiopulmonary, peripheral
◆ Risk for imbalanced fluid volume
◆ Risk for infection
◆ Risk for injury

EXPECTED OUTCOMES

The patient will:
◆ express feelings of comfort and decreased pain
◆ use support systems to assist with anxiety and fear
◆ maintain adequate cardiac output and hemodynamic stability
◆ verbalize the importance of balancing activity, as tolerated, with rest
◆ verbalize feelings of fear and anxiety
◆ maintain temperature within normal limits
◆ achieve adequate nutritional intake
◆ maintain adequate ventilation and oxygenation
◆ maintain skin integrity
◆ demonstrate effective coping mechanisms
◆ maintain acceptable tissue perfusion and cellular oxygenation
◆ maintain fluid balance
◆ experience no further signs or symptoms of infection
◆ avoid complications.

NURSING INTERVENTIONS

◆ Give drugs and I.V. fluids, as prescribed.
◆ If pneumonic plague, use standard and droplet precautions.
◆ Provide adequate nutrition.
◆ Maintain a patent airway and adequate oxygenation.
◆ Apply warm, moist compresses to buboes.
◆ Provide meticulous skin care.
◆ Prevent further injury to necrotic tissue areas.
◆ Institute seizure precautions.
◆ Report suspected plague cases to local public health department.

MONITORING

◆ Vital signs
◆ Intake and output
◆ Skin integrity
◆ Pulmonary status
◆ Cardiovascular status
◆ Nutritional status
◆ Seizures
◆ Complications
◆ Abnormal bleeding
◆ Mentation

PATIENT TEACHING

GENERAL

Be sure to cover:
◆ the disorder, diagnosis, and treatment
◆ drug administration, dosage, and possible adverse effects
◆ isolation procedures
◆ personal protective measures
◆ avoidance of contact with sick or dead wild animals and the need to wear gloves when handling animal carcasses
◆ importance of insect and rodent population control
◆ use of repellents, insecticides, and protective clothing when at risk for exposure to rodents' fleas
◆ elimination of rodent food and habitats
◆ insecticide control of fleas.

RESOURCES

Organizations

Centers for Disease Control and Prevention: *www.cdc.gov*
National Center for Infectious Diseases: *www.cdc.gov/ncidod*

Selected references

Dennis, D.T., and Chow, C.C. "Plague," *Pediatric Infectious Disease Journal* 23(1):69-71, January 2004.
Drumm, C., et al. "Plague Comes to New York: Visitors from New Mexico Test a Big-City Hospital's Emergency Preparedness," *AJN* 104(8):61-64, August 2004.
Khasnis, A.A., and Nettleman, M.D. "Global Warming and Infectious Disease," *Archives of Medical Research* 36(6):689-96, November-December 2005.
Mwengee, W., et al. "Treatment of Plague with Gentamicin or Doxycycline in a Randomized Clinical Trial in Tanzania," *Clinical Infectious Diseases* 42(5):614-21, March 2006.
Snow, M. "Preparing for a Plague Outbreak," *Nursing* 35(12):14, December 2005.

Pleural effusion and empyema

- Fluid accumulation in the pleural space; the fluid may be extracellular, pus (empyema), blood (hemothorax), chyle (chylothorax), or bilious
- Effusion classified as transudative or exudative

PATHOPHYSIOLOGY
- Typically, fluid and other blood components migrate through the walls of intact capillaries bordering the pleura.
- In transudative effusion, fluid is watery and diffuses out of the capillaries if hydrostatic pressure increases or capillary oncotic pressure decreases.
- In exudative effusion, inflammatory processes increase capillary permeability. Exudative effusion is less watery and contains high concentrations of white blood cells (WBCs) and plasma proteins.
- Empyema occurs when pulmonary lymphatics become blocked, leading to outpouring of contaminated lymphatic fluid into the pleural space.

CAUSES
Empyema
- Infected wound
- Intra-abdominal infection
- Lung abscess
- Pulmonary infection
- Thoracic surgery

Exudative pleural effusion
- Pleural infection
- Pleural inflammation
- Pleural malignancy

Transudative pleural effusion
- Cardiovascular disease
- Hepatic disease
- Hypoproteinemia
- Renal disease

INCIDENCE
- The disorder can occur at any age.
- It affects both sexes equally.

COMPLICATIONS
- Atelectasis
- Infection
- Hypoxemia
- Pneumothorax

HISTORY
- Underlying pulmonary disease
- Shortness of breath
- Chest pain
- Malaise

PHYSICAL FINDINGS
- Fever
- Trachea deviated away from the affected side
- Dullness and decreased tactile fremitus over the effusion
- Diminished or absent breath sounds
- Pleural friction rub
- Bronchial breath sounds
- In empyema, foul-smelling sputum

LABORATORY
- Pleural fluid analysis findings:
- In transudative effusion: specific gravity is below 1.015; less than 3 g/dl of protein is present.
- In exudative effusion: ratio of protein in pleural fluid to protein in serum is 0.5 or higher; lactate dehydrogenase (LD) level is 200 IU or higher; ratio of LD in pleural fluid to LD in serum is 0.6 or higher.
- In empyema: microorganisms are present, WBC count is increased, and glucose level is decreased.
- In esophageal rupture or pancreatitis: pleural fluid amylase levels exceed serum amylase levels.

IMAGING
- Chest X-rays may show pleural effusions; lateral decubitus films may show loculated pleural effusions or small pleural effusions not visible on standard chest X-rays.
- Computed tomography scan of the thorax shows pleural effusions.

DIAGNOSTIC PROCEDURES
- Thoracentesis obtains pleural fluid specimens for analysis.

OTHER
- Tuberculin skin test may be positive for tuberculosis.
- Pleural biopsy may be positive for carcinoma.

TREATMENT

GENERAL
◆ Thoracentesis to remove fluid
◆ Possible chest tube insertion
◆ Possible chemical pleurodesis (usually for recurrent pleural effusions)

DIET
◆ High-calorie

ACTIVITY
◆ As tolerated

MEDICATIONS
◆ Antibiotics
◆ Oxygen

SURGERY
◆ Removal of thick coating over lung (decortication)

NURSING CONSIDERATIONS

NURSING DIAGNOSES
◆ Acute pain
◆ Anxiety
◆ Fatigue
◆ Impaired gas exchange
◆ Ineffective airway clearance
◆ Ineffective breathing pattern
◆ Ineffective coping
◆ Risk for infection

EXPECTED OUTCOMES
The patient will:
◆ report feelings of comfort and reduced pain
◆ report reduced levels of anxiety
◆ verbalize the importance of balancing activity with adequate rest periods
◆ maintain adequate ventilation and oxygenation
◆ maintain a patent airway
◆ maintain an effective breathing pattern
◆ use support systems and develop adequate coping mechanisms
◆ remain free from signs and symptoms of infection.

NURSING INTERVENTIONS
◆ Give prescribed drugs and oxygen.
◆ Assist during thoracentesis.
◆ Encourage the patient to use incentive spirometry.
◆ Encourage deep-breathing exercises.
◆ Provide meticulous chest tube care.
◆ Ensure chest tube patency.
◆ Keep petroleum gauze at the bedside.

MONITORING
◆ Vital signs
◆ Intake and output
◆ Respiratory status
◆ Pulse oximetry
◆ Signs and symptoms of pneumothorax
◆ Chest tube drainage

PATIENT TEACHING

GENERAL
Be sure to cover:
◆ the disorder, diagnosis, and treatment
◆ drug administration, dosage, and possible adverse effects
◆ how thoracentesis is performed
◆ chest tube insertion and drainage
◆ signs and symptoms of infection
◆ signs and symptoms of pleural fluid reaccumulation
◆ when to notify the practitioner.

DISCHARGE PLANNING
◆ Provide a home health referral for follow-up care.
◆ Refer the patient to a smoking-cessation program if indicated.

RESOURCES
Organizations
American Association for Respiratory Care: *www.aarc.org*
American Thoracic Society: *www.thoracic.org*

Selected references
Guyton, A.C., and Hall, J.E. *Textbook of Medical Physiology,* 11th ed. Philadelphia: W.B. Saunders Co., 2006.
Kunyoshi, V., et al. "Complicated Pneumonias with Empyema and/or Pneumatocele in Children," *Pediatric Surgery International* 22(2):186-90, February 2006.
Ruiz, E., et al. "Angiogenic Factors and Angiogenesis Inhibitors in Exudative Pleural Effusions," *Lung* 183(3):185-95, May-June 2005.
Schiza, S.E., et al. "Pharmacotherapy in Complicated Parapneumonic Pleural Effusions and Thoracic Empyema," *Pulmonary Pharmacology & Therapeutics* 18(6):381-89, 2005.
Soriano, T., et al. "Factors Influencing Length of Hospital Stay in Patients with Bacterial Pleural Effusion," *Respiration* 72(6):587-93, November-December 2005.

Pleurisy

OVERVIEW

- Inflammation of the visceral and parietal pleurae that line the inside of the thoracic cage and envelop the lungs
- Also called *pleuritis*

PATHOPHYSIOLOGY

- The pleurae become swollen and congested.
- As a result, pleural fluid transport is hampered, and friction between the pleural surfaces increases.

CAUSES

- Cancer
- Certain drugs, such as methotrexate or penicillin
- Chest trauma
- Dressler's syndrome
- Heart failure
- Human immunodeficiency virus
- Kidney disease
- Pathologic rib fractures
- Pneumonia
- Pneumothorax
- Pulmonary embolism
- Radiation therapy
- Rheumatoid arthritis
- Sickle cell disease
- Systemic lupus erythematosus
- Tuberculosis
- Viruses

INCIDENCE

- The disorder affects both sexes equally.

COMPLICATIONS

- Adhesions
- Pleural effusion
- Chronic pain or shortness of breath

ASSESSMENT

HISTORY

- Sudden dull, aching, burning, or sharp pain that worsens on inspiration
- Predisposing factor
- Cough
- Shortness of breath
- Fever

PHYSICAL FINDINGS

- Characteristic late-inspiration and early-expiration pleural friction rub
- Coarse vibration on palpation of the affected area

DIAGNOSTIC TEST RESULTS

IMAGING

- Chest X-rays show absence of pneumonia.

DIAGNOSTIC PROCEDURES

- Electrocardiography shows absence of ischemic heart disease.

TREATMENT

GENERAL
◆ Treatment of symptoms
◆ Possible intercostal nerve block

DIET
◆ As tolerated

ACTIVITY
◆ Bed rest

MEDICATIONS
◆ Anti-inflammatory agents
◆ Analgesics
◆ Antibiotics, if caused by infection

SURGERY
◆ Thoracentesis

NURSING CONSIDERATIONS

NURSING DIAGNOSES
◆ Activity intolerance
◆ Acute pain
◆ Anxiety
◆ Impaired gas exchange
◆ Ineffective airway clearance
◆ Ineffective breathing pattern
◆ Ineffective coping

EXPECTED OUTCOMES
The patient will:
◆ demonstrate energy conservation techniques
◆ express feelings of increased comfort and relief of pain
◆ verbalize strategies to reduce anxiety
◆ maintain adequate ventilation and oxygenation
◆ maintain a patent airway
◆ maintain respiratory rate within five breaths of baseline
◆ use support systems to assist with coping.

NURSING INTERVENTIONS
◆ Give prescribed drugs.
◆ Encourage deep breathing and coughing.
◆ Encourage the patient to use incentive spirometry.
◆ Assist the patient in splinting the affected side.
◆ Position the patient in high Fowler's position.
◆ Plan care to allow frequent rest periods.
◆ Assist with passive range-of-motion (ROM) exercises.
◆ Encourage active ROM exercises.
◆ Provide comfort measures.
◆ Assist with thoracentesis.
◆ Encourage verbalization and provide emotional support.

MONITORING
◆ Vital signs
◆ Intake and output
◆ Response to treatment
◆ Pain control
◆ Complications
◆ Breath sounds
◆ Respiratory status

PATIENT TEACHING

GENERAL
Be sure to cover:
◆ the disorder, diagnosis, and treatment
◆ drug administration, dosage, and possible adverse effects
◆ how to perform splinting and deep-breathing exercises
◆ importance of regular rest periods
◆ signs and symptoms of possible complications
◆ when to notify the practitioner.

RESOURCES
Organizations
American Association for Respiratory Care: *www.aarc.org*
National Heart, Lung, and Blood Institute: *www.nhlbi.nih.gov*

Selected references
Diseases, 4th ed. Philadelphia: Lippincott Williams & Wilkins, 2006.
Gorg, C., et al. "Contrast-enhanced Sonography for Differential Diagnosis of Pleurisy and Focal Pleural Lesions of Unknown Cause," *Chest* 128(6):3894-99, December 2005.
Guyton, A.C., and Hall, J.E. *Textbook of Medical Physiology,* 11th ed. Philadelphia: W.B. Saunders Co., 2006.
Yoshida, H., et al. "Imidapril-induced Eosinophilic Pleurisy. Case Report and Review of the Literature," *Respiration* 72(4):423-26, July-August 2005.

Pneumocystis carinii pneumonia LIFE-THREATENING DISORDER

OVERVIEW

- Communicable, opportunistic lung infection commonly associated with human immunodeficiency virus (HIV)
- A leading cause of opportunistic infection and death among patients with acquired immunodeficiency syndrome (AIDS) in industrialized countries
- Also known as *PCP*

PATHOPHYSIOLOGY

- The infecting organism invades the lungs bilaterally, multiplies extracellularly, and fills alveoli with organisms and exudate.
- As a result, gas exchange is impaired.
- Alveoli hypertrophy and thicken, eventually leading to extensive consolidation.

RISK FACTORS

- Immunocompromised state

CAUSES

- *P. carinii;* spreads mainly through the air (although part of the normal flora in most healthy people, this organism becomes an aggressive pathogen in immunocompromised patients)
- Possible role of B-cell function defects

INCIDENCE

- *P. carinii* pneumonia is most common in premature or malnourished infants, children with primary immunodeficiency disease, patients receiving immunosuppressive therapy, and those with HIV or AIDS.

COMPLICATIONS

- Disseminated infection
- Hypoxemia
- Respiratory failure
- Pneumothorax
- Death

ASSESSMENT

HISTORY

- Immunodepression, as from HIV infection, leukemia, lymphoma, or organ transplantation

PHYSICAL FINDINGS

- Low-grade, intermittent fever
- Tachypnea
- Dyspnea
- Accessory muscle use for breathing
- Cyanosis (with acute illness)
- Dullness on percussion (with consolidation)
- Crackles
- Decreased breath sounds

DIAGNOSTIC TEST RESULTS

LABORATORY

- Histologic sputum specimen studies show *P. carinii*.
- Arterial blood gas (ABG) values indicate hypoxia and an increased A-a gradient.

IMAGING

- Chest X-rays may show slowly progressing, fluffy infiltrates, occasional nodular lesions, or spontaneous pneumothorax.
- Gallium scan may show increased uptake over the lungs.

DIAGNOSTIC PROCEDURES

- Fiber-optic bronchoscopy is the most commonly used study to confirm PCP.
- Transbronchial biopsy is an invasive procedure less commonly performed to confirm diagnosis.
- Open lung biopsy is an invasive procedure rarely performed to confirm diagnosis.

TREATMENT

GENERAL
◆ Supportive care
◆ Mechanical ventilation

DIET
◆ High-calorie, high-protein
◆ Nutritional supplements as needed
◆ Small, frequent meals
◆ Increased fluid intake

ACTIVITY
◆ Rest periods when fatigued

MEDICATIONS
◆ Co-trimoxazole (may be given prophylactically to AIDS and other high-risk patients)
◆ Oxygen
◆ Immunosuppressants
◆ Antibiotics

NURSING CONSIDERATIONS

NURSING DIAGNOSES
◆ Activity intolerance
◆ Deficient fluid volume
◆ Fear
◆ Hyperthermia
◆ Imbalanced nutrition: Less than body requirements
◆ Impaired gas exchange
◆ Impaired social interaction
◆ Ineffective breathing pattern
◆ Powerlessness

EXPECTED OUTCOMES
The patient will:
◆ perform activities of daily living to the fullest extent possible
◆ maintain adequate fluid volume
◆ verbalize fears, feelings, and concerns
◆ remain afebrile
◆ experience no further weight loss
◆ regain normal ABG values and maintain adequate ventilation and oxygenation
◆ demonstrate effective social interaction skills
◆ maintain an effective breathing pattern
◆ participate in self-care and make decisions about care.

NURSING INTERVENTIONS
◆ Implement standard precautions.
◆ Give prescribed drugs and oxygen.
◆ Encourage ambulation, deep-breathing exercises, and use of incentive spirometry.
◆ Provide adequate rest periods.
◆ Encourage the patient to express fears, feelings, and concerns.
◆ Provide emotional support.

MONITORING
◆ Respiratory status
◆ ABG values
◆ Fluid and electrolyte status

PATIENT TEACHING

GENERAL
Be sure to cover:
◆ the disorder, diagnosis, and treatment
◆ drug administration, dosage, and possible adverse effects
◆ energy conservation techniques
◆ prevention (for HIV-infected patients and other immunocompromised individuals)
◆ home oxygen therapy if indicated.

DISCHARGE PLANNING
◆ Refer the patient to a pulmonologist or an infectious diseases specialist for follow-up care, as needed.
◆ If the patient has AIDS or HIV, provide information about resources and support organizations.

RESOURCES

Organizations
Centers for Disease Control and Prevention: *www.cdc.gov*
Harvard Medical School's Consumer Health Information: *www.intelihealth.com*
National Health Information Center: *www.health.gov/nhic/*
National Institute of Allergy and Infectious Diseases: *www.niaid.nih.gov*
National Library of Medicine: *www.nlm.nih.gov*

Selected references
Ioannidis, J., and Wilkinson, D. "HIV: Prevention of Opportunistic Infections," *Clinical Evidence* (13):834-53, June 2005.
Kasper, D.L., et al, eds. *Harrison's Principles of Internal Medicine*, 16th ed. New York: McGraw-Hill Book Co., 2005.
Pop, S.M., et al. "Pneumocystis: Immune Recognition and Evasion," *International Journal of Biochemistry & Cell Biology* 38(1):17-22, January 2006.
Wells, J., et al. "Complement and Fc Function Are Required for Optimal Antibody Prophylaxis against *Pneumocystis Carinii* Pneumonia," *Infection and Immunity* 74(1):390-93, January 2006.

Pneumonia

- Acute infection of the lung parenchyma that impairs gas exchange
- May be classified by etiology, location, or type

PATHOPHYSIOLOGY

- A gel-like substance forms as microorganisms and phagocytic cells break down.
- This substance consolidates within the lower airway structure.
- Inflammation involves the alveoli, alveolar ducts, and interstitial spaces surrounding the alveolar walls.
- In lobar pneumonia, inflammation starts in one area and may extend to the entire lobe. In bronchopneumonia, it starts simultaneously in several areas, producing patchy, diffuse consolidation. In atypical pneumonia, inflammation is confined to the alveolar ducts and interstitial spaces.

CAUSES

Aspiration pneumonia
- Caustic substance entering airway

Bacterial and viral pneumonia
- Abdominal and thoracic surgery
- Alcoholism
- Aspiration
- Atelectasis
- Bacterial or viral respiratory infections
- Cancer
- Chronic illness and debilitation
- Chronic respiratory disease
- Endotracheal intubation or mechanical ventilation
- Exposure to noxious gases
- Immunosuppressive therapy
- Influenza
- Malnutrition
- Sickle cell disease
- Tracheostomy

RISK FACTORS

- Advanced age
- Debilitation
- Nasogastric (NG) tube feedings
- Impaired gag reflex
- Poor oral hygiene
- Decreased level of consciousness
- Immobility
- History of smoking

INCIDENCE

- Pneumonia affects both sexes and all ages.
- There are more than 4 million cases annually in the United States.

 AGE FACTOR *Incidence and mortality are highest in elderly patients.*

COMPLICATIONS

- Septic shock
- Hypoxemia
- Respiratory failure
- Empyema
- Bacteremia
- Endocarditis
- Pericarditis
- Meningitis
- Lung abscess
- Pleural effusion

ASSESSMENT

HISTORY

Aspiration pneumonia
- Fever
- Weight loss
- Malaise

Bacterial pneumonia
- Sudden onset of:
  – Pleuritic chest pain
  – Cough
  – Purulent sputum production
  – Chills

Viral pneumonia
- Nonproductive cough
- Constitutional symptoms
- Fever

PHYSICAL FINDINGS

- Fever
- Sputum production
- Dullness over the affected area
- Crackles, wheezing, or rhonchi
- Decreased breath sounds
- Decreased fremitus
- Tachypnea
- Use of accessory muscles

DIAGNOSTIC TEST RESULTS

LABORATORY

- Complete blood count shows leukocytosis.
- Blood cultures are positive for the causative organism.
- Arterial blood gas (ABG) values show hypoxemia.
- Fungal or acid-fast bacilli cultures identify the etiologic agent.
- Assay for legionella soluble antigen in urine detects presence of antigen.
- Sputum culture, Gram stain, and smear reveal the infecting organism.

IMAGING

- Chest X-rays generally show patchy or lobar infiltrates.

DIAGNOSTIC PROCEDURES

- Bronchoscopy or transtracheal aspiration specimens identify the etiologic agent.

OTHER

- Pulse oximetry may reveal decreased oxygen saturation.

TREATMENT

GENERAL

- Mechanical ventilation (positive end-expiratory pressure) for respiratory failure

DIET

- High-calorie, high-protein
- Adequate fluids

ACTIVITY

- Bed rest initially; progress as tolerated

MEDICATIONS

- Antibiotics
- Humidified oxygen
- Antitussives
- Analgesics
- Bronchodilators

SURGERY

◆ Drainage of parapneumonic pleural effusion or lung abscess

NURSING CONSIDERATIONS

NURSING DIAGNOSES

◆ Acute pain
◆ Anxiety
◆ Hyperthermia
◆ Imbalanced nutrition: Less than body requirements
◆ Impaired gas exchange
◆ Ineffective airway clearance
◆ Ineffective coping
◆ Risk for deficient fluid volume
◆ Risk for infection

EXPECTED OUTCOMES

The patient will:
◆ express feelings of increased comfort and relief from pain
◆ identify measures to reduce anxiety
◆ maintain a normal body temperature
◆ maintain adequate caloric intake
◆ maintain adequate ventilation and oxygenation
◆ maintain a patent airway
◆ demonstrate effective coping strategies
◆ maintain fluid balance
◆ remain free from signs and symptoms of infection.

NURSING INTERVENTIONS

◆ Give prescribed drugs.
◆ Give prescribed I.V. fluids and electrolyte replacement.
◆ Maintain a patent airway and adequate oxygenation.
◆ Give prescribed supplemental oxygen. Give oxygen cautiously if the patient has chronic lung disease.
◆ Suction the patient as needed.
◆ Obtain sputum specimens as needed.
◆ Provide a high-calorie, high-protein diet of soft foods.
◆ Give supplemental oral feedings, NG tube feedings, or parenteral nutrition, if needed.
◆ Take steps to prevent aspiration during NG feedings.
◆ Dispose of secretions properly.

◆ Provide a quiet, calm environment with frequent rest periods.
◆ Include the patient in care decisions whenever possible.

MONITORING

◆ Vital signs
◆ Intake and output
◆ Daily weight
◆ Sputum production
◆ Respiratory status
◆ Breath sounds
◆ Pulse oximetry
◆ ABG values

Preventing pneumonia

◆ Urge bedridden and postoperative patients to perform deep-breathing and coughing exercises frequently. Position these patients properly to promote full aeration and secretion drainage.
◆ Advise patients to avoid using antibiotics indiscriminately for minor infections. Doing so could produce upper airway colonization with antibiotic-resistant bacteria. If pneumonia develops, the causative organisms may require treatment with more toxic antibiotics.
◆ Encourage high-risk patients to ask the practitioner about an annual influenza vaccination and pneumococcal pneumonia vaccination. A single dose of pneumococcal vaccine is recommended for most patients age 54 and older; certain patients may need one booster dose after 5 years.
◆ Discuss ways to avoid spreading the infection to others. Remind patients to sneeze and cough into tissues and to dispose of tissues in a waxed or plastic bag. Advise patients to wash their hands thoroughly after handling contaminated tissues.

PATIENT TEACHING

GENERAL

Be sure to cover:
◆ the disorder, diagnosis, and treatment
◆ drug administration, dosage, and possible adverse effects
◆ need for adequate fluid intake
◆ importance of adequate rest
◆ deep-breathing and coughing exercises
◆ adequate fluid intake
◆ chest physiotherapy
◆ avoidance of irritants that stimulate secretions
◆ when to notify the practitioner
◆ home oxygen therapy if required
◆ ways to prevent pneumonia. (See *Preventing pneumonia.*)

DISCHARGE PLANNING

◆ Refer the patient to a smoking-cessation program if indicated.

RESOURCES

Organizations

American Lung Association: *www.lungusa.org*
Centers for Disease Control and Prevention: *www.cdc.gov*
National Institute of Allergy and Infectious Diseases: *www.niaid.nih.gov*

Selected references

Andriesse, G.I., and Verhoef, J. "Nosocomial Pneumonia: Rationalizing the Approach to Empirical Therapy," *Treatments in Respiratory Medicine* 5(1):11-30, 2006.
Diseases, 4th ed. Philadelphia: Lippincott Williams & Wilkins, 2006.
Dunn, L. "Pneumonia: Classification, Diagnosis and Nursing Management," *Nursing Standard* 19(42):50-54, June-July 2005.
Loeb, M.B. "Pneumonia in Nursing Homes and Long-term Facilities," *Seminars in Respiratory and Critical Care Medicine* 26(6):650-55, December 2005.
Micek, S.T., et al. "Optimizing Antibiotic Treatment for Ventilator-associated Pneumonia," *Pharmacotherapy* 26(2):204-13, February 2006.

Pneumothorax LIFE-THREATENING DISORDER

OVERVIEW

- Accumulation of air or gas between the parietal and visceral pleurae, leading to lung collapse
- Degree of lung collapse determined by amount of trapped air or gas
- Most common pneumothorax types: open, closed, and tension

PATHOPHYSIOLOGY

- Air accumulates and separates the visceral and parietal pleurae.
- Negative pressure is eliminated, affecting elastic recoil forces.
- The lung recoils and collapses toward the hilus.
- In open pneumothorax, atmospheric air flows directly into the pleural cavity, collapsing the lung on the affected side.
- In closed pneumothorax, air enters the pleural space from within the lung, increasing pleural pressure and preventing lung expansion.
- In tension pneumothorax, air in the pleural space is under higher pressure than air in the adjacent lung. Air enters the pleural space from a pleural rupture only on inspiration. This air pressure exceeds barometric pressure, causing compression atelectasis. Increased pressure may displace the heart and great vessels and cause mediastinal shift.

CAUSES

Closed pneumothorax

- Barotrauma
- Blunt chest trauma
- Clavicle fracture
- Congenital bleb rupture
- Emphysematous bullae rupture
- Erosive tubercular or cancerous lesions
- Interstitial lung disease
- Rib fracture

Open pneumothorax

- Central venous catheter insertion
- Chest surgery
- Penetrating chest injury
- Percutaneous lung biopsy
- Thoracentesis
- Transbronchial biopsy

Tension pneumothorax

- Chest tube occlusion or malfunction
- High positive end-expiratory pressures, causing rupture of alveolar blebs
- Lung or airway puncture from positive-pressure ventilation
- Mechanical ventilation after chest injury
- Penetrating chest wound

INCIDENCE

- The disorder occurs in 9,000 people in the United States annually.

COMPLICATIONS

- Pulmonary and circulatory impairment
- Death

ASSESSMENT

HISTORY

- May not produce symptoms (with small pneumothorax)
- Sudden, sharp, pleuritic pain
- Pain that worsens with chest movement, breathing, and coughing
- Shortness of breath

PHYSICAL FINDINGS

- Asymmetrical chest wall movement
- Overexpansion and rigidity on the affected side
- Possible cyanosis
- Subcutaneous emphysema
- Hyperresonance on the affected side
- Decreased or absent breath sounds on the affected side
- Decreased tactile fremitus over the affected side

Tension pneumothorax

- Distended jugular veins
- Pallor
- Anxiety
- Tracheal deviation away from the affected side
- Weak, rapid pulse
- Hypotension
- Tachypnea
- Cyanosis

DIAGNOSTIC TEST RESULTS

LABORATORY

- Arterial blood gas analysis may show hypoxemia.

IMAGING

- Chest X-ray shows air in the pleural space and, possibly, a mediastinal shift.

OTHER

- Pulse oximetry may show decreased oxygen saturation.

TREATMENT

GENERAL
- Conservative treatment of spontaneous pneumothorax with no signs of increased pleural pressure, less than 30% lung collapse, and no obvious physiologic compromise
- Chest tube insertion
- Needle thoracostomy

DIET
- As tolerated

ACTIVITY
- Bed rest

MEDICATIONS
- Oxygen
- Analgesics

SURGERY
- Thoracotomy, pleurectomy for recurring spontaneous pneumothorax
- Repair of traumatic pneumothorax
- Doxycycline or talc installation into pleural space

NURSING CONSIDERATIONS

NURSING DIAGNOSES
- Acute pain
- Anxiety
- Fear
- Impaired gas exchange
- Ineffective breathing pattern
- Ineffective coping
- Ineffective tissue perfusion: Cardiopulmonary
- Risk for infection

EXPECTED OUTCOMES
The patient will:
- express feelings of increased comfort and a decrease in pain
- identify strategies to reduce anxiety
- discuss fears and concerns
- maintain adequate ventilation and oxygenation
- maintain a respiratory rate within five breaths of baseline
- use support systems to assist with coping
- maintain adequate cardiopulmonary perfusion
- remain free from signs and symptoms of infection.

NURSING INTERVENTIONS
- Give prescribed drugs.
- Assist with chest tube insertion.

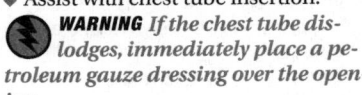 **WARNING** *If the chest tube dislodges, immediately place a petroleum gauze dressing over the opening.*

- Provide comfort measures.
- Encourage deep-breathing and coughing exercises.
- Offer reassurance as appropriate.
- Include the patient and family members in care decisions whenever possible.

MONITORING
- Vital signs
- Intake and output
- Respiratory status
- Breath sounds
- Chest tube system
- Complications
- Pneumothorax recurrence

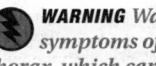 **WARNING** *Watch for signs and symptoms of tension pneumothorax, which can be fatal. These include anxiety, hypotension, tachycardia, tachypnea, and cyanosis.*

PATIENT TEACHING

GENERAL
Be sure to cover:
- the disorder, diagnosis, and treatment
- drug administration, dosage, and possible adverse effects
- chest tube insertion
- deep-breathing exercises
- signs and symptoms of recurrent spontaneous pneumothorax and when to notify the practitioner.

DISCHARGE PLANNING
- Refer the patient to a smoking-cessation program if appropriate.

RESOURCES
Organizations
American Lung Association: *www.lungusa.org*
National Heart, Lung, and Blood Institute: *www.nhlbi.nih.gov*

Selected references

Jenner, R., and Sen, A. "Chest Drains in Traumatic Occult Pneumothorax," *Emergency Medicine Journal* 23(2):138-39, February 2006.

Ong, Y.E., et al. "Radiotherapy: A Novel Treatment for Pneumothorax," *European Respiratory Journal* 27(2):427-29, February 2006.

Trevisanuto, D., et al. "Neonatal Pneumothorax: Comparison between Neonatal Transfers and Inborn Infants," *Journal of Perinatal Medicine* 33(5):449-54, October 2005.

Yamamoto, L., et al. "Thoracic Trauma: The Deadly Dozen," *Critical Care Nursing Quarterly* 28(1):22-40, January-March 2005.

Zhan, C., et al. "Accidental Iatrogenic Pneumothorax in Hospitalized Patients," *Medical Care* 44(2):182-86, February 2006.

Polycystic kidney disease

OVERVIEW

- Growth of multiple, bilateral, grape-like clusters of fluid-filled cysts in the kidneys
- May progress slowly even after renal insufficiency symptoms appear
- Has two distinct forms: infantile form, which causes stillbirth or early neonatal death; and adult form, which has insidious onset but usually becomes obvious between ages 30 and 50
- Usually fatal within 4 years of uremic symptom onset, unless dialysis begins
- Carries a widely varying prognosis in adults
- Also known as *PKD*

PATHOPHYSIOLOGY

- Cysts enlarge the kidneys, compressing and eventually replacing functioning renal tissue.
- Renal deterioration results; deterioration is more gradual in adults than in infants.
- The condition progresses relentlessly to fatal uremia.

CAUSES

- Adult form inherited as an autosomal dominant trait
- Familial
- Infantile form inherited as an autosomal recessive trait

RISK FACTORS

- Autosomal dominant PKD in one parent: 50% chance the disease will pass to a child
- Autosomal recessive PKD: if both parents carry the abnormal gene and pass the gene to their child, risk is 1 in 4 that disease will pass to a child

INCIDENCE

- The disease affects both sexes equally.
- Infantile form of the disease occurs in 1 of 6,000 to 40,000 infants.
- Adult form occurs in 1 of 50 to 1,000 adults.

COMPLICATIONS

- Hepatic failure
- Renal failure
- Respiratory failure
- Heart failure
- Recurrent hematuria
- Life-threatening retroperitoneal bleeding
- Proteinuria

ASSESSMENT

HISTORY
Adult polycystic disease

- Family history
- Polyuria
- Urinary tract infections
- Headaches
- Pain in back or flank area
- Gross hematuria
- Abdominal pain, usually worsened on exertion and eased by lying down

PHYSICAL FINDINGS
Infantile form

- Pronounced epicanthal folds
- Pointed nose
- Small chin
- Floppy, low-set ears (Potter facies)
- Huge, bilateral, symmetrical flank masses that are tense and can't be transilluminated
- Signs of respiratory distress, heart failure and, eventually, uremia and renal failure
- Signs of portal hypertension (bleeding varices)

Adult form

- Hypertension
- Signs of an enlarging kidney mass
- Grossly enlarged kidneys (in advanced stages)

DIAGNOSTIC TEST RESULTS

LABORATORY

- Urinalysis may show hematuria or bacteria or protein.
- Creatinine clearance test results may show renal insufficiency or failure.
- Tests may reveal sodium loss or retention.

IMAGING

- Excretory or retrograde urography reveals enlarged kidneys, with pelvic elongation, flattening of the calyces, and indentations caused by cysts. In a neonate, excretory urography shows poor excretion of contrast medium.
- Ultrasonography, tomography, and radioisotopic scans show kidney enlargement and cysts.
- Tomography, computed tomography scan, and magnetic resonance imaging show multiple areas of cystic damage.

TREATMENT

GENERAL
◆ Monitoring of renal function
◆ Dialysis

DIET
◆ Low-protein and, possibly, low-sodium
◆ Fluid restriction (in renal failure)

ACTIVITY
◆ Avoidance of contact sports

MEDICATIONS
◆ Analgesics
◆ Antibiotics for urinary tract infection
◆ Antihypertensive agents for hypertension

SURGERY
◆ Kidney transplantation
◆ Surgical drainage for cystic abscess or retroperitoneal bleeding

NURSING CONSIDERATIONS

NURSING DIAGNOSES
◆ Acute pain
◆ Deficient fluid volume
◆ Fatigue
◆ Impaired urinary elimination
◆ Ineffective coping
◆ Ineffective tissue perfusion: Renal
◆ Interrupted family processes
◆ Risk for infection
◆ Risk for injury

EXPECTED OUTCOMES
The patient (or family) will:
◆ report feelings of increased comfort
◆ maintain fluid balance
◆ verbalize the importance of balancing activity with adequate rest periods
◆ demonstrate skill in managing the urinary elimination problem
◆ demonstrate adaptive coping behaviors
◆ modify lifestyle to minimize risk of decreased tissue perfusion
◆ discuss the impact of the patient's condition on the family unit
◆ remain free from signs and symptoms of infection
◆ avoid or minimize complications.

NURSING INTERVENTIONS
◆ Give prescribed drugs.
◆ Provide supportive care to minimize symptoms.
◆ Individualize patient care accordingly.

MONITORING
◆ Urine (for blood, cloudiness, calculi, and granules)
◆ Intake and output
◆ Electrolytes
◆ Vital signs
◆ Access site for dialysis

PATIENT TEACHING

GENERAL
Be sure to cover:
◆ the disorder, diagnosis, and treatment
◆ drug administration, dosage, and possible adverse effects
◆ follow-up with the practitioner for severe or recurring headaches
◆ signs and symptoms of urinary tract infection and prompt notification of the practitioner
◆ importance of blood pressure control
◆ possible need for dialysis or transplantation.

DISCHARGE PLANNING
◆ Refer a young adult patient or the parents of an infant with polycystic kidney disease for genetic counseling.

RESOURCES
Organizations
American Association of Kidney Patients: *www.aakp.org*
National Institute of Diabetes & Digestive & Kidney Diseases: *www.niddk.nih.gov*
Polycystic Kidney Research Foundation: *www.pkdcure.org*

Selected references
Bisceglia, M., et al. "Renal Cystic Diseases: A Review," *Advances in Anatomic Pathology* 13(1):26-56, January 2006.
Diseases, 4th ed. Philadelphia: Lippincott Williams & Wilkins, 2006.
Fuller, T.F., et al. "End Stage Polycystic Kidney Disease: Indications and Timing of Native Nephrectomy Relative to Kidney Transplantation," *Journal of Urology* 174(6):2284-88, December 2005.
Thivierge, C., et al. "Overexpression of PKD1 Causes Polycystic Kidney Disease," *Molecular and Cellular Biology* 26(4):1538-48, February 2006.
Torres, V.E. "Vasopressin Antagonists in Polycystic Kidney Disease," *Kidney International* 68(5):2405-18, November 2005.

Polycystic ovarian syndrome

- Metabolic disorder characterized by multiple ovarian cysts
- Prognosis good for ovulation and fertility with appropriate treatment
- Also known as *PCOS* or *Stein-Leventhal syndrome*

PATHOPHYSIOLOGY

- A general feature of all anovulation syndromes is a lack of pulsatile release of gonadotropin-releasing hormone.
- Initial ovarian follicle development is normal.
- Many small follicles begin to accumulate because no dominant follicle is selected.
- These follicles may respond abnormally to hormonal stimulation, causing an abnormal pattern of estrogen secretion during the menstrual cycle.
- Endocrine abnormalities may be the cause of polycystic ovarian syndrome or cystic abnormalities; muscle and adipose tissue are resistant to the effects of insulin, and lipid metabolism is abnormal.

CAUSES

- Exact cause unknown
- Abnormal enzyme activity (may trigger excessive androgen secretion)
- Endocrine abnormalities

INCIDENCE

- Polycystic ovarian syndrome occurs in 6% to 10% of women in the United States; 50% to 80% of these women are obese.
- Among women who seek treatment for infertility, more than 75% have some degree of polycystic ovarian syndrome, usually manifested by anovulation alone.
- Women of reproductive age are affected.
- Mothers or sisters of affected women are also frequently affected.

COMPLICATIONS

- Endometrial cancer
- Increased risk of cardiovascular disease and type 2 diabetes mellitus
- Secondary amenorrhea
- Oligomenorrhea
- Infertility
- Addison's disease
- Hypertension
- Ovarian atrophy
- Coronary artery disease

ASSESSMENT

HISTORY

- Diabetes
- Mild pelvic discomfort
- Lower back pain
- Dyspareunia
- Abnormal uterine bleeding secondary to disturbed ovulatory pattern
- Infertility
- Amenorrhea

PHYSICAL FINDINGS

- Obesity
- Hirsutism
- Decreased breast size
- Acne
- Male-pattern hair loss
- Hyperpigmentation of the skin

DIAGNOSTIC TEST RESULTS

LABORATORY

- Urine 17-ketosteroid level is slightly elevated.
- Anovulation is confirmed.
- Estrogen action is unopposed during menstrual cycle due to anovulation.
- Ratio of luteinizing hormone to follicle-stimulating hormone is elevated (usually 3:1 or greater).
- Testosterone and androstenedione levels are elevated.

IMAGING

- Ultrasonography permits visualization of the ovary.
- Magnetic resonance imaging reveals enlarged ovaries.

OTHER

- Laparoscopy permits direct visualization of the ovary.
- Surgery may confirm ovarian cysts.

TREATMENT

GENERAL
- Lifestyle modifications
- Hair removal

DIET
- Weight-loss
- Diabetic

ACTIVITY
- Daily exercise program

MEDICATIONS
- Clomiphene
- Spironolactone
- Low-dose hormonal contraceptives
- Metformin
- Flutamide

SURGERY
- Ovarian wedge resection
- Laparoscopic surgery to create focal areas of damage in the ovarian cortex and stoma

NURSING CONSIDERATIONS

NURSING DIAGNOSES
- Acute pain
- Anxiety
- Deficient fluid volume
- Ineffective coping
- Ineffective sexuality patterns
- Risk for infection

EXPECTED OUTCOMES
The patient will:
- report feelings of increased comfort
- identify strategies to reduce anxiety
- maintain a normal fluid volume
- demonstrate effective coping mechanisms
- express feelings with partner about the condition and its effect on their sexual relationship
- remain free from signs and symptoms of infection.

NURSING INTERVENTIONS
- Postoperatively, encourage frequent movement in bed and early ambulation.
- Provide emotional support.
- Encourage weight reduction if appropriate.
- Provide guidelines for exercise program.

MONITORING
Preoperatively
- Signs of cyst rupture

Postoperatively
- Vital signs
- Signs of infection

PATIENT TEACHING

GENERAL
Be sure to cover:
- the disorder, diagnosis, and treatment
- diabetic diet if appropriate
- low-calorie diet
- importance of regular follow-up care.

DISCHARGE PLANNING
- Refer the patient to a reproductive endocrinologist.
- Refer the patient to supportive services as appropriate.

RESOURCES
Organizations
The Hormone Foundation: *www.hormone.org/learn/pcos.html*
Mayo Clinic: *www.mayoclinic.org*
The Polycystic Ovarian Syndrome Association: *www.pcosupport.org*

Selected references
Allemand, M.C., et al. "Diagnosis of Polycystic Ovaries by Three-Dimensional Transvaginal Ultrasound," *Fertility and Sterility* 85(1):214-19, January 2006.

Franks, S., et al. "Development of Polycystic Ovary Syndrome: Involvement of Genetic and Environmental Factors," *International Journal of Andrology* 29(1):278-85, February 2006.

Lane, D.E. "Polycystic Ovary Syndrome and its Differential Diagnosis," *Obstetrical & Gynecological Survey* 61(2):125-35, February 2006.

Mohlig, M., et al. "Predictors of Abnormal Glucose Metabolism in Women with Polycystic Ovary Syndrome," *European Journal of Endocrinology* 154(2):295-301, February 2006.

Snyder, B.S. "Polycystic Ovary Syndrome (PCOS) in the Adolescent Patient: Recommendations for Practice," *Pediatric Nursing* 31(5):416-21, September-October 2005.

Polycythemia vera

- Chronic, myeloproliferative disorder of increased red blood cell (RBC) mass, leukocytosis, thrombocytosis, and increased hemoglobin concentration
- Also called *primary polycythemia, erythema, polycythemia rubra vera, splenomegalic polycythemia, Budd-Chiari syndrome,* and *Osler-Vaquez disease*

PATHOPHYSIOLOGY

- Uncontrolled and rapid cellular reproduction and maturation cause proliferation or hyperplasia of all bone marrow cells.
- Increased RBC mass makes the blood abnormally viscous and inhibits blood flow to the microcirculation.
- Diminished blood flow and thrombocytosis set the stage for intravascular thrombosis.

CAUSES

- Unknown

INCIDENCE

- Onset of the disease is usually between ages 50 and 70.
- The disease is common among Jewish men but also affects all ethnic groups.
- It's rare in children and blacks.

COMPLICATIONS

- Hemorrhage
- Vascular thromboses
- Uric acid calculi
- Myelofibrosis
- Acute leukemia

HISTORY

- Vague feeling of fullness in the head or rushing in the ears
- Tinnitus
- Headache
- Dizziness, vertigo
- Epistaxis
- Night sweats
- Epigastric and joint pain
- Vision alterations, such as scotomas, double vision, and blurred vision
- Pruritus
- Abdominal fullness

PHYSICAL FINDINGS

- Congestion of the conjunctiva, retina, and retinal veins
- Oral mucous membrane congestion
- Hypertension
- Ruddy cyanosis
- Ecchymosis
- Hepatosplenomegaly

LABORATORY

- Uric acid level is increased.
- Increased RBC mass (total greater than 36 ml/kg in males and 32 ml/kg in females) and normal arterial oxygen saturation confirm diagnosis with splenomegaly or two of the following:
  - platelet count above 400,000/μl (thrombocytopenia)
  - white blood cell count above 12,000/μl in adults
  - elevated leukocyte alkaline phosphatase level
  - serum vitamin B_{12} levels greater than 900 pg/ml or B_{12}-binding capacity greater than 2200 pg/ml.
- Arterial oxygen saturation is 92% or higher.

IMAGING

- Computed tomography of abdomen shows enlarged spleen.

DIAGNOSTIC PROCEDURES

- Bone marrow biopsy shows panmyelosis.

GENERAL

- Phlebotomy
- Pheresis
- Sequential compression stockings, if deep vein thrombosis isn't present

MEDICATIONS

- Myelosuppressive agents
- Radioactive phosphorus
- Chemotherapy

SURGERY

- Splenectomy, as needed

NURSING CONSIDERATIONS

NURSING DIAGNOSES
- Activity intolerance
- Acute pain
- Anxiety
- Fatigue
- Imbalanced nutrition: Less than body requirements
- Ineffective tissue perfusion: Peripheral
- Risk for impaired skin integrity
- Risk for infection
- Risk for injury

EXPECTED OUTCOMES
The patient will:
- verbalize the importance of balancing activity, as tolerated, with rest
- express feelings of increased comfort and decreased pain
- verbalize measures to reduce anxiety level
- express feelings of increased energy
- maintain daily calorie requirements
- maintain strong peripheral pulses
- maintain skin integrity
- remain free from evidence of infection
- remain free from complications.

NURSING INTERVENTIONS
- Keep the patient active and ambulatory.
- If bed rest is needed, start daily active and passive range-of-motion exercises, and apply sequential compression stockings as appropriate.
- Encourage additional fluid intake.
- If the patient has symptom-producing splenomegaly, suggest or provide small, frequent meals followed by a rest period.
- If the patient has pruritus, give prescribed drugs.
- Encourage the patient to express concerns about the disease and its treatment.

WARNING *Report acute abdominal pain immediately. It may signal splenic infarction, renal calculus formation, or abdominal organ thrombosis.*

During and after phlebotomy
- Make sure the patient is lying down comfortably. Stay alert for tachycardia, clamminess, and complaints of vertigo. If these effects occur, the procedure should be stopped.
- Immediately after phlebotomy, have the patient sit up for about 5 minutes before letting him walk. Give 24 oz (709.8 ml) of juice or water.

During myelosuppressive chemotherapy
- If nausea and vomiting occur, begin antiemetic therapy and adjust the patient's diet.
- During treatment with radioactive phosphorus, obtain a blood sample for complete blood cell (CBC) count and platelet count before starting treatment. (Personnel who administer radioactive phosphorus should take radiation precautions to prevent contamination.)
- Have the patient lie down during I.V. administration and for 15 to 20 minutes afterward.

MONITORING
- Vital signs
- Adverse reactions to drugs
- CBC and platelet count before and during therapy
- Complications
- Signs and symptoms of impending stroke
- Hypertension
- Signs and symptoms of heart failure
- Signs and symptoms of bleeding

PATIENT TEACHING

GENERAL
Be sure to cover:
- the disorder, diagnosis, and treatment
- importance of staying as active as possible
- use of an electric razor to prevent accidental cuts
- ways to minimize falls and contusions at home
- avoidance of high altitudes
- common bleeding sites, if the patient has thrombocytopenia

- importance of reporting abnormal bleeding promptly
- phlebotomy procedure (if scheduled) and its effects
- symptoms of iron deficiency to report
- possible adverse reactions to myelosuppressive therapy
- instructions on infection prevention for an outpatient who develops leukopenia (including avoiding crowds and watching for infection symptoms)
- radioactive phosphorus administration procedure (if scheduled) and the possible need for repeated phlebotomies
- dental care
- use of gloves when outdoors if temperature is below 50° F (10° C).

RESOURCES
Organizations
The Leukemia and Lymphoma Society: *www.leukemia.org*
Mayo Clinic: *www.mayoclinic.org*
The Merck Manuals Online Medical Library: *www.merck.com/mmhe*
National Heart, Lung, and Blood Institute: *www.nhlbi.nih.gov*

Selected references
Kasper, D.L., et al, eds. *Harrison's Principles of Internal Medicine,* 16th ed. New York: McGraw-Hill Book Co., 2005.
Munson, B.L. "Myths & Facts...about Polycythemia Vera," *Nursing* 35(5):28, May 2005.
Silver, R.T. "Treatment of Polycythemia Vera with Recombinant Interferon Alpha (rIFNalpha) or Imatinib Mesylate," *Current Hematology Reports* 4(3):235-37, May 2005.
Tierney, L., et al. *Current Medical Diagnosis & Treatment 2006.* New York: McGraw-Hill Book Co., 2006.
Wu, C.F., et al. "Polycythaemia Vera Presenting as ST-elevation Myocardial Infarction," *Heart, Lung & Circulation* 14(1):51-53, March 2005.

Polyps, intestinal

OVERVIEW

- A small, tumorlike growth that projects from a mucous membrane surface
- May develop in the colon or rectum, where they protrude into the GI tract

PATHOPHYSIOLOGY

- Masses of tissue resulting from unrestrained cell growth in the upper epithelium rise above the mucosal membrane and protrude into the GI tract.
- They may be described by their appearance:
- pedunculated: attached by a stalk to the intestinal wall
- sessile: attached to the intestinal wall with a broad base and no stalk.
- Polyps are classified according to tissue type:
- adenomatous polyps, such as tubular adenoma, tubulovillous adenoma, and villous adenoma
- nonadenomatous polyps, such as hyperplastic polyps, inflammatory polyps, and juvenile polyps.
- Most polyps are benign. However, villous and familial polyps show a marked inclination to become malignant.

  ⚡ **WARNING** *Familial polyposis is commonly linked to rectosigmoid adenocarcinoma.*

CAUSES

- Unknown

RISK FACTORS

- Heredity
- Age
- High-fat, low-fiber diet

INCIDENCE

- Villous adenomas are most prevalent in men older than age 55.
- Common polypoid adenomas are most prevalent in white women between ages 45 and 60.
- Incidence in both sexes increases after age 70.
- Juvenile polyps are most common in children younger than age 10.

COMPLICATIONS

- Anemia
- Bowel obstruction
- Rectal bleeding
- Intussusception
- Colorectal cancer (villous adenomas and familial polyps)
- Electrolyte imbalance

ASSESSMENT

HISTORY

- Diarrhea
- Bloody stools
- Painful defecation
- Changes in bowel habits

PHYSICAL FINDINGS

- Polyp felt during digital rectal examination

DIAGNOSTIC TEST RESULTS

LABORATORY

- Occult blood is present in the stools.
- Hemoglobin level is low.
- Hematocrit level (with anemia) is low.
- Serum electrolyte levels are imbalanced (with villous adenomas).

IMAGING

- Barium enema identifies polyps that are located high in the colon.

DIAGNOSTIC PROCEDURES

- Sigmoidoscopy, colonoscopy, and rectal biopsy identify polyps.

TREATMENT

GENERAL
- Smoking cessation

DIET
- Low-fat, high-fiber
- Minimal red meat
- Alcohol avoidance

ACTIVITY
- As tolerated

MEDICATIONS
- Analgesics

SURGERY
- Polypectomy, commonly by fulguration (destruction by high-frequency electricity) during endoscopy
- Abdominoperineal resection, low anterior resection, ileostomy, colostomy
- Biopsy
- Snare removal during colonoscopy

NURSING CONSIDERATIONS

NURSING DIAGNOSES
- Acute pain
- Anxiety
- Diarrhea
- Risk for imbalanced fluid volume
- Risk for infection

EXPECTED OUTCOMES
The patient will:
- express increased comfort
- identify strategies to reduce anxiety
- return to normal bowel habits
- attain and maintain normal fluid and electrolyte balance
- remain free from signs and symptoms of infection.

NURSING INTERVENTIONS
- Observe the amount and character of stools.
- Prepare the patient with precancerous or familial lesions for colonoscopy or abdominoperineal resection.
- Provide emotional support.

MONITORING
- Electrolyte levels
- Rectal bleeding
- Vital signs
- Intake and output

After surgery
- Signs of bleeding
- Wound condition

PATIENT TEACHING

GENERAL
Be sure to cover:
- the disorder, diagnosis, and treatment
- wound care if appropriate
- enterostomal therapy and care.

DISCHARGE PLANNING
- If the patient has benign polyps, stress the need for routine follow-up studies to check for new polypoid growth.

RESOURCES
Organizations
American Gastroenterological Association: *www.gastro.org*
The Merck Manuals Online Medical Library: *www.merck.com/mmhe*
National Digestive Diseases Information Clearinghouse: *www.niddk.nih.gov/health/digest/nddic.htm*

Selected references
Hassan, C., et al. "Histologic Risk Factors and Clinical Outcome in Colorectal Malignant Polyp: A Pooled-Data Analysis," *Diseases of the Colon and Rectum* 48(8):1588-96, August 2005.
Summers, R.M., et al. "Computed Tomographic Virtual Colonoscopy Computer-aided Polyp Detection in a Screening Population," *Gastroenterology* 129(6):1832-44, December 2005.
Wayne, J.D. "Advanced Polypectomy," *Gastrointestinal Endoscopy Clinics of North America* 15(4):733-56, October 2005.

Porphyrias

- Umbrella term for a group of metabolic disorders that affect the biosynthesis of heme (a hemoglobin component), resulting in excessive porphyrin production
- Classified by the site of excessive porphyrin production as erythropoietic, hepatic, or erythrohepatic porphyria

PATHOPHYSIOLOGY

- Various metabolic disorders affect heme biosynthesis.
- This leads to excessive production and excretion of porphyrins or their precursors.

CAUSES

- Inherited as an autosomal dominant trait, except Günther disease (inherited as an autosomal recessive trait)
- Lead ingestion or exposure (toxic-acquired porphyria)

RISK FACTORS

- Certain medications
- Hormonal changes
- Infection
- Malnutrition

INCIDENCE

- The disorder is more common in Whites than in Blacks or Asians.

COMPLICATIONS

- With hepatic porphyria: neurologic and hepatic dysfunction
- With acute intermittent porphyria: flaccid paralysis, respiratory paralysis, and death
- With erythropoietic porphyria: hemolytic anemia

HISTORY

- Mild or severe abdominal pain
- Photosensitivity
- Paresthesia
- Neuritic pain

PHYSICAL FINDINGS

- Wide variation, depending on the type of porphyria
- Psychosis
- Seizures
- Skin lesions
- Darkening of urine left in the light or air
- Neurologic signs of wristdrop or footdrop
- Muscle weakness
- Fever (with an acute attack)
- Splenomegaly (if hemolytic anemia is present)
- Wheezing and dyspnea (with acute intermittent porphyria)

LABORATORY

- Urine aminolevulinic acid is present in the ion-exchange chromatography test.
- In acute intermittent porphyria, urine porphobilinogen (as shown by the Watson-Schwartz test), leukocytosis, elevated bilirubin and alkaline phosphatase levels, and hyponatremia are present.
- In variegate porphyria, protoporphyrin and coproporphyrin are present in stools.
- In hereditary coproporphyria, abundant coproporphyrin is present in stools and, to a lesser extent, in urine.
- In porphyria cutanea tarda, uroporphyrin excretion is increased, with varying amounts of fecal porphyrins.
- In Günther disease, urine porphyrins are present.
- In erythropoietic protoporphyria, protoporphyrin is present in red blood cells.
- In toxic acquired porphyria, urine lead level is 0.2 mg/L or higher.
- In porphyria cutanea tarda, serum iron levels are increased.

TREATMENT

GENERAL
◆ Avoidance of direct sun exposure

DIET
◆ High-carbohydrate
◆ Fluid restriction
◆ No alcohol

MEDICATIONS
◆ Beta-carotene supplements
◆ Chlorpromazine I.V.
◆ Analgesics
◆ Hematin
◆ Sunscreen preparations

SURGERY
◆ In hemolytic anemia: splenectomy

Drugs that aggravate porphyria

Make sure the patient with porphyria doesn't receive any of the following drugs, which are known to trigger signs and symptoms of porphyria:
◆ barbiturates
◆ carbamazepine (Tegretol)
◆ carisoprodol (Vanadom)
◆ chloramphenicol (Chloromycetin)
◆ chlordiazepoxide (Librium)
◆ danazol
◆ diazepam (Valium)
◆ ergot alkaloids
◆ estrogens
◆ griseofulvin
◆ imipramine (Tofranil)
◆ methsuximide (Celontin)
◆ methyldopa (Aldomet)
◆ pentazocine (Talwin)
◆ phenytoin (Dilantin)
◆ progesterones
◆ sulfonamides
◆ tolbutamide.

NURSING CONSIDERATIONS

NURSING DIAGNOSES
◆ Acute pain
◆ Constipation
◆ Impaired gas exchange
◆ Impaired skin integrity
◆ Risk for injury

EXPECTED OUTCOMES
The patient will:
◆ express feelings of increased comfort
◆ regain normal bowel movements
◆ maintain adequate ventilation and oxygenation
◆ maintain skin integrity
◆ avoid complications.

NURSING INTERVENTIONS
◆ Check the patient's history for use of medications that can trigger an acute attack. (See *Drugs that aggravate porphyria*.)
◆ Give prescribed drugs.
◆ Perform passive and active range-of-motion exercises.
◆ Encourage the patient to express feelings and concerns about the disease.
◆ Provide emotional support.

MONITORING
◆ Respiratory status
◆ GI motility
◆ Vital signs
◆ Response to treatment

PATIENT TEACHING

GENERAL
Be sure to cover:
◆ the disorder, diagnosis, and treatment
◆ avoidance of excessive sun exposure
◆ importance of wearing medical identification
◆ lead sources (if the patient has toxic-acquired porphyria)
◆ precipitating factors, including crash diets, fasting, and use of alcohol, estrogens, and barbiturates
◆ stress-management techniques
◆ ways to prevent infection
◆ value of a high-carbohydrate diet.

DISCHARGE PLANNING
◆ For toxic-acquired porphyria, refer the patient and family to resources that can help identify lead sources in the home.

RESOURCES
Organizations
American Porphyria Foundation: *www.porphyriafoundation.com*
National Organization for Rare Disorders: *www.rarediseases.org*

Selected references
Chen, H.W., et al. "Effects of Diabetes on the ED Presentation of Acute Intermittent Porphyria," *American Journal of Emergency Medicine* 23(4):571-72, July 2005.

Dombeck, T.A., and Satonik, R.C. "The Porphyrias," *Emergency Medicine Clinics of North America* 23(3):885-99, August 2005.

Herrick, A.L., and McColl, K.E. "Acute Intermittent Porphyria," *Best Practice & Research - Clinical Gastroenterology* 19(2):235-49, April 2005.

Millward, L.M., et al. "Anxiety and Depression in the Acute Porphyrias," *Journal of Inherited Metabolic Disease* 28(6):1099-107, 2005.

Posttraumatic stress disorder

- Development of psychological symptoms, such as intense fear and feelings of hopelessness and loss of control, after exposure to extreme trauma
- Can be acute, chronic, or delayed
- Also known as *PTSD*

PATHOPHYSIOLOGY

- The alpha$_2$-adrenergic receptor response that inhibits stress-induced release of norepinephrine is impaired.
- Progressive behavioral sensitization results, with generalization to stimulus cues from the original trauma.
- Consequently, responses of increased sympathetic activity occur.

CAUSES

- An event that the patient views as traumatic (typically an event outside the range of usual human experience)

RISK FACTORS

- History of psychopathology
- Neurotic and extroverted characteristics
- History of child abuse or neglect

INCIDENCE

- PTSD affects 30% of trauma victims.
- The disorder occurs in up to 15% of people in the United States at some time in their lives.
- It's more common in women than in men.
- PTSD can occur at any age.

COMPLICATIONS

- Increased risk of other anxiety, mood, and substance-related disorders
- Substance abuse
- Feelings of detachment or estrangement, which may damage interpersonal relationships
- Suicide

HISTORY

- Difficulty falling or staying asleep
- Aggressive outbursts on awakening
- Panic attacks
- Phobic avoidance of situations that arouse memories of the traumatic event
- Early life experiences, interpersonal factors, military experiences, or other incidents that suggest the traumatic event
- Symptoms that began immediately or soon after the trauma (although in some cases, symptoms don't develop until months or years later)
- Pangs of painful emotions and unwelcome thoughts
- Traumatic reexperiencing of the traumatic event
- Chronic anxiety
- Rage and survivor guilt
- Use of violence to solve problems
- Depression and suicidal thoughts
- Fantasies of retaliation

PHYSICAL FINDINGS

- Emotional numbing (diminished or constricted response)
- Memory impairment
- Difficulty concentrating
- Signs of substance abuse
- Physiologic reactivity on exposure to internal or external cues that symbolize or resemble an aspect of the traumatic event

DSM-IV-TR *criteria*

Diagnosis is confirmed when the patient meets the following criteria:

- Exposure to a traumatic event that included both of the following:
- actual or threatened death or serious injury or threat to the physical integrity of self or others
- a response of intense fear, helplessness, or horror.
- Persistent reexperiencing of this traumatic event in at least one of these ways:
- recurrent and intrusive distressing recollections of the event
- recurrent distressing dreams of the event
- flashbacks of the event
- intense psychological distress at exposure to events
- physiologic reactivity on exposure to events.
- Persistent avoidance of stimuli associated with the trauma, or numbing of general responsiveness not present before the trauma, as indicated by at least three of these criteria:
- efforts to avoid thoughts or feelings associated with the traumatic event
- efforts to avoid activities or situations that arouse recollections of the traumatic event
- inability to recall an important aspect of the event
- sharply decreased interest in significant activities
- feeling of detachment or estrangement from others
- restricted range of effect
- sense of a foreshortened future.
- Persistent symptoms of increased arousal (not previously present) as indicated by two or more of these criteria:
- difficulty falling or staying asleep
- irritability or outbursts of anger
- difficulty concentrating
- hypervigilance
- exaggerated startle response.
     The disturbance must have lasted at least 1 month and must cause significant distress or impairment of social, occupational, or other important areas of functioning.

GENERAL

- Mental status examination results fit the *DSM-IV-TR* criteria.

TREATMENT

GENERAL
- Supportive or expressive psycho-therapy
- Behavior therapies
- Support groups
- Rehabilitation programs in physical, social, and occupational areas
- Treatment of alcohol or drug abuse, as needed
- Active avoidance of stimuli that trigger memories of the traumatic event

MEDICATIONS
- Benzodiazepines (short-term use)
- Tricyclic antidepressants
- Monoamine oxidase inhibitors
- Selective serotonin-reuptake inhibitors
- Sedating antidepressants
- Anticonvulsants

NURSING CONSIDERATIONS

NURSING DIAGNOSES
- Anxiety
- Chronic low self-esteem
- Disturbed personal identity
- Disturbed sleep pattern
- Fear
- Impaired social interaction
- Ineffective coping
- Ineffective role performance
- Powerlessness
- Risk for posttrauma syndrome

EXPECTED OUTCOMES
The patient will:
- verbalize strategies to reduce anxiety
- use available support systems
- express feelings related to personal identity
- report feeling well-rested
- use effective coping mechanisms to reduce fear
- maintain or reestablish adaptive social interactions with family members
- use effective coping mechanisms
- resume usual roles and responsibilities
- participate in self-care and the decision-making process
- express feelings and fears related to the traumatic event.

NURSING INTERVENTIONS
- Encourage the patient to express feelings of grief, mourning, and anger.
- Practice crisis intervention techniques as needed.
- Assume a positive, consistent, honest, and nonjudgmental attitude.
- Help the patient evaluate behavior.

MONITORING
- Response to drug therapy
- Suicidal tendencies or thoughts

PATIENT TEACHING

GENERAL
Be sure to cover:
- the disorder, diagnosis, and treatment
- healing process
- importance of identifying and avoiding cues that worsen symptoms
- problem-solving skills
- relaxation and breathing techniques
- drug administration, dosage, and possible adverse effects.

DISCHARGE PLANNING
- Refer the patient to support services.
- Refer the patient for psychotherapy.
- Refer the patient to physical, social, and occupational rehabilitation programs, as indicated.
- Refer the patient to drug treatment programs as appropriate.

RESOURCES
Organizations
American Psychiatric Association: *www.psych.org*
American Psychological Association: *www. apa.org*
National Center for Posttraumatic Stress Disorder: *www.ncptsd.org*

Selected references
Diagnostic and Statistical Manual of Mental Disorders, Fourth Edition, Text Revision. Washington, D.C.: American Psychiatric Association, 2000.
Gross, R., and Neria, Y. "Posttraumatic Stress among Survivors of Bioterrorism," *JAMA* 292(5):566, August 2004.
Kashdan, T.B., et al. "Anhedonia and Emotional Numbing in Combat Veterans with PTSD," *Behaviour Research and Therapy* 44(3):457-67, March 2006.
Kasper, D.L., et al, eds. *Harrison's Principles of Internal Medicine,* 16th ed. New York: McGraw-Hill Book Co., 2005.
Olszewski, T.M., and Varrasse, J.F. "The Neurobiology of PTSD: Implications for Nurses," *Journal of Psychosocial Nursing and Mental Health Services* 43(6):40-47, June 2005.

Precocious puberty

- Early sexual maturity (before age 10 in males and age 8 in females)
- True precocious puberty: early maturation of the hypothalamic-pituitary-gonadal axis, development of secondary sex characteristics, gonadal development, and spermatogenesis
- Pseudoprecocious puberty: development of secondary sex characteristics without gonadal development

PATHOPHYSIOLOGY

- In males, precocious puberty results from pituitary or hypothalamic intracranial lesions that cause excessive secretion of gonadotropin.
- In females, it results from early development and activation of the endocrine glands without corresponding abnormality.

CAUSES
In males
True precocious puberty
- Genetically transmitted as a dominant gene
- Idiopathic

Pseudoprecocious puberty
- Congenital adrenogenital syndrome
- Testicular tumors

In females
True precocious puberty
- Central nervous system (CNS) disorders
- Idiopathic

Pseudoprecocious puberty
- Estrogen or androgen ingestion
- Increased end-organ sensitivity to low levels of circulating sex hormones
- Ovarian and adrenocortical tumors

IRISK FACTORS
- Heridity, in males (autosomal dominant)

INCIDENCE
- Precocious puberty is five times more common in females than in males.

AGE FACTOR *Males as young as 7 with true precocious puberty have fathered children.*

COMPLICATIONS
- Testicular tumor (males)
- Ovarian or adrenal malignancy (females)

HISTORY
- Rapid growth spurt
- Early muscle development (males)
- Aggressive behavior (males)
- Early menarche (females)

PHYSICAL FINDINGS
- Enlarged penis or testicles (males)
- Enlarged breasts (females)
- Pubic hair
- Underarm hair
- Acne

LABORATORY
In males with true precocious puberty
- Plasma testosterone levels are elevated.
- Ejaculate shows live spermatozoa.
- Levels of luteinizing and follicle-stimulating hormones and corticotropins are elevated.

In males with pseudoprecocious puberty
- Chromosomal karyotype analysis shows abnormal pattern of autosomes and sex chromosomes.
- Levels of 24-hour urine 17-ketosteroids and other steroids are elevated.

In females with true precocious puberty
- Estradiol level may be elevated.
- Adrenocorticotrophic hormone (ACTH) level is elevated 30 to 60 minutes after ACTH is injected.

In females with pseudoprecocious puberty
- Vaginal smear shows estrogen secretion.
- Urine tests show gonadotropic activity and excretion of 17-ketosteroids.
- Levels of luteinizing and follicle-stimulating hormones are elevated.

IMAGING
- X-rays of the hands, wrists, knees, and hips determine bone age and possibly premature epiphyseal closure.
- Ultrasound verifies suspected abdominal lesion.
- X-rays may show CNS tumors.

TREATMENT

GENERAL
- Based on underlying cause
- Supportive psychological counseling

MEDICATIONS
- Medroxyprogesterone (females)
- Gonadotropin-releasing hormone agonists

SURGERY
- Removal of ovarian or adrenal tumors
- Removal of thyroid gland

NURSING CONSIDERATIONS

NURSING DIAGNOSES
- Chronic low self-esteem
- Disturbed body image
- Impaired adjustment
- Ineffective coping
- Deficient knowledge (sexual maturity)

EXPECTED OUTCOMES
The patient (or family) will:
- voice feelings related to self-esteem
- express positive feelings about body
- express feelings of acceptance and adjustment to early sexual development
- agree to seek help from peer support groups or professional counselors to increase adaptive coping behaviors

NURSING INTERVENTIONS
- Provide emotional support.

MONITORING
- Complications
- Medication reactions

PATIENT TEACHING

GENERAL
Be sure to cover:
- the disorder, diagnosis, and treatment
- drug administration, dosage, and possible adverse effects
- the need to continue social and emotional support
- information about body functions related to sexual maturity.

DISCHARGE PLANNING
- Patient and family should follow up with practitioner for bone-age growth and medication-related changes.

RESOURCES
Organizations
American Academy of Pediatrics: *www.aap.org*
Mayo Clinic: *www.mayoclinic.org*
National Institute of Child Health & Human Development: *www.nichd.nih.gov*

Selected references
Ibanez, L., et al. "Early Puberty-Menarche after Precocious Pubarche: Relation to Prenatal Growth," *Pediatrics* 117(1): 117-21, January 2006.
Parent, A.S., et al. "Early Onset of Puberty: Tracking Genetic and Environmental Factors," *Hormone Research* 64(Suppl 2):41-47, 2005.
Phillip, M., and Lazar, L. "Precocious Puberty: Growth and Genetics," *Hormone Research* 64(Suppl 2):56-61, 2005.
Tremblay, L., and Frigon, J.Y. "Precocious Puberty in Adolescent Girls: A Biomarker of Later Psychosocial Adjustment Problems," *Child Psychiatry and Human Development* 36(1):73-94, Fall 2005.

Premenstrual syndrome

OVERVIEW

- Group of somatic, behavioral, cognitive, and mood-related symptoms occurring 1 to 14 days before menses and usually subsiding with menses onset
- Causes effects that range from minimal discomfort to severe, disruptive symptoms
- Also known as *PMS* and *premenstrual dysphoric disorder (PMDD)* (see *Premenstrual dysphoric disorder*)

PATHOPHYSIOLOGY

- PMS may result from a progesterone deficiency during the luteal phase of the ovarian cycle.
- Hormone levels and patterns in women with PMS don't differ significantly from those in women who don't experience PMS.

CAUSES

- Physiologic, psychological, and sociocultural factors
- Possible progesterone deficiency in the luteal phase
- Possible serotonin or norepinephrine deficiency

INCIDENCE

- PMS affects 30% of women in the United States.
- Moderate to severe symptoms occur in 14% to 88% of adolescent girls.
- PMS usually occurs between ages 25 and 45.
- The condition affects women in their 40s most severely.
- PMS resolves completely at menopause.

COMPLICATIONS

- Psychosocial problems
- Reduced self-esteem
- Depression
- Inability to function (in PMDD)

ASSESSMENT

HISTORY

- Behavioral changes
- Breast tenderness or swelling
- Abdominal tenderness or bloating
- Joint pain
- Headache
- Edema
- Diarrhea or constipation
- Worsening of skin, respiratory, or neurologic problems
- Lower back pain

PHYSICAL FINDINGS

- Possible edema

DIAGNOSTIC TEST RESULTS

LABORATORY

- Blood studies rule out anemia, thyroid disease, or other hormonal imbalances.

OTHER

- A daily symptom calendar aids diagnosis of PMS.
- Psychological evaluation may be used to rule out or detect an underlying psychiatric disorder.

Premenstrual dysphoric disorder

Premenstrual dysphoric disorder (PMDD) is a severe form of premenstrual syndrome (PMS) that has a cyclical occurrence of psychiatric symptoms that starts after ovulation (usually the week before the onset of menstruation) and ends within the first day or two of menses. Its underlying cause and pathophysiology remain unclear. However, researchers theorize that normal cyclic changes in the body cause abnormal responses to neurotransmitters, such as serotonin, resulting in physical and behavioral signs and symptoms.

PMDD affects as many as 1 in 20 American women who have regular menstrual periods. It's unclear why some women are affected whereas others aren't.

HOW PMDD AND PMS DIFFER

PMDD is characterized by severe monthly mood swings and physical signs and symptoms that interfere with everyday life. Compared with PMS, its signs and symptoms are abnormal and unmanageable. Although depression, anxiety, and sadness are common with PMS, in patients with PMDD, these symptoms are extreme. Some women may feel the urge to hurt or kill themselves or others.

The *DSM-IV-TR* sets these criteria for diagnosing PMDD:

- functional impairment
- predominant mood symptoms, with one being affective
- symptoms beginning 1 week before the onset of menstruation
- symptoms that don't result from any underlying primary mood disorder.

In addition, at least five of the following symptoms must be present:

- appetite changes
- decreased interests
- difficulty concentrating
- fatigue
- feelings of being overwhelmed
- insomnia or hypersomnia
- irritability
- "low mood"
- mood swings
- physical symptoms
- tension.

TREATMENT

GENERAL
- Symptom relief
- Stress reduction
- Relaxation techniques

DIET
- Low in simple sugars, caffeine intake, animal fat, and sodium
- Increased calcium and complex carbohydrate intake

ACTIVITY
- Aerobic exercise

MEDICATIONS
- Antidepressants
- Vitamins (such as B complex)
- Progestins
- Prostaglandin inhibitors
- Monophasic birth control pills
- Nonsteroidal anti-inflammatory drugs
- Pituitary-ovarian axis supplements
- Gonadotropin-releasing hormone agonists

NURSING CONSIDERATIONS

NURSING DIAGNOSES
- Acute pain
- Anxiety
- Disturbed body image
- Excess fluid volume
- Hopelessness
- Impaired social interaction
- Ineffective coping
- Ineffective role performance
- Ineffective sexuality patterns
- Interrupted family processes
- Situational low self-esteem

EXPECTED OUTCOMES
The patient will:
- express feelings of increased comfort
- identify strategies to reduce anxiety
- express positive feelings about self
- maintain a normal fluid balance
- become actively involved in planning own care
- use available support systems, such as family, friends, and groups, to develop and maintain effective coping skills
- identify effective and ineffective coping techniques
- resume usual roles and responsibilities
- express the effects of the condition on sexuality patterns
- express the effects of the condition on the family unit
- express feelings about self-esteem.

NURSING INTERVENTIONS
- Encourage adequate fluid intake.
- Provide comfort measures.
- Offer emotional support and reassurance.
- Encourage the patient to express feelings.
- Help the patient develop effective coping strategies.
- Instruct the patient to chart symptoms daily for two cycles.

MONITORING
- Response to treatment
- Coping skills

PATIENT TEACHING

GENERAL
Be sure to cover:
- the disorder, diagnosis, and treatment
- physiologic basis of PMS
- beneficial lifestyle changes
- relaxation and stress-reduction techniques
- dietary management.

DISCHARGE PLANNING
- Refer the patient to a self-help group for women with PMS.
- Refer the patient for psychological counseling as indicated.
- Refer the patient to a dietitian as needed.

RESOURCES
Organizations
American College of Obstetricians and Gynecologists: *www.acog.org*
National Association for Premenstrual Syndrome: *www.pms.org.uk*

Selected references
Chou, P.B., and Morse, C.A. "Understanding Premenstrual Syndrome from a Chinese Medicine Perspective," *Journal of Alternative and Complementary Medicine* 11(2):355-61, April 2005.

Dowd, S.M. "Premenstrual Dysphoric Disorder. A Clinical Trial Approach to Assessment," *Advance for Nurse Practitioners* 13(2):57-59, February 2005.

Martin, V.T., et al. "Symptoms of Premenstrual Syndrome and Their Association with Migraine Headache," *Headache* 46(1):125-37, January 2006.

Steiner, M., et al. "Expert Guidelines for the Treatment of Severe PMS, PMDD, and Comorbidities: The Role of SSRIs," *Journal of Women's Health* 15(1):57-69, January-February 2006.

Pressure ulcers

- Localized areas of ischemic tissue caused by pressure, shearing, or friction
- Most common over bony prominences, especially the sacrum, ischial tuberosities, greater trochanter, heels, malleoli, and elbows
- May be superficial, caused by localized skin irritation (with subsequent surface maceration), or deep, arising in underlying tissue (Deep lesions may go undetected until they penetrate the skin.)
- Also called *decubitus ulcers*, *pressure sores*, or *bedsores*

PATHOPHYSIOLOGY

- Impaired skin capillary pressure results in local tissue anoxia.
- Anoxia leads to edema and multiple capillary thromboses.
- An inflammatory reaction results in ulceration and necrosis of ischemic cells.

CAUSES

- Friction
- Local tissue compression
- Shearing force

RISK FACTORS

- Poor nutrition
- Diabetes mellitus
- Immobility or paralysis
- Cardiovascular disorders
- Advanced age
- Incontinence
- Obesity
- Edema
- Anemia
- Poor hygiene
- Exposure to chemicals
- Steroids

INCIDENCE

- Pressure ulcers affect about 10% of hospitalized patients and 20% to 40% of patients in long-term care facilities.

COMPLICATIONS

- Secondary bacterial infection
- Septicemia
- Gangrene

ASSESSMENT

HISTORY

- One or more risk factors

PHYSICAL FINDINGS

- Shiny, erythematous superficial lesion (early) (see *Four stages of pressure ulcers*)
- Small blisters or erosions with progression of superficial erythema
- Possible necrosis and ulceration with deeper erosions and ulcerations
- Malodorous, purulent discharge (suggesting secondary bacterial infection)
- Black eschar around and over the lesion

Four stages of pressure ulcers

To protect the patient from pressure ulcer complications, learn to recognize the four stages of ulcer formation.

STAGE I

The skin is red and intact and doesn't blanch with external pressure. (A black person's skin may look purple.) The skin feels warm and firm. Usually, the sore reverses after pressure is removed.

STAGE II

Skin breaks appear and discoloration may occur. Penetrating to the subcutaneous fat layer, the sore is painful and visibly swollen. The ulcer may be characterized as an abrasion, blister, or shallow crater. If pressure is removed, the sore may heal within 1 to 2 weeks.

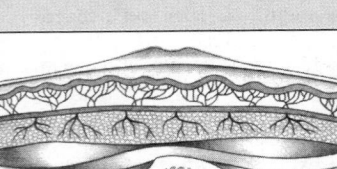

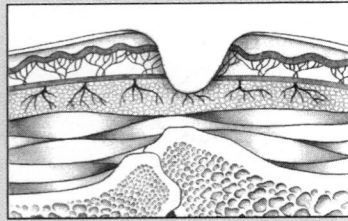

STAGE III

A hole develops that oozes foul-smelling yellow or green fluid. The ulcer extends into the muscle and may develop a black, leathery crust, or eschar, at its edges and eventually, at the center. Undermining may be present. The ulcer isn't painful, but healing may take months.

STAGE IV

The ulcer destroys tissue from the skin to the bone and becomes necrotic. Findings include foul drainage and deep tunnels that extend from the ulcer. The ulcer may take months or even a year to heal.

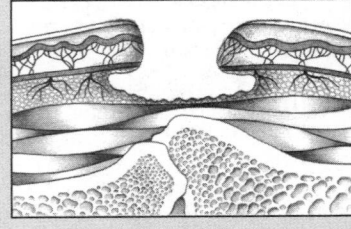

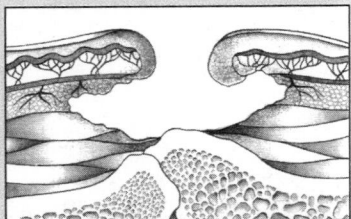

DIAGNOSTIC TEST RESULTS

LABORATORY
- Infecting organism is identified by wound culture and sensitivity testing of exudate.
- Total serum protein is decreased.

OTHER
- Diagnosis is typically made from inspection.

TREATMENT

GENERAL
- Measures to prevent pressure ulcers
- Relief of pressure on the affected area
- Meticulous skin care
- Devices such as pads, mattresses, and special beds
- Moist wound therapy dressings
- Whirlpool baths

DIET
- High in protein, iron, and vitamin C (unless contraindicated)

ACTIVITY
- As tolerated
- Active and passive range-of-motion (ROM) exercises
- Frequent turning and repositioning

MEDICATIONS
- Enzymatic ointments
- Healing ointments
- Antibiotics if indicated

SURGERY
- Debridement of necrotic tissue
- Skin grafting (in severe cases)

NURSING CONSIDERATIONS

NURSING DIAGNOSES
- Imbalanced nutrition: Less than body requirements
- Impaired physical mobility
- Impaired skin integrity
- Impaired tissue integrity
- Risk for infection

EXPECTED OUTCOMES
The patient will:
- maintain adequate daily caloric intake
- maintain joint mobility and ROM
- exhibit improved or healed lesions or wounds
- have reduced redness, swelling, and pain at the site of impaired tissue
- avoid infection and other complications.

NURSING INTERVENTIONS
- Give prescribed drugs.
- Apply dressings appropriate for the ulcer stage.
- Encourage adequate food and fluid intake.
- Reposition the bedridden patient at least every 2 hours.
- Elevate the head of the bed 30 degrees or less.
- Perform passive ROM exercises.
- Encourage active ROM exercises if possible.
- Use pressure-relief aids on the bed.
- Provide meticulous skin care.

MONITORING
- Changes in skin color, turgor, temperature, sensation, and drainage
- Change in the ulcer stage
- Laboratory results
- Complications
- Response to treatment
- Intake and output

PATIENT TEACHING

GENERAL
Be sure to cover:
- disorder, diagnosis, and treatment
- techniques for changing positions
- active and passive ROM exercises
- avoidance of skin-damaging agents
- debridement procedures
- skin graft surgery if required
- signs and stages of healing
- importance of a well-balanced diet and adequate fluid intake
- drug administration, dosage, and possible adverse effects
- importance of reporting signs and symptoms of infection to the practitioner.

DISCHARGE PLANNING
- Refer the patient to a wound care specialist if indicated.

RESOURCES
Organizations
American Academy of Dermatology: *www.aad.org*
Dermatology Foundation: *www.dermfnd.org*
National Decubitus Foundation: *www.decubitus.org*

Selected references
Domini, L.M., et al. "Nutritional Status and Evolution of Pressure Sores in Geriatric Patients," *Journal of Nutrition, Health & Aging* 9(6):446-54, November-December 2005.

Jones, J. "Evaluation of Pressure Ulcer Prevention Devices: A Critical Review of the Literature," *Journal of Wound Care* 14(9):422-25, October 2005.

Lepisto, M., et al. "Developing a Pressure Ulcer Risk Assessment Scale for Patients in Long-term Care," *Ostomy/Wound Management* 52(2):34-46, February 2006.

Moore, Z. "Pressure Ulcer Grading," *Nursing Standard* 19(52):56-64, September 2005.

Thomas, D.R. "Prevention and Treatment of Pressure Ulcers," *Journal of the American Medical Directors Association* 7(1):46-59, January-February 2006.

Prostate cancer

OVERVIEW

- Proliferation of cancer cells that usually take the form of adenocarcinomas and typically originate in the posterior prostate gland
- May progress to widespread bone metastasis and death
- Leading cause of cancer death in men

PATHOPHYSIOLOGY

- Slow-growing prostatic cancer seldom causes signs and symptoms until it's well advanced.
- Typically, when a primary prostatic lesion spreads beyond the prostate gland, it invades the prostatic capsule and spreads along ejaculatory ducts in the space between the seminal vesicles or perivesicular fascia.
- Endocrine factors may play a role, leading researchers to suspect that androgens speed tumor growth.
- Malignant prostatic tumors seldom result from the benign hyperplastic enlargement that commonly develops around the prostatic urethra in older men.

CAUSES

- Unknown

RISK FACTORS

- Older than age 40
- Infection
- Vasectomy
- Family history
- Heavy metal exposure

INCIDENCE

- Prostate cancer is most common in Blacks; least common in Asians.
- The incidence isn't affected by socioeconomic status or fertility.
- It's the most common tumor found in men older than age 50.

COMPLICATIONS

- Spinal cord compression
- Deep vein thrombosis
- Pulmonary emboli
- Myelophthisis
- Death

ASSESSMENT

HISTORY

- Symptoms rare in early stages
- Later, urinary problems, such as difficulty initiating a urinary stream, dribbling, and urine retention

PHYSICAL FINDINGS

- In early stages: nonraised, firm, nodular mass with a sharp edge
- In advanced disease: edema of the scrotum or leg; a hard lump in the prostate region

DIAGNOSTIC TEST RESULTS

LABORATORY

- Serum prostate-specific antigen (PSA) level is elevated (may indicate cancer with or without metastasis).

IMAGING

- Transrectal prostatic ultrasonography shows prostate size and presence of abnormal growths.
- Bone scan and excretory urography determines the disease's extent.
- Magnetic resonance imaging and computed tomography scan defines the extent of the tumor.

OTHER

- Digital rectal examination and PSA test identify cancer (recommended yearly by the American Cancer Society for men older than age 40).

TREATMENT

GENERAL
- Varies with cancer stage
- Radiation therapy or internal beam radiation

DIET
- Well-balanced

MEDICATIONS
- Hormonal therapy
- Chemotherapy

SURGERY
- Prostatectomy
- Orchiectomy
- Radical prostatectomy
- Transurethral resection of prostate
- Cryosurgical ablation

NURSING CONSIDERATIONS

NURSING DIAGNOSES
- Acute pain
- Anxiety
- Fear
- Impaired urinary elimination
- Ineffective coping
- Risk for infection
- Sexual dysfunction

EXPECTED OUTCOMES
The patient will:
- express feelings of increased comfort
- use support systems to assist with anxiety and fear
- verbalize fears and concerns
- maintain an adequate urine output
- demonstrate effective coping mechanisms
- remain free from signs and symptoms of infection
- express feelings about potential or actual changes in sexual activity.

NURSING INTERVENTIONS
- Give prescribed drugs.
- Encourage the patient to express his feelings.
- Provide emotional support.

MONITORING
- Pain level
- Wound site
- Postoperative complications
- Medication effects

PATIENT TEACHING

GENERAL
Be sure to cover:
- the disorder, diagnosis, and treatment
- perineal exercises that decrease incontinence
- follow-up care
- drug administration, dosage, and possible adverse effects.

DISCHARGE PLANNING
- Refer the patient to appropriate resources and support services.

RESOURCES
Organizations
American Cancer Society:
www.cancer.org
Guide to Internet Resources for Cancer:
www.cancerindex.org
National Cancer Institute:
www.cancer.gov

Selected references
Atlas of Pathophysiology, 2nd ed. Philadelphia: Lippincott Williams & Wilkins, 2005.

Baillargeon, J., and Rose, D.P. "Obesity, Adipokines, and Prostate Cancer (Review)," *International Journal of Oncology* 28(3):737-45, March 2006.

Mitchell, R.E., et al. "Does Year of Radical Prostatectomy Independently Predict Outcome in Prostate Cancer?" *Urology* 67(2):368-72, February 2006.

Nishiyama, T., et al. "Stepping-Stone to the Further Advancement of Androgen-Deprivation Therapy for Prostate Cancer," *Expert Review of Anticancer Therapy* 6(2):259-68, February 2006.

Yu, G., et al. "CSR1 Suppresses Tumor Growth and Metastasis of Prostate Cancer," *American Journal of Pathology* 168(2):597-607, February 2006.

Prostatitis

- Inflammation of the prostate gland
- Occurs in acute, chronic, and several other forms

ACUTE PROSTATITIS
- Easily recognized and treated

CHRONIC PROSTATITIS
- Most common cause of recurrent urinary tract infection (UTI) in men
- More difficult to recognize than acute prostatitis

OTHER PROSTATITIS FORMS
- Granulomatous prostatitis (also called *tuberculous prostatitis*)
- Nonbacterial prostatitis
- Prostatodynia (painful prostate)

PATHOPHYSIOLOGY
- Infectious organism spreads to the prostate gland by the hematogenous route, an ascending urethral infection, invasion of rectal bacteria via lymphatic vessels, or reflux of infected bladder urine into prostate ducts.
- Inflammation results.

CAUSES
- Bacterial prostatitis: *Escherichia coli* (80% of cases); *Klebsiella, Enterobacter, Proteus, Pseudomonas, Serratia, Streptococcus, Staphylococcus,* and diphtheroids (20% of cases)
- Chronic prostatitis: bacterial invasion from urethra
- Granulomatous prostatitis: miliary spread of *Mycobacterium tuberculosis*
- Nonbacterial prostatitis: *Mycoplasma, Ureaplasma, Chlamydia,* or *Trichomonas vaginalis,* or a virus
- Prostatodynia: unknown

RISK FACTORS
- Invasive urethral procedures
- Infrequent or excessive sexual intercourse

INCIDENCE
- Chronic prostatitis affects up to 35% of men older than age 50.
- Chronic prostatitis and nonbacterial prostatitis are each diagnosed in 5 of 1,000 outpatients.
- Bacterial prostatitis is diagnosed in 2 of 10,000 outpatients.

COMPLICATIONS
- UTI
- Prostatic abscess
- Acute urine retention
- Pyelonephritis
- Epididymitis

HISTORY
- Sudden fever, chills
- Lower back pain
- Perineal fullness
- Arthralgia, myalgia
- Urinary urgency and frequency
- Dysuria, nocturia
- Transient erectile dysfunction

Chronic bacterial prostatitis
- May not produce symptoms
- Usually causes same urinary symptoms as the acute form, but to a lesser degree
- Hemospermia
- Persistent urethral discharge
- Painful ejaculation

Nonbacterial prostatitis
- Dysuria
- Mild perineal or lower back pain
- Frequent nocturia

Prostatodynia
- Perineal, lower back, or pelvic pain

PHYSICAL FINDINGS
- Cloudy urine
- Distended bladder
- Prostatic tenderness, induration, swelling, firmness, and warmth
- Crepitation (if prostatic calculi present)

Chronic bacterial prostatitis
- Stony, hard induration of the prostate

LABORATORY
- Urine culture identifies infectious organism.
- In nonbacterial prostatitis, inflammatory cells are found in smears of prostatic secretion.
- In prostatodynia, negative urine cultures and absence of inflammatory cells are found in smears of prostatic secretions.

DIAGNOSTIC PROCEDURES
- In granulomatous prostatitis: prostate tissue biopsy shows *M. tuberculosis.*
- Urodynamic evaluation reveals detrusor hyperreflexia and pelvic floor myalgia (from chronic spasms).

OTHER
- Rectal examination findings may suggest prostatitis.

TREATMENT

GENERAL
- Sitz baths
- Prostatic massage

DIET
- Increased oral fluids

ACTIVITY
- Bed rest until the condition improves
- Regular, protected sexual intercourse

After surgery
- Avoidance of lifting, strenuous exercise, and long automobile rides
- No sexual activity for several weeks after discharge

MEDICATIONS
- Analgesics
- Antipyretics

Acute prostatitis
- Systemic antibiotic therapy

Chronic prostatitis
- Oral antibiotics

Granulomatous prostatitis
- Antitubercular drug combinations

Nonbacterial prostatitis
- Oral antibiotics
- Anticholinergics

Prostatodynia
- Muscle relaxants
- Alpha-adrenergic blocking agents

SURGERY
- Transurethral resection of the prostate or total prostatectomy, if drug therapy unsuccessful

NURSING CONSIDERATIONS

NURSING DIAGNOSES
- Acute pain
- Impaired urinary elimination
- Ineffective coping
- Ineffective sexuality patterns
- Risk for infection
- Sexual dysfunction
- Situational low self-esteem

EXPECTED OUTCOMES
The patient will:
- express feelings of increased comfort
- demonstrate skill in managing urinary elimination problems
- use available counseling, referrals, or support groups
- resume sexual activity to the fullest extent possible
- remain free from signs or symptoms of infection
- express his feelings about potential or actual changes in sexual activity
- express feelings related to self-esteem.

NURSING INTERVENTIONS
- Give prescribed drugs.
- Ensure bed rest and adequate hydration.
- Give sitz baths.
- Avoid rectal examinations.

MONITORING
After surgery
- Intake and output
- Catheter function and drainage
- Signs of infection
- Pain control

PATIENT TEACHING

GENERAL
Be sure to cover:
- the disorder, diagnosis, and treatment
- drug administration, dosage, and possible adverse effects
- importance of increased fluid intake
- benefits of regular sexual activity (with chronic prostatitis)
- prescribed activity limits
- importance of getting immediate medical attention for fever, inability to void, or bloody urine.

RESOURCES
Organizations
American Association of Kidney Patients: *www.aakp.org*
National Institute of Diabetes & Digestive & Kidney Diseases: *www.niddk.nih.gov*

Selected references
Chen, W.M., et al. "Combination Regimen in the Treatment of Chronic Prostatitis," *Archives of Andrology* 52(2):117-21, March-April 2006.
Diseases, 4th ed. Philadelphia: Lippincott Williams & Wilkins, 2006.
Habermacher, G.M., et al. "Prostatitis/Chronic Pelvic Pain Syndrome," *Annual Review of Medicine* 57:195-206, 2006.
Propert, K.J., et al. "A Prospective Study of Symptoms and Quality of Life in Men with Chronic Prostatitis/Chronic Pelvic Pain Syndrome: The National Institutes of Health Chronic Prostatitis Cohort Study," *Journal of Urology* 175(2):619-23, February 2006.

Pseudomembranous enterocolitis

OVERVIEW

- Acute inflammation and necrosis of the small and large intestines
- Usually affects the mucosa but may extend into the submucosa and, rarely, into other layers
- Marked by severe diarrhea
- Can be fatal in 1 to 7 days from severe dehydration or from toxicity, peritonitis, or perforation

PATHOPHYSIOLOGY

- Pseudomembranous enterocolitis is associated with antibiotic use.
- The balance of normal intestinal flora is altered, permitting an overgrowth of certain organisms.
- Necrotic mucosa is replaced by a pseudomembrane filled with staphylococci, leukocytes, mucus, fibrin, and inflammatory cells.

CAUSES

- Unknown
- Possible role of *Clostridium difficile*

RISK FACTORS

- Antibiotic therapy
- Recent abdominal surgery
- Cancer chemotherapy
- Compromised immune system
- Advanced age
- Bone-marrow transplantation
- Intestinal ischemia
- Uremia
- Burns

INCIDENCE

- The disorder affects both sexes equally.
- It's most common in nursing home and hospital patients.
- It affects 6 of 100,000 people treated with antibiotics.

COMPLICATIONS

- Severe dehydration
- Electrolyte imbalance
- Hemorrhage
- Hypotension
- Hypovolemia
- Sepsis
- Shock
- Colonic perforation
- Peritonitis
- Toxic megacolon
- Death

ASSESSMENT

HISTORY

- Current or recent antibiotic treatment
- Sudden onset of copious, watery, or bloody diarrhea
- Cramping abdominal pain
- Low-grade fever
- Nausea
- Vomiting

PHYSICAL FINDINGS

- Abdominal tenderness

DIAGNOSTIC TEST RESULTS

LABORATORY

- White blood cell count is elevated.
- Hypoalbuminemia is present.
- Stool culture identifies *C. difficile*.

IMAGING

- Abdominal X-ray reveals mucosal edema.
- Computed tomography scan may show distention as well as diffuse and focal thickening of the colon wall.

DIAGNOSTIC PROCEDURES

- Rectal biopsy through sigmoidoscopy confirms pseudomembranous enterocolitis.
- Endoscopy reveals characteristic pseudomembranes.

TREATMENT

GENERAL
- Discontinuation of offending antibiotics
- Avoidance of opioids and antidiarrheals
- Supportive treatment
- I.V. fluids (if the condition is severe)
- Enteric precautions

DIET
- Nothing by mouth until bowel recovery occurs (if the condition is severe)

ACTIVITY
- Bed rest until recovery begins

MEDICATIONS
- Oral metronidazole or oral vancomycin
- Electrolyte replacement

SURGERY
- Diverting ileostomy or bowel resection (with perforation or toxic megacolon)
- Early subtotal colectomy

NURSING CONSIDERATIONS

NURSING DIAGNOSES
- Acute pain
- Deficient fluid volume
- Diarrhea
- Imbalanced nutrition: Less than body requirements
- Ineffective tissue perfusion: GI
- Risk for infection

EXPECTED OUTCOMES
The patient will:
- express feelings of increased comfort
- maintain normal fluid volume
- regain normal bowel function
- maintain adequate caloric intake
- exhibit signs of adequate GI perfusion
- remain free from signs and symptoms of infection.

NURSING INTERVENTIONS
- Give prescribed drugs and I.V. fluids.
- Keep the patient as comfortable as possible.
- Maintain precautions to prevent the infection from spreading to other patients.

MONITORING
- Vital signs
- Fluid and nutritional status
- Skin integrity
- Bowel function
- Electrolytes

PATIENT TEACHING

GENERAL
Be sure to cover:
- the disorder, diagnosis, and treatment
- drug administration, dosage, and possible adverse effects
- signs and symptoms of a recurrence
- importance of cautioning future prescribers (if the disorder was antibiotic-related).

RESOURCES
Organizations
Digestive Disease National Coalition: *www.ddnc.org*
National Digestive Diseases Information Clearinghouse: *www.niddk.nih.gov/health/digest/nddic.htm*

Selected references
Handbook of Diseases, 3rd ed. Philadelphia: Lippincott Williams & Wilkins, 2004.
McNally, P. *GI/Liver Secrets*, 3rd ed. Philadelphia: Hanley & Belfus, Inc., 2006.
Morales, C.R., et al. "Pseudomembranous Colitis Associated with Chemotherapy with 5-Fluorouracil," *Clinical & Translational Oncology* 7(6):358-61, July 2005.
Tierney, L., et al. *Current Medical Diagnosis & Treatment 2006*. New York: McGraw-Hill Book Co., 2006.
Wolf, P.L., and Kasyan, A. "Images in Clinical Medicine. Pseudomembranous Colitis Associated with Clostridium Difficile," *New England Journal of Medicine* 353(23):2491, December 2005.

Psoriasis

- Hereditary chronic skin disease marked by epidermal proliferation
- Causes lesions of erythematous papules and plaques covered with silvery scales (Lesions vary widely in severity and distribution.)
- Involves recurring remissions and exacerbations
- Exacerbations unpredictable, but usually controllable with therapy

PATHOPHYSIOLOGY

- Psoriatic skin cells have a shortened maturation time as they migrate from the basal membrane to the surface or stratum corneum.
- As a result, the stratum corneum develops thick, scaly plaques (the cardinal manifestation of psoriasis).

CAUSES

- Beta-hemolytic streptococci infection
- Genetic predisposition
- Physical trauma
- Possible autoimmune process

RISK FACTORS

- Pregnancy
- Endocrine changes
- Cold weather
- Emotional stress

INCIDENCE

- Psoriasis affects about 2% of people in the United States.
- The disorder affects both sexes equally.
- It can occur at any age.
- It's more common among whites.
- There are two periods of onset: early (young adulthood) and late (middle adulthood).

COMPLICATIONS

- Infection
- Altered self-image
- Social isolation
- Depression

HISTORY

- Family history of psoriasis
- Risk factors
- Pruritus and burning
- Arthritic symptoms such as morning joint stiffness
- Remissions and exacerbations

PHYSICAL FINDINGS

- Erythematous, well-demarcated papules and plaques covered with silver scales, typically appearing on the scalp, chest, elbows, knees, back, and buttocks
- In mild psoriasis: plaques scattered over a small skin area
- In moderate psoriasis: plaques more numerous and larger (up to several centimeters in diameter)
- In severe psoriasis: plaques covering at least one-half of the body
- Friable or adherent scales
- Fine bleeding points or Auspitz sign after attempts to remove scales
- Thin, erythematous guttate lesions, alone or with plaques, and with few scales (see *Identifying types of psoriasis*)
- Small indentations or pits, and yellow or brown discoloration of fingernails or toenails
- In severe cases, separation of nail from nail bed

LABORATORY

- Serum uric acid level is elevated.
- In early-onset familial psoriasis, human leukocyte antigens Cw6, B13, and Bw57 are found.

DIAGNOSTIC PROCEDURES

- Skin biopsy can help rule out other diseases.

Identifying types of psoriasis

Psoriasis occurs in various forms, ranging from one or two localized plaques that seldom require long-term medical attention to widespread lesions and crippling arthritis.

ERYTHRODERMIC PSORIASIS

This type is marked by extensive flushing all over the body, which may result in scaling. The rash may develop rapidly, signaling new psoriasis or gradually in chronic psoriasis. Sometimes the rash occurs as an adverse drug reaction.

GUTTATE PSORIASIS

This type typically affects children and young adults. Erupting in drop-size plaques over the trunk, arms, legs and, sometimes, the scalp, this rash generalizes in several days. It's commonly associated with upper respiratory streptococcal infections.

INVERSE PSORIASIS

Smooth, dry, bright-red plaques characterize inverse psoriasis. Located in skin folds (armpits and groin, for example), the plaques fissure easily.

PSORIASIS VULGARIS

This psoriasis type is the most common. It begins with red, dotlike lesions that gradually enlarge and produce dry, silvery scales. The plaques usually appear symmetrically on the knees, elbows, extremities, genitalia, scalp, and nails.

PUSTULAR PSORIASIS

This type features an eruption of local or extensive small, raised, pus-filled plaques. Possible triggers include emotional stress, sweating, infections, and adverse drug reactions.

TREATMENT

GENERAL
- Depends on the psoriasis type, extent, and effect on the patient's quality of life
- Lesion management
- Lukewarm baths
- Ultraviolet B light or natural sunlight
- Smoking cessation
- Avoidance of aggravating medications

DIET
- No alcohol

MEDICATIONS
- Topical corticosteroid creams and ointments
- Antihistamines
- Analgesics
- Nonsteroidal anti-inflammatory agents
- Occlusive ointment bases
- Urea or salicylic acid preparations
- Coal tar preparations
- Vitamin D analogs
- Emollients
- Kerolytic agents
- Methotrexate for severe, unresponsive psoriasis
- Potent retinoic acid derivative for resistant psoriasis
- Cyclosporine for severe, widespread psoriasis

SURGERY
- Surgical nail removal to treat severely disfigured or damaged nails caused by psoriasis

NURSING CONSIDERATIONS

NURSING DIAGNOSES
- Acute pain
- Disturbed body image
- Impaired skin integrity
- Ineffective therapeutic regimen management
- Powerlessness
- Social isolation

EXPECTED OUTCOMES
The patient will:
- report feelings of increased comfort
- verbalize feelings about changed body image
- exhibit improved or healed lesions
- demonstrate understanding of proper skin care regimen
- express feelings of control over his condition and well-being
- maintain family and peer relationships.

NURSING INTERVENTIONS
- Give prescribed drugs.
- Apply topical medications using a downward motion.
- Encourage the patient to verbalize his feelings.
- Provide emotional support.
- Involve family members in the treatment regimen.

MONITORING
- Response to treatment
- Lipid profile results
- Liver function tests
- Renal function
- Blood pressure
- Signs and symptoms of hepatic or bone marrow toxicity

PATIENT TEACHING

GENERAL
Be sure to cover:
- the disorder, diagnosis, and treatment
- risk factors
- incommunicability of psoriasis
- likelihood of exacerbations and remissions
- drug administration, dosage, and possible adverse effects
- how to apply prescribed ointments, creams, and lotions
- importance of avoiding scratching plaques
- measures to relieve pruritus
- importance of avoiding sun exposure
- stress-reduction techniques
- safety precautions
- relationship between psoriasis and arthritis
- when to notify the practitioner.

DISCHARGE PLANNING
- Refer the patient to the National Psoriasis Foundation.

RESOURCES
Organizations
National Psoriasis Foundation:
www.psoriasis.org
The Psoriasis Association:
www.psoriasis-association.org.uk
Psoriasis Support:
www.psoriasissupport.com

Selected references
Cooper, M. "Diseases of the Epidermis: Psoriasis," *Dermatology Nursing* 17(5):381, October 2005.

Melton, L.P. "Psoriasis in the War Zone," *AJN* 105(3):52-56, March 2005.

Nemeth, M., et al. "Psoriatic Arthritis: A Holistic Approach to Management," *Advance for Nurse Practitioners* 13(11):29-34, November 2005.

Van de Kerkhof, P.C. "Perceptions on the Treatment of Psoriasis," *Journal of Dermatological Treatment* 16(5-6):255-56, 2005.

Pulmonary edema LIFE-THREATENING DISORDER

OVERVIEW

- Accumulation of fluid in the extravascular spaces of the lung
- Common complication of cardiovascular disorders
- May be chronic or acute
- Can become fatal rapidly

PATHOPHYSIOLOGY

- Pulmonary edema results from either increased pulmonary capillary hydrostatic pressure or decreased colloid osmotic pressure. Normally, the two pressures are in balance.
- If pulmonary capillary hydrostatic pressure increases, the compromised left ventricle needs higher filling pressures to maintain adequate output; these pressures are transmitted to the left atrium, pulmonary veins, and pulmonary capillary bed. Fluids and solutes are then forced from the intravascular compartment into the lung interstitium. With fluid overloading the interstitium, some fluid floods peripheral alveoli and impairs gas exchange.
- If colloid osmotic pressure decreases, the pulling force that contains intravascular fluids is lost, and nothing opposes the hydrostatic force. Fluid flows freely into the interstitium and alveoli, causing pulmonary edema.

CAUSES

- Heart disease or injury
- Lung disease or injury

RISK FACTORS

- Acute myocardial ischemia and infarction
- Arrhythmias
- Barbiturate or opiate poisoning
- Diastolic dysfunction
- Fluid overload
- Impaired pulmonary lymphatic drainage
- Inhalation of irritating gases
- Left atrial myxoma
- Left-sided heart failure
- Pneumonia
- Pulmonary veno-occlusive disease
- Valvular heart disease

INCIDENCE

- Pulmonary edema is more common in middle-aged and elderly people.
- It can affect both sexes equally.

COMPLICATIONS

- Respiratory and metabolic acidosis
- Cardiac or respiratory arrest
- Death

ASSESSMENT

HISTORY

- Predisposing risk factor
- Persistent cough
- Dyspnea on exertion
- Paroxysmal nocturnal dyspnea
- Orthopnea

PHYSICAL FINDINGS

- Restlessness and anxiety
- Rapid, labored breathing
- Intense, productive cough
- Frothy, bloody sputum
- Mental status changes
- Jugular vein distention
- Sweaty, cold, clammy skin
- Wheezing
- Crackles
- S_3
- Tachycardia
- Hypotension
- Thready pulse
- Peripheral edema
- Hepatomegaly

DIAGNOSTIC TEST RESULTS

LABORATORY

- Arterial blood gas (ABG) analysis shows hypoxemia, hypercapnia, or acidosis.

IMAGING

- Chest X-rays show diffuse haziness of the lung fields, cardiomegaly, and pleural effusion.

DIAGNOSTIC PROCEDURES

- Pulse oximetry may show decreased oxygen saturation.
- Pulmonary artery catheterization may reveal increased pulmonary artery wedge pressures.
- Electrocardiography may show valvular disease and left ventricular hypokinesis or akinesis.

TREATMENT

GENERAL
- Fluid overload reduction
- Improved gas exchange and myocardial function
- Correction of underlying condition
- Mechanical ventilation

DIET
- Sodium-restricted
- Fluid restriction

ACTIVITY
- As tolerated

MEDICATIONS
- Supplemental oxygen
- Diuretics
- Antiarrhythmics
- Morphine

⚡ **WARNING** *Be aware that morphine can further compromise respirations in a patient with respiratory distress. Keep resuscitation equipment at hand in case the patient stops breathing.*

- Preload-reducing agents
- Afterload-reducing agents
- Bronchodilators
- Positive inotropic agents
- Vasopressors

SURGERY
- Valve repair or replacement or myocardial revascularization if appropriate to correct the underlying cause

NURSING CONSIDERATIONS

NURSING DIAGNOSES
- Anxiety
- Excess fluid volume
- Fear
- Impaired gas exchange
- Ineffective coping
- Ineffective tissue perfusion: Cardiopulmonary

EXPECTED OUTCOMES
The patient will:
- verbalize decreased anxiety and fear
- maintain adequate fluid balance
- discuss fears and concerns
- maintain adequate ventilation
- develop adequate coping mechanisms
- maintain adequate cardiac output and circulation.

NURSING INTERVENTIONS
- Give prescribed drugs and oxygen.
- Place the patient in high Fowler's position.
- Restrict fluids and sodium intake.
- Promote rest and relaxation.
- Provide emotional support.

MONITORING
- Vital signs
- Intake and output
- Daily weight
- Respiratory status
- Response to treatment
- Complications
- Heart rhythm
- ABG values
- Pulse oximetry values
- Hemodynamic values

PATIENT TEACHING

GENERAL
Be sure to cover:
- the disorder, diagnosis, and treatment
- drug administration, dosage, and possible adverse effects
- fluid and sodium restrictions
- daily weight
- signs and symptoms of fluid overload
- energy conservation strategies
- avoidance of alcohol
- when to notify the practitioner.

DISCHARGE PLANNING
- Refer the patient to a cardiac rehabilitation program if indicated
- Refer the patient to a smoking-cessation program if indicated.

RESOURCES
Organizations
American Thoracic Society: *www.thoracic.org*
National Heart, Lung, and Blood Institute: *www.nhlbi.nih.gov*

Selected references
Patroniti, N., et al. "Measurement of Pulmonary Edema in Patients with Acute Respiratory Distress Syndrome," *Critical Care Medicine* 33(11):2547-54, November 2005.

Poole, J.H., and Spreen, D.T. "Acute Pulmonary Edema in Pregnancy," *Journal of Perinatal & Neonatal Nursing* 19(4):316-31, October-December 2005.

Remo, E.F. "Heart Failure Management. Prevention of Pulmonary Edema is Essential," *Advance for Nurse Practitioners* 13(12):27-28, 30, 62, December 2005.

Ware, L.B., and Matthay, M.A. "Clinical Practice. Acute Pulmonary Edema," *New England Journal of Medicine* 353(26):2788-96, December 2005.

Pulmonary embolism
LIFE-THREATENING DISORDER

OVERVIEW

- Obstruction of the pulmonary arterial bed occurring when a mass (such as a dislodged thrombus) lodges in the main pulmonary artery or branch, partially or completely obstructing it
- Most thrombi originate in deep veins of the leg
- May not produce symptoms, but sometimes causes rapid death from pulmonary infarction

PATHOPHYSIOLOGY
- Thrombus formation results from vascular wall damage, venous stasis, or blood hypercoagulability.
- Trauma, clot dissolution, sudden muscle spasm, intravascular pressure changes, or peripheral blood flow changes can cause the thrombus to loosen or fragmentize.
- The thrombus (now an embolus) floats to the heart's right side and enters the lung through the pulmonary artery. There, the embolus may dissolve, continue to fragmentize, or grow.

- By occluding the pulmonary artery, the embolus prevents alveoli from producing enough surfactant to maintain alveolar integrity. Alveoli collapse and atelectasis develops.
- If the embolus enlarges, it may occlude most or all of the pulmonary vessels and cause death.

CAUSES
- Deep vein thrombosis
- Pelvic, renal, and hepatic vein thrombosis
- Rarely, other types of emboli, such as bone, air, fat, amniotic fluid, tumor cells, or a foreign body
- Right heart thrombus
- Upper extremity thrombosis
- Valvular heart disease

RISK FACTORS
- Various disorders and treatments (see *Who's at risk for pulmonary embolism?*)

INCIDENCE
- Pulmonary embolism develops in 600,000 to 700,000 people annually.
- It affects both sexes equally.

- It's more common with advancing age.

COMPLICATIONS
- Respiratory failure
- Pulmonary infarction
- Pulmonary hypertension
- Embolic extension
- Hepatic congestion and necrosis
- Pulmonary abscess
- Shock
- Acute respiratory distress syndrome
- Massive atelectasis
- Right-sided heart failure
- Ventilation-perfusion mismatch
- Death

ASSESSMENT

HISTORY
- Predisposing risk factor
- Shortness of breath for no apparent reason
- Pleuritic pain or angina

PHYSICAL FINDINGS
- Tachycardia
- Low-grade fever
- Weak, rapid pulse
- Hypotension
- Productive cough, possibly with blood-tinged sputum
- Warmth, tenderness, and edema of the lower leg
- Restlessness
- Transient pleural friction rub
- Crackles
- S_3 and S_4 with increased intensity of the pulmonic component of S_2
- With a large embolus: cyanosis, syncope, distended neck veins

DIAGNOSTIC TEST RESULTS

LABORATORY
- Arterial blood gas (ABG) values show hypoxemia.
- D-dimer level is elevated.

IMAGING
- Lung ventilation perfusion scan shows a ventilation-perfusion mismatch.

Who's at risk for pulmonary embolism?

Many disorders and treatments heighten the risk of pulmonary embolism. At particular risk are surgical patients. The anesthetic used during surgery can injure lung vessels, and surgery or prolonged bed rest can promote venous stasis, which compounds the risk.

PREDISPOSING DISORDERS
- Cardiac arrhythmia (especially atrial fibrillation)
- Lung disorders, especially chronic types
- Cardiac disorders
- Infection
- Diabetes mellitus
- History of thromboembolism, thrombophlebitis, or vascular insufficiency
- Sickle cell disease
- Autoimmune hemolytic anemia
- Polycythemia
- Osteomyelitis
- Long-bone fracture
- Manipulation or disconnection of central lines

VENOUS STASIS
- Prolonged bed rest or immobilization
- Obesity
- Older than age 40
- Burns
- Recent childbirth
- Orthopedic casts

VENOUS INJURY
- Surgery, particularly of the legs, pelvis, abdomen, or thorax
- Leg or pelvic fractures or injuries
- I.V. drug abuse
- I.V. therapy

INCREASED BLOOD COAGULABILITY
- Cancer
- Use of high-estrogen hormonal contraceptives

- Pulmonary angiography shows a pulmonary vessel filling defect or an abrupt vessel ending and reveals the location and extent of pulmonary embolism.
- Chest X-rays may show a small infiltrate or effusion.
- Spiral chest computed tomography scan may show central pulmonary emboli.

DIAGNOSTIC PROCEDURES
- Electrocardiography may reveal right axis deviation and right bundle-branch block; it also may show atrial fibrillation.

TREATMENT

GENERAL
- Maintenance of adequate cardiovascular and pulmonary function
- Mechanical ventilation if indicated

DIET
- Possible fluid restriction

ACTIVITY
- Bed rest during the acute phase

MEDICATIONS
- Oxygen therapy
- Thrombolytics
- Anticoagulation
- Corticosteroids (controversial)
- Diuretics
- Antiarrhythmics
- Vasopressors (for hypotension)
- Antibiotics (for septic embolus)

SURGERY
- Vena caval interruption
- Vena caval filter placement
- Pulmonary embolectomy

NURSING CONSIDERATIONS

NURSING DIAGNOSES
- Acute pain
- Anxiety
- Decreased cardiac output
- Fear

- Imbalanced nutrition: Less than body requirements
- Impaired gas exchange
- Ineffective airway clearance
- Ineffective coping
- Ineffective tissue perfusion: Cardiopulmonary
- Risk for injury

EXPECTED OUTCOMES
The patient will:
- verbalize feelings of increased comfort and relief of pain
- identify strategies to reduce anxiety
- maintain adequate cardiac output
- discuss fears and concerns
- consume required daily caloric intake
- maintain adequate ventilation and oxygenation
- maintain a patent airway
- use support systems to assist with coping
- maintain adequate cardiopulmonary perfusion
- remain free from complications.

NURSING INTERVENTIONS
- Give prescribed drugs.
- Avoid I.M. injections.
- Encourage active and passive range-of-motion exercises, unless contraindicated.
- Avoid massage of the lower legs.
- Apply antiembolism stockings.
- Provide adequate nutrition.
- Assist with ambulation as soon as the patient is stable.
- Encourage use of incentive spirometry.

MONITORING
- Vital signs
- Intake and output
- Respiratory status
- Pulse oximetry
- ABG values
- Signs of deep vein thrombosis
- Complications
- Coagulation study results
- Abnormal bleeding
- Stools for occult blood

PATIENT TEACHING

GENERAL
Be sure to cover:
- the disease, diagnosis, and treatment
- drug administration, dosage, and possible adverse effects
- ways to prevent deep vein thrombosis and pulmonary embolism
- signs and symptoms of abnormal bleeding
- prevention of abnormal bleeding
- how to monitor anticoagulant effects
- dietary sources of vitamin K
- when to notify the practitioner.

DISCHARGE PLANNING
- Refer the patient to a weight-management program, if indicated.

RESOURCES
Organizations
American Lung Association: *www.lungusa.org*
National Heart, Lung, and Blood Institute: *www.nhlbi.nih.gov*

Selected references
Bonde, P., and Graham, A. "Surgical Management of Pulmonary Embolism," *Journal of Thoracic and Cardiovascular Surgery* 131(2):503-04, February 2006.
Kucher, N., et al. "Massive Pulmonary Embolism," *Circulation* 113(4):577-82, January 2006.
Roy, P.M., et al. "Appropriateness of Diagnostic Management and Outcomes of Suspected Pulmonary Embolism," *Annals of Internal Medicine* 144(3):157-64, February 2006.
Yang, J.C. "Prevention and Treatment of Deep Vein Thrombosis and Pulmonary Embolism in Critically Ill Patients," *Critical Care Nursing Quarterly* 28(1):72-79, January-March 2005.

Pulmonary hypertension LIFE-THREATENING DISORDER

OVERVIEW

- Pulmonary condition in which there's increased pressure in the pulmonary artery
- Occurs in a primary form (rare) and a secondary form
- In both forms, resting systolic pulmonary artery pressure (PAP) above 30 mm Hg and mean PAP above 20 mm Hg
- Primary form also known as *PPH*

PATHOPHYSIOLOGY

- In primary pulmonary hypertension, the intimal lining of the pulmonary arteries thickens for no apparent reason. This narrows the artery and impairs distensibility, increasing vascular resistance.
- Secondary pulmonary hypertension occurs from hypoxemia caused by conditions involving alveolar hypoventilation, vascular obstruction, or left-to-right shunting.

CAUSES
Primary pulmonary hypertension
- Unknown
- Associated with portal hypertension
- Possible altered autoimmune mechanisms
- Possible hereditary factors

Secondary pulmonary hypertension
- Lung disease

RISK FACTORS
Secondary pulmonary hypertension
- Chronic obstructive pulmonary disease
- Congenital cardiac defects
- Diffuse interstitial pneumonia
- Hypoventilation syndromes
- Kyphoscoliosis
- Left atrial myxoma
- Malignant metastasis
- Mitral stenosis
- Obesity
- Pulmonary embolism
- Sarcoidosis
- Scleroderma
- Sleep apnea
- Use of some diet drugs
- Vasculitis

INCIDENCE

- Primary pulmonary hypertension is most common in women ages 20 to 40.
- It's more prevalent in people with collagen disease.

COMPLICATIONS
- Cor pulmonale
- Heart failure
- Cardiac arrest
- Death

ASSESSMENT

HISTORY
- Shortness of breath with exertion
- Weakness, fatigue
- Pain during breathing
- Near-syncope

PHYSICAL FINDINGS
- Ascites
- Jugular vein distention
- Peripheral edema
- Restlessness and agitation
- Mental status changes
- Decreased diaphragmatic excursion
- Apical impulse displaced beyond mid-clavicular line
- Right ventricular lift
- Reduced carotid pulse
- Hepatomegaly
- Tachycardia
- Systolic ejection murmur
- Widely split S_2
- S_3 and S_4
- Hypotension
- Decreased breath sounds
- Tubular breath sounds

DIAGNOSTIC TEST RESULTS

LABORATORY
- Arterial blood gas (ABG) values show hypoxemia.

IMAGING
- Ventilation-perfusion lung scan may show a ventilation-perfusion mismatch.
- Pulmonary angiography may reveal filling defects in the pulmonary vasculature.

DIAGNOSTIC PROCEDURES
- Electrocardiography may reveal right-axis deviation.
- Pulmonary artery catheterization shows increased PAP, with systolic pressure above 30 mm Hg; increased pulmonary artery wedge pressure; decreased cardiac output; and decreased cardiac index.
- Pulmonary function tests may show decreased flow rates and increased residual volume or reduced total lung capacity.
- Echocardiography may show valvular heart disease or atrial myxoma.

OTHER
- Lung biopsy may show tumor cells.

TREATMENT

GENERAL
- Based on underlying disease
- Symptom relief
- Smoking cessation

DIET
- Low-sodium
- Fluid restriction (in right-sided heart failure)

ACTIVITY
- Bed rest during acute phase

MEDICATIONS
- Oxygen therapy
- Cardiac glycosides
- Diuretics
- Vasodilators
- Calcium channel blockers
- Bronchodilators
- Beta-adrenergic blockers
- Epoprostenol

SURGERY
- Heart-lung transplantation if indicated

NURSING CONSIDERATIONS

NURSING DIAGNOSES
- Activity intolerance
- Anxiety
- Decreased cardiac output
- Fatigue
- Fear
- Impaired gas exchange
- Ineffective coping

EXPECTED OUTCOMES
The patient will:
- demonstrate skill in conserving energy while carrying out daily activities to tolerance level
- verbalize strategies to reduce anxiety
- maintain adequate cardiac output
- express feelings of energy and decreased fatigue
- discuss fears and concerns
- maintain adequate ventilation and oxygenation
- use support systems to assist with coping.

NURSING INTERVENTIONS
- Give prescribed drugs and oxygen.
- Implement comfort measures.
- Provide adequate rest periods.
- Offer emotional support.

MONITORING
- Vital signs
- Intake and output
- Daily weight
- Respiratory status
- Signs and symptoms of right-sided heart failure
- Heart rhythm
- ABG values
- Hemodynamic values

PATIENT TEACHING

GENERAL
Be sure to cover:
- the disorder, diagnosis, and treatment
- drug administration, dosage, and possible adverse effects
- dietary restrictions
- frequent rest periods
- signs and symptoms of right-sided heart failure
- when to notify the practitioner.

DISCHARGE PLANNING
- Refer the patient to a smoking-cessation program, if indicated.

RESOURCES
Organizations
American Lung Association: *www.lungusa.org*
American Thoracic Society: *www.thoracic.org*
National Heart, Lung, and Blood Institute: *www.nhlbi.nih.gov*

Selected references
Holcomb, S.S. "Understanding Pulmonary Arterial Hypertension," *Nursing* 34(9):50-54, September 2004.
Steinbis, S. "What You Should Know about Pulmonary Hypertension," *Nurse Practitioner* 29(4):8, April 2004.
Thistlethwaite, P.A., et al. "Outcomes of Pulmonary Endarterectomy for Treatment of Extreme Thromboembolic Pulmonary Hypertension," *Journal of Thoracic and Cardiovascular Surgery* 131(2):307-13, February 2006.

Pulmonary insufficiency

OVERVIEW

- Heart condition in which blood ejected into the pulmonary artery during systole flows back into the right ventricle during diastole
- Also called *pulmonary regurgitation*

PATHOPHYSIOLOGY
- Pulmonic valve is incompetent.
- Incompetency is caused by:
- dilation of the pulmonic valve ring
- acquired alteration of pulmonic cusp morphology
- congenital absence or malformation.
- Blood flows back into the right ventricle from the pulmonary artery.
- Fluid overload occurs in the ventricle.
- Chronic backflow causes ventricular hypertrophy and right-sided heart failure.

CAUSES
- Carcinoid heart disease
- Dilated cardiomyopathy
- Infective endocarditis
- Pulmonary hypertension
- Rheumatic heart disease
- Tetralogy of Fallot

INCIDENCE
- Pulmonary insufficiency occurs at various ages.
- Pulmonary insufficiency affects both males and females.

COMPLICATIONS
- Heart failure
- Pulmonary edema
- Thromboembolism
- Endocarditis
- Arrhythmias

ASSESSMENT

HISTORY
- Pulmonary hypertension
- Infective endocarditis
- Tetralogy of Fallot
- Rheumatic heart disease
- Carcinoid heart disease
- Orthopnea
- Dyspnea
- Fatigue
- Angina
- Palpitations

PHYSICAL FINDINGS
- Tachycardia
- Crackles in the lungs
- Hepatomegaly (right-sided failure)
- Jugular vein distention
- Palpable right ventricular systolic pulsation at left lower sternal border
- S_3 or S_4 at left mid-to-lower sternal border
- Hemoptysis

DIAGNOSTIC TEST RESULTS

IMAGING
- Chest X-rays reveal cardiomegaly, right-sided heart enlargement, and pulmonary hypertension.
- Echocardiography shows right ventricular hypertrophy and dilation.

DIAGNOSTIC PROCEDURES
- Electrocardiography may show incomplete right bundle-branch block and right axis deviation.
- Cardiac catheterization may determine underlying etiology.

TREATMENT

GENERAL
- Correction of underlying condition
- Symptom relief

DIET
- Low-sodium

ACTIVITY
- As tolerated

MEDICATIONS
- Diuretics
- Inotropic agent
- Angiotensin-converting enzyme inhibitors
- Oxygen
- Prophylactic antibiotics before and after surgery or dental care to prevent endocarditis

SURGERY
- Annuloplasty or valvuloplasty to reconstruct or repair the valve
- Valve replacement with a prosthetic valve

Identifying the murmur of pulmonary insufficiency

A high-pitched, blowing decrescendo murmur at Erb's point characterizes pulmonary insufficiency.

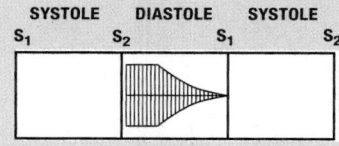

SYSTOLE	DIASTOLE	SYSTOLE	
S_1	S_2	S_1	S_2

NURSING CONSIDERATIONS

NURSING DIAGNOSES
- Activity intolerance
- Decreased cardiac output
- Excess fluid volume
- Fatigue
- Impaired gas exchange
- Impaired physical mobility
- Ineffective coping
- Ineffective tissue perfusion: Cardiopulmonary
- Risk for infection

EXPECTED OUTCOMES
The patient will:
- perform activities of daily living without weakness or fatigue
- maintain hemodynamic stability, have no arrhythmias, and maintain adequate cardiac output
- develop no complications of excess fluid volume
- verbalize the importance of balancing activity with adequate rest periods
- maintain adequate ventilation and oxygenation
- maintain joint mobility and range of motion
- demonstrate adaptive coping behaviors
- maintain adequate cardiopulmonary perfusion
- remain free from signs and symptoms of infection.

NURSING INTERVENTIONS
- Give prescribed oxygen.
- Watch for signs of heart failure or pulmonary edema.

MONITORING
- Vital signs and pulse oximetry
- Cardiac status (see *Identifying the murmur of pulmonary insufficiency*)
- Pulmonary artery catheter readings
- Intake and output
- Adverse effects of drug therapy

PATIENT TEACHING

GENERAL
Be sure to cover:
- the disorder, diagnosis, and treatment
- dietary restrictions
- drug administration, dosage, and possible adverse effects.

DISCHARGE PLANNING
- Encourage follow-up care with a cardiologist.

RESOURCES
Organizations
American Heart Association: *www.americanheart.org*
American Lung Association: *www.lungusa.org*
National Heart, Lung, and Blood Institute: *www.nhlbi.nih.gov*

Selected references
Bouzas, B., et al. "Pulmonary Regurgitation: Not a Benign Lesion," *European Heart Journal* 26(5):433-39, March 2005.
Davlouros, P.A., et al. "Timing and Type of Surgery for Severe Pulmonary Regurgitation after Repair of Tetralogy of Fallot," *International Journal of Cardiology* 97(Suppl 1):91-101, December 2004.
Diseases, 4th ed. Philadelphia: Lippincott Williams & Wilkins, 2006.
Gaynor, J.W. "Severe Pulmonary Insufficiency Should Be Conservatively Treated," *Cardiology in the Young* 15(Suppl 1):68-71, February 2005.

Pulmonary stenosis

OVERVIEW

- Heart condition in which obstructed right ventricular outflow causes right ventricular hypertrophy, eventually resulting in right-sided heart failure

PATHOPHYSIOLOGY

- Dynamic or fixed obstruction affects blood flow from the right ventricle to the pulmonary arteriole vasculature.
- Chronic obstruction may result in right-sided heart failure.

CAUSES

- Aortic graft aneurysm
- Carcinoid heart disease
- Congenital defect
- Rheumatic heart disease
- Sinus of Valsalva aneurysm

INCIDENCE

- Pulmonary stenosis affects females slightly more than males.

COMPLICATIONS

- Heart failure
- Pulmonary edema
- Thromboembolism
- Endocarditis
- Arrhythmias

ASSESSMENT

HISTORY

- Congenital defect
- Sinus of Valsalva aneurysm
- Aortic graft aneurysm
- Rheumatic heart disease
- Carcinoid heart disease
- Orthopnea
- Exertional dyspnea
- Fatigue
- Angina
- Palpitations

PHYSICAL FINDINGS

- Palpable impulse from the right ventricle along the left parasternal border
- Peripheral edema
- Split S_2
- Systolic ejection click
- Crackles in the lungs
- Hepatomegaly (right-sided failure)
- Jugular vein distention

DIAGNOSTIC TEST RESULTS

IMAGING

- Chest X-rays reveal prominence of the main, right, or left pulmonary arteries.
- Echocardiography shows thickening of the valves, characteristic doming of nondysplastic valves, and right ventricular hypertrophy.
- Cardiac ultrasonography reveals thickening of valves, characteristic doming of nondysplastic valves, and right-ventricular hypertrophy.

DIAGNOSTIC PROCEDURES

- Electrocardiography may show mild right axis deviation.

TREATMENT

GENERAL
- Based on underlying cause
- Symptom relief

DIET
- Low-sodium

ACTIVITY
- Avoidance of vigorous physical activity

MEDICATIONS
- Diuretics
- Inotropic agents
- Angiotensin-converting enzyme inhibitors
- Oxygen
- Prophylactic antibiotics before and after surgery or dental care to prevent endocarditis

SURGERY
- Balloon valvoplasty
- Pulmonary artery balloon angioplasty
- Valvotomy

Identifying the murmur of pulmonary stenosis

A medium-pitched, harsh crescendo-decrescendo murmur in the area of the pulmonary valve characterizes pulmonary stenosis.

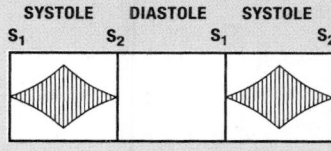

SYSTOLE	DIASTOLE	SYSTOLE
S₁	S₂	S₁ S₂

NURSING CONSIDERATIONS

NURSING DIAGNOSES
- Activity intolerance
- Decreased cardiac output
- Excess fluid volume
- Fatigue
- Impaired gas exchange
- Impaired physical mobility
- Ineffective coping
- Ineffective tissue perfusion: Cardiopulmonary
- Risk for infection

EXPECTED OUTCOMES
The patient will:
- perform activities of daily living without weakness or fatigue
- maintain hemodynamic stability, have no arrhythmias, and maintain adequate cardiac output
- develop no complications of excess fluid volume
- verbalize the importance of balancing activity with adequate rest periods
- maintain adequate ventilation and oxygenation
- maintain joint mobility and range of motion
- demonstrate adaptive coping behaviors
- maintain adequate cardiopulmonary perfusion
- remain free from signs and symptoms of infection.

NURSING INTERVENTIONS
- Give prescribed oxygen.
- Watch for signs of heart failure or pulmonary edema.
- Encourage verbalization and provide support.
- Give prescribed drugs.

MONITORING
- Vital signs and pulse oximetry
- Cardiac status (see *Identifying the murmur of pulmonary stenosis*)
- Pulmonary artery catheter readings
- Intake and output
- Adverse effects of drug therapy

PATIENT TEACHING

GENERAL
Be sure to cover:
- the disorder, diagnosis, and treatment
- dietary restrictions
- activity restrictions
- drug administration, dosage, and possible adverse effects.

DISCHARGE PLANNING
- Encourage follow-up care with a cardiologist.

RESOURCES
Organizations
American Heart Association: *www.americanheart.org*
American Lung Association: *www.lungusa.org*
National Heart, Lung, and Blood Institute: *www.nhlbi.nih.gov*

Selected references
Earing, M.G., et al. "Long-term Follow-up of Patients after Surgical Treatment for Isolated Pulmonary Valve Stenosis," *Mayo Clinic Proceedings* 80(7):871-76, July 2005.
Ross-Hesselink, J.W., et al. "Long-term Outcome after Surgery for Pulmonary Stenosis (A Longitudinal Study of 22-33 Years)," *European Heart Journal* 27(4):482-88, February 2006.
Ucar, T., et al. "Bilateral Coronary Artery Dilatation and Supravalvular Pulmonary Stenosis in a Child with Noonan Syndrome," *Pediatric Cardiology* 26(6):848-50, November-December 2005.

Q fever

- Acute systemic disease that affects people exposed to cattle, sheep, or goats
- Rare human-to-human transmission; possible sexual transmission
- May be acute or chronic

PATHOPHYSIOLOGY

- *Coxiella burnetii* is excreted in urine, milk, and feces of infected animals.
- Once ingested, it proliferates in macrophages (in the acidic phagolysosome vacuole) and then gains access to the blood, producing a transient bacteremia.
- It may invade many organs, most commonly the lungs and liver.
- Inflammation occurs, manifested by granulomas in the liver, spleen, and bone marrow. These classic doughnut-shaped granulomas disappear with convalescence.

CAUSES

- *Coxiella burnetii* infection

RISK FACTORS

- Prolonged or frequent exposure to animals
- Immunocompromised condition
- History of heart valve abnormality

INCIDENCE

- Q fever affects men more than women because men are more likely to be exposed to livestock.
- The disease most commonly affects people ages 25 to 40.

COMPLICATIONS

- Chronic fatigue syndrome
- Heart failure
- Endocarditis (see *Treating Q fever endocarditis*)
- Pneumonia
- Hepatitis

HISTORY

- Exposure to cattle, sheep, or goats
- Headache
- Mylagia
- Chills, fever

PHYSICAL FINDINGS

- Crackles (pneumonia)
- Hepatomegaly and jaundice (hepatitis)
- Heart murmur, signs of heart failure (endocarditis)

Treating Q fever endocarditis

Chronic Q fever endocarditis usually requires the use of multiple drugs to treat effectively. Two different drug treatment protocols have been evaluated:
- doxycycline with quinolones, for at least 4 years
- doxycycline with hydroxychloroquine, for 1½ to 3 years.

The second drug treatment protocol causes fewer relapses but requires routine eye examinations to detect accumulation of chloroquine.

Some patients with *Coxiella burnetii* endocarditis require surgery to remove damaged valves.

LABORATORY

- Patients with acute form may have an elevated white blood cell count, transient thrombocytopenia, and elevated transaminases and alkaline phosphatase.
- Cerebrospinal fluid evaluation reveals lymphocytosis, elevated protein level, and normal glucose level.
- Complement fixation reveals antephase II antibody titers of 40 or more (acute disease) and antiphase I antibody titers of 200 of more (chronic disease).
- Microimmunofluorescence reveals immunoglobulin (Ig) G antiphase II antibody titers of 200 or more and IgM antephase II antibody titers of 50 or more (acute). (The presence of antephase I antibodies indicates chronic Q fever; the presence of IgG antephase I antibody titers of 800 or more is highly predictive of endocarditis.)

IMAGING

- Chest X-rays may show segmental or lobar opacities, multiple round opacities, and pleural effusion.
- Echocardiography may show pericardial effusion with pericarditis.

DIAGNOSTIC PROCEDURES

- Electrocardiography shows T-wave abnormalities with myocarditis and pericarditis.

TREATMENT

GENERAL
- Symptom relief

DIET
- As tolerated

ACTIVITY
- As tolerated

MEDICATIONS
- Antibiotics
- Antimalarials

SURGERY
- Possible valve replacement

NURSING CONSIDERATIONS

NURSING DIAGNOSES
- Decreased cardiac output
- Fatigue
- Impaired gas exchange
- Risk for injury

EXPECTED OUTCOMES
The patient will:
- maintain adequate cardiac output and hemodynamic stability
- express feelings of increased energy and decreased fatigue
- maintain adequate ventilation and oxygenation
- avoid complications.

NURSING INTERVENTIONS
- Provide emotional support.
- Give prescribed drugs.

MONITORING
- Vital signs
- Cardiac status
- Respiratory status
- Response to treatment

PATIENT TEACHING

GENERAL
Be sure to cover:
- the disorder, diagnosis, and treatment
- the importance of follow-up care and compliance with long-term therapy
- dosage, administration, and possible adverse effects of prescribed medications.

RESOURCES
Organizations
Centers for Disease Control and Prevention Division of Viral and Rickettsial Diseases: *www.cdc.gov/ncidod/dvrd*

Selected references
Daya, M, and Nakamura, Y. "Pulmonary Disease from Biological Agents: Anthrax, Plague, Q fever, and Tularemia," *Critical Care Clinics* 21(4):747-63, vii, October 2005.

Milazzo, A., et al. "Q Fever Vaccine Uptake in South Australian Meat Processors Prior to the Introduction of the National Q Fever Management Program," *Communicable Diseases Intelligence* 29(4):400-06, 2005.

Reina-Serrano, S., et al. "Q Fever Related Cholecystitis: A Missed Entity?" *Lancet Infectious Diseases* 5(12):734-35, December 2005.

Tsironi, M., et al. "Acute Q Fever Lobar Pneumonia: A Case Report," *Journal of Infection* 51(3):e89-91, October 2005.

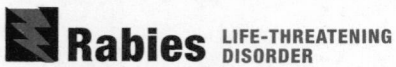

Rabies LIFE-THREATENING DISORDER

OVERVIEW

- An acute central nervous system (CNS) infection usually transmitted by animal bite
- Incubation period usually 20 to 90 days, possibly up to 19 years
- 70% of cases in the United States from raccoon, skunk, fox, or bat bite; vaccinations have reduced transmission from dogs
- Almost always fatal if symptoms occur, although prompt treatment may prevent fatal CNS invasion

PATHOPHYSIOLOGY

- The rabies virus is transmitted through the bite of an infected animal that introduces the virus through the skin or mucous membrane.
- The virus begins to replicate in the striated muscle cells at the bite site.
- It then travels up the nerves to the CNS and replicates in the brain.
- Finally, it moves through the nerves into other tissues, including the salivary glands.

CAUSES

- Airborne droplet transmission (occasionally)
- Bite from a rabid animal
- Infected tissue transplants (occasionally)

RISK FACTORS

- Occupation with exposure to potentially rabid animals
- Travel to areas with poor rabies control

INCIDENCE

- Rabies can affect anyone at any age.
- Annually, rabies causes an estimated 35,000 to 50,000 deaths worldwide.

COMPLICATIONS

- Paralysis
- Coma
- Death

ASSESSMENT

HISTORY

- Animal bite
- Fever
- Malaise

PHYSICAL FINDINGS

- Burning at wound site
- Tachycardia
- Excessive salivation
- Shallow respirations
- Dilated pupils and photophobia

DIAGNOSTIC TEST RESULTS

LABORATORY

- Virus is isolated from the patient's saliva or throat; examination of blood shows fluorescent rabies antibody (FRA).
- White blood cell count is elevated with increased polymorphonuclear and large mononuclear cells.
- Urinary glucose, acetone, and protein levels are elevated.

OTHER

- Animal should be confined and observed for 10 days by a veterinarian. (If the animal appears rabid, it should be killed and its brain tissues tested for FRA and Negri bodies.)

First aid for animal bites

- Immediately wash the bite vigorously with soap and water for at least 10 minutes to remove the animal's saliva.
- Flush the wound with an antiviral, followed by a clear-water rinse.
- Apply a sterile dressing.
- If possible, don't suture the wound, and don't immediately stop the bleeding (unless it's massive) because blood flow helps to clean the wound.
- Question the patient about the bite. Ask whether he provoked the animal (if so, chances are it isn't rabid) and whether he can identify it or its owner. (The animal may be confined for observation.)
- Consult local public health authorities for treatment information.

TREATMENT

GENERAL
- Immediate wound treatment (see *First aid for animal bites*)

MEDICATIONS
- Tetanus-diphtheria prophylaxis, if needed
- Passive immunization with rabies immune globulin and active immunization with human diploid cell vaccine as soon as possible (if not previously immunized)
- Vaccine booster (if already immunized)

NURSING CONSIDERATIONS

NURSING DIAGNOSES
- Anxiety
- Decreased cardiac output
- Hyperthermia
- Imbalanced nutrition: Less than body requirements
- Impaired swallowing
- Impaired tissue integrity
- Ineffective breathing pattern
- Risk for deficient fluid volume
- Risk for infection

EXPECTED OUTCOMES
The patient will:
- identify strategies to reduce anxiety
- maintain adequate cardiac output and hemodynamic stability
- remain afebrile
- achieve adequate nutritional intake
- swallow without pain or aspiration
- maintain tissue integrity with reduced redness and swelling
- maintain respiratory rate within 5 breaths/minute of baseline
- maintain normal fluid balance
- experience no further signs or symptoms of infection.

NURSING INTERVENTIONS
- When injecting the rabies vaccine, rotate injection sites on the upper arm or thigh.
- Cooperate with public health authorities to determine the animal's vaccination status. If the animal is proven rabid, help identify others at risk.
- Provide aggressive supportive care (even after onset of coma).
- Follow standard precautions.
- Provide emotional support.

MONITORING
- Injection site reactions
- Cardiac and pulmonary function

PATIENT TEACHING

GENERAL
Be sure to cover:
- the need for vaccination of household pets that may be exposed to rabid wild animals
- importance of not touching wild animals, especially if they appear ill or overly docile (a possible sign of rabies)
- prophylactic rabies vaccine for high-risk people, such as farm workers, forest rangers, spelunkers (cave explorers), and veterinarians.

RESOURCES
Organizations
National Center for Infectious Diseases: *www.cdc.gov/ncidod*
Rabies.com: *www.rabies.com*
World Health Organization: *www.who.int*

Selected references
Goudsmit, J., et al. "Comparison of an Anti-rabies Human Monoclonal Antibody Combination with Human Polyclonal Anti-rabies Immune Globulin," *Journal of Infectious Diseases* 193(6):796-801, March 2006.

Lembo, T. "Evaluation of a Direct, Rapid Immunohistochemical Test for Rabies Diagnosis," *Emerging Infectious Diseases* 12(2):310-13, February 2006.

Repasky, T.M., and Soskis, E. "Designing a Rabies Postexposure Prophylaxis Program with Emphasis on Staff and Patient Education," *Journal of Emergency Nursing* 31(2):173-77, April 2005.

Yamada, K., et al. "Multigenic Relation to the Attenuation of Rabies Virus," *Microbiology and Immunology* 50(1):25-32, 2006.

Radiation exposure

OVERVIEW

- Exposure to excessive radiation that causes tissue damage
- Damage varies with amount of body area exposed, length of exposure, dosage absorbed, distance from the source, and presence of protective shielding
- Can result from cancer radiotherapy, working in a radiation facility, or other exposure to radioactive materials
- Can be acute or chronic

PATHOPHYSIOLOGY

- Ionization occurs in the molecules of living cells.
- Electrons are removed from atoms. Charged atoms or ions form and react with other atoms to cause cell damage.
- Rapidly dividing cells are the most susceptible to radiation damage. Highly differentiated cells are more resistant to radiation.

CAUSES

- Exposure to radiation through inhalation, ingestion, or direct contact

RISK FACTORS

- Cancer
- Employment in a radiation facility

INCIDENCE

- The incidence of radiation exposure is unknown.

COMPLICATIONS

- Leukemia
- Thyroid cancer
- Fetal growth retardation or genetic defects in offspring (from exposure during childbearing years)
- Decreased fertility
- Shortened life span
- Anemia
- Malignant neoplasms
- Bone necrosis and fractures

ASSESSMENT

HISTORY
Acute hematopoietic radiation toxicity

- Bleeding from the skin, genitourinary tract, and GI tract due to thrombocytopenia (initial response)
- Pancytopenia with no apparent signs and symptoms (latent period)
- Nosebleeds, hemorrhage, and increased susceptibility to infection (after latent period)

GI radiation toxicity

- Intractable nausea, vomiting, and diarrhea

Cerebral radiation toxicity

- Nausea, vomiting, and diarrhea
- Lethargy

Cardiovascular radiation toxicity

- Chest pain
- Irregular heartbeat

PHYSICAL FINDINGS
Generalized radiation exposure

- Signs of hypothyroidism
- Cataracts
- Skin dryness, erythema, atrophy, and malignant lesions
- Alopecia
- Brittle nails

Acute hematopoietic radiation toxicity

- Petechiae
- Pallor
- Weakness
- Oropharyngeal abscesses

GI radiation toxicity

- Mouth and throat ulcers and infection
- Circulatory collapse and death

Cerebral radiation toxicity

- Tremors
- Seizures
- Confusion
- Coma and death

Cardiovascular radiation toxicity

- Cardiac arrhythmia
- Hypotension
- Signs of cardiogenic shock

DIAGNOSTIC TEST RESULTS

LABORATORY

- White blood cell, platelet, and lymphocyte counts are decreased.
- Serum potassium and chloride levels are decreased.

IMAGING

- X-rays may reveal bone necrosis.

DIAGNOSTIC PROCEDURES

- Bone marrow studies may show blood dyscrasia.

OTHER

- Geiger counter helps determine if radioactive material was ingested or inhaled and evaluates the amount of radiation in open wounds.
- Electrocardiography reveals cardiac arrhythmia or cardiac damage.

TREATMENT

GENERAL
- Management of life-threatening injuries
- Symptomatic and supportive treatment
- Based on the type and extent of radiation injury

DIET
- High-protein, high-calorie

ACTIVITY
- As tolerated

MEDICATIONS
- Chelating agents
- Potassium iodide
- Aluminum phosphate gel
- Barium sulfate

NURSING CONSIDERATIONS

NURSING DIAGNOSES
- Anxiety
- Decreased intracranial adaptive capacity
- Deficient fluid volume
- Imbalanced nutrition: Less than body requirements
- Impaired oral mucous membrane
- Impaired skin integrity
- Risk for infection

EXPECTED OUTCOMES
The patient will:
- verbalize feelings of anxiety and fear
- remain oriented to person, place, and time
- maintain normal fluid volume
- maintain an acceptable weight
- remain free from complications related to trauma to oral mucous membranes
- experience skin healing without complications
- remain free from signs and symptoms of infection.

NURSING INTERVENTIONS
- Implement appropriate respiratory and cardiac support measures.
- Give prescribed I.V. fluids and electrolytes.
- For skin contamination, wash the patient's body thoroughly with mild soap and water.
- Debride and irrigate open wounds, as ordered.
- For ingested radioactive material, perform gastric lavage and whole-bowel irrigation, and administer activated charcoal, as ordered.
- Dispose of contaminated clothing properly.
- Dispose of contaminated excrement and body fluids according to facility policy.
- Use strict sterile technique.

MONITORING
- Intake and output
- Fluid and electrolyte balance
- Vital signs
- Signs and symptoms of hemorrhage
- Nutritional status

PATIENT TEACHING

GENERAL
Be sure to cover:
- the injury process, diagnosis, and treatment
- effects of radiation exposure
- how to prevent a recurrence
- skin care
- wound care
- need for follow-up care.

DISCHARGE PLANNING
- Refer the patient to resource and support services.
- If the patient was exposed to significant amounts of radiation, refer him to genetic counseling resources.

RESOURCES
Organizations
Environmental Protection Agency: *www.epa.gov/radiation*
National Center for Injury Prevention and Control: *www.cdc.gov/ncipc*
National Institutes of Health: *www.nih.gov*
United States Nuclear Regulatory Commission—Radiation Exposure Information and Reporting System (REIRS) for Radiation Workers: *www.reirs.com*

Selected references
Hendrix, C. "Radiation Guidelines for Radioimmunotherapy with Yttrium 90 Ibritumomab Tiuxetan," *Clinical Journal of Oncology Nursing* 8(1):31-34, February 2004.
Thieden, E., et al. "Ultraviolet Radiation Exposure Pattern in Winter Compared With Summer Based on Time-stamped Personal Dosimeter Readings," *British Journal of Dermatology* 154(1):133-38, January 2006.
Valentin, J., International Commission on Radiological Protection. "Protecting People Against Radiation Exposure in the Event of a Radiological Attack. A Report of The International Commission on Radiological Protection," *Annals of the ICRP* 35(1):1-110, iii-iv, 2005.
Wolfson, A.B., et al. *Harwood-Nuss' Clinical Practice of Emergency Medicine,* 4th ed. Philadelphia: Lippincott Williams & Wilkins, 2005.

Rape-trauma syndrome

- ◆ Syndrome that occurs after rape (sexual intercourse without consent) or attempted rape and causes varying degrees of physical and psychological trauma
- ◆ Refers to the victim's short- and long-term reactions and the methods used to cope with trauma
- ◆ Carries a good prognosis if the victim receives physical and emotional support and counseling to help deal with feelings

PATHOPHYSIOLOGY

- ◆ Rape causes psychological and physiologic reactions.
- ◆ Early stage (short-term) and late stage (long-term) reactions can occur.

CAUSES

- ◆ Rape or attempted rape

INCIDENCE

- ◆ Rape-trauma syndrome affects all ages (reported victims from ages 2 months to 97 years).
- ◆ The syndrome is most common in women ages 16 to 19 (about 8% of American women experience rape or attempted rape).

COMPLICATIONS

- ◆ Lasting psychiatric problems, such as depression, guilt, anxiety, and suicidal ideation
- ◆ Sexually transmitted disease (STD)
- ◆ Unwanted pregnancy

ASSESSMENT

HISTORY

- ◆ Early stage
- – Disbelief
- – Panic
- – Severe anxiety
- – Anger
- – Self-blame
- – Humiliation
- – Depression
- ◆ Late stage
- – Anxiety
- – Nightmares
- – Flashbacks
- – Depression
- – Anger
- – Disinterest in sex
- – Anorgasmia
- – Suicidal ideation
- ◆ Rape or attempted rape
- ◆ Time the victim arrived at the facility; time of examination
- ◆ Date and time of alleged rape
- ◆ Whether the victim was pregnant at the time of the attack
- ◆ Date of last menstrual period
- ◆ Details of obstetric and gynecologic history
- ◆ Victim's statements (recorded in the first person, using quotation marks)
- ◆ Objective information provided by others

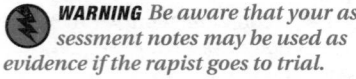 **WARNING** *Be aware that your assessment notes may be used as evidence if the rapist goes to trial.*

PHYSICAL FINDINGS

- ◆ Sore throat
- ◆ Difficulty swallowing
- ◆ Vaginal pain
- ◆ Rectal pain
- ◆ Pain from other injuries incurred during the assault
- ◆ Early stage
- – Reddened (sore) throat
- – Mouth irritation
- – Ecchymoses
- – Rectal pain and bleeding
- – Lacerations, contusions, and abrasions to vulva, cervix, and vaginal walls
- – Lacerations and contusions to anus and perineum
- – Outward calm

- – Compliance
- – Glibness
- – Talkativeness

DIAGNOSTIC TEST RESULTS

LABORATORY

- ◆ STD screening test result may be positive.
- ◆ Rapid plasma reagin card test result may be positive for syphilis.
- ◆ Urine pregnancy test result may be positive 0 to 3 weeks after missed period.
- ◆ Serum human chorionic gonadotropin test result becomes positive 24 to 48 hours after implantation.
- ◆ Result of drug screen (if symptoms warrant) may be positive.
- ◆ Serum ethanol level (if symptoms warrant) may be elevated.

WARNING *If the rape occurred within 7 days, the following specimens may be obtained for legal purposes: blood; samples for deoxyribonucleic acid testing (should be collected within 48 hours); hairs of a different color than the victim's or that are obviously out of place; fibers; soiled or torn material; body fluids, such as blood or semen, that don't belong to the victim; and specimens from the cervical canal, throat, or rectum.*

TREATMENT

GENERAL
- Treatment of physical injuries
- Crisis intervention and counseling
- Follow-up gynecologic examination after 7 to 14 days; for male patient, follow-up urologic examination
- Emergency contraception such as the Copper-T intrauterine device

ACTIVITY
- Based on injuries

MEDICATIONS
- Tetanus prophylaxis
- STD prophylaxis
- Emergency contraceptive pills

NURSING CONSIDERATIONS

NURSING DIAGNOSES
- Acute pain
- Anxiety
- Disturbed body image
- Disturbed sleep pattern
- Impaired oral mucous membrane
- Ineffective coping
- Powerlessness
- Rape-trauma syndrome
- Risk for infection
- Situational low self-esteem

EXPECTED OUTCOMES
The patient will:
- achieve pain relief with analgesia or other measures
- report absence of or reduction in anxiety
- express positive feelings about self
- appear well rested and verbalize feelings as such
- not exhibit complications related to trauma to oral mucous membranes
- use support systems and exhibit adequate coping behaviors
- identify methods to achieve control over personal situation
- recognize signs and symptoms of rape-trauma syndrome and demonstrate healthy coping behaviors
- remain free from signs and symptoms of infection
- discuss feelings related to the rape and its effect on self-esteem.

NURSING INTERVENTIONS
- Don't leave the patient alone unless requested.
- Place the patient's clothing in paper, not plastic, bags. Label each bag and its contents.
- Collect and label fingernail scrapings and foreign material obtained by combing the patient's pubic hair.
- Label all specimens with the patient's name, practitioner's name, and site from which the specimen was obtained.
- Note the name of the person to whom specimens were given.
- Report the rape if required by state law.
- Encourage the patient to express feelings.
- Provide emotional support.

MONITORING
- Mental status
- Vital signs
- Signs and symptoms of shock

PATIENT TEACHING

GENERAL
Be sure to cover:
- the disorder, diagnosis, and treatment
- verbal and written instructions regarding treatment
- medication administration, dosage, and possible adverse effects.

DISCHARGE PLANNING
- Encourage the patient to get follow-up care.
- Refer the patient to resource and support services.

RESOURCES
Organizations
Arming Women Against Rape and Endangerment: *www.aware.org*
National Institutes of Health: *www.nih.gov*
Women Organized Against Rape: *www.woar.org*

Selected references
Burgess, A.W., et al. "Forensic Markers in Elder Female Sexual Abuse Cases," *Clinics in Geriatric Medicine* 21(2):399-412, May 2005.

Lessing, J.E. "Primary Care Provider Interventions for the Delayed Disclosure of Adolescent Sexual Assault," *Journal of Pediatric Health Care* 19(1):17-24, January-February 2005.

Mancino, P., et al. "Introducing Colposcopy and Vulvovaginoscopy as Routine Examinations for Victims of Sexual Assault," *Clinical and Experimental Obstetrics & Gynecology* 30(1):40-42, 2003.

Wolfson, A.B., et al. *Harwood-Nuss' Clinical Practice of Emergency Medicine*, 4th ed. Philadelphia: Lippincott Williams & Wilkins, 2005.

Raynaud's disease

- Primary arteriospastic disorder
- Causes episodic vasospasms in the small peripheral arteries and arterioles in response to cold exposure or stress
- Typically occurs in three phases
- Exclusion of secondary causes needed for diagnosis
- Also called *vasospastic arterial disease*

PATHOPHYSIOLOGY

- Blood flow to digits decreases in response to stress or cold.
- Proposed explanations for decreased digital blood flow include an antigen-antibody immune response (most probable theory), intrinsic vascular wall hyperactivity to cold, ineffective basal heat production, and increased vasomotor tone from sympathetic stimulation or stress.

CAUSES

- Raynaud's disease has no underlying cause.
- Raynaud's phenomenon has the same pathophysiology as Raynaud's disease but has an identified underlying cause. (See *Causes of Raynaud's phenomenon*.)

INCIDENCE

- Raynaud's disease is more common in females, particularly between late adolescence and age 40.

COMPLICATIONS

- Ischemia
- Gangrene
- Amputation

HISTORY

- Altered skin color in response to cold or stress (in all stages)
- Numbness and tingling (in first stage)
- Throbbing, burning, painful sensation (in third stage)

PHYSICAL FINDINGS

- First stage — marked pallor of affected skin areas
- Second stage — cyanosis of affected skin areas
- Third stage — red, warm skin
- Between attacks — normal appearance of affected areas (occasionally, coolness and excessive perspiration of these areas)
- In long-standing disease — trophic changes, such as sclerodactylia and ulcerations

DIAGNOSTIC PROCEDURES

- Arteriography and digital photo-plethysmography may aid diagnosis.

Causes of Raynaud's phenomenon

Raynaud's phenomenon may be caused by the following diseases and conditions as well as the use of certain drugs.

COLLAGEN VASCULAR DISEASE
- Dermatomyositis
- Polymyositis
- Rheumatoid arthritis
- Scleroderma
- Systemic lupus erythematosus

ARTERIAL OCCLUSIVE DISEASE
- Acute arterial occlusion
- Atherosclerosis of the extremities
- Thoracic outlet syndrome
- Thromboangiitis obliterans

NEUROLOGIC DISORDERS
- Carpal tunnel syndrome
- Stroke
- Intervertebral disk disease
- Poliomyelitis
- Spinal cord tumors
- Syringomyelia

BLOOD DYSCRASIAS
- Cold agglutinins
- Cryofibrinogenemia
- Myeloproliferative disorders
- Waldenström's disease

TRAUMA
- Cold injury

- Electric shock
- Hammering
- Keyboarding
- Piano playing
- Vibration injury

DRUGS
- Betaadrenergic blockers
- Bleomycin
- Cisplatin
- Ergot derivatives such as ergotamine
- Methysergide
- Vinblastine

OTHER
- Pulmonary hypertension

TREATMENT

GENERAL
- Smoking cessation
- Biofeedback therapy

ACTIVITY
- Avoidance of activities involving exposure to cold and mechanical or chemical injury

MEDICATIONS
- Calcium channel blockers
- Alpha blockers
- Vasodilators

SURGERY
- Sympathectomy, if conservative treatment fails to prevent ischemic ulcers
- Amputation of fingers or toes if gangrene develops (rare)

NURSING CONSIDERATIONS

NURSING DIAGNOSES
- Acute pain
- Impaired skin integrity
- Impaired tissue integrity
- Ineffective coping
- Ineffective role performance
- Ineffective thermoregulation
- Ineffective tissue perfusion: Peripheral

EXPECTED OUTCOMES
The patient will:
- describe feeling increased comfort and decreased pain
- maintain skin integrity
- experience reduced tissue redness, swelling, and pain
- demonstrate effective coping skills
- continue to function in usual roles as much as possible
- maintain adequate skin temperature in affected areas
- maintain tissue perfusion and oxygenation.

NURSING INTERVENTIONS
- Evaluate the patient's occupation and its effect on symptom occurrence.
- Help the patient identify stress triggers and use effective coping strategies.
- Provide psychological support and reassurance.

MONITORING
- Response to treatment
- Signs and symptoms of skin breakdown
- Signs and symptoms of infection

PATIENT TEACHING

GENERAL
Be sure to cover:
- avoidance of exposure to cold
- importance of wearing mittens or gloves in cold weather and when handling cold items or defrosting the freezer
- avoidance of stress and cigarette smoking
- need to inspect skin frequently and to seek immediate care for evidence of skin breakdown or infection
- prescribed medications and possible adverse reactions, including which ones to report to the practitioner
- importance of follow-up care.

DISCHARGE PLANNING
- Refer the patient to a smoking-cessation program or a support group, as indicated.

RESOURCES
Organizations
Mayo Clinic: *www.mayoclinic.com*
National Institute of Arthritis and Musculoskeletal and Skin Diseases: *www.nih.gov/niams/healthinfo*

Selected references
Anderson, J.E., et al. "Raynaud's Phenomenon of the Nipple: A Treatable Cause of Painful Breastfeeding," *Pediatrics* 113(4):e360-64, April 2004.

Cooke, J.P., and Marshall, J.M. "Mechanisms of Raynaud's Disease," *Vascular Medicine* 10(4):293-307, November 2005.

Fries, R., et al. "Sildenafil in the Treatment of Raynaud's Phenomenon Resistant to Vasodilatory Therapy," *Circulation* 112(19):2980-85, November 2005.

Kasper, D.L., et al., eds. *Harrison's Principles of Internal Medicine,* 16th ed. New York: McGraw-Hill Book Co., 2005.

The Merck Manual of Diagnosis & Therapy, 18th ed., Whitehouse Station, N.J.: Merck & Co., Inc., 2006.

Summers, A. "From White to Blue to Red: Raynaud's Phenomenon," *Emergency Nurse* 13(7):18-20, November 2005.

Reiter's syndrome

OVERVIEW

- Self-limiting syndrome associated with polyarthritis, urethritis, mucocutaneous lesions, and conjunctivitis (or, less commonly, uveitis)

PATHOPHYSIOLOGY

- Infection is thought to trigger an aberrant and hyperactive immune response that causes inflammation in involved target organs.

CAUSES

- Exact cause unknown

RISK FACTORS

- Genetic susceptibility
- Typically follows venereal or enteric infection, especially with *Mycoplasma, Shigella, Campylobacter, Salmonella, Yersinia*, or *Chlamydia*

INCIDENCE

- Reiter's syndrome is most common in men ages 20 to 40, especially those positive for human immunodeficiency virus.
- The syndrome is rare in women and children.

COMPLICATIONS

- Ankylosing spondylitis
- Persistent joint pain and swelling
- Anterior uveitis, glaucoma, blindness
- Prostatitis and hemorrhagic cystitis
- Cardiomyopathy, pericarditis
- Pulmonary edema
- Vertebral inflammation
- Foot deformity and chronic heel pain

ASSESSMENT

HISTORY

- Initially, dysuria, hematuria, urinary urgency and frequency, and mucopurulent penile discharge with swelling and reddening of the urethral meatus
- Possible suprapubic pain, fever, and anorexia with weight loss

PHYSICAL FINDINGS

- Small, painless ulcers on glans penis
- Asymmetrical and extremely variable polyarticular arthritis, usually in weight-bearing joints of the legs and sometimes in the lower back or sacroiliac joints
- Warm, erythematous, painful joints
- Muscle wasting near affected joints
- Swollen, sausagelike appearance of fingers and toes
- Skin lesions (keratoderma blennorrhagicum)
- Thick, opaque, brittle nails with keratic debris accumulation under nails
- Painless, transient ulcerations on the buccal mucosa, palate, and tongue
- Patches of scaly skin on the palms, soles, scalp, or trunk
- Ophthalmologic symptoms such as photophobia, eye pain, excessive tearing, erythema, and burning

DIAGNOSTIC TEST RESULTS

LABORATORY

- Human leukocyte antigen (HLA) test result is positive for HLA B27.
- Complete blood count and anemia panel show mild anemia.
- White blood cell (WBC) count and erythrocyte sedimentation rate are elevated.
- Many WBCs (mostly polymorphonuclear leukocytes) appear in urethral discharge and synovial fluid.
- Synovial fluid is grossly purulent with high complement and protein levels.
- Cultures of urethral discharge and synovial fluid are used to rule out other possible causes of symptoms.

IMAGING

- During the first few weeks of the syndrome, X-rays are normal. Later they may show osteoporosis in inflamed areas. If inflammation persists, X-rays may show small joint erosion, periosteal proliferation (new bone formation) of involved joints, and calcaneal spurs.

TREATMENT

GENERAL
- Physical therapy
- Padded or supportive shoes

DIET
- High-calorie, high-protein

ACTIVITY
- During acute stages, weight-bearing restrictions or complete bed rest

MEDICATIONS
- Nonsteroidal anti-inflammatory drugs (NSAIDs)
- Analgesics
- Cytotoxic agents
- Corticosteroids
- Antibiotics (for underlying infection)

SURGERY
- Surgical reconstruction of joints if medical management doesn't prevent severe joint damage

NURSING CONSIDERATIONS

NURSING DIAGNOSES
- Acute pain
- Disturbed sensory perception (visual)
- Fatigue
- Imbalanced nutrition: Less than body requirements
- Impaired oral mucous membrane
- Impaired physical mobility
- Impaired skin integrity
- Impaired tissue integrity
- Impaired urinary elimination
- Ineffective role performance
- Ineffective sexuality patterns
- Risk for infection

EXPECTED OUTCOMES
The patient will:
- express feelings of increased comfort and decreased pain
- maintain optimal functioning within the confines of the vision impairment
- express feelings of increased energy
- maintain weight or achieve ideal weight
- maintain adequate oral mucous membranes
- attain the highest degree of mobility possible within confines of the disease
- experience healing of wounds and lesions without complications
- experience reduced tissue pain, redness, and swelling
- maintain adequate urine output
- recognize limitations imposed by the illness and express feelings about these limitations
- verbalize feelings about altered sexuality patterns
- remain free from signs or symptoms of infection.

NURSING INTERVENTIONS
- Follow standard precautions.
- Give prescribed analgesics as needed.
- Provide a high-calorie, high-protein diet.
- Provide frequent rest periods.
- Develop an exercise regimen with the physical therapist.
- Maintain a nonjudgmental attitude.

MONITORING
- Response to medications
- Complications
- Pain control
- Joint mobility

PATIENT TEACHING

GENERAL
Be sure to cover:
- the disorder, diagnosis, and treatment
- importance of using condoms and avoiding multiple sex partners
- how to avoid exposure to enteric pathogens (such as via anal intercourse)
- drug dosages and possible adverse reactions
- importance of taking NSAIDs with meals or milk
- maintaining normal daily activities and moderate exercise
- good posture and body mechanics
- use of a firm mattress.

DISCHARGE PLANNING
- If the patient has severe or chronic joint impairment, arrange for occupational counseling.

RESOURCES
Organizations
Arthritis Foundation: *www.arthritis.org*
National Institute of Arthritis and Musculoskeletal and Skin Diseases: *www.nih.gov/niams/healthinfo*
Reiter's Information and Support Group: *www.risg.org*

Selected references
Eapen, B.R. "A New Insight into the Pathogenesis of Reiter's Syndrome Using Bioinformatics Tools," *International Journal of Dermatology* 42(3):242-43, March 2003.

Kohnke, S.J. "Reactive Arthritis. A Clinical Approach," *Orthopaedic Nursing* 23(4):274-80, July-August 2004.

Liao, C.H., et al. "Juvenile Reiter's Syndrome: A Case Report," *Journal of Microbiology, Immunology, and Infection* 37(6):379-81, December 2004.

The Merck Manual of Diagnosis & Therapy, 18th ed., Whitehouse Station, N.J.: Merck & Co., Inc., 2006.

Relapsing fever

OVERVIEW

- An acute infectious disease caused by *Borrelia* spirochetes
- Transmitted to humans by lice or ticks and characterized by relapses and remissions
- Primary *Borrelia* reservoirs in rodents and other wild animals
- Secondary reservoir possible in people, requiring no transmission by ordinary contagion and allowing possible congenital infection and transmission by contaminated blood
- Mortality for untreated louse-borne relapsing fever usually above 10%, possibly up to 50% in an epidemic
- With treatment, excellent prognosis for both louse-borne and tick-borne relapsing fevers
- Also called *tick, fowl-nest, cabin,* or *vagabond fever* or *bilious typhoid*

PATHOPHYSIOLOGY

- Inoculation takes place when the victim crushes the louse, causing its infected blood or body fluid to enter victim's bitten or abraded skin or mucous membranes.
- Because tick bites are virtually painless and most *Ornithodoros* ticks feed at night but don't imbed themselves in the victim's skin, many people are bitten unknowingly.

CAUSES

- Bite from body louse (*Pediculus humanus corporis*) that carries *Borrelia* spirochete, which typically occurs in epidemics during wars, famines, and mass migrations
- Bite from tick that carries one of three species of *Borrelia* most closely identified with tick carriers: *B. hermsii* (associated with *Ornithodoros hermsi*), *B. turicatae* (associated with *O. turicata*), or *B. parkeri* (associated with *O. parkeri*)

RISK FACTORS

- Cold weather and crowded living conditions, which favor the spread of body lice

INCIDENCE

- Relapsing fever is most common in indigent victims already suffering from other infections and malnutrition.
- Louse-borne disease is most common in North and Central Africa, Europe, Asia, and South America; there have been no cases in the United States since 1900.
- Tick-borne disease in the United States is most prevalent in Texas and other western states, usually during the summer, when ticks and their hosts (chipmunks, goats, and prairie dogs) are most active; occasional cold-weather outbreaks in people such as campers who sleep in tick-infested cabins.
- Louse-borne disease is slightly more common in females; tick-borne, in males.

COMPLICATIONS

- Nephritis
- Bronchitis
- Pneumonia
- Endocarditis
- Seizures
- Cranial nerve lesions
- Paralysis
- Coma
- Bleeding
- Death

ASSESSMENT

HISTORY

- Recent travel to an epidemic or louse-infested area
- Recent exposure to tick-infested area
- Fever
- Headache
- Malaise
- Arthralgia
- Attacks that subside and recur

PHYSICAL FINDINGS

- Splenomegaly
- Hepatomegaly
- Lymphadenopathy
- Transient petechial rash over torso during febrile periods
- Nuchal rigidity
- Jaundice

DIAGNOSTIC TEST RESULTS

LABORATORY

- During febrile periods, spirochetes may appear in blood smears using Wright's or Giemsa stain.
- In severe infection, spirochetes appear in urine and cerebrospinal fluid.
- White blood cell count may reach 25,000/µl; lymphocytes and erythrocyte sedimentation rate may increase.
- Syphilis test may show a false-positive result.

TREATMENT

GENERAL
◆ Supportive therapy

DIET
◆ As tolerated

ACTIVITY
◆ As tolerated

MEDICATIONS
◆ Antipyretics
◆ Antibiotics

⚡ **WARNING** *Antibiotics shouldn't be given at the height of a severe febrile attack because they may cause Jarisch-Herxheimer reaction, resulting in malaise, rigors, leukopenia, flushing, fever, tachycardia, rising respiratory rate, and hypotension. This reaction, which is caused by toxic by-products from massive spirochete destruction, can mimic septic shock and may prove fatal. Antibiotics should be postponed until the fever subsides.*

NURSING CONSIDERATIONS

NURSING DIAGNOSES
◆ Acute pain
◆ Decreased cardiac output
◆ Deficient fluid volume
◆ Diarrhea
◆ Hyperthermia
◆ Impaired skin integrity

EXPECTED OUTCOMES
The patient will:
◆ express increased comfort and decreased pain
◆ maintain adequate cardiac output and hemodynamic stability
◆ maintain adequate fluid volume
◆ experience return to normal bowel movements
◆ maintain a normal body temperature
◆ exhibit healed or improved lesions or wounds.

NURSING INTERVENTIONS
◆ Give tepid sponge baths and antipyretics.
◆ Encourage fluid intake.
◆ Administer antibiotics carefully. Document and report any hypersensitive reactions (rash, fever, anaphylaxis), especially a Jarisch-Herxheimer reaction.
◆ Report all cases of louse-borne or tick-borne relapsing fever to the local public health department as required by law.

MONITORING
◆ Vital signs
◆ Level of consciousness

PATIENT TEACHING

GENERAL
Be sure to cover:
◆ symptoms of relapsing fever in family members and in others who may have been exposed to ticks or lice along with the victim
◆ proper hand-washing technique
◆ prevention for travelers going to tick-infested areas, such as wearing clothing that covers as much skin as possible and tucking pant legs into boots or socks.

RESOURCES
Organizations
Lyme Disease Foundation, Inc.:
www.lyme.org
National Center for Infectious Diseases:
www.cdc.gov/ncidod

Selected references
Buckingham, S.C. "Tick-borne Infections in Children: Epidemiology, Clinical Manifestations, and Optimal Management Strategies," *Paediatric Drugs* 7(3):163-76, 2005.
Bunikis, J., et al. "Typing of *Borrelia* Relapsing Fever Group Strains," *Emerging Infectious Diseases* 10(9):1661-664, September 2004.
Londono, D., et al. "Cardiac Apoptosis in Severe Relapsing Fever Borreliosis," *Infection and Immunity* 73(11):7669-676, November 2005.
Roscoe, C., and Epperly, T. "Tick-borne Relapsing Fever," *American Family Physician* 72(10):2039-2044, November 2005.

Renal agenesis LIFE-THREATENING DISORDER

OVERVIEW

- Congenital absence of one (unilateral renal agenesis [URA]) or both (bilateral renal agenesis [BRA]) kidneys at birth
- Lack of amniotic fluid (oligohydramnios) with BRA, causing complications such as impaired fetal lung development, thoracic compression, limb contractures, and other abnormalities
- BRA is always fatal
- Formerly called *Potter's syndrome*

PATHOPHYSIOLOGY
- Ureteric bud fails to develop.

CAUSES
- Exact cause unknown
- Genetics, possibly autosomal dominant

RISK FACTORS
- Parent with kidney malformation, especially absence of one kidney
- Uncontrolled diabetes during pregnancy (renal agenesis in fetus)

INCIDENCE
- Renal agenesis occurs in about 1 per 3,000 to 10,000 births in the United States.
- BRA is more common in males than females (2:1).
- URA is more common than BRA.

COMPLICATIONS
- Death

ASSESSMENT

HISTORY
- Fetuses with BRA: oligohydramnios, plus nonvisualization (with maternal sonogram) of fetal kidneys, ureters, and bladder

PHYSICAL FINDINGS
- Neonates with BRA: low-set, floppy ears and a broad, flat nose; underdeveloped lungs

DIAGNOSTIC TEST RESULTS

IMAGING
- Maternal sonography reveals oligohydramnios, along with nonvisualization of fetal kidneys, ureters, and bladder, confirming BRA.
- Maternal sonography has more difficulty detecting URA.
- Doppler studies may distinguish BRA from severe intrauterine growth retardation.

TREATMENT

GENERAL
- Supportive care to parents of fetus with BRA
- Comfort measures for infant with BRA

NURSING CONSIDERATIONS

NURSING DIAGNOSES
- Anticipatory grieving
- Deficient fluid volume
- Impaired gas exchange
- Ineffective airway clearance
- Interrupted family processes
- Risk for disproportionate growth

EXPECTED OUTCOMES
The patient (or family) will:
- seek support systems and exhibit adequate coping behaviors
- exhibit signs of adequate amniotic fluid
- maintain optimal gas exchange, with adequate ventilation and oxygenation
- maintain a patent airway
- express understanding of the disorder, and use support systems to assist with coping
- express understanding of norms for growth and development.

NURSING INTERVENTIONS
- Provide support and encourage verbalization.

MONITORING
- Vital signs
- Respiratory status
- Renal status (with URA)

PATIENT TEACHING

GENERAL
Be sure to cover (with the parents):
- the disorder, diagnosis, and treatment.

DISCHARGE PLANNING
- Refer the family to support services, as needed.

RESOURCES

Organizations
American Academy of Pediatrics: *www.aap.org*
American Association of Kidney Patients: *www.aakp.org*
National Institute of Diabetes & Digestive & Kidney Diseases: *www.niddk.nih.gov*

Selected references
Bacanli, A., et al. "Nevoid Basal Cell Carcinoma Syndrome Associated With Unilateral Renal Agenesis: Acceleration of Basal Cell Carcinomas Following Radiotherapy," *Journal of the European Academy of Dermatology & Venereology* 19(4):510-11, July 2005.

Esra Onal, E., et al. "Tubular Skin Appendage, Renal Agenesis and Popliteal Web: A Further Example of the Human Homologue of Disorganization (Ds)," *Clinical Dysmorphology* 14(2):89-91, April 2005.

Gonzalez, E., et al. "Factors Influencing the Progression of Renal Damage in Patients With Unilateral Renal Agenesis and Remnant Kidney," *Kidney International* 68(1):263-70, July 2005.

Renal calculi

- Formation of calculi (*stones*) anywhere in the urinary tract
- Most common in the renal pelvis or calyces
- Vary in size; may be single or multiple (see *Variations in renal calculi*)
- Necessitate hospitalization in roughly 1 of every 1,000 Americans

PATHOPHYSIOLOGY

- Calculi form when substances normally dissolved in the urine, such as calcium oxalate and calcium phosphate, precipitate.
- Large, rough calculi may occlude the opening to the ureteropelvic junction.
- The frequency and force of peristaltic contractions increase, causing pain.

CAUSES

- Unknown

RISK FACTORS

- Dehydration
- Infection
- Urine pH changes
- Urinary tract obstruction
- Immobilization
- Metabolic factors
- Family member with history of renal calculi

INCIDENCE

- Renal calculi affect more men than women.
- This disorder is rare in blacks and in children.
- The disorder affects men and women mostly age 35 to 45 but can occur at any age.

COMPLICATIONS

- Renal parenchymal damage
- Renal cell necrosis
- Hydronephrosis
- Complete ureteral obstruction

HISTORY

- Classic renal colic pain — severe pain that travels from the costovertebral angle to the flank and then to the suprapubic region and external genitalia
- With calculi in the renal pelvis and calyces — relatively constant, dull pain
- Pain of fluctuating intensity; may be excruciating at its peak
- Nausea, vomiting
- Fever, chills
- Anuria (rare)

PHYSICAL FINDINGS

- Hematuria
- Abdominal distention
- Costovertebral tenderness on palpation
- Tachycardia
- Elevated blood pressure

LABORATORY

- A 24-hour urine collection shows calcium oxalate, phosphorus, and uric acid excretion levels.
- Urinalysis shows increased urine specific gravity, hematuria, crystals, casts, and pyuria.

IMAGING

- Kidney-ureter-bladder (KUB) radiography reveals most renal calculi.
- Excretory urography helps confirm the diagnosis and determines calculi size and location.
- I.V. pyelography and abdominal computed tomography may reveal stones or obstruction of the ureter.
- Kidney ultrasonography can detect obstructive changes and radiolucent calculi not seen on KUB.

Variations in renal calculi

Renal calculi vary in size and type. Small calculi may remain in the renal pelvis or pass down the ureter. A staghorn calculus (a cast of the calyceal and pelvic collecting system) may develop from a calculus that stays in the kidney.

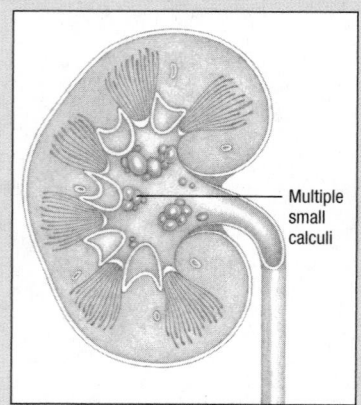

Multiple small calculi

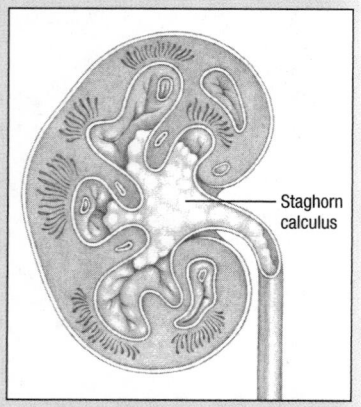

Staghorn calculus

TREATMENT

GENERAL
- Percutaneous ultrasonic lithotripsy
- Extracorporeal shock wave lithotripsy
- Vigorous hydration (more than 3 qt [3 L]/day)

DIET
- Restrictions based on stone composition

MEDICATIONS
- Antibiotics
- Analgesics
- Diuretics
- Methenamine mandelate
- Allopurinol (for uric acid calculi)
- Ascorbic acid
- Nonsteroidal anti-inflammatory drug ketorolac (Toradol)
- Desmopressin (DDAVP)

SURGERY
- Cystoscopy
- Ureteral stent
- Percutaneous nephrostomy

NURSING CONSIDERATIONS

NURSING DIAGNOSES
- Acute pain
- Impaired urinary elimination
- Ineffective tissue perfusion: Renal
- Risk for imbalanced fluid volume
- Risk for infection
- Risk for injury

EXPECTED OUTCOMES
The patient will:
- report increased comfort and decreased pain
- demonstrate the ability to manage urinary elimination problems
- maintain adequate urine output
- maintain fluid balance
- remain free from signs and symptoms of infection
- avoid or minimize complications.

NURSING INTERVENTIONS
- Provide I.V. fluids, as ordered; force fluids as needed.
- Strain all urine and save solid material for analysis.
- Encourage ambulation to aid spontaneous calculus passage.

MONITORING
- Intake and output
- Daily weight
- Pain control
- Catheter function and drainage
- Signs and symptoms of infection

PATIENT TEACHING

GENERAL
Be sure to cover:
- the disorder, diagnosis, and treatment
- prescribed diet and importance of compliance
- drug therapy
- ways to prevent recurrences
- how to strain urine for stones
- immediate return visit to hospital for fever, uncontrolled pain, or vomiting.

DISCHARGE PLANNING
- Patients who don't meet admission criteria should arrange for a follow-up visit with a urologist in 2 to 3 days.

RESOURCES
Organizations
American Association of Kidney Patients: *www.aakp.org*
National Institute of Diabetes & Digestive & Kidney Diseases: *www.niddk.nih.gov*
National Kidney Foundation: *www.kidney.org*

Selected references
Colella, J., et al. "Urolithiasis/Nephrolithiasis: What's it All About?" *Urologic Nursing* 25(6):427-48, 475, 449, December 2005.
Diseases, 4th ed. Philadelphia: Lippincott Williams & Wilkins, 2006.
Moe, O.W. "Kidney Stones: Pathophysiology and Medical Management," *Lancet* 367(9507):333-44, January 2006.
Thomas, J.C., et al. "Pediatric Ureteroscopic Stone Management," *Journal of Urology* 174(3):1072-1074, September 2005.

Renal failure, acute

- Sudden interruption of renal function resulting from obstruction, reduced circulation, or renal parenchymal disease
- Classified as prerenal failure, intrarenal failure (also called intrinsic or parenchymal failure), or postrenal failure
- Usually reversible with medical treatment
- If not treated, may progress to end-stage renal disease, uremia, and death
- Normally occurs in three distinct phases: oliguric, diuretic, and recovery

Oliguric phase
- May last a few days or several weeks
- Urine output less than 400 ml/day
- Fluid volume excess, azotemia, and electrolyte imbalance
- Local mediators released, causing intrarenal vasoconstriction
- Medullary hypoxia causing cellular swelling and adherence of neutrophils to capillaries and venules
- Hypoperfusion
- Cellular injury and necrosis
- Reperfusion causing reactive oxygen species to form, leading to further cellular injury

Diuretic phase
- Renal function recovering
- Urine output gradually increasing
- Glomerular filtration rate improving, although tubular transport systems remain abnormal

Recovery phase
- May last 3 to 12 months, or longer
- Gradual return to normal or near normal renal function

PATHOPHYSIOLOGY
Prerenal failure
- Prerenal failure is caused by impaired blood flow.
- Decrease in filtration pressure causes decline in glomerular filtration rate.

- Failure to restore blood volume or blood pressure may cause acute tubular necrosis (ATN) or acute cortical necrosis.

Intrarenal failure
- A severe episode of hypotension, commonly associated with hypovolemia, is often a significant contributing event.
- Cell swelling, injury, and necrosis — a form of reperfusion injury that may also be caused by nephrotoxins — results from ischemia-generated toxic oxygen-free radicals and anti-inflammatory mediators.

Postrenal failure
- Postrenal failure usually occurs with urinary tract obstruction that affects the kidneys bilaterally such as prostatic hyperplasia.

CAUSES
Prerenal failure
- Hemorrhagic blood loss
- Hypotension or hypoperfusion
- Hypovolemia
- Loss of plasma volume
- Water and electrolyte losses

Intrarenal failure
- ATN
- Coagulation defects
- Glomerulopathies
- Malignant hypertension

Postrenal failure
- Bladder neck obstruction
- Obstructive uropathies, usually bilateral
- Ureteral destruction

INCIDENCE
- Acute renal failure is seen in 5% of hospitalized patients.

COMPLICATIONS
- Renal shutdown
- Electrolyte imbalance
- Metabolic acidosis
- Acute pulmonary edema
- Hypertensive crisis
- Infection

HISTORY
- Predisposing disorder
- Recent fever, chills, or central nervous system problem
- Recent GI problem

PHYSICAL FINDINGS
- Oliguria or anuria
- Tachycardia
- Bibasilar crackles
- Irritability, drowsiness, or confusion
- Altered level of consciousness
- Bleeding abnormalities
- Dry, pruritic skin
- Dry mucous membranes
- Uremic breath odor

LABORATORY
- Blood urea nitrogen, serum creatinine, and potassium levels are elevated.
- Hematocrit, blood pH, bicarbonate, and hemoglobin levels are decreased.
- Urine casts and cellular debris are present, and specific gravity is decreased.
- In glomerular disease, proteinuria and urine osmolality are close to serum osmolality level.
- Urine sodium level is less than 20 mEq/L, caused by decreased perfusion in oliguria.
- Urine sodium level is greater than 40 mEq/L from an intrarenal problem in oliguria.
- Urine creatinine clearance is used to measure glomerular filtration rate and estimate the number of remaining functioning nephrons.

IMAGING
The following imaging tests may show the cause of renal failure:
- kidney ultrasonography
- kidney-ureter-bladder radiography
- excretory urography renal scan
- retrograde pyelography
- computed tomography scan
- nephrotomography.

DIAGNOSTIC PROCEDURES
◆ Electrocardiography shows tall, peaked T waves; a widening QRS complex; and disappearing P waves if hyperkalemia is present.

TREATMENT

GENERAL
◆ Hemodialysis or peritoneal dialysis (if appropriate)

DIET
◆ High-calorie, low-protein, low-sodium, and low-potassium
◆ Fluid restriction

ACTIVITY
◆ Rest periods when fatigued

MEDICATIONS
◆ Diuretics
◆ In hyperkalemia, hypertonic glucose-and-insulin infusions, sodium bicarbonate, sodium polystyrene sulfonate

SURGERY
◆ Insertion of vascular access for hemodialysis

NURSING CONSIDERATIONS

NURSING DIAGNOSES
◆ Activity intolerance
◆ Decreased cardiac output
◆ Risk for imbalanced fluid volume
◆ Fatigue
◆ Fear
◆ Imbalanced nutrition: Less than body requirements
◆ Impaired urinary elimination
◆ Ineffective tissue perfusion: Renal
◆ Interrupted family processes
◆ Risk for infection
◆ Risk for injury

EXPECTED OUTCOMES
The patient (or family) will:
◆ perform activities of daily living without excessive fatigue or exhaustion
◆ maintain hemodynamic stability
◆ maintain fluid balance

◆ remain free from signs and symptoms of circulatory overload
◆ express the importance of balancing activities with adequate rest periods
◆ discuss fears or concerns
◆ verbalize appropriate food choices
◆ demonstrate the ability to manage urinary elimination problems
◆ maintain adequate urine output
◆ verbalize the effect the patient's condition has on the family unit
◆ remain free from signs or symptoms of infection
◆ avoid or minimize complications.

NURSING INTERVENTIONS
◆ Give prescribed drugs.
◆ Encourage the patient to express feelings.
◆ Provide emotional support.
◆ Identify patients at risk for and take steps to prevent ATN. (See *Preventing acute tubular necrosis*.)

MONITORING
◆ Intake and output
◆ Daily weight
◆ Renal function studies
◆ Vital signs
◆ Effects of excess fluid volume
◆ Dialysis access site

Preventing acute tubular necrosis

Acute tubular necrosis occurs mainly in elderly hospitalized patients. Contributing causes include aminoglycoside therapy and exposure to industrial chemicals, heavy metals, and contrast media. Patients who have been exposed must receive adequate hydration; monitor their urinary output closely.

To prevent acute tubular necrosis, make sure every patient is well hydrated before surgery or after X-rays that use a contrast medium. Administer mannitol, as ordered, to a high-risk patient before and during these procedures. Carefully monitor a patient receiving a blood transfusion, and stop the transfusion immediately if signs of transfusion reaction (fever, rash, and chills) occur.

PATIENT TEACHING

GENERAL
Be sure to cover:
◆ disorder, diagnosis, and treatment
◆ administration, dosages, and possible adverse reactions to medications
◆ recommended fluid allowance
◆ compliance with diet and drug regimen
◆ importance of immediately reporting weight changes of 3 lb or more
◆ signs and symptoms of edema and importance of reporting them.

DISCHARGE PLANNING
◆ Encourage follow-up care with nephrologist.

RESOURCES
Organizations
American Association of Kidney Patients: *www.aakp.org*
National Institute of Diabetes & Digestive & Kidney Diseases: *www.niddk.nih.gov*
National Kidney Foundation: *www.kidney.org*

Selected references
Chan, V., et al. "Valve Replacement Surgery Complicated by Acute Renal Failure — Predictors of Early Mortality," *Journal of Cardiac Surgery* 21(2):139-43, March-April 2006.
Diseases, 4th ed. Philadelphia: Lippincott Williams & Wilkins, 2006.
Francisco, A.L., and Pinera, C. "Challenges and Future of Renal Replacement Therapy," *Hemodialysis International* 10 Suppl 1:S19-23, January 2006.
Perkins, C., and Kisel, M. "Utilizing Physiological Knowledge to Care for Acute Renal Failure," *British Journal of Nursing* 14(14):768-73, July-August 2005.
Uchino, S., et al. "Acute Renal Failure in Critically Ill Patients: A Multinational, Multicenter Study," *JAMA* 294(7):813-18, August 2005.

Renal failure, chronic

OVERVIEW

- The end result of gradually progressive loss of renal function
- Symptoms sparse until more than 75% of glomerular filtration lost, worsening as renal function declines
- Fatal unless treated; to sustain life, may require maintenance dialysis or kidney transplantation

PATHOPHYSIOLOGY

- Nephron destruction eventually causes irreversible renal damage.
- Disease may progress through the following stages: reduced renal reserve, renal insufficiency, renal failure, and end-stage renal disease.

CAUSES

- Chronic glomerular disease
- Chronic infections such as chronic pyelonephritis
- Collagen diseases such as systemic lupus erythematosus
- Congenital anomalies such as polycystic kidney disease
- Endocrine disease
- Nephrotoxic agents
- Obstructive processes such as calculi
- Vascular diseases

INCIDENCE

- Chronic renal failure affects about 2 in 100,000 people.
- The disorder can occur at any age but it's more common in adults.
- Chronic renal failure affects more men than women.
- It affects more Blacks than Whites.

COMPLICATIONS

- Anemia
- Peripheral neuropathy
- Lipid disorders
- Platelet dysfunction
- Pulmonary edema
- Electrolyte imbalances
- Sexual dysfunction

ASSESSMENT

HISTORY

- Predisposing factor
- Dry mouth
- Fatigue
- Nausea
- Hiccups
- Muscle cramps
- Fasciculations, twitching
- Infertility, decreased libido
- Amenorrhea
- Impotence
- Pathologic fractures

PHYSICAL FINDINGS

- Decreased urine output
- Hypotension or hypertension
- Altered level of consciousness
- Peripheral edema
- Cardiac arrhythmias
- Bibasilar crackles
- Pleural friction rub
- Gum ulceration and bleeding
- Uremic fetor
- Abdominal pain on palpation
- Poor skin turgor
- Pale, yellowish bronze skin color
- Thin, brittle fingernails and dry, brittle hair
- Growth retardation (in children)

DIAGNOSTIC TEST RESULTS

LABORATORY

- Blood urea nitrogen, serum creatinine, sodium, and potassium levels are elevated.
- Arterial blood gas (ABG) values show decreased arterial pH and bicarbonate levels.
- Hematocrit and hemoglobin level are low; red blood cell (RBC) survival time decreases.
- Mild thrombocytopenia and platelet defects appear.
- Aldosterone secretion is increased.
- Hyperglycemia and hypertriglyceridemia occur.
- High-density lipoprotein levels are decreased.
- ABG values show metabolic acidosis.
- Urine specific gravity is fixed at 1.010.
- Patient has proteinuria, glycosuria, and urinary RBCs, leukocytes, casts, and crystals.

IMAGING

- Kidney-ureter-bladder radiography, excretory urography, nephrotomography, renal scan, and renal arteriography show reduced kidney size.

DIAGNOSTIC PROCEDURES

- Renal biopsy allows histologic identification of the underlying pathology.
- Electroencephalography shows changes suggesting metabolic encephalopathy.

TREATMENT

GENERAL
◆ Hemodialysis or peritoneal dialysis

DIET
◆ Low-protein (with peritoneal dialysis, high protein), high-calorie, low-sodium, low-phosphorus, and low-potassium
◆ Fluid restriction

ACTIVITY
◆ Rest periods when fatigued

MEDICATIONS
◆ Loop diuretics
◆ Cardiac glycosides
◆ Antihypertensives
◆ Antiemetics
◆ Iron and folate supplements
◆ Erythropoietin
◆ Antipruritics
◆ Supplementary vitamins and essential amino acids

SURGERY
◆ Creation of vascular access for dialysis
◆ Possible kidney transplant

NURSING CONSIDERATIONS

NURSING DIAGNOSES
◆ Acute pain
◆ Decreased cardiac output
◆ Disabled family coping
◆ Excess fluid volume
◆ Imbalanced nutrition: Less than body requirements
◆ Impaired gas exchange
◆ Impaired oral mucous membrane
◆ Impaired urinary elimination
◆ Ineffective coping
◆ Ineffective sexuality patterns
◆ Ineffective tissue perfusion: Renal
◆ Interrupted family processes
◆ Powerlessness
◆ Risk for infection
◆ Risk for injury

EXPECTED OUTCOMES
The patient (or family) will:
◆ report increased comfort and decreased pain
◆ maintain hemodynamic stability
◆ demonstrate adaptive coping behaviors
◆ maintain fluid balance
◆ verbalize appropriate food choices according to the prescribed diet
◆ maintain adequate ventilation and oxygenation
◆ maintain intact oral mucous membranes
◆ demonstrate the ability to manage urinary elimination problems
◆ use support resources and exhibit adaptive coping behaviors
◆ resume sexual activity to the fullest extent possible
◆ maintain adequate urine output
◆ verbalize the effect the patient's condition has on the family unit
◆ verbalize feelings of control over condition and own well-being
◆ remain free from signs or symptoms of infection
◆ avoid or minimize complications.

NURSING INTERVENTIONS
◆ Give prescribed drugs.
◆ Perform meticulous skin care.
◆ Encourage the patient to express feelings.
◆ Provide emotional support.

MONITORING
◆ Renal function studies
◆ Vital signs
◆ Intake and output
◆ Daily weight
◆ Signs and symptoms of fluid overload
◆ Signs and symptoms of bleeding

PATIENT TEACHING

GENERAL
Be sure to cover:
◆ the disorder, diagnosis, and treatment
◆ dietary changes
◆ fluid restrictions
◆ dialysis site care, as appropriate
◆ importance of wearing or carrying medical identification.

DISCHARGE PLANNING
◆ Refer the patient to resource and support services.

RESOURCES
Organizations
American Association of Kidney Patients: *www.aakp.org*
National Institute of Diabetes & Digestive & Kidney Diseases: *www.niddk.nih.gov*
National Kidney Foundation: *www.kidney.org*

Selected references
Campoy, S., and Elwell, R. "Pharmacology and CKD: How Chronic Kidney Disease and Its Complications Alter Drug Response," *AJN* 105(9):60-71, September 2005.
Castner, D., and Douglas, C. "Now on Stage: Chronic Kidney Disease," *Nursing* 35(12):58-63, December 2005.
Diseases, 4th ed. Philadelphia: Lippincott Williams & Wilkins, 2006.
Harwood, L., et al. "Preparing for Hemodialysis: Patient Stressors and Responses," *Nephrology Nursing Journal* 32(3):295-302, May-June 2005.
Lim, W.H., et al. "Renal Transplantation Reverses Functional Deficiencies in Circulating Dendritic Cell Subsets in Chronic Renal Failure Patients," *Transplantation* 81(2):160-68, January 2006.

Respiratory acidosis LIFE-THREATENING DISORDER

OVERVIEW

- Acid-base disturbance characterized by reduced alveolar ventilation, as shown by hypercapnia (partial pressure of arterial carbon dioxide [$Paco_2$] above 45 mm Hg)
- Carries varying prognosis, depending on the severity of the underlying disturbance and the patient's general condition
- Can be acute or chronic

PATHOPHYSIOLOGY

- Depressed ventilation causes respiratory acidosis.
- Carbon dioxide is then retained, and hydrogen ion concentration increases.
- Respiratory acidosis results.

CAUSES

- Elevated carbon dioxide levels resulting from respiratory or metabolic failure

RISK FACTORS

- Airway obstruction
- Asthma
- Central nervous system (CNS) trauma
- Chronic bronchitis
- Chronic metabolic alkalosis
- Chronic obstructive pulmonary disease
- CNS-depressant drugs
- Extensive pneumonia
- Large pneumothorax
- Neuromuscular disease
- Parenchymal lung disease
- Pulmonary edema
- Severe acute respiratory distress syndrome

INCIDENCE

- Respiratory acidosis affects males and females equally.

COMPLICATIONS

- Shock
- Respiratory arrest
- Cardiac arrest

ASSESSMENT

HISTORY

- Predisposing risk factor
- Headache
- Shortness of breath
- Nausea and vomiting

PHYSICAL FINDINGS

- Diaphoresis
- Bounding pulses
- Rapid, shallow respirations
- Tachycardia and other arrhythmias
- Hypotension
- Papilledema
- Mental status changes
- Asterixis (tremor)
- Depressed deep tendon reflexes

DIAGNOSTIC TEST RESULTS

LABORATORY

- Arterial blood pH is below 7.35, and $Paco_2$ is above 45 mm Hg (hypercapnia).

IMAGING

- Chest X-ray may reveal lung disease or illness.

OTHER

- Pulmonary function tests may help diagnose underlying respiratory disease.

TREATMENT

GENERAL
- Correction of the condition causing alveolar hypoventilation
- Possible mechanical ventilation
- Possible dialysis
- I.V. fluid administration
- Smoking cessation
- Chest tube insertion for pneumothorax

DIET
- Possible need for parenteral nutrition

ACTIVITY
- As tolerated

MEDICATIONS
- Oxygen
- Bronchodilators
- Antibiotics
- Sodium bicarbonate
- Drug therapy for the underlying condition

SURGERY
- Bronchoscopy

NURSING CONSIDERATIONS

NURSING DIAGNOSES
- Anxiety
- Decreased cardiac output
- Fear
- Impaired gas exchange
- Ineffective airway clearance
- Ineffective coping
- Risk for deficient fluid volume

EXPECTED OUTCOMES
The patient will:
- identify measures to reduce anxiety
- maintain adequate cardiac output
- discuss fears or concerns
- maintain adequate ventilation and oxygenation
- maintain a patent airway
- use support systems to assist with coping
- maintain fluid balance.

NURSING INTERVENTIONS
- Give prescribed drugs and oxygen.
- Provide adequate fluids.
- Maintain a patent airway.
- Perform tracheal suctioning, as needed.

MONITORING
- Vital signs
- Intake and output
- Neurologic status
- Respiratory status
- Arterial blood gas values
- Serum electrolyte values
- Mechanical ventilator settings

⚡ **WARNING** *Be aware that pulse oximetry, used to monitor oxygen saturation, won't reveal increasing carbon dioxide levels.*

PATIENT TEACHING

GENERAL
Be sure to cover:
- the disorder, diagnosis, and treatment
- supplemental oxygen
- prescribed drugs and possible adverse effects
- how to perform coughing and deep-breathing exercises
- signs and symptoms of acid-base imbalance and when to notify the practitioner.

DISCHARGE PLANNING
- Refer the patient for home oxygen therapy, if indicated.
- Refer the patient to a smoking-cessation program, if appropriate.

RESOURCES
Organizations
American Association for Respiratory Care: *www.aarc.org*
American Lung Association: *www.lungusa.org*

Selected references
Broccard, A.F. "Respiratory Acidosis and Acute Respiratory Distress Syndrome: Time to Trade in a Bull Market?" *Critical Care Medicine* 34(1):229-31, January 2006.

Diseases, 4th ed. Philadelphia: Lippincott Williams & Wilkins, 2006.

Doerr, C.H., et al. "Hypercapnic Acidosis Impairs Plasma Membrane Wound Resealing in Ventilator-injured Lungs," *American Journal of Respiratory and Critical Care Medicine* 171(12):1371-377, June 2005.

Kregenow, D.A., et al. "Hypercapnic Acidosis and Mortality in Acute Lung Injury," *Critical Care Medicine* 34(1):1-7, January 2006.

Respiratory distress syndrome

OVERVIEW

- Respiratory disorder that involves widespread alveolar collapse
- Most common cause of neonatal death
- If mild, subsides slowly after about 3 days
- Also called *RDS* or *hyaline membrane disease*

PATHOPHYSIOLOGY

- In neonates born before the 27th week of gestation, immaturity of alveoli and capillary blood supply lead to alveolar collapse from lack of surfactant (a lipoprotein normally present in alveoli and respiratory bronchioles).
- Surfactant deficiency causes widespread atelectasis, resulting in inadequate alveolar ventilation and shunting of blood through collapsed lung areas.
- Hypoxia and acidosis result.
- Compensatory grunting occurs, producing positive end-expiratory pressure (PEEP) that helps prevent further alveolar collapse.

CAUSES

- Surfactant deficiency stemming from preterm birth

RISK FACTORS

- Diabetes in mother during pregnancy
- Stress during preterm delivery

INCIDENCE

- RDS almost exclusively affects neonates born before the 27th gestational week; it occurs in about 60% of those born before the 28th week.
- RDS is most common in neonates of mothers with diabetes, neonates delivered by cesarean birth, and neonates delivered suddenly after antepartum hemorrhage.

COMPLICATIONS

- Respiratory insufficiency
- Shock
- Bronchopulmonary dysplasia
- Death

ASSESSMENT

HISTORY

- Preterm birth
- Cesarean birth
- Maternal history of diabetes or antepartum hemorrhage

PHYSICAL FINDINGS

- Rapid, shallow respirations
- Intercostal, subcostal, or sternal retractions
- Nasal flaring
- Audible expiratory grunting
- Pallor
- Frothy sputum
- Low body temperature
- Diminished air entry and crackles
- Possible hypotension, peripheral edema, and oliguria
- Possible apnea, bradycardia, and cyanosis

DIAGNOSTIC TEST RESULTS

LABORATORY

- Partial pressure of arterial oxygen (Pao_2) is decreased; partial pressure of arterial carbon dioxide ($Paco_2$) may be normal, decreased, or increased; and arterial pH is decreased.
- Lecithin-sphingomyelin ratio shows prenatal lung development and RDS risk.

IMAGING

- Chest X-rays may show a fine reticulonodular pattern and dark streaks, indicating air-filled, dilated bronchioles.

TREATMENT

GENERAL

- Mechanical ventilation with PEEP or continuous positive airway pressure (CPAP)
- For a neonate who can't maintain adequate gas exchange, high-frequency oscillation ventilation
- Radiant warmer or Isolette

DIET

- Tube feedings or total parenteral nutrition

MEDICATIONS

- I.V. fluids
- Sodium bicarbonate
- Pancuronium bromide
- Prophylactic antibiotics
- Diuretics
- Surfactant replacement therapy
- Vitamin E
- Antenatal corticosteroids
- Oxygen therapy

SURGERY

- Possible tracheostomy

NURSING DIAGNOSES

- Impaired gas exchange
- Impaired skin integrity
- Ineffective airway clearance
- Risk for infection
- Risk for injury

EXPECTED OUTCOMES

The patient (or family) will:
- maintain adequate ventilation and oxygenation
- maintain skin integrity
- maintain a patent airway
- remain free from signs and symptoms of infection
- identify factors that increase the risk of neonatal injury.

NURSING INTERVENTIONS

- Give prescribed drugs.
- Suction, as necessary.
- Change the transcutaneous Pao_2 monitor lead placement site every 2 to 4 hours.
- Adjust PEEP or CPAP settings as indicated by arterial blood gas (ABG) values.
- Implement measures to prevent infection.
- Provide mouth care every 2 hours.
- Encourage parents to participate in the infant's care.
- Encourage parents to ask questions and to express their fears and concerns.
- Advise parents that full recovery may take up to 12 months.
- Offer emotional support.

WARNING *In a neonate on a mechanical ventilator, watch carefully for signs of barotrauma and accidental disconnection from the ventilator. Check ventilator settings and alarms frequently. Be alert for signs of complications of PEEP or CPAP therapy, such as decreased cardiac output, pneumothorax, and pneumomediastinum.*

MONITORING

- Vital signs
- ABG values
- Intake and output
- Central venous pressure
- Signs and symptoms of infection
- Thrombosis
- Decreased peripheral circulation
- Pulse oximetry
- Daily weight
- Skin color
- Respiratory status
- Skin integrity

WARNING *Watch for evidence of complications from oxygen therapy: lung capillary damage, decreased mucus flow, impaired ciliary functioning, and widespread atelectasis. Also be alert for signs of patent ductus arteriosus, heart failure, retinopathy, pulmonary hypertension, necrotizing enterocolitis, and neurologic abnormalities.*

GENERAL

Be sure to cover (with the parents):
- the disorder, diagnosis, and treatment
- drugs and possible adverse effects
- explanations of respiratory equipment, alarm sounds, and mechanical noise
- potential complications
- when to notify the practitioner.

DISCHARGE PLANNING

- Refer the parents to pastoral counselors and social worker, as indicated.
- Refer the patient for follow-up care with a neonatal ophthalmologist, as indicated.

RESOURCES

Organizations

American Academy of Pediatrics: *www.aap.org*
American Association for Respiratory Care: *www.aarc.org*
American Lung Association: *www.lungusa.org*
National Heart, Lung, and Blood Institute: *www.nhlbi.nih.gov*

Selected references

Boyd, S. "Causes and Treatment of Neonatal Respiratory Distress Syndrome," *Nursing Times* 100(30):40-44, July-August 2004.

Burnes, S.M. "Mechanical Ventilation of Patients with Acute Respiratory Distress Syndrome and Patients Requiring Weaning: The Evidence Guiding Practice," *Critical Care Nurse* 25(4):14-23, August 2005.

Fan, E., et al. "Ventilatory Management of Acute Lung Injury and Acute Respiratory Distress Syndrome," *JAMA* 294(22):2889-896, December 2005.

Rebmann, T. "Severe Acute Respiratory Distress Syndrome: Implications for Perinatal and Neonatal Nurses," *Journal of Perinatal & Neonatal Nursing* 19(4):332-45, October-December 2005.

Respiratory syncytial virus infection

- Virus that's the leading cause of lower respiratory tract infection in infants and young children and upper respiratory infections in adults
- Suspected cause of fatal respiratory diseases in infants
- Can cause serious illness in immunocompromised adults, institutionalized elderly people, and patients with underlying cardiopulmonary disease
- Also known as *RSV*

PATHOPHYSIOLOGY

- The virus attaches to cells, eventually resulting in necrosis of the bronchiolar epithelium; in severe infection, peribronchiolar infiltrate of lymphocytes and mononuclear cells occurs.
- Intra-alveolar thickening and filling of the alveolar spaces with fluid results.
- Narrowing of the airway passages on expiration prevents air from leaving the lungs, causing progressive overinflation.

CAUSES

- Respiratory syncytial virus, a subgroup of myxoviruses resembling paramyxovirus

RISK FACTORS

- Day care attendance
- Contact with school-age children
- Low birth weight
- Crowded living conditions
- Environmental air pollutants

INCIDENCE

- RSV almost exclusively affects infants and young children, especially those in day-care settings.
- The incidence is highest among infants ages 1 to 6 months, peaking between ages 2 and 3 months.
- Annual RSV epidemics occur during winter and spring.

COMPLICATIONS

- Pneumonia and progressive pneumonia
- Bronchiolitis
- Croup
- Otitis media
- Respiratory failure
- Sudden infant death syndrome
- Residual lung damage

ASSESSMENT

HISTORY

- Nasal congestion
- Coughing
- Wheezing
- Malaise
- Sore throat
- Earache
- Dyspnea
- Fever

PHYSICAL FINDINGS

- Nasal and pharyngeal inflammation
- Otitis media
- Severe respiratory distress (nasal flaring, retraction, cyanosis, and tachypnea)
- Wheezes, rhonchi, and crackles

DIAGNOSTIC TEST RESULTS

LABORATORY

- Cultures of nasal and pharyngeal secretions show RSV.
- Serum RSV antibody titers are elevated.
- Arterial blood gas values show hypoxemia and respiratory acidosis.
- In dehydration, blood urea nitrogen levels are elevated.

TREATMENT

GENERAL
- Respiratory support
- Symptomatic treatment

DIET
- Adequate nutrition
- Avoidance of overhydration

ACTIVITY
- Rest periods when fatigued

MEDICATIONS
- Ribavirin
- Oxygen (for severe infection)
- I.V. fluids (for severe infection)

SURGERY
- Possible tracheostomy

NURSING CONSIDERATIONS

NURSING DIAGNOSES
- Activity intolerance
- Compromised family coping
- Imbalanced nutrition: Less than body requirements
- Impaired gas exchange
- Impaired social interaction
- Ineffective airway clearance
- Ineffective breathing pattern
- Risk for aspiration
- Risk for deficient fluid volume
- Risk for infection

EXPECTED OUTCOMES
The patient (or family) will:
- return to previous activity level
- demonstrate effective coping strategies for handling their child's illness
- maintain adequate nutritional intake
- express or indicate feelings of increased comfort while maintaining adequate air exchange
- demonstrate effective social interactions in both one-on-one and group settings
- maintain a patent airway, cough effectively, and expectorate mucus
- maintain an effective breathing pattern and a respiratory rate within 5 breaths/minute of baseline
- not develop aspiration pneumonia
- maintain adequate fluid volume
- experience no further signs or symptoms of infection.

NURSING INTERVENTIONS
- Institute contact isolation.
- Perform percussion, drainage, and suction when necessary.
- Give prescribed oxygen.
- Use a croup tent, as needed.
- Place the patient in semi-Fowler's position.
- Observe for signs and symptoms of dehydration, and administer I.V. fluids accordingly.
- Promote bed rest.
- Offer diversional activities tailored to the patient's condition and age.

MONITORING
- Respiratory status
- Fluid and electrolyte status

PATIENT TEACHING

GENERAL
Be sure to cover (with the parents):
- the disorder, diagnosis, and treatment
- how the infection spreads
- preventive measures (RSV immune globulin)
- drugs and possible adverse effects
- importance of a nonsmoking environment in the home
- follow-up care.

RESOURCES
Organizations
American Lung Association: *www.lungusa.org*
Mayo Clinic: *www.mayoclinic.com*
National Center for Infectious Diseases: *www.cdc.gov/ncidod*
National Institute of Allergy and Infectious Diseases: *www.niaid.nih.gov*
The RSV Info Center: *www.rsvinfo.com*

Selected references
Blanco, J.C., et al. "Prospects of Antiviral and Anti-Inflammatory Therapy for Respiratory Syncytial Virus Infection," *Expert Review of Anti-Infective Therapy* 3(6):945-55, December 2005.

Kasper, D.L., et al., eds. *Harrison's Principles of Internal Medicine,* 16th ed. New York: McGraw-Hill Book Co., 2005.

Lauts, N.M. "RSV: Protecting the Littlest Patients," *RN* 68(12):46-51, December 2005.

Mejias, A., et al. "Respiratory Syncytial Virus Infections: Old Challenges and New Opportunities," *Pediatric Infectious Disease Journal* 24(11 Suppl):S189-96, November 2005.

Nagayama, Y., et al. "Gender Analysis in Acute Bronchiolitis Due to Respiratory Syncytial Virus," *Pediatric Allergy and Immunology* 17(1):29-36, February 2006.

Pruitt, B. "Keeping Respiratory Syncytial Virus at Bay," *Nursing* 35(11): 62-64, November 2005.

Retinal detachment

OVERVIEW

- Partial or complete separation of the sensory retina from the underlying pigment epithelium
- May be primary or secondary
- Commonly occurs spontaneously
- Usually involves only one eye; may occur in the other eye later
- Rarely heals spontaneously; usually can be reattached successfully with surgery
- Carries varying prognosis depending on the retinal area affected

PATHOPHYSIOLOGY

- A hole or tear in the retina allows the liquid vitreous to seep between the retinal layers.
- Liquid separates the sensory retinal layer from its choroidal blood supply. (See *Understanding retinal detachment*.)

CAUSES

- Age-related degenerative changes
- Hereditary factors, usually related to myopia
- Intraocular inflammation
- Systemic disease
- Traction placed on the retina by vitreous bands or membranes
- Trauma
- Tumors

 AGE FACTOR *In a child, retinal detachment can result from retinopathy of prematurity, tumors (retinoblastomas), or trauma.*

RISK FACTORS

- Myopia
- Cataract surgery
- Trauma
- History of uncontrolled diabetes

INCIDENCE

- Retinal detachment affects twice as many men as women.
- This disorder is more common with increased age.

COMPLICATIONS

- Severe vision impairment
- Blindness

ASSESSMENT

HISTORY

- Sensation of seeing floaters and flashes
- Painless vision loss, described as sensation of looking through a veil, curtain, or cobweb (which may obscure objects in a particular area of the visual field)

PHYSICAL FINDINGS

- Visual field loss

DIAGNOSTIC TEST RESULTS

IMAGING

- Ocular ultrasonography, used to examine the retina if the lens is opaque, shows intraocular and intraorbital pathology; also commonly detects retinal detachments, characteristically producing a dense, sheetlike echo on a B-mode scan.

DIAGNOSTIC PROCEDURES

- Direct ophthalmoscopy shows folds or discoloration in the usually transparent retina.
- Indirect ophthalmoscopy shows retinal tears.

Understanding retinal detachment

Traumatic injury or degenerative changes cause retinal detachment by allowing the retina's sensory tissue layers to separate from the retinal pigment epithelium. This permits fluid — from the vitreous, for example — to seep into the space between the retinal pigment epithelium and the rods and cones of the tissue layers.

The pressure, which results from the fluid entering the space, balloons the retina into the vitreous cavity away from choroidal circulation. Separated from its blood supply, the retina can't function. Without prompt repair, the detached retina can cause permanent vision loss.

GENERAL
- Varies with location and severity of detachment

DIET
- Nothing by mouth before surgery

ACTIVITY
- Bed rest before surgery
- Restriction of eye movements before surgery, by patching affected eye
- Prevent further separation before surgery, by positioning the patient's head to allow gravity to pull the detached retina closer to the choroid

MEDICATIONS
- Antiemetics
- Analgesics
- Mydriatics
- Cycloplegics
- Corticosteroid eyedrops
- Antibiotic eyedrops

SURGERY
- Cryothermy
- Laser therapy
- Scleral buckling (may be followed by vitreous replacement with silicone, oil, air, or gas)
- Diathermy

NURSING DIAGNOSES
- Anxiety
- Disturbed sensory perception (visual)
- Impaired tissue integrity
- Ineffective health maintenance
- Risk for infection
- Risk for injury

EXPECTED OUTCOMES
The patient will:
- verbalize strategies to reduce anxiety
- regain the previous level of visual functioning
- regain adequate perfusion to the retina
- maintain current health status
- show no signs or symptoms of infection
- avoid injury and complications.

NURSING INTERVENTIONS
- Prepare the patient for surgery.
- Give prescribed antibiotics and cycloplegic or mydriatic eyedrops.
- In macular involvement, maintain bed rest to prevent further retinal detachment.
- Postoperatively, position the patient as directed.
- Give prescribed antiemetics as indicated.
- Give prescribed analgesics.
- Discourage activities that increase intraocular pressure.
- With retrobulbar injection, apply a protective eye patch.
- Apply cold compresses.
- Avoid putting pressure on the eye.
- Provide encouragement and emotional support.

MONITORING
- Localized corneal edema and perilimbal congestion after laser therapy
- Persistent pain
- Vital signs
- Visual acuity
- Response to treatment

GENERAL
Be sure to cover:
- the disorder, diagnosis, and treatment
- leg and deep-breathing exercises
- possible persistence of blurred vision for several days after laser therapy
- importance of avoiding driving, bending, heavy lifting, and other activities that affect intraocular pressure for several days after surgery
- avoidance of activities that could cause eye trauma
- how to instill eyedrops
- importance of wearing sunglasses
- applying cold compresses
- drugs and possible adverse effects
- signs and symptoms of increasing ocular pressure and infection
- early symptoms of retinal detachment.

RESOURCES
Organizations
American Academy of Ophthalmology: *www.aao.org*
National Eye Institute: *www.nei.nih.gov*
Prevent Blindness America: *www.preventblindness.org*
Vision Council of America: *www.visionsite.org*

Selected references
Boyd-Monk, H. "Bringing Common Eye Emergencies into Focus," *Nursing* 35(12):46-51, December 2005.
Church, J.R., and Winder, S.M. "Surgical Repair of a Retinal Detachment in a Patient with Osteogenesis Imperfecta," *Retina* 26(2):242-43, February 2006.
Sonoda, Y., et al. "Endoscopy-guided Subretinal Fluid Drainage in Vitrectomy for Retinal Detachment," *Ophthalmologica* 220(2):83-86, 2006.
Yuen, K.S., et al. "Bilateral Exudative Retinal Detachments as the Presenting Features of Idiopathic Orbital Inflammation," *Clinical & Experimental Ophthalmology* 33(6):671-74, December 2005.

Reye's syndrome

OVERVIEW

- An acute childhood illness that causes fatty infiltration of the liver with concurrent hyperammonemia, encephalopathy, and increased intracranial pressure (ICP)
- Possible fatty infiltration of the kidneys, brain, and myocardium
- Variable prognosis depending on the severity of central nervous system depression

PATHOPHYSIOLOGY

- Damaged hepatic mitochondria disrupt the urea cycle, which normally changes ammonia to urea for excretion from the body.
- This results in hyperammonemia, hypoglycemia, and an increase in serum short-chain fatty acids, leading to encephalopathy.
- Simultaneously, fatty infiltration is found in renal tubular cells, neuronal tissue, and muscle tissue, including the heart.

CAUSES

- Aspirin use
- Viral infection (such as varicella or influenza)

INCIDENCE

- The incidence of Reye's syndrome usually increases during influenza outbreaks.
- Reye's syndrome occurs more often after aspirin ingestion.
  - **AGE FACTOR** *Reye's syndrome is most common in children ages 4 to 12, with peak incidence at age 6.*

COMPLICATIONS

- Increased ICP
- Coma
- Seizures
- Respiratory failure

ASSESSMENT

HISTORY

- Viral infection
- Aspirin use
- Vomiting
- Change in mental status

PHYSICAL FINDINGS

- Hyperactive reflexes
- Increased blood pressure
- Tachycardia
- Lethargy

DIAGNOSTIC TEST RESULTS

LABORATORY

- Low or absent serum salicylate level rules out aspirin overdose.
- Liver-function studies show aspartate aminotransferase and alanine aminotransferase levels elevated to twice normal; bilirubin level is usually normal.
- Cerebrospinal fluid (CSF) analysis reveals a white blood cell count of less than 10; with coma, CSF pressure increases.
- Coagulation studies result in prolonged prothrombin and partial thromboplastin times.
- Blood values show elevated serum ammonia levels; normal or, in 15% of cases, low serum glucose levels; and increased serum fatty acid and lactate levels.

DIAGNOSTIC PROCEDURES

- Liver biopsy reveals fatty droplets uniformly distributed throughout cells.

OTHER

- History of a recent viral disorder with typical signs and symptoms strongly suggests Reye's syndrome.

TREATMENT

- Dictated by stage of the syndrome (see *Stages of treatment for Reye's syndrome*)

NURSING DIAGNOSES
◆ Anxiety
◆ Fear
◆ Impaired gas exchange
◆ Impaired physical mobility
◆ Ineffective breathing pattern
◆ Ineffective tissue perfusion: Cerebral
◆ Risk for impaired skin integrity

EXPECTED OUTCOMES
The patient (or family) will:
◆ express reduced levels of anxiety
◆ discuss fears and concerns
◆ maintain adequate ventilation and oxygenation
◆ maintain joint mobility and range of motion
◆ maintain respiratory rate within 5 breaths/minute of baseline
◆ maintain orientation to environment without evidence of deficit
◆ maintain skin integrity.

NURSING INTERVENTIONS
◆ Maintain seizure precautions.
◆ Provide skin and mouth care.
◆ Perform or assist with range-of-motion exercises.

MONITORING
◆ Vital signs
◆ Intake and output
◆ ICP
◆ Respiratory status
◆ Cardiovascular status
◆ Level of consciousness

GENERAL
Be sure to cover:
◆ using a nonsalicylate analgesic and an antipyretic such as acetaminophen for children.

DISCHARGE PLANNING
◆ Refer parents to the National Reye's Syndrome Foundation for more information.

RESOURCES
Organizations
American Liver Foundation: *www.liverfoundation.org*
Mayo Clinic: *www.mayoclinic.com*
National Institute of Neurological Disorders and Stroke: *www.ninds.nih.gov*
National Reye's Syndrome Foundation: *www.reyessyndrome.org*

Selected references
Ramonet, M.D., et al. "Epidemiologic Overview of Reye's Syndrome," *Journal of Pediatric Gastroenterology & Nutrition* 39 (Suppl 1):S159, June 2004.
Rice, S. "Reye's Syndrome Isn't Just Child's Play," *Nursing* 33(9):32hn1-32hn4, September 2003.
Waller, P., and Suvarna, R. "Is Aspirin a Cause of Reye's Syndrome?" *Drug Safety* 27(1):71-74, 2004.
Wei C., et al. "Reye's syndrome Developing in an Infant on Treatment of Kawasaki Syndrome," *Journal of Paediatrics & Child Health* 41(5-6):303-304, May-June 2005.
Wittenstein, B., et al. "'African Medicine' and Reye's Syndrome," *Lancet* 363(9412):860, March 2004.

Stages of treatment for Reye's syndrome

SIGNS AND SYMPTOMS	BASELINE TREATMENT
Stage I Vomiting, lethargy, hepatic dysfunction	◆ To decrease intracranial pressure (ICP) and brain edema, give I.V. fluids at two-thirds of the maintenance dose. Also give an osmotic diuretic or furosemide (Lasix). ◆ To treat hypoprothrombinemia, give vitamin K; if vitamin K proves unsuccessful, give fresh frozen plasma. ◆ Monitor serum ammonia and blood glucose levels and plasma osmolality every 4 to 8 hours to check progress.
Stage II Hyperventilation, delirium, hepatic dysfunction, hyperactive reflexes	◆ Continue baseline treatment.
Stage III Coma, hyperventilation, decorticate rigidity, hepatic dysfunction	◆ Continue baseline and seizure treatment. ◆ Monitor ICP with a subarachnoid screw or other invasive device. ◆ Provide endotracheal intubation and mechanical ventilation to control partial pressure of carbon dioxide. A paralyzing agent, such as pancuronium I.V. may help maintain ventilation. ◆ Give mannitol I.V. or glycerol by nasogastric tube.
Stage IV Deepening coma; decerebrate rigidity; large, fixed pupils; minimal hepatic dysfunction	◆ Continue baseline and supportive care. ◆ If all previous measures fail, some pediatric centers use barbiturate coma, decompressive craniotomy, hypothermia, or an exchange transfusion.
Stage V Seizures, loss of deep tendon reflexes, flaccidity, respiratory arrest, ammonia level greater than 300 mg/dl	◆ Continue baseline and supportive care.

Rhabdomyolysis

OVERVIEW

- Breakdown of skeletal muscle tissue, causing myoglobinuria
- Usually follows major muscle trauma, especially a muscle crush injury
- Good prognosis if contributing causes are stopped or disease is checked before damage is irreversible

PATHOPHYSIOLOGY

- Muscle trauma that compresses tissue causes ischemia and necrosis.
- The ensuing local edema further increases compartment pressure and tamponade; pressure from severe swelling causes blood vessels to collapse, leading to tissue hypoxia, muscle infarction, neural damage in the area of the fracture, and release of myoglobin from the necrotic muscle fibers into the circulation.

CAUSES

- Skeletal muscle damage

RISK FACTORS

- Anesthetics that cause intraoperative rigidity
- Cardiac arrhythmias
- Electrolyte disturbances
- Excessive muscular activity associated with status epilepticus, electroconvulsive therapy, or high-voltage electrical shock
- Familial tendency
- Hyperthermia
- Infection, especially severe infection
- Prescription and nonprescription drugs (see *Drugs that may cause rhabdomyolysis*)
- Strenuous exertion such as long-distance running
- Traumatic injury

RISK FACTORS

- Alcohol use
- Recent soft tissue compression
- Seizure activity

INCIDENCE

- Rhabdomyolysis occurs more often in males than in females.
- The disorder may occur at any age.

COMPLICATIONS

- Acute renal failure
- Acute tubular necrosis

ASSESSMENT

HISTORY

- Muscle trauma or breakdown
- Muscle pain
- Presence of any risk factors

PHYSICAL FINDINGS

- Dark, reddish-brown urine
- Tense, tender muscle compartment (compartment syndrome)

DIAGNOSTIC TEST RESULTS

LABORATORY

- Urine myoglobin level exceeds 0.5 mg/dl (evident with only 200 g of muscle damage).
- Creatinine kinase level is elevated (0.5 to 0.95 mg/dl) from muscle damage.
- Serum potassium, phosphate, creatinine, and creatine levels are elevated.
- Hypocalcemia occurs in early stages, hypercalcemia in later stages.
- Intracompartmental venous pressure measurements (using a wick catheter, needle, or slit catheter inserted into the muscle) are elevated.

IMAGING

- Computed tomography, magnetic resonance imaging, and bone scintigraphy are used to detect muscle necrosis.

Drugs that may cause rhabdomyolysis

The use of these drugs may cause rhabdomyolysis:

- amphetamines
- antilipemics
- antipsychotics
- anesthetic and paralytic agents
- antihistamines
- cocaine
- corticosteroids
- cyclic antidepressants
- emetics
- fibric acid derivatives
- laxatives
- neuroleptics
- salicylates
- sedative-hypnotics
- selective serotonin reuptake inhibitors.

TREATMENT

GENERAL
- For underlying disorder
- Prevention of renal failure

DIET
- Increased fluid intake

ACTIVITY
- Bed rest

MEDICATIONS
- Anti-inflammatories
- Corticosteroids (in extreme cases)
- Analgesics
- I.V. fluids
- Diuretics
- Sodium bicarbonate

SURGERY
- Immediate fasciotomy and debridement if compartment venous pressure exceeds 25 mm Hg

NURSING CONSIDERATIONS

NURSING DIAGNOSES
- Acute pain
- Excess fluid volume
- Hyperthermia
- Impaired urinary elimination

EXPECTED OUTCOMES
The patient will:
- express increased comfort and decreased pain
- exhibit signs of normal fluid balance
- maintain a normal body temperature
- maintain normal renal function and urine output.

NURSING INTERVENTIONS
- Give prescribed I.V. fluids and medication.
- Measure intake and output accurately.
- Promote comfort measures.

MONITORING
- Intake and output
- Urine myoglobins
- Renal studies
- Pain control

PATIENT TEACHING

GENERAL
Be sure to cover:
- the disorder, diagnosis, and treatment
- the need for prolonged, low-intensity training as opposed to short bursts of intense exercise.

RESOURCES
Organizations
American Association of Kidney Patients: *www.aakp.org*
National Institute of Diabetes & Digestive & Kidney Diseases: *www.niddk.nih.gov*
Rhabdomyolysis Kidney Failure and Damage: *www.rhabdomyolysis.org*

Selected references
Betten, D.P., et al. "Massive Honey Bee Envenomation-induced Rhabdomyolysis in an Adolescent," *Pediatrics* 117(1):231-35, January 2006.

Hansen, K.E., et al. "Outcomes of 45 Patients with Statin-Associated Myopathy," *Archives of Internal Medicine* 165(22):2671-676, December 2005.

Kring, D. "Outmuscling Rhabdomyolysis," *Nursing Management* Suppl:24, 26, 29, 2005.

Ocana, J., et al. "Rhabdomyolysis," *American Journal of Kidney Diseases* 47(1):A32, e1-2, January 2006.

Vasudevan, A.R., et al. "Safety of Statins: Effects on Muscle and the Liver," *Cleveland Clinic Journal of Medicine* 72(11):990-93, 996-1001, November 2005.

Rheumatic fever and rheumatic heart disease

OVERVIEW

- Systemic inflammatory disease of childhood that occurs 2 to 6 weeks after an inadequately treated upper respiratory tract infection with group A beta-hemolytic streptococci
- Principally involves the heart, joints, central nervous system, skin, and subcutaneous tissues
- In rheumatic heart disease, early acute phase that may affect endocardium, myocardium, or pericardium, possibly followed later by chronic valvular disease
- Commonly recurs

PATHOPHYSIOLOGY

- Rheumatic fever appears to be a hypersensitivity reaction in which antibodies produced to combat streptococci react and produce lesions at specific tissue sites.
- Antigens of group A streptococci bind to receptors in the heart, muscle, brain, and synovial joints, causing an autoimmune response.
- Because the antigens are similar to the body's own cells, antibodies may attack healthy body cells by mistake.

CAUSES

- Group A beta-hemolytic streptococcal pharyngitis

INCIDENCE

- In the United States, incidence of rheumatic heart disease and rheumatic fever is most common in the northern states.
- Worldwide, 15 to 20 million new cases occur each year.

COMPLICATIONS

- Destruction of mitral and aortic valves
- Severe pancarditis
- Pericardial effusion
- Heart failure
- Systemic emboli

AGE FACTOR *In children, mitral insufficiency is the major consequence of rheumatic heart disease.*

ASSESSMENT

HISTORY

- Recent streptococcal infection
- Recent history of low-grade fever spiking to at least 100.4° F (38° C) in late afternoon, along with unexplained epistaxis and abdominal pain
- Migratory joint pain (polyarthritis)

PHYSICAL FINDINGS

- Swelling, redness, and signs of effusion, most commonly in the knees, ankles, elbows, and hips
- With pericarditis: sharp, sudden pain that usually starts over the sternum and radiates to the neck, shoulders, back, and arms; increases with deep inspiration and decreases when the patient sits up and leans forward
- With heart failure caused by severe rheumatic carditis: dyspnea, right upper quadrant pain, and a hacking, nonproductive cough
- Skin lesions, such as erythema marginatum, typically on the trunk and extremities
- Subcutaneous nodules, 3 mm to 2 cm in diameter, that are firm, movable, and nontender occurring near tendons or bony prominences of joints, persisting for several days to weeks
- With left-sided heart failure: edema and tachypnea, bibasilar crackles, and ventricular or atrial gallop
- Transient chorea up to 6 months after original streptococcal infection
- Pericardial friction rub
- Heart murmurs and gallops

DIAGNOSTIC TEST RESULTS

LABORATORY

- During acute phase, white blood cell count and erythrocyte sedimentation rate are elevated.
- During inflammation, complete blood count shows slight anemia.
- C-reactive protein test result is positive, especially during acute phase.
- In severe carditis, cardiac enzyme levels are increased.
- Antistreptolysin-O titer is elevated in 95% of patients within 2 months of onset.
- Throat cultures show group A beta-hemolytic streptococci.

IMAGING

- Chest X-rays show normal heart size (except with myocarditis, heart failure, and pericardial effusion).
- Echocardiography helps evaluate valvular damage, chamber size, and ventricular function and detects pericardial effusion.

DIAGNOSTIC PROCEDURES

- Electrocardiography reveals no diagnostic changes, but 20% of patients show a prolonged PR interval.
- Cardiac catheterization evaluates valvular damage and left ventricular function in severe cardiac dysfunction.

TREATMENT

GENERAL
◆ Symptomatic treatment

DIET
◆ Sodium restriction, if indicated

ACTIVITY
◆ Bed rest during acute phase
◆ Gradual activity increase, as tolerated

MEDICATIONS
◆ Antibiotics
◆ Anti-inflammatories

SURGERY
◆ Commissurotomy, valvuloplasty, or heart valve replacement

NURSING DIAGNOSES

◆ Activity intolerance
◆ Acute pain
◆ Anxiety
◆ Decreased cardiac output
◆ Deficient diversional activity
◆ Fatigue
◆ Impaired gas exchange
◆ Ineffective role performance
◆ Risk for infection

EXPECTED OUTCOMES
The patient will:
◆ carry out activities of daily living without weakness or fatigue
◆ express feelings of comfort
◆ cope with medical condition without demonstrating severe signs of anxiety
◆ maintain hemodynamic stability, have no arrhythmias, and maintain adequate cardiac output
◆ identify appropriate diversionary activities to partake in while on bed rest
◆ verbalize the importance of balancing activity with adequate rest periods
◆ maintain adequate ventilation and oxygenation
◆ express feelings about diminished capacity to perform usual roles

◆ remain free from signs and symptoms of infection.

NURSING INTERVENTIONS
◆ Find out if the patient has ever had a hypersensitivity reaction to penicillin. Warn the parents (if appropriate) that such a reaction is possible.
◆ Give prescribed antibiotics on time.
◆ Stress the importance of bed rest. Provide a bedside commode.
◆ Position the patient upright.
◆ Provide analgesics and oxygen, as needed.
◆ Allow the patient to express feelings and concerns.
◆ Help the parents overcome any guilt feelings they may have about their child's illness.
◆ Encourage the parents and child to vent their frustrations during the long recovery. If the child has severe carditis, help them prepare for permanent changes in the child's lifestyle.

MONITORING
◆ Vital signs
◆ Heart rhythm
◆ Heart and breath sounds

PATIENT TEACHING

GENERAL
Be sure to cover:
◆ the disorder, diagnosis, and treatment
◆ the importance of resuming activities of daily living slowly and scheduling frequent rest periods as instructed by the practitioner
◆ what to do if signs of an allergic reaction to penicillin occur
◆ the importance of reporting early signs and symptoms of left-sided heart failure, such as dyspnea and a hacking, nonproductive cough, and immediately reporting signs of recurrent streptococcal infection
◆ keeping the child away from people with respiratory tract infections
◆ transient nature of chorea
◆ compliance with prolonged antibiotic therapy and follow-up care
◆ the need for prophylactic antibiotics before any dental work or invasive procedures.

RESOURCES
Organizations
American Heart Association: *www.americanheart.org*
National Heart, Lung, and Blood Institute: *www.nhlbi.nih.gov*

Selected references
Carapetis, J.R., et al. "Acute Rheumatic Fever," *Lancet* 366(9480):155-68, July 2005.
Kasper, D.L., et al., eds. *Harrison's Principles of Internal Medicine,* 16th ed. New York: McGraw-Hill Book Co., 2005.
Lee, G.M., and Wessels, M.R. "Changing Epidemiology of Acute Rheumatic Fever in the United States," *Clinical Infectious Diseases* 42(4):448-50, February 2006.
The Merck Manual of Diagnosis & Therapy, 18th ed., Whitehouse Station, N.J.: Merck & Co., Inc., 2006.
Mota, C. "Limitations and Perspectives with the Approach to Rheumatic Fever and Rheumatic Heart Disease," *Cardiology in the Young* 15(6):580-82, December 2005.

Rheumatoid arthritis

- Chronic, systemic, symmetrical inflammatory disease
- Primarily attacks peripheral joints and surrounding muscles, tendons, ligaments, and blood vessels
- Marked by spontaneous remissions and unpredictable exacerbations
- Potentially crippling

PATHOPHYSIOLOGY

- Cartilage damage resulting from inflammation triggers further immune responses, including complement activation.
- Complement, in turn, attracts polymorphonuclear leukocytes and stimulates release of inflammatory mediators, which exacerbates joint destruction.

CAUSES

- Exact cause unknown
- Possible link to viral or bacterial infection, hormonal factors, and lifestyle

INCIDENCE

- Rheumatoid arthritis strikes three times as many women as men.
- The disorder can occur at any age, with peak onset between ages 35 and 50.

COMPLICATIONS

- Fibrous or bony ankylosis
- Soft-tissue contractures
- Joint deformities
- Sjögren's syndrome
- Spinal cord compression
- Carpal tunnel syndrome
- Osteoporosis
- Recurrent infections
- Hip joint necrosis

ASSESSMENT

HISTORY

- Insidious onset of nonspecific symptoms, including fatigue, malaise, anorexia, persistent low-grade fever, weight loss, and vague articular symptoms
- Later, more specific localized articular symptoms, commonly in the fingers
- Bilateral and symmetrical symptoms, which may extend to the wrists, elbows, knees, and ankles
- Stiff joints
- Stiff, weak, or painful muscles
- Numbness or tingling in the feet or weakness or loss of sensation in the fingers
- Pain on inspiration
- Shortness of breath

PHYSICAL FINDINGS

- Joint deformities and contractures
- Painful, red, swollen arms
- Foreshortened hands
- Boggy wrists
- Rheumatoid nodules
- Leg ulcers
- Eye redness
- Joints that are warm to the touch
- Pericardial friction rub
- Positive Babinski's sign

DIAGNOSTIC TEST RESULTS

LABORATORY

- Rheumatoid factor test is positive in 75% to 80% of patients, as indicated by a titer of 1:160 or higher.
- Synovial fluid analysis shows increased volume and turbidity but decreased viscosity and complement (C3 and C4) levels, with white blood cell count possibly exceeding 10,000/µl.
- Serum globulin levels are elevated.
- Erythrocyte sedimentation rate is elevated.
- Complete blood count shows moderate anemia and slight leukocytosis.

IMAGING

- In early stages, X-rays show bone demineralization and soft-tissue swelling. Later, they help determine the extent of cartilage and bone destruction, erosion, subluxations, and deformities and show the characteristic pattern of these abnormalities.
- Magnetic resonance imaging and computed tomography scan may show the extent of damage.

OTHER

- Synovial tissue biopsy shows inflammation.

TREATMENT

GENERAL

- Moist heat application
- Adequate sleep
- Splinting

ACTIVITY

- Range-of-motion (ROM) exercises and carefully individualized therapeutic exercises
- Frequent rest periods

MEDICATIONS

- Salicylates
- Nonsteroidal anti-inflammatory drugs
- Antimalarials (hydroxychloroquine)
- Gold salts
- Penicillamine
- Corticosteroids
- Antineoplastics
- Monoclonal antibody therapy, such as infliximab (Remicade)

SURGERY

- Metatarsal head and distal ulnar resectional arthroplasty and insertion of Silastic prosthesis between the metacarpophalangeal and proximal interphalangeal joints
- Arthrodesis (joint fusion)
- Synovectomy
- Osteotomy
- Repair of ruptured tendon
- In advanced disease, joint reconstruction or total joint arthroplasty

NURSING DIAGNOSES
- Activity intolerance
- Bathing or hygiene self-care deficit
- Chronic pain
- Energy field disturbance
- Fatigue
- Hopelessness
- Impaired physical mobility
- Ineffective health maintenance
- Ineffective role performance
- Ineffective tissue perfusion: Peripheral
- Powerlessness
- Risk for impaired skin integrity
- Risk for infection

EXPECTED OUTCOMES
The patient will:
- verbalize the importance of balancing activity, as tolerated, with rest
- participate in activities of daily living to the fullest extent possible
- express feelings of increased comfort and decreased pain
- express an increased sense of well-being
- express feelings of increased energy
- make decisions on own behalf
- attain the highest degree of mobility possible within the confines of the disease
- continue to receive treatments that promote relaxation and inner well-being
- recognize limitations imposed by the illness and express feelings about these limitations
- maintain adequate peripheral perfusion, as evidenced by palpable pulses and warm extremities
- express feelings of control over condition
- maintain skin integrity
- exhibit no signs or symptoms of infection.

NURSING INTERVENTIONS
- Give prescribed analgesics, and monitor effects.
- Perform meticulous skin care.
- Supply adaptive devices, such as a zipper-pull, easy-to-open beverage cartons, lightweight cups, and unpackaged silverware.

After total knee or hip arthroplasty
- Give prescribed blood products and antibiotics.
- Have the patient perform active dorsiflexion; immediately report inability to do so.
- Supervise isometric exercises every 2 hours.
- After total hip arthroplasty, check traction for pressure areas and keep the head of the bed raised 30 to 45 degrees.
- Change or reinforce dressings, as needed, using aseptic technique.
- Have the patient turn, cough, and breathe deeply every 2 hours.
- After total knee arthroplasty, keep the leg extended and slightly elevated.
- After total hip arthroplasty, keep the hip in abduction. Watch for and immediately report inability to rotate the hip or bear weight on it, increased pain, or a leg that appears shorter.
- Assist patient in activities, keeping the weight on the unaffected side.

MONITORING
- Joint mobility and pain level
- Skin integrity
- Vital signs and daily weight
- Hematocrit and serum electrolyte and hemoglobin levels
- Activity tolerance
- Laboratory values

GENERAL
Be sure to cover:
- the disorder, diagnosis, and treatment
- chronic nature of rheumatoid arthritis and possible need for major lifestyle changes
- importance of a balanced diet and weight control
- importance of adequate sleep
- sexual concerns.

If the patient requires total knee or hip arthroplasty, be sure to cover:
- preoperative and surgical procedures
- postoperative exercises
- deep-breathing and coughing exercises to perform after surgery
- performing frequent ROM leg exercises after surgery
- use of a constant-passive-motion device after total knee arthroplasty, or placement of an abduction pillow between the legs after total hip arthroplasty
- how to use a trapeze to move about in bed
- drug dosages and possible adverse effects.

DISCHARGE PLANNING
- Refer the patient for physical and occupational therapy.
- Refer the patient to the Arthritis Foundation.

RESOURCES
Organizations
Arthritis Foundation: *www.arthritis.org*
Johns Hopkins Arthritis Center: *www.hopkins-arthritis.som.jhmi.edu*
National Institute of Arthritis and Musculoskeletal and Skin Diseases: *www.nih.gov/niams/healthinfo*
The Arthritis Society: *www.arthritis.ca*

Selected references
Bathon, J.M., et al. "Safety and Efficacy of Etanercept Treatment in Elderly Subjects with Rheumatoid Arthritis," *Journal of Rheumatology* 33(2):234-43, February 2006.
Firestein, G.S. "Inhibiting Inflammation in Rheumatoid Arthritis," *New England Journal of Medicine* 354(1):80-82, January 2006.
Kasper, D.L., et al., eds. *Harrison's Principles of Internal Medicine,* 16th ed. New York: McGraw-Hill Book Co., 2005.
Mitka, M. "Early Rheumatoid Arthritis Treatments Weighed," *JAMA* 294(24): 3073-3074, December 2005.

Rocky Mountain spotted fever

OVERVIEW

- Acute infectious, febrile, rash-producing illness associated with outdoor activities
- Fatal in about 5% of patients

PATHOPHYSIOLOGY

- Infecting organism multiplies in endothelial cells and spreads via the bloodstream.
- Focal areas of infiltration lead to thrombosis and leakage of red blood cells into surrounding tissue.

CAUSES

- Occasionally, inhalation of or contact of abraded skin with tick excreta or tissue juices
- *Rickettsia rickettsii*, transmitted by the wood tick (*Dermacentor andersoni*) in the western United States and by the dog tick (*D. variabilis*) in the eastern United States

RISK FACTORS

- Recent hiking

INCIDENCE

- Rocky Mountain spotted fever is endemic throughout the continental United States.
- The disease is particularly prevalent in children ages 5 to 9.
- The disease occurs with increased frequency in spring and summer.

COMPLICATIONS

- Lobar pneumonia
- Disseminated intravascular coagulation
- Renal failure
- Meningoencephalitis
- Hepatic injury
- Death
- Cardiac or respiratory failure

ASSESSMENT

HISTORY

- Recent exposure to ticks or tick-infested areas, or a known tick bite
- Abrupt symptom onset, including persistent fever (temperature of 102° to 104° F [38.9° to 40° C]); generalized, excruciating headache; and aching in bones, muscles, joints, and back

PHYSICAL FINDINGS

- Erythematous macules, 1 to 5 mm in diameter, becoming maculopapules that blanch with pressure
- Frank hemorrhage at the center of maculopapules, creating petechia that don't blanch with pressure
- Bronchial cough
- Tachypnea
- Altered level of consciousness
- Decreased urine output; dark urine
- Tachycardia
- Hypotension
- Hepatomegaly, splenomegaly
- Generalized pitting edema
- Abdominal tenderness

DIAGNOSTIC TEST RESULTS

LABORATORY

- Serologic test results may be negative in initial stages.
- Indirect immunofluorescence assay has diagnostic titer of 64 or greater, detectable between days 7 and 14 of the illness.
- Latex agglutination diagnostic titer is 128 or greater 1 week after onset.
- Platelet count, white blood cell count (WBC), and fibrinogen levels are decreased.
- Prothrombin time and partial thromboplastin time are prolonged.
- Serum protein levels (especially albumin) are decreased.
- Hyponatremia and hypochloremia occur, related to increased aldosterone excretion.
- Serum creatinine, blood urea nitrogen, and potassium levels are elevated.
- Hepatic function is abnormal.
- Cerebrospinal fluid analysis shows mild mononuclear pleocytosis with slightly elevated protein content.
- Immunohistologic examination of cutaneous biopsy of a rash lesion shows *R. rickettsii*.

TREATMENT

GENERAL
- Careful tick removal
- Careful fluid administration
- Intubation and mechanical ventilation, if needed
- Hemodialysis, if needed
- Treatment of hemorrhage and thrombocytopenia, if needed

DIET
- Small, frequent meals
- Parenteral nutrition, if the patient can't receive oral intake

ACTIVITY
- Bed rest until condition improves

MEDICATIONS
- Doxycycline (drug of choice), tetracycline, or chloramphenicol (in pregnant women)
- Anticonvulsants
- Oxygen therapy

NURSING CONSIDERATIONS

NURSING DIAGNOSES
- Activity intolerance
- Acute pain
- Decreased cardiac output
- Deficient fluid volume
- Hyperthermia
- Imbalanced nutrition: Less than body requirements
- Impaired skin integrity
- Ineffective tissue perfusion: Cardiopulmonary
- Risk for infection

EXPECTED OUTCOMES
The patient will:
- resume normal activity level during recovery
- report increased comfort and decreased pain
- maintain adequate cardiac output
- maintain adequate fluid volume
- remain afebrile
- maintain adequate nutritional intake
- exhibit improved or healed lesions or wounds
- maintain hemodynamic stability
- maintain normal WBC count and differential.

NURSING INTERVENTIONS
- Give prescribed drugs.
- Provide oxygen therapy and assisted ventilation for pulmonary complications as ordered.
- Offer mentholated lotions if the rash itches.
- Turn the patient frequently.
- Encourage incentive spirometry and deep breathing.
- Plan care to promote adequate rest periods.

MONITORING
- Vital signs
- Fluid and electrolyte status
- Respiratory status
- Neurologic status
- Skin integrity

PATIENT TEACHING

GENERAL
Be sure to cover:
- the disorder, diagnosis, and treatment
- importance of reporting recurrent symptoms immediately
- preventive strategies, including avoiding tick-infested areas, whole-body inspection (including scalp) every 3 to 4 hours for attached ticks, protective clothing, and insect repellent
- correct tick removal technique using tweezers or forceps and steady traction.

DISCHARGE PLANNING
- Refer the patient to an infectious disease specialist if needed.

RESOURCES
Organizations
Harvard University Consumer Health Information: *www.intelihealth.com*
Lyme Disease Foundation, Inc.: *www.lyme.org*
Mayo Clinic: *www.mayoclinic.com*
The Merck Manuals Online Medical Library: *www.merck.com/mmhe*
National Center for Infectious Diseases: *www.cdc.gov/ncidod*

Selected references
Gunther, G., and Haglund, M. "Tick-borne Encephalopathies: Epidemiology, Diagnosis, Treatment and Prevention," *CNS Drugs* 19(12):1009-32, 2005.
Kasper, D.L., et al., eds. *Harrison's Principles of Internal Medicine,* 16th ed. New York: McGraw-Hill Book Co., 2005.
Paddock, C.D., et al. "*Rickettsia parkeri:* A Newly Recognized Cause of Spotted Fever Rickettsiosis in the United States," *Clinical Infectious Diseases* 38(6):805-11, March 2004.
Raoult, D., and Paddock, C.D. "*Rickettsia Parkeri* Infection and Other Spotted Fevers in the United States," *New England Journal of Medicine* 353(6):626-27, August 2005.
Razzaq, S., and Schutze, G.E. "Rocky Mountain Spotted Fever: A Physician's Challenge," *Pediatrics in Review/American Academy of Pediatrics* 26(4):125-30, April 2005.

Rosacea

- Chronic adult skin disorder that affects the skin and eyes
- Produces flushing and dilation of small blood vessels in the face, especially the nose and cheeks
- May cause papules and pustules but without the characteristic comedones of acne vulgaris
- Usually spreads slowly; rarely subsides spontaneously
- Usually associated with rhinophyma (dilated follicles and thickened, bulbous skin on the nose)

PATHOPHYSIOLOGY

- Vascular reactivity leads to varying degrees of papules, pustules, and hyperplasia of the sebaceous glands.

CAUSES

- Exact cause unknown

RISK FACTORS

- Drinking hot beverages
- Using tobacco or alcohol
- Eating spicy foods
- Engaging in physical activity
- Being exposed to extreme heat or cold or to sunlight
- Stress

INCIDENCE

- Rosacea is most common in white women ages 30 to 50.
- Rosacea is usually more severe in men than in women.

COMPLICATIONS

- Decreased self-esteem
- Rosacea fulminans

With ocular involvement

- Blepharitis
- Conjunctivitis
- Uveitis
- Keratitis
- Recurrent chalazion

HISTORY

- Facial flushing
- Gritty feeling in eyes
- Facial edema
- Predisposing or aggravating factors
- Complaints of burning or stinging of face

PHYSICAL FINDINGS

- Flushed areas on the cheeks, nose, forehead, and chin, usually starting across the central oval of the face (see *Lupoid or granulomatous rosacea*)
- Telangiectasia with pustules and papules
- Rhinophyma (thickened and disfigured noses) (in severe rosacea)
- Dry skin appearance
- Facial edema
- Ocular rosacea:
- Conjunctival infection
- Chalazion
- Episcleritis

DIAGNOSTIC PROCEDURES

- Skin biopsy may rule out other diseases such as lupus erythematosus.

OTHER

- Rosacea is confirmed by observation of typical vascular and acneiform lesions without comedones.

Lupoid or granulomatous rosacea

Firm yellow, brownish, or reddish cutaneous papules or nodules characterize the variant form called lupoid or granulomatous rosacea. The lesions are less inflammatory than those of rosacea. Often the surrounding skin is relatively normal looking, but sometimes it's red and thickened diffusely. Usually, the lesions are monomorphic in each patient, affecting the cheeks and periorificial areas. Other signs or symptoms of rosacea aren't needed to make the diagnosis of this form of rosacea. Diascopy with a glass spatula reveals the lupoid character of the infiltrations. Lupoid or granulomatous rosacea may scar the skin.

TREATMENT

GENERAL
◆ Facial massage

DIET
◆ Identification and avoidance of aggravating factors, such as hot beverages, alcohol, and spicy foods

ACTIVITY
◆ Avoidance of physical activities involving sunlight or exposure to extreme heat or cold

MEDICATIONS
◆ Topical azelaic acid
◆ Topical sodium sulfacetamide
◆ Topical metronidazole
◆ Oral doxycycline (for ocular involvement)
◆ Topical corticosteroids

SURGERY
◆ Electrosurgery
◆ Laser therapy

NURSING CONSIDERATIONS

NURSING DIAGNOSES
◆ Disturbed body image
◆ Impaired skin integrity
◆ Risk for infection
◆ Situational low self-esteem

EXPECTED OUTCOMES
The patient will:
◆ voice feelings about changed body image
◆ exhibit improved or healed wounds or lesions
◆ avoid or minimize the risk of secondary infection
◆ report feelings of improved self-image.

NURSING INTERVENTIONS
◆ Give prescribed drugs.
◆ Encourage patient to express feelings.
◆ Offer emotional support and reassurance.
◆ Assist with identification of triggers.

MONITORING
◆ Adverse reactions to prescribed drugs
◆ Complications
◆ Response to treatment

PATIENT TEACHING

GENERAL
Be sure to cover:
◆ the disorder, diagnosis, and treatment
◆ drugs and possible adverse effects
◆ aggravating factors
◆ stress-reduction techniques
◆ meticulous hand washing and personal hygiene
◆ ways to prevent infection
◆ signs and symptoms of infection
◆ when to notify the practitioner
◆ use of noncomedogenic, high-factor sunscreen when exposed to sunlight and wind.

RESOURCES
Organizations
American Academy of Dermatology: *www.aad.org*
Dermatology Foundation: *www.dermfnd.org*
International Rosacea Foundation: *www.internationalrosaceafoundation.org*
National Rosacea Society: *www.rosacea.org*

Selected references
Butterwick, K.J., et al. "Laser and Light Therapies for Acne Rosacea," *Journal of Drugs in Dermatology* 5(1):35-39, January 2006.

Katz, B., and Patel, V. "Photodynamic Therapy for the Treatment of Erythema, Papules, Pustules, and Severe Flushing Consistent with Rosacea," *Journal of Drugs in Dermatology* 5(2 Suppl):6-8, February 2006.

Lindow, K.B. "Rosacea. An Overview of Diagnosis and Management," *Advance for Nurse Practitioners* 12(12):27-32, December 2004.

Lindow, K.B., et al. "Perception of Self in Persons with Rosacea," *Dermatology Nursing* 17(4):249-54, 314, August 2005.

Roebuck, H.L. "Face Up to Rosacea," *Nurse Practitioner* 30(9):24-30, 35, September 2005.

Roseola infantum

OVERVIEW

- Common acute, benign, presumably viral illness characterized by fever with subsequent rash (see *Incubation and duration of common rash-producing infections*)
- Also known as *exanthema subitum*

PATHOPHYSIOLOGY

- Human herpesvirus type 6B (HHV-6B), which causes the disorder, is similar to cytomegalovirus.
- HHV-6B shows persistent and intermittent or chronic shedding in the normal population, resulting in the unusually early infection of children.
- HHV-6B is thought to be latent in salivary glands and blood.

CAUSES

- HHV-6B
- Transmission by saliva and possibly by genital secretions

INCIDENCE

- Roseola infantum affects infants and young children, typically from age 6 months to 3 years.
- The disease affects both sexes equally.
- It occurs year-round, but it's most common in spring and fall.

COMPLICATIONS

- Encephalopathy
- Thrombocytopenic purpura
- Febrile seizures
- Meningitis
- Hepatitis

ASSESSMENT

HISTORY

- Abruptly increasing, unexplainable fever that peaks between 103° and 105° F (39.4° and 40.5° C) for 3 to 5 days and then drops suddenly
- Anorexia
- Irritability
- Listlessness
- Cough

PHYSICAL FINDINGS

- When temperature drops abruptly, maculopapular, nonpruritic rash appears that blanches with pressure.
- Profuse rash on the trunk, arms, and neck; mild rash on the face and legs occurs and fades within 24 hours.
- Nagayama spots (red papules on soft palate and uvula) occur.
- Periorbital edema occurs.

DIAGNOSTIC TEST RESULTS

LABORATORY

- Causative organism is present in saliva.
- HHV-6B is isolated in peripheral blood.
- Complete blood count shows leukopenia and relative lymphocytosis as temperature increases.
- Immunofluorescence or enzyme immunoassays may show seroconversion during the convalescent phase.

OTHER

- Usually, roseola infantum is diagnosed from clinical observation.

Incubation and duration of common rash-producing infections

INFECTION	INCUBATION (DAYS)	DURATION (DAYS)
Roseola	5 to 15	3 to 6
Varicella	10 to 14	7 to 14
Rubeola	13 to 17	5
Rubella	6 to 18	3
Herpes simplex	2 to 12	7 to 21

TREATMENT

GENERAL
◆ Supportive and symptomatic

DIET
◆ Increased fluid intake

ACTIVITY
◆ Rest until fever subsides

MEDICATIONS
◆ Antipyretics
◆ Anticonvulsants

NURSING CONSIDERATIONS

NURSING DIAGNOSES
◆ Deficient fluid volume
◆ Hyperthermia
◆ Imbalanced nutrition: Less than body requirements
◆ Impaired skin integrity

EXPECTED OUTCOMES
The patient will:
◆ maintain adequate fluid volume
◆ regain a normal body temperature
◆ achieve adequate nutritional intake
◆ exhibit improved or healed lesions or wounds.

NURSING INTERVENTIONS
◆ Give tepid sponge baths and prescribed antipyretics.
◆ Replace fluids and electrolytes, as needed.
◆ Institute seizure precautions.
◆ Provide emotional support to parents.

MONITORING
◆ Neurologic status
◆ Fluid and electrolyte status
◆ Vital signs, especially temperature

PATIENT TEACHING

GENERAL
Be sure to cover:
◆ the disorder, diagnosis, and treatment
◆ methods to reduce fever:
– tepid sponge baths
– dressing the child in lightweight clothing
– keeping a comfortable room temperature
– use of antipyretics
◆ importance of adequate fluid intake
◆ no need for isolation
◆ reassurance that brief febrile seizures won't cause brain damage and will stop as the fever subsides.

RESOURCES
Organizations
American Academy of Dermatology: *www.aad.org*
American Academy of Neurology: *www.aan.com*
American Academy of Pediatrics: *www.aap.org*
Dermatology Foundation: *www.dermfnd.org*
National Institute of Allergy and Infectious Diseases: *www.niaid.nih.gov*

Selected references
Kasper, D.L., et al., eds. *Harrison's Principles of Internal Medicine,* 16th ed. New York: McGraw-Hill Book Co., 2005.
Ohsaka, M., et al. "Acute Necrotizing Encephalopathy Associated with Human Herpesvirus-6 Infection," *Pediatric Neurology* 34(2):160-63, February 2006.
Tamiya, H., et al. "Generalized Eruptive Histiocytoma with Rapid Progression and Resolution Following Exanthema Subitum," *Clinical and Experimental Dermatology* 30(3):300-301, May 2005.
Zerr, D.M., et al. "A Population-based Study of Primary Human Herpesvirus 6 Infection," *New England Journal of Medicine* 352(8):768-76, February 2005.

Rotavirus

OVERVIEW

◆ Self-limiting intestinal illness that causes mild to severe diarrhea in children

PATHOPHYSIOLOGY
◆ Rotavirus invades and damages the cells of the intestinal mucosa.
◆ Damage decreases viable absorptive surface, causing an imbalance of secretion and absorption that results in diarrhea.

CAUSES
◆ Infection with rotavirus, a member of the *Reoviridae* family
◆ Transmitted primarily by the fecal-oral route through ingestion of contaminated water or food or through contact with contaminated surfaces (see *Spreading rotavirus infection*)

INCIDENCE
◆ The incidence of rotavirus is highest among infants and young children; it affects most children in the United States by age 2.
◆ A winter seasonal pattern occurs in the United States and other temperate climate countries, with annual epidemics from November to April.
◆ Annually, rotavirus causes hospitalization of about 55,000 children in the United States and kills more than 600,000 children worldwide.

COMPLICATIONS
◆ Severe dehydration and shock
◆ Skin breakdown
◆ Worsening of other conditions such as cystic fibrosis

ASSESSMENT

HISTORY
◆ Fever, nausea, and vomiting followed by diarrhea

PHYSICAL FINDINGS
◆ Diarrhea
◆ Signs of dehydration, such as:
– Tachycardia
– Hypotension
– Dry mucous membranes
– Concentrated urine
– Poor tear production
– Poor skin turgor
– Oliguria
– Sunken eyeballs
– Sunken anterior fontanel
◆ Rectal excoriation

DIAGNOSTIC TEST RESULTS

LABORATORY
◆ Rapid antigen detection shows rotavirus in stool.

Spreading rotavirus infection

Rotavirus infection is contagious. Rotavirus particles pass in the stool of infected persons before and after they have symptoms of the illness. A child can catch a rotavirus infection if he puts his fingers in his mouth after touching something that has been contaminated by the stool of an infected person. Usually this happens when the child forgets to wash his hands often enough, especially before eating and after using the toilet. Because of the widespread nature of rotavirus and the fact that almost 100% of children get rotavirus illness, total prevention of the spread of rotavirus is nearly impossible.

TREATMENT

GENERAL
- Skin care
- Symptomatic

DIET
- Small, frequent meals
- Increased fluid intake

ACTIVITY
- Rest periods when fatigued

MEDICATIONS
- None (antibiotics and antimotility drugs contraindicated)

NURSING CONSIDERATIONS

NURSING DIAGNOSES
- Activity intolerance
- Acute pain
- Fatigue
- Hyperthermia
- Imbalanced nutrition: Less than body requirements
- Impaired skin integrity
- Risk for deficient fluid volume

EXPECTED OUTCOMES
The patient will:
- return to previous activity level
- report decreased levels or absence of pain
- verbalize or demonstrate increased energy
- remain afebrile
- maintain adequate nutritional status
- exhibit improved or healed lesions or wounds
- maintain normal fluid volume and electrolyte balance.

NURSING INTERVENTIONS
- Institute enteric precautions.
- Enforce strict hand washing and careful cleaning of all equipment, including toys.
- Implement measures to ensure adequate hydration.
- Clean the patient's perineum thoroughly to prevent skin breakdown.
- Be aware that breast-fed infants can continue to breast-feed without restrictions. Bottle-fed infants can use lactose-free soybean formulas.

MONITORING
- Intake and output (including stools)
- Skin integrity

PATIENT TEACHING

GENERAL
Be sure to cover (with the parents):
- the disorder, diagnosis, and treatment
- proper hand-washing technique
- instructions on diaper changing and thorough cleaning of the perineum and all affected surfaces
- the importance of notifying the practitioner of increased diarrhea or signs of dehydration.

RESOURCES
Organizations
National Center for Infectious Diseases: *www.cdc.gov/ncidod*
National Institute of Allergy and Infectious Diseases: *www.niaid.nih.gov*
Rotavirus Vaccine Program: *www.rotavirusvaccine.org*
World Health Organization: *www.who.int*

Selected references
Haupt, R.M., et al. "Physician's Knowledge and Attitudes about Rotavirus Gastroenteritis and Rotavirus Vaccine," *Pediatric Annals* 35(1):54-61, January 2006.

Kasper, D.L., et al., eds. *Harrison's Principles of Internal Medicine*, 16th ed. New York: McGraw-Hill Book Co., 2005.

Lowenthal, A., et al. "Secondary Bacteremia after Rotavirus Gastroenteritis in Infancy," *Pediatrics* 117(1):224-26, January 2006.

Parashar, U.D. "Rotavirus and Severe Childhood Diarrhea," *Emerging Infectious Diseases* 12(2):304-306, February 2006.

Ruiz-Palacios, G.M., et al. "Safety and Efficacy of an Attenuated Vaccine Against Severe Rotavirus Gastroenteritis," *New England Journal of Medicine* 354(1):11-22, January 2006.

Rubella

- Acute, mildly contagious viral disease that causes a distinctive maculo-papular rash (resembling measles or scarlet fever) and lymphadenopathy
- Self-limiting with an excellent prognosis, except for congenital rubella, which can have disastrous consequences
- Transmitted through contact with blood, urine, stools, or nasopharyngeal secretions of an infected person; can also be transmitted transplacentally
- Communicable from about 10 days before until 5 days after rash appears
- Also called *German measles* and *three-day measles*

PATHOPHYSIOLOGY

- A ribonucleic acid virus enters the bloodstream, usually through the respiratory route.
- The incubation period lasts 18 days, with a duration of 12 to 23 days.
- The rash is thought to result from virus dissemination to the skin.

CAUSES

- Rubella virus (a togavirus), spread by direct contact or contaminated airborne respiratory droplets

RISK FACTORS

- Exposure to active case without immunization

INCIDENCE

- Rubella occurs worldwide.
- The disease is most common among children ages 5 to 9, adolescents, and young adults.
- Epidemics occur in institutions, colleges, and military populations.
- Rubella flourishes during spring, with limited outbreaks in schools and workplaces.

COMPLICATIONS

- Arthritis
- Postinfectious encephalitis
- Thrombocytopenic purpura
- Congenital rubella

In fetal infection (rare after 20th week of gestation)

- Intrauterine death
- Spontaneous abortion
- Congenital malformations of major organ systems

ASSESSMENT

HISTORY

- Inadequate immunization, exposure to a person with rubella infection within the previous 2 to 3 weeks, or recent travel to an endemic area without reimmunization
- In a child, absence of prodromal symptoms
- In an adolescent or adult, headache, malaise, anorexia, coryza, sore throat, and cough preceding rash onset
- Polyarthralgias and polyarthritis (in some adults)

PHYSICAL FINDINGS

- Rash accompanied by low-grade fever (99° to 101° F [37.2° to 38.3° C]) that may reach 104° F (40° C)
- Exanthematous, maculopapular, mildly pruritic rash; typically begins on the face, and spreads rapidly, covering the trunk and limbs within hours
- Small, red, petechial macules on the soft palate (Forschheimer spots) preceding or accompanying the rash
- Coryza
- Conjunctivitis
- Suboccipital, postauricular, and postcervical lymph node enlargement

DIAGNOSTIC TEST RESULTS

LABORATORY

- Cultures of throat, blood, urine, and cerebrospinal fluid isolate the rubella virus; convalescent serum shows a fourfold increase in antibody titers.
- Enzyme-linked immunosorbent assay for immunoglobulin (Ig) M antibodies reveals rubella-specific IgM antibody.
- In congenital rubella, rubella-specific IgM antibody is present in umbilical cord blood.

OTHER

- Usually, the diagnosis is made from clinical observation.

GENERAL
◆ Skin care
◆ Isolation precautions

DIET
◆ Small, frequent meals
◆ Increased fluid intake

ACTIVITY
◆ Rest until fever subsides

MEDICATIONS
◆ Antipyretics
◆ Analgesics

Giving the rubella vaccine

Know how to manage rubella immunization before giving the vaccine. First, ask about allergies, especially to neomycin. If the person has this allergy or has had a reaction to any immunization in the past, check with the practitioner before giving the vaccine.

If the person is a woman of childbearing age, ask if she's pregnant. If she is or thinks she may be, don't give the vaccine.

Give the vaccine at least 3 months after any administration of immune globulin or blood. These substances may have antibodies that could neutralize the vaccine.

Don't vaccinate an immunocompromised person, a person with immunodeficiency disease, or a person receiving immunosuppressant, radiation, or corticosteroid therapy. Instead, administer immune serum globulin, as ordered, to prevent or reduce infection.

NURSING DIAGNOSES
◆ Activity intolerance
◆ Acute pain
◆ Compromised family coping
◆ Hyperthermia
◆ Impaired skin integrity
◆ Risk for infection

EXPECTED OUTCOMES
The patient will:
◆ perform self-care activities to tolerance level
◆ express feelings of comfort and relief from pain
◆ demonstrate adaptive coping behaviors
◆ remain afebrile
◆ exhibit improvement or healing of lesions or wounds
◆ experience no further signs or symptoms of infection.

NURSING INTERVENTIONS
◆ Give prescribed drugs.
◆ Institute isolation precautions until 5 days after the rash disappears. Keep an infant with congenital rubella in isolation for 3 months, until three throat cultures are negative.
◆ Keep the patient's skin clean and dry.
◆ Make sure that the patient receives care only from nonpregnant hospital workers who aren't at risk for rubella. As ordered, administer immune globulin to nonimmunized people who visit the patient. (See *Giving the rubella vaccine*.)
◆ Report confirmed rubella cases to local public health officials.

MONITORING
◆ Vital signs
◆ Skin for signs of exanthem
◆ Auditory impairment in congenital rubella

GENERAL
Be sure to cover (with the parents):
◆ the disorder, diagnosis, and treatment
◆ ways to reduce fever
◆ devastating effects of rubella on an unborn fetus
◆ importance of people with rubella avoiding pregnant women
◆ avoidance of aspirin in a child receiving rubella vaccine.

DISCHARGE PLANNING
◆ Refer the patient to an infectious disease specialist if congenital rubella is confirmed.
◆ Provide parents of an infant with congenital rubella with support, counseling, and referrals, as needed.

RESOURCES
Organizations
Centers for Disease Control and Prevention: *www.cdc.gov*
Mayo Clinic: *www.mayoclinic.com*
National Institute of Allergy and Infectious Diseases: *www.niaid.nih.gov*
World Health Organization: *www.who.int*

Selected references
Bedford, H., and Tookey, P. "Rubella and the MMR Vaccine," *Nursing Times* 102(5):55-57, January-February 2006.
Corcoran, C., and Hardie, D.R. "Serologic Diagnosis of Congenital Rubella: A Cautionary Tale," *Pediatric Infectious Disease Journal* 24(3):286-87, March 2005.
Kasper, D.L., et al., eds. *Harrison's Principles of Internal Medicine*, 16th ed. New York: McGraw-Hill Book Co., 2005.
Singh, R., et al. "Measles, Mumps and Rubella - The Urologist's Perspective," *International Journal of Clinical Practice* 60(3):335-39, March 2006.

Rubeola

- Acute, highly contagious infection causing a characteristic rash
- In the United States, prognosis usually excellent
- Can be severe or fatal in patients with impaired cell-mediated immunity
- Mortality highest in children younger than age 2 and in adults
- Also called *measles* or *morbilli*

PATHOPHYSIOLOGY

- Virus invades the respiratory epithelium and spreads via the bloodstream to the reticuloendothelial system, infecting all types of white blood cells.
- Viremia and viruria develop, leading to infection of the entire respiratory tract, which spreads to the integumentary system.
- In measles encephalitis, focal hemorrhage, congestion, and perivascular demyelination occur.

RISK FACTORS

- Lack of immunization

CAUSES

- Rubeola virus
- Spread by direct contact or by contaminated airborne respiratory droplets, with portal of entry in the upper respiratory tract

INCIDENCE

- Rubeola affects mostly preschool children.
- In temperate zones, the disease most commonly occurs in late winter and early spring.

COMPLICATIONS

- Secondary bacterial infection
- Autoimmune reaction
- Bronchitis
- Otitis media
- Pneumonia
- Encephalitis

HISTORY

- Inadequate immunization and exposure to someone with measles in the past 14 days
- Photophobia
- Malaise
- Anorexia
- Coryza
- Hoarseness
- Hacking cough

PHYSICAL FINDINGS

- Temperature peaking at 103° to 105° F (39.4°C to 40.5° C)
- Periorbital edema
- Conjunctivitis
- Koplik's spots (tiny, bluish-gray specks, surrounded by red halo) on oral mucosa opposite the molars, which may bleed
- Pruritic rash starting as faint macules behind the ears and on the neck and cheeks, becoming papular and erythematous, and rapidly spreading over the face, neck, eyelids, arms, chest, back, abdomen, and thighs
- Fading of rash when it reaches the feet 2 to 3 days later, occurring in the same sequence it appeared, leaving brown discoloration that disappears in 7 to 10 days
- Severe cough
- Rhinorrhea
- Lymphadenopathy

LABORATORY

- The rubeola virus appears in blood, nasopharyngeal secretions, and urine during the febrile period.
- Serum antibodies appear within 3 days after rash onset and reach peak titers 2 to 4 weeks later.

TREATMENT

GENERAL
- Respiratory isolation precautions
- Use of vaporizer
- Warm environment
- Skin care

DIET
- Small, frequent meals
- Increased fluid intake

ACTIVITY
- Rest until symptoms improve

MEDICATIONS
- Antipyretics

NURSING CONSIDERATIONS

NURSING DIAGNOSES
- Activity intolerance
- Disturbed sensory perception (visual)
- Hyperthermia
- Imbalanced nutrition: Less than body requirements
- Impaired oral mucous membrane
- Impaired skin integrity
- Risk for infection

EXPECTED OUTCOMES
The patient (or family) will:
- perform self-care activities to tolerance level
- maintain level of visual acuity
- remain afebrile
- communicate an understanding of the patient's special dietary needs
- remain free from complications related to trauma to oral mucous membranes
- exhibit improved or healed lesions or wounds
- experience no further signs or symptoms of infection.

NURSING INTERVENTIONS
- Institute respiratory isolation measures for 4 days after rash onset.
- Follow standard precautions.
- Give prescribed drugs.
- Encourage bed rest during the acute period.
- If photophobia occurs, darken the room or provide sunglasses.
- To prevent disease spread, administer measles vaccine, as ordered and needed.
- Report measles cases to local public health authorities.

MONITORING
- Vital signs
- Skin for signs of exanthem
- Eyes for conjunctivitis
- Mental status
- Signs and symptoms of pneumonia
- Ears for otitis media

PATIENT TEACHING

GENERAL
Be sure to cover (with the parents):
- the disorder, diagnosis, and treatment
- supportive measures, isolation, bed rest, and increased fluids
- instructions on cleaning a vaporizer (if used) and the importance of changing the water every 8 hours
- early signs and symptoms of complications that should be reported.

RESOURCES
Organizations
Mayo Clinic: *www.mayoclinic.com*
National Center for Infectious Diseases: *www.cdc.gov/ncidod*
National Institute of Allergy and Infectious Diseases: *www.niaid.nih.gov*
World Health Organization: *www.who.int*

Selected references
Bedford, H. "Measles and the Importance of Maintaining Vaccination Levels," *Nursing Times* 100(26):52-55, June-July 2004.
Kasper, D.L., et al., eds. *Harrison's Principles of Internal Medicine*, 16th ed. New York: McGraw-Hill Book Co., 2005.
Ovsyannikova, I.G., et al. "Human Leukocyte Antigen Haplotypes in the Genetic Control of Immune Response to Measles-Mumps-Rubella Vaccine," *Journal of Infectious Diseases* 193(5):655-63, March 2006.
Yoshida, M., et al. "Development of Follicular Rash in Measles," *British Journal of Dermatology* 153(6):1226-228, December 2005.

Saint Louis encephalitis LIFE-THREATENING DISORDER

OVERVIEW

- Acute inflammatory disease of short duration that involves the brain, spinal cord, and meninges following the bite of an infected mosquito (mosquitoes infective for life)
- Usually produces no symptoms, but severe infection may have acute onset
- Incubation period of 4 to 21 days
- No person-to-person transmission
- No chronic infection or reports of relapsing infection
- Also known as *SEV, SLEV, mosquito-borne encephalitis, arbovirus,* and *viral encephalitis*

PATHOPHYSIOLOGY

- The virus is found in common birds, such as sparrows, finches, blue jays, robins, and doves.
- Culex mosquitoes feed on these birds, contract the virus, and then pass it on to human hosts through a bite.
- A primary viremia follows reproduction of the virus at the site of inoculation.
- In subclinical disease, the pathogen is cleared by the liver, spleen, and lymph nodes before invasion of the central nervous system (CNS).
- Secondary viremia occurs with continued viral replication, which overwhelms the liver, spleen, and lymph nodes.
- The virus then invades the CNS, including the brain and spinal cord.

CAUSES

- Laboratory-acquired infections possible through infected blood, cerebrospinal fluid (CSF), urine, and exudates
- Transmission by the bite of an infected mosquito

RISK FACTORS

- Human immunodeficiency virus infection
- Age older than 70 (10-fold increased risk of clinical illness)
- Travel to endemic areas
- Participation in outdoor activities
- Low socioeconomic status

INCIDENCE

- St. Louis encephalitis occurs in North, South, and Central America and the Caribbean; it's a major health problem in the United States.
- The highest incidence in late summer or early fall.
- Incidence is higher in males than in females, probably because of more outdoor exposure.
- Highly susceptible individuals include elderly people, those living in crowded conditions, those living in low-income areas, and those working outside or participating in outdoor activities in endemic areas.

COMPLICATIONS

- Acute encephalitis
- Death
- Movement disorders and motor deficits
- Seizures and coma
- Cranial nerve palsies

⚡ **WARNING** *Patients with atherosclerosis, heart disease, and hypertension have an increased risk of death from this infection.*

ASSESSMENT

HISTORY

- Exposure to infected insect
- Onset of encephalitis characterized by:
  – Malaise
  – Fever
  – Cough and sore throat, followed by common symptoms of headache, nausea, vomiting, confusion, disorientation, irritability, tremors, and possible seizures

PHYSICAL FINDINGS

- Temperature elevation
- Normal neurologic examination
- A deep coma in 5% of patients
- Cranial nerve palsies in about 25% of patients
- Possibly ataxia
- Possibly seizures (infrequent, but more common in children)

DIAGNOSTIC TEST RESULTS

LABORATORY

- One of the following will be present: A fourfold increase in the antivirus antibody titer between the acute and the convalescent periods; virus isolation from tissue, blood, or CSF; or specific immunoglobulin M antibody.
- Pyuria or proteinuria occurs.
- Sodium level is decreased.
- CSF pressure is normal to mildly elevated, blood glucose level is normal, and protein level is normal to mildly elevated; CSF white blood cell count usually is less than 200/µl.

TREATMENT

GENERAL
- Supportive
- Management of seizures or neurologic symptoms

DIET
- As tolerated

ACTIVITY
- Bed rest

MEDICATIONS
- Antipyretics
- Analgesics

NURSING CONSIDERATIONS

NURSING DIAGNOSES
- Fatigue
- Hyperthermia
- Imbalanced nutrition: Less than body requirements
- Impaired physical mobility
- Ineffective tissue perfusion: Cerebral
- Risk for injury

EXPECTED OUTCOMES
The patient will:
- verbalize the importance of balancing activity, as tolerated, with rest
- maintain normal body temperature
- maintain adequate nutrition and fluid intake
- maintain joint mobility and range of motion (ROM)
- exhibit signs of maintaining adequate cerebral perfusion
- remain safe from falls caused by ataxia or seizures.

NURSING INTERVENTIONS
- Give prescribed drugs.
- Encourage nutritional intake.
- Encourage fluids and lying flat after lumbar puncture.
- Assist with ambulation, as needed.
- Frequently reposition the unconscious patient.
- Encourage ROM exercises (passive ROM exercises if the patient is unconscious).

MONITORING
- Vital signs
- Level of consciousness
- Skin breakdown
- Seizure activity
- Complications of lumbar puncture, if performed

PATIENT TEACHING

GENERAL
Be sure to cover:
- the disorder, diagnosis, and treatment
- mosquito bite prevention, such as:
- staying inside between dusk and dark
- wearing long pants and long-sleeved shirts when outside
- spraying exposed skin with insect repellent
- avoiding areas of standing water where mosquitoes congregate.

DISCHARGE PLANNING
- Encourage follow-up appointments, as needed.

RESOURCES
Organizations
American Academy of Neurology: *www.aan.com*
American Neurological Association: *www.aneuroa.org*
National Center for Infectious Diseases: *www.cdc.gov/ncidod*
World Health Organization: *www.who.int*

Selected references
Sejvar, J.J., et al. "Post-infectious Encephalomyelitis Associated with St. Louis Encephalitis Virus Infection," *Neurology* 63(9):1719-721, November 2004.
Shaman, J. "Achieving Operational Hydrologic Monitoring of Mosquito-Borne Disease," *Emerging Infectious Diseases* 11(9):1343-50, September 2005.
Weaver, S.C. "Host Range, Amplification and Arboviral Disease Emergence," *Archives of Virology*. Supplementum. (19):33-44, 2005.
Wootton, S.H., et al. "St. Louis Encephalitis in Early Infancy," *Pediatric Infectious Disease Journal* 23(10):951-54, October 2004.

Salmonella infection

- One of the most common intestinal infections in the United States
- Occurs as enterocolitis, bacteremia, localized infection, typhoid fever, or paratyphoid fever
- Nontyphoid forms, usually mild to moderate illness with low mortality
- Typhoid fever most severe form; usually lasts from 1 to 4 weeks and confers lifelong immunity, although patient may become a carrier

PATHOPHYSIOLOGY

- Invasion occurs across the small intestinal mucosa, altering the plasma membrane and entering the lamina propria.
- Invasion activates cell-signaling pathways, which alter electrolyte transport, and may cause diarrhea.
- Some salmonella produce a molecule that increases electrolyte and fluid secretion.

CAUSES

- Gram-negative bacilli of the genus *Salmonella* (member of the *Enterobacteriaceae* family)
- Typhoid fever: *S. typhi*
- Enterocolitis: *S. enteritidis*
- Bacteremia: *S. choleresis*

RISK FACTORS

- Nontyphoidal infection — usually, ingestion of contaminated water or food or inadequately processed food, especially eggs, chicken, turkey, and duck
- Contact with infected person or animal
- Ingestion of contaminated dry milk, chocolate bars, or pharmaceuticals of animal origin
- **AGE FACTOR** *Salmonella infection may occur in children younger than age 5 and from fecal-oral spread.*
- Typhoid fever — usually, drinking water contaminated by excretions of a carrier

INCIDENCE

- Incidence is increasing in the United States due to travel to endemic areas, especially the borders of Mexico.
- Paratyphoid fever is rare in the United States.

COMPLICATIONS

- Dehydration
- Hypovolemic shock
- Abscess formation
- Sepsis
- Toxic megacolon

HISTORY

- With enterocolitis, possible report of contaminated food eaten 6 to 48 hours before onset of symptoms
- With bacteremia, patient usually reveals immunocompromised condition, especially acquired immunodeficiency syndrome
- With typhoid fever, possible ingestion of contaminated food or water, typically 1 to 2 weeks before symptoms develop

PHYSICAL FINDINGS

- Fever
- Abdominal pain
- With enterocolitis, severe diarrhea
- With typhoidal infection, headache, increasing fever, and constipation

LABORATORY

- Blood culture in typhoid or paratyphoid fever and bacteremia shows causative organism in most cases.
- Stool culture in typhoid or paratyphoid fever and enterocolitis shows causative organism.
- Other culture specimens (urine, bone marrow, pus, and vomitus) show causative organism.
- Presence of *S. typhi* in stools 1 or more years after treatment indicates that the patient is a carrier (about 3% of patients).
- Widal's test, an agglutination reaction against somatic and flagellar antigens, suggests typhoid fever with a fourfold increase in titer.
- Complete blood count (CBC) shows transient leukocytosis during the first week of typhoidal salmonella infection.
- CBC shows leukopenia during the third week of typhoidal salmonella infection.
- CBC shows leukocytosis with local infection.

Preventing recurrence of salmonella infection

To prevent salmonella infection from recurring, follow these teaching guidelines:

- Explain the causes of salmonella infection.
- Show the patient how to wash his hands by wetting them under running water, lathering with soap and scrubbing, rinsing under running water with his fingers pointing down, and drying with a clean towel or paper towel.
- Tell the patient to wash his hands after using the bathroom and before eating.
- Tell him to cook foods thoroughly — especially eggs and chicken — and to refrigerate them at once.
- Teach him how to avoid cross-contaminating foods by cleaning preparation surfaces with hot, soapy water and drying them thoroughly after use; cleaning surfaces between foods when preparing more than one food; and washing his hands before and after handling each food.
- Tell the patient with a positive stool culture to avoid handling food and to use a separate bathroom or clean the bathroom after each use.
- Tell the patient to report dehydration, bleeding, or recurrence of signs of salmonella infection.

TREATMENT

GENERAL
◆ Usually no treatment
◆ Possible hospitalization for severe diarrhea

DIET
◆ Fluid and electrolyte replacement
◆ High-calorie fluids

ACTIVITY
◆ As tolerated

MEDICATIONS
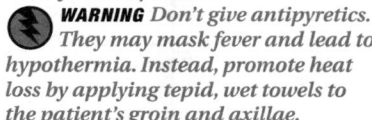 **WARNING** *Avoid antidiarrheals because their use may prolong the infectious process.*

WARNING *Don't give antipyretics. They may mask fever and lead to hypothermia. Instead, promote heat loss by applying tepid, wet towels to the patient's groin and axillae.*

SURGERY
◆ Surgical drainage of localized abscesses

NURSING CONSIDERATIONS

NURSING DIAGNOSES
◆ Activity intolerance
◆ Acute pain
◆ Deficient fluid volume
◆ Diarrhea
◆ Hyperthermia
◆ Imbalanced nutrition: Less than body requirements
◆ Risk for infection

EXPECTED OUTCOMES
The patient will:
◆ demonstrate skill in conserving energy while carrying out daily activities to tolerance level
◆ report adequate pain relief with analgesia or other measures
◆ regain and maintain fluid and electrolyte balance
◆ return to a normal elimination pattern
◆ remain afebrile
◆ experience no further weight loss
◆ experience no further signs or symptoms of infection.

NURSING INTERVENTIONS
◆ Follow enteric precautions until three consecutive stool cultures are negative.
◆ Watch closely for signs of bowel perforation.
◆ Maintain adequate I.V. fluid and electrolyte therapy, as ordered.
◆ Provide good skin and mouth care.
◆ Apply mild heat to relieve abdominal cramps.
◆ Report salmonella cases to local public health officials.

MONITORING
◆ Fluid and electrolyte status
◆ Vital signs
◆ Daily weight

PATIENT TEACHING

GENERAL
Be sure to cover:
◆ the disorder, diagnosis, and treatment
◆ the need for close contacts to obtain a medical examination and treatment if cultures are positive
◆ how to prevent salmonella infections
◆ the need to be vaccinated (for those at high risk for contracting typhoid fever, such as laboratory workers and travelers)
◆ the importance of proper hand washing
◆ the need to avoid preparing food or pouring water for others until salmonella infection is eliminated.

DISCHARGE PLANNING
◆ Arrange for follow-up with an infectious disease specialist or a gastroenterologist as needed. (See *Preventing recurrence of salmonella infection.*)

RESOURCES
Organizations
National Center for Infectious Diseases: *www.cdc.gov/ncidod*
The Merck Manuals Online Medical Library: *www.merck.com/mmhe*
World Health Organization: *www.who.int*

Selected references
Feder, H.M., and Zempsky, W. "Neonatal Salmonella Orchitis," *Infectious Diseases in Clinical Practice* 13(6):313-14, November 2005.
Hosoglu, S., et al. "Risk Factors for Enteric Perforation in Patients with Typhoid Fever," *American Journal of Epidemiology* 160(1):46-50, July 2004.
Kilby, J.M. "Salmonella Infections in the Setting of AIDS: A Serpentine Course," *Southern Medical Journal* 98(11):1066-67, November 2005.
Kasper, D.L., et al., eds. *Harrison's Principles of Internal Medicine*, 16th ed. New York: McGraw-Hill Book Co., 2005.

Sarcoidosis

OVERVIEW

- A multisystemic, granulomatous disorder that characteristically produces lymphadenopathy, pulmonary infiltration, and skeletal, liver, eye, or skin lesions
- May be acute (usually resolves within 2 years) or chronic
- Chronic, progressive sarcoidosis (uncommon) associated with pulmonary fibrosis and progressive pulmonary disability

PATHOPHYSIOLOGY

- An excessive inflammatory process begins in the alveoli, bronchioles, and blood vessels of the lungs.
- Monocyte-macrophages accumulate in the target tissue where they induce the inflammatory process.
- CD4+ T-lymphocytes and sensitized immune cells form a ring around the inflamed area.
- Fibroblasts, mast cells, collagen fibers, and proteoglycans encase the inflammatory and immune cells, causing granuloma formation.

CAUSES

- Exact cause unknown
- Possible causes:
- Hypersensitivity response to atypical mycobacteria, fungi, and pine pollen
- Chemicals
- T-cell abnormalities
- Lymphokine production abnormalities

INCIDENCE

- Sarcoidosis is most common in people ages 20 to 40.
- In the United States, it predominantly occurs among blacks.
- It affects twice as many women as men.
- Incidence is slightly higher in families, suggesting genetic predisposition.

COMPLICATIONS

- Pulmonary fibrosis
- Pulmonary hypertension
- Cor pulmonale

ASSESSMENT

HISTORY

- Pain in the wrists, ankles, and elbows
- General fatigue and malaise
- Unexplained weight loss
- Breathlessness and dyspnea
- Nonproductive cough
- Substernal pain

PHYSICAL FINDINGS

- Erythema nodosum
- Punched out lesions on the fingers and toes
- Cranial or peripheral nerve palsies
- Extensive nasal mucosal lesions
- Anterior uveitis
- Glaucoma and blindness occasionally in advanced disease
- Bilateral hilar and paratracheal lymphadenopathy
- Splenomegaly
- Arrhythmias

DIAGNOSTIC TEST RESULTS

LABORATORY

- Arterial blood gas (ABG) analysis shows a decreased partial pressure of arterial oxygen and increased carbon dioxide levels.

IMAGING

- Chest X-rays show bilateral hilar and right paratracheal adenopathy, with or without diffuse interstitial infiltrates.

DIAGNOSTIC PROCEDURES

- Kveim Siltzbach skin test shows granuloma development at the injection site in 2 to 4 weeks when positive.
- Lymph node, skin, or lung biopsy shows noncaseating granulomas with negative cultures for mycobacteria and fungi.
- Pulmonary function tests show decreased total lung capacity and compliance and reduced diffusing capacity.

GENERAL
- None needed for sarcoidosis that produces no symptoms
- Protection from sunlight

DIET
- Low-calcium for hypercalcemia
- Reduced-sodium, high-calorie
- Adequate fluids

ACTIVITY
- As tolerated

MEDICATIONS
- Corticosteroids

NURSING CONSIDERATIONS

NURSING DIAGNOSES
- Activity intolerance
- Anxiety
- Dysfunctional grieving
- Fear
- Imbalanced nutrition: Less than body requirements
- Impaired gas exchange
- Risk for infection

EXPECTED OUTCOMES
The patient will:
- perform activities of daily living within confines of the illness
- identify strategies to reduce anxiety
- use support systems to assist with coping
- discuss fears and concerns
- maintain adequate nutrition and hydration
- maintain adequate ventilation and oxygenation
- remain free from signs and symptoms of infection.

NURSING INTERVENTIONS
- Give prescribed drugs.
- Administer supplemental oxygen.
- Provide a nutritious, high-calorie diet.
- Encourage oral fluid intake.
- Provide a low-calcium diet for hypercalcemia.

- Provide emotional support.
- Provide comfort measures.
- Include the patient in care decisions whenever possible.

MONITORING
- Vital signs
- Intake and output
- Daily weight
- Respiratory status
- Chest X-ray results
- Sputum production
- ABG results
- Cardiac rhythm

WARNING *Because corticosteroids may induce or worsen diabetes mellitus, test the patient's blood by fingersticks for glucose and acetone at least every 12 hours at the beginning of corticosteroid therapy. Also, watch for other adverse effects, such as fluid retention, electrolyte imbalance (especially hypokalemia), moon face, hypertension, and personality changes.*

PATIENT TEACHING

GENERAL
Be sure to cover:
- the disorder, diagnosis, and treatment
- drugs and possible adverse effects
- when to notify the practitioner
- steroid therapy
- the need for regular follow-up examinations
- the importance of wearing a medical identification bracelet
- infection prevention.

DISCHARGE PLANNING
- Refer a patient with failing vision to community support and resource groups such as the American Foundation for the Blind, if necessary.

RESOURCES
Organizations
American Lung Association:
www.lungusa.org
American Thoracic Society:
www.thoracic.org
National Sarcoidosis Resource Center:
www.nsrc-global.net
Sarcoidosis Center:
www.sarcoidcenter.com

Selected references
Alazemi, S., and Campos, M.A. "Interferon-induced Sarcoidosis," International Journal of Clinical Practice 60(2):201-11, February 2006.

Caca, I., et al. "Conjunctival Deposits as the First Sign of Systemic Sarcoidosis in a Pediatric Patient," *European Journal of Ophthalmology* 16(1):160-62, January-February 2006.

Choi, H.J., et al. "Papular Sarcoidosis Limited to the Knees: A Clue for Systemic Sarcoidosis," *International Journal of Dermatology* 45(2); 169-70, February 2006.

Doughan, A.R., and Williams, B.R. "Cardiac Sarcoidosis," *Heart* 92(2):282-88, February 2006.

Gurrieri, C., et al. "Cytokines, Chemokines and Other Biomolecular Markers in Sarcoidosis," *Sarcoidosis, Vasculitis, and Diffuse Lung Diseases* 22 (Suppl 1):S9-14, December 2005.

Scabies

- Transmissible skin infestation with *Sarcoptes scabiei var. hominis* (itch mite)
- Characterized by burrows, severe pruritus, and excoriations

PATHOPHYSIOLOGY
- Mites burrow into the skin on contact, progressing 2 to 3 mm per day.
- Females live about 4 to 6 weeks and lay about 40 to 50 eggs, which hatch in 3 to 4 days.
- Pruritus occurs only after sensitization to the mite develops. With initial infestation, sensitization requires several weeks. With reinfestation, sensitization develops within 24 hours.
- Dead mites, eggs, larvae, and their excrement trigger an inflammatory eruption of the skin in infested areas.

CAUSES
- Direct (skin to skin) contact or contact with contaminated articles for up to 48 hours (see *Scabies: Cause and effect*)

RISK FACTORS
- Overcrowded living conditions
- Poor hygiene
- Sexual promiscuity
- Day-care or institutional settings

INCIDENCE
- Scabies is common in children, young adults, elderly, and debilitated patients.
- It occurs worldwide.
- It can be endemic.

COMPLICATIONS
- Excoriations
- Secondary bacterial infection
- Abscess formation
- Septicemia

HISTORY
- Predisposing risk factors
- May not produce symptoms, initially
- Intense pruritus that's more severe at night

PHYSICAL FINDINGS
- Characteristic gray-brown, threadlike burrows (0.5 to 1 cm long) with tiny papule or vesicle at one end
- Common sites: flexor surfaces of wrists, elbows, axillary folds, waistline, nipples in females, and genitalia

AGE FACTOR *In infants, the burrows may appear on the head and neck.*

- Papules, vesicles, crusting, abscess formation, and cellulites with secondary infection

LABORATORY
- Wound culture demonstrates secondary bacterial infection.

DIAGNOSTIC PROCEDURES
- Mineral oil burrow-scraping reveals mites, nits, or eggs, and feces or scybala.
- Punch biopsy may help to confirm the diagnosis.

OTHER
- Resolution of infestation with therapeutic trial of a pediculicide confirms the diagnosis.

Scabies: Cause and effect

Infestation with *Sarcoptes scabiei* — the itch mite — causes scabies. This mite (shown enlarged below) has a hard shell and measures a microscopic 0.1 mm.

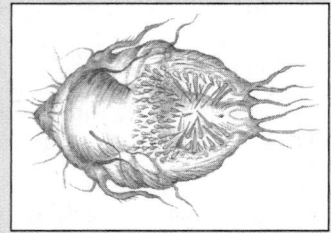

TREATMENT

GENERAL
- Bathing with soap and water
- Performing skin care
- Decontaminating environment and clothing

MEDICATIONS
- Scabicides
- 6% to 10% sulfur solution
- Systemic antibiotics
- Antipruritics

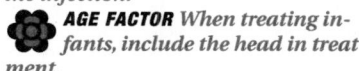 **WARNING** *Avoid the use of topical steroids, which may potentiate the infection.*

AGE FACTOR *When treating infants, include the head in treatment.*

NURSING CONSIDERATIONS

NURSING DIAGNOSES
- Acute pain
- Disturbed body image
- Impaired skin integrity
- Ineffective therapeutic regimen management
- Risk for infection

EXPECTED OUTCOMES
The patient (or family) will:
- report feelings of increased comfort
- voice feelings about change in body image
- exhibit improved or healed wounds or lesions, and resolution of the infestation
- demonstrate understanding of proper skin care regimen
- avoid or minimize secondary infection.

NURSING INTERVENTIONS
- Trim patient's fingernails short.
- Give prescribed drugs.
- Isolate the patient until treatment is completed.
- Practice meticulous hand washing.
- Sterilize blood pressure cuffs in a gas autoclave before using on other patients.
- Decontaminate linens, towels, clothing, and personal articles.
- Disinfect the patient's room after discharge.
- If the patient is a child, notify his school of the infestation.
- Encourage verbalization of feelings.
- Observe wound and skin precautions for 24 hours after treatment with a scabicide.

MONITORING
- Response to treatment
- Complications
- Neurologic status

WARNING *Prolonged use of scabicides may lead to excessive central nervous system stimulation and seizures.*

PATIENT TEACHING

GENERAL
Be sure to cover:
- the disorder, diagnosis, and treatment
- identification of characteristic lesions
- modes of transmission
- mite resistance to scabicides
- assessment of close personal contacts for infestation
- successful treatment for infestation with good hygiene and scabicides
- prevention of transmission and recurrence
- proper application of the prescribed scabicide.

RESOURCES
Organizations
American Academy of Dermatology: *www.aad.org*
Dermatology Foundation: *www.dermfnd.org*
National Center for Infectious Diseases: *www.cdc.gov/ncidod*

Selected references
Almeida, H.L. Jr. "Treatment of Steroid-resistant Nodular Scabies with Topical Pimecrolimus," *Journal of the American Academy of Dermatology* 53(2):357-58, August 2005.

Cestari, T.F., and Martignago, B.F. "Scabies, Pediculosis, Bedbugs, and Stinkbugs: Uncommon Presentations," *Clinical Dermatology* 23(6):545-54, November-December 2005.

Krohn, B. "Scabies in Long-term Care Settings. Expedient Diagnosis and Treatment Are Essential," *Advance for Nurse Practitioners* 12(12):35-36, December 2004.

Pannell, R.S., et al. "The Incidence of Molluscum Contagiosum, Scabies and Lichen Planus," *Epidemiology and Infection* 133(6):985-91, December 2005.

Siderits, R., et al. "Preparation and Use of a Scabies Skin Scraping Kit," *Advances in Skin & Wound Care* 19(1):22-25, January-February 2006.

Scarlet fever

- A hypersensitivity reaction that usually follows streptococcal pharyngitis
- May follow other streptococcal infections, such as wound infections, urosepsis, and puerperal sepsis
- Also known as *scarlatina*

PATHOPHYSIOLOGY

- After infection, an erythrogenic toxin is produced, resulting in a hypersensitivity reaction.
- Replication site is the tonsils and pharynx.
- Inflammatory reaction occurs.

CAUSES

- Group A beta-hemolytic streptococci transmitted by direct contact with infected person or droplet spread; indirectly by contact with contaminated articles or ingestion of contaminated food

INCIDENCE

- The disease is most common in children ages 3 to 15, peaking in those ages 4 to 8.
- Infection rate is increased in overcrowded situations.
- Males and females are affected equally.

COMPLICATIONS

- Severe disseminated toxic illness
- Septicemia
- Rheumatic heart disease
- Liver damage
- Otitis media
- Peritonsillar and retropharyngeal abscess
- Sinusitis
- Glomerulonephritis
- Meningitis
- Brain abscess

HISTORY

- Possible contact with person with a sore throat
- Sore throat
- Headache
- Chills
- Anorexia
- Abdominal pain
- Malaise
- Likely high temperature (100° to 103° F [37.8° to 39.4° C])
- Characteristic rash 12 to 48 hours after onset of fever

PHYSICAL FINDINGS

- Inflamed and heavily coated tongue, progressing to strawberry-like tongue
- Tongue that peels and becomes beefy red, returning to normal by the end of week 2
- Red and edematous uvula, tonsils, and posterior oropharynx, with mucopurulent exudate
- Fine, erythematous rash, appears first on the upper chest and back, spreading to the neck, abdomen, legs, and arms
- Rash resembling sunburn with goose bumps; blanches with pressure
- Flushed face; circumoral pallor
- Tachycardia

LABORATORY

- Pharyngeal culture is positive for group A beta-hemolytic streptococci.
- Complete blood count reveals increased white blood cell count and eosinophilia during the second week.

OTHER

- Findings from physical examination aid in the diagnosis.

TREATMENT

GENERAL
- Appropriate skin care
- Isolation for 24 hours after starting antibiotics

DIET
- Increased fluid intake

ACTIVITY
- Rest periods when fatigued

MEDICATIONS
- Antibiotics
- Antipyretics

NURSING CONSIDERATIONS

NURSING DIAGNOSES
- Acute pain
- Hyperthermia
- Impaired oral mucous membrane
- Impaired skin integrity
- Impaired swallowing
- Risk for infection

EXPECTED OUTCOMES
The patient will:
- express feelings of increased comfort or absence of pain at rest
- remain afebrile
- have moist and pink mucous membranes without lesions
- maintain skin integrity
- chew and swallow without discomfort
- experience no further signs or symptoms of infection.

NURSING INTERVENTIONS
- Implement respiratory secretion precautions for 24 hours after starting antibiotic therapy.
- Offer frequent oral fluids and oral hygiene.
- Give prescribed drugs.
- Provide skin care to relieve discomfort from the rash.
- Provide warm liquids or cold foods to ease sore throat pain.
- Use a cool mist humidifier to keep the air moist and prevent the throat from getting too dry and more sore.

MONITORING
- Adverse drug reactions
- Response to treatment
- Complications
- Body temperature
- Rash
- Nutritional status
- Signs and symptoms of dehydration

PATIENT TEACHING

GENERAL
Be sure to cover:
- the disorder, diagnosis, and treatment
- the need to take oral antibiotics for the prescribed length of time to prevent serious complications
- proper disposal of purulent discharge
- follow-up care
- when to notify the practitioner
- drugs and possible adverse effects
- prevention of scarlet fever and strep throat.

RESOURCES
Organizations
American Academy of Dermatology: *www.aad.org*
American Academy of Pediatrics: *www.aap.org*
Harvard University Consumer Health Information: *www.intelihealth.com*
National Center for Infectious Diseases: *www.cdc.gov/ncidod*

Selected references
Diseases, 4th ed. Philadelphia: Lippincott Williams & Wilkins, 2006.
Kasper, D.L., et al., eds. *Harrison's Principles of Internal Medicine*, 16th ed. New York: McGraw-Hill Book Co., 2005.
Vargas, M.H. "Ecological Association between Scarlet Fever and Asthma," *Respiratory Medicine* 100(2):363-66, February 2006.

Schizophrenia

OVERVIEW

- Disturbances in thought content and form, perception, affect, language, social activity, sense of self, volition, interpersonal relationships, and psychomotor behavior
- Five types recognized by the *DSM-IV-TR*: catatonic, paranoid, disorganized, residual, and undifferentiated
- Insidious onset and poor outcome
- Can progress to social withdrawal, perceptual distortions, chronic delusions, and hallucinations
- Up to one-third of patients having only one psychotic episode
- Some patients having no disability between periods of exacerbation; others needing continuous institutional care
- Worsening prognosis with each acute episode

PATHOPHYSIOLOGY

- A biochemical hypothesis holds that schizophrenia results from excessive activity at dopaminergic synapses.
- Other neurotransmitter alterations may also contribute to schizophrenic symptoms.
- Structural abnormalities of the intraventricular system, temporal lobe abnormalities, decreased volume of the amygdala and hippocampus of the limbic system, structural changes in prefrontal white matter, and increased volume of the basal ganglia have been found.

CAUSES

- Exact cause unknown
- May result from a combination of genetic, biological, cultural, and psychological factors

RISK FACTORS

- Familial history
- Gestational and birth complications
- Prenatal nutritional deficiencies

INCIDENCE

- The disease affects about 0.85% of people worldwide, with a lifetime prevalence of 1% to 1.5%.
- Close relatives of patients are up to 50 times more likely to develop schizophrenia; the closer the degree of biological relatedness, the higher the risk.
- Incidence is higher among lower socioeconomic groups.

AGE FACTOR *The onset of schizophrenia usually occurs during late adolescence.*

COMPLICATIONS

- Suicide
- Impairment of health
- Impairment of social functioning

ASSESSMENT

HISTORY

- Possible long-standing psychiatric illness with repeated episodes
- Decreased social functioning

PHYSICAL FINDINGS

- Decreased emotional expression
- Impaired concentration

DSM-IV-TR *criteria*

Diagnosis depends on identifying two or more of the following signs and symptoms for a significant portion of time during a 1-month period (or only one symptom if delusions are bizarre, hallucinations consist of a voice issuing a running commentary, or hallucinations consist of two or more voices conversing with each other):

- delusions
- prominent hallucinations
- disorganized speech
- grossly disorganized or catatonic behavior
- negative symptoms (flat affect or inability to make decisions or speak).

In addition, one or more major areas of functioning (work, relationships, and self-care) are markedly below previous level, and the disturbance isn't due to a substance, medical condition, or schizoaffective or mood disorder.

DIAGNOSTIC TEST RESULTS

GENERAL

- Diagnosis is based on mental status examination findings that fit *DSM-IV-TR* criteria for schizophrenia.

TREATMENT

GENERAL
- Psychotherapy
- Social skills training
- Family therapy
- Vocational counseling

MEDICATIONS
- Antipsychotic drugs (neuroleptic drugs)
- Antidepressants
- Anxiolytics

NURSING CONSIDERATIONS

NURSING DIAGNOSES
- Anxiety
- Bathing or hygiene self-care deficit
- Disabled family coping
- Disturbed body image
- Disturbed personal identity
- Disturbed sensory perception (auditory, visual, kinesthetic)
- Disturbed sleep pattern
- Dressing or grooming self-care deficit
- Fear
- Hopelessness
- Imbalanced nutrition: Less than body requirements
- Impaired home maintenance
- Impaired social interaction
- Impaired verbal communication
- Ineffective coping
- Ineffective role performance
- Powerlessness
- Risk for injury
- Risk for other-directed violence
- Risk for self-directed violence
- Social isolation

EXPECTED OUTCOMES
The patient (or family) will:
- consider an alternative interpretation of a situation without becoming unduly hostile or anxious
- perform bathing and hygiene activities to the fullest extent possible
- demonstrate adaptive coping behaviors
- verbalize positive feelings about self
- identify internal and external factors that trigger delusional episodes
- maintain maximal functioning within the limits of his auditory, visual, or kinesthetic impairment
- resume appropriate rest and activity patterns
- perform dressing and grooming activities to the fullest extent possible
- express fears and concerns
- participate in care and prescribed therapies
- remain free from signs of malnutrition
- maintain usual roles and responsibilities to the fullest extent possible
- demonstrate effective social interaction skills in both one-on-one and group settings
- express needs
- develop effective coping behaviors
- recognize limitations imposed by the illness and express feelings about these limitations
- gradually join in self-care and the decision-making process
- remain free from injury
- not harm others
- not harm self
- maintain family and peer relationships.

NURSING INTERVENTIONS
- Evaluate the patient's ability to carry out activities of daily living.
- Maintain a safe environment, minimizing stimuli.
- Give prescribed drugs.
- Adopt an accepting and consistent approach.
- Avoid promoting dependence.
- Reward positive behavior.
- Provide reality-based explanations for distorted body images or hypochondriacal complaints.
- Set limits on inappropriate behavior.
- Offer simple and matter-of-fact explanations about environmental safeguards, drugs, and policies.
- Build trust; be honest and dependable. Don't threaten, and don't promise what you can't fulfill.

MONITORING
- Suicidal ideation
- Homicidal ideation
- Effects of drug regimen
- Weight

PATIENT TEACHING

GENERAL
Be sure to cover:
- the disorder, diagnosis, and treatment
- drug administration, dosage, and possible adverse effects
- how family members can recognize an impending relapse, and ways to manage symptoms.

DISCHARGE PLANNING
- Refer the patient to appropriate community resources and support services.

RESOURCES
Organizations
American Psychiatric Association: *www.psych.org*
American Psychological Association: *www.apa.org*
National Alliance for the Mentally Ill: *www.nami.org*
National Alliance for Research on Schizophrenia and Depression: *www.narsad.org*

Selected references
Bilder, R.M., et al. "Cognitive Development in Schizophrenia: Follow-Back from the First Episode," *Journal of Clinical and Experimental Neuropsychology* 28(2):270-82, February 2006.

Chur-Hansen, A., et al. "Mental Health Nurses' and Psychiatrists' Views on the Prognosis of Schizophrenia and Depression: An Exploratory, Qualitative Investigation," *Journal of Psychiatric and Mental Health Nursing* 12(5):607-13, October 2005.

Diagnostic and Statistical Manual of Mental Disorders, Fourth Edition, Text Revision. Washington, D.C.: American Psychiatric Association, 2000.

Honer, W.G., et al. "Clozapine Alone Versus Clozapine and Risperidone with Refractory Schizophrenia," *New England Journal of Medicine* 354(5):472-82, February 2006.

Moser, D.J., et al. "Informed Consent in Medication-Free Schizophrenia Research," *American Journal of Psychiatry* 162(2):1209-11, June 2005.

Scleroderma

- Connective tissue disease characterized by inflammatory, degenerative, and fibrotic changes in skin, blood vessels, synovial membranes, skeletal muscles, and internal organs; thickening of tissues
- May affect the visceral organs or remain localized to the skin when the connective tissues of many organs, including the heart, kidney, GI tract, and lungs, are involved
- Cutaneous lesions usually on the face, hands, neck, and upper chest
- Also known as *systemic sclerosis*

PATHOPHYSIOLOGY

- The skin atrophies, and infiltrates containing CD4+ T cells surround the blood vessels; inflamed collagen fibers become edematous, losing strength and elasticity.
- The dermis becomes tightly bound to the underlying structures, resulting in atrophy of the affected dermal appendages and destruction of the distal phalanges by osteoporosis.
- As the disease progresses, atrophy can affect other areas.

CAUSES

- Unknown
- Possible causes:
- Systemic exposure to silica dust, polyvinyl chloride, or organic solvents
- Anticancer agents such as bleomycin or nonopioid analgesics such as pentazocine
- Fibrosis due to an abnormal immune system response
- Underlying vascular cause with tissue changes initiated by inconsistent perfusion
- Viral infection

INCIDENCE

- Scleroderma rarely occurs in children or men younger than age 35.
- It affects women three to four times more often than men, especially between ages 30 and 50.
- Peak incidence is from ages 50 to 60.

COMPLICATIONS

- Related to thickening of tissues:
- Slowly healing ulcerations on fingertips or toes leading to gangrene
- Decreased food intake and weight loss due to GI symptoms
- Arrhythmias and dyspnea
- Malignant hypertension
- Respiratory failure
- Renal failure
- Esophageal or intestinal obstruction or perforation
- Raynaud's phenomenon
- Pulmonary fibrosis

HISTORY

- Pain, stiffness, and swelling of fingers and joints (later symptoms)
- Frequent reflux, heartburn, dysphagia, and bloating after meals due to GI dysfunction
- Diarrhea, constipation, and malodorous floating stool

PHYSICAL FINDINGS

- Skin thickening, commonly limited to the distal extremities and face, but possibly involving internal organs
- CREST syndrome (a benign subtype of limited systemic sclerosis): calcinosis, Raynaud's phenomenon, esophageal dysfunction, sclerodactyly, and telangiectasia
- Patchy skin changes with a teardrop-like appearance known as morphea (localized scleroderma)
- Band of thickened skin on the face or extremities that severely damages underlying tissues, causing atrophy and deformity (linear scleroderma)
- Raynaud's phenomenon (blanching, cyanosis, and erythema of the fingers and toes); progressive phalangeal resorption that may shorten the fingers (early symptoms)
- Taut, shiny skin over the entire hand and forearm due to skin thickening
- Tight and inelastic facial skin, causing a masklike appearance and "pinching" of the mouth
- Thickened skin over proximal limbs and trunk (diffuse systemic sclerosis)
- Abdominal distention

LABORATORY

- Erythrocyte sedimentation rate is slightly elevated, rheumatoid factor is positive in 25% to 35% of patients, and antinuclear antibody is positive.
- Urinalysis shows proteinuria, microscopic hematuria, and casts.

IMAGING

- Hand X-rays show terminal phalangeal tuft resorption, subcutaneous calcification, and joint space narrowing and erosion.
- Chest X-rays show bilateral basilar pulmonary fibrosis.
- GI X-rays show distal esophageal hypomotility and stricture, duodenal loop dilation, small-bowel malabsorption pattern, and large diverticula.

DIAGNOSTIC PROCEDURES

- Pulmonary function studies show decreased diffusion and vital capacity.
- Electrocardiography shows nonspecific abnormalities related to myocardial fibrosis and possible arrhythmias.
- Skin biopsy shows changes consistent with disease progression, such as marked thickening of the dermis and occlusive vessel changes.

GENERAL

- Physical therapy
- Heat therapy
- Hemodialysis
- Lanolin emollients for skin care

DIET

- Soft, bland foods
- Possible enteral feedings

ACTIVITY

- Regular exercise, as tolerated
- Frequent rest periods

MEDICATIONS

- Immunosuppressants
- Vasodilators
- Antihypertensives
- Antacids
- Histamine-2 receptor antagonist or proton pump inhibitor
- Broad-spectrum antibiotics
- Angiotensin-converting enzyme inhibitor
- Oxygen therapy

SURGERY

- Digital sympathectomy or, rarely, cervical sympathetic blockade
- Digital plaster cast
- Possible surgical debridement
- Renal transplant

NURSING CONSIDERATIONS

NURSING DIAGNOSES

- Activity intolerance
- Acute pain
- Decreased cardiac output
- Diarrhea
- Disabled family coping
- Disturbed body image
- Fatigue
- Fear
- Imbalanced nutrition: Less than body requirements
- Impaired gas exchange
- Impaired physical mobility
- Impaired skin integrity
- Ineffective coping
- Ineffective tissue perfusion: Peripheral
- Risk for infection

EXPECTED OUTCOMES

The patient (or family) will:

- verbalize the importance of balancing activity, as tolerated, with rest
- express feelings of increased comfort and decreased pain
- maintain adequate cardiac output
- regain normal bowel function
- demonstrate effective coping behaviors
- express positive feelings about self
- express feelings of increased energy
- discuss fears and concerns
- achieve adequate nutritional intake

- maintain adequate ventilation and oxygenation
- attain the highest degree of mobility possible within the confines of disease
- exhibit improved or healed wounds or lesions
- use support systems to help cope with the disease
- maintain adequate peripheral perfusion, as evidenced by palpable pulses and warm extremities
- remain free from signs or symptoms of infection.

NURSING INTERVENTIONS

- Avoid using fingersticks for blood tests.
- Provide heat therapy to relieve joint stiffness.
- Elevate the head of the bed to help relieve GI symptoms.
- Provide meticulous skin care.
- Encourage oral fluid intake.
- Provide a soft, bland diet with frequent small meals.
- Administer oxygen, as ordered, for pulmonary complications.

MONITORING

- Intake and output
- Possible adverse reactions to prescribed drugs
- Daily weight
- End organ damage such as renal failure
- Skin integrity
- Nutritional status
- Vital signs, especially blood pressure
- Renal function
- Electrocardiograms
- Pulmonary function
- Abdominal distention

PATIENT TEACHING

GENERAL

Be sure to cover:

- the disorder, diagnosis, and treatment
- how to assess skin for changes
- avoiding cold weather and cigarette smoking
- reporting abnormal bleeding or

bruising and any nonhealing abrasions

- the importance of staying as active as possible, with frequent rest periods
- follow-up care.

DISCHARGE PLANNING

- Refer the patient to physical therapy and occupational therapy as needed.
- Refer the patient to a smoking-cessation program, if needed.
- Refer the patient to the Scleroderma Foundation.

RESOURCES

Organizations

American Academy of Dermatology: *www.aad.org*
Arthritis Foundation: *www.arthritis.org*
National Institute of Allergy and Infectious Diseases: *www.niaid.nih.gov*
Raynaud's & Scleroderma Association: *www.raynauds.org.uk*
The Scleroderma Foundation: *www.scleroderma.org*
Scleroderma Research Foundation: *www.srfcure.org*

Selected references

Chang, B., et al. "Natural History of Mild-Moderate Pulmonary Hypertension and the Risk Factors for Severe Pulmonary Hypertension in Scleroderma," *Journal of Rheumatology* 33(2):269-74, February 2006.

Joslin, N. "Early Identification Key to Scleroderma Treatment," *Nurse Practitioner* 29(7):24-39, July 2004.

Kasper, D.L., et al., eds. *Harrison's Principles of Internal Medicine*, 16th ed. New York: McGraw-Hill Book Co., 2005.

Melani, L., et al. "A Case of Nodular Scleroderma," *Journal of Dermatology* 32(12):1028-31, December 2005.

Pope, J.E., et al. "Scleroderma Treatment Differs Between Experts and General Rheumatologists," *Arthritis and Rheumatism* 55(1):138-45, February 2006.

The Merck Manual of Diagnosis & Therapy, 18th ed., Whitehouse Station, N.J.: Merck & Co., Inc., 2006.

Scoliosis

OVERVIEW

- Lateral curvature of the spine that's apparent on frontal projection, measures greater than 10 degrees, and is associated with vertebral rotation
- Right thoracic curve most common
- Classified as nonstructural or funcitonal (flexible spinal curve, with temporary straightening when patient leans sideways) or structural (fixed deformity)

PATHOPHYSIOLOGY

- The vertebrae rotate, forming the convex part of the curve.
- The rotation causes rib prominence along the thoracic spine and waistline asymmetry in the lumbar spine.
- Severity of spinal deformity dictates physiological impairment.

CAUSES

- Local inflammation and infection
- Neurofibromatosis (Recklinghausen's disease)
- Neuromuscular scoliosis: may be caused by muscular dystrophy, polio, cerebral palsy, or spinal muscular atrophy
- Nonstructural scoliosis: may result from acute disk disease, leg length discrepancies, paraspinal inflammation, or poor posture
- Structural scoliosis: no known cause
- Traumatic scoliosis: may result from vertebral fractures or disk disease

  AGE FACTOR *Degenerative scoliosis may develop in older patients with osteoporosis and degenerative joint disease of the spine.*

RISK FACTORS

- Congenital or neuromuscular problem
- Aging process

INCIDENCE

- Less than 1% of school-age children are affected.
- The disorder is seen at growth spurts between ages 10 and 13.
- It affects females 7 times more than males.
- Infantile scoliosis is most common in boys ages 1 to 3.
- Juvenile scoliosis affects boys and girls ages 3 to 10 about equally.
- Adolescent scoliosis occurs after age 10 and during adolescence.

COMPLICATIONS

- Debilitating back pain
- Severe deformity
- With thoracic curve exceeding 60 degrees, possible reduced pulmonary function
- With thoracic curve exceeding 80 degrees, increased risk of cor pulmonale in middle age
- Disturbed self-image

ASSESSMENT

HISTORY

- Familial history
- Detected during community or school scoliosis screening
- Hemlines look uneven
- Pant legs appear unequal in length
- One hip higher than the other
- Backache, fatigue, and dyspnea

PHYSICAL FINDINGS

- Signs of scoliosis (see *Testing for scoliosis*)

Testing for scoliosis

When assessing the patient for an abnormal spinal curve, use this screening test for scoliosis. Have the patient remove her shirt and stand as straight as she can with her back to you. Instruct her to distribute her weight evenly on each foot. While the patient does this, observe both sides of her back from neck to buttocks. Look for these signs:

- uneven shoulder height and shoulder blade prominence
- unequal distance between the arms and the body
- asymmetrical waistline
- uneven hip height
- a sideways lean.

  With the patient's back still facing you, ask the patient to do the "forward-bend" test. In this test, the patient places her palms together and slowly bends forward, remembering to keep her head down. As she complies, check for these signs:

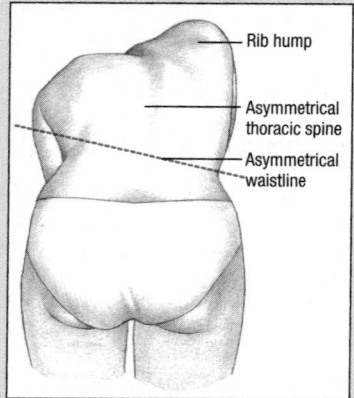

- Rib hump
- Asymmetrical thoracic spine
- Asymmetrical waistline

- asymmetrical thoracic spine or prominent rib cage (rib hump) on either side
- asymmetrical waistline.

DIAGNOSTIC TEST RESULTS

IMAGING
◆ Spinal X-ray studies confirm scoliosis and determine the degree of curvature and flexibility of the spine; they also determine skeletal maturity, predict remaining bone growth, and differentiate nonstructural from structural scoliosis.

OTHER
◆ Bone growth studies may help determine skeletal maturity.

TREATMENT

GENERAL
◆ Close observation
◆ Brace
◆ Spinal orthoses
◆ Functional strengthening program

ACTIVITY
◆ Gradually increased activity
◆ No vigorous sports
◆ Prescribed exercise regimen
◆ Swimming, but no diving

SURGERY
◆ Posterior spinal fusion and internal stabilization (rods and spinal hardware)

NURSING CONSIDERATIONS

NURSING DIAGNOSES
◆ Anxiety
◆ Chronic pain
◆ Disturbed body image
◆ Fear
◆ Impaired physical mobility
◆ Risk for injury

EXPECTED OUTCOMES
The patient will:
◆ identify strategies to reduce anxiety
◆ experience feelings of increased comfort and decreased pain
◆ express positive feelings about self
◆ discuss fears and concerns
◆ maintain joint mobility and range of motion (ROM) within the confines of the disease
◆ demonstrate measures to prevent injury to self.

NURSING INTERVENTIONS
◆ Promote self-care while allowing adequate time.
◆ Provide emotional support.
◆ Encourage deep-breathing exercises.
◆ Promote active ROM arm exercises.

MONITORING
◆ Sensation, movement, color, and pulses
◆ Intake and output
◆ Activity level
◆ Pain control after surgery

PATIENT TEACHING

GENERAL
Be sure to cover:
◆ the disorder, diagnosis, and treatment
◆ brace care
◆ skin care
◆ safe body mechanics
◆ relaxation techniques
◆ strengthening exercises.

RESOURCES
Organizations
American Academy of Orthopaedic Surgeons: *www.aaos.org*
American College of Obstetricians and Gynecologists: *www.acog.org*
National Scoliosis Foundation: *www.scoliosis.org*
Scoliosis Association, Inc.: *www.scoliosisassoc.org*
Scoliosis Research Society: *www.srs.org*

Selected references
Diseases, 4th ed. Philadelphia: Lippincott Williams & Wilkins, 2006.
Gillingham, B.L., et al. "Early Onset Idiopathic Scoliosis," *Journal of the American Academy of Orthopaedic Surgeons* 14(2):101-12, February 2006.
Handbook of Pathophysiology, 2nd ed. Philadelphia: Lippincott Williams & Wilkins, 2005.
Larsson, E.L., et al. "Long-term Follow-up of Functioning after Spinal Surgery in Patients with Neuromuscular Scoliosis," *Spine* 30(19):2145-152, October 2005.
Lonstein, J.E. "Scoliosis: Surgical Versus Nonsurgical Treatment," *Clinical Orthopaedics and Related Research* 443:248-59, February 2006.

Secondary polycythemia

OVERVIEW

- Excessive production of circulating red blood cells (RBCs) due to hypoxia, tumor, or disease
- Also called *reactive polycythemia*

PATHOPHYSIOLOGY

- The disorder may result from increased production of the hormone erythropoietin.
- Bone marrow is stimulated to produce RBCs. (Increased production of erythropoietin is possibly an inappropriate pathologic response to renal, central nervous system, or endocrine disorders or to certain neoplasms.)
- It may result as a compensatory response to several conditions, such as:
- hypoxemia
- hemoglobin abnormalities
- heart failure
- right-to-left shunting of blood in the heart
- central or peripheral alveolar hypoventilation
- low oxygen content at high altitudes.
- The disorder may be an inappropriate (pathologic) response to renal disease, central nervous system disease, neoplasms, or endocrine disorders.

CAUSES

- Increased production of erythropoietin

RISK FACTORS

- Conditions that cause prolonged tissue hypoxia, such as shock or compression of major blood vessels
- Recessive genetic trait

INCIDENCE

- The disorder occurs in 2 of every 100,000 people living at or near sea level.
- A greater incidence occurs among those living at high altitudes.

COMPLICATIONS

- Hemorrhage
- Thromboembolism

ASSESSMENT

HISTORY

- Emphysema
- Headaches
- Lethargy

PHYSICAL FINDINGS

- Clubbed fingers
- Ruddy skin
- Cyanosis
- Splenomegaly
- Shortness of breath
- Hypoxemia

DIAGNOSTIC TEST RESULTS

LABORATORY

- RBC mass is increased.
- Hematocrit and hemoglobin level are elevated.
- Mean corpuscular volume and mean corpuscular hemoglobin level are elevated.
- Urinary erythropoietin count is elevated
- Blood histamine level is elevated.
- Arterial oxygen saturation level is normal to low.

DIAGNOSTIC PROCEDURES

- Bone marrow biopsy reveals hyperplasia confined to the erythroid series.

TREATMENT

GENERAL
◆ Correction of underlying disease or environmental condition
◆ Phlebotomy
◆ Plasmapheresis
◆ Smoking cessation

DIET
◆ Low-sodium
◆ High in fluids

ACTIVITY
◆ As tolerated

MEDICATIONS
◆ Analgesics
◆ Low-flow oxygen therapy

NURSING CONSIDERATIONS

NURSING DIAGNOSES
◆ Activity intolerance
◆ Anxiety
◆ Fatigue
◆ Fear
◆ Impaired gas exchange
◆ Ineffective coping
◆ Ineffective protection
◆ Risk for deficient fluid volume
◆ Risk for infection
◆ Risk for injury

EXPECTED OUTCOMES
The patient will:
◆ verbalize the importance of balancing activity, as tolerated, with rest
◆ identify strategies to reduce anxiety
◆ express feelings of increased energy
◆ verbalize fears and concerns
◆ maintain adequate ventilation
◆ demonstrate effective coping skills
◆ demonstrate use of protective measures, including conservation of energy, maintenance of balanced diet, and attainment of adequate rest
◆ maintain normal fluid balance
◆ remain free from signs and symptoms of infection
◆ state safety and preventive measures.

NURSING INTERVENTIONS
◆ Promote optimal activity.
◆ Before and after phlebotomy, check the patient's blood pressure with him lying down. After the procedure, have the patient drink about 24 oz (710 ml) of water or juice. To prevent syncope, have him sit up for about 5 minutes before walking.
◆ Encourage verbalization and provide support.
◆ Give prescribed drugs.

MONITORING
◆ Signs of thrombosis
◆ Respiratory status
◆ Vital signs

PATIENT TEACHING

GENERAL
Be sure to cover:
◆ the disorder, diagnosis, and treatment
◆ symptoms of recurring polycythemia and the importance of reporting them promptly
◆ the importance of regular blood studies (every 2 to 3 months), even after the disease is controlled
◆ the need for relocation if altitude is a contributing factor
◆ dietary restrictions
◆ using an electric razor
◆ maintaining a safe environment
◆ alternating rest periods and activity.

DISCHARGE PLANNING
◆ Refer the patient to social services as appropriate.

RESOURCES
Organizations
American Heart Association: *www.americanheart.org*
National Heart, Lung, and Blood Institute: *www.nhlbi.nih.gov*

Selected references
Carey, P.M., et al. "Automated Red Cell Reduction on Polycythemia Using a Non-Therapeutic Apheresis Instrument," *Transfusion* 44 Supplement 1:13a, September 2004.
Diseases, 4th ed. Philadelphia: Lippincott Williams & Wilkins, 2006.
Jefferson, J.A., et al. "Increased Oxidative Stress Following Acute and Chronic High Altitude Exposure," *High Altitude Medicine & Biology* 5(1):61-69, Spring 2004.
Rosenkrantz, T.S. "Polycythemia and Hyperviscosity in the Newborn," *Seminars in Thrombosis & Hemostasis. The Hyperviscosity Syndromes.* 29(5):515-28, 2003.

Seizure disorder

- Neurologic condition characterized by recurrent seizures
- Doesn't affect intelligence
- In about 80% of patients, good seizure control with strict adherence to prescribed treatment
- Also known as *epilepsy*

PATHOPHYSIOLOGY

- Seizures are paroxysmal events involving abnormal electrical discharges of neurons in the brain and cell membrane potential.
- On stimulation, the neuron fires, the discharge spreads to surrounding cells, and stimulation continues to one side or both sides of the brain, resulting in seizure activity.

CAUSES

- 50% of cases idiopathic

Nonidiopathic seizure disorder

- Anoxia
- Apparent familial incidence in some seizure disorders
- Birth trauma
- Brain tumors or other space-occupying lesions
- Genetic abnormalities (tuberous sclerosis and phenylketonuria)
- Ingestion of toxins, such as mercury, lead, or carbon monoxide
- Meningitis, encephalitis, or brain abscess
- Metabolic abnormalities (hypoglycemia, pyridoxine deficiency, hypoparathyroidism)
- Perinatal infection
- Perinatal injuries
- Stroke
- Traumatic injury

INCIDENCE

- The first seizure usually occurs during childhood or after age 50.
- Seizure disorder affects 1% to 2% of the population.

COMPLICATIONS

- Anoxia
- Traumatic injury

HISTORY

- Anoxia
- Seizure occurrence unpredictable and unrelated to activities
- Precipitating factors or events possibly reported
- Headache
- Head trauma
- Drug use
- Family history of seizure disorder
- Muscle contractions
- Mood changes
- Lethargy
- Myoclonic jerking
- Description of an aura
- Pungent smell
- GI distress
- Rising or sinking feeling in the stomach
- Dreamy feeling
- Unusual taste in the mouth
- Vision disturbance

PHYSICAL FINDINGS

- Findings possibly normal while patient isn't having a seizure and when the cause is idiopathic
- Findings related to underlying cause of the seizure

LABORATORY

- Serum glucose and calcium study results rule out other diagnoses.

IMAGING

- Computed tomography scan and magnetic resonance imaging may indicate abnormalities in internal structures.
- Skull radiography may show certain neoplasms within the brain substance or skull fractures.
- Brain scan may show malignant lesions when X-ray findings are normal or questionable.
- Cerebral angiography may show cerebrovascular abnormalities, such as aneurysm or tumor.

OTHER

- Electroencephalography (EEG) shows paroxysmal abnormalities. (A negative EEG doesn't rule out epilepsy because paroxysmal abnormalities occur intermittently.)
- Lumbar puncture may reveal abnormal cerebrospinal fluid pressure, indicating an infection.

TREATMENT

GENERAL

- Airway protection during seizure
- Vagal nerve stimulation (see *Vagal nerve stimulation*)
- A detailed presurgical evaluation to characterize seizure type, frequency, site of onset, psychological functioning, and degree of disability to select candidates for surgery in medically intractable patients
- Safety measures

DIET

- No restrictions

ACTIVITY

- As tolerated

MEDICATIONS

- Anticonvulsants

SURGERY

- Removal of a demonstrated focal lesion
- Correction of the underlying problem

Vagal nerve stimulation

The vagal nerve stimulator, or *VNS*, is a Food and Drug Administration–approved method to treat medically refractory seizure disorder. The stimulator device is about the size of a pacemaker and is surgically placed in a pocket under the skin in the upper chest. Leadwires from the stimulator are tunneled under the skin to a neck incision where the vagal nerve has been exposed. The electrode coils are then placed around the nerve. The treating physician has a computer, which can be used to alter the stimulation parameters, thereby optimizing the treatment of seizures.

The VNS device stimulates the vagal nerve for 30 seconds every 5 minutes to prevent seizure occurrence. A magnet over the area can activate the device to give extra, on-demand stimulation if the patient feels a seizure coming on. Adverse effects are voice change, throat discomfort, shortness of breath, and coughing and are usually experienced only when the device is on.

NURSING CONSIDERATIONS

NURSING DIAGNOSES

- Anxiety
- Fear
- Ineffective coping
- Risk for injury
- Social isolation

EXPECTED OUTCOMES

The patient will:

- express feelings of decreased anxiety
- discuss fears and concerns
- use support systems and develop adequate coping
- remain free from injury
- maintain usual participation in social situations and activities.

NURSING INTERVENTIONS

- Institute seizure precautions.
- Prepare the patient for surgery if indicated.
- Give prescribed anticonvulsants.
- Protect the patient from injury.
- Maintain a patent airway.
- Promote the patient's self-esteem.

MONITORING

- Response to anticonvulsants
- Vital signs
- Seizure activity
- Respiratory status
- Adverse drug reactions
- Associated injuries

PATIENT TEACHING

GENERAL

Be sure to cover:

- the disorder, diagnosis, and treatment
- maintaining a normal lifestyle
- compliance with the prescribed drug schedule
- adverse drug effects
- care during a seizure
- the importance of regular meals and checking with the practitioner before dieting
- the importance of carrying a medical identification card or wearing medical identification jewelry.

DISCHARGE PLANNING

- Refer the patient to the Epilepsy Foundation of America.
- Refer the patient to his state's motor vehicle department for information about a driver's license.

RESOURCES

Organizations

The American Academy of Pediatrics: *www.aap.org*
Epilepsy Foundation of America: *www.efa.org*
National Institutes of Health: *www.nih.gov*

Selected references

Crawford, P. "Best Practice Guidelines for the Management of Women with Epilepsy," *Epilepsia* 46:117-24, 2005.

Diseases, 4th ed. Philadelphia: Lippincott Williams & Wilkins, 2006.

Handbook of Pathophysiology, 2nd ed. Philadelphia: Lippincott Williams & Wilkins, 2005.

Leppik, I.E., Epilepsy Foundation of America. "Choosing an Antiepileptic. Selecting Drugs for Older Patients with Epilepsy," *Geriatrics* 60(11):42-47, November 2005.

Shackleton, D.P., et al. "Living with Epilepsy: Long-term Prognosis and Psychosocial Outcomes," *Neurology* 61(1):64-70, July 2003.

Smy, J. "Improving the Lives of Epilepsy Patients," *Nursing Times* 101(27):44-45, July 2005.

Septic arthritis

OVERVIEW

- Inflammation of a synovial membrane
- Usually caused by bacteria
- Usually affects a single joint
- May have sudden onset
- Also known as *infectious arthritis*

PATHOPHYSIOLOGY

- Bacteria invade a joint, and inflammation of the synovial lining results.
- Organisms invade the joint cavity, and effusion and pyogenesis follow.
- Eventual bone and cartilage destruction result.

CAUSES

- Bacteria spread from a primary site of infection
- *Escherichia coli*
- Fungi or mycobacteria (rare cause)
- Gram-negative bacilli
- Gram-positive or -negative cocci
- *Haemophilus influenzae*
- *Neisseria gonorrhoeae*
- *Pseudomonas*
- *Salmonella*
- *Staphylococcus aureus*
- *Streptococcus pneumoniae*
- *Streptococcus pyogenes*
- *Streptococcus viridans*

RISK FACTORS

- Concurrent bacterial infection
- Serious chronic illness
- Alcoholism
- Advanced age
- Immune system depression
- History of immunosuppressive therapy
- I.V. drug abuse
- Recent articular trauma
- Arthroscopy and joint surgery
- Intra-articular injections
- Local joint abnormalities

INCIDENCE

- Septic arthritis caused by gram-positive cocci is more common in children age 2 and older and adults.
- Septic arthritis caused by *H. influenzae* is most common in children younger than age 2.

COMPLICATIONS

- Osteomyelitis
- Loss of joint cartilage
- Ankylosis
- Fatal septicemia

ASSESSMENT

HISTORY

- Abrupt onset of intense pain in the affected joint
- Fever and chills

PHYSICAL FINDINGS

- Affected joint kept in a flexed position
- Redness and edema over the affected joint
- Severely reduced range of motion (ROM)
- Warmth and extreme tenderness over the involved joint
- Chills

DIAGNOSTIC TEST RESULTS

LABORATORY

- Synovial fluid analysis shows pus or watery, cloudy fluid of decreased viscosity, typically with 50,000/µl or more white blood cells (WBCs) containing primarily neutrophils; and a low glucose level.
- Gram stain or culture of the fluid identifies the causative organism.
- Countercurrent immunoelectrophoresis measures bacterial antigens in body fluids and guides treatment.
- Positive blood cultures confirm the diagnosis even with negative synovial culture.
- WBC count is elevated with many polymorphonuclear cells.
- Erythrocyte sedimentation rate is increased.
- C-reactive protein level is elevated.
- Lactic assay distinguishes septic from nonseptic arthritis.

IMAGING

- X-rays may show distention of the joint capsule, narrowing of the joint space, and erosion of bone.
- Radioisotope joint scan may show infection or inflammation, especially in less accessible joints.

DIAGNOSTIC PROCEDURES

- Arthrocentesis allows collection of a synovial fluid specimen for analysis.
- Biopsy of the synovial membrane confirms the diagnosis and identifies the causative organism.

TREATMENT

GENERAL
- Based on antimicrobial susceptibilities and the patient's age
- Drainage by repeated closed-needle aspiration, arthroscopy, or arthrotomy
- Joint immobilization

ACTIVITY
- Exercise, as tolerated

MEDICATIONS
- Analgesics
- Parenteral antibiotics

SURGERY
- Reconstructive surgery for severe joint damage
- Possible open surgical drainage

NURSING CONSIDERATIONS

NURSING DIAGNOSES
- Acute pain
- Anxiety
- Dressing or grooming self-care deficit
- Fear
- Impaired physical mobility
- Risk for infection

EXPECTED OUTCOMES
The patient will:
- express feelings of increased comfort and decreased pain
- identify measures to reduce anxiety
- perform activities of daily living within the confines of the disorder
- discuss fears and concerns
- maintain joint mobility and ROM
- remain free from signs and symptoms of infection.

NURSING INTERVENTIONS
- Practice strict sterile technique.
- Check splints or traction regularly.
- Maintain proper alignment.
- Assist with ROM exercises.
- Give prescribed drugs for pain.
- Allow adequate time for and promote self-care.

MONITORING
- Signs and symptoms of joint inflammation
- Vital signs and fever pattern
- Pain levels
- Response to pain medications
- Condition after joint aspiration

PATIENT TEACHING

GENERAL
Be sure to cover:
- the disorder, diagnosis, and treatment
- the etiology of the disease
- the role of I.V. drug use
- the prevention of recurrence
- prescribed drugs
- adverse drug reactions
- the exercise regimen
- rest periods
- home I.V. therapy, if required
- avoiding aggravating factors.

DISCHARGE PLANNING
- Refer the patient to drug counseling, if appropriate.

RESOURCES
Organizations
Arthritis Foundation: *www.arthritis.org*
National Institute of Arthritis and Musculoskeletal and Skin Diseases: *www.nih.gov/niams/healthinfo*

Selected references
Butbul-Aviel, Y., et al. "Procalcitonin as a Diagnostic Aid in Osteomyelitis and Septic Arthritis," *Pediatric Emergency Care* 21(12):828-32, December 2005.
Diseases, 4th ed. Philadelphia: Lippincott Williams & Wilkins, 2006.
Handbook of Pathophysiology, 2nd ed. Philadelphia: Lippincott Williams & Wilkins, 2005.
Lu, J.J., et al. "Septic Arthritis Caused by Vancomycin-Intermediate *Staphylococcus Aureus*," *Journal of Clinical Microbiology* 43(8):4156-158, August 2005.
Ross, J.J. "Septic Arthritis," *Infectious Disease Clinics of North America* 19(4):799-817, December 2005.
Zicat, B., et al. "Septic Arthritis of the Acromioclavicular Joint: Tc-99m Leukocyte Imaging," *Clinical Nuclear Medicine* 31(3):145-46, March 2006.

Severe acute respiratory syndrome

LIFE-THREATENING DISORDER

OVERVIEW

- Severe viral infection that may progress to pneumonia
- Believed to be less infectious than influenza
- Incubation period estimated to range from 2 to 7 days (average, 3 to 5 days)
- Not highly contagious when protective measures are used
- Also known as *SARS*

PATHOPHYSIOLOGY

- Coronaviruses cause diseases in pigs, birds, and other animals.
- A theory suggests that a coronavirus may have mutated, allowing transmission to and infection of humans.

CAUSES

- A new type of coronavirus known as *SARS-associated coronavirus (SARS-CoV)*

RISK FACTORS

- Close contact with aerosolized (exhaled) droplets and bodily secretions from an infected person
- Travel to endemic areas

INCIDENCE

- SARS is more common in adults than children.
- Outbreaks are prevalent in China, Hong Kong, Toronto, Singapore, Taiwan, and Vietnam; many other countries report smaller numbers of cases.
- It affects all races.
- It affects both sexes equally.

COMPLICATIONS

- Respiratory difficulties
- Severe thrombocytopenia (low platelet count)
- Heart failure
- Liver failure
- Death

ASSESSMENT

HISTORY

- Contact with a person known to have SARS
- Travel to an endemic area
- Flulike symptoms
- Headache
- Diarrhea
- Nausea and vomiting

PHYSICAL FINDINGS

- Nonproductive cough
- Rash
- High fever
- Respiratory distress in later stages

DIAGNOSTIC TEST RESULTS

LABORATORY

- Antibodies to coronavirus are detected.
- Sputum Gram stain and culture isolates coronavirus.
- Platelet count may be low.

IMAGING

- Changes in chest X-rays indicate pneumonia (infiltrates).

DIAGNOSTIC PROCEDURES

- SARS-specific polymerase chain reaction test detects SARS-CoV ribonucleic acid.
- Antibody testing via enzyme-linked immunosorbent assay and the immunofluorescent antibody test is in development.

GENERAL
- Symptomatic treatment
- Isolation for hospitalized patients
- Strict respiratory and mucosal barrier precautions
- Quarantine of exposed people to prevent spread
- Global surveillance and reporting of suspected cases to national health authorities
- Intubation and mechanical ventilation, if indicated

DIET
- As tolerated

ACTIVITY
- As tolerated

MEDICATIONS
- Antivirals
- Combination of steroids and antimicrobials
- Oxygen therapy

NURSING DIAGNOSES
- Activity intolerance
- Anxiety
- Dysfunctional grieving
- Fear
- Imbalanced nutrition: Less than body requirements
- Impaired gas exchange
- Risk for infection

EXPECTED OUTCOMES
The patient will:
- perform activities of daily living as tolerated
- identify strategies to reduce anxiety
- use support systems to assist with coping
- discuss fears and concerns
- maintain adequate nutrition and hydration
- maintain adequate ventilation and oxygenation
- remain free from signs and symptoms of infection.

NURSING INTERVENTIONS
- Give prescribed drugs.
- Encourage adequate nutritional intake.
- Observe, record, and report nature of rash.
- Maintain proper isolation technique.
- Collect laboratory specimens, as needed.

MONITORING
- Vital signs
- Nutritional status
- Respiratory status
- Complications

GENERAL
Be sure to cover:
- the importance of frequent hand washing
- covering mouth and nose when coughing or sneezing
- avoiding close personal contact with friends and family
- the importance of not going to work, school, or other public places until 10 days after fever and respiratory symptoms resolve
- wearing a surgical mask when around other people or, if the patient can't wear one, mask wearing by those in contact with the patient
- not sharing silverware, towels, or bedding until they have been washed in soap and hot water
- using disposable gloves and household disinfectant to clean any surface that might have been exposed to the patient's body fluids.

DISCHARGE PLANNING
- Refer the patient for follow-up, as needed.

RESOURCES
Organizations
Centers for Disease Control and Prevention: *www.cdc.gov*
Occupational Safety & Health Administration: *www.osha.gov/dep/sars/*
World Health Organization: *www.who.int*

Selected references
Chan, P.K., et al. "SARS: Clinical Presentation, Transmission, Pathogenesis and Treatment Options," *Clinical Science* 110(2):193-204, February 2006.
Chu, C.M., et al. "Viral Load Distribution in SARS Outbreak," *Emerging Infectious Diseases* 11(12):1882-886, December 2005.
Rebmann, T. "Severe Acute Respiratory Syndrome: Implications for Perinatal and Neonatal Nurses," *Journal of Perinatal & Neonatal Nursing* 19(4):332-45, October-December 2005.
Tseng, H.C., et al. "SARS: Key Factors in Crisis Management," *Journal of Nursing Research* 13(1):58-65, March 2005.

Severe combined immunodeficiency disease

LIFE-THREATENING DISORDER

OVERVIEW

- Disorder that involves deficient or absent cell-mediated (T cell) and humoral (B cell) immunity
- Predisposes patient to infection from all classes of microorganisms during infancy
- Also known as *SCID* and *graft-versus-host disease*

PATHOPHYSIOLOGY

- Three types of SCID have been identified:
- reticular dysgenesis, the most severe type, in which the hematopoietic stem cell fails to differentiate into lymphocytes and granulocytes
- Swiss-type agammaglobulinemia, in which the hematopoietic stem cell fails to differentiate into lymphocytes alone
- enzyme deficiency, such as adenosine deaminase deficiency, in which the buildup of toxic products in the lymphoid tissue causes damage and subsequent dysfunction.

CAUSES

- Failure of thymus or bursa equivalent to develop normally or possible defect in thymus and bone marrow (responsible for T- and B-cell development)
- Possible enzyme deficiency
- Transmitted as autosomal recessive trait but may be X linked

RISK FACTORS

- Family history of SCID

INCIDENCE

- SCID affects more males than females.
- The disease occurs in 1 of 100,000 to 500,000 births.
- The onset is usually about age 2 months.

COMPLICATIONS

- Without treatment, infection within 1 year of birth causes death
- Pneumonia
- Oral ulcers
- Failure to thrive
- Dermatitis

ASSESSMENT

HISTORY

- Extreme susceptibility to infection within the first few months after birth, but probably no sign of gram-negative infection until about age 6 months because of protection by maternal immunoglobulin G

PHYSICAL FINDINGS

- Emaciated appearance and failure to thrive
- Assessment findings dependent on the type and site of infection
- Signs of chronic otitis media and sepsis
- Signs of the usual childhood diseases such as chickenpox

DIAGNOSTIC TEST RESULTS

GENERAL

- Defective humoral immunity is difficult to detect before an infant reaches age 5 months.

LABORATORY

- Tests show a severely diminished or absent T-cell number and function.

IMAGING

- A chest X-ray characteristically shows bilateral pulmonary infiltrates.

DIAGNOSTIC PROCEDURES

- Lymph node biopsy showing an absence of lymphocytes confirms diagnosis.

TREATMENT

GENERAL

- Strict protective isolation (germ-free environment)
- Gene therapy (experimental)

DIET

- No dietary restrictions

ACTIVITY

- As tolerated

MEDICATIONS

- Immunoglobulin
- Antibiotics

SURGERY

- Histocompatible bone marrow transplantation
- Fetal thymus and liver transplantation
- Stem cell transplant

NURSING DIAGNOSES

- Acute pain
- Anxiety
- Delayed growth and development
- Diarrhea
- Disabled family coping
- Impaired gas exchange
- Impaired oral mucous membrane
- Impaired skin integrity
- Ineffective protection
- Risk for impaired parent/infant/child attachment
- Risk for infection

EXPECTED OUTCOMES

The patient (or parents) will:
- exhibit signs of increased comfort and decreased pain
- verbalize strategies to reduce anxiety
- demonstrate age-appropriate skills and behaviors
- regain normal bowel function
- develop adequate coping mechanisms and support systems
- maintain adequate ventilation and oxygenation
- maintain intact oral mucous membranes
- maintain skin integrity
- demonstrate protective measures, including conserving energy, maintaining a balanced diet, and getting plenty of rest
- establish eye, physical, and verbal contact with the infant or child
- not experience chills, fever, and other signs or symptoms of illness.

NURSING INTERVENTIONS

- If infection develops, provide prompt and aggressive drug therapy and supportive care, as ordered.
- Watch for adverse effects of any drugs given.
- Avoid vaccinations, and give only irradiated blood products if a transfusion is ordered.

   AGE FACTOR *Although SCID infants must remain in strict protective isolation, try to provide a stimulating atmosphere to promote growth and development.*

- Encourage parents to visit their child often, to hold him, and to bring him toys that can be easily sterilized.
- Maintain a normal day and night routine, and talk to the child as much as possible.
- If parents can't visit, call them often to report on the infant's condition.
- Provide emotional support for the family.

MONITORING

- Signs and symptoms of infection
- Growth and development
- Skin integrity
- Respiratory status
- Response to treatment
- Complications
- Signs and symptoms of transplant rejection
- Social interaction

GENERAL

Be sure to cover:
- the disorder, diagnosis, and treatment
- the proper technique for strict protective isolation
- the signs and symptoms of infection and the need to notify a practitioner promptly
- drug administration, dosage, purpose, and adverse effects.

DISCHARGE PLANNING

- Encourage the parents to seek genetic counseling.

RESOURCES

Organizations

Centers for Disease Control and Prevention: *www.cdc.gov*
The Merck Manuals Online Medical Library: *www.merck.com/mmhe*

Selected references

Grunebaum, E., et al. "Bone Marrow Transplantation for Severe Combined Immune Deficiency," *JAMA* 295(5):508-18, February 2006.

Kasper, D.L., et al., eds. *Harrison's Principles of Internal Medicine*, 16th ed. New York: McGraw-Hill Book Co., 2005.

McGhee, S.A., et al. "Potential Costs and Benefits of Newborn Screening for Severe Combined Immunodeficiency," *Journal of Pediatrics* 147(5):603-608, November 2005.

The Merck Manual of Diagnosis & Therapy, 18th ed., Whitehouse Station, N.J.: Merck & Co., Inc., 2006.

Pesu, M., et al. "Jak3, Severe Combined Immunodeficiency, and a New Class of Immunosuppressive Drugs," *Immunological Reviews* 203:127-42, February 2005.

Shigellosis

OVERVIEW

- An acute intestinal infection caused by the bacteria *Shigella*, a short, non-motile, gram-negative rod
- Can be classified into four groups:
- Group A, caused by *S. dysenteriae;* most common in Central America; causes particularly severe infection and septicemia
- Group B, is caused by *S. flexneri;* together with group D responsible for 90% of shigellosis cases
- Group C, caused by *S. boydii;* occurs internationally
- Group D, caused by *S. sonnei*
- Also known as *bacillary dysentery*

PATHOPHYSIOLOGY

- Highly contagious aerobic, non-motile, glucose-fermenting, gram-negative rods cause diarrhea after ingestion of as few as 180 organisms.
- Rods invade the colonic epithelium and produce enterotoxin, which enhances virulence.

CAUSES

- Occasional transmission by housefly vector
- Transmission of *Shigella* bacteria through the fecal-oral route, by direct contact with contaminated objects, or through ingestion of contaminated food or water

INCIDENCE

- Shigellosis is most common in children ages 1 to 4; many adults acquire the illness from children.
- The disease is endemic in North America, Europe, and the tropics; in the United States, about 23,000 cases occur annually, usually in children or elderly, debilitated, or malnourished people.
- Shigellosis commonly occurs among confined populations, such as those in mental institutions and hospitals.

COMPLICATIONS

- Electrolyte imbalance (especially hypokalemia)
- Metabolic acidosis
- Shock

ASSESSMENT

HISTORY

- Crowded living conditions
- Close contact with someone who has acute diarrhea
- Fever
- Diarrhea
- Tenesmus

PHYSICAL FINDINGS

- Pus in stools
- Signs of dehydration
- Decreased blood pressure
- Hyperactive bowel sounds
- Abdominal tenderness
- Abdominal distention
- Rapid, thready pulse

DIAGNOSTIC TEST RESULTS

LABORATORY

- Microscopic examination of stools reveals mucus, red blood cells, and polymorphonuclear leukocytes.
- Direct immunofluorescence with specific antisera may reveal *Shigella*.

DIAGNOSTIC PROCEDURES

- Sigmoidoscopy or proctoscopy may reveal typical superficial ulcerations.

TREATMENT

GENERAL
◆ Enteric precautions

DIET
◆ Low-residue
◆ Replacement of fluids and electrolytes with I.V. infusions of normal saline solution (with electrolytes)

MEDICATIONS
◆ Antibiotics (of questionable value but may be used)

⚡ **WARNING** *Antidiarrheals that slow intestinal motility are contraindicated in shigellosis because they delay fecal excretion of Shigella and prolong fever and diarrhea.*

⚡ **WARNING** *A vaccine to help prevent shigellosis is currently being developed.*

◆ I.V. fluids

NURSING CONSIDERATIONS

NURSING DIAGNOSES
◆ Acute pain
◆ Deficient fluid volume
◆ Diarrhea
◆ Hyperthermia
◆ Imbalanced nutrition: Less than body requirements
◆ Risk for infection

EXPECTED OUTCOMES
The patient will:
◆ report adequate pain relief with analgesia or other measures
◆ regain and maintain normal fluid and electrolyte balance
◆ regain normal bowel elimination pattern
◆ remain afebrile
◆ maintain adequate nutrition and hydration
◆ exhibit no further signs or symptoms of infection.

NURSING INTERVENTIONS
◆ Give prescribed I.V. fluids.
◆ Maintain enteric precautions until microscopic bacteriologic studies confirm that the stool specimen is negative.

MONITORING
◆ Vital signs
◆ Comfort level
◆ Intake and output

PATIENT TEACHING

GENERAL
Be sure to cover:
◆ the disorder, diagnosis, and treatment
◆ prevention of infecting others.

RESOURCES
Organizations
National Center for Infectious Diseases: *www.cdc.gov/ncidod*
National Digestive Diseases Information Clearinghouse: *www.niddk.nih.gov/ health/digest/nddic.htm*
World Health Organization: *www.who.int*

Selected references

Amieva, M.R. "Important Bacterial Gastrointestinal Pathogens in Children: A Pathogenesis Perspective," *Pediatric Clinics of North America* 52(3):749-77, vi, June 2005.

Ekdahl, K., and Andersson, Y. "The Epidemiology of Travel-Associated Shigellosis — Regional Risks, Seasonality and Serogroups," *Journal of Infection* 51(3):222-29, October 2005.

Ford, T. "Emerging Issues in Water and Health Research," *Journal of Water and Health* 4 Suppl 1:59-65, 2006.

Grinblat, J., et al. "Diarrhea in Elderly Patients Due to *Clostridium Difficile* Associated with *Salmonella* and *Shigella* Infection," *Archives of Gerontology and Geriatrics* 39(3):277-82, November-December 2004.

Niyogi, S.K. "Shigellosis," *Journal of Microbiology* 43(2):133-43, April 2005.

Shock, cardiogenic
LIFE-THREATENING DISORDER

OVERVIEW

- A condition of diminished cardiac output that severely impairs tissue perfusion
- The most lethal form of shock
- Sometimes called *pump failure*

PATHOPHYSIOLOGY

- Left ventricular dysfunction initiates a series of compensatory mechanisms that attempt to increase cardiac output.
- As cardiac output decreases, aortic and carotid baroreceptors activate sympathetic nervous responses.
- Responses increase heart rate, left ventricular filling pressure, and peripheral resistance to flow to enhance venous return to the heart.
- This action initially stabilizes the patient but later causes deterioration with increasing oxygen demands on the already compromised myocardium.
- These events consist of a cycle of low cardiac output, sympathetic compensation, myocardial ischemia, and even lower cardiac output.

CAUSES

- Acute mitral or aortic insufficiency
- End-stage cardiomyopathy
- Myocardial infarction (MI) (most common)
- Myocardial ischemia
- Myocarditis
- Papillary muscle dysfunction
- Ventricular aneurysm
- Ventricular septal defect

INCIDENCE

- The condition typically affects patients in whom the area of MI involves 40% or more of left ventricular muscle mass (a group in which mortality may exceed 85%).

COMPLICATIONS

- Multiple organ dysfunction
- Death

ASSESSMENT

HISTORY

- Disorder, such as MI or cardiomyopathy, that severely decreases left ventricular function
- Anginal pain

PHYSICAL FINDINGS

- Urine output less than 20 ml/hour
- Pale, cold, clammy skin
- Decreased sensorium
- Rapid, shallow respirations
- Rapid, thready pulse
- Mean arterial pressure of less than 60 mm Hg in adults
- Gallop rhythm, faint heart sounds and, possibly, a holosystolic murmur
- Jugular vein distention
- Severe anxiety
- Decreased level of consciousness (LOC)
- Pulmonary crackles

DIAGNOSTIC TEST RESULTS

LABORATORY

- Serum enzyme measurements show elevated levels of creatine kinase, lactate dehydrogenase, aspartate aminotransferase, and alanine aminotransferase.
- Troponin levels are elevated.

IMAGING

- Cardiac catheterization and echocardiography may reveal other conditions that can lead to pump dysfunction and failure, such as cardiac tamponade, papillary muscle infarct or rupture, ventricular septal rupture, pulmonary emboli, venous pooling, and hypovolemia.

DIAGNOSTIC PROCEDURES

- Pulmonary artery pressure monitoring reveals increased pulmonary artery pressure and pulmonary artery wedge pressure, reflecting an increase in left ventricular end diastolic pressure (preload) and heightened resistance to left ventricular emptying (afterload) caused by ineffective pumping and increased peripheral vascular resistance.
- Invasive arterial pressure monitoring shows systolic arterial pressure less than 80 mm Hg caused by impaired ventricular ejection.
- Arterial blood gas (ABG) analysis may show metabolic and respiratory acidosis and hypoxia.
- Electrocardiography demonstrates possible evidence of acute MI, ischemia, or ventricular aneurysm.

TREATMENT

GENERAL

- Intra-aortic balloon pump (IABP)
- Symptomatic
- Intubation and mechanical ventilation, if indicated

DIET

- Possible parenteral nutrition or tube feedings

ACTIVITY

- Bed rest

MEDICATIONS

- Vasopressors
- Inotropics
- Analgesics; sedatives
- Osmotic diuretics
- Vasodilators
- Oxygen
- Antiarrhythmics

SURGERY

- Possible ventricular assist device
- Possible heart transplant

NURSING CONSIDERATIONS

NURSING DIAGNOSES
- Anxiety
- Decreased cardiac output
- Excess fluid volume
- Fear
- Hopelessness
- Impaired gas exchange
- Impaired physical mobility
- Ineffective coping
- Ineffective tissue perfusion: Cardiopulmonary

EXPECTED OUTCOMES
The patient will:
- verbalize strategies to reduce anxiety
- maintain adequate cardiac output and hemodynamic stability
- develop no complications of fluid volume excess
- discuss fears and concerns
- make decisions on own behalf
- maintain adequate ventilation and oxygenation
- maintain joint mobility and muscle strength
- express feelings and develop adequate coping mechanisms
- maintain adequate cardiopulmonary perfusion.

NURSING INTERVENTIONS
- Administer oxygen therapy.
- Follow IABP protocols and policies.

  WARNING *When a patient is on an IABP, move him as little as possible. Never place the patient in a sitting position higher than 45 degrees (including for chest X-rays) because the balloon may tear through the aorta and cause immediate death. Assess pedal pulses and skin temperature and color. Check the dressing on the insertion site frequently for bleeding, and change it according to facility protocol. Also check the site for hematoma or signs of infection, and culture any drainage.*
- Monitor the patient for cardiac arrhythmias.

- Plan your care to allow frequent rest periods, and provide as much privacy as possible. Allow the patient's family to visit and comfort him as much as possible.
- Provide explanations and reassurance for the patient and his family as appropriate.
- Prepare the patient and his family for a possibly fatal outcome, and help them find effective coping strategies.

MONITORING
- ABG levels (acid-base balance) and pulse oximetry
- Complete blood count and electrolyte levels
- Vital signs and peripheral pulses
- Cardiac status
- Hemodynamics
- Intake and output
- Respiratory status
- LOC

PATIENT TEACHING

GENERAL
Be sure to cover:
- the disorder, diagnosis, and treatment
- explanations and reassurance for patient and his family
- the possibly fatal outcome.

RESOURCES
Organizations
American Heart Association: *www.americanheart.org*
National Heart, Lung, and Blood Institute: *www.nhlbi.nih.gov*

Selected references
Ellis, T.C., et al. "Therapeutic Strategies for Cardiogenic Shock, 2006." *Current Treatment Options in Cardiovascular Medicine* 8(1):79-94, February 2006.
Jolly, S., et al. "Effect of Vasopressin on Hemodynamics in Patients with Refractory Cardiogenic Shock Complicating Acute Myocardial Infarction," *American Journal of Cardiology* 96(12):1617-20, December 2005.
Nanda, U., et al. "Modified Release Verapamil Induced Cardiogenic Shock," *Emergency Medicine Journal* 22(11):832-33, November 2005.
Nettina, S.M. *Lippincott Manual of Nursing Practice,* 8th ed. Philadelphia: Lippincott Williams & Wilkins, 2006.
Revelly, J.P., et al. "Lactate and Glucose Metabolism in Severe Sepsis and Cardiogenic Shock," *Critical Care Medicine* 33(10):2235-40, October 2005.

Shock, hypovolemic
LIFE-THREATENING DISORDER

- Reduced intravascular blood volume causing circulatory dysfunction and inadequate tissue perfusion resulting from loss of blood, plasma, or fluids
- Potentially life-threatening

PATHOPHYSIOLOGY

- When fluid is lost from the intravascular space, venous return to the heart is reduced.
- This decreases ventricular filling, which leads to a drop in stroke volume.
- Cardiac output falls, causing reduced perfusion to tissues and organs.
- Tissue anoxia prompts a shift in cellular metabolism from aerobic to anaerobic pathways.
- This produces an accumulation of lactic acid, resulting in metabolic acidosis.

CAUSES

- Acute blood loss (about one-fifth of total volume)
- Acute pancreatitis
- Ascites
- Burns
- Dehydration, as from excessive perspiration, severe diarrhea, protracted vomiting, diabetes insipidus, diuresis, or inadequate fluid intake
- Diuretic abuse
- Intestinal obstruction
- Peritonitis

INCIDENCE

- The incidence of hypovolemic shock depends on its cause.
- Hypovolemic shock affects all ages.
- It affects males and females equally.
- Hypovolemic shock occurs more frequently and is less likely to be tolerated in elderly patients.

COMPLICATIONS

- Acute respiratory distress syndrome
- Acute tubular necrosis and renal failure
- Disseminated intravascular coagulation
- Multiple organ dysfunction

HISTORY

- Disorders or conditions that reduce blood volume, such as GI hemorrhage, trauma, and severe diarrhea and vomiting
- Patient with cardiac disease: possible anginal pain because of decreased myocardial perfusion and oxygenation

PHYSICAL FINDINGS

- Pale, cool, clammy skin
- Decreased sensorium
- Rapid, shallow respirations
- Urine output usually less than 20 ml/hour
- Rapid, thready pulse
- Mean arterial pressure less than 60 mm Hg in adults (in chronic hypotension, mean pressure may fall below 50 mm Hg before signs of shock)
- Orthostatic vital signs and tilt test results consistent with hypovolemic shock (see *Checking for early hypovolemic shock*)

Checking for early hypovolemic shock

Orthostatic vital signs and tilt test results can help in assessing for the possibility of impending hypovolemic shock.

ORTHOSTATIC VITAL SIGNS

Measure the patient's blood pressure and pulse rate while he's lying in a supine position, sitting, and standing. Wait at least 1 minute between each position change. A systolic blood pressure decrease of 10 mm Hg or more between positions or a pulse rate increase of 10 beats/minute or more is a sign of volume depletion and impending hypovolemic shock.

TILT TEST

With the patient lying in a supine position, raise his legs above heart level. If his blood pressure increases significantly, the test is positive, indicating volume depletion and impending hypovolemic shock.

LABORATORY

- Hematocrit is low, and hemoglobin levels and red blood cell and platelet counts are decreased.
- Serum potassium, sodium, lactate dehydrogenase, creatinine, and blood urea nitrogen levels are elevated.
- Urine specific gravity (greater than 1.020) and urine osmolality are increased.
- pH and partial pressure of arterial oxygen are decreased, and partial pressure of arterial carbon dioxide is increased.
- Aspiration of gastric contents through a nasogastric tube identifies internal bleeding.
- Occult blood tests are positive.
- Coagulation studies show coagulopathy from disseminated intravascular coagulation.

IMAGING

- Chest or abdominal X-rays help to identify internal bleeding sites.

DIAGNOSTIC PROCEDURES

- Gastroscopy helps to identify internal bleeding sites.
- Invasive hemodynamic monitoring shows reduced central venous pressure, right atrial pressure, pulmonary artery pressure, pulmonary artery wedge pressure, and cardiac output.

TREATMENT

GENERAL
- In severe cases, an intra-aortic balloon pump, ventricular assist device, or pneumatic antishock garment
- Bleeding control by direct application of pressure and related measures
- Intubation and mechanical ventilation, if indicated

DIET
- Possible parenteral nutrition or tube feedings

ACTIVITY
- Bed rest

MEDICATIONS
- Prompt and vigorous blood and fluid replacement
- Positive inotropics
- Oxygen therapy

SURGERY
- Possibly, to correct underlying problem

NURSING CONSIDERATIONS

NURSING DIAGNOSES
- Anxiety
- Decreased cardiac output
- Deficient fluid volume
- Disabled family coping
- Impaired gas exchange
- Ineffective tissue perfusion: Cardiopulmonary, renal, cerebral
- Risk for infection
- Risk for injury

EXPECTED OUTCOMES
The patient (or family) will:
- verbalize strategies to reduce anxiety
- maintain adequate cardiac output and hemodynamic stability
- maintain adequate fluid volume
- express feelings and develop adequate coping mechanisms
- maintain adequate ventilation and oxygenation
- maintain adequate cardiopulmonary, renal, and cerebral perfusion as evidenced by palpable pulses, no signs of respiratory distress, normal urine output, and normal mentation
- remain free from signs and symptoms of infection
- avoid complications or injury.

NURSING INTERVENTIONS
- Check for a patent airway and adequate circulation. If blood pressure and heart rate are absent, start cardiopulmonary resuscitation.
- Obtain type and cross match, as ordered. In an emergency situation when there isn't time for cross matching, give type O-negative blood, which can be given to anyone.
- Give prescribed I.V. solutions or blood products.
- Insert an indwelling urinary catheter.
- Give prescribed oxygen.
- Provide emotional support to the patient and family.

MONITORING
- Vital signs and peripheral pulses
- Cardiac rhythm
- Coagulation studies for signs of impending coagulopathy
- Complete blood count and electrolyte measurements
- Arterial blood gas levels
- Intake and output
- Hemodynamics

PATIENT TEACHING

GENERAL
Be sure to cover:
- the disorder, diagnosis, and treatment
- procedures and their purpose
- the risks associated with blood transfusions
- the purpose of all equipment such as mechanical ventilation
- dietary restrictions
- drugs and possible adverse effects.

RESOURCES
Organizations
American Heart Association: *www.americanheart.org*
National Heart, Lung, and Blood Institute: *www.nhlbi.nih.gov*

Selected references
Kelley, D.M. "Hypovolemic Shock: An Overview," *Critical Care Nursing Quarterly* 28(1):2-19, January-March 2005.
Muhlberg, A.H., and Ruth-Sahd, L. "Holistic Care: Treatment and Interventions for Hypovolemic Shock Secondary to Hemorrhage," *Dimensions of Critical Care Nursing* 23(2):55-59, March/April 2004.
Nettina, S.M. *Lippincott Manual of Nursing Practice,* 8th ed. Philadelphia: Lippincott Williams & Wilkins, 2006.
Yanagawa, Y., et al. "Early Diagnosis of Hypovolemic Shock by Sonographic Measurement of Inferior Vena Cava in Trauma Patients," *Journal of Trauma-Injury Infection & Critical Care* 58(4):825-29, April 2005.

Shock, septic LIFE-THREATENING DISORDER

OVERVIEW

- Low systemic vascular resistance and an elevated cardiac output
- Probably a response to infections that release microbes or an immune mediator

PATHOPHYSIOLOGY

- Initially, the body's defenses activate chemical mediators in response to the invading organisms.
- The release of these mediators results in low systemic vascular resistance and increased cardiac output.
- Blood flow is unevenly distributed in the microcirculation, and plasma leaking from capillaries causes functional hypovolemia.
- Diffuse increase in capillary permeability occurs.
- Eventually, cardiac output decreases, and poor tissue perfusion and hypotension cause multisystem dysfunction syndrome and death.

CAUSES

- Any pathogenic organism
- Gram-negative bacteria, such as *Escherichia coli, Klebsiella pneumoniae, Serratia, Enterobacter,* and *Pseudomonas,* most common causes (up to 70% of cases)

RISK FACTORS

- Impaired immunity
- Young or old age

INCIDENCE

- About two-thirds of the cases of septic shock occur in hospitalized patients (most of whom have underlying diseases).

COMPLICATIONS

- Disseminated intravascular coagulation
- Renal failure
- Heart failure
- GI ulcers
- Abnormal liver function
- Death

ASSESSMENT

HISTORY

- Possible disorder or treatment that can cause immunosuppression
- Possibly, previous invasive tests or treatments, surgery, or trauma
- Possible fever and chills (although 20% of patients may be hypothermic)

PHYSICAL FINDINGS

Hyperdynamic or warm phase

- Peripheral vasodilation
- Skin possibly pink and flushed or warm and dry
- Altered level of consciousness (LOC) reflected in agitation, anxiety, irritability, and shortened attention span
- Respirations rapid and shallow
- Urine output below normal
- Rapid, full, bounding pulse
- Blood pressure normal or slightly elevated

Hypodynamic or cold phase

- Peripheral vasoconstriction and inadequate tissue perfusion
- Pale skin and possible cyanosis
- Decreased LOC; possible obtundation and coma
- Respirations possibly rapid and shallow
- Urine output possibly less than 25 ml/hour or absent
- Rapid, weak, thready pulse
- Irregular pulse if arrhythmias are present
- Cold, clammy skin
- Hypotension
- Crackles or rhonchi if pulmonary congestion is present

DIAGNOSTIC TEST RESULTS

LABORATORY

- Blood cultures are positive for the causative organism.
- Complete blood count shows the presence or absence of anemia and leukopenia, severe or absent neutropenia, and usually the presence of thrombocytopenia.
- Blood urea nitrogen and creatinine levels are increased, and creatinine clearance is decreased.
- Prothrombin time and partial thromboplastin time are abnormal.
- Serum lactate dehydrogenase levels are elevated, with metabolic acidosis.
- Urine studies show increased specific gravity (more than 1.02), increased osmolality, and decreased sodium levels.
- Arterial blood gas (ABG) analysis demonstrates increased blood pH and partial pressure of arterial oxygen and decreased partial pressure of arterial carbon dioxide with respiratory alkalosis in early stages.

DIAGNOSTIC PROCEDURES

- Invasive hemodynamic monitoring shows:
- – increased cardiac output and decreased systemic vascular resistance in warm phase
- – decreased cardiac output and increased systemic vascular resistance in cold phase.

TREATMENT

GENERAL
- Removal or replacement of I.V., intra-arterial, or urinary drainage catheters whenever possible
- In patients immunosuppressed from drug therapy, drugs discontinued or reduced, if possible
- Mechanical ventilation if respiratory failure occurs
- Fluid volume replacement

DIET
- Possible parenteral nutrition or tube feedings

ACTIVITY
- Bed rest

MEDICATIONS
- Antimicrobial
- Granulocyte transfusions
- Colloid or crystalloid infusions
- Oxygen
- Diuretics
- Vasopressors
- Antipyretics
- Drotrecogin alpha (Xigris)
- I.V. fluids

NURSING CONSIDERATIONS

NURSING DIAGNOSES
- Anxiety
- Decreased cardiac output
- Deficient fluid volume
- Disabled family coping
- Impaired gas exchange
- Ineffective tissue perfusion: Cardiopulmonary, renal
- Risk for imbalanced body temperature
- Risk for infection
- Risk for injury

EXPECTED OUTCOMES
The patient (or family) will:
- verbalize strategies to reduce anxiety
- maintain adequate cardiac output and hemodynamic stability
- maintain adequate fluid volume
- express feelings and develop adequate coping mechanisms
- maintain adequate ventilation and oxygenation
- maintain adequate cardiopulmonary and renal perfusion
- maintain a normal body temperature
- remain free from signs and symptoms of infection
- avoid complications or injury.

NURSING INTERVENTIONS
- Remove or replace I.V., intra-arterial, or urinary drainage catheters, and send them to the laboratory to culture for the presence of the causative organism.
- Give prescribed I.V. fluids and blood products.

  ⚡ **WARNING** *A progressive drop in blood pressure accompanied by a thready pulse usually signals inadequate cardiac output from reduced intravascular volume. Notify a practitioner immediately and increase the infusion rate.*
- Administer appropriate antimicrobial I.V. drugs.
- Notify a practitioner if urine output is less than 30 ml/hour.
- Administer prescribed oxygen.
- Provide emotional support to the patient and his family.
- Document the occurrence of a nosocomial infection, and report it to the infection control practitioner.

MONITORING
- ABG levels and pulse oximetry
- Intake and output
- Vital signs and peripheral pulses
- Hemodynamics
- Cardiac rhythm
- Heart and breath sounds

PATIENT TEACHING

GENERAL
Be sure to cover:
- the disorder, diagnosis, and treatment
- all procedures and their purpose (to ease the patient's anxiety)
- risks associated with blood transfusions
- all equipment and its purpose
- drugs and possible adverse effects
- possible complications.

RESOURCES
Organizations
American Heart Association: *www.americanheart.org*
National Heart, Lung, and Blood Institute: *www.nhlbi.nih.gov*

Selected references
Hernandez, G., et al. "Implementation of a Norepinephrine-based Protocol for Management of Septic Shock: A Pilot Feasibility Study," *Journal of Trauma* 60(1):77-81, January 2006.
Nettina, S.M. *Lippincott Manual of Nursing Practice*, 8th ed. Philadelphia: Lippincott Williams & Wilkins, 2006.
Rivers, E.P. "Early Goal-Directed Therapy in Severe Sepsis and Septic Shock: Converting Science to Reality," *Chest* 129(2):217-18, February 2006.
Sutherland, A.M., et al. "Are Vasopressin Levels Increased or Decreased in Septic Shock?" *Critical Care Medicine* 34(2):542-43, February 2006.

Silicosis

- Progressive pneumoconiosis disease characterized by nodular lesions, commonly leading to fibrosis
- Classified according to severity of pulmonary disease and rapidity of onset and progression
- Usually a simple illness that produces no symptoms
- Considered an industrial disease
- Prognosis good unless complications occur

PATHOPHYSIOLOGY

- Small particles of mineral dust are inhaled and deposited in the respiratory bronchioles, alveolar ducts, and alveoli.
- The surface of these particles generates silicon-based radicals that lead to the production of hydroxy, hydrogen peroxide, and other oxygen radicals that damage cell membranes and inactivate essential cell proteins.
- Alveolar macrophages ingest the particles, become activated, and release cytokines, such as tumor necrosis factor and others that attract other inflammatory cells.
- The inflammation damages resident cells and the extracellular matrix.
- Fibroblasts are stimulated to produce collagen, resulting in fibrosis.

CAUSES

- Silica dust due to:
- manufacture of ceramics (flint) and building materials (sandstone)
- mining of gold, lead, zinc, and iron
- mixed form in construction materials (cement)
- powder form (silica flour), in paints, porcelain, scouring soaps, and wood fillers.

RISK FACTORS

- Occupational exposure to silica dust

INCIDENCE

- The highest incidence of silicosis occurs in those who work around silica dust, such as foundry workers, boiler scalers, and stonecutters.

- Acute silicosis is possible after 1 to 3 years in sand blasters, tunnel workers, and others exposed to high levels of respirable silica.
- Accelerated silicosis is possible in those exposed to lower concentrations of free silica, usually after about 10 years of exposure.
- Silicosis is more common in those ages 40 to 75.
- Silicosis is more common in males than in females.

COMPLICATIONS

- Pulmonary fibrosis
- Cor pulmonale
- Cardiac or respiratory failure
- Pulmonary tuberculosis
- Lung infection
- Pneumothorax

HISTORY

- Long-term exposure to silica dust
- Dyspnea on exertion
- Dry cough, especially in the morning

PHYSICAL FINDINGS

- Decreased chest expansion
- Tachypnea
- Lethargy
- Decreased mentation
- Areas of increased and decreased resonance
- Medium crackles, wheezing
- Diminished breath sounds

⚡ **WARNING** *Assess patient for the presence of an intensified ventricular gallop on inspiration, which is a hallmark of cor pulmonale.*

- Hemoptysis

LABORATORY

- Arterial blood gas analysis shows:
- normal partial pressure of oxygen in simple silicosis (may be significantly decreased in late stages or complicated disease)
- normal partial pressure of carbon dioxide in early stages of the disease. (Hyperventilation may cause it to decrease; partial pressure of arterial carbon dioxide may increase if restrictive lung disease develops.)

IMAGING

- Chest X-rays in simple silicosis show small, discrete, nodular lesions distributed throughout both lung fields, although they typically concentrate in the upper lung.
- Lung nodes may appear enlarged and show eggshell calcification.
- Chest X-rays in complicated silicosis show one or more conglomerate masses of dense tissue.

DIAGNOSTIC PROCEDURES

- Pulmonary function tests show:
- reduced forced vital capacity (FVC) in complicated silicosis
- reduced forced expiratory volume in 1 second (FEV_1) with obstructive disease
- reduced FEV_1 with a normal or high ratio of FEV_1 to FVC in complicated silicosis
- reduced diffusing capacity for carbon monoxide when fibrosis destroys alveolar walls and obliterates pulmonary capillaries or when it thickens the alveolocapillary membrane.

TREATMENT

GENERAL
- Relief of respiratory symptoms
- Management of hypoxia and cor pulmonale
- Prevention of respiratory tract infections
- Steam inhalation and chest physiotherapy

DIET
- Increased fluid intake
- High-calorie, high-protein

ACTIVITY
- Regular exercise program, as tolerated

MEDICATIONS
- Bronchodilators
- Oxygen
- Antibiotics
- Anti-inflammatories

SURGERY
- Possible tracheostomy
- Possible lung transplantation
- Whole lung lavage

NURSING CONSIDERATIONS

NURSING DIAGNOSES
- Fatigue
- Imbalanced nutrition: Less than body requirements
- Impaired gas exchange
- Ineffective breathing pattern
- Interrupted family processes
- Risk for infection

EXPECTED OUTCOMES
The patient (or family) will:
- use energy-conservation techniques
- consume required daily caloric intake
- maintain adequate ventilation and oxygenation
- maintain a respiratory rate within 5 breaths/minute of baseline
- identify and contact available resources as needed
- verbalize the importance of complying with routine screenings for tuberculosis.

NURSING INTERVENTIONS
- Give prescribed drugs.
- Perform chest physiotherapy.
- Provide a high-calorie, high-protein diet.
- Provide small, frequent meals.
- Provide frequent mouth care.
- Ensure adequate hydration.
- Encourage daily exercise as tolerated.
- Provide diversional activities as appropriate.
- Provide frequent rest periods.
- Help with adjustment to the lifestyle changes associated with a chronic illness.
- Include the patient and family in care decisions whenever possible.

MONITORING
- Vital signs
- Intake and output
- Daily weight
- Respiratory status
- Activity tolerance
- Complications
- Changes in mentation
- Sputum production
- Breath sounds

PATIENT TEACHING

GENERAL
Be sure to cover:
- disorder, diagnosis, and treatment
- drugs and possible adverse effects
- when to notify a practitioner
- the need to avoid crowds and people with known infections
- home oxygen therapy, if needed
- transtracheal catheter care, if needed
- postural drainage, chest percussion
- coughing, deep-breathing exercises
- the need to consume a high-calorie, high-protein diet
- adequate hydration
- the risk of tuberculosis
- energy-conservation techniques.

DISCHARGE PLANNING
- Refer the patient for influenza and pneumococcus immunizations, as needed.
- Refer the patient to a smoking-cessation program, if indicated.

RESOURCES
Organizations
Mine Safety and Health Administration: *www.msha.gov*
National Institute for Occupational Safety and Health: *www.cdc.gov/niosh*
World Health Organization: *www.who.int*

Selected references
Collins, J.F., et al. "Development of a Chronic Inhalation Reference Level for Respirable Crystalline Silica," *Regulatory Toxicology and Pharmacology* 43(3):292-300, December 2005.
Lahiri, S., et al. "The Cost Effectiveness of Occupational Health Interventions: Prevention of Silicosis," *American Journal of Industrial Medicine* 48(6):503-14, December 2005.
McDonald, J.C., et al. "Mortality from Lung and Kidney Disease in a Cohort of North American Industrial Sand Workers: An Update," *Annals of Occupational Hygiene* 49(5):367-73, July 2005.
Rosenberg, B., et al. "Change in the World of Occupational Health: Silica Control, Then and Now," *Journal of Public Health Policy* 26(2):192-202, July 2005.

Sinusitis

OVERVIEW

- Inflammation of the paranasal sinuses
- Usually follows upper respiratory infections
- May be acute, subacute, chronic, allergic, or hyperplastic
- In hyperplastic sinusitis, a combination of purulent acute sinusitis and allergic sinusitis or rhinitis
- For all types, prognosis good

PATHOPHYSIOLOGY

- Impairment in drainage of sinuses and retention of secretions result in inflammation.

CAUSES

- Allergic rhinitis
- Any condition that interferes with sinus drainage and ventilation
- Bacterial infections (common)
- Blood dyscrasias
- Diabetes
- Endotracheal intubation
- Fungal infections (uncommon)
- Immunocompromised states
- Orofacial trauma
- Swimming in contaminated conditions
- Viral infections

RISK FACTORS

- Anatomic abnormalities
- Viral upper respiratory infection
- Allergies
- Overuse of topical decongestants
- Asthma

INCIDENCE

- Sinusitis affects 16% of population annually.
- It affects all ages.
- It affects both sexes equally.

COMPLICATIONS

- Meningitis
- Cavernous and sinus thrombosis
- Bacteremia or septicemia
- Brain abscess
- Osteomyelitis
- Mucocele
- Orbital cellulitis or abscess

ASSESSMENT

HISTORY

- Nasal congestion
- Nasal discharge, clear turning purulent
- Sore throat
- Localized headache
- Generalized malaise; fatigue
- Pain specific to the affected sinus (see *Locating the paranasal sinuses*)
- Vague facial discomfort
- Nonproductive cough

PHYSICAL FINDINGS

- Edematous nasal mucosa
- Low-grade fever
- Edema over sinuses
- Enlarged turbinates
- Mucosal lining thickening
- Mucosal polyps (hyperplastic sinusitis)
- Pain and pressure over affected sinus areas with palpation

DIAGNOSTIC TEST RESULTS

LABORATORY

- Culture and sensitivity testing of purulent nasal drainage shows the causative bacterial organism.

IMAGING

- Sinus X-rays show cloudiness in affected sinus, air-fluid levels, or thickened mucosal lining.
- Ultrasonography and computed tomography scans show recurrent or chronic sinusitis, unresolved sinusitis.

DIAGNOSTIC PROCEDURES

- Transillumination of sinuses may be diminished.
- Sinus endoscopy shows purulent nasal drainage, nasal edema, and obstruction of ostia.

Locating the paranasal sinuses

The location of a patient's sinusitis pain indicates the affected sinus. For example, an infected maxillary sinus can cause tooth pain. (*Note:* The sphenoid sinus, which lies under the eye and above the soft palate, isn't depicted here.)

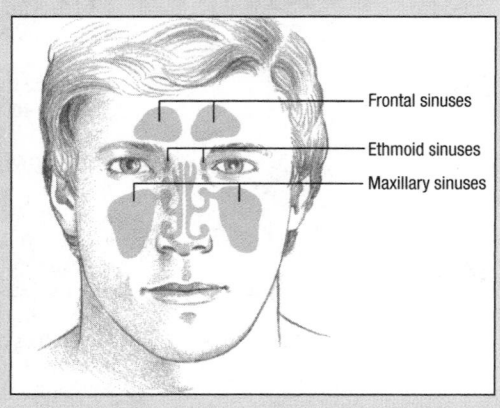

- Frontal sinuses
- Ethmoid sinuses
- Maxillary sinuses

GENERAL

- Based on type of sinusitis
- Indirect drainage of ethmoid and sphenoid sinuses
- Steam inhalation
- Local heat applications

ACTIVITY

- Adequate rest periods

MEDICATIONS

- Antibiotics
- Analgesics
- Vasoconstrictors
- Corticosteroids
- Antihistamines

SURGERY

- Antral puncture to remove purulent material
- Sinus irrigation

NURSING CONSIDERATIONS

NURSING DIAGNOSES

- Acute pain
- Anxiety
- Disturbed sensory perception (olfactory)
- Impaired oral mucous membrane
- Ineffective airway clearance
- Ineffective breathing pattern
- Risk for infection

EXPECTED OUTCOMES

The patient will:

- express feelings of increased comfort
- identify strategies to reduce anxiety
- regain a normal sense of smell
- experience healed oral mucous membranes without complications
- maintain a patent airway
- exhibit an effective breathing pattern
- remain free from signs and symptoms of infection.

NURSING INTERVENTIONS

- Encourage oral fluid intake.
- Elevate head of the bed no more than 30 degrees.
- Encourage expression of concerns.

- Apply warm compresses.
- Give prescribed drugs.
- Encourage use of humidifiers.

 WARNING *Watch for and report vomiting, chills, fever, edema of the forehead or eyelids, blurred or double vision, and personality changes.*

After surgery

- Place the patient in semi-Fowler's position.
- Apply ice compresses over the nose and iced saline gauze over the eyes for 24 hours.
- Frequently change the mustache dressing or drip pad.
- Provide meticulous and frequent mouth care.

MONITORING

- Complications
- Response to treatment
- Pain control
- Nasal discharge

After surgery

- Excessive drainage or bleeding
- Consistency, amount, and color of drainage
- Vital signs

GENERAL

Be sure to cover:

- the disorder, diagnosis, and treatment
- prescribed drugs
- potential adverse reactions
- cautions against driving a motor vehicle or consuming alcohol while taking antihistamines or analgesics
- the need to complete the full course of prescribed antibiotics
- the need to leave nasal packing in place for 12 to 24 hours after surgery
- the need to breathe through the mouth and refrain from blowing the nose and sneezing
- the need to refrain from smoking for at least 2 or 3 days after surgery
- signs and symptoms of complications
- importance of medical follow-up
- proper hand-washing technique
- avoidance of bending and stooping during the acute phase
- avoidance of contact with an infected person.

RESOURCES

Organizations

American Academy of Allergy, Asthma & Immunology: *www.aaaai.org*

Asthma and Allergy Foundation of America: *www.aafa.org*

Selected references

Costa Carvalho, B.T., et al. "Immunological Evaluation of Allergic Respiratory Children with Recurrent Sinusitis," *Pediatric Allergy & Immunology* 16(6):534-38, September 2005.

Landsberg, R., et al. "A Targeted Endoscopic Approach to Chronic Isolated Frontal Sinusitis," *Otolarygology – Head and Neck Surgery* 134(1):28-32, January 2006.

Slavin, R.G., et al. "The Diagnosis and Management of Sinusitis: A Practice Parameter Update," *Journal of Allergy and Clinical Immunology* 116(6 Suppl):S13-47, December 2005.

Stein M., and Caplan, E.S. "Nosocomial Sinusitis: A Unique Subset of Sinusitis," *Current Opinion in Internal Medicine* 4(3):239-42, June 2005.

Sjögren's syndrome

OVERVIEW

- Connective tissue disease that's the most common autoimmune disorder after rheumatoid arthritis
- May be primary disorder or associated with other inflammatory connective tissue disorders

PATHOPHYSIOLOGY

- Lymphocytic infiltration of exocrine glands causes tissue damage resulting in xerostomia and dry eyes.
- Immunologic system is activated.

CAUSES

- Exact cause unknown
- Immunologic activation
- Possible genetic and environmental factors

INCIDENCE

- Sjögren's syndrome affects more women (about 90%) than men.
- The mean age of onset is 50.

COMPLICATIONS

- Corneal ulceration or perforation
- Epistaxis
- Deafness
- Otitis media
- Splenomegaly
- Renal tubular necrosis

ASSESSMENT

HISTORY

- Xerophthalmia or xerostomia
- Gritty, sandy eye along with redness, burning, photosensitivity, eye fatigue, itching, and mucoid discharge
- Difficulty swallowing and talking; an abnormal taste or smell sensation (or both); thirst; ulcers of the tongue, mouth, and lips (especially at the corners of the mouth); and severe dental caries
- Possible epistaxis, hoarseness, chronic nonproductive cough, recurrent otitis media, and frequent respiratory tract infections
- Possible dyspareunia
- Generalized itching, fatigue, recurrent low-grade fever, and arthralgia or myalgia

PHYSICAL FINDINGS

- Mouth ulcers, dental caries and, possibly, enlarged salivary glands
- Palpable purpura
- Palpable lymph node enlargement
- Dry, sticky, erythematous oral mucosa

DIAGNOSTIC TEST RESULTS

LABORATORY

- Erythrocyte sedimentation rate is elevated in more than 90% of patients.
- Complete blood count shows mild anemia and leukopenia in about 30% of patients.
- Serum protein electrophoresis shows hypergammaglobulinemia in about 50% of patients.
- Typically, 75% to 90% of patients test positive for rheumatoid factor, and between 50% and 80% of patients test positive for antinuclear antibodies.

DIAGNOSTIC PROCEDURES

- For a diagnosis of Sjögren's syndrome, symptoms must meet specific criteria. (See *Diagnosing Sjögren's syndrome.*)
- Tests supporting the diagnosis include measuring eye involvement with the Schirmer's test and a slit-lamp examination with rose bengal dye.
- Labial biopsy (to detect lymphoid foci), a simple procedure with minimal risk, is the only specific diagnostic technique.
- Salivary gland involvement may be evaluated by measuring the volume of parotid saliva, by secretory sialography, and by salivary scintigraphy.
- Salivary gland biopsy results typically show lymphocytic infiltration in Sjögren's syndrome; lower lip biopsy findings show salivary gland infiltration by lymphocytes.

Diagnosing Sjögren's syndrome

For a diagnosis of Sjögren's syndrome, the patient must have:

- keratoconjunctivitis sicca
- diminished salivary gland flow
- a positive salivary gland biopsy, showing mononuclear cell infiltration
- the presence of autoantibodies in a serum sample, indicating a systemic autoimmune process.

TREATMENT

GENERAL
◆ Meticulous oral hygiene
◆ Humidifier
◆ Unscented skin lotions
◆ Frequent dental care

DIET
◆ Avoidance of sugar, tobacco, alcohol, and spicy, salty, or highly acidic foods
◆ Increased oral fluid intake for mouth dryness

MEDICATIONS
◆ Pilocarpine and cevimeline
◆ Preservative-free artificial tears and sustained-release cellulose capsules
◆ Artificial saliva
◆ Glucocorticoids or other immuno-suppressives for extraglandular manifestations such as systemic vasculitis
◆ Saline nasal sprays
◆ Vaginal lubricants
◆ Nonsteroidal anti-inflammatory drugs
◆ Antifungals
◆ Ophthalmic lubricants
◆ Cyclosporin eyedrops (Restasis)
◆ Antimalarial such as hydroxychloroquine (Plaquenil)

NURSING CONSIDERATIONS

NURSING DIAGNOSES
◆ Acute pain
◆ Disturbed body image
◆ Disturbed sensory perception (visual)
◆ Fatigue
◆ Impaired oral mucous membrane
◆ Impaired skin integrity
◆ Impaired swallowing
◆ Impaired tissue integrity
◆ Ineffective sexuality patterns
◆ Ineffective therapeutic regimen management
◆ Risk for deficient fluid volume
◆ Risk for infection
◆ Risk for injury
◆ Sexual dysfunction

EXPECTED OUTCOMES
The patient will:
◆ express feelings of increased comfort
◆ verbalize feelings regarding a change in body image
◆ maintain optimal functioning within the limits of the vision impairment
◆ express feelings of increased energy
◆ have pink and moist oral mucosa
◆ exhibit improved or healed wounds or lesions
◆ exhibit no signs of aspiration
◆ experience reduced redness, swelling, and pain at the site of impaired tissue
◆ express feelings related to altered sexuality patterns
◆ demonstrate good oral hygiene practices
◆ maintain adequate fluid balance
◆ remain free from signs and symptoms of infection
◆ avoid complications
◆ acknowledge problems in sexual function.

NURSING INTERVENTIONS
◆ Instill artificial tears as often as every 30 minutes to prevent eye damage, and instill an eye ointment at bedtime.
◆ Provide plenty of fluids, especially water, for the patient to drink, and sugarless chewing gum or candy.

MONITORING
◆ Response to treatment
◆ Extraglandular manifestations
◆ Complications

PATIENT TEACHING

GENERAL
Be sure to cover:
◆ disorder, diagnosis, and treatment
◆ instilling eyedrops and ointments
◆ need for sunglasses to protect eyes
◆ need to keep the face clean and to avoid rubbing the eyes
◆ avoidance of saliva-decreasing drugs, such as atropine derivatives, antihistamines, anticholinergics, and antidepressants
◆ meticulous oral hygiene and regular dental visits
◆ high-calorie, protein-rich liquid supplements to prevent malnutrition if mouth lesions make eating painful
◆ the need for a nutritious diet
◆ avoidance of sugar, tobacco, alcohol, and spicy, salty, or highly acidic foods
◆ the need to humidify the home and work environments
◆ use of normal saline solution to relieve nasal dryness
◆ avoidance of prolonged hot showers and baths and the use of moisturizing lotions on dry skin.

RESOURCES
Organizations
American College of Rheumatology: *www.rheumatology.org*
Arthritis Foundation: *www.arthritis.org*
Sjögren's Syndrome Foundation: *www.sjogrens.org*
National Institute of Neurological Disorders and Stroke: *www.ninds.nih.gov*

Selected references
Hansen, A., et al. "Immunopathogenesis of Primary Sjögren's Syndrome: Implications for Disease Management and Therapy," *Current Opinion in Rheumatology* 17(5):558-65, September 2005.
Larche, M.J. "A Short Review of the Pathogenesis of Sjögren's Syndrome," *Autoimmunity Reviews* 5(2):132-35, February 2006.
Ohlsson, V., et al. "Renal Tubular Necrosis, Arthritis and Autoantibodies: Primary Sjögren's Syndrome in Childhood," *Rheumatology* 45(2):238-40, February 2006.

Skull fracture

- Break in the integrity of the skull bone
- May be simple (closed) or compound (open)
- May displace bone fragments
- May be linear (common hairline break, without displacement of structures), comminuted (splintering or crushing the bone into several fragments), or depressed (a fracture that pushes the bone toward the brain)

⚡ **WARNING** *Because possible damage to the brain is the first concern, rather than the fracture itself, a skull fracture is considered a neurosurgical condition.*

- Classified according to location, such as cranial vault fracture and basilar fractures

⚡ **WARNING** *Because of the danger of grave cranial complications and meningitis, basilar fractures are usually far more serious than vault fractures.*

PATHOPHYSIOLOGY

- Trauma to the head causes a fracture at certain anatomic sites:
- parietal bone
- squama of temporal bone
- foramen magnum
- petrous temporal ridge
- inner parts of the sphenoid wings at the skull base
- middle cranial fossa
- cribriform plate
- roof of orbits in the anterior cranial fossa
- bony areas between the mastoid and dural sinuses in the posterior cranial fossa

CAUSES

- Head trauma

RISK FACTORS

- Participation in contact sports
- Reckless behavior
- Involvement in an abusive relationship
- Young age

INCIDENCE

- A simple linear skull fracture is the most common type, especially in children younger than age 5.
- A skull fracture may occur at any age.

COMPLICATIONS

- Epilepsy
- Hydrocephalus
- Organic brain syndrome
- Headaches, giddiness, fatigability, neuroses, and behavior disorders
- Respiratory failure

ASSESSMENT

HISTORY

- Head trauma
- Headache
- Loss of consciousness

PHYSICAL FINDINGS

- Decreased pulse and respirations
- Altered level of consciousness (LOC)
- Scalp wound
- Bleeding in the periorbital area, nose, pharynx, ears, or under the conjunctivae
- Cerebrospinal fluid (CSF) leakage from the nose or ears; halo sign on pillowcase (a blood-tinged spot surrounded by a lighter ring)

DIAGNOSTIC TEST RESULTS

LABORATORY

- Reagent strips turn blue if CSF is present.

IMAGING

- Computed tomography scan and magnetic resonance imaging show fracture, intracranial hemorrhage from ruptured blood vessels, and swelling.

TREATMENT

GENERAL
◆ Based on type and severity of fracture
◆ Supportive
◆ Cleaning and debridement of wounds

DIET
◆ As tolerated; nothing by mouth if surgery needed

ACTIVITY
◆ Limited, based on severity of fracture

MEDICATIONS
◆ Mild analgesics
◆ Prophylactic antibiotics
◆ Dexamethasone (basilar and vault fractures)

⚡ **WARNING** *Don't give the patient opioids or sedatives because they may depress respirations, increase carbon dioxide levels, lead to increased intracranial pressure, and mask changes in neurologic status.*

SURGERY
◆ Craniotomy to elevate or remove fragments that have been driven into the brain and to extract foreign bodies and necrotic tissue, thereby reducing the risk of infection and further brain damage (severe injury)

NURSING CONSIDERATIONS

NURSING DIAGNOSES
◆ Acute pain
◆ Anxiety
◆ Decreased intracranial adaptive capacity
◆ Disturbed sensory perception (visual)
◆ Imbalanced nutrition: Less than body requirements
◆ Impaired skin integrity
◆ Ineffective breathing pattern
◆ Ineffective coping
◆ Risk for infection
◆ Risk for injury
◆ Risk for posttrauma syndrome

EXPECTED OUTCOMES
The patient will:
◆ express increased comfort and decreased pain
◆ express feelings of decreased anxiety
◆ maintain a stable neurologic state
◆ achieve optimal visual functioning within the limits of the vision impairment
◆ maintain adequate nutritional intake orally or through I.V. fluids
◆ experience wound healing without complications
◆ maintain an effective breathing pattern
◆ develop adequate coping mechanisms and support systems
◆ exhibit no signs or symptoms of infection
◆ remain free from further injury
◆ relate fears and feelings related to traumatic event.

NURSING INTERVENTIONS
◆ Establish and maintain a patent airway.

⚡ **WARNING** *Nasal airways are contraindicated in patients with possible basilar skull fractures. Intubation may be necessary.*

◆ Suction through the mouth, not the nose, to prevent the introduction of bacteria.
◆ Position the patient with a head injury for proper secretion drainage. Elevate the head of the bed 30 degrees if intracerebral injury is suspected.
◆ Apply appropriate dressings; control bleeding as necessary.
◆ Institute seizure precautions.

MONITORING
◆ Vital signs
◆ Neurologic status
◆ Comfort level

PATIENT TEACHING

GENERAL
Be sure to cover:
◆ preoperative and postoperative care, if appropriate
◆ need to watch closely for changes in mental status, LOC, or respirations
◆ use of mild analgesics as opposed to opioids
◆ wound care.

RESOURCES
Organizations
American Academy of Neurology: *www.aan.com*
American Academy of Orthopaedic Surgeons: *www.aaos.org*
American Orthopaedic Association: *www.aoassn.org*

Selected references
Dijkstra, P.U., et al. "Function Impairment and Pain after Closed Treatment of Fractures of the Mandibular Condyle," *Journal of Trauma* 59(2):424-30, August 2005.
Holsti, M., et al. "Pediatric Closed Head Injuries Treated in an Observation Unit," *Pediatric Emergency Care* 21(10):639-44, October 2005.
Hung, K.L., et al. "Rational Management of Simple Depressed Skull Fractures in Infants," *Journal of Neurosurgery* 103(1 Suppl):69-72, July 2005.
Kienstra, M.A., and Van Loveren, H. "Anterior Skull Base Fractures," *Facial Plastic Surgery* 21(3):180-86, August 2005.

Smallpox LIFE-THREATENING DISORDER

OVERVIEW

- Acute, highly contagious infectious disease caused by *Poxvirus variola*
- Associated with tremendous morbidity and mortality
- Two related viruses:
- Variola major (classic smallpox), with a case mortality rate of 20% to 50%
- Variola minor (alastrim), a clinically milder form with mortality less than 1%
- Eliminated worldwide in 1980 (World Health Organization declaration) as a result of a global vaccination and eradication program; routine smallpox vaccination stopped; variola virus, preserved in two research laboratories, remains unlikely but potential source of infection (humans' sole reservoir of infection; no carrier state)
- Potential for use in bioterrorism and biological warfare; classified as category A biological disease, transmitted human to human with no known treatment
- Also known as *variola*

PATHOPHYSIOLOGY

- Poxviruses are characterized by a large double-stranded deoxyribonucleic acid (DNA) genome and a brick-shaped morphology.
- Poxviruses are the only DNA viruses that replicate in cytoplasm.
- The virus is spread through direct contact or inhalation of respiratory droplets.
- The incubation period is 7 to 19 days. Illness onset is in 10 to 14 days, with onset of the characteristic rash in 2 to 4 days. Fever and macular rash appear after an average incubation period of 12 days, with a progression to typical vesicular and pustular lesions over 1 or 2 weeks.
- It's most contagious during the first week of illness (before the eruptive period) and during the time between lesion development and scab disappearance.

CAUSES

- *Poxvirus variola*

RISK FACTORS

- Lack of immunization with exposure to active virus

INCIDENCE

- The last known case of smallpox in the United States was in 1949.
- The last case of endemic smallpox was in Africa in 1977.
- The disease affects people of all ages.
- In temperate zones, the incidence of smallpox was highest in the winter.
- In tropical zones, the incidence was highest during hot, dry months.

COMPLICATIONS

- Secondary bacterial infections
- Encephalitis
- Bleeding abnormalities
- Blindness
- Death

ASSESSMENT

HISTORY

- Influenza-type symptoms
- High fever, chills
- Rash
- Malaise
- Headache, backache
- Abdominal pain
- Nausea, vomiting

PHYSICAL FINDINGS

- After average incubation period of 12 days:
- Fever
- Macular rash
- Progression to typical vesicular and pustular lesions, and then crusted scabs
- Centrifugal distribution to rash; starts on the face and extremities; moves to the trunk

DIAGNOSTIC TEST RESULTS

LABORATORY

- Culture of aspirate from vesicles and pustules shows presence of variola.
- Electron microscopy of vesicular scrapings shows presence of variola.

TREATMENT

GENERAL
- Home treatment if possible to reduce spread
- No current treatment other than supportive
- Strict isolation

DIET
- As tolerated

ACTIVITY
- As tolerated

MEDICATIONS
- Antibiotics
- Antipruritics
- Antihistamines
- Analgesics
- I.V. fluids

NURSING CONSIDERATIONS

NURSING DIAGNOSES
- Acute pain
- Anxiety
- Disturbed body image
- Hyperthermia
- Imbalanced nutrition: Less than body requirements
- Impaired skin integrity
- Ineffective coping

EXPECTED OUTCOMES
The patient will:
- express feelings of comfort and relief from pain
- verbalize feelings of fear and anxiety
- verbalize positive feelings regarding self and body image
- remain afebrile
- maintain adequate nutrition and hydration
- exhibit healed or improved lesions or wounds
- demonstrate effective coping mechanisms.

NURSING INTERVENTIONS
- Give prescribed drugs.
- Report any case of smallpox to the appropriate public health office.
- Institute strict exposure precautions, including isolation and airborne, contact, and standard precautions.
- Autoclave laundry and hospital waste before laundering or incinerating.
- Provide meticulous skin care.
- Encourage verbalization of fears and concerns.
- Provide adequate hydration.
- Provide a well-balanced diet.
- Assist in the development of effective coping mechanisms.
- Provide adequate rest periods.

MONITORING
- Vital signs
- Intake and output
- Complications
- Fluid and electrolyte status
- Signs and symptoms of secondary bacterial infection

PATIENT TEACHING

GENERAL
Be sure to cover:
- disorder, diagnosis, and treatment
- drugs and possible adverse effects
- when to notify the practitioner
- isolation precautions
- hydration
- skin lesion care.

DISCHARGE PLANNING
- Refer those in direct contact with an infected person for pre-exposure and postexposure vaccination if more than 3 years have passed since last vaccination.

RESOURCES
Organizations
National Center for Infectious Diseases: *www.cdc.gov/ncidod*
United States Department of Health & Human Services: *www.hhs.gov*
World Health Organization: *www.who.int*

Selected references
Beasley, A., et al. "Treating Patients with Smallpox in the Operating Room," *AORN Journal* 80(4):681-85, 688-89, October 2004.

Jahrling, P.B., et al. "Countermeasures to the Bioterrorist Threat of Smallpox," *Current Molecular Medicine* 5(8):817-26, December 2005.

Mack, K. "Oncology Nursing Implications Related to Smallpox Bioterrorism Preparations," *Clinical Journal of Oncology Nursing* 8(1):51-55, February 2004.

Milgrom, H., et al. "Smallpox Vaccination: A Conundrum of Risks and Outcomes," *Current Opinion in Allergy & Clinical Immunology* 5(3):207-209, June 2005.

Moore, Z.S., et al. "Smallpox," *Lancet* 367(9508):425-35, February 2006.

Murphy, F.A., and Osburn, B.I. "Adventitious Agents and Smallpox Vaccine in Strategic National Stockpile," *Emerging Infectious Diseases* 11(7):1086-1089, July 2005.

Seguin, D., and Stoner, H.J. "Triage of a Febrile Patient with a Rash: A Comparison of Chickenpox, Monkeypox, and Smallpox," *Disaster Management & Response* 2(3):81-86, July-September 2004.

Spinal injury

- Fractures, contusions, dislocations, or compressions of the spine
- Most common sites: C5, C6, C7, T12, and L1 vertebrae

PATHOPHYSIOLOGY

- Injury causes microscopic hemorrhages.
- All of the gray matter is filled with blood.
- Necrosis results.
- Edema causes spinal cord compression.
- Blood supply is further decreased.
- Long-term scarring and meningeal thickening occur.
- Nerves are blocked or tangled.
- Sensory and motor deficits occur.

CAUSES

- Trauma to the spine

RISK FACTORS

- Diving into shallow water
- Fall
- Gunshot and related wound
- Motor vehicle accident
- Improper lifting of heavy object
- Neoplastic lesion
- Osteoporosis

INCIDENCE

- Spinal injury is most common between ages 15 and 35.

COMPLICATIONS

- Paralysis
- Death
- Autonomic dysreflexia
- Spinal shock
- Neurogenic shock

HISTORY

- Muscle spasm
- Back or neck pain
- In cervical fractures, point tenderness
- Predisposing risk factors

PHYSICAL FINDINGS

- Level of injury and any spinal cord damage located by neurologic assessment
- Limited movement and activities that cause pain
- Surface wounds
- Pain location
- Loss of sensation below the level of injury
- Deformity

IMAGING

- Spinal X-rays, myelography, computed tomography scans, and magnetic resonance imaging can indicate the location of the fracture and the site of the compression.

GENERAL

- Stabilization of spine and prevention of cord damage
- Hemodynamic support
- Application of a hard cervical collar
- Wound care (if appropriate)
- Chemotherapy and radiation for neoplastic lesion
- Aspiration precautions
- Skeletal traction with skull tongs
- Rotation bed with cervical traction (if appropriate)
- Splinting: thoracic lumbar sacral orthotics
- Intubation and mechanical ventilation, if indicated

ACTIVITY

- Bed rest on a firm surface
- Physical therapy, as appropriate

MEDICATIONS

- Corticosteroids
- Analgesics
- Muscle relaxants
- Chemotherapy for neoplastic lesion
- Oxygen therapy

SURGERY

- Decompression of spinal cord
- Stabilization of spinal column

NURSING DIAGNOSES
- Acute pain
- Anxiety
- Autonomic dysreflexia
- Deficient diversional activity
- Deficient fluid volume
- Disturbed body image
- Dressing or grooming self-care deficit
- Hopelessness
- Impaired physical mobility
- Ineffective airway clearance
- Ineffective breathing pattern
- Ineffective coping
- Risk for aspiration
- Risk for disuse syndrome
- Risk for impaired skin integrity
- Risk for infection
- Risk for posttrauma syndrome

EXPECTED OUTCOMES
The patient will:
- express feelings of increased comfort and decreased pain
- express feelings of decreased anxiety
- show no signs or symptoms of autonomic dysreflexia
- participate in interests and activities unrelated to the illness or confinement
- maintain adequate fluid volume
- express positive feelings about self
- participate in self-care activities at the highest level possible within the confines of the injury
- recognize choices and alternatives and make decisions on own behalf
- attain the highest degree of mobility possible within the confines of the injury
- maintain a patent airway
- maintain adequate ventilation and oxygenation
- develop effective coping mechanisms
- show no signs of aspiration
- maintain muscle strength and joint range of motion to the highest degree possible within the confines of the injury
- maintain skin integrity with no signs or symptoms of breakdown

- show no signs or symptoms of infection
- express feelings and fears about the traumatic event.

NURSING INTERVENTIONS
- Apply a hard cervical collar.
- Immobilize the patient.
- Perform ROM exercises of the extremities, as appropriate.
- Comfort and reassure the patient.
- Give prescribed drugs.
- Provide wound care, if appropriate.
- Provide diversionary activities.
- Provide proper skin care.

MONITORING
- Neurologic changes
- Respiratory status
- Changes in skin sensation and loss of muscle strength
- Skin integrity
- Hydration and nutritional status
- Pain control

GENERAL
Be sure to cover:
- the disorder, diagnosis, and treatment
- traction methods used
- exercises to maintain physical mobility
- drug administration, dosage, and possible adverse effects
- the prescribed home care regimen
- the importance of follow-up examinations.

DISCHARGE PLANNING
- Refer the patient to the appropriate rehabilitation center.
- Refer the patient to resource and support services.

RESOURCES
Organizations
American Academy of Neurology: *www.aan.com*
American Spinal Injury Association: *www.asia-spinalinjury.org*
Christopher Reeve Foundation: *www.christopherreeve.org*
National Spinal Cord Injury Association: *www.spinalcord.org*

Selected references
Atlas of Pathophysiology, 2nd ed. Philadelphia: Lippincott Williams & Wilkins, 2005.

Cotton, B.A., et al. "Respiratory Complications and Mortality Risk Associated with Thoracic Spine Injury," *Journal of Trauma* 59(6):1400-407, December 2005.

Hayes, J.S., and Arriola, T. "Pediatric Spinal Injuries," *Pediatric Nursing* 31(6):464-67, November-December 2005.

Lemke, D.M. "Vertebroplasty and Kyphoplasty for Treatment of Painful Osteoporotic Compression Fractures," *Journal of the American Academy of Nurse Practitioners* 17(7):268-76, July 2005.

Wilson, J.B., et al. "Spinal Injuries in Contact Sports," *Current Sports Medicine Reports* 5(1):50-55, February 2006.

Sprains and strains

OVERVIEW

- Sprain — complete or incomplete tear in supporting ligaments surrounding a joint caused by a twisting or wrenching motion
- Strain — acute or chronic injury to a muscle or tendinous attachment caused by stress, overuse, or overstretching
- Classified as mild, moderate, or severe (see *Classifying sprains and strains*)

PATHOPHYSIOLOGY

Sprain
- A ligament tear causes bleeding.
- A hematoma forms.
- Inflammatory exudates follow.
- Granulation tissue develops.
- Collagen forms.
- Swelling or stretching of nerves or vessels occurs.
- Persistent laxity and chronic joint instability result.

Strain
- Strains result from the same process as sprains.
- New tendon or muscle eventually becomes strong enough to withstand normal muscle strain.

CAUSES
- Excessive or new exercise
- Fall
- Motor vehicle accident
- Sport injury
- Trauma

RISK FACTORS
- Participation in sports
- Strenuous exercise

INCIDENCE
- Sprains and strains are more common in athletes (occurs in 80% of athletes).
- These disorders are more common in men than in women.

COMPLICATIONS

Sprain
- Avulsion fracture

Strain
- Complete rupture of muscle tendon unit
- Deep vein thrombosis

ASSESSMENT

HISTORY
- Physical activity
- Similar past injury
- Systemic disease with high risk factors
- Local pain that worsens during joint movement
- Loss of mobility
- Sharp, transient pain and rapid swelling
- Stiffness, soreness, and generalized tenderness

PHYSICAL FINDINGS
- Ecchymosis
- Swelling
- Point tenderness

DIAGNOSTIC TEST RESULTS

IMAGING
- X-ray results are used to rule out fractures and confirm damage to ligaments.

Classifying sprains and strains

The guide below will help you classify the severity of sprains and strains.

SPRAINS
- Grade 1 (mild): minor or partial ligament tear with normal joint stability and function
- Grade 2 (moderate): partial tear with mild joint laxity and some function loss
- Grade 3 (severe): complete tear or incomplete separation of ligament from bone, causing total joint laxity and function loss

STRAINS
- Grade 1 (mild): microscopic muscle or tendon tear (or both) with no loss of strength
- Grade 2 (moderate): incomplete tear with bleeding into muscle tissue and some loss of strength
- Grade 3 (severe): complete rupture, usually resulting from separation of muscle from muscle, muscle from tendon, or tendon from bone (usually stems from sudden, violent movement or direct injury)

GENERAL

◆ RICE — *rest, ice,* compression (wrapping in an elastic bandage), and *ele*vation of affected area

DIET

◆ Nothing by mouth if surgery scheduled

ACTIVITY

◆ Rehabilitation or exercise program
◆ Limited activity and weight bearing to injured area, based on extent of injury
◆ Elevation of affected joint above the level of the heart for 48 to 72 hours
◆ Range-of-motion (ROM) exercises

MEDICATIONS

◆ Vitamin C supplements
◆ Nonsteroidal anti-inflammatory drugs
◆ Analgesics
◆ Cox-2 inhibitors

SURGERY

◆ Based on extent of injury

NURSING DIAGNOSES

◆ Acute pain
◆ Impaired physical mobility
◆ Risk for injury

EXPECTED OUTCOMES

The patient will:
◆ express feelings of increased comfort and decreased pain
◆ attain the highest possible level of mobility
◆ identify factors that increase the potential for injury.

NURSING INTERVENTIONS

◆ Apply ice intermittently.
◆ Apply an elastic bandage or air cast.
◆ Give prescribed drugs.
◆ Elevate the extremity.

MONITORING

◆ Edema
◆ Response to treatment
◆ Pain control
◆ Complications
◆ Adverse effects of drugs
◆ ROM

GENERAL

Be sure to cover:
◆ the disorder, diagnosis, and treatment
◆ how to apply ice intermittently for the first 12 to 48 hours
◆ how to reapply elastic bandage or air cast
◆ crutch gait training
◆ avoidance of further injury to the joint
◆ drug administration, dosage, and possible adverse effects.

RESOURCES

Organizations

American Academy of Orthopaedic Surgeons: *www.aaos.org*
American Orthopaedic Society for Sports Medicine: *www.sportsmed.org*
National Institute of Arthritis and Musculoskeletal and Skin Diseases: *www.nih.gov/niams/healthinfo*

Selected references

Atlas of Pathophysiology, 2nd ed. Philadelphia: Lippincott Williams & Wilkins, 2005.
Crites, B.M. "Ankle Sprains," *Current Opinion in Orthopedics* 16(2):117-19, April 2005.
Paget S.A., et al. *Hospital for Special Surgery Manual of Rheumatology and Outpatient Orthopedic Disorders,* 5th ed. Philadelphia: Lippincott Williams & Wilkins, 2006.
Willems, T.M., et al. "Intrinsic Risk Factors for Inversion Ankle Sprains in Females—A Prospective Study," *Scandinavian Journal of Medicine & Science in Sports* 15(5):336-45, October 2005.

Spurious polycythemia

- Blood disorder characterized by an increased hematocrit and a normal or low red blood cell (RBC) total mass
- Results from diminished plasma volume and subsequent hemoconcentration
- Also known as *relative polycythemia, stress erythrocytosis, stress polycythemia, benign polycythemia, Gaisböck's disease,* or *pseudopolycythemia*

PATHOPHYSIOLOGY

- Conditions that promote severe fluid loss decrease plasma volume and lead to hemoconcentration.
- Nervous stress causes hemoconcentration by an unknown mechanism. This form of erythrocytosis (chronically elevated hematocrit) is particularly common in the middle-aged man who is a chronic smoker and has a type A personality (tense, hard-driving, and anxious).
- In many patients, an increased hematocrit merely reflects a normally high RBC mass and low plasma volume. This is particularly common in patients who don't smoke, aren't obese, and have no history of hypertension.

CAUSES

- Dehydration
- Hemoconcentration from stress
- High-normal RBC mass and low-normal plasma volume
- Hypertension
- Thromboembolic disease
- Elevated serum cholesterol and uric acid
- Familial tendency
- Pregnancy

INCIDENCE

- Spurious polycythemia usually affects middle-age people.
- This disorder is more common in men than in women.

COMPLICATIONS

- Thromboemboli

HISTORY

- Headaches
- Dizziness
- Cardiac or pulmonary disease
- Fatigue
- Diaphoresis
- Dyspnea
- Claudication

PHYSICAL FINDINGS

- Ruddy appearance
- Short neck
- Hepatosplenomegaly
- Slight hypertension
- Hypoventilation when recumbent

LABORATORY

- Hemoglobin level and hematocrit are increased.
- RBC count is increased.
- RBC mass is normal or decreased.
- Arterial oxygen saturation is normal.
- Bone marrow is normal.
- Plasma volume is decreased or normal.
- Hyperlipidemia may be present.
- Uricosuria may be present.

TREATMENT

GENERAL
◆ Appropriate fluids and electrolytes to correct dehydration

DIET
◆ Cessation of dietary diuretics such as caffeine
◆ Low-cholesterol, low-fat
◆ Adequate hydration

ACTIVITY
◆ Adequate exercise

MEDICATIONS
◆ Antidiarrheals, if needed
◆ I.V. fluids

NURSING CONSIDERATIONS

NURSING DIAGNOSES
◆ Activity intolerance
◆ Acute pain
◆ Anxiety
◆ Deficient fluid volume
◆ Fatigue
◆ Impaired gas exchange
◆ Ineffective breathing pattern
◆ Ineffective tissue perfusion: Peripheral

EXPECTED OUTCOMES
The patient will:
◆ verbalize the importance of balancing activity, as tolerated, with rest
◆ express feelings of increased comfort and decreased pain
◆ verbalize measures to reduce anxiety
◆ maintain normal fluid volume
◆ express feelings of increased energy
◆ exhibit adequate ventilation and oxygenation
◆ maintain a respiratory rate within 5 breaths of baseline
◆ maintain adequate peripheral perfusion, as evidenced by palpable pulses and warm extremities.

NURSING INTERVENTIONS
◆ Give prescribed I.V. fluids.
◆ Encourage adequate fluid intake.
◆ Encourage activity.
◆ Provide emotional support.
◆ Provide dietary counseling, if appropriate.

MONITORING
◆ Intake and output
◆ Blood studies
◆ Response to treatment

PATIENT TEACHING

GENERAL
Be sure to cover:
◆ the disorder, diagnosis, and treatment
◆ changing the patient's work habits, if appropriate
◆ the need for proper relaxation
◆ dietary restrictions
◆ importance of proper hydration
◆ recognizing and reporting of signs and symptoms of increasing polycythemia and thromboembolism.

DISCHARGE PLANNING
◆ Refer the patient to a smoking-cessation program, if necessary.
◆ Emphasize the need for follow-up examinations every 3 to 4 months after leaving the hospital.

RESOURCES
Organizations
National Heart, Lung, and Blood Institute: *www.nhlbi.nih.gov*
National Library of Medicine: *www.nlm.nih.gov*

Selected references
Diseases, 4th ed. Philadelphia: Lippincott Williams & Wilkins, 2006.
Sevastos, N., et al. "Pseudohyperkalemia in Patients with Increased Cellular Components of Blood," *American Journal of the Medical Sciences* 331(7):17-21, January 2006.
Sirhan, S., et al. "Red Cell Mass and Plasma Volume Measurements in Polycythemia: Evaluation of Performance and Practical Utility," *Cancer* 104(1): 213-15, July 2005.

Squamous cell carcinoma

◆ Invasive tumor arising from keratinizing epidermal cells

PATHOPHYSIOLOGY

◆ Transformation from a premalignant lesion to squamous cell carcinoma may begin with induration and inflammation of an existing lesion.
◆ When squamous cell carcinoma arises from normal skin, the nodule grows slowly on a firm, indurated base. If untreated, this nodule eventually ulcerates and invades underlying tissues. (See *Squamous cell carcinoma nodule.*)

CAUSES

◆ Exact cause unknown
◆ Actinic damage from solar ultraviolet (UV) radiation
◆ Burns, scars
◆ Chemical carcinogens
◆ Ionizing radiation
◆ Ulcerations

RISK FACTORS

◆ Overexposure to the sun's UV rays
◆ Radiation therapy
◆ Ingestion of herbicides containing arsenic
◆ Chronic skin irritation and inflammation
◆ Exposure to local carcinogens (such as tar and oil)
◆ Hereditary diseases (such as xeroderma pigmentosum and albinism)
◆ Presence of premalignant lesions (such as actinic keratosis or Bowen's disease)
◆ Rarely, develops on site of smallpox vaccination, psoriasis, or chronic discoid hippus erythematosus
◆ Outdoor employment
◆ Residence in sunny, warm climate

INCIDENCE

◆ Squamous cell carcinoma is most common in fair-skinned, light-eyed, and light-haired people.

COMPLICATIONS

◆ Lymph node involvement
◆ Visceral metastasis

ASSESSMENT

HISTORY

◆ Areas of chronic ulceration, especially on sun-damaged skin
◆ Pain, malaise, anorexia, fatigue, and weakness

PHYSICAL FINDINGS

◆ Lesions on the face, ears, or dorsa of the hands and forearms, and on other areas of sun-damaged skin (lesions possibly scaly and keratotic with raised, irregular borders; in late disease, lesions growing outward or exophytic and friable and tending toward chronic crusting)

DIAGNOSTIC TEST RESULTS

DIAGNOSTIC PROCEDURES

◆ Excisional biopsy allows a definitive diagnosis.

Squamous cell carcinoma nodule

An ulcerated nodule with an indurated base and a raised, irregular border is a typical lesion in squamous cell carcinoma.

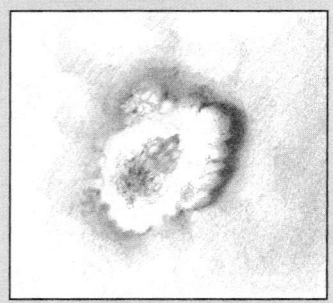

TREATMENT

GENERAL
- Determined by size, shape, location, and invasiveness of tumor and condition of underlying tissue
- Radiation therapy for older or debilitated patients

DIET
- High-protein, high-calorie

MEDICATIONS
- Chemotherapy
- Topical corticosteroids
- Analgesics

SURGERY
- Wide surgical excision, curettage, and electrodesiccation
- Cryosurgery

NURSING CONSIDERATIONS

NURSING DIAGNOSES
- Acute pain
- Anxiety
- Disturbed body image
- Fatigue
- Fear
- Imbalanced nutrition: Less than body requirements
- Impaired skin integrity
- Ineffective coping

EXPECTED OUTCOMES
The patient will:
- express feelings of increased comfort
- use support systems to assist with anxiety and fear.
- express positive feelings about self
- experience feelings of increased energy
- express concerns and fears related to the diagnosis and condition
- maintain adequate nutrition and hydration
- exhibit improved or healed lesions or wounds
- demonstrate positive coping behaviors.

NURSING INTERVENTIONS
- Encourage verbalization and provide emotional support.
- Deliver appropriate wound care.
- Provide periods of rest between procedures if the patient fatigues easily.
- Provide small, frequent meals and a high-protein, high-calorie diet.

MONITORING
- Wound site
- Adverse effects of radiation therapy, such as nausea, vomiting, hair loss, malaise, and diarrhea
- Pain control

PATIENT TEACHING

GENERAL
Be sure to cover:
- the disorder, diagnosis, and treatment
- drug administration, dosage, and possible adverse effects
- information about skin examination
- the importance of follow-up skin surveillance
- avoidance of excessive sun exposure to prevent recurrence; the need to use strong sunscreen.

DISCHARGE PLANNING
- Refer the patient to resource and support services.

RESOURCES
Organizations
American Academy of Dermatology: *www.aad.org*
American Cancer Society: *www.cancer.org*
Guide to Internet Resources for Cancer: *www.cancerindex.org*
National Cancer Institute: *www.cancer.gov*

Selected references
Atlas of Pathophysiology, 2nd ed. Philadelphia: Lippincott Williams & Wilkins, 2005.
Casciato, D.A. *Manual of Clinical Oncology,* 5th ed. Philadelphia: Lippincott Williams & Wilkins, 2004.
Kanitakis, J., et al. "Squamous Cell Carcinoma of the Skin Complicating Lupus Vulgaris," *Journal of the European Academy of Dermatology & Venereology* 20(1):114-16, January 2006.
Kurt, M., et al. "Malignant Fibrous Histiocytoma, Malignant Melanoma, and Squamous Cell Carcinoma Arising from Different Areas in an Adult," *Southern Medical Journal* 98(12):1228-229, December 2005.
Lim, Y.C., et al. "Level IIb Lymph Node Metastasis in Laryngeal Squamous Cell Carcinoma," *Laryngoscope* 116(2):268-72, February 2006.

Staphylococcal scalded skin syndrome

- Severe skin disorder marked by epidermal erythema, peeling, and necrosis that gives the skin a scaled appearance
- Follows a consistent three-stage pattern of progression
- Full recovery in most patients, with residual scarring unlikely

PATHOPHYSIOLOGY

- Infecting organism is group 2 *Staphylococcus aureus*.
- Penicillinase-producing organism releases epidermolytic toxins that are widely disseminated from a systemic site.

CAUSES

- Group 2 *Staphylococcus aureus*, primarily phage type 71

RISK FACTORS

- Impaired immunity
- Renal insufficiency
- Neonates (due to immature immune and renal systems)
- Adults undergoing immunosuppressant therapy

INCIDENCE

- This disease is most prevalent in infants ages 1 to 3 months but may develop in children younger than age 5 years.
- Staphylococcal scalded skin syndrome is uncommon in adults.

COMPLICATIONS

- Fluid and electrolyte loss
- Sepsis
- Death
- Septicemia
- Secondary infections

HISTORY

- Prodromal upper respiratory tract infection, possibly with concomitant purulent conjunctivitis
- Characteristic lesions, tender to palpation
- Exfoliation within 24 to 48 hours
- Fever

PHYSICAL FINDINGS

- Profoundly ill appearance
- Cutaneous changes progressing through the three phases of erythema, exfoliation (24 to 48 hours later), and desquamation.

Erythema

- Visible around mouth and other orifices
- Spreads in widening circles over entire body surface

Exfoliation

- Superficial erosions and minimal crusting, usually around body orifices
- In severe disease, large, flaccid bullae erupt and may spread to cover extensive body areas
- When ruptured, bullae expose sections of tender, oozing, denuded skin

Desquamation

- Affected areas dry and powdery scales form
- Normal skin replaces scales in 5 to 7 days
- Residual scarring rare

DIAGNOSTIC PROCEDURES

- Isolation of group 2 *S. aureus* on cultures of skin lesions confirms diagnosis.
- Exfoliative cytology and biopsy aid in differential diagnosis, ruling out erythema multiforme and drug-induced toxic epidermal necrolysis (which are similar to staphylococcal scalded skin syndrome).
- Blood cultures recover causative organism in very ill patients.

OTHER

- Careful observation of three-stage disease progression helps confirm diagnosis.

TREATMENT

GENERAL
◆ Fluid and electrolyte replacement

DIET
◆ As tolerated

ACTIVITY
◆ As tolerated

MEDICATIONS
◆ Systemic antibiotic (usually penicillinase-resistant penicillin)

NURSING CONSIDERATIONS

NURSING DIAGNOSES
◆ Acute pain
◆ Disturbed body image
◆ Impaired skin integrity
◆ Ineffective therapeutic regimen management
◆ Ineffective thermoregulation
◆ Risk for deficient fluid volume
◆ Risk for infection

EXPECTED OUTCOMES
The patient (or family) will:
◆ report feelings of increased comfort
◆ voice feelings about change in body image
◆ exhibit improved or healed wounds or lesions
◆ demonstrate the appropriate skin care regimen
◆ maintain a normal body temperature
◆ maintain a normal fluid balance
◆ avoid or minimize the risk of secondary infection.

NURSING INTERVENTIONS
◆ Maintain skin integrity using strict aseptic technique to prevent secondary infection.
◆ Leave affected areas uncovered or loosely covered to prevent friction and sloughing of skin.
◆ Place cotton between severely affected fingers and toes to prevent webbing.
◆ Administer warm baths and soaks during the recovery period.
◆ Gently debride exfoliated areas.

🌸 **AGE FACTOR** *Provide special care for the neonate, if required, including placement in an Isolette to maintain body temperature and provide isolation.*

MONITORING
◆ Skin integrity
◆ Vital signs
◆ Intake and output
◆ Fluid and electrolyte status
◆ Complications

PATIENT TEACHING

GENERAL
Be sure to cover:
◆ the disorder, diagnosis, and treatment
◆ meticulous hand-washing and aseptic techniques when changing dressings and providing comfort measures, such as warm soaks and baths
◆ the importance of avoiding friction on the skin surface during the exfoliation stage
◆ the importance of avoiding picking or rubbing scales during the desquamation stage
◆ that complications are rare and residual scars are unlikely.

DISCHARGE PLANNING
◆ Instruct parents to contact the practitioner if adverse reactions to antibiotic therapy occur.
◆ Explain the importance of completing the prescribed course of antibiotic therapy, even after the lesions appear to have healed.

RESOURCES
Organizations
American Academy of Dermatology: *www.aad.org*
Dermatology Foundation: *www.dermfnd.org*
National Center for Infectious Diseases: *www.cdc.gov/ncidod*
The Merck Manuals Online Medical Library: *www.merck.com/mmhe*

Selected references
Baartmans, M.G., et al. "Neonate with Staphylococcal Scalded Skin Syndrome," *Archives of Disease in Childhood. Fetal and Neonatal Edition* 91(1):F25, January 2006.
Chi, C.Y., et al. "A Clinical and Microbiological Comparison of *Staphylococcus Aureus* Toxic Shock and Scalded Skin Syndromes in Children," *Clinical Infectious Diseases* 42(2):181-85, January 2006.
Diseases, 4th ed. Philadelphia: Lippincott Williams & Wilkins, 2006.
Patel, G.K. "Treatment of Staphylococcal Scalded Skin Syndrome," *Expert Review of Anti-Infective Therapy* 2(4):575-87, August 2004.

Stomatitis

OVERVIEW

- Inflammation of oral mucosa; may extend to the buccal mucosa, lips, palate, and tongue
- Common infection occurring alone or as part of systemic disease
- Two main types: acute herpetic stomatitis and aphthous stomatitis
- Usually heals spontaneously, without scarring, in 10 to 14 days

PATHOPHYSIOLOGY

- Stomatitis is an inflammatory reaction that may cause loss of the oral epithelium as a protective barrier.

CAUSES

Acute herpetic stomatitis
- Herpes simplex virus

Aphthous stomatitis
- Unknown (autoimmune and psychosomatic causes under investigation)

RISK FACTORS

- Smoking
- Poor oral hygiene
- Stress
- Poor nutrition
- Chemotherapy
- Immunosuppression

INCIDENCE

- Acute herpetic stomatitis is common in children ages 1 to 3.
- Aphthous stomatitis is common in young girls and female adolescents.

COMPLICATIONS

- Dysphagia
- Sepsis (in immunocompromised patient)
- Ocular or central nervous system involvement (herpetic stomatitis)

ASSESSMENT

HISTORY

- Burning mouth pain
- Malaise
- Lethargy
- Anorexia
- Irritability
- Fever
- Extreme tenderness of the oral mucosa
- Predisposing risk factors

PHYSICAL FINDINGS

Herpetic stomatitis
- Bleeding and swollen gums
- Papulovesicular ulcers in the mouth and throat
- Submaxillary lymphadenitis

Aphthous stomatitis
- Slight swelling of the mucous membrane
- Single or multiple shallow ulcers with whitish centers and red borders, about 2 to 5 mm in diameter (see *Looking at aphthous stomatitis*)

DIAGNOSTIC TEST RESULTS

LABORATORY

- Smear of ulcer exudate identifies the causative organism in Vincent's angina (painful pseudomembranous ulceration of gums, oral mucous membranes, pharynx, and tonsils).
- Viral cultures performed on fluid and herpetic vesicles in acute herpetic stomatitis identify the virus.

OTHER

- Physical assessment helps confirm diagnosis.

Looking at aphthous stomatitis

In aphthous stomatitis, numerous small, round vesicles appear. They soon break and leave shallow ulcers with red areolae.

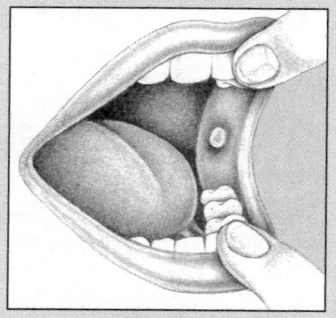

TREATMENT

GENERAL
- Symptom relief
- Nonantiseptic warm water mouth rinses
- Ice
- Soft-bristled toothbrush
- Smoking cessation

DIET
- Soft, pureed, or liquid, as tolerated; avoidance of salty, spicy foods

ACTIVITY
- As tolerated

MEDICATIONS
- I.V. fluids (severe cases)

Acute herpetic stomatitis
- Topical anesthetic solutions
- Topical corticosteroids
- Acyclovir

Aphthous stomatitis
- Topical anesthetic coating agent

NURSING CONSIDERATIONS

NURSING DIAGNOSES
- Acute pain
- Imbalanced nutrition: Less than body requirements
- Impaired oral mucous membrane
- Ineffective health maintenance
- Risk for infection

EXPECTED OUTCOMES
The patient will:
- express feelings of increased comfort and decreased pain
- maintain adequate nutritional intake
- show improvement or complete healing of lesions or wounds
- demonstrate good oral hygiene practices
- exhibit no further signs or symptoms of infection.

NURSING INTERVENTIONS
- Advise using a sponge instead of a toothbrush for brushing teeth.
- Suggest rinsing with hydrogen peroxide or normal saline mouthwash.
- Give prescribed analgesics.
- Develop a meal plan based on soft, liquid, or pureed foods.
- Offer iced drinks.

MONITORING
- Lesion state
- Response to treatment
- Complications

PATIENT TEACHING

GENERAL
Be sure to cover:
- the infection and expected course
- the importance of good oral hygiene
- the proper application of topical drugs
- recommended dietary changes
- adverse effects of prescribed drugs
- (with aphthous stomatitis) the need to avoid such precipitating factors as stress and fatigue.

DISCHARGE PLANNING
- Refer the patient to a smoking-cessation program, if appropriate.

RESOURCES
Organizations
National Digestive Diseases Information Clearinghouse: *www.niddk.nih.gov/health/digest/nddic.htm*
National Institute of Diabetes & Digestive & Kidney Diseases: *www.niddk.nih.gov*

Selected references
Albanidou-Farmaki, E., et al. "Outcome Following Treatment for *Helicobacter Pylori* in Patients with Recurrent Aphthous Stomatitis," *Oral Diseases* 11(1):22-26, January 2005.
Handbook of Diseases, 3rd ed. Philadelphia: Lippincott Williams & Wilkins, 2004.
Jurge, S., et al. "Number VI Recurrent Aphthous Stomatitis," *Oral Diseases* 12(1):1-21, January 2006.
Shulman, J.D., et al. "Risk Factors Associated with Denture Stomatitis in the United States," *Journal of Oral Pathology & Medicine* 34(6):340-46, July 2005.

Streptococcus pneumoniae infection, drug-resistant

OVERVIEW

- Infections caused by *Streptococcus pneumoniae* among leading causes of illness and death among people who are young, old, and debilitated
- Seven serotypes (6A, 6B, 9V, 14, 19A, 19F, and 23F) accounting for most drug-resistant *S. pneumoniae*
- Vaccine available for the 23 most common serotypes
- Commonly resistant to penicillin; also resistant to erythromycin, co-trimoxazole, vancomycin, tetracycline, chloramphenicol, and ofloxacin
- In pneumonias caused by resistant strains, death rate twice as high as in those sensitive to antibiotics
- Also known as *DRSP*

PATHOPHYSIOLOGY

- DRSP can affect people by colonization or infection.
- People who carry *S. pneumoniae* as part of their normal flora but remain asymptomatic may unknowingly spread the infection.
- Disease results when bacteria multiply locally (otitis media), multiply after aspiration (pneumonia), or invade a sterile site (central nervous system or blood).

CAUSES

- Abuse of antimicrobial agents
- Increasing prevalence of strains resistant to multiple drug classes

RISK FACTORS

- Contact with infected respiratory droplets or direct or indirect contact with objects freshly soiled with respiratory discharge
- Populations at risk:
- Elderly people
- Children age 2 and older
- Blacks
- Native Americans
- People with autoimmune disorders
- Nursing home residents
- Child-care workers

AGE FACTOR *The Advisory Committee on Immunization Practices recommends the* S. pneumoniae *vaccine be given to people age 2 and older with certain medical conditions and to all people age 65 and older.*

INCIDENCE

- DRSP causes 3% to 35% of pneumococcal illness.

COMPLICATIONS

- Colonized people not commonly detected or treated
- Treatment failures, prolonged hospitalization, recurrent disease, and increased cost
- Death in 14% of adults with invasive disease
- Neurologic sequelae after meningitis
- Hearing impairment from recurrent otitis media
- Developmental delay in children with recurrent otitis media

ASSESSMENT

HISTORY

- Member of high-risk population
- Recent exposure to respiratory secretions of infected person
- Recent antimicrobial use

PHYSICAL FINDINGS
In meningitis

- Fever
- Stiff neck
- Drowsiness
- Rash
- Seizures
- Increased white blood cells in cerebrospinal fluid (CSF)

In otitis media

- High fever (101.3° F [38.5° C])
- Irritability
- Possibly effusion
- Bulging tympanic membrane that's red, opaque, white, yellow, or purple and immobile on pneumatic otoscope
- Pain in the affected ear

In pneumonia

- Fluid-filled tissue and lobes
- Shaking chills
- Cough
- Rust- or green-colored mucus
- High fever
- Diaphoresis
- Elevated pulse and respirations
- Bluish lips and nail beds
- Confusion or delirium

DIAGNOSTIC TEST RESULTS

LABORATORY
◆ Bacteria are isolated from a fluid sample (blood, CSF, sputum, respiratory drops, ear).

IMAGING
◆ Chest X-rays display pneumonia.

DIAGNOSTIC PROCEDURES
◆ Lumbar puncture is performed for suspected meningitis.

TREATMENT

GENERAL
◆ Supportive, symptomatic care

DIET
◆ As tolerated

ACTIVITY
◆ As tolerated

MEDICATIONS
◆ Analgesics
◆ Antibiotics
◆ Vancomycin (meningitis)

NURSING CONSIDERATIONS

NURSING DIAGNOSES
◆ Acute pain
◆ Anxiety
◆ Fatigue
◆ Hyperthermia
◆ Imbalanced nutrition: Less than body requirements
◆ Impaired gas exchange
◆ Ineffective airway clearance
◆ Ineffective coping
◆ Risk for deficient fluid volume
◆ Risk for infection

EXPECTED OUTCOMES
The patient will:
◆ express feelings of comfort and relief of pain
◆ identify measures to reduce anxiety
◆ express feelings of increased energy
◆ maintain a normal body temperature
◆ achieve adequate nutritional intake
◆ maintain adequate ventilation and oxygenation
◆ maintain a patent airway
◆ use support systems to assist with coping
◆ maintain adequate fluid balance
◆ remain free from signs and symptoms of infection.

NURSING INTERVENTIONS
◆ Give prescribed drugs.
◆ Provide rest periods as needed.
◆ Provide emotional support.

MONITORING
◆ Seizures
◆ Vital signs
◆ Intake and output
◆ Complications after lumbar puncture

PATIENT TEACHING

GENERAL
Be sure to cover:
◆ the importance of covering the mouth and nose while sneezing or coughing
◆ regular hand washing
◆ taking the entire prescription of antibiotic for any infection
◆ never giving a prescribed antibiotic to anyone else
◆ importance of reporting to a practitioner a change in symptoms.

DISCHARGE PLANNING
◆ Refer the patient for follow-up, as needed.
◆ Recommend to the patient that close contacts receive the *S. pneumoniae* vaccine.

RESOURCES
Organizations
National Center for Infectious Diseases: *www.cdc.gov/ncidod*
National Library of Medicine: *www.nlm.nih.gov*

Selected references
Fuller, J.D., et al. "Drug-resistant Pneumococcal Pneumonia: Clinical Relevance and Approach to Management," *European Journal of Clinical Microbiology & Infectious Diseases* 24(12):780-88, December 2005.

Lynch, J.P. 3rd, and Zhanel, G.G. "Escalation of Antimicrobial Resistance among Streptococcus Pneumoniae: Implications for Therapy," *Seminars in Respiratory and Critical Care Medicine* 26(6):575-616, December 2005.

Sherpa, T.Y., and Leaf, H.L. "Pneumococcal Vaccination in Adults," *Current Infectious Disease Reports* 7(3):211-17, May 2005.

Stroke LIFE-THREATENING DISORDER

OVERVIEW

- Sudden impairment of blood circulation to the brain
- Third most common cause of death in the United States
- Affects 500,000 people each year, causing death in half
- Most common cause of neurologic disability
- About 50% of stroke survivors permanently disabled
- Recurrences possible within weeks, months, or years
- Also known as *cerebrovascular accident* or *brain attack*

PATHOPHYSIOLOGY

- The oxygen supply to the brain is interrupted or diminished.
- In thrombotic or embolic stroke, neurons die from lack of oxygen.
- In hemorrhagic stroke, impaired cerebral perfusion causes infarction.

CAUSES

Cerebral thrombosis
- Most common cause of stroke
- Obstruction of a blood vessel in the extracerebral vessels
- Site possibly intracerebral

Cerebral embolism
- Cardiac arrhythmias
- Endocarditis
- History of rheumatic heart disease
- Open heart surgery
- Posttraumatic valvular disease
- Second most common cause of stroke

Cerebral hemorrhage
- Arteriovenous malformation
- Cerebral aneurysms
- Chronic hypertension
- Third most common cause of stroke

RISK FACTORS

- History of transient ischemic attack
- Heart disease
- Smoking
- Familial history of cerebrovascular disease
- Obesity
- Alcohol use
- Cardiac arrhythmias
- Diabetes mellitus
- Hypertension
- Use of hormonal contraceptives in conjunction with smoking and hypertension
- High red blood cell count
- High serum triglyceride levels
- Elevated cholesterol and triglycerides

INCIDENCE

- Stroke mostly affects older adults but can strike at any age.
- Stroke is more common in men than in women.
- Stroke affects Blacks and Hispanics more commonly than other groups.

COMPLICATIONS

- Malnutrition
- Infections
- Sensory impairment
- Aspiration
- Contractures
- Skin breakdown
- Deep vein thrombosis
- Pulmonary emboli
- Depression
- Seizures

ASSESSMENT

HISTORY

- Varying clinical features, depending on artery affected, severity of damage, and extent of collateral circulation
- One or more risk factors present
- Sudden onset of hemiparesis or hemiplegia
- Gradual onset of dizziness, mental disturbances, or seizures
- Loss of consciousness or sudden aphasia

PHYSICAL FINDINGS

- With stroke in left hemisphere, signs and symptoms on right side
- With stroke in right hemisphere, signs and symptoms on left side
- With stroke that causes cranial nerve damage, signs and symptoms on same side
- Change in level of consciousness
- With conscious patient, anxiety along with communication and mobility difficulties
- Urinary incontinence
- Loss of voluntary muscle control
- Hemiparesis or hemiplegia on one side of the body
- Decreased deep tendon reflexes
- Hemianopsia on the affected side of the body
- With left-sided hemiplegia, problems with visuospatial relations
- Sensory losses

DIAGNOSTIC TEST RESULTS

LABORATORY

- Laboratory tests, including anticardiolipin antibodies, antiphospholipid, factor V mutation, antithrombin III, protein S, and protein C, may show increased thrombotic risk.

IMAGING

- Magnetic resonance imaging and angiography allow for evaluation of the location and size of the lesion.
- Cerebral angiography details the disruption of cerebral circulation and is the test of choice for examining the entire cerebral blood flow.
- Computed tomography scan detects structural abnormalities.
- Positron emission tomography provides data on cerebral metabolism and on cerebral blood flow changes.

OTHER

- Transcranial Doppler studies evaluate the velocity of blood flow.
- Carotid Doppler measures flow through the carotid arteries.
- Two-dimensional echocardiography evaluates the heart for dysfunction.
- Cerebral blood flow studies measure blood flow to the brain.
- Electrocardiography evaluates electrical activity in cortical infarction.

TREATMENT

GENERAL

- Careful blood pressure management
- Helping patient adapt to specific deficits
- Physical, speech, and occupational rehabilitation

◆ Supportive, symptomatic treatment

DIET
◆ Pureed dysphagia diet or tube feedings, if indicated

MEDICATIONS
◆ Tissue plasminogen activator when the cause isn't hemorrhagic (emergency care within 3 hours of onset of the symptoms)
◆ Anticonvulsants
◆ Stool softeners
◆ Anticoagulants
◆ Analgesics
◆ Antidepressants
◆ Antiplatelets
◆ Lipid-lowering agents
◆ Antihypertensives

SURGERY
◆ Craniotomy
◆ Endarterectomy
◆ Extracranial intracranial bypass
◆ Ventricular shunts

NURSING CONSIDERATIONS

NURSING DIAGNOSES
◆ Anxiety
◆ Bathing or hygiene self-care deficit
◆ Disturbed sensory perception (tactile)
◆ Dressing or grooming self-care deficit
◆ Impaired gas exchange
◆ Impaired physical mobility
◆ Impaired verbal communication
◆ Ineffective airway clearance
◆ Ineffective coping
◆ Ineffective tissue perfusion: Cerebral
◆ Powerlessness
◆ Risk for aspiration
◆ Risk for disuse syndrome
◆ Risk for impaired skin integrity
◆ Risk for infection
◆ Risk for injury
◆ Situational low self-esteem
◆ Toileting self-care deficit
◆ Total urinary incontinence

EXPECTED OUTCOMES
The patient (or family) will:
◆ identify strategies to reduce anxiety
◆ perform bathing and hygiene activities to the fullest extent possible
◆ report signs and symptoms of impaired sensation
◆ perform dressing and grooming activities to the fullest extent possible
◆ maintain adequate ventilation and oxygenation
◆ achieve maximum mobility possible
◆ effectively communicate needs verbally or through an alternate means of communication
◆ maintain a patent airway
◆ develop adequate coping mechanisms and support systems
◆ exhibit signs of adequate cerebral perfusion
◆ express feelings of control over health and well-being
◆ remain free from signs of aspiration
◆ maintain joint mobility and range of motion
◆ maintain intact skin with no signs of breakdown
◆ remain free from injury and from signs or symptoms of infection
◆ verbalize feelings about self-esteem
◆ perform toileting needs to the fullest extent possible.

NURSING INTERVENTIONS
◆ Maintain a patent airway and oxygenation.
◆ Offer urinal or bedpan every 2 hours.
◆ Insert an indwelling urinary catheter, if necessary.
◆ Ensure adequate nutrition.
◆ Follow the physical therapy program, and assist the patient with exercise.
◆ Establish and maintain patient communication.
◆ Provide psychological support.
◆ Set realistic, short-term goals.
◆ Protect the patient from injury and complications.
◆ Provide careful positioning to prevent aspiration and contractures.
◆ Give prescribed drugs.

MONITORING
◆ Neurologic, GI, and respiratory status
◆ Vital signs
◆ Fluid, electrolyte, and nutritional intake
◆ Development of deep vein thrombosis and pulmonary embolus

PATIENT TEACHING

GENERAL
Be sure to cover:
◆ disorder, diagnosis, and treatment
◆ occupational and speech therapy programs
◆ the dietary and drug regimens
◆ adverse drug reactions
◆ stroke prevention.

DISCHARGE PLANNING
◆ Refer the patient to home care, outpatient, and speech and occupational rehabilitation programs as needed.

RESOURCES
Organizations
American Academy of Neurology: *www.aan.com*
American Heart Association: *www.americanheart.org*
American Neurological Association: *www.aneuroa.org*
American Stroke Association: *www.strokeassociation.org*
National Aphasia Association: *www.aphasia.org*
National Stroke Association: *www.stroke.org*

Selected references
Bakas, T., et al. "Outcomes among Family Caregivers of Aphasic versus Nonaphasic Stroke Survivors," *Rehabilitation Nursing* 31(1):33-42, January-February 2006.
Gardner, M.R. "Outcomes in Children Experiencing Neurologic Insults as Preterm Neonates," *Pediatric Nursing* 31(6):448, 451-56, November-December 2005.
Handbook of Pathophysiology, 2nd ed. Philadelphia: Lippincott Williams & Wilkins, 2005.
Kasper, D.L., et al., eds. *Harrison's Principles of Internal Medicine,* 16th ed. New York: McGraw-Hill Book Co., 2005.
King, J.E., and Ezell, J. "How Do I Manage Stroke in a Menstruating Woman?" *Nursing* 36(1):22, January 2006.
Koenig, M.A., et al. "Safety of Induced Hypertension Therapy in Patients with Acute Ischemic Stroke," *Neurocritical Care* 4(1):3-7, 2006.
Professional Guide to Diseases, 8th ed. Philadelphia: Lippincott Williams & Wilkins, 2005.

◣ Subdural hematoma

- Meningeal hemorrhage resulting from accumulation of blood in subdural space
- May be acute (less than 72 hours old), subacute (3 to 20 days old), or chronic (older than 20 days)
- May be unilateral or bilateral

PATHOPHYSIOLOGY

Acute

- Blunt impact to the skull may cause a tear in connecting veins (rarely, arteries) in the cerebral cortex.

Chronic

- Chronic subdural hematoma begins as a separation in the dura-arachnoid interface, which then is filled by cerebrospinal fluid (CSF).
- Dural border cells proliferate around this CSF collection to produce a neomembrane.
- Fragile new vessels grow into the membrane and hemorrhage.

CAUSE

- Head trauma
- Fragile blood vessels

RISK FACTORS

Acute

- Anticoagulation therapy
- Age

Chronic

- Alcoholism
- Epilepsy
- Coagulopathy
- Arachnoid cysts
- Anticoagulant therapy (including aspirin)
- Cardiovascular disease (hypertension, arteriosclerosis)
- Thrombocytopenia
- Diabetes

INCIDENCE

- The acute type of subdural hematoma occurs in 5% to 25% of patients with severe head injuries.
- The acute type is most common in people older than age 40; the chronic type is most common in people older than age 50.
- Both types occur more frequently in men than in women.

COMPLICATIONS

- Neurologic impairment
- Coma
- Death

HISTORY

- Head trauma
- Headache
- Change in level of consciousness (LOC)
- Predisposing risk factors

PHYSICAL FINDINGS

- Dilated, nonreactive pupil ipsilateral to the hematoma
- Hemiparesis contralateral to the hematoma
- Balance problems
- Altered LOC

LABORATORY

- CSF is yellow with relatively low protein (chronic subdural hematoma).
- Coagulation studies may be abnormal.

IMAGING

- Computed tomography scan, X-rays, and arteriography reveal mass and altered blood flow in the area.

TREATMENT

GENERAL
- Supportive treatment
- Wound care
- Fresh frozen plasma (to correct coagulation)
- Intubation and mechanical ventilation, as indicated

DIET
- Adequate hydration
- Based on extent of injury
- Nothing by mouth if surgery is needed

ACTIVITY
- Bed rest initially, then as tolerated
- Flat bed after evacuation of hematoma

MEDICATIONS
- If coagulation studies are abnormal, vitamin K, fresh frozen plasma, platelets, or clotting products
- Analgesics (after extent of injury is determined)
- Osmotic diuretics
- Anticonvulsants
- Prophylactic antibiotics (with surgery)
- Oxygen therapy

SURGERY
- Burr holes
- Craniotomy

NURSING CONSIDERATIONS

NURSING DIAGNOSES
- Acute pain
- Anxiety
- Decreased intracranial adaptive capacity
- Impaired skin integrity
- Ineffective coping
- Ineffective tissue perfusion: Cerebral
- Risk for infection
- Risk for injury

EXPECTED OUTCOMES
The patient will:
- express feelings of increased comfort and decreased pain
- identify strategies to reduce anxiety
- remain neurologically stable
- maintain skin integrity
- seek support systems and exhibit adequate coping behaviors
- exhibit signs of adequate cerebral perfusion
- remain free from signs or symptoms of infection
- avoid injury or complications.

NURSING INTERVENTIONS
- Provide appropriate wound care.
- Give prescribed drugs.
- Provide emotional support.
- Institute seizure precautions.

MONITORING
- Vital signs
- Neurologic status
- Wound healing
- Seizure activity
- Respiratory status

PATIENT TEACHING

GENERAL
Be sure to cover:
- importance of reporting changes in neurologic status
- avoiding aspirin as a pain treatment
- observing for CSF drainage and signs of infection.

DISCHARGE PLANNING
- Refer the patient to physical therapy, occupational therapy, and speech therapy, as appropriate.
- Refer the patient to social services, as appropriate.

RESOURCES
Organizations
American Academy of Neurology: *www.aan.com*
American Neurological Association: *www.aneuroa.org*
Harvard University Consumer Health Information: *www.intelihealth.com*
National Institute of Neurological Disorders and Stroke: *www.ninds.nih.gov*

Selected references
Effron, D., et al. "Subdural Hematoma," *Journal of Emergency Medicine* 30(1):93-94, January 2006.
Erol, F.S., et al. "Irrigation vs. Closed Drainage in the Treatment of Chronic Subdural Hematoma," *Journal of Clinical Neuroscience* 12(3): 261-63, April 2005.
Horn, E.M., et al. "Bedside Twist Drill Craniostomy for Chronic Subdural Hematoma: A Comparative Study," *Surgical Neurology* 65(2);150-53, February 2006.
Nolan, S. "Traumatic Brain Injury: A Review," *Critical Care Nursing Quarterly* 28(2):188-94, April-June 2005.
Scuibba, D.M., et al. "Acute Intracranial Subdural Hematoma Following a Lumbar CSF Leak Caused by Spine Surgery," *Spine* 30(24):E730-E732, December 2005.

Substance abuse and dependence

- Use of a legal or illegal substance that causes physical, mental, emotional, or social harm, such as opioids, stimulants, depressants, antianxiolytics, and hallucinogens
- Number one health problem in the United States

PATHOPHYSIOLOGY
- Tolerance develops when a drug is administered long term, with cross-tolerance developing.
- Withdrawal occurs with abrupt discontinuation or administration of an antagonist due to rebound noradrenergic activity in the central nervous system (CNS).

CAUSES
- Combination of low self-esteem, peer pressure, inadequate coping skills, and curiosity
- May follow the use of prescribed drugs to relieve physical pain

RISK FACTORS
- Male gender
- History of depression
- History of other substance abuse disorders
- Familial history
- Peer pressure
- Low socioeconomic status

INCIDENCE
- Substance abuse and dependence can occur at any age.
- Experimentation with substances is common, beginning in adolescence and preadolescence.
- The disorder affects more than 18 million Americans who use alcohol and 5 million who use illicit drugs (fewer than one-fourth treated).

COMPLICATIONS
- Cardiac and respiratory arrest
- Intracranial hemorrhage
- Acquired immunodeficiency syndrome
- Subacute bacterial endocarditis
- Hepatitis
- Cirrhosis
- Vasculitis
- Septicemia
- Thrombophlebitis
- Pulmonary emboli
- Gangrene
- Malnutrition and GI disturbances
- Respiratory infections
- Musculoskeletal dysfunction
- Trauma
- Depression and increased risk of suicide
- Psychosis
- Toxic or allergic reactions
- Impaired social and occupational functioning

ASSESSMENT

HISTORY
- Abdominal pain, nausea, or vomiting
- Painful injury or chronic illness
- Feigned illnesses
- Overdose
- High tolerance to potentially addictive drugs
- Amenorrhea
- Suggestive behavior patterns or the presence of known risk factors
- Mood swings, anxiety, impaired memory, sleep disturbances, flashbacks, slurred speech, depression, and thought disorders

PHYSICAL FINDINGS
- Lacrimation (with opiate withdrawal)
- Nystagmus (with CNS depressants and phencyclidine intoxication)
- Drooping eyelids (with opiate or CNS depressant use)
- Constricted pupils (with opiate use or withdrawal)
- Dilated pupils (with hallucinogens or amphetamines)
- Rhinorrhea (with opiate withdrawal or cocaine abuse)
- Inflammation, atrophy, or perforation of the nasal mucosa (with drug sniffing)
- Sweating (with opiates or CNS stimulants or drug withdrawal)
- Sensation of bugs crawling on the skin (with alcohol withdrawal)
- Excoriated skin
- Needle marks or tracks
- Cellulitis or abscesses
- Thrombophlebitis
- Fascial infection
- Bilateral crackles and rhonchi (with smoking and inhaling drugs or by opiate overdose)
- Cardiopulmonary signs of overdose (respiratory depression and hypotension)
- Acute onset hypertension
- Cardiac arrhythmias
- Hemorrhoids
- Tremors, hyperreflexia, hyporeflexia, and seizures
- Uncooperative, disruptive, or violent behavior

DSM-IV-TR *criteria*
- Diagnosis is confirmed with at least three of the following criteria (some symptoms must have persisted for at least 1 month or have occurred repeatedly over a longer time):
- substance often taken in larger amounts or for a longer time than the patient intended
- persistent desire or one or more unsuccessful efforts to cut down or control substance use
- excessive time devoted to activities necessary to obtain the substance
- frequent intoxication or withdrawal symptoms when expected to fulfill major obligations at work, school, or home or when substance use is physically hazardous
- impaired social, occupational, or recreational activities
- continued substance use despite the recognition of a persistent or recurrent social, psychological, or physical problem that's caused or exacerbated by the use of the substance
- marked tolerance
- characteristic withdrawal symptoms
- substance commonly taken to relieve or avoid withdrawal symptoms.

DIAGNOSTIC TEST RESULTS

LABORATORY
- Serum or urine drug screen reveals the substance.
- Serum protein electrophoresis shows elevated serum globulin levels.

- Serum glucose measurement shows hypoglycemia.
- Complete blood count (CBC) shows leukocytosis.
- Liver function is abnormal.
- CBC shows elevated mean corpuscular hemoglobin levels.
- Uric acid levels are elevated.
- Blood urea nitrogen levels are decreased.

OTHER
- Mental status examination findings fit *DSM-IV-TR* criteria.

TREATMENT

GENERAL
- Symptomatic treatment based on the drug ingested
- Fluid replacement therapy
- Symptomatic treatment for complications
- Gastric lavage, induced emesis, activated charcoal instillation, forced diuresis and, possibly, hemoperfusion or hemodialysis
- Detoxification (inpatient or outpatient)
- Psychotherapy
- Relaxation techniques
- Rehabilitation

DIET
- Well-balanced

ACTIVITY
- Monitored, for safety

MEDICATIONS
- Detoxification with the same drug or a pharmacologically similar drug
- Sedatives
- Anticholinergics
- Antidiarrheal agents
- Antianxiety drugs
- Anticonvulsants
- Nutritional and vitamin supplements

NURSING CONSIDERATIONS

NURSING DIAGNOSES
- Anxiety

- Bathing or hygiene self-care deficit
- Compromised family coping
- Dressing or grooming self-care deficit
- Dysfunctional family processes: Alcoholism
- Hopelessness
- Imbalanced nutrition: Less than body requirements
- Impaired social interaction
- Ineffective coping
- Ineffective role performance
- Powerlessness
- Risk for deficient fluid volume
- Risk for injury
- Risk for other-directed violence
- Situational low self-esteem

EXPECTED OUTCOMES
The patient (or family) will:
- verbalize strategies to reduce anxiety
- develop adequate coping mechanisms and support systems
- acknowledge that the patient has a problem and needs treatment
- consume regular, nutritious meals
- engage in social interactions with others
- acknowledge the effects of his condition on his usual roles and responsibilities
- gradually join in self-care and the decision-making process
- maintain an adequate fluid balance
- avoid injury
- not harm others
- express his feelings related to self-esteem.

NURSING INTERVENTIONS
- Maintain a quiet, safe environment.
- Institute seizure precautions.
- Set limits for dealing with demanding, manipulative behavior.

MONITORING
- Vital signs
- Suicide ideation
- Visitors
- Signs of complications
- Nutrition
- Effects of pharmacologic therapy

PATIENT TEACHING

GENERAL
Be sure to cover:
- the disorder, diagnosis, and treatment
- detoxification and rehabilitation, as appropriate
- measures for preventing human immunodeficiency virus infection and hepatitis
- measures for safer sex and birth control.

DISCHARGE PLANNING
- Recommend participation in a drug-oriented self-help group.
- Refer the patient to support services.

RESOURCES
Organizations
Alcoholics Anonymous: *www.alcoholics-anonymous.org*
Nar-Anon: *www.naranon.com*
Narcotics Anonymous: *www.na.org*
National Council on Alcoholism and Drug Dependence: *www.ncadd.org*

Selected references
Collins, E.D., et al. "Anesthesia-assisted vs. Buprenorphine- or Clonidine-assisted Heroin Detoxification and Naltrexone Induction: A Randomized Trial," *JAMA* 294(8):903-13, August 2005.

Diagnostic and Statistical Manual of Mental Disorders, Fourth Editiion, Text Revision. Washington, D.C.: American Psychiatric Association, 2000.

Fazel S., et al. "Substance Abuse and Dependence in Prisoners: A Systematic Review," *Addiction* 101(2):181-91, February 2006.

Letizia, M., and Reinbolz, M. "Identifying and Managing Acute Alcohol Withdrawal in the Elderly," *Geriatric Nursing* 26(3):176-83, May-June 2005.

McClelland, G.T. "The Effects and Management of Crack Cocaine Dependence," *Nursing Times* 101(29):26-27, July 2005.

Sudden infant death syndrome LIFE-THREATENING DISORDER

OVERVIEW

- Sudden death of an infant younger than age 1 year without identifiable cause
- Also known as *SIDS* and *crib death*

PATHOPHYSIOLOGY
Hypotheses
- The infant may have damage to the respiratory control center in the brain from chronic hypoxemia.
- The infant may not respond to increasing carbon dioxide levels. During an episode of apnea, carbon dioxide levels increase, but the child isn't stimulated to breathe. As apnea continues, high levels of carbon dioxide further suppress the ventilatory effort until the infant stops breathing.
- The infant may have periods of sleep apnea and eventually die during one of these episodes.

CAUSES
- Possibly viral
- Hypoxia theory
- Apnea theory
- Possible *Clostridium botulinum* toxin
- Possibly associated with diphtheria, tetanus, and pertussis vaccines

INCIDENCE
- About 7,000 SIDS deaths occur annually in the United States.
- The incidence is 2 in every 1,000 live births; about 60% are male.
- **AGE FACTOR** *SIDS occurs mostly between ages 1 and 4 months. Incidence declines rapidly between ages 4 and 12 months.*
- Incidence is increased in non–breast-fed infants.
- It occurs most often in fall and winter.
- There's a slightly higher incidence in:
  - preterm neonates
  - Inuit neonates
  - disadvantaged black neonates
  - neonates of mothers younger than age 20
  - multiple birth neonates.

COMPLICATIONS
- Always fatal

ASSESSMENT

HISTORY
- Occasionally, respiratory tract infection
- Possible abnormal hepatic or pancreatic function
- Previous near-miss respiratory event in 60% of cases
- With infant wedged in a crib corner or with blankets wrapped around head, suffocation ruled out by autopsy as the cause of death
- With frothy, blood-tinged sputum found around infant's mouth or on crib sheets revealing a patent airway, aspiration of vomitus ruled out by autopsy as cause of death
- No crying or signs of disturbed sleep by infant

PHYSICAL FINDINGS
- Postmortem examination may show:
  - changes indicating chronic hypoxia, hypoxemia, and large airway obstruction
  - bruising; possible fractured ribs
  - blood in the infant's mouth, nose, or ears
  - mottled complexion; extremely cyanotic lips and fingertips
  - pooled blood in legs and feet
  - diaper possibly wet and full of stool.

DIAGNOSTIC TEST RESULTS

DIAGNOSTIC PROCEDURES
- Autopsy may show:
  - small or normal adrenal glands
  - enlarged thymus
  - petechiae over the visceral surfaces of the pleura, within the thymus, and in the epicardium
  - well-preserved lymphoid structures
  - signs of chronic hypoxemia
  - increased pulmonary artery smooth muscle
  - edematous, congestive, and fully expanded lungs
  - liquid blood in the heart
  - stomach curd inside the trachea.

GENERAL
◆ Emotional support for the family
◆ Prevention for any surviving infant found apneic and any sibling with apnea; assessment with home apnea monitor until the at-risk infant passes age of vulnerability

NURSING CONSIDERATIONS

NURSING DIAGNOSES
◆ Dysfunctional grieving
◆ Fear
◆ Hopelessness
◆ Interrupted family processes
◆ Risk for sudden infant death syndrome
◆ Spiritual distress

EXPECTED OUTCOMES
The family will:
◆ seek appropriate support persons for assistance
◆ use available support systems to assist in coping
◆ identify feelings of hopelessness regarding the current situation
◆ share feelings about the event
◆ verbalize measures to prevent SIDS
◆ use effective coping strategies to ease spiritual discomfort.

NURSING INTERVENTIONS
◆ Make sure that both parents are present when the child's death is confirmed.
◆ Stay calm and allow the parents to express their feelings.
◆ Reassure the parents that they aren't to blame.
◆ Allow the parents to see the infant in a private room and to express their grief. Stay in the room with them, if appropriate.
◆ Offer to call clergy, friends, or relatives.
◆ Return the infant's belongings to the parents.
◆ Make sure that the parents receive the autopsy report promptly.

MONITORING
◆ Parents' reactions and coping mechanisms

PATIENT TEACHING

GENERAL
Be sure to cover:
◆ the need for an autopsy to confirm the diagnosis
◆ basic facts about SIDS
◆ information to help parents cope with pregnancy and the first year of a new infant's life, if they decide to have another child.

DISCHARGE PLANNING
◆ Refer the parents and family to community and health care facility support services.
◆ Refer the parents to a local SIDS parents' group.
◆ Advise the parents to contact the SIDS hot line (1-800-221-SIDS).
◆ Refer the parents to cardiopulmonary resuscitation classes, if appropriate.
◆ Refer the family to a home health nurse for continued support, if indicated.

RESOURCES
Organizations
American Academy of Pediatrics: *www.aap.org*
American Sudden Infant Death Syndrome Institute: *www.sids.org*
Association of SIDS and Infant Mortality Programs: *www.asip1.org*
National Institute of Child Health and Human Development: *www.nichd.nih.gov*
SIDS Alliance: *www.sidsalliance.org*

Selected references
Heinig, M.J., and Banuelos, J. "American Academy of Pediatrics Task Force on Sudden Infant Death Syndrome (SIDS) Statement on SIDS Reduction: Friend or Foe of Breastfeeding?" *Journal of Human Lactation* 22(1):7-10, November 2005.
Maindonald, E. "Helping Parents Reduce the Risk of SIDS," *Nursing* 35(7):50-52, July 2005.
Makielski, J.C. "SIDS: Genetic and Environmental Influences May Cause Arrhythmia in This Silent Killer," *Journal of Clinical Investigation* 116(2):297-99, February 2006.
Menihan, C.A., et al. "Fetal Heart Rate Patterns and Sudden Infant Death Syndrome," *Journal of Obstetrics, Gynecologic, and Neonatal Nursing* 35(1):116-22, January-February 2006.
Thompson, D.G. "Safe Sleep Practices for Hospitalized Infants," *Pediatric Nursing* 31(5):400-403, 409, September-October 2005.

Syndrome of inappropriate antidiuretic hormone

OVERVIEW

OVERVIEW

- Disease of the posterior pituitary marked by excessive release of antidiuretic hormone (ADH) (vasopressin)
- Prognosis depends on underlying disorder and response to treatment
- Also known as *SIADH*

PATHOPHYSIOLOGY

- Excessive ADH secretion occurs in the absence of normal physiologic stimuli for its release.
- Excessive water reabsorption from the distal convoluted tubule and collecting ducts results in hyponatremia and normal to slightly increased extracellular fluid volume. (See *Understanding SIADH*.)

CAUSES

- Central nervous system disorders
- Drugs
- Miscellaneous conditions, such as myxedema and psychosis
- Neoplastic diseases
- Oat cell carcinoma of the lung
- Pulmonary disorders

INCIDENCE

- SIADH is a common cause of hospital-acquired hyponatremia.

COMPLICATIONS

- Water intoxication
- Cerebral edema
- Severe hyponatremia
- Heart failure
- Seizures
- Coma
- Death

ASSESSMENT

HISTORY

- Possible clue to the cause
- Cerebrovascular disease
- Cancer
- Pulmonary disease
- Recent head injury
- Anorexia, nausea, vomiting
- Weight gain
- Lethargy, headaches, emotional and behavioral changes

PHYSICAL FINDINGS

- Tachycardia
- Disorientation
- Seizures and coma
- Sluggish deep tendon reflexes
- Muscle weakness

DIAGNOSTIC TEST RESULTS

LABORATORY

- Serum osmolality levels are less than 280 mOsm/kg.
- Serum sodium levels are less than 123 mEq/L.
- Urine sodium levels are more than 20 mEq/L without diuretics.
- Renal function tests are normal.

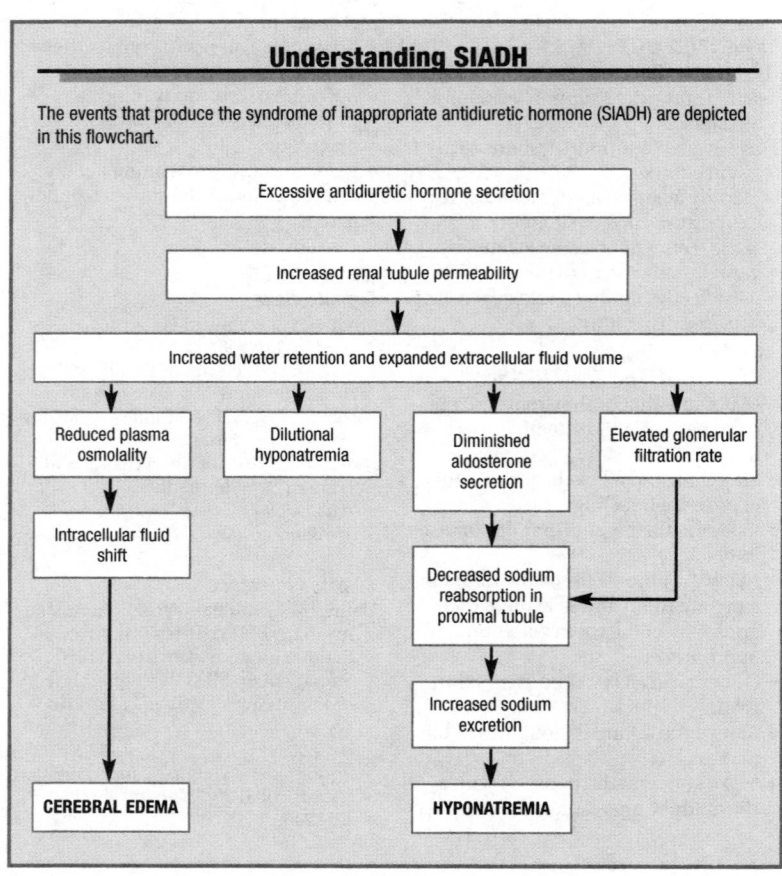

Understanding SIADH

The events that produce the syndrome of inappropriate antidiuretic hormone (SIADH) are depicted in this flowchart.

TREATMENT

GENERAL
◆ Based primarily on symptoms
◆ Correction of the underlying cause

DIET
◆ Restricted water intake (500 to 1,000 ml/day)
◆ High-salt, high-protein or urea supplements to enhance water excretion

ACTIVITY
◆ As tolerated

MEDICATIONS
◆ Demeclocycline or lithium for long-term treatment
◆ Loop diuretics if fluid overload, history of heart failure, or resistance to treatment
◆ 3% sodium chloride solution if serum sodium level is less than 120 mEq/L or if the patient is having seizures

SURGERY
◆ To treat underlying cause such as cancer

NURSING CONSIDERATIONS

NURSING DIAGNOSES
◆ Anxiety
◆ Excess fluid volume
◆ Fear
◆ Risk for injury

EXPECTED OUTCOMES
The patient will:
◆ identify strategies to reduce anxiety
◆ maintain adequate fluid balance
◆ discuss fears and concerns
◆ avoid complications.

NURSING INTERVENTIONS
◆ Restrict fluids.
◆ Provide comfort measures for thirst.
◆ Reduce unnecessary environmental stimuli.
◆ Orient as needed.
◆ Provide a safe environment.
◆ Institute seizure precautions as needed.
◆ Give prescribed drugs.

MONITORING
◆ Intake and output
◆ Vital signs
◆ Daily weight
◆ Serum electrolytes, especially sodium
◆ Response to treatment
◆ Breath sounds
◆ Heart sounds
◆ Neurologic checks
◆ Changes in level of consciousness

WARNING *Watch closely for signs and symptoms of heart failure, which may occur because of fluid overload.*

PATIENT TEACHING

GENERAL
Be sure to cover:
◆ the disorder, diagnosis, and treatment
◆ fluid restriction
◆ methods to decrease discomfort from thirst
◆ prescribed drugs and possible adverse effects
◆ self-monitoring techniques for fluid retention such as daily weight
◆ signs and symptoms that require immediate medical intervention.

RESOURCES
Organizations
American Cancer Society: *www.cancer.org*
Endocrine and Metabolic Diseases Information Service: *www.endocrine.niddk.nih.gov*
Endocrine Society: *www.endo-society.org*

Selected references
Diseases, 4th ed. Philadelphia: Lippincott Williams & Wilkins, 2006.
Feldman, B.J., et al. "Nephrogenic Syndrome of Inappropriate Antidiuresis," *New England Journal of Medicine* 352(18):1884-890, May 2005.
Huang, E.A., et al. "Oral Urea for the Treatment of Chronic Syndrome of Inappropriate Antidiuresis in Children," *Journal of Pediatrics* 148(1):128-31, January 2006.
Nakazato, Y., et al. "Unpleasant Sweet Taste: A Symptom of SIADH Caused by Lung Cancer," *Journal of Neurology, Neurosurgery & Psychiatry* 77(3):405-406, March 2006.
Nettina, S.M. *Lippincott Manual of Nursing Practice,* 8th ed. Philadelphia: Lippincott Williams & Wilkins, 2006.

Syphilis

OVERVIEW

- Chronic, infectious, sexually transmitted disease (STD)
- Untreated, progresses in four stages: primary, secondary, latent, and late (formerly called tertiary)

PATHOPHYSIOLOGY

- The infecting organism penetrates intact mucous membranes or abrasions in the skin, entering lymphatics and blood.
- Systemic infection and systemic foci precede primary lesion development at the site of inoculation.
- Organ involvement occurs from dissemination.

CAUSES

- The spirochete *Treponema pallidum*
- Transmission primarily through sexual contact during the primary, secondary, and early latent stages of infection
- Prenatal transmission possible
- Transmission by way of fresh blood transfusion (rare)

RISK FACTORS

- Unsafe sexual practices

INCIDENCE

- In the United States, incidence of syphilis is highest in urban populations, especially in people between ages 15 and 39.
- About 34,000 cases, in primary and secondary stages, are reported in the United States annually.

COMPLICATIONS

- Cardiovascular disease
- Irreversible neurologic disease
- Irreversible organ damage
- Membranous glomerulonephritis
- With fetal infection:
- Spontaneous abortion
- Stillbirth
- Low birth weight
- Deafness

ASSESSMENT

HISTORY

- Unprotected sexual contact with an infected person or with multiple or anonymous sexual partners

PHYSICAL FINDINGS

Primary syphilis

- One or more chancres (small, fluid-filled lesions) on the genitalia; others on the anus, fingers, lips, tongue, nipples, tonsils, or eyelids
- In female patient, possible chancres on cervix or vaginal wall
- Unilateral or bilateral adenopathy

Secondary syphilis

- Headache, malaise
- Nausea, vomiting
- Anorexia, weight loss
- Sore throat, slight fever
- Symmetrical mucocutaneous lesions
- Rash possibly macular, papular, pustular, or nodular
- Lesions uniform, well defined, and generalized
- Macules typically erupting between rolls of fat on the trunk and proximally on the arms, palms, soles, face, and scalp
- In warm, moist body areas, lesions enlarged and eroding, producing highly contagious, pink or grayish white lesions (condylomata lata)
- Alopecia
- Brittle and pitted nails
- Generalized lymphadenopathy

Latent syphilis

- Physical signs and symptoms absent except for possible recurrence of mucocutaneous lesions that resemble those of secondary syphilis

Late syphilis

- Findings that vary with the involved organ
- Three subtypes:
- Neurosyphilis affecting meningovascular tissues: headache, vertigo, insomnia, hemiplegia, seizures, and psychological difficulties; if parenchymal tissue affected: paresis, alteration in intellect, paranoia, illusions, and hallucinations; in addition, Argyll Robertson pupil (a small, irregular pupil that's nonreactive to light but accommodates for vision), ataxia, slurred speech, trophic joint changes, positive Romberg's sign, and a facial tremor
- Late benign: gummas (lesions that develop between 1 and 10 years after infection and may be a chronic, superficial nodule or a deep, granulomatous lesion that's solitary, asymmetrical, painless, indurated, and large or small) visible on the skin and mucocutaneous tissues; commonly affect bones and can develop in any organ
- Cardiovascular: decreased cardiac output that may cause decreased urine output and decreased sensorium related to hypoxia, pulmonary congestion

DIAGNOSTIC TEST RESULTS

LABORATORY

- Dark-field microscopy identifies *T. pallidum* from lesion exudate to provide an immediate syphilis diagnosis. (See *Identifying syphilis by dark-field microscopy.*)
- Non-treponemal serologic tests include the Venereal Disease Research Laboratory (VDRL) slide test, the rapid plasma reagin (RPR) test, and the automated reagin test, detecting nonspecific antibodies.
- Treponemal serologic studies include the fluorescent treponemal antibody absorption test, the *T. pallidum* hemagglutination assay, and the microhemagglutination assay, detecting the specific antitreponemal antibody and confirming positive screening results.
- Cerebrospinal fluid examination identifies neurosyphilis when the total protein level is above 40 mg/dl, the VDRL slide test is reactive, and the white blood cell count exceeds 5 mononuclear cells/μl.

TREATMENT

GENERAL
◆ Immediate examination of all sexual contacts
◆ Avoidance of pregnancy until a good response to therapy demonstrated
◆ Hospitalization for symptomatic late syphilis

ACTIVITY
◆ No sexual activity until cured

MEDICATIONS
◆ Antibiotics (penicillin the treatment of choice)

NURSING CONSIDERATIONS

NURSING DIAGNOSES
◆ Acute pain
◆ Disturbed body image
◆ Impaired physical mobility
◆ Impaired skin integrity
◆ Ineffective sexuality patterns
◆ Risk for infection
◆ Risk for injury
◆ Sexual dysfunction

Identifying syphilis by dark-field microscopy

The presence of spiral-shaped bacteria (*Treponema pallidum*) on dark-field examination confirms the diagnosis of syphilis.

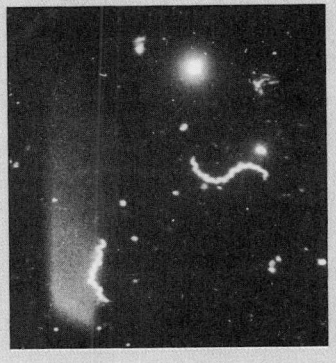

EXPECTED OUTCOMES
The patient will:
◆ express feelings of increased comfort and decreased pain
◆ express concern about self-concept, self-esteem, and body image
◆ maintain joint mobility and muscle strength
◆ exhibit improved or healed lesions or wounds
◆ voice feelings about potential or actual changes in sexual activity
◆ state infection risk factors and experience no further signs or symptoms of infection
◆ avoid or minimize complications
◆ verbalize methods to protect against future STD infection.

NURSING INTERVENTIONS
◆ Follow standard precautions.
◆ Give prescribed drugs.
◆ Promote rest and adequate nutrition.
◆ In secondary syphilis, keep lesions clean and dry; dispose of contaminated materials properly.
◆ Report all syphilis cases to the appropriate public health authorities.

MONITORING
◆ Neurologic status
◆ Cardiovascular status
◆ Complications
◆ Response to treatment
◆ Compliance with treatment

PATIENT TEACHING

GENERAL
Be sure to cover:
◆ the disorder, diagnosis, and treatment
◆ the need to complete the course of therapy even after symptoms subside
◆ the importance of informing, testing, and treating sexual partners
◆ the need to refrain from sexual activity until treatment is completed and follow-up VDRL/RPR test results are normal
◆ information for patient and sexual partners about human immunodeficiency virus infection

◆ risks to the fetus if the patient is contemplating pregnancy
◆ following safer sex practices.

DISCHARGE PLANNING
◆ As needed, obtain a physical or occupational therapy consultation.
◆ Refer the patient for contact tracing.
◆ Refer the patient to a specialist if congenital syphilis is suspected.
◆ Consult a social worker to determine home care needs.

RESOURCES
Organizations
Centers for Disease Control and Prevention: *www.cdc.gov*
Harvard University Consumer Health Information: *www.intelihealth.com*
Mayo Clinic: *www.mayoclinic.com*
National Health Information Center: *www.health.gov/nhic*

Selected references
Ferguson, L.A., and Varnado, J.W. "Syphilis: An Old Enemy Still Lurks," *Journal of the American Academy of Nurse Practitioners* 18(2):49-55, February 2006.
Ghanem, K.G., et al. "Doxycycline Compared with Benzathine Penicillin for the Treatment of Early Syphilis," *Clinical Infectious Diseases* 42(6):e45-49, March 2006.
Heymann, W.R. "The History of Syphilis," *Journal of the American Academy of Dermatology* 54(2):322-23, February 2006.
Hyman, E.L. "Syphilis," *Pediatrics in Review* 27(1):37-39, January 2006.
Kasper, D.L., et al., eds. *Harrison's Principles of Internal Medicine,* 16th ed. New York: McGraw-Hill Book Co., 2005.
Taylor M.L., et al. "Prostate Cancer and Sexually Transmitted Diseases: A Meta-Analysis," *Family Medicine* 37(7):506-12, July-August 2005.

Systemic lupus erythematosus

OVERVIEW

- A chronic inflammatory autoimmune disorder that affects connective tissues
- Two forms: discoid lupus erythematosus (DLE) and systemic lupus erythematosus (SLE)
- Only the skin affected by DLE

PATHOPHYSIOLOGY

- The body produces antibodies, such as antinuclear antibodies (ANAs), against its own cells.
- The formed antigen antibody complexes suppress the body's normal immunity and damage tissues.
- Patients with SLE produce antibodies against many different tissue components, such as red blood cells (RBCs), neutrophils, platelets, lymphocytes, and almost any organ or tissue in the body.

CAUSES

- Unknown

RISK FACTORS

- Stress
- Streptococcal or viral infections
- Exposure to sunlight or ultraviolet light
- Injury
- Surgery
- Exhaustion
- Emotional upsets
- Immunization, pregnancy
- Abnormal estrogen metabolism

INCIDENCE

- SLE affects women eight times more often than men (15 times more often during childbearing years).
- SLE occurs worldwide, and it's most prevalent among Asians and Blacks.

COMPLICATIONS

- Pleurisy
- Pleural effusions
- Pericarditis, myocarditis, endocarditis
- Coronary atherosclerosis
- Renal failure
- Seizures and mental dysfunction

ASSESSMENT

HISTORY

- Possible fever, anorexia, weight loss, malaise, fatigue, abdominal pain, nausea, vomiting, diarrhea, constipation, rash, and polyarthralgia
- Possible drug history with one of 25 drugs that can cause SLE-like reaction
- Irregular menstruation or amenorrhea, particularly during flare-ups
- Chest pain and dyspnea
- Emotional instability, psychosis, organic brain syndrome, headaches, irritability, and depression
- Oliguria, urinary frequency, dysuria, and bladder spasms

PHYSICAL FINDINGS

- Joint involvement that resembles rheumatoid arthritis
- Raynaud's phenomenon
- Skin eruptions provoked or aggravated by sunlight or ultraviolet light
- Tachycardia, central cyanosis, and hypotension
- Altered level of consciousness, weakness of the extremities, and speech disturbances
- Skin lesions
- Butterfly rash over nose and cheeks
- Patchy alopecia (common)
- Vasculitis
- Lymph node enlargement (diffuse or local and nontender)
- Pericardial friction rub

DIAGNOSTIC TEST RESULTS

LABORATORY

- Complete blood count with differential shows anemia and a reduced white blood cell (WBC) count, decreased platelet count, and elevated erythrocyte sedimentation rate; serum electrophoresis shows hypergammaglobulinemia.
- ANA, anti–deoxyribonucleic acid, and lupus erythematosus cell test findings are positive in most patients with active SLE, but these are only slightly useful in diagnosing the disease. (ANA test is sensitive but not specific for SLE.)
- Urine studies show RBCs, WBCs, urine casts, sediment, and significant protein loss (more than 3.5 g in 24 hours).
- Blood studies demonstrate decreased serum complement (C3 and C4) levels, indicating active disease. (Leukopenia, mild thrombocytopenia, and anemia are also seen during active disease.)
- C-reactive protein level is increased during flare-ups.
- Rheumatoid factor is positive in 30% to 40% of patients.

IMAGING

- Chest X-rays may disclose pleurisy or lupus pneumonitis.

DIAGNOSTIC PROCEDURES

- Central nervous system (CNS) involvement may account for abnormal EEG results in about 70% of patients, but brain and magnetic resonance imaging scans may be normal in patients with SLE despite CNS disease.
- Electrocardiography may show a conduction defect with cardiac involvement or pericarditis.
- Renal biopsy shows progression of SLE and the extent of renal involvement.
- Skin biopsy shows immunoglobulin and complement deposition in the dermal-epidermal junction in 90% of patients.

TREATMENT

GENERAL

- Use of sunscreen with sun protection factor of at least 15

DIET

- No restrictions unless renal failure occurs

ACTIVITY

- Regular exercise program

MEDICATIONS

- Nonsteroidal anti-inflammatory drugs
- Topical corticosteroid creams
- Fluorinated steroids
- Antimalarials
- Corticosteroids
- Cytotoxic drugs
- Antihypertensives

SURGERY

- Possible joint replacement

NURSING CONSIDERATIONS

NURSING DIAGNOSES

- Acute pain
- Constipation
- Decreased cardiac output
- Diarrhea
- Disturbed body image
- Fatigue
- Imbalanced nutrition: Less than body requirements
- Impaired oral mucous membrane
- Impaired physical mobility
- Impaired skin integrity
- Impaired tissue integrity
- Impaired urinary elimination
- Ineffective breathing pattern
- Risk for infection
- Risk for peripheral neurovascular dysfunction

EXPECTED OUTCOMES

The patient will:

- express feelings of increased comfort and decreased pain
- pass soft, regular stool without straining
- maintain adequate cardiac output
- resume a normal bowel elimination pattern
- verbalize feelings about a changed body image
- express feelings of increased energy
- maintain daily calorie requirements
- maintain intact oral mucous membrane
- maintain joint mobility and range of motion (ROM)
- maintain skin integrity
- have reduced pain, redness, and swelling at the site of impaired tissue

- maintain fluid balance: intake will equal output
- maintain a respiratory rate within 5 breaths/minute of baseline
- remain free from signs and symptoms of infection
- report alterations in sensation or pain in the extremities.

NURSING INTERVENTIONS

- Provide a mouth rinse of normal saline solution after meals to assist healing of oral lesions.
- Apply heat packs to relieve joint pain and stiffness.
- Encourage regular exercise to maintain full ROM.
- Explain the expected benefit of prescribed drugs, and watch for adverse effects.
- Institute seizure precautions if you suspect CNS involvement.
- Warm and protect the patient's hands and feet if the patient has Raynaud's phenomenon.
- Support the patient's self-image.

MONITORING

- Signs and symptoms of organ involvement
- Urine, stools, and GI secretions for blood
- Scalp for hair loss and skin and mucous membranes for petechiae, bleeding, ulceration, pallor, and bruising
- Response to treatment
- Complications
- Nutritional status
- Joint mobility
- Seizure activity

PATIENT TEACHING

GENERAL

Be sure to cover:

- the disorder, diagnosis, and treatment
- ROM exercises and body alignment and postural techniques
- ways to avoid infection, such as avoiding crowds and people with known infections
- the need to notify a practitioner if fever, cough, or rash occurs or if

chest, abdominal, muscle, or joint pain worsens
- the importance of eating a balanced diet and the restrictions associated with prescribed drugs
- prescribed drugs
- the importance of good skin care
- the benefits of exercise
- the importance of keeping regular follow-up appointments and contacting a practitioner if flare-ups occur
- the need to wear protective clothing and use a sunscreen
- how to perform meticulous mouth care.

DISCHARGE PLANNING

- Arrange for a physical therapy and occupational therapy consultation if musculoskeletal involvement compromises mobility.

RESOURCES

Organizations

Arthritis Foundation: *www.arthritis.org*
Lupus Foundation of America: *www.lupus.org*

Selected references

Burt, R.K., et al. "Nonmyeloablative Hematopoietic Stem Cell Transplantation for Systemic Lupus Erythematosus," *JAMA* 295(5):527-35, February 2006.

Kasper, D.L., et al., eds. *Harrison's Principles of Internal Medicine,* 16th ed. New York: McGraw-Hill Book Co., 2005.

Kyttaris, V.C., et al. "Gene Therapy in Systemic Lupus Erythematosus," *Current Gene Therapy* 5(6):677-84, December 2005.

Lash, A.A., and Lusk, B. "Systemic Lupus Erythematosus in the Intensive Care Unit," *Critical Care Nurse* 24(2):56-60, 62-65, April 2004.

The Merck Manual of Diagnosis & Therapy, 18th ed., Whitehouse Station, N.J.: Merck & Co., Inc., 2006.

Petri, M. "Systemic Lupus Erythematosus: 2006 Update," *Journal of Clinical Rheumatology* 12(1):37-40, February 2006.

Taeniasis

- A parasitic infestation by *Taenia saginata* (beef tapeworm), *T. solium* (pork tapeworm), *Diphyllobothrium latum* (fish tapeworm), or *Hymenolepis nana* (dwarf tapeworm)
- Usually a chronic, benign intestinal disease; dangerous systemic and central nervous system symptoms possible if *T. solium* larvae invade the brain or striated muscle of vital organs
- Also called *tapeworm disease* and *cestodiasis*

PATHOPHYSIOLOGY
- Gastric acid activates larvae after ingestion of undercooked, bacteria-infested beef or pork.
- Mature tapeworms fasten to the intestinal wall and produce ova that are passed in the feces.
- A single tapeworm produces an average of 50,000 eggs per day and may live 25 years.

CAUSES
T. saginata
- Uncooked or undercooked beef

T. solium
- Uncooked or undercooked pork

D. latum
- Uncooked or undercooked freshwater fish, such as pike, trout, salmon, and turbot

H. nana
- Inadequate hand-washing facilities
- No intermediate host
- Person-to-person transmission via ova passed in stool

INCIDENCE
T. saginata
- This type of taeniasis occurs worldwide but is most prevalent in Europe and East Africa.

T. solium
- Incidence of this type of taeniasis is highest in Mexico and Latin America.
- The lowest incidence is among Muslims and Jews.

D. latum
- This type of taeniasis is most prevalent in Finland, parts of the former Soviet Union, Japan, Alaska, Australia, the Great Lakes region of the United States, Switzerland, Chile, and Argentina.

H. nana
- *H. nana* is the most common tapeworm in humans.
- *H. nana* is particularly prevalent among institutionalized mentally retarded children and in underdeveloped countries.

COMPLICATIONS
- Appendicitis
- Obstruction of bile ducts and pancreatic duct

ASSESSMENT

HISTORY
- Ingestion of raw or undercooked beef or pork
- Occasionally, worm segments exiting through the anus and appearing on bed clothes
- Increased hunger
- Weight loss
- Nausea
- Abdominal pain (usually in the morning) relieved by eating
- Pruritus ani

PHYSICAL FINDINGS
- Weight loss
- Intraocular larvae

DIAGNOSTIC TEST RESULTS

LABORATORY
- Tapeworm ova or body segments may be observed in feces (may require multiple specimens).

DIET
◆ As tolerated

ACTIVITY
◆ As tolerated

MEDICATIONS
◆ Anthelmintics
◆ High-dose glucocorticosteroids

⚡ **WARNING** *During treatment for T. solium, other health-related measures, such as laxative use and induced vomiting, are contraindicated because of the danger of autoinfection and systemic disease.*

SURGERY
◆ Possible if complications develop

NURSING DIAGNOSES
◆ Diarrhea
◆ Imbalanced nutrition: Less than body requirements
◆ Risk for deficient fluid volume
◆ Risk for infection

EXPECTED OUTCOMES
The patient will:
◆ return to a normal elimination pattern
◆ maintain adequate nutrition and hydration
◆ maintain an adequate fluid balance
◆ experience no further signs or symptoms of infection.

NURSING INTERVENTIONS
◆ Dispose of the patient's excretions carefully. Wear gloves when giving personal care and handling fecal excretions, bedpans, and bed linens; wash your hands thoroughly and instruct the patient to do the same.
◆ Tell the patient not to consume anything after midnight on the day niclosamide therapy begins because the drug must be taken on an empty stomach.
◆ After giving niclosamide, document passage of strobilae.

MONITORING
◆ Stool specimens
◆ Daily weight
◆ Response to treatment

GENERAL
Be sure to cover:
◆ the disorder, diagnosis, and treatment
◆ expected response to treatment
◆ preventing reinfection by washing hands thoroughly and cooking meat and fish thoroughly.

DISCHARGE PLANNING
◆ After drug treatment, all types of tapeworm infestation require a follow-up laboratory examination of stool specimens during the next 3 to 5 weeks to check for any remaining ova or worm segments.
◆ Persistent infestation typically requires a second course of medication.

RESOURCES
Organizations
National Center for Infectious Diseases: *www.cdc.gov/ncidod*
World Health Organization: *www.who.int*

Selected references
Campbell, G., et al. "Genetic Variation in *Taenia Solium*," *Parasitology International* 55(Suppl):S121-126, 2006.
Montresor, A., and Palmer, K. "Taeniasis/Cysticercosis Trend Worldwide and Rationale for Control," *Parasitology International* 55 (Suppl):S301-303, December 2006.
Nunes, C.M., et al. "*Taenia Saginata*: Differential Diagnosis of Human Taeniasis by Polymerase Chain Reaction-Restriction Fragment Length Polymorphism Assay," *Experimental Parasitology* 110(4):412-15, August 2005.

Tay-Sachs disease LIFE-THREATENING DISORDER

OVERVIEW

- Lipid storage disease that results from a congenital enzyme deficiency
- Leads to progressive mental and motor deterioration
- Always fatal, usually before age 5
- Rare form occurs in patients between ages 20 and 30
- No known cure

PATHOPHYSIOLOGY

- In this autosomal recessive disorder, the enzyme hexosaminidase A is absent or deficient.
- Without hexosaminidase A, lipid pigments (ganglioside GM2) accumulate and progressively destroy and demyelinate central nervous system cells.
- The juvenile form typically appears between ages 2 and 5 as a progressive deterioration of psychomotor skills and gait.

CAUSES

- Autosomal recessive disorder

INCIDENCE

- This disease affects fewer than 100 infants born yearly in the United States.
- This disease is about 100 times more common (about 1 in 3,600 live births) in those with Ashkenazi Jewish ancestry than in the general population.
- About 1 in 30 Ashkenazi Jews, French Canadians, and American Cajuns are heterozygous carriers of the gene for this disorder.

COMPLICATIONS

- Recurrent bronchopneumonia
- Dementia
- Blindness
- Seizures
- Paralysis
- Death

ASSESSMENT

HISTORY

- Familial history of Tay-Sachs disease
- Normal appearance at birth (possibly with exaggerated Moro's reflex)
- Onset of clinical signs and symptoms between ages 5 and 6 months
- Progressive deterioration
- Psychomotor retardation
- Blindness
- Dementia

PHYSICAL FINDINGS

- In 3- to 6-month-old infant:
- Apathetic appearance
- Augmented response to loud sounds
- Progressive weakness of the neck, trunk, arm, and leg muscles that prevents child from sitting up or lifting head
- Difficulty turning over
- Inability to grasp objects
- Progressive vision loss
- By age 18 months:
- Possible seizures
- Generalized paralysis
- Spasticity
- Blindness
- Holding eyes wide open and rolling eyeballs
- Pupils always dilated
- Decerebrate rigidity
- Complete vegetative state
- Head circumference possibly showing enlargement
- Pupils nonreactive to light
- Ophthalmoscopic examination possibly showing optic nerve atrophy and a distinctive cherry-red spot on the retina
- In a child who survives bouts of recurrent bronchopneumonia:
- Possible ataxia and progressive motor retardation between ages 2 and 8

DIAGNOSTIC TEST RESULTS

LABORATORY

- A serum analysis may show deficient hexosaminidase A.
- An amniocentesis or chorionic villus sampling will allow prenatal diagnosis of hexosaminidase A deficiency.

TREATMENT

GENERAL
◆ Supportive care
◆ Suctioning
◆ Postural drainage to remove secretions
◆ Meticulous skin care
◆ Long-term care in special facility

DIET
◆ Tube feedings with nutritional supplements

ACTIVITY
◆ As tolerated
◆ Active and passive range-of-motion exercises

MEDICATIONS
◆ Mild laxatives
◆ Anticonvulsants

NURSING CONSIDERATIONS

NURSING DIAGNOSES
◆ Anticipatory grieving
◆ Disabled family coping
◆ Impaired physical mobility
◆ Ineffective airway clearance
◆ Risk for impaired skin integrity
◆ Risk for injury

EXPECTED OUTCOMES
The patient (or family) will:
◆ express appropriate feelings of guilt
◆ seek outside sources to assist with coping and adjustment to the patient's condition
◆ maintain muscle strength and joint range of motion
◆ maintain a patent airway
◆ maintain skin integrity
◆ avoid complications.

NURSING INTERVENTIONS
◆ Help the patient's family deal with progressive illness and death.
◆ Prevent skin breakdown.
◆ Provide adequate nutrition.
◆ Maintain a patent airway.
◆ Implement seizure precautions.
◆ Give drug treatments.
◆ Stress the importance of amniocentesis in future pregnancies.

MONITORING
◆ Vital signs
◆ Intake and output
◆ Respiratory status
◆ Nutritional status
◆ Neurologic status
◆ Response to treatment

PATIENT TEACHING

GENERAL
Be sure to cover:
◆ disorder, diagnosis, and treatment
◆ how to perform suctioning
◆ how to perform postural drainage
◆ how to give tube feedings
◆ need for proper skin care to prevent breakdown.

DISCHARGE PLANNING
◆ Refer parents for genetic counseling.
◆ Refer parents to National Tay-Sachs and Allied Diseases Association.
◆ Refer the parents for psychological counseling, if indicated.
◆ Refer the siblings for screening to determine whether they're carriers.
◆ If the siblings are adult carriers, refer them for genetic counseling; stress that the disease isn't transmitted to offspring unless both parents are carriers.

RESOURCES
Organizations
National Institute of Neurological Disorders and Stroke: *www.ninds.nih.gov*
National Organization for Rare Disorders: *www.rarediseases.org*
National Tay-Sachs and Allied Diseases Association: *www.ntsad.org*

Selected references
Bembi, B., et al. "Substrate Reduction Therapy in the Infantile Form of Tay-Sachs Disease," *Neurology* 66(2):278-80, January 2006.
Gason, A.A., et al. "Tay Sachs Disease Carrier Screening in Schools: Educational Alternatives and Cheekbrush Sampling," *Genetics in Medicine* 7(9):626-32, November-December 2005.
Leib, J.R., et al. "Carrier Screening Panels for Ashkenazi Jews: Is More Better?" *Genetics in Medicine* 7(3):185-90, March 2005.
Neudorfer, O., et al. "Late-Onset Tay-Sachs Disease: Phenotypic Characterization and Genotypic Correlations in 21 Affected Patients," *Genetics in Medicine* 7(2):119-23, February 2005.
Rucker, J.C., et al. "Neuro-ophthalmology of Late-Onset Tay-Sachs Disease (LOTS)," *Neurology* 63(10):1918-26, November 2004.

Tendinitis and bursitis

Tendinitis

◆ Inflammation affecting the tendons and tendon-muscle attachments
◆ Most common sites:
– Shoulder rotator cuff
– Hip
– Achilles' tendon
– Hamstring
– Elbow

Bursitis

◆ Painful inflammation of one or more bursae
◆ Most common sites:
– Subdeltoid
– Subacromial
– Olecranon
– Trochanteric
– Calcaneal
– Prepatellar
◆ May be septic, calcific, acute, or chronic

PATHOPHYSIOLOGY
Tendinitis

◆ Inflammation causes localized pain around the affected area.
◆ Joint movement is restricted.
◆ Swelling results from fluid accumulation.
◆ Calcium deposits form in and around the tendon.
◆ Further swelling and immobility result in and around the tendon.

Bursitis

◆ Bursae sacs hold lubricating synovial fluid.
◆ Inflammation causes gradual pain and limits joint motion.

CAUSES
Tendinitis

◆ Abnormal body development
◆ Hypermobility in calcific tendinitis
◆ Musculoskeletal disorders: Rheumatic diseases and congenital defects
◆ Postural malalignment
◆ Trauma, such as a strain during sports activity

Bursitis

◆ Common stressors:
– Repetitive kneeling
– Jogging in worn-out shoes on hard asphalt surfaces
– Prolonged sitting with crossed legs on hard surfaces
◆ Recurring trauma from an inflammatory joint disease
◆ Septic bursitis: Wound infection or bacterial invasion (see *Anatomy of tendons and bursae*)

INCIDENCE

◆ These disorders are more common in elderly people.
◆ These disorders are also common in those who perform activities that overstress a tendon or repeatedly stress a joint.

COMPLICATIONS

◆ Scar tissue with subsequent disability

HISTORY
Tendinitis

◆ Traumatic injury or strain from athletic activity
◆ Concurrent musculoskeletal disorder
◆ Palpable tenderness over the affected site
◆ Referred tenderness in the related segment
◆ Shoulder:
– Localized pain that's most severe at night
– Pain that usually interferes with sleep
– Pain aggravated by heat
◆ Elbow: pain when grasping objects or twisting the elbow
◆ Hamstring: pain in the posterolateral aspect of the knee
◆ Foot: pain over the Achilles' tendon and on dorsiflexion

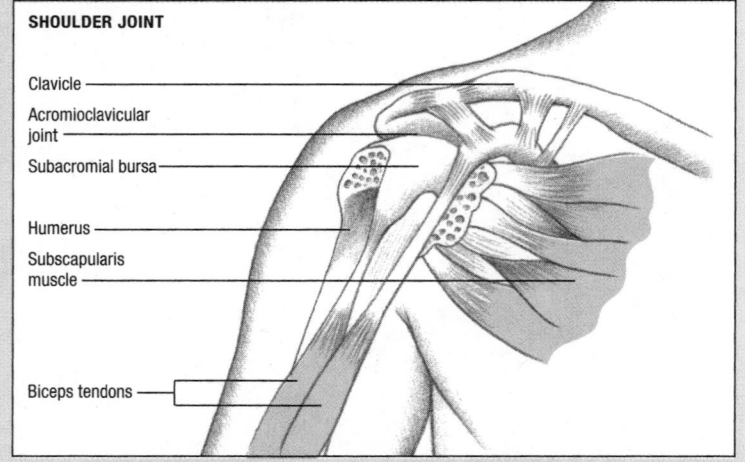

Anatomy of tendons and bursae

Tendons, like stiff rubber bands, hold the muscles in place and enable them to move the bones. Bursae are located at friction points around joints and between tendons, cartilage, or bone. Bursae keep these body parts lubricated so they move freely.

SHOULDER JOINT

Clavicle
Acromioclavicular joint
Subacromial bursa
Humerus
Subscapularis muscle
Biceps tendons

Bursitis
◆ Unusual strain or injury 2 to 3 days before pain began
◆ Pain that develops suddenly or gradually
◆ Pain that may limit movement
◆ Work or leisure activity that may involve repetitive action

PHYSICAL FINDINGS
Tendinitis
◆ Shoulder: restricted shoulder movement (especially abduction)
◆ Elbow: tenderness over the lateral epicondyle
◆ Hamstring: palpable tenderness when knee flexed at a 90-degree angle
◆ Foot: crepitus when the patient moves his foot

Bursitis
◆ Tenderness over the affected site
◆ Swelling with severe bursitis

DIAGNOSTIC TEST RESULTS

LABORATORY
◆ Various serum and urine test results rule out other disorders.

IMAGING
◆ X-rays in tendinitis may show bony fragments, osteophyte sclerosis, or calcium deposits.
◆ X-rays in calcific bursitis may show calcium deposits in the joint.
◆ Arthrography is usually normal in tendinitis with minor irregularities on the tendon under the surface.

DIAGNOSTIC PROCEDURES
◆ Arthrocentesis may identify causative microorganisms and other causes of inflammation.

TREATMENT

GENERAL
◆ Cold, heat, or ultrasound applications

DIET
◆ No restrictions

ACTIVITY
◆ Resting the affected joint
◆ Range-of-motion (ROM) exercises

MEDICATIONS
◆ Nonsteroidal anti-inflammatory drugs (NSAIDs)
◆ Local anesthetics
◆ Corticosteroids
◆ Oral anti-inflammatories
◆ Short-term analgesics

NURSING CONSIDERATIONS

NURSING DIAGNOSES
◆ Anxiety
◆ Chronic pain
◆ Dressing or grooming self-care deficit
◆ Impaired physical mobility

EXPECTED OUTCOMES
The patient will:
◆ develop adequate coping mechanisms and decreased anxiety
◆ have increased comfort and decreased pain
◆ perform dressing and grooming activities to the fullest extent possible
◆ maintain joint mobility and ROM.

NURSING INTERVENTIONS
◆ Apply cold or heat therapies, as ordered.
◆ Promote self-care.
◆ Give drug therapy.
◆ Encourage use of active ROM exercises.

MONITORING
◆ Severity and pattern of pain
◆ Response to treatment
◆ ROM

PATIENT TEACHING

GENERAL
Be sure to cover:
◆ the disorder, diagnosis, and treatment
◆ how to minimize GI distress from NSAIDs
◆ adverse drug reactions
◆ activities that promote rest and relaxation
◆ strengthening exercises
◆ prescribed exercise regimen
◆ need for proper sports equipment, shoes, and playing surfaces
◆ use of cushioned shoes
◆ application of cold packs
◆ proper body mechanics.

DISCHARGE PLANNING
◆ Refer the patient to a weight-management program, as appropriate.

RESOURCES
Organizations
American College of Rheumatology: *www.rheumatology.org*
American Orthopaedic Association: *www.aoassn.org*
Arthritis Foundation: *www.arthritis.org*

Selected references
Chen, M.J., et al. "Ultrasound-Guided Shoulder Injections in the Treatment of Subacromial Bursitis," *American Journal of Physical Medicine & Rehabilitation* 85(1):31-35, January 2006.
Diseases, 4th ed. Philadelphia: Lippincott Williams & Wilkins, 2006.
Handbook of Pathophysiology, 2nd ed. Philadelphia: Lippincott Williams & Wilkins, 2005.
Llinas, L. et al. "Osteomyelitis Resulting from Chronic Filamentous Fungus Olecranon Bursitis," *Journal of Clinical Rheumatology* 11(5):280-82, October 2005.
Meislin, R.J., et al. "Persistent Shoulder Pain: Epidemiology, Pathophysiology, and Diagnosis," *American Journal of Orthopedics* 34(12 Suppl):5-9, December 2005.
Small, L.N., and Ross, J.J. "Suppurative Tenosynovitis and Septic Bursitis," *Infectious Disease Clinics of North America* 19(4):991-1005, xi, December 2005.

Testicular cancer

- Proliferation of cancerous cells in the testicles
- Most originating from germinal cells and about 40% becoming seminomas
- Prognosis dependent on cancer cell type and stage; with treatment, a more than 5-year survival rate

PATHOPHYSIOLOGY

- Testicular cancer spreads through the lymphatic system to the iliac, para-aortic, and mediastinal nodes.
- Metastases affect the lungs, liver, viscera, and bone.

CAUSES

- Exact cause unknown

RISK FACTORS

- Cryptorchidism (see *Cryptorchidism and testicular cancer*)
- Mumps orchitis
- Inguinal hernia in childhood
- Maternal use of diethylstilbestrol (DES) or other estrogen-progestin combinations during pregnancy

INCIDENCE

- Testicular cancer is most common in men ages 20 to 40.
- This disease is rare in nonwhite men.
- This disease accounts for less than 1% of all male cancer deaths.
- This disease is rare in children.

COMPLICATIONS

- Back or abdominal pain from retroperitoneal adenopathy
- Metastasis
- Ureteral obstruction

HISTORY

- Previous injury to the scrotum
- Viral infection, such as mumps
- Use of DES or other estrogen-progestin drugs by the patient's mother during pregnancy
- Feeling of heaviness or a dragging sensation in the scrotum
- Weight loss; late sign
- Fatigue and weakness; late sign

PHYSICAL FINDINGS

- Enlarged testes
- Gynecomastia
- Lethargic, thin, and pallid appearance; later stages
- Palpable firm, smooth testicular mass
- Enlarged lymph nodes in surrounding areas

LABORATORY

- Elevated levels of the proteins human chorionic gonadotropin (HCG) and alpha-fetoprotein (AFP), which are tumor markers, suggest testicular cancer and can differentiate a seminoma from a nonseminoma.
- Elevated HCG and AFP levels indicate a nonseminoma.
- Elevated HCG and normal AFP levels indicate a seminoma.

DIAGNOSTIC PROCEDURES

- A biopsy confirms the diagnosis and can be used to stage the disease.

Cryptorchidism and testicular cancer

In men with cryptorchidism (the failure of a testicle to descend into the scrotum), testicular tumors are about 50 times more common than in men with normal anatomic structure. A simple surgical procedure, called orchiopexy, can bring the testicle to its normal position in the scrotum and reduce the testicular cancer risk. Nevertheless, testicular tumors occur more commonly in a surgically descended testicle than in a naturally descended one.

WHAT HAPPENS IN ORCHIOPEXY

In orchiopexy, the surgeon incises the groin area and separates the testicle and its blood supply from surrounding abdominal structures. Then, he creates a "tunnel" into the scrotum to accommodate the descent of the testicle.

REDUCING THE RISK FURTHER

After orchiopexy, urge the patient to examine his testicles monthly to detect a tumor at its earliest stage.

TREATMENT

GENERAL
- Varies with tumor cell type and stage
- Radiation therapy
- Autologous bone marrow transplantation for patients nonresponsive to standard therapy

DIET
- Well-balanced

MEDICATIONS
- Chemotherapy
- Hormonal therapy

SURGERY
- Orchiectomy and retroperitoneal node dissection

NURSING CONSIDERATIONS

NURSING DIAGNOSES
- Acute pain
- Anxiety
- Disturbed body image
- Fear
- Impaired oral mucous membrane
- Ineffective coping
- Ineffective role performance
- Risk for infection
- Sexual dysfunction

EXPECTED OUTCOMES
The patient will:
- report feeling less pain
- express feelings of decreased anxiety
- express positive feelings about himself
- express concerns and fears related to his diagnosis and condition
- maintain intact oral mucous membranes
- demonstrate positive coping mechanisms
- continue to function in usual roles to the greatest degree possible
- avoid infection and other complications
- express feelings and perceptions about change in sexual performance.

NURSING INTERVENTIONS
- Encourage verbalization and provide support.
- Administer drug therapy.
- Apply an ice pack to the scrotum.

MONITORING
- Wound site
- Vital signs
- Hydration and nutritional status
- Pain control
- Effects of medication
- Postoperative complications

PATIENT TEACHING

GENERAL
Be sure to cover:
- the disorder, diagnosis, and treatment
- sperm-banking procedures before the patient begins treatment, especially if he'll be having bilateral orchiectomy
- that infertility and impotence usually don't follow unilateral orchiectomy
- testicular self-examination.

DISCHARGE PLANNING
- Refer the patient to available resource and support services.

RESOURCES
Organizations
American Cancer Society: *www.cancer.org*
Guide to Internet Resources for Cancer: *www.cancerindex.org*
National Cancer Institute: *www.cancer.gov*
Testicular Cancer Information & Support: *www.tc-cancer.com*
The Testicular Cancer Resource Center: *www.tcrc.acor.org/*

Selected references
Atlas of Pathophysiology, 2nd ed. Philadelphia: Lippincott Williams & Wilkins, 2005.

Gleason, A.M. "Racial Disparities in Testicular Cancer: Impact on Health Promotion," *Journal of Transcultural Nursing* 17(1):58-64, January 2006.

Kleier, J.A. "Nurse Practitioners' Behavior Regarding Teaching Testicular Self-examination," *Journal of the American Academy of Nurse Practitioners* 16(5):206-208, 210, 212 passim, May 2004.

Richie, J.P. "Fertility Gonadal and Sexual Function in Survivors of Testicular Cancer," *Journal of Urology* 175(3 Pt 1):961-62, March 2006.

Stevenson, T.D., and McNeill, J.A. "Surgical Management of Testicular Cancer," *Clinical Journal of Oncology Nursing* 8(4):355-60, August 2004.

van den Belt-Dusebout, A.W., et al. "Long-term Risk of Cardiovascular Disease in 5-year Survivors of Testicular Cancer," *Journal of Clinical Oncology* 24(3):467-75, January 2006.

Testicular torsion

◆ An abnormal twisting of the spermatic cord caused by rotation of a testis or the mesorchium (a fold in the area between the testis and epididymis)
◆ Causes strangulation and eventual infarction of the testis if untreated
◆ 90% of cases unilateral

PATHOPHYSIOLOGY

◆ Normally, the tunica vaginalis envelops the testis and attaches to the epididymis and spermatic cord.
◆ Intravaginal torsion is the most common type of testicular torsion in adolescents.
◆ Testicular twisting in intravaginal torsion may result from an abnormality of the tunica, in which the testis is abnormally positioned, or from a narrowing of the mesentery support.
◆ In extravaginal torsion, most common in neonates, loose attachment of the tunica vaginalis to the scrotal lining causes spermatic cord rotation above the testis. A sudden forceful contraction of the cremaster muscle may precipitate this condition. (See *Extravaginal torsion.*)

CAUSES

◆ Congenital anomaly
◆ Exercise
◆ Sexual activity
◆ Trauma
◆ Undescended testicle

INCIDENCE

◆ This disease occurs most commonly between the ages of 12 and 18, but may occur at any age.

COMPLICATIONS

◆ Loss of testicle
◆ Infarction of testicle
◆ Infection

HISTORY

◆ Previous episodes of intermittent testicular pain that resolved spontaneously
◆ Sudden scrotal pain
◆ Nausea and vomiting
◆ Abdominal pain
◆ Fever

PHYSICAL FINDINGS

◆ Scrotal swelling
◆ Painful testicle
◆ Horizontal lie of the testicle
◆ Scrotal erythema
◆ Ipsilateral loss of the cremasteric reflex

DIAGNOSTIC PROCEDURES

◆ Doppler ultrasonography helps distinguish testicular torsion from strangulated hernia, undescended testes, or epididymitis.

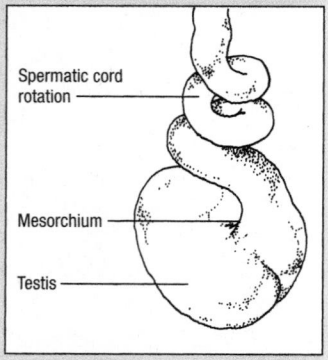

Extravaginal torsion

In extravaginal torsion, rotation of the spermatic cord above the testis causes strangulation and, eventually, infarction of the testis.

Spermatic cord rotation

Mesorchium

Testis

TREATMENT

GENERAL
◆ Manual detorsion

DIET
◆ Nothing by mouth before surgery; as tolerated after surgery

ACTIVITY
◆ As tolerated after surgery

MEDICATIONS
◆ Analgesics

SURGERY
◆ Immediate surgical repair by orchiopexy (fixation of a viable testis to the scrotum) or orchiectomy (excision of a nonviable testis); as with ovarian torsion in the female, preservation of the organ preferred

NURSING CONSIDERATIONS

NURSING DIAGNOSES
◆ Acute pain
◆ Anxiety
◆ Risk for infection
◆ Risk for injury
◆ Situational low self-esteem

EXPECTED OUTCOMES
The patient will:
◆ report increased comfort and decreased pain
◆ report feelings of decreased anxiety
◆ minimize risks for infection
◆ avoid or minimize complications
◆ express positive feelings about self.

NURSING INTERVENTIONS
◆ Promote the patient's comfort before and after surgery.
◆ After surgery, administer drugs for pain.
◆ Apply an ice bag with a cover to reduce edema.
◆ Protect the wound from contamination.

MONITORING
◆ Voiding
◆ Scrotal swelling
◆ Pain control

PATIENT TEACHING

GENERAL
Be sure to cover:
◆ the disorder, diagnosis, and treatment
◆ wound care.

RESOURCES
Organizations
American Urological Association: *www.auanet.org*
Harvard University Consumer Health Information: *www.intelihealth.com*
The Merck Manuals Online Medical Library: *www.merck.com/mmhe*

Selected references
Antao, B., and MacKinnon, A.E. "Axial Fixation of Testes for Prevention of Recurrent Testicular Torsion," *Surgeon* 4(1):20-21, 62, February 2006.

Eaton, S.H., et al. "Intermittent Testicular Torsion: Diagnostic Features and Management Outcomes," *Journal of Urology* 174(4 Pt 2):1532-535, October 2005.

Mansbach, J.M., et al. "Testicular Torsion and Risk Factors for Orchiectomy," *Archives of Pediatric & Adolescent Medicine* 159(12):1167-171, December 2005.

Yerkes, E.B., et al. "Management of Perinatal Torsion: Today, Tomorrow or Never?" *Journal of Urology* 174(4 Pt 2):1579-82, October 2005.

Tetanus LIFE-THREATENING DISORDER

OVERVIEW

- An acute exotoxin-mediated infection
- Usually systemic, but possibly localized
- Up to 60% fatal in unimmunized patients
- Also known as *lockjaw*

PATHOPHYSIOLOGY

- After the organism enters the body, local infection and tissue necrosis result.
- Toxins enter the bloodstream and lymphatics, eventually spreading to central nervous system tissues.
- The incubation period is 3 to 21 days.

CAUSES

- Anaerobic, spore-forming, gram-positive bacillus *Clostridium tetani*
- Transmission through puncture wounds, burns, or minor wounds contaminated by soil, dust, or animal excreta containing *C. tetani*

INCIDENCE

- Tetanus occurs worldwide but is more prevalent in agricultural regions and developing countries that lack mass immunization programs.
- Tetanus is one of the most common causes of neonatal deaths in developing countries.
- In the United States, about 110 cases occur each year; all are in patients who aren't immunized or whose immunization has expired.
- About 75% of cases occur between April and September.

COMPLICATIONS

- Pneumonia
- Airway obstruction
- Respiratory arrest
- Heart failure
- Fractures
- Cardiac arrhythmias
- Rhabdomyolysis
- Death

ASSESSMENT

HISTORY

- Inadequate immunization
- Recent wound or burn
- Pain or paresthesia at the site of injury
- Complaints of difficulty chewing or swallowing food

PHYSICAL FINDINGS

- Spasm and increased muscle tone near the wound (local infection)
- Irregular heartbeat and tachycardia
- Marked muscle hypertonicity
- Hyperactive deep tendon reflexes
- Profuse sweating, low-grade fever
- Painful, involuntary muscle contractions
- Rigid neck and facial muscles, resulting in lockjaw and a grotesque, grinning expression (risus sardonicus)
- Rigid somatic muscles causing arched back rigidity (opisthotonos)
- Intermittent tonic seizures

DIAGNOSTIC TEST RESULTS

LABORATORY

- Blood cultures and tetanus antibody tests are negative in tetanus patients.
- Wound culture is positive in one-third of all tetanus patients.

DIAGNOSTIC PROCEDURES

- A lumbar puncture (spinal tap) may show elevated cerebrospinal fluid pressure.

TREATMENT

GENERAL
◆ Airway maintenance

DIET
◆ Enteral or parenteral feeding

ACTIVITY
◆ Bed rest until recovery

MEDICATIONS
◆ Tetanus immune globulin
◆ Tetanus antitoxin
◆ Tetanus toxoid immunization
◆ Muscle relaxants
◆ Neuromuscular blockers
◆ Antibiotics

NURSING CONSIDERATIONS

NURSING DIAGNOSES
◆ Acute pain
◆ Imbalanced nutrition: Less than body requirements
◆ Impaired physical mobility
◆ Ineffective airway clearance
◆ Ineffective breathing pattern
◆ Ineffective tissue perfusion: Cerebral, peripheral
◆ Risk for deficient fluid volume
◆ Risk for injury

EXPECTED OUTCOMES
The patient will:
◆ express feelings of increased comfort and decreased pain
◆ maintain adequate nutrition and hydration
◆ resume normal physical mobility during recovery
◆ maintain a patent airway
◆ maintain adequate ventilation and oxygenation
◆ maintain tissue perfusion and cellular oxygenation
◆ maintain adequate fluid balance
◆ remain free from injury during severe spasming or seizure activity.

NURSING INTERVENTIONS
◆ Debride and clean the injury site.
◆ Check the immunization history.
◆ Maintain an adequate airway and ventilation.
◆ Keep emergency airway equipment on standby.
◆ Administer I.V. therapy as prescribed.
◆ Minimize stimulation.
◆ Perform range-of-motion exercises.

MONITORING
◆ Response to treatment
◆ Fluid and electrolyte status
◆ Respiratory status
◆ Cardiovascular status
◆ Injury site
◆ Complications
◆ Deep tendon reflexes
◆ Muscle tone

PATIENT TEACHING

GENERAL
Be sure to cover:
◆ the disorder, diagnosis, and treatment
◆ importance of getting a booster dose of tetanus toxoid every 10 years
◆ importance of tetanus prophylaxis in case of a skin injury or burn
◆ importance of avoiding external stimulation (evokes muscle spasms) and to keep the room dark and quiet
◆ potential outcomes.

RESOURCES
Organizations
Centers for Disease Control and Prevention: *www.cdc.gov*
Mayo Clinic: *www.mayoclinic.com*
U.S. Food and Drug Administration: *www.fda.gov*

Selected references
Burton, T., and Crane, S. "Unnecessary Tetanus Boosters in the ED," *Emergency Medicine Journal* 22(8):609-10, August 2005.

Gonzalez-Forero, D., et al. "Transynaptic Effects of Tetanus Neurotoxin in the Oculomotor System," *Brain* 128(9): 2175-88, September 2005.

Hoel, T., et al. "Combined Diphtheria-Tetanus-Pertussis Vaccine for Tetanus-Prone Wound Management in Adults," *European Journal of Emergency Medicine* 13(2):67-71, April 2006.

Kasper, D.L., et al., eds. *Harrison's Principles of Internal Medicine*, 16th ed. New York: McGraw-Hill Book Co., 2005.

Rhee, P., et al. "Tetanus and Trauma: A Review and Recommendations," *Journal of Trauma-Injury Infection & Critical Care* 58(5):1082-1088, May 2005.

Sheffield, J.S., and Ramin, S.M. "Tetanus in Pregnancy," *American Journal of Perinatology* 21(4):173-82, May 2004.

Tetralogy of Fallot

OVERVIEW

- A combination of four cardiac defects: ventricular septal defect (VSD); right ventricular outflow tract obstruction (pulmonary stenosis); right ventricular hypertrophy; and dextroposition of the aorta, with overriding of the VSD

PATHOPHYSIOLOGY

- Blood shunts right to left through the VSD, permitting unoxygenated blood to mix with oxygenated blood, resulting in cyanosis.
- This condition sometimes coexists with other congenital heart defects, such as patent ductus arteriosus or atrial septal defect.

CAUSES

- Exact cause unknown
- Associated with fetal alcohol syndrome and thalidomide use during pregnancy

INCIDENCE

- This disorder accounts for about 10% of all congenital heart diseases.
- This disorder occurs equally in males and females.

COMPLICATIONS

- Cerebral abscesses
- Pulmonary thrombosis
- Venous thrombosis
- Cerebral embolism
- Infective endocarditis
- In females with tetralogy of Fallot who live to childbearing age, increased risk of spontaneous abortion, premature births, and low birth weight

ASSESSMENT

HISTORY

- Blue spells
- Diminished exercise tolerance
- Increasing dyspnea on exertion
- Growth retardation
- Eating difficulties

PHYSICAL FINDINGS

- Clubbing
- Cyanosis
- Dyspnea on exertion
- Loud systolic heart murmur (best heard along the left sternal border), which may diminish or obscure the pulmonic component of S_2
- Cardiac thrill at the left sternal border and an obvious right ventricular impulse
- Prominent inferior sternum

DIAGNOSTIC TEST RESULTS

LABORATORY

- Arterial oxygen saturation is diminished in patients with this disorder.
- Polycythemia is present in patients with this disorder. Hematocrit levels may be more than 60%.

IMAGING

- Chest X-rays may demonstrate decreased pulmonary vascular marking, depending on the severity of the pulmonary obstruction, and a boot-shaped cardiac silhouette.
- Echocardiography identifies septal overriding of the aorta, the VSD, and pulmonary stenosis and detects the hypertrophied walls of the right ventricle.

DIAGNOSTIC PROCEDURES

- An electrocardiogram may show right ventricular hypertrophy, right axis deviation and, possibly, right atrial hypertrophy.
- Cardiac catheterization confirms the diagnosis by showing pulmonary stenosis, the VSD, and the overriding aorta and ruling out other cyanotic heart defects.

TREATMENT

GENERAL
- Prevention and treatment of complications
- During cyanotic spells, knee-chest position and administration of oxygen and morphine to improve oxygenation

MEDICATIONS
- Beta-adrenergic blockers
- Prophylactic antibiotics

SURGERY
- Palliative surgery performed on infants with potentially fatal hypoxic spells; goal of surgery is to enhance blood flow to lungs to reduce hypoxia, commonly accomplished by joining the subclavian artery to the pulmonary artery (Blalock-Taussig procedure)
- Complete corrective surgery relieves pulmonary stenosis, closes VSD; left ventricular outflow directed to aorta

NURSING CONSIDERATIONS

NURSING DIAGNOSES
- Decreased cardiac output
- Delayed growth and development
- Disabled family coping
- Impaired gas exchange

EXPECTED OUTCOMES
The patient (or family) will:
- maintain adequate cardiac output, hemodynamic stability, and have no arrhythmias
- demonstrate age-appropriate skills and behaviors to the extent possible
- agree to seek help from peer support groups or professional counselors to ensure adaptive coping behaviors
- maintain adequate ventilation and oxygenation.

NURSING INTERVENTIONS
- Provide postoperative care.
- Administer drug therapy.
- Explain the disorder and its treatment to the patient's parents. Inform them that their child will set his own exercise limits and will know when to rest.

MONITORING
- Vital signs
- Blue spells
- Oxygenation levels
- Intake and output

PATIENT TEACHING

GENERAL
Be sure to cover:
- how to recognize serious hypoxic spells, which can cause dramatically increased cyanosis; deep, sighing respirations; and loss of consciousness
- preventing infective endocarditis and other infections, and keeping the child away from people with infections
- following good dental hygiene, and watching for ear, nose, and throat infections and dental caries, all of which require immediate treatment.

RESOURCES
Organizations
American Academy of Pediatrics: *www.aap.org*
American Heart Association: *www.americanheart.org*
Mayo Clinic: *www.mayoclinic.com*
National Heart, Lung, and Blood Institute: *www.nhlbi.nih.gov*

Selected references
Chong, W.Y., et al. "Aortic Root Dilation and Aortic Elastic Properties in Children after Repair of Tetralogy of Fallot," *American Journal of Cardiology* 97(6):905-909, March 2006.
McRae, M.E. "Repaired Tetralogy of Fallot in the Adult," *Progress in Cardiovascular Nursing* 20(3):104-10, Summer 2005.
Meijer, J.M., et al. "Pregnancy, Fertility, and Recurrence Risk in Corrected Tetralogy of Fallot," *Heart* 91(6):801-805, June 2005.
Oosterhof, T., et al. "Cardiovascular Magnetic Resonance in the Follow-Up of Patients with Corrected Tetralogy of Fallot: A Review," *American Heart Journal* 151(2):265-72, February 2006.

Thalassemia

OVERVIEW

OVERVIEW

- Group of genetic disorders; characterized by defective synthesis in one or more of polypeptide chains needed for hemoglobin production
- Most commonly occur as a result of reduced or absent production of alpha or beta chains
- Affects hemoglobin production and impairs red blood cell (RBC) synthesis

PATHOPHYSIOLOGY
In beta-thalassemia
- The fundamental defect in thalassemia is the uncoupling of alpha- and beta-chain synthesis.
- Beta-chain production is depressed, moderately in beta-thalassemia minor and severely in beta-thalassemia major (also called *Cooley's anemia*).
- The depression of beta-chain synthesis results in erythrocytes with reduced hemoglobin and accumulations of free-alpha chains.
- The free-alpha chains are unstable and easily precipitate in the cell; most erythroblasts that contain precipitates are destroyed by mononuclear phagocytes in the marrow, resulting in ineffective erythropoiesis and anemia.
- Some precipitate-carrying cells mature and enter the bloodstream but are destroyed prematurely in the spleen, resulting in mild hemolytic anemia.

In alpha-thalassemia
- Four forms exist:
- – alpha trait (the carrier trait), in which a single alpha-chain–forming gene is defective
- – alpha-thalassemia minor, in which two genes are defective
- – hemoglobin H disease, in which three genes are defective
- – alpha-thalassemia major, in which all four alpha-chain–forming genes are defective; death is inevitable because alpha chains are absent and oxygen can't be released to the tissues.

CAUSES
- Inherited autosomal recessive disorder

INCIDENCE
- Thalassemia is the second most common cause of microcytic anemia.
- Alpha-thalassemia is more common in Blacks and Asians.
- Beta-thalassemia is more common in Mediterranean populations.

COMPLICATIONS
- Iron overload from RBC transfusions
- Pathologic fractures
- Cardiac arrhythmias
- Liver failure
- Heart failure
- Death

Skull changes in thalassemia major

This illustration of an X-ray shows a characteristic skull abnormality in thalassemia major: diploetic fibers extending from internal lamina and resembling hair standing on end.

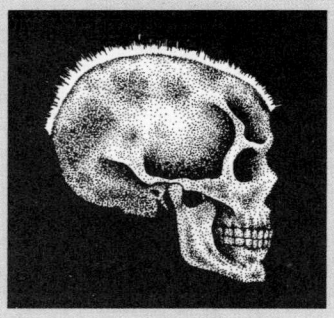

ASSESSMENT

HISTORY
- Severity of anemia and symptoms range from mild to severe; symptoms include fatigue, shortness of breath, headache, angina

PHYSICAL FINDINGS
- Pallor or bronze appearance
- Dyspnea on exertion
- Splenomegaly
- Hepatomegaly
- Tachycardia
- Systolic murmur (in moderate or severe anemia)

DIAGNOSTIC TEST RESULTS

LABORATORY
- A complete blood count may show decreased hemoglobin, hematocrit, and mean corpuscular volume.
- The serum iron level is normal or increased.
- The serum ferritin level is normal or increased.
- The total iron-binding capacity is normal.
- The reticulocyte count is normal or increased.
- A hemoglobin electrophoresis may show decreased alpha- or beta-hemoglobulin chains.

IMAGING
- In thalassemia major, X-rays of the skull and long bones may show a thinning and widening of the marrow space because of overactive bone marrow. Long bones may show areas of osteoporosis. The phalanges may also be deformed (rectangular or biconvex). The bones of the skull and vertebrae may appear granular. (See *Skull changes in thalassemia major.*)

TREATMENT

GENERAL
- No treatment for mild or moderate forms
- Iron supplements contraindicated in all forms

DIET
- Avoidance of iron-rich foods

ACTIVITY
- Avoidance of strenuous activities

MEDICATIONS
- Transfusions of packed RBCs
- Desferal (chelation therapy)

SURGERY
- Splenectomy
- Bone marrow transplantation

NURSING CONSIDERATIONS

NURSING DIAGNOSES
- Activity intolerance
- Delayed growth and development
- Disturbed body image
- Ineffective tissue perfusion: Cardiopulmonary
- Interrupted family processes
- Risk for infection

EXPECTED OUTCOMES
The patient (or family) will:
- verbalize the importance of balancing activity, as tolerated, with frequent rest periods
- demonstrate age-appropriate skills and behaviors to the extent possible
- express positive feelings about himself
- maintain hemodynamic stability and develop no arrhythmias
- discuss how the patient's condition has affected the family's daily life
- remain free from signs and symptoms of infection.

NURSING INTERVENTIONS
- Administer blood transfusions, and watch for adverse reactions.
- Provide an adequate diet, and encourage oral fluid intake.
- Provide emotional support to help the patient and family cope with the chronic nature of the illness and the need for lifelong transfusions.

MONITORING
- Transfusion reaction
- Signs and symptoms of iron overload
- Complications
- Cardiac arrhythmias
- Anemia symptom severity
- Response to treatment

PATIENT TEACHING

GENERAL
Be sure to cover:
- the disorder, diagnosis, and treatment
- importance of good nutrition
- signs and symptoms of iron overload
- follow-up care
- various options for healthy physical and creative outlets with the parents of a young patient. Such a child must avoid strenuous athletic activity. Reassure the parents that the child may be allowed to participate in less stressful activities.

DISCHARGE PLANNING
- Refer the patient to a hematologist.
- Refer the patient for genetic counseling.

RESOURCES
Organizations
Cooley's Anemia Foundation: *www.cooleysanemia.org*
Iron Disorders Institute: *www.irondisorders.org*
National Heart, Lung, and Blood Institute: *www.nhlbi.nih.gov*
Thalassaemia International Federation: *www.thalassaemia.org.cy*

Selected references
Aessopos, A., et al. "Cardiac Status in Well-Treated Patients with Thalassemia Major," *European Journal of Haematology* 73(5):359-66, November 2004.

Aydinok, Y., et al. "Psychosocial Implications of Thalassemia Major," *Pediatrics International* 47(1):84-89, February 2005.

Chui, D.H., et al. "Screening and Counseling for Thalassemia," *Blood* 107(4):1735-37, February 2005.

Kasper, D.L., et al., eds. *Harrison's Principles of Internal Medicine,* 16th ed. New York: McGraw-Hill Book Co., 2005.

Tierney, L., et al. *Current Medical Diagnosis & Treatment 2006.* New York: McGraw-Hill Book Co., 2006.

Thrombocytopenia

OVERVIEW

- A deficient number of circulating platelets
- The most common cause of hemorrhagic disorders

PATHOPHYSIOLOGY

- A lack of platelets can cause inadequate hemostasis.
- Four mechanisms are responsible for the lack of platelets: decreased platelet production, decreased platelet survival, pooling of blood in the spleen, and intravascular dilation of circulating platelets.
- Megakaryocytes are giant cells in bone marrow that produce the marrow. Platelet production decreases when the number of megakaryocytes is reduced or when platelet production becomes dysfunctional.

CAUSES

- Decreased or defective platelet production in the bone marrow
- Increased platelet destruction outside the marrow caused by an underlying disorder (such as cirrhosis of the liver, disseminated intravascular coagulation, or severe infection)
- May be congenital or acquired
- Sequestration (hypersplenism, hypothermia) or platelet loss
- Transient occurrence after a viral infection or infectious mononucleosis

INCIDENCE

- The acquired form of this condition is more common.

COMPLICATIONS

Severe thrombocytopenia
- Hemorrhage
- Death

ASSESSMENT

HISTORY

- Sudden onset of petechiae and ecchymoses or bleeding into mucous membranes (GI, urinary, vaginal, or respiratory)
- Malaise, fatigue, and general weakness, with or without accompanying blood loss
- In acquired thrombocytopenia, possible use of one or several offending drugs
- Menorrhagia

PHYSICAL FINDINGS

- Petechiae and ecchymoses, along with slow, continuous bleeding from any injuries or wounds
- In adults, blood-filled bullae in the mouth

DIAGNOSTIC TEST RESULTS

LABORATORY

- Platelet count is diminished to less than 100,000/µl in adults with this disease.
- Bleeding time is prolonged.
- Prothrombin and partial thromboplastin times are normal.

DIAGNOSTIC PROCEDURES

- In severe thrombocytopenia, a bone marrow study will show the number, sizes, and cytoplasmic maturity of the megakaryocytes (bone marrow cells that release mature platelets); the study may show ineffective platelet production as the cause of thrombocytopenia and be used to rule out a malignant disease process.

TREATMENT

GENERAL

- Removal of the offending agents in drug-induced thrombocytopenia

DIET

- Well-balanced

ACTIVITY

- Rest periods between activities
- During active bleeding, strict bed rest

MEDICATIONS

- Platelet transfusions
- Corticosteroids
- Immune globulin

SURGERY

- Splenectomy

NURSING CONSIDERATIONS

NURSING DIAGNOSES
◆ Activity intolerance
◆ Anxiety
◆ Disturbed body image
◆ Fatigue
◆ Impaired skin integrity
◆ Ineffective coping
◆ Ineffective protection
◆ Risk for infection
◆ Risk for injury

EXPECTED OUTCOMES
The patient will:
◆ verbalize the importance of balancing activity, as tolerated, with rest
◆ state measures to reduce levels of anxiety
◆ express positive feelings about self
◆ express feelings of increased energy
◆ exhibit improved or healed wounds or lesions
◆ demonstrate effective coping skills
◆ demonstrate use of protective measures, including conserving energy, maintaining a balanced diet, and getting adequate rest
◆ experience no fever, chills, or other signs or symptoms of illness
◆ incur no injuries.

NURSING INTERVENTIONS
◆ Provide emotional support.
◆ Provide rest periods between activities.
◆ Provide a stool softener if necessary.
◆ Protect all areas of ecchymosis and petechiae from further injury.
◆ Take precautions against bleeding; protect the patient from trauma.
◆ Avoid invasive procedures.
◆ During active bleeding, maintain strict bed rest; keep the head of the bed elevated.

MONITORING
◆ Daily platelet count
◆ Bleeding
◆ Ecchymoses and petechiae
◆ Occult blood in stool, urine, and emesis
◆ During corticosteroid therapy, fluid and electrolyte balance and signs and symptoms of infection, pathologic fractures, and mood changes

PATIENT TEACHING

GENERAL
Be sure to cover:
◆ disorder and its cause, if known, and, if appropriate, reassuring the patient that thrombocytopenia commonly resolves spontaneously
◆ how to recognize and report signs of intracranial bleeding and other signs of bleeding
◆ avoidance of straining with stools and coughing, both of which can lead to increased intracranial pressure
◆ function of platelets
◆ importance of understanding that even minor bumps or scrapes may result in bleeding if thrombocytopenia is severe
◆ how to control local bleeding
◆ importance of avoiding the offending drug in drug-induced thrombocytopenia
◆ importance of watching for and reporting cushingoid symptoms and discontinuing corticosteroids gradually in patients who must receive long-term corticosteroid therapy
◆ avoidance of aspirin in any form as well as other drugs that impair coagulation
◆ using a humidifier at night if the patient experiences frequent nosebleeds
◆ how to examine the skin for ecchymoses and petechiae
◆ how to test stools for occult blood
◆ importance of wearing medical identification jewelry.

RESOURCES
Organizations
Harvard University Consumer Health Information: *www.intelihealth.com*
Mayo Clinic: *www.mayoclinic.com*
The Merck Manuals Online Medical Library: *www.merck.com/mmhe*
National Heart, Lung, and Blood Institute: *www.nhlbi.nih.gov*

Selected references
Begelman, S.M., et al. "Heparin-induced Thrombocytopenia from Venous Thromboembolism Treatment," *Journal of Internal Medicine* 258(6):563-72, December 2005.
Francis, J.L., and Drexler, A.J. "Striking Back at Heparin-induced Thrombocytopenia," *Nursing* 35(9):48-51, September 2005.
Gyamfi, C., and Eddleman, K.A. "Alloimmune Thrombocytopenia," *Clinical Obstetrics & Gynecology* 48(4):897-909, December 2005.
Kasper, D.L., et al., eds. *Harrison's Principles of Internal Medicine,* 16th ed. New York: McGraw-Hill Book Co., 2005.
Tierney, L., et al. *Current Medical Diagnosis & Treatment 2006.* New York: McGraw-Hill Book Co., 2006.

Thrombophlebitis

- Development of a thrombus that may cause vessel occlusion or embolization
- An acute condition characterized by inflammation and thrombus formation
- May occur in deep or superficial veins (see *Major venous pathways of the leg*)
- Typically occurs at the valve cusps because venous stasis encourages accumulation and adherence of platelet and fibrin

PATHOPHYSIOLOGY

- Alterations in the epithelial lining cause platelet aggregation and fibrin entrapment of red blood cells, white blood cells, and additional platelets.
- The thrombus initiates a chemical inflammatory process in the vessel epithelium that leads to fibrosis, which may occlude the vessel lumen or embolize.

CAUSES

- Fracture of the spine, pelvis, femur, or tibia
- Hormonal contraceptives such as estrogens
- May be idiopathic
- Neoplasms
- Pregnancy and childbirth
- Prolonged bed rest
- Surgery
- Trauma
- Venous stasis
- Venulitis

INCIDENCE

- The incidence of this disorder is increasing with the use of subclavian vein catheters.
- The risk for developing deep vein thrombophlebitis dramatically increases after age 40.

COMPLICATIONS

- Pulmonary embolism
- Chronic venous insufficiency

HISTORY

- Asymptomatic in up to 50% of patients with deep vein thrombophlebitis
- Possible tenderness, aching, or severe pain in the affected leg or arm; fever, chills, and malaise

PHYSICAL FINDINGS

- Redness, swelling, and tenderness of the affected leg or arm
- Possible positive Homans' sign
- Positive cuff sign
- Possible warm feeling in affected leg or arm
- Lymphadenitis in case of extensive vein involvement

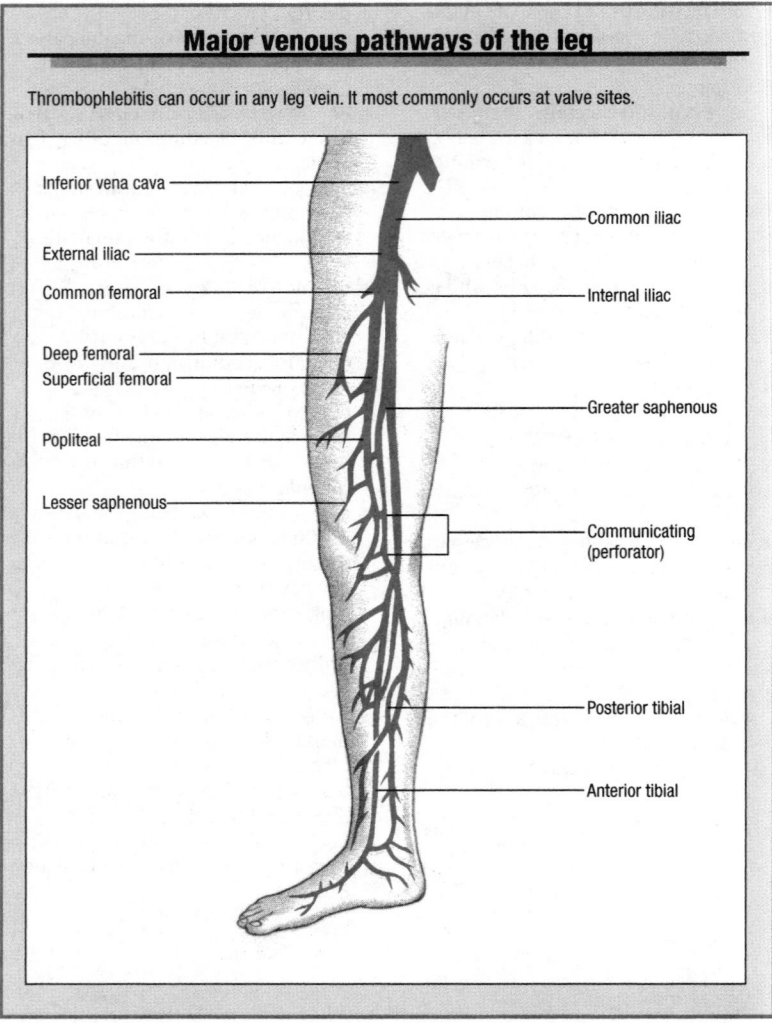

Major venous pathways of the leg

Thrombophlebitis can occur in any leg vein. It most commonly occurs at valve sites.

- Inferior vena cava
- External iliac
- Common femoral
- Deep femoral
- Superficial femoral
- Popliteal
- Lesser saphenous
- Common iliac
- Internal iliac
- Greater saphenous
- Communicating (perforator)
- Posterior tibial
- Anterior tibial

DIAGNOSTIC TEST RESULTS

DIAGNOSTIC PROCEDURES
◆ Doppler ultrasonography may show a reduced blood flow to a specific area and any obstruction to the venous flow, particularly in iliofemoral deep vein thrombophlebitis.
◆ Plethysmography may show a decreased circulation distal to the affected area; this test is more sensitive than ultrasonography in detecting deep vein thrombophlebitis.
◆ Phlebography confirms the diagnosis and may show filling defects and a diverted blood flow.

TREATMENT

GENERAL
◆ Application of warm, moist compresses to the affected area
◆ Antiembolism stockings

ACTIVITY
◆ Bed rest, with elevation of the affected extremity

MEDICATIONS
◆ Anticoagulants
◆ Thrombolytics
◆ Analgesics

SURGERY
◆ Simple ligation to vein plication, or clipping
◆ Embolectomy
◆ Caval interruption with transvenous placement of a vena cava filter

NURSING CONSIDERATIONS

NURSING DIAGNOSES
◆ Activity intolerance
◆ Acute pain
◆ Impaired skin integrity
◆ Ineffective tissue perfusion: Cardiopulmonary, peripheral
◆ Risk for infection
◆ Risk for injury

EXPECTED OUTCOMES
The patient will:
◆ reduce metabolic demands
◆ express feelings of increased comfort and decreased pain
◆ maintain normal skin color and temperature
◆ maintain tissue perfusion and cellular oxygenation
◆ develop no signs or symptoms of infection
◆ remain free from complications.

NURSING INTERVENTIONS
◆ Enforce bed rest and elevate the patient's affected arm or leg, but avoid compressing the popliteal space.
◆ Apply warm compresses or a covered aquathermia pad.
◆ Give prescribed analgesics.
◆ Mark, measure, and record the circumference of the affected arm or leg daily, and compare this measurement with that of the other arm or leg.
◆ Give prescribed anticoagulants.
◆ Perform or encourage range-of-motion exercises.
◆ Use pneumatic compression devices.
◆ Apply antiembolism stockings.
◆ Encourage early ambulation.

MONITORING
◆ Signs and symptoms of bleeding
◆ Vital signs
◆ Partial thromboplastin time for patient on heparin therapy
◆ Prothrombin time for patient on warfarin
◆ Signs and symptoms of heparin-induced thrombocytopenia
◆ Signs and symptoms of pulmonary embolism
◆ Response to treatment

PATIENT TEACHING

GENERAL
Be sure to cover:
◆ the disorder, diagnosis, and treatment
◆ importance of follow-up blood studies to monitor anticoagulant therapy
◆ how to give injections, if necessary
◆ avoidance of prolonged sitting or standing
◆ proper application and use of antiembolism stockings
◆ importance of adequate hydration
◆ use of an electric razor
◆ avoidance of products that contain aspirin.

RESOURCES
Organizations
Harvard University Consumer Health Information: *www.intelihealth.com*
Mayo Clinic: *www.mayoclinic.com*
The Merck Manuals Online Medical Library: *www.merck.com/mmhe*
National Heart, Lung, and Blood Institute: *www.nhlbi.nih.gov*

Selected references
Chirinos, J.A., et al. "Septic Thrombophlebitis: Diagnosis and Management," *American Journal of Cardiovascular Drugs* 6(1):9-14, 2006.
Comp, P.C. "Should Coagulation Tests Be Used to Determine which Oral Contraceptive Users Have an Increased Risk of Thrombophlebitis?" *Contraception* 73(1):4-5, January 2006.
Craig, A. "Pain, Inflammation and a Nodule after IV Medication," *Advance for Nurse Practitioners* 13(7):21-22, July 2005.
Decousus, H., and Leizorovicz, A. "Superficial Thrombophlebitis of the Legs: Still a Lot to Learn," *Journal of Thrombosis and Haemostasis* 3(6):1149-151, June 2005.
Kasper, D.L., et al., eds. *Harrison's Principles of Internal Medicine*, 16th ed. New York: McGraw-Hill Book Co., 2005.
The Merck Manual of Diagnosis & Therapy, 18th ed., Whitehouse Station, N.J.: Merck & Co., Inc., 2006.

Thyroid cancer

- Proliferation of cancer cells in the thyroid gland
- The most common endocrine malignancy
- Papillary carcinomas: 80% of all cases
- Medullary cancer: may be associated with pheochromocytoma; curable when detected before it causes symptoms

PATHOPHYSIOLOGY

- Papillary cancer is usually multifocal and bilateral. It metastasizes slowly into regional nodes of the neck, mediastinum, lungs, and other distant organs.
- Papillary cancer is the least virulent form of thyroid cancer.
- Follicular cancer is less common but is more likely to recur and metastasize to the regional lymph nodes and spread through blood vessels into the bones, liver, and lungs.
- Medullary (solid) carcinoma originates in the parafollicular cells derived from the last branchial pouch and contains amyloid and calcium deposits. It can produce calcitonin, histaminase, corticotropin (producing Cushing's syndrome), and prostaglandin E2 and F3. Untreated medullary cancer grows rapidly, commonly metastasizing to bones, liver, and kidneys.
- Anaplastic carcinoma (giant and spindly cell cancer) resists radiation and is almost never curable by resection. This cancer metastasizes rapidly, causing death by invading the trachea and compressing adjacent structures.

CAUSES

- Previous exposure to radiation treatment in the neck area
- Prolonged secretion of thyroid-stimulating hormone (radiation or heredity)

RISK FACTORS

- Familial predisposition (possibly inherited as an autosomal dominant trait)
- Chronic goiter

INCIDENCE

- Thyroid cancer occurs in 1 to 3 per 100,000 men.
- Thyroid cancer occurs in 2 to 4 per 100,000 women.
- This disease occurs in Iceland and Hawaii nearly twice as often as in Canada and the U.S. mainland.
- Thyroid cancer is particularly common among Chinese males and Filipino females.
- Thyroid cancer is rare in children.

COMPLICATIONS

- Dysphagia
- Stridor
- Hormone alterations
- Distant metastasis

HISTORY

- Sensitivity to cold and mental apathy (hypothyroidism)
- Sensitivity to heat, restlessness, and overactivity (hyperthyroidism)
- Diarrhea
- Dysphagia
- Anorexia
- Irritability
- Ear pain

PHYSICAL FINDINGS

- Hard, painless nodule in an enlarged thyroid gland or palpable lymph nodes with thyroid enlargement
- Hoarseness and vocal stridor
- Disfiguring thyroid mass
- Bruits

LABORATORY

- A calcitonin assay may identify silent medullary carcinoma. Measuring the calcitonin level in a resting state and during calcium infusion (15 mg/kg over 4 hours) may show an elevated fasting calcitonin level and an abnormal response to calcium stimulation, indicating medullary cancer.

IMAGING

- A thyroid scan differentiates functional nodes, which are rarely malignant, from hypofunctional nodes, which are commonly malignant.
- An ultrasonography may show changes in the sizes of thyroid nodules after thyroxine suppression therapy. It's also used to guide fine-needle aspiration and detect recurrent disease.
- Magnetic resonance imaging and computed tomography scans provide a basis for treatment planning by showing the extent of the disease in the thyroid and surrounding structures.

DIAGNOSTIC PROCEDURES

- A fine-needle aspiration biopsy differentiates benign from malignant thyroid nodules.
- A histologic analysis stages the disease and thereby guides treatment plans.

GENERAL
◆ Radioisotope (^{131}I) therapy with external radiation (sometimes postoperatively in lieu of radical neck excision) or alone (for metastasis)

DIET
◆ Soft diet with small frequent meals if dysphagia occurs

MEDICATIONS
◆ Suppressive thyroid hormone therapy
◆ Chemotherapy

SURGERY
Papillary or follicular cancer
◆ Total or subtotal thyroidectomy with modified node dissection (bilateral or homolateral) on the side of the primary cancer

Medullary or anaplastic cancer
◆ Total thyroidectomy and radical neck excision

NURSING CONSIDERATIONS

NURSING DIAGNOSES
◆ Acute pain
◆ Anxiety
◆ Diarrhea
◆ Disturbed body image
◆ Imbalanced nutrition: Less than body requirements
◆ Impaired gas exchange
◆ Impaired skin integrity
◆ Impaired swallowing
◆ Impaired verbal communication
◆ Ineffective airway clearance
◆ Risk for aspiration

EXPECTED OUTCOMES
The patient will:
◆ express feelings of increased comfort and decreased pain
◆ express feelings of decreased anxiety
◆ resume a normal elimination pattern
◆ express positive feelings about self
◆ maintain current weight without further loss
◆ maintain adequate ventilation and oxygenation
◆ maintain skin integrity
◆ maintain the ability to swallow
◆ express feelings and needs without frustration
◆ maintain a patent airway
◆ not aspirate.

NURSING INTERVENTIONS
◆ Encourage verbalization and provide support.

Before surgery
◆ Prepare the patient for scheduled surgery.
◆ Establish a way to communicate postoperatively.

After surgery
◆ Keep the patient in semi-Fowler's position, with adequate neck support.
◆ Keep a tracheotomy set and oxygen equipment nearby in case of respiratory obstruction.

MONITORING
◆ Vital signs
◆ Wound site
◆ Pain control
◆ Serum calcium levels (if the parathyroid glands were removed)
◆ Postoperative complications
◆ Hydration and nutritional status

PATIENT TEACHING

GENERAL
Be sure to cover:
◆ the disorder, diagnosis, and treatment
◆ surgical and postoperative procedures and positioning
◆ treatments and home care
◆ drug administration, dosage, and possible adverse effects.

DISCHARGE PLANNING
◆ Refer the patient to available resource and support services.

RESOURCES
Organizations
American Cancer Society:
www.cancer.org
Guide to Internet Resources for Cancer:
www.cancerindex.org
National Cancer Institute:
www.cancer.gov

Selected references
Atlas of Pathophysiology, 2nd ed. Philadelphia: Lippincott Williams & Wilkins, 2005.

Clark, J.R., et al. "Variables Predicting Distant Metastases in Thyroid Cancer," *Laryngoscope* 115(4):661-67, April 2005.

Hameed, R., and Zacharin, M.R. "Changing Face of Paediatric and Adolescent Thyroid Cancer," *Journal of Paediatrics & Child Health* 41(11):572-74, November 2005.

Kumar, V., et al. "Anaplastic Thyroid Cancer and Hyperthyroidism," *Endocrine Pathology* 16(3):245-50, Fall 2005.

Pacilio, M., et al. "Management of ^{131}I Therapy for Thyroid Cancer: Cumulative Dose from In-Patients, Discharge Planning and Personnel Requirements," *Nuclear Medicine Communications* 26(7):623-31, July 2005.

Patel, K.N., and Shaha, A.R. "Locally Advanced Thyroid Cancer," *Current Opinion in Otolaryngology & Head & Neck Surgery* 13(2):112-16, April 2005.

Thyroiditis

- Several disorders that involve inflammation of the thyroid gland
- Autoimmune (Hashimoto's) thyroiditis: the most common chronic inflammatory disease of the thyroid gland
- Postpartum thyroiditis: a form of autoimmune thyroiditis that occurs within 1 year of delivery
- Subacute thyroiditis: a transient inflammation of the thyroid gland that's probably viral in origin
- Riedel's thyroiditis: a rare condition with unknown etiology that may be a variant of Hashimoto's thyroiditis
- Supportive thyroiditis: an uncommon bacterial or fungal infection of the thyroid that's potentially very serious
- Silent thyroiditis: a transient hyperthyroid condition that's characterized by a small painless goiter and may be autoimmune in origin

PATHOPHYSIOLOGY

- The inflammatory process has varying effects on thyroid hormone levels; levels may be low, normal, or high. Also, lymphocytes and leukocytes may infiltrate thyroid tissue.
- Hashimoto's thyroiditis is thought to result from lymphocytic infiltration of the thyroid gland and formation of antibodies to thyroid antigens in the blood.
- Riedel's thyroiditis causes intense fibrosis of the thyroid and surrounding structures.

CAUSES

- Actinomycosis
- Bacterial infection
- Influenza, coxsackievirus, or adenovirus infections
- Mumps
- Sarcoidosis and amyloidosis
- Syphilis
- Tuberculosis

INCIDENCE

- Thyroiditis is more common in women than in men.

- Autoimmune thyroiditis is most common in middle-age women and is the most common cause of sporadic goiter in children.
- Postpartum thyroiditis occurs within 1 year of delivery.

COMPLICATIONS

- Depending on type of inflammation:
- Non-Hodgkin's lymphoma of the thyroid gland
- Permanent hypothyroid or hyperthyroid condition
- Abscess formation and rupture
- Tracheal or esophageal compression, necrosis, and hemorrhage

ASSESSMENT

HISTORY

- Recent viral or bacterial infection
- Disorder, such as systemic lupus erythematosus, rheumatoid arthritis, pernicious anemia, or Graves' disease
- Gradual onset of hypothyroid-like symptoms
- Occasionally, symptoms of hyperthyroidism
- Local pain or pain referred to the lower jaw, ear, or occiput
- Dysphagia
- Dyspnea
- Asthenia, malaise

PHYSICAL FINDINGS

- Enlargement of the thyroid gland (goiter)
- Reddened skin over the thyroid gland
- Indurated neck tissues
- Small, firm, and finely nodular thyroid gland with a characteristic bandlike depression circling the gland
- A small lymph node in the midline above the isthmus
- Nodularity
- Swelling and warmth of the overlying skin
- Woody, hard enlargement that feels "anchored" to surrounding structures
- Stridor

DIAGNOSTIC TEST RESULTS

LABORATORY

- In autoimmune processes, serum thyroglobulin and microsomal antibody levels are increased.

Hashimoto's thyroiditis

- The thyroid-stimulating hormone (TSH) level is increased.
- The triiodothyronine and thyroxine levels are normal or decreased.
- The antimicrosomal and antithyroglobulin antibodies are increased.

Subacute thyroiditis

- Thyroid hormone levels may be elevated, suppressed, or normal depending on the phase of the disorder.
- Protein-bound iodine levels are increased.
- TSH levels are decreased in the thyrotoxic phase, failing to respond to thyrotropin-releasing hormone; in the hypothyroid phase, TSH levels are increased.
- Radioactive iodine (^{131}I) uptake is decreased.
- Erythrocyte sedimentation rate, white blood cell count, and hepatic enzyme levels are increased.
- Thyroid antibody levels are transiently low.
- Thyroglobin levels are increased.

Riedel's thyroiditis

- ^{131}I uptake is normal or decreased.
- Antimicrosomal antibody levels are increased.

IMAGING

- Thyroid scan may show isolated areas of function or total failure to visualize the gland.

DIAGNOSTIC PROCEDURES

- Fine-needle thyroid gland biopsy offers histologic confirmation.

TREATMENT

GENERAL
- Varies with the type of thyroiditis

ACTIVITY
- As tolerated

MEDICATIONS
- Thyroid hormone
- Analgesics
- Anti-inflammatory drugs
- Beta-adrenergic blockers
- Corticosteroids
- Antibiotics

SURGERY
- Partial thyroidectomy

NURSING CONSIDERATIONS

NURSING DIAGNOSES
- Acute pain
- Disturbed body image
- Imbalanced nutrition: Less than body requirements
- Impaired swallowing
- Ineffective airway clearance
- Ineffective coping

EXPECTED OUTCOMES
The patient will:
- express feelings of increased comfort
- express positive feelings about self
- consume adequate daily caloric intake
- swallow without coughing or choking
- maintain a patent airway
- demonstrate adaptive coping behaviors.

NURSING INTERVENTIONS
- Administer drug therapy.
- Elevate the head of the bed 90 degrees during mealtimes and for 30 minutes afterward.
- Keep suction equipment readily available.
- Consult the dietitian.
- Provide frequent mouth care.
- Provide meticulous skin care.
- Provide comfort measures.
- Encourage oral fluid intake.
- Encourage verbalization of feelings.
- Offer emotional support.
- Help develop effective coping strategies.

⚡ **WARNING** *After a thyroidectomy, watch for signs of tetany, caused by accidental parathyroid injury during surgery. Keep 10% calcium gluconate available for I.V. use if needed. Check dressings frequently for excessive bleeding. Watch for signs of airway obstruction, such as difficulty talking or increased swallowing, and keep tracheotomy equipment handy.*

MONITORING
- Vital signs
- Intake and output
- Daily weight
- Respiratory status
- Signs and symptoms of hyperthyroidism or hypothyroidism
- Neck circumference

PATIENT TEACHING

GENERAL
Be sure to cover:
- the disorder, diagnosis, and treatment
- drug administration, dosage, and possible adverse effects
- when to notify the physician
- signs and symptoms of respiratory distress
- signs and symptoms of hyperthyroidism and hypothyroidism
- long-term hormone replacement therapy after thyroidectomy
- importance of wearing or carrying medical identification.

DISCHARGE PLANNING
- Refer the patient to a mental health professional for additional counseling if indicated.

RESOURCES
Organizations
American Foundation of Thyroid Patients: *www.thyroidfoundation.org*
American Thyroid Association: *www.thyroid.org*
Endocrine and Metabolic Diseases Information Service: *www.endocrine.niddk.nih.gov*
Endocrine Society: *www.endo-society.org*
Thyroid Foundation of American: *www.tsh.org*

Selected references
Cipolla, C., et al. "Hashimoto Thyroiditis Coexistent with Papillary Thyroid Carcinoma," *The American Surgeon* 71(10):874-78, October 2005.

Erdem, F., et al. "Autoimmune Thyroiditis during Thalidomide Treatment," *American Journal of Hematology* 81(2):152, February 2006.

Goldani, L.Z., et al. "Fungal Thyroiditis: An Overview," *Mycopathologia* 161(3):129-39, March 2006.

Lucas, A., et al. "Postpartum Thyroiditis: Long-term Follow-up," *Thyroid* 15(10):1177-181, October 2005.

Stagi, S., et al. "Thyroid Function, Autoimmune Thyroiditis and Coeliac Disease in Juvenile Idiopathic Arthritis," *Rheumatology* 44(4):517-20, April 2005.

Tonsillitis

OVERVIEW

- Inflammation of the tonsils
- May be acute or chronic
- Typical viral infection: Mild and of limited duration

PATHOPHYSIOLOGY

- The inflammatory response to cell damage by viruses or bacteria may result in hyperemia and fluid exudation.

CAUSES

- Bacterial infection (group A beta-hemolytic streptococci)
- Viral infection

INCIDENCE

- Tonsillitis is more common in children than adults.
- Viral tonsillitis is more common than bacterial tonsillitis.
- Bacterial infection occurs more frequently in the winter.

  AGE FACTOR *Tonsillitis common-ly affects children between ages 5 and 10. Tonsils tend toward hyper-trophy during childhood and atrophy after puberty.*

COMPLICATIONS

- Chronic upper airway obstruction
- Sleep disturbance, sleep apnea
- Cor pulmonale
- Failure to thrive
- Eating or swallowing disorders
- Speech abnormalities
- Febrile seizures
- Otitis media
- Cardiac valvular disease
- Peritonsillar abscesses
- Glomerulonephritis
- Bacterial endocarditis
- Cervical lymph node abscesses

ASSESSMENT

HISTORY

- Mild to severe sore throat
- Young child possibly stops eating
- Muscle and joint pain
- Chills
- Malaise
- Headache
- Pain, commonly referred to the ears
- Constant urge to swallow
- Constricted feeling in the back of the throat

PHYSICAL FINDINGS

- Fever
- Swollen, tender submandibular lymph nodes
- Generalized inflammation of pharyngeal wall
- Swollen tonsils projecting from between the pillars of the fauces and exuding white or yellow follicles
- Purulent drainage with application of pressure to tonsillar pillars
- Uvula possibly edematous and inflamed

DIAGNOSTIC TEST RESULTS

LABORATORY

- A throat culture may reveal the infecting organism.
- A serum white blood cell count usually reveals leukocytosis.

TREATMENT

GENERAL

- Symptom relief

DIET

- Adequate fluid intake

ACTIVITY

- Rest periods as needed

MEDICATIONS

- Aspirin or acetaminophen
- Antibiotics

SURGERY

- Possible tonsillectomy

NURSING DIAGNOSES

◆ Acute pain
◆ Anxiety
◆ Impaired swallowing
◆ Ineffective breathing pattern
◆ Risk for aspiration
◆ Risk for deficient fluid volume

EXPECTED OUTCOMES

The patient will:
◆ express feelings of increased comfort
◆ express feelings of decreased anxiety
◆ swallow without pain or aspiration
◆ maintain an effective breathing pattern, with a respiratory rate within 5 breaths/minute of baseline
◆ show no signs of aspiration
◆ have adequate fluid volume, with balanced intake and output.

NURSING INTERVENTIONS

Before surgery

◆ Encourage oral fluids.
◆ Offer a child ice cream and flavored drinks and ices.
◆ Provide humidification.
◆ Encourage gargling to soothe the throat and remove debris from tonsillar crypts.

After surgery

◆ Maintain a patent airway.
◆ Prevent aspiration by side positioning.
◆ Keep suction equipment readily available.
◆ Provide water after gag reflex returns.
◆ Later, encourage nonirritating oral fluids.
◆ Avoid milk products and salty or irritating foods.
◆ Provide analgesics for pain relief.
◆ Encourage deep-breathing exercises.

MONITORING

◆ Hydration status
◆ Effect of pain medication

Before surgery

◆ Bleeding abnormalities

After surgery

◆ Vital signs
◆ Signs and symptoms of bleeding
◆ Respiratory status

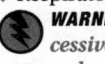 **WARNING** *Immediately report excessive bleeding, increased pulse rate, or decreasing blood pressure.*

 WARNING *The greatest risk of bleeding is 7 to 10 days after surgery.*

GENERAL

Be sure to cover:
◆ the disorder, diagnosis, and treatment
◆ importance of completing the entire course of antibiotics
◆ avoidance of irritants
◆ importance of eating soft foods for about 3 weeks after surgery to decrease the risk of rebleeding
◆ medications, dosages, and possible adverse effects
◆ possibility of throat discomfort and some bleeding after surgery
◆ expecting a white scab to form in the throat 5 to 10 days after surgery
◆ importance of reporting bleeding, ear discomfort, or a fever that lasts 3 days or more.

RESOURCES

Organizations

American Academy of Allergy, Asthma & Immunology: *www.aaaai.org*
Harvard University Consumer Health Information: *www.intelihealth.com*
Mayo Clinic: *www.mayoclinic.com*
National Institute of Allergy and Infectious Diseases: *www.niaid.nih.gov*

Selected references

Deason, J., and Hope, B. "A 23-year-old Man with Chest Pressure, Pallor, Tachypnea, and Tonsillitis," *Journal of Emergency Nursing* 31(2):199-202, April 2005.

Giger, R., et al. "Hemorrhage Risk after Quinsy Tonsillectomy," *Otolaryngology — Head and Neck Surgery* 133(5): 729-34, November 2005.

Ohashi, M., et al. "Severe Acute Tonsillitis Caused by Rothia Dentocariosa in a Healthy Child," *Pediatric Infectious Disease Journal* 24(5):466-67, May 2005.

Webb, C.J., et al. "Tonsillar Size Is an Important Indicator of Recurrent Acute Tonsillitis," *Clinical Otolaryngology & Allied Sciences* 29(4):369-71, August 2004.

Toxic shock syndrome LIFE-THREATENING DISORDER

OVERVIEW

- An inflammatory response syndrome linked to bacterial infections
- An acute and life-threatening condition
- Often associated with menstruation
- Also called *TSS*

PATHOPHYSIOLOGY

- Toxic exoproteins are produced by infecting organisms.
- TSST-1 is the most common toxin; staphylococcal enterotoxin B is the second most common.
- For the illness to develop, the patient must be infected with a toxigenic strain of *Staphylococcus aureus* and lack antibodies to that strain.

CAUSES

- Penicillin-resistant *S. aureus*

RISK FACTORS

- Tampon use
- Varicella infection
- Streptococcal pharyngitis
- Childbirth
- Abortion

INCIDENCE

- Toxic shock syndrome affects 1 in 100,000 people.
- TSS primarily affects young people.
- Half of all cases of TSS occur in settings other than menstruation.
- TSS affects both sexes and all ages.

COMPLICATIONS

- Septic abortion
- Musculoskeletal and respiratory infections
- Staphylococcal bacteremia
- Renal and myocardial dysfunction
- Acute respiratory distress syndrome
- Desquamation of the skin
- Peripheral gangrene
- Muscle weakness
- Neuropsychiatric dysfunction

ASSESSMENT

HISTORY

- Possible recent streptococcal infection
- Possible tampon usage or menstruation
- Intense myalgia, headache
- Nausea, vomiting, and diarrhea
- Sore throat
- Dizziness

PHYSICAL FINDINGS

- Sudden onset of fever (104° F [40° C] or higher)
- Pharyngeal infection, strawberry tongue
- Hypotension
- Altered mental status
- Macular erythroderma (generalized or local)
- Peripheral edema
- Vaginal hyperemia, purulent vaginal discharge

DIAGNOSTIC TEST RESULTS

LABORATORY

- The isolation of *S. aureus* from vaginal discharge or the infection site supports the diagnosis. (See *Guidelines for diagnosing toxic shock syndrome.*)
- The blood urea nitrogen examination may show azotemia.
- A urinalysis may show pyuria.
- Serum albumin levels may reveal hypoalbuminemia.
- Serum calcium levels may reveal hypocalcemia.
- Serum phosphorus levels may reveal hypophosphatemia.
- Complete blood count may show leukocytosis or leukopenia.
- Platelet count may show thrombocytopenia.
- Serum creatinine level is increased.

Guidelines for diagnosing toxic shock syndrome

Toxic shock syndrome is typically diagnosed based on the following criteria.
- Fever 102° F (38.9° C) or higher
- Diffuse macular erythrodermal rash (sunburn rash)
- Hypotension (systolic blood pressure 90 mm Hg or less in adults or below the 5th percentile for age)
- Involvement of at least three organ systems:
  – GI (vomiting, diarrhea)
  – Muscular (myalgias or liver function test at least twice normal upper limit)
  – Mucous membrane hyperemia (conjunctiva, vagina, oropharyngeal)
  – Renal (blood urea nitrogen or creatinine level at least twice normal upper limit, or pyuria)
  – Hepatic (total serum bilirubin or aminotransferase level twice normal level)
  – Hematologic (thrombocytopenia)
  – Central nervous system (disorientation or change in level of consciousness)
- Desquamation, especially of palms and soles, 1 or 2 weeks after onset of illness
- Other conditions ruled out

TREATMENT

GENERAL
- Aggressive fluid resuscitation
- Correction of electrolyte imbalances
- Supportive treatment such as possible ventilatory support
- Identification and decontamination of toxin production site
- Bed rest until acute phase resolved

MEDICATIONS
- Antibiotics
- Inotropics
- Vasopressors
- I.V. immunoglobulin

SURGERY
- Examination and irrigation of recent surgical wounds

NURSING CONSIDERATIONS

NURSING DIAGNOSES
- Acute pain
- Decreased cardiac output
- Deficient fluid volume
- Hyperthermia
- Impaired tissue integrity
- Ineffective tissue perfusion: Renal, cerebral, cardiopulmonary, GI, or peripheral

EXPECTED OUTCOMES
The patient will:
- report feelings of comfort and decreased pain
- maintain adequate cardiac output
- maintain adequate fluid volume
- remain afebrile
- maintain collateral circulation
- maintain tissue perfusion and cellular oxygenation.

NURSING INTERVENTIONS
- Administer drug therapy.
- Assess fluid balance and replace fluids intravenously, as needed.
- Reorient the patient as needed.
- Use appropriate safety measures to prevent injury.
- Use standard precautions for vaginal discharge and lesion drainage.

MONITORING
- Cardiovascular status
- Fluid and electrolyte status
- Neurologic status
- Vital signs
- Pulmonary status
- Response to treatment
- Complications

PATIENT TEACHING

GENERAL
Be sure to cover:
- the disorder, diagnosis, and treatment
- importance of avoiding tampons, especially superabsorbent ones, because of the risk of recurrence
- TSS prevention.

RESOURCES
Organizations
Mayo Clinic: *www.mayoclinic.com*
National Center for Infectious Diseases — Division of Bacterial and Mycotic Diseases: *www.cdc.gov/ncidod/dbmd*
Toxic Shock Syndrome Information Service: *www.toxicshock.com*
U.S. Food and Drug Administration: *www.fda.gov*

Selected references
Arora, S. "A Case of Non-Menstrual Staphylococcal Toxic Shock Syndrome," *Journal of General Internal Medicine* 19(Suppl 1):24-25, April 2004.
Chuang, Yu-Yu, et al. "Toxic Shock Syndrome in Children: Epidemiology, Pathogenesis, and Management," *Pediatric Drugs* 7(1):11-25, 2005.
Hidalgo-Carballal, A., and Suarez-Mier, M.P. "Sudden Unexpected Death in a Child with Varicella Caused by Necrotizing Fasciitis and Streptococcal Toxic Shock Syndrome," *American Journal of Forensic Medicine & Pathology* 27(1):93-96, March 2006.
Kasper, D.L., et al., eds. *Harrison's Principles of Internal Medicine*, 16th ed. New York: McGraw-Hill Book Co., 2005.

Toxoplasmosis

OVERVIEW

- One of the most common parasitic infectious diseases
- Usually causes localized infection
- May produce significant generalized infection, especially in an immuno-deficient patient
- Once infected, organism carried for life and acute infection can reactivate
- Congenital type characterized by lesions in the central nervous system (CNS); may result in stillbirth or serious birth defects

PATHOPHYSIOLOGY

- After ingestion, parasites are released from latent cysts by the digestive process; they then invade the GI tract and multiply.
- Parasites disseminate to various organs, especially lymphatic tissue, skeletal muscle, myocardium, retina, placenta, and the CNS.
- The parasite infects host cells, replicates, and then invades adjoining cells, resulting in cell death and focal necrosis surrounded by an acute inflammatory response.

CAUSES

- Congenital toxoplasmosis from transplacental transmission
- The protozoan *Toxoplasma gondii*, which exists in trophozoite forms in the acute stages of infection and in cystic forms (tissue cysts and oocysts) in latent stages
- Transmitted by ingestion of tissue cysts in raw or undercooked meat or by fecal oral contamination from infected cats

INCIDENCE

- Up to 70% United States residents have been infected with the Toxoplasma organism. Most develop no signs or symptoms and will develop immunity.
- This disease occurs worldwide but is less common in cold or hot, arid climates and at high elevations.

COMPLICATIONS

- Seizure disorder
- Vision loss (see *Ocular toxoplasmosis*)
- Mental retardation
- Deafness
- Generalized infection
- Stillbirth
- Congenital toxoplasmosis

ASSESSMENT

HISTORY

- Possible immunocompromised state, exposure to cat feces, or ingestion of poorly cooked meat
- Malaise
- Fatigue
- Myalgia
- Headache
- Sore throat
- Vomiting

PHYSICAL FINDINGS

- Fever (if generalized, possibly 106° F [41.1° C])
- Cough
- Dyspnea
- Cyanosis
- Coarse crackles
- Delirium, seizures
- Diffuse maculopapular rash (except on the palms, soles, and scalp)
- In an infant with congenital toxoplasmosis:
- Epilepsy, mental retardation
- Hydrocephalus or microcephalus
- Jaundice, purpura, rash
- Lymphadenopathy, splenomegaly, and hepatomegaly
- Strabismus, blindness

Ocular toxoplasmosis

Ocular toxoplasmosis (active chorioretinitis) is characterized by focal necrotizing retinitis. It accounts for about 25% of all cases of granulomatous uveitis. Although usually the result of a congenital infection, it may not appear until adolescence or young adulthood, when infection is reactivated.

Symptoms include blurred vision, scotoma, pain, photophobia, and impairment or loss of central vision. Vision improves as inflammation subsides but usually without recovery of lost visual acuity. Ocular toxoplasmosis may subside after treatment with prednisone.

DIAGNOSTIC TEST RESULTS

LABORATORY
◆ Specimens, such as bronchoalveolar lavage material from immunocompromised patients or a lymph node biopsy, contain parasites.
◆ Intraperitoneal inoculation with blood or other body fluids into mice or tissue cultures may show an isolation of parasites.
◆ A polymerase chain reaction detects the parasite's genetic material, especially in detecting congenital infections in utero.

TREATMENT

GENERAL
◆ No treatment in otherwise healthy patient who isn't pregnant
◆ Seizure precautions

ACTIVITY
◆ Rest periods when fatigued

MEDICATIONS
◆ Pyrimethamine plus sulfadiazine with leucovorin

NURSING CONSIDERATIONS

NURSING DIAGNOSES
◆ Activity intolerance
◆ Acute pain
◆ Deficient fluid volume
◆ Fatigue
◆ Hyperthermia
◆ Impaired skin integrity
◆ Ineffective breathing pattern
◆ Risk for injury

EXPECTED OUTCOMES
The patient will:
◆ return to previous activity level
◆ report decrease or absence of pain
◆ have an adequate fluid volume
◆ report an increased energy level
◆ remain afebrile
◆ maintain skin integrity
◆ maintain respiratory rate within 5 breaths/minute of baseline
◆ develop no complications.

NURSING INTERVENTIONS
◆ Give tepid sponge baths to decrease fever.
◆ Administer drug therapy.
◆ Provide chest physiotherapy, and administer oxygen, as needed. Assist ventilations if needed.
◆ Institute seizure precautions.

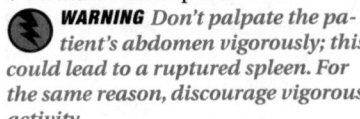 **WARNING** *Don't palpate the patient's abdomen vigorously; this could lead to a ruptured spleen. For the same reason, discourage vigorous activity.*
◆ Report all cases of toxoplasmosis to the local public health department.

MONITORING
◆ Neurologic status
◆ Response to treatment
◆ Complications

PATIENT TEACHING

GENERAL
Be sure to cover:
◆ the disorder, diagnosis, and treatment
◆ necessary drugs, including the need for frequent blood tests
◆ importance of regularly scheduled follow-up care
◆ prevention of toxoplasmosis (washing hands after working with soil, cooking meat thoroughly and freezing promptly, covering children's sandboxes, and keeping flies away from food)
◆ need for pregnant women to avoid cleaning and handling cat litter boxes, or to wear gloves.

DISCHARGE PLANNING
◆ Refer the patient for follow-up with a neurologist or infectious disease specialist if needed.

RESOURCES
Organizations
National Center for Infectious Diseases: *www.cdc.gov/ncidod*
National Institute of Allergy and Infectious Diseases: *www.niaid.nih.gov*

Selected references
Dzitko, K., et al. "Toxoplasma Gondii: Serological Recognition of Reinfection," *Experimental Parasitology* 112(2):134-37, February 2006.
Kasper, D.L., et al., eds. *Harrison's Principles of Internal Medicine,* 16th ed. New York: McGraw-Hill Book Co., 2005.
Many, A., and Koren, G. "Toxoplasmosis during Pregnancy," *Canadian Family Physician* 52:29-30, 32, January 2006.
Sukthana, Y. "Toxoplasmosis: Beyond Animals to Humans," *Trends in Parasitology* 22(3):137-42, March 2006.

Tracheoesophageal fistula and esophageal atresia

OVERVIEW

- Tracheoesophageal fistula: a developmental anomaly characterized by an abnormal connection between the trachea and the esophagus; usually accompanies esophageal atresia, in which the esophagus is closed off at some point
- Malformations have numerous anatomic variations, most commonly, esophageal atresia with fistula to the distal segment
- Two of the most serious surgical emergencies in neonates; requires immediate diagnosis and correction

PATHOPHYSIOLOGY

- Tracheoesophageal fistula and esophageal atresia result from failure of the embryonic esophagus and trachea to develop and separate correctly.
- Respiratory system development begins at about day 26 of gestation.
- Abnormal development of the septum during this time can lead to tracheoesophageal fistula.
- The most common abnormality is type C tracheoesophageal fistula with esophageal atresia, in which the upper section of the esophagus terminates in a blind pouch, and the lower section ascends from the stomach and connects with the trachea by a short fistulous tract. (See *Types of tracheoesophageal anomalies*)
- In type A atresia, both esophageal segments are blind pouches, and neither is connected to the airway.
- In types B and D, the upper portion of the esophagus opens into the trachea; infants with this anomaly may experience life-threatening aspiration of saliva or food.
- In type E (or H-type) tracheoesophageal fistula without atresia, the fistula may occur anywhere between the level of the cricoid cartilage and the midesophagus but usually is higher in the trachea than in the esophagus. Such a fistula may be as small as a pinpoint.

CAUSES

- Commonly found in infants with other anomalies, such as:
  – Congenital heart disease
  – Genitourinary abnormalities
  – Imperforate anus
  – Intestinal atresia
- Congenital anomalies

INCIDENCE

- Esophageal atresia occurs in about 1 of 4,000 live births; about one-third of these neonates are born prematurely.

COMPLICATIONS

- Aspiration of secretions into the lungs leading to respiratory distress, pneumonia, or cessation of breathing
- Death if untreated

After surgery

- Abnormal esophageal motility
- Recurrent fistulas
- Pneumothorax
- Esophageal stricture

ASSESSMENT

HISTORY

- Coughing and choking after eating

PHYSICAL FINDINGS

- Respiratory distress
- Drooling

DIAGNOSTIC TEST RESULTS

IMAGING

- Chest X-rays demonstrate the position of the catheter and can also show a dilated, air-filled upper esophageal pouch, pneumonia in the right upper lobe, or bilateral pneumonitis. Both pneumonia and pneumonitis suggest aspiration.
- Abdominal X-rays may show gas in the bowel in a distal fistula (type C) but not in a proximal fistula (type B) or atresia without a fistula (type A).
- Cinefluorography allows visualization on a fluoroscopic screen. After a

Types of tracheoesophageal anomalies

The American Academy of Pediatrics classifies tracheoesophageal anomalies as shown below:

TYPE A (7.7%)	TYPE B (0.8%)	TYPE C (86.5%)	TYPE D (0.7%)	TYPE E OR H (4.2%)
Esophageal atresia without fistula	Esophageal atresia with tracheoesophageal fistula to the proximal segment	Esophageal atresia with fistula to the distal segment only	Esophageal atresia with fistula to both segments	Tracheoesophageal fistula without atresia

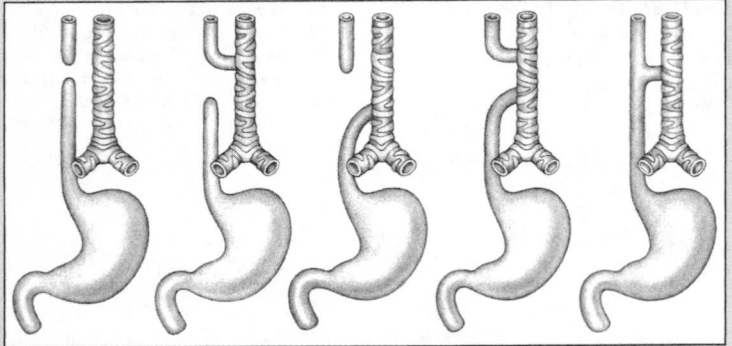

size 10 or 12 French catheter is passed through the patient's nostril into the esophagus, a small amount of contrast medium is instilled to define the tip of the upper pouch and to differentiate between overflow aspiration from a blind end (atresia) and aspiration from passage of liquids through a tracheoesophageal fistula.

Other
◆ A size 6 or 8 French catheter passed through the nose meets an obstruction (esophageal atresia) about 4″ to 5″ (10 to 12.5 cm) distal to the nostrils. Aspiration of the gastric contents is less acidic than normal.

TREATMENT

GENERAL
◆ I.V. fluids
◆ Supine position with the head low to facilitate drainage or with the head elevated to prevent aspiration
◆ After surgery: placement of a suction catheter in the upper esophageal pouch to control secretions and prevent aspiration

MEDICATIONS
◆ Antibiotics for superimposed infection

SURGERY
◆ Type and timing of surgical procedure depends on nature of anomaly, patient's general condition, and presence of coexisting congenital defects; both disorders usually considered surgical emergencies
◆ In premature neonates (nearly 33% of infants with this anomaly) who are poor surgical risks, correction of combined tracheoesophageal fistula and esophageal atresia done in two stages:
– Gastrostomy and closure of the fistula (for gastric decompression, prevention of reflux, and feeding)
– Anastomosis of the esophagus
◆ Correction of esophageal atresia alone requiring anastomosis of proximal and distal esophageal segments in one or two stages:

– End-to-end anastomosis (commonly produces postoperative stricture)
– End-to-side anastomosis (less likely to produce postoperative stricture)
◆ If esophageal ends widely separated, a colonic interposition or elongation of the proximal segment of the esophagus by bougienage

NURSING CONSIDERATIONS

NURSING DIAGNOSES
◆ Compromised family coping
◆ Imbalanced nutrition: Less than body requirements
◆ Ineffective airway clearance
◆ Risk for aspiration
◆ Risk for impaired parent/infant/child attachment
◆ Risk for infection
◆ Risk for injury

EXPECTED OUTCOMES
The patient (or family) will:
◆ seek support systems and exhibit adequate coping behaviors
◆ maintain adequate weight
◆ maintain a patent airway and develop no respiratory complications
◆ show no signs of aspiration
◆ exhibit signs of positive parent/infant/child bonding
◆ remain free from signs and symptoms of infection
◆ avoid or minimize complications.

NURSING INTERVENTIONS
◆ Administer oxygen as needed.
◆ Perform pulmonary physiotherapy and suctioning, as needed.
◆ Provide a humid environment.
◆ Give antibiotics and parenteral fluids.
◆ Maintain gastrostomy tube feedings.
◆ Offer the parents support and guidance in dealing with their infant's acute illness. Encourage them to participate in care and to hold and touch the infant as much as possible to facilitate bonding.

MONITORING
◆ Respiratory status
◆ Intake and output

After surgery
◆ Chest tubes
◆ Signs of complications

PATIENT TEACHING

GENERAL
Be sure to cover:
◆ the disorder, diagnosis, and treatment
◆ feeding procedures
◆ recognizing and reporting complications
◆ proper positioning.

DISCHARGE PLANNING
◆ Instruct the parents that X-rays are required about 10 days after surgery, and again 1 and 3 months later, to evaluate the effectiveness of surgical repair.

RESOURCES
Organizations
American Academy of Pediatrics: *www.aap.org*
Digestive Disease National Coalition: *www.ddnc.org*
The Merck Manuals Online Medical Library: *www.merck.com/mmhe*
National Digestive Diseases Information Clearinghouse: *www.niddk.nih.gov/health/digest/nddic.htm*

Selected references
Allen, S.R., et al. "The Effect of a Right-Sided Aortic Arch on Outcome in Children with Esophageal Atresia and Tracheoesophageal Fistula," *Journal of Pediatric Surgery* 41(3):479-83, March 2006.
Brunner, H.G., and van Bokhoven, H. "Genetic Players in Esophageal Atresia and Tracheoesophageal Fistula," *Current Opinion in Genetics & Development* 15(3):341-47, June 2005.
Katsura, S., et al. "Esophageal Atresia with Double Tracheoesophageal Fistula — A Case Report and Review of the Literature," *European Journal of Pediatric Surgery* 15(5):354-57, October 2005.
Rothenberg, S.S. "Thoracoscopic Repair of Esophageal Atresia and Tracheo-Esophageal Fistula," *Seminars in Pediatric Surgery* 14(1):2-7, February 2005.

Transposition of the great arteries

OVERVIEW

- Congenital heart defect in which the great arteries are reversed: aorta arising from right ventricle and pulmonary artery from left ventricle, producing two noncommunicating circulatory systems
- Commonly coexists with other congenital heart defects: Ventricular septal defect (VSD), VSD with pulmonary stenosis (PS), atrial septal defect (ASD), patent ductus arteriosus (PDA)

PATHOPHYSIOLOGY

- In transposition, oxygenated blood returning to the left side of the heart is carried back to the lungs by a transposed pulmonary artery; unoxygenated blood returning to the right side of the heart is carried to the systemic circulation by a transposed aorta.
- Communication between the pulmonary and systemic circulations is necessary for survival. In infants with isolated transposition, blood mixes only at the patent foramen ovale and at the PDA, resulting in slight mixing of unoxygenated systemic blood and oxygenated pulmonary blood.
- In infants with concurrent cardiac defects, greater mixing of blood occurs.

CAUSES

- Faulty embryonic development

INCIDENCE

- This disorder accounts for about 5% of all congenital heart defects.
- This disorder affects males two to three times more than females.

COMPLICATIONS

- Heart failure
- Cardiac arrhythmia
- Eisenmenger's syndrome (irreversible and progressive pulmonary vascular obstructive disease)

ASSESSMENT

HISTORY

- Diminished exercise tolerance
- Fatigability
- Coughing

PHYSICAL FINDINGS

- Cyanosis
- Clubbing of nailbeds
- Pronounced murmurs if ASD, VSD, PDA, or PS is present

DIAGNOSTIC TEST RESULTS

LABORATORY

- Arterial blood gas (ABG) measurements indicate hypoxia and secondary metabolic acidosis.

IMAGING

- Chest X-rays are normal in the first days of life. Within days to weeks, right atrial and right ventricular enlargements characteristically cause the heart to appear oblong. X-rays also show increased pulmonary vascular markings, except when PS coexists.
- Echocardiography demonstrates the reversed position of the aorta and pulmonary artery and records echoes from both semilunar valves simultaneously, due to aortic valve displacement. It also detects other cardiac defects.

DIAGNOSTIC PROCEDURES

- An electrocardiogram typically reveals a right axis deviation and right ventricular hypertrophy; it may be normal in a neonate.
- Cardiac catheterization reveals decreased oxygen saturation in left ventricular blood and aortic blood; increased right atrial, right ventricular, and pulmonary artery oxygen saturation; and right ventricular systolic pressure equal to systemic pressure. Dye injection reveals the transposed vessels and the presence of any other cardiac defects.

GENERAL
◆ Atrial balloon septostomy (Rashkind procedure) during cardiac catheterization

DIET
◆ Increased caloric density before correction; no restrictions after correction

ACTIVITY
◆ As tolerated

MEDICATIONS
◆ Inotropic agents
◆ Loop diuretics
◆ Prostaglandins
◆ Prophylactic antibiotics

SURGERY
One of three surgical procedures can correct transposition, depending on the defect's physiology:
◆ Mustard procedure replacing the atrial septum with a Dacron or pericardial partition, allowing systemic venous blood to be channeled to the pulmonary artery
◆ Senning procedure using the atrial septum to create partitions to redirect blood flow
◆ Arterial switch, or Jatene procedure, in which transposed arteries are surgically anastomosed to the correct ventricle; left ventricle must be used to pump at systemic pressure

NURSING DIAGNOSES
◆ Activity intolerance
◆ Decreased cardiac output
◆ Excess fluid volume
◆ Fatigue
◆ Impaired gas exchange
◆ Ineffective tissue perfusion: Cardiopulmonary
◆ Risk for infection

EXPECTED OUTCOMES
The patient will:
◆ attain the highest degree of mobility possible
◆ maintain adequate cardiac output and have no arrhythmias
◆ avoid complications of excess fluid
◆ exhibit signs of increased energy
◆ maintain adequate ventilation and oxygenation
◆ maintain hemodynamic stability
◆ remain free from signs and symptoms of infection.

NURSING INTERVENTIONS
◆ Offer emotional support.
◆ Give digoxin and I.V. fluids, being careful to avoid fluid overload.
◆ Watch for signs of baffle obstruction such as marked facial edema after Mustard or Senning procedures.

MONITORING
◆ Vital signs
◆ ABG values
◆ Intake and output
◆ Central venous pressure
◆ Signs of heart failure

GENERAL
Be sure to cover (with the parents):
◆ the disorder, diagnosis, and treatment
◆ how to recognize signs of heart failure and digoxin toxicity (poor feeding and vomiting)
◆ importance of regular checkups to monitor cardiovascular status
◆ protecting the infant from infection and giving antibiotics.

RESOURCES
Organizations
American Academy of Pediatrics: *www.aap.org*
American Heart Association: *www.americanheart.org*
American Lung Association: *www.lungusa.org*

Selected references
Diseases, 4th ed. Philadelphia: Lippincott Williams & Wilkins, 2006.
Gregoric, I.D., et al. "Left Ventricular Assist Device Implantation in a Patient with Congenitally Corrected Transposition of the Great Arteries," *Texas Heart Institute Journal* 32(4):567-69, 2005.
McQuillen, P.S., et al. "Balloon Atrial Septostomy is Associated with Preoperative Stroke in Neonates with Transposition of the Great Arteries," *Circulation* 113(2):280-85, January 2006.
Ou, P., et al. "Detection of Coronary Complications after the Arterial Switch Operation for Transposition of the Great Arteries: First Experience with Multislice Computed Tomography in Children," *Journal of Thoracic and Cardiovascular Surgery* 131(3):639-43, March 2006.
Paladini, D., et al. "Diagnosis, Characterization and Outcome of Congenitally Corrected Transposition of the Great Arteries in the Fetus: A Multicenter Series of 30 Cases," *Ultrasound in Obstetrics & Gynecology* 27(3):281-85, March 2006.

Trichinosis

- Infection caused by larvae of intestinal roundworm *Trichinella spiralis*
- May produce multiple symptoms, such as respiratory, central nervous system (CNS), cardiovascular complications and, rarely, death
- Also known as *trichiniasis* or *trichinellosis*

PATHOPHYSIOLOGY

- *T. spiralis* cysts are found primarily in swine, less commonly in dogs, cats, bears, foxes, wolves, and marine animals. These cysts result from the animals' ingestion of similarly contaminated flesh. In swine, such infection results from eating table scraps or raw garbage.
- After gastric juices free the worm from the cyst capsule, it reaches sexual maturity in a few days.
- The female roundworm burrows into the intestinal mucosa and reproduces.
- Larvae are then transported through the lymphatic system and the bloodstream. They become embedded as cysts in striated muscle, especially in the diaphragm, chest, arms, and legs.
- Human-to-human transmission doesn't take place.

CAUSES

- Ingestion of uncooked or undercooked meat that contains *T. spiralis* cysts

INCIDENCE

- Trichinosis occurs worldwide, especially in populations that eat pork or bear meat.
- This disorder affects both sexes equally.

COMPLICATIONS

- Meningitis
- Subcortical infarcts
- Encephalitis
- Myocarditis with heart failure
- Nephritis
- Glomerulonephritis
- Sinusitis
- Pneumonia

HISTORY

- Ingestion of raw or improperly cooked pork or pork products
- Myalgia
- Abdominal discomfort
- Diarrhea
- Constipation
- Anorexia
- Nausea

PHYSICAL FINDINGS

- Diffuse weakness
- Dyspnea on exertion
- Hoarseness
- Cough
- Abdominal distention
- Macular or petechial rash
- Periorbital edema

LABORATORY

- Stools may contain mature worms and larvae during the invasion stage of trichinosis.
- Diagnosis of trichinosis is confirmed by elevated acute and convalescent antibody titers (determined by flocculation tests 3 to 4 weeks after infection).
- Aspartate aminotransferase, alanine aminotransferase, creatine kinase, and lactate dehydrogenase levels are increased during the acute stages of this disorder, and the eosinophil count is increased (up to 15,000/µl).
- The cerebrospinal fluid lymphocyte level (to 300/µl) is normal or increased, and protein levels are increased, indicating CNS involvement.

DIAGNOSTIC PROCEDURES

- Skeletal muscle biopsies can show encysted larvae 10 days after ingestion; if available, analyses of contaminated meat also show larvae.
- Skin testing may show a positive histamine-like reactivity 15 minutes after intradermal injection of the antigen (within 17 to 20 days after ingestion); however, such a result may remain positive for up to 5 years after exposure.

GENERAL
◆ Supportive care as indicated

DIET
◆ As tolerated

ACTIVITY
◆ Initially, bed rest with increased activity as tolerated

MEDICATIONS
◆ Antipyretics
◆ Anthelmintics
◆ Glucocorticoids
◆ Analgesics

NURSING DIAGNOSES
◆ Acute pain
◆ Diarrhea
◆ Disturbed sensory perception (visual)
◆ Fatigue
◆ Hyperthermia
◆ Impaired physical mobility
◆ Impaired skin integrity
◆ Impaired swallowing
◆ Ineffective breathing pattern
◆ Risk for deficient fluid volume

EXPECTED OUTCOMES
The patient will:
◆ report increased comfort and decreased pain
◆ return to a normal elimination pattern
◆ maintain optimal functioning within the limits of the visual impairment
◆ express feelings of increased energy
◆ maintain a normal body temperature
◆ maintain muscle strength and joint range of motion
◆ avoid skin breakdown or infection
◆ swallow without pain or discomfort
◆ maintain an effective breathing pattern
◆ maintain an adequate fluid balance.

NURSING INTERVENTIONS
◆ Reduce fever with alcohol rubs, tepid baths, hypothermia blankets, or antipyretics.
◆ Relieve muscle pain with analgesics, enforced bed rest, and proper body alignment.
◆ Frequently reposition the patient, and gently massage bony prominences to prevent pressure ulcers.
◆ Report all cases of trichinosis to local public health authorities.

MONITORING
◆ Response to treatment
◆ Vital signs
◆ Respiratory status

GENERAL
Be sure to cover:
◆ proper cooking and storing methods for all meat from carnivores
◆ importance of avoiding pork consumption when traveling to foreign countries or to poor areas of the United States; swine in these areas are commonly fed raw garbage.

RESOURCES
Organizations
Centers for Disease Control and Prevention — Division of Parasitic Diseases: *www.cdc.gov/ncidod/dpd*
The Merck Manuals Online Medical Library: *www.merck.com/mmhe*
U.S. Food and Drug Administration: *www.fda.gov*

Selected references
Astudillo, L.M., and Arlet, P.M. "Images in Clinical Medicine. The Chemosis of Trichinosis," *New England Journal of Medicine* 351(5):487, July 2004.
Diseases, 4th ed. Philadelphia: Lippincott Williams & Wilkins, 2006.
Kolodziej-Sobocinska, M. et al. "Trichinella Spiralis: Macrophage Activity and Antibody Response in Chronic Murine Infection," *Experimental Parasitology* 112(1):52-62, January 2006.
Ozdemir, D., et al. "Acute Trichinellosis in Children Compared with Adults," *Pediatric Infectious Disease Journal* 24(10):897-900, October 2005.

Trichomoniasis

- A protozoal infection of the lower genitourinary tract
- May be acute or chronic in females
- Risk of recurrence minimized when sexual partners are treated concurrently

PATHOPHYSIOLOGY

- *Trichomonas vaginalis* (a tetraflagellated, motile protozoan) causes trichomoniasis in females by infecting the vagina, the urethra and, possibly, the endocervix, bladder, Bartholin's glands, or Skene's glands. In males, it infects the lower urethra and, possibly, the prostate gland, seminal vesicles, or epididymis.
- *T. vaginalis* grows best when the vaginal mucosa is more alkaline than normal (pH about 5.5 to 5.8).

CAUSES

- Usually transmitted by sexual intercourse; less commonly, by contaminated douche equipment or moist washcloths

RISK FACTORS

- Factors that raise the vaginal pH:
- – Use of hormonal contraceptives
- – Pregnancy
- – Bacterial overgrowth
- – Exudative cervical or vaginal lesions
- – Frequent douching, which disturbs lactobacilli that normally live in the vagina and maintain acidity

INCIDENCE

- This disorder affects about 15% of sexually active females and 10% of sexually active males.

COMPLICATIONS

- With pregnant women: preterm or low–birth-weight neonate
- Prostatitis
- Epididymitis
- Urethral stricture disease
- Infertility

HISTORY

- Severe itching
- Dyspareunia
- Dysuria
- Urinary frequency
- Postcoital spotting, menorrhagia, or dysmenorrhea

PHYSICAL FINDINGS

- Vaginal erythema, edema, and frank excoriation
- Frothy, malodorous, greenish yellow vaginal discharge
- Rarely, a thin, gray pseudomembrane over the vagina

LABORATORY

- Direct microscopic examination of vaginal or seminal discharge is decisive when it reveals *T. vaginalis*, a motile, pear-shaped organism. Examination of clear urine specimens may also reveal *T. vaginalis*.

OTHER

- Cervical examination demonstrates punctate cervical hemorrhages, giving the cervix a strawberry appearance that's almost pathognomonic for this disorder.

GENERAL
- Abstinence from sexual intercourse until cured
- Sitz baths to help relieve symptoms

MEDICATIONS
- Single 2-g dose of oral metronidazole given to both sexual partners

NURSING DIAGNOSES
- Acute pain
- Anxiety
- Deficient fluid volume
- Impaired skin integrity
- Impaired urinary elimination
- Ineffective sexuality patterns
- Sexual dysfunction

EXPECTED OUTCOMES
The patient will:
- express feelings of increased comfort and decreased pain
- identify strategies to reduce anxiety
- maintain fluid balance; intake will equal output
- experience lesion and wound healing without complications
- maintain a normal urinary output
- discuss the impact of the disorder on self and significant others
- acknowledge a problem or potential problem in sexual function.

NURSING INTERVENTIONS
- Instruct the patient to avoid using tampons.
- Provide emotional support.
- Practice standard precautions.

MONITORING
- Response to treatment

GENERAL
Be sure to cover:
- importance of referring all sexual partners for treatment
- importance of avoiding alcohol while taking metronidazole because alcohol may cause a reaction of confusion, headache, cramps, vomiting, and seizures
- possibility that metronidazole may turn urine dark brown
- importance of avoiding over-the-counter douches and vaginal sprays because they can alter vaginal pH
- benefits of wearing loose-fitting, cotton underwear, which reduce the risk of genitourinary bacterial growth by allowing ventilation.

RESOURCES
Organizations
American Association of Kidney Patients: *www.aakp.org*
American College of Obstetricians and Gynecologists: *www.acog.org*
Centers for Disease Control and Prevention: *www.cdc.gov*
Harvard University Consumer Health Information: *www.intelihealth.com*

Selected references
Miller, W.C., et al. "The Prevalence of Trichomoniasis in Young Adults in the United States," *Sexually Transmitted Diseases* 32(10):593-98, October 2005.

Nanda, N., et al. "Trichomoniasis and Its Treatment," *Expert Review of Anti-Infective Therapy* 4(1):125-35, February 2006.

Sobel, J.D. "What's New in Bacterial Vaginosis and Trichomoniasis?" *Infectious Disease Clinics of North America* 19(2):387-406, June 2005.

Van Der Pol, B., et al. "Prevalence, Incidence, Natural History, and Response to Treatment of Trichomonas Vaginalis Infection among Adolescent Women," *Journal of Infectious Diseases* 192(12):2039-2044, December 2005.

Tricuspid insufficiency

OVERVIEW

- Heart condition in which the tricuspid valve doesn't function properly
- Also called *tricuspid regurgitation*

PATHOPHYSIOLOGY

- The tricuspid valve is incompetent.
- Blood flows back into the right atrium.
- Fluid overload occurs in the atrium.
- Heart failure occurs, and impedance to the pulmonary vasculature may result in hypoxemia, cyanosis, and polycythemia.

CAUSES

- Carcinoid heart disease
- Connective tissue disease
- Endocarditis
- Epstein's anomaly
- Papillary muscle dysfunction
- Prolapse
- Rheumatic heart disease
- Trauma

INCIDENCE

- Tricuspid insufficiency affects both sexes equally.
- This disorder usually occurs in childhood.

COMPLICATIONS

- Heart failure
- Pulmonary edema
- Thromboembolism
- Endocarditis
- Arrhythmias

ASSESSMENT

HISTORY

- Occurrence of one of listed causes
- Orthopnea, dyspnea
- Fatigue
- Angina
- Palpitations

PHYSICAL FINDINGS

- Tachycardia
- Crackles in the lungs
- Hepatomegaly (right-sided failure)
- Jugular vein distention
- S_3
- Diminished peripheral pulses
- Ascites
- Atrial fibrillation
- Peripheral edema
- Pansystolic murmur (see *Identifying the murmur of tricuspid insufficiency*)

DIAGNOSTIC TEST RESULTS

IMAGING

- Chest X-rays may show right atrial and ventricular enlargement.
- Echocardiography may reveal right ventricular dilation and prolapse or flailing of the tricuspid leaflets.

DIAGNOSTIC PROCEDURES

- An electrocardiogram may show right atrial hypertrophy, right or left ventricular hypertrophy, atrial fibrillation, and incomplete right bundle-branch block.
- Right-sided heart catheterization shows high atrial pressure, tricuspid insufficiency, and decreased or normal output.

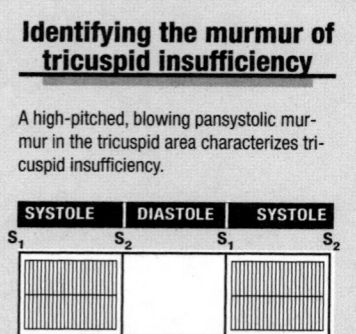

Identifying the murmur of tricuspid insufficiency

A high-pitched, blowing pansystolic murmur in the tricuspid area characterizes tricuspid insufficiency.

SYSTOLE	DIASTOLE	SYSTOLE	
S_1	S_2	S_1	S_2

TREATMENT

GENERAL
- Underlying cause

DIET
- Low sodium
- Fluid restriction

ACTIVITY
- As tolerated

MEDICATIONS
- Diuretics
- Cardiac glycosides
- Anticoagulants
- Angiotensin-converting enzyme inhibitors
- Oxygen
- Prophylactic antibiotics before and after surgery or dental care to prevent endocarditis

SURGERY
- Annuloplasty or valvuloplasty to reconstruct or repair the valve
- Valve replacement with a prosthetic valve

NURSING CONSIDERATIONS

NURSING DIAGNOSES
- Activity intolerance
- Decreased cardiac output
- Excess fluid volume
- Fatigue
- Impaired gas exchange
- Impaired physical mobility
- Ineffective coping
- Ineffective tissue perfusion: Cardiopulmonary
- Risk for infection

EXPECTED OUTCOMES
The patient will:
- carry out activities of daily living without weakness or fatigue
- maintain adequate cardiac output and hemodynamic stability and exhibit no arrhythmias
- exhibit no complications of excess fluid volume
- verbalize the importance of balancing activity with adequate rest periods
- maintain adequate ventilation and oxygenation
- maintain joint mobility and range of motion
- demonstrate adaptive coping behaviors
- maintain adequate cardiopulmonary perfusion
- remain free from signs and symptoms of infection.

NURSING INTERVENTIONS
- Administer oxygen.
- Watch for signs of heart failure or pulmonary edema.
- Alternate periods of activity and rest.
- Keep patient's legs elevated to improve venous return to the heart.

MONITORING
- Vital signs and pulse oximetry
- Cardiac rhythm
- Pulmonary artery catheter readings
- Intake and output
- Adverse effects of drug therapy

PATIENT TEACHING

GENERAL
Be sure to cover:
- the disorder, diagnosis, and treatment
- dietary restrictions and drugs
- signs and symptoms that should be reported
- importance of consistent follow-up care
- importance of elevating both legs when sitting.

RESOURCES
Organizations
American Heart Association: *www.americanheart.org*
National Heart, Lung, and Blood Institute: *www.nhlbi.nih.gov*

Selected references
Lin, C.H. "Traumatic Tricuspid Regurgitation Resulting in Protein-Losing Enteropathy: A Case Report," *Journal of Heart Valve Disease* 14(6):852-54, November 2005.

Matsunaga, A., and Duran, C.M. "Progression of Tricuspid Regurgitation after Repaired Functional Ischemic Mitral Regurgitation," *Circulation* 112(9 Suppl):I453-57, August 2005.

Messing, B., et al. "Mild Tricuspid Regurgitation: A Benign Fetal Finding at Various Stages of Pregnancy," *Ultrasound in Obstetrics & Gynecology* 26(6):606-609, November 2005.

Tatebe, S., et al. "Posttraumatic Tricuspid Insufficiency Successfully Repaired by Conventional Technique," *Journal of Cardiac Surgery* 20(4):356-57, July-August 2005.

Wang, J., et al. "Selective Annuloplasty for Tricuspid Regurgitation in Children," *Annals of Thoracic Surgery* 79(3):937-41, March 2005.

Tricuspid stenosis

OVERVIEW

- Heart condition in which the tricuspid valve improperly functions, allowing backflow of blood into the right atrium and causing right atrial enlargement

PATHOPHYSIOLOGY

- Alterations in the structure of the tricuspid valve cause incompetence of the valve.
- Restriction of blood flow into the right ventricle and, subsequently, to the pulmonary vasculature occurs.
- Obstructed venous return results in hepatic enlargement, decreased pulmonary blood flow, peripheral edema, and right atrial enlargement.

CAUSES

- Carcinoid heart disease
- Endomyocardial fibrosis
- Infective endocarditis
- Mitral and aortic valve disorders
- Rheumatic heart disease
- Systemic lupus erythematosus
- Tricuspid atresia

INCIDENCE

- Tricuspid stenosis affects females slightly more commonly than males.

COMPLICATIONS

- Heart failure
- Pulmonary edema
- Thromboembolism
- Endocarditis
- Arrhythmias

ASSESSMENT

HISTORY

- Orthopnea
- Dyspnea
- Fatigue
- Angina
- Palpitations

PHYSICAL FINDINGS

- Diastolic murmur (see *Identifying the murmur of tricuspid stenosis*)
- Split S_1
- Crackles in the lungs
- Hepatomegaly (with right-sided failure)
- Ascites

DIAGNOSTIC TEST RESULTS

IMAGING

- A chest X-ray may reveal cardiomegaly.
- Echocardiography may reveal structure of the valves.

DIAGNOSTIC PROCEDURES

- An electrocardiogram may show atrial fibrillation.

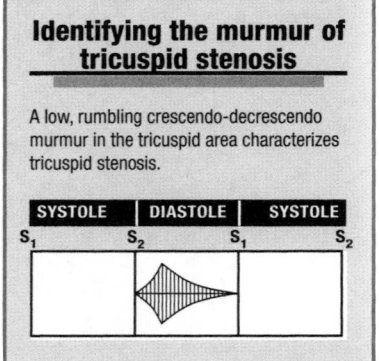

Identifying the murmur of tricuspid stenosis

A low, rumbling crescendo-decrescendo murmur in the tricuspid area characterizes tricuspid stenosis.

SYSTOLE	DIASTOLE	SYSTOLE	
S_1	S_2	S_1	S_2

TREATMENT

GENERAL
◆ Underlying cause

DIET
◆ Low sodium
◆ Fluid restriction

ACTIVITY
◆ As tolerated

MEDICATIONS
◆ Diuretics
◆ Inotropic agent
◆ Angiotensin-converting enzyme inhibitors
◆ Oxygen
◆ Antibiotics before and after surgery or if infection is present

SURGERY
◆ Balloon valvoplasty
◆ Pulmonary artery balloon angioplasty
◆ Valvotomy

NURSING CONSIDERATIONS

NURSING DIAGNOSES
◆ Activity intolerance
◆ Decreased cardiac output
◆ Excess fluid volume
◆ Fatigue
◆ Fear
◆ Impaired gas exchange
◆ Impaired physical mobility
◆ Ineffective coping
◆ Ineffective tissue perfusion: Cardiopulmonary
◆ Risk for infection

EXPECTED OUTCOMES
The patient will:
◆ carry out activities of daily living without weakness or fatigue
◆ maintain adequate cardiac output and hemodynamic stability and exhibit no arrhythmias
◆ exhibit no complications of excess fluid volume
◆ verbalize the importance of balancing activity with adequate rest periods
◆ discuss fears or concerns
◆ maintain adequate ventilation and oxygenation
◆ maintain joint mobility and range of motion
◆ demonstrate adaptive coping behaviors
◆ maintain adequate cardiopulmonary perfusion
◆ remain free from signs and symptoms of infection.

NURSING INTERVENTIONS
◆ Administer oxygen.
◆ Watch for signs of heart failure or pulmonary edema.
◆ Alternate periods of activity and rest.
◆ When sitting in a chair, elevate legs to improve venous return to the heart.
◆ Elevate the head of the bed.
◆ Keep the patient on a low-sodium diet.
◆ If the patient has surgery, watch for hypotension, arrhythmias, and thrombus formation.

MONITORING
◆ Vital signs and pulse oximetry
◆ Cardiac rhythm
◆ Pulmonary artery catheter readings
◆ Intake and output
◆ Adverse effects of drug therapy

PATIENT TEACHING

GENERAL
Be sure to cover:
◆ the disorder, diagnosis, and treatment
◆ dietary restrictions
◆ prescribed drugs
◆ signs and symptoms that should be reported
◆ importance of consistent follow-up care.

RESOURCES
Organizations
American Heart Association: *www.americanheart.org*
National Heart, Lung, and Blood Institute: *www.nhlbi.nih.gov*

Selected references
Diseases, 4th ed. Philadelphia: Lippincott Williams & Wilkins, 2006.
Faletra, F., et al. "Three-Dimensional Transthoracic Echocardiography Images of Tricuspid Stenosis," *Heart* 91(4):499, April 2005.
Sharieff, S., et al. "Concurrent Percutaneous Valvuloplasty of Mitral and Tricuspid Valve Stenoses," *Journal of Invasive Cardiology* 17(6):340-42, June 2005.
Uribe-Etxebarria, N., et al. "Reversible Tricuspid Valve Stenosis due to a Metastatic Dissemination of a Noncardiac Sarcoma," *Annals of Thoracic Surgery* 80(1):e1-2, July 2005.

Trigeminal neuralgia

OVERVIEW

- Painful disorder of the 5th cranial (trigeminal) nerve
- Right side of face affected more commonly than left
- Can subside spontaneously
- Remissions last from several months to years
- Also known as *tic douloureux*

PATHOPHYSIOLOGY

- The trigeminal nerve has multiple branches. This nerve affects chewing movements and sensations of the face, scalp, and teeth. (See *Trigeminal nerve function and distribution*.)
- A trigger zone is stimulated, and interaction or short circuiting of touch and pain fibers occurs.
- Paroxysmal attacks of excruciating facial pain result.

CAUSES

- Exact cause unknown
- Afferent reflex phenomenon
- Compression of the nerve root by:
- Middle fossa tumors
- Posterior fossa tumors
- Vascular lesions
- Herpes zoster
- Multiple sclerosis

INCIDENCE

- Patients older than age 40 are most affected by trigeminal neuralgia.
- About 25% more women than men are affected with trigeminal neuralgia.

COMPLICATIONS

- Excessive weight loss
- Depression
- Social isolation

ASSESSMENT

HISTORY

- Searing or burning facial pain that occurs in lightning-like jabs
- Lasts from 1 to 15 minutes (usually 1 or 2 minutes)
- Localized in an area innervated by the trigeminal nerve
- Initiated by a light touch to a hypersensitive area
- Attacks may follow:
- draft of air
- exposure to heat or cold
- eating, smiling, and talking
- drinking hot or cold beverages
- a period that's free from pain.

PHYSICAL FINDINGS

- Favoring (splinting) of affected area
- Affected side of the face unwashed and unshaven
- Patient never touches affected area
- No impairment of sensory or motor function

DIAGNOSTIC TEST RESULTS

IMAGING

- Skull X-rays, computed tomography scan, and magnetic resonance imaging results rule out sinus or tooth infections and tumors.

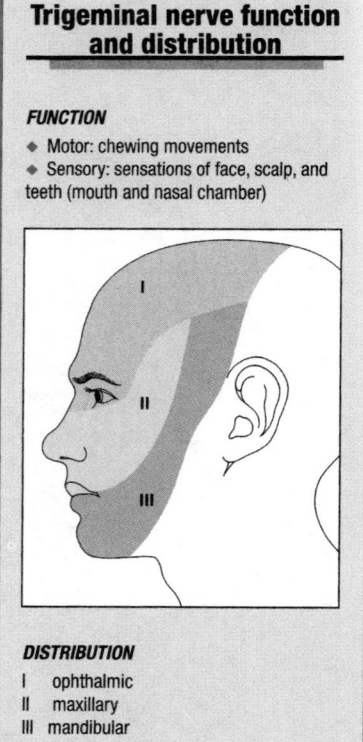

Trigeminal nerve function and distribution

FUNCTION

- Motor: chewing movements
- Sensory: sensations of face, scalp, and teeth (mouth and nasal chamber)

DISTRIBUTION

I   ophthalmic
II maxillary
III mandibular

TREATMENT

GENERAL
◆ Clinical trials investigating use of transmitter-receptor or ion channel-specific drugs

DIET
◆ No restrictions

ACTIVITY
◆ No restrictions

MEDICATIONS
◆ Anticonvulsants
◆ Analgesics

SURGERY
◆ Microsurgery
◆ Radiosurgery with stereotactic technique
◆ Gamma radiosurgery to trigeminal root (noninvasive)

NURSING CONSIDERATIONS

NURSING DIAGNOSES
◆ Activity intolerance
◆ Acute pain
◆ Anxiety
◆ Fatigue
◆ Imbalanced nutrition: Less than body requirements
◆ Ineffective coping
◆ Ineffective role performance

EXPECTED OUTCOMES
The patient will:
◆ perform activities of daily living within confines of the disorder
◆ express feelings of increased comfort and decreased pain
◆ express feelings of decreased anxiety
◆ express feelings of increased energy and decreased fatigue
◆ consume required caloric intake daily
◆ demonstrate adaptive coping behaviors
◆ perform routine roles within the confines of the disorder.

NURSING INTERVENTIONS
◆ Provide emotional support.
◆ Provide nutritional management.
◆ Administer drug therapy.
◆ After microsurgery, provide postcraniotomy care.

MONITORING
◆ Characteristics of each attack
◆ Precipitating factors of each attack
◆ Response to medications
◆ Postoperatively, neurologic function and vital signs

PATIENT TEACHING

GENERAL
Be sure to cover:
◆ the disorder, diagnosis, and treatment
◆ preoperative teaching if indicated
◆ drugs and possible adverse effects
◆ nutritional management
◆ prevention of neuralgia attacks.

RESOURCES
Organizations
American Chronic Pain Association: *www.theacpa.org*
American Pain Foundation: *www.painfoundation.org*
Trigeminal Neuralgia Association: *www.tna-support.org*

Selected references
Aryan, H.E., et al. "Multimodality Treatment of Trigeminal Neuralgia: Impact of Radiosurgery and High Resolution Magnetic Resonance Imaging," *Journal of Clinical Neuroscience* 13(2):239-44, February 2006.
Cox, C.L., et al. "Cranial Nerve Damage," *Emergency Nurse* 12(2):14-21, May 2004.
Cruccu, G., et al. "Diagnostic Accuracy Of Trigeminal Reflex Testing In Trigeminal Neuralgia," *Neurology* 66(1):139-41, January 2006.
Diseases, 4th ed. Philadelphia: Lippincott Williams & Wilkins, 2006.
Handbook of Pathophysiology, 2nd ed. Philadelphia: Lippincott Williams & Wilkins, 2005.
Lin, Y.W., et al. "Fatal Paranasal Sinusitis Presenting as Trigeminal Neuralgia," *Headache* 46(1):174-78, January 2006.
Truini, A., et al. "New Insight into Trigeminal Neuralgia," *Journal of Headache and Pain* 6(4):237-39, September 2005.

Trisomy 13 syndrome LIFE-THREATENING DISORDER

OVERVIEW

- Third most common multiple malformation syndrome
- In most affected infants, full trisomy 13 is present at birth; rarely, mosaic partial trisomy 13 syndrome (with varying phenotypes) or translocation types will appear
- Brain and facial abnormalities; major cardiac, GI, and limb malformations are typical
- Full trisomy 13 syndrome fatal
- Also known as *Patau's syndrome*

PATHOPHYSIOLOGY

- About 75% of all cases result from chromosomal nondisjunction.
- About 20% of all cases result from chromosomal translocation, involving a rearrangement of chromosome 13 with another chromosome.
- About 5% of all cases are estimated to be mosaics; the clinical effects in these cases may be less severe.

CAUSES

- Chromosomal abnormality

RISK FACTORS

- Advanced maternal age (mean maternal age about 31)

INCIDENCE

- Many trisomic zygotes spontaneously abort.
- Of the infants affected with this disorder, 50% to 70% die within 1 month after birth and 85% die by the end of their first year
- Only isolated cases of survival beyond age 5 exist for full trisomy 13 patients; in all survivors, profound mental retardation is present.
- This disorder is estimated to affect 1 in 4,000 to 10,000 neonates.

COMPLICATIONS

- Congenital heart defects: hypoplastic left heart, ventricular septal defect, patent ductus arteriosus, or dextroposition, which may significantly contribute to the cause of death
- Musculoskeletal abnormalities
- Microphthalmia, cataracts, and other eye abnormalities

ASSESSMENT

HISTORY

- Failure to thrive
- Seizures
- Apnea
- Feeding difficulties

PHYSICAL FINDINGS

- Sloping forehead with wide sutures and fontanel
- Scalp defect at the vertex
- Bilateral cleft lip with associated cleft palate
- Flat, broad nose
- Low-set ears and inner ear abnormalities
- Polydactyl hands and feet
- Clubfoot
- Omphaloceles
- Neural tube defects
- Cystic hygroma
- Genital abnormalities

DIAGNOSTIC TEST RESULTS

LABORATORY

- A karyotype, done either prenatally or on peripheral blood lymphocytes or skin fibroblasts in a neonate or an aborted fetus, is diagnostic.
- Results are abnormal in multiple-marker maternal serum screening tests involving different combinations of alpha-fetoprotein, human chorionic gonadotropin (HCG) or free beta-HCG in some laboratories, and unconjugated estriol.

IMAGING

- An ultrasound usually reveals multiple abnormalities in the fetus.

GENERAL
◆ Supportive care

NURSING DIAGNOSES
◆ Compromised family coping
◆ Decreased cardiac output
◆ Delayed growth and development
◆ Impaired gas exchange
◆ Risk for imbalanced fluid volume

EXPECTED OUTCOMES
The patient (or family) will:
◆ seek support systems and exhibit adequate coping behaviors
◆ maintain adequate cardiac output and hemodynamic stability
◆ function at the highest level possible and appear comfortable
◆ maintain adequate ventilation and oxygenation
◆ maintain an adequate fluid balance.

NURSING INTERVENTIONS
◆ Maintain the infant's fluid balance.
◆ Position the infant comfortably.
◆ Allow adequate time for the parents to bond with and hold their child.
◆ Provide emotional support to the family.

MONITORING
◆ Intake and output
◆ Safety
◆ Growth

GENERAL
Be sure to cover:
◆ the disorder, diagnosis, and treatment
◆ activities that can be carried out with the child
◆ safety factors.

DISCHARGE PLANNING
◆ Refer the parents of an affected infant for genetic counseling to explore the cause of the disorder and to discuss the risk of recurrence in future pregnancies.
◆ Refer the parents to a social worker or grief counselor for additional support if needed.
◆ Refer the parents to the Support Organization for Trisomy 18, 13, and Related Disorders (S.O.F.T.) national support program to allow them to interact with other parents of infants with trisomy 18 and trisomy 13.
◆ Refer the family to pediatric hospice service, if available.

RESOURCES
Organizations
Living with Trisomy 13:
www.livingwithtrisomy13.org
Support Organization for Trisomy 18, 13, and Related Disorders (S.O.F.T.):
www.trisomy.org

Selected references
Bdolah, Y, et al. "Circulating Angiogenic Proteins in Trisomy 13," *American Journal of Obstetrics & Gynecology* 194(1):239-45, January 2006.
Matsui, T., et al. "Temporal Bone Histopathology in Trisomy 13," *Otology & Neurotology* 26(3):545, May 2005.
Papageorghiou, A.T., et al. "Sonographic Screening for Trisomy 13 at 11 to 13+6 Weeks of Gestation," *American Journal of Obstetrics & Gynecology* 194(2):397-401, February 2006.

Trisomy 18 syndrome LIFE-THREATENING DISORDER

OVERVIEW

- Second most common multiple malformation syndrome
- Full trisomy 18 involves extra (third) copy of chromosome 18 in each cell; partial trisomy 18 with varying phenotypes and translocation types also reported
- Intrauterine growth retardation, congenital heart defects, microcephaly, and other malformations in most infants with this disorder
- Full trisomy 18 syndrome generally fatal; 30% to 50% of infants die within the first 2 months, 90% die within the first year
- Most surviving patients profoundly mentally retarded
- Also known as *Edwards' syndrome*

PATHOPHYSIOLOGY

- Most cases of trisomy 18 result from spontaneous meitotic nondisjunction, affecting the extra copy of chromosome 18 in each cell.

CAUSES

- Chromosomal abnormality

RISK FACTORS

- Typically increases with maternal age (mean maternal age 32½)

INCIDENCE

- Incidence ranges from 1 in 3,000 to 8,000 neonates, with three to four females affected for every male.

COMPLICATIONS

- Congenital heart defects (in 80% to 90% of patients), such as ventricular septal defect, tetralogy of Fallot, and transposition of the great vessels, which may be the cause of death in many infants
- Other congenital anomalies, such as diaphragmatic hernia, various renal defects, omphalocele, neural tube defects, genital and perineal abnormalities (including imperforate anus), and oligohydramnios

ASSESSMENT

HISTORY

- Growth retardation, which begins in utero and remains significant after birth

PHYSICAL FINDINGS

- Short, narrow nose with upturned nares
- Low-set, simplified ears
- Conspicuous clenched hand with overlapping fingers (commonly seen on ultrasound)
- Cystic hygroma
- Choroid plexus cysts (also seen in some normal infants)

DIAGNOSTIC TEST RESULTS

LABORATORY

- A karyotype, done either prenatally or on peripheral blood lymphocytes or skin fibroblasts in a neonate or an aborted fetus, is diagnostic.
- Results are abnormal in multiple-marker maternal serum screening tests involving different combinations of alpha-fetoprotein, human chorionic gonadotropin, and unconjugated estriol.

IMAGING

- An ultrasound commonly reveals variable abnormalities in the fetus.

TREATMENT

GENERAL
◆ Emotional support for the family

DIET
◆ Nutrition maintenance using gavage feedings

NURSING CONSIDERATIONS

NURSING DIAGNOSES
◆ Compromised family coping
◆ Decreased cardiac output
◆ Delayed growth and development
◆ Impaired gas exchange
◆ Risk for imbalanced fluid volume

EXPECTED OUTCOMES
The patient (or family) will:
◆ seek support systems and exhibit adequate coping behaviors
◆ maintain adequate cardiac output
◆ function at the highest level possible and appear comfortable
◆ maintain adequate ventilation and oxygenation
◆ maintain an adequate fluid balance.

NURSING INTERVENTIONS
◆ Allow adequate time for the parents to bond with and hold their child.
◆ Provide emotional support to the family.

MONITORING
◆ Intake and output
◆ Growth

PATIENT TEACHING

GENERAL
Be sure to cover:
◆ the disorder, diagnosis, and treatment
◆ home care and feeding techniques.

DISCHARGE PLANNING
◆ Refer the parents of a child affected with trisomy 18 syndrome for genetic counseling to explore the cause of the disorder and discuss the risk of recurrence in a future pregnancy.
◆ Refer the parents to a social worker or grief counselor for additional support if needed.
◆ Refer the parents to the Support Organization for Trisomy 18, 13, and Related Disorders (S.O.F.T.) national support program to allow them to interact with other parents of infants with trisomy 18 and trisomy 13.
◆ Refer the family to pediatric hospice service, if available.

RESOURCES
Organizations
Support Organization for Trisomy 18, 13, and Related Disorders (SOFT): *www.trisomy.org*
Trisomy 18 Foundation: *www.trisomy18.org*

Selected references
Bobrowski, R., et al. "What Is the Real Risk for Trisomy 18?" *American Journal of Obstetrics & Gynecology* 189(6) Supplement 1:S233, December 2003.
Moyano, D., et al. "Fetal Echocardiography in Trisomy 18," *Archives of Disease in Childhood Fetal & Neonatal Edition* 90(6):520-22, November 2005.
Oyelese, Y., et al. "Evaluation of the Significance of a Positive Serum Screen for Trisomy 18," *American Journal of Obstetrics & Gynecology* 193(Suppl 6):S162, February 2006.
Tran, S.H., et al. "Ethnic Variation in the Prevalence of Choroid Plexus Cysts and the Association with Trisomy 18," *Obstetrics & Gynecology* 105(4) Suppl:51S, April 2005.

Tuberculosis

OVERVIEW

- Acute or chronic lung infection characterized by pulmonary infiltrates and the formation of granulomas with caseation, fibrosis, and cavitation
- Prognosis excellent with proper treatment and compliance
- Also known as *TB*

PATHOPHYSIOLOGY

- Multiplication of the bacillus *mycobacterium tuberculosis* causes an inflammatory process where deposited.
- A cell-mediated immune response follows, usually containing the infection within 4 to 6 weeks.
- The T-cell response results in the formation of granulomas around the bacilli, making them dormant. This confers immunity to subsequent infection.
- Bacilli within granulomas may remain viable for many years, resulting in a positive purified protein derivative or other skin test for TB.
- Active disease develops in 5% to 15% of those infected.
- Transmission occurs when an infected person coughs or sneezes.

CAUSES

- Exposure to *M. tuberculosis*
- Exposure to other strains of mycobacteria (sometimes)

RISK FACTORS

- Close contact with newly diagnosed TB patient
- History of prior TB exposure
- Multiple sexual partners
- Recent immigration from Africa, Asia, Mexico, or South America
- Gastrectomy
- History of silicosis, diabetes, malnutrition, cancer, Hodgkin's disease, or leukemia
- Drug and alcohol abuse
- Residence in nursing home, mental health facility, or prison
- Immunosuppression and use of corticosteroids
- Homelessness

INCIDENCE

- The overall incidence rate for TB has decreased but is greater among high-risk populations.
- TB is twice as common in men as in women.
- TB is four times as common in non-whites as in Whites.
- There is higher incidence in Black and Hispanic men between ages 25 and 44.
- The highest incidence occurs in people who live in crowded, poorly ventilated, unsanitary conditions.

COMPLICATIONS

- Massive pulmonary tissue damage
- Respiratory failure
- Bronchopleural fistulas
- Pneumothorax
- Pleural effusion
- Pneumonia
- Infection of other body organs by small mycobacterial foci
- Liver involvement disease secondary to drug therapy

ASSESSMENT

HISTORY
In primary infection
- May be asymptomatic after a 4- to 8-week incubation period
- Weakness and fatigue
- Anorexia, weight loss
- Low-grade fever
- Night sweats

In reactivated infection
- Chest pain
- Productive cough for blood, or mucopurulent or blood-tinged sputum
- Low-grade fever

PHYSICAL FINDINGS
- Dullness over the affected area
- Crepitant crackles
- Bronchial breath sounds
- Wheezes
- Whispered pectoriloquy

DIAGNOSTIC TEST RESULTS

LABORATORY

- Tuberculin skin test result is positive in active and inactive tuberculosis.
- Stains and cultures of sputum, cerebrospinal fluid, urine, abscess drainage, or pleural fluid show heat-sensitive, nonmotile, aerobic, acid-fast bacilli.

IMAGING

- Chest X-rays show nodular lesions, patchy infiltrates, cavity formation, scar tissue, and calcium deposits.
- Computed tomography or magnetic resonance imaging shows presence and extent of lung damage.

DIAGNOSTIC PROCEDURES

- Bronchoscopy specimens show heat-sensitive, nonmotile, aerobic, acid-fast bacilli in specimens.

TREATMENT

GENERAL

- When disease no longer infectious (in 2 to 4 weeks), resumption of normal activities while continuing to take medication

DIET
- Well-balanced, high-calorie

ACTIVITY
- Rest, initially; then as tolerated

MEDICATIONS

- Antitubercular therapy for at least 6 months with daily oral doses of isoniazid, rifampin, and pyrazinamide, plus ethambutol in some cases.
- Second-line drugs include:
- capreomycin
- streptomycin
- aminosalicylic acid (para-aminosalicylic acid)
- pyrazinamide
- cycloserine.

SURGERY
- For some complications

NURSING CONSIDERATIONS

NURSING DIAGNOSES
- Fatigue
- Imbalanced nutrition: Less than body requirements
- Impaired gas exchange
- Ineffective airway clearance
- Ineffective coping
- Ineffective therapeutic regimen management
- Risk for injury

EXPECTED OUTCOMES
The patient will:
- identify measures to prevent or reduce fatigue
- consume required daily caloric intake
- maintain adequate ventilation and oxygenation
- maintain a patent airway
- use support systems to assist with coping
- express an understanding of the illness and comply with treatment modalities
- remain free from complications.

NURSING INTERVENTIONS
- Administer drug therapy.
- Isolate the patient in a quiet, properly ventilated room, and maintain tuberculosis precautions.
- Provide diversional activities.
- Properly dispose of secretions.
- Provide adequate rest periods.
- Provide well-balanced, high-calorie foods.
- Provide small, frequent meals.
- Consult with dietitian if oral supplements are needed.
- Perform chest physiotherapy.
- Provide supportive care.
- Include the patient in care decisions.

MONITORING
- Vital signs
- Intake and output
- Daily weight
- Complications
- Adverse reactions
- Visual acuity if taking ethambutol
- Liver and kidney function tests

PATIENT TEACHING

GENERAL
Be sure to cover:
- the disorder, diagnosis, and treatment
- drugs and potential adverse effects
- when to notify the physician
- need for isolation
- postural drainage and chest percussion
- coughing and deep-breathing exercises
- regular follow-up examinations
- signs and symptoms of recurring TB
- possible decreased hormonal contraceptive effectiveness while taking rifampin
- need for a high-calorie, high-protein, balanced diet
- TB prevention. (See *Preventing tuberculosis.*)

DISCHARGE PLANNING
- Refer anyone exposed to an infected patient for testing and follow-up.
- Refer patient to a support group, such as the American Lung Association.
- Refer patient to a smoking-cessation program, if indicated.

Preventing tuberculosis

Explain respiratory and standard precautions to a hospitalized patient with tuberculosis. Before discharge, tell him that he must take precautions to prevent spreading the disease, such as wearing a mask around others, until his physician tells him he's no longer contagious. He should tell all health care providers he sees, including his dentist and optometrist, that he has tuberculosis so that they can institute infection control precautions.

Teach the patient other specific precautions to avoid spreading the infection. Tell him to cough and sneeze into tissues and to dispose of the tissues properly. Stress the importance of washing his hands thoroughly in hot, soapy water after handling his own secretions. Also instruct him to wash his eating utensils separately in hot, soapy water.

RESOURCES

Organizations
American Lung Association: *www.lungusa.org*
Centers for Disease Control and Prevention: *www.cdc.gov*
National Institute of Allergy and Infectious Diseases: *www.niaid.nih.gov*
U.S. Department of Labor Occupational Safety & Health Administration: *www.osha.gov*
World Health Organization: *www.who.int*

Selected references
Forget, E.J., and Menzies, D. "Adverse Reactions to First-Line Antituberculosis Drugs," *Expert Opinion on Drug Safety* 5(2):231-49, March 2006.

Glickman, S.W., et al. "Medicine. A Portfolio of Drug Development for Tuberculosis," *Science* 311(5765):1246-247, March 2006.

Jereb, J.A., et al. "Commentary on the Risk of Active Tuberculosis," *Archives of Pediatrics & Adolescent Medicine* 160(3): 317-18, March 2006.

Kaufmann, S.H. "Robert Koch, the Nobel Prize, and the Ongoing Threat of Tuberculosis," *New England Journal of Medicine* 353(23):2423-426, December 2005.

Rubin, E.J. "Toward a New Therapy for Tuberculosis," *New England Journal of Medicine* 352(9):933-34, March 2005.

Williams, V.G. "Tuberculosis: Clinical Features, Diagnosis and Management," *Nursing Standard* 20(22):49-53, February 2006.

Tularemia

OVERVIEW

- *Francisella tularensis* organism, a gram-negative pleomorphic bacterium, causing disease in humans and animals
- As few as 10 organisms able to cause disease
- Incubation period 3 to 4 days
- Six forms:
  - Ulceroglandular
  - Glandular
  - Oculoglandular
  - Oropharyngeal
  - Pneumonic
  - Septicemic

PATHOPHYSIOLOGY

- The organism gains access to the host by skin or mucous membrane inoculation, inhalation, or ingestion.
- After inoculation a papule, which eventually evolves into an ulcer, and high fever develop.

CAUSES

- Bites of ticks and deerflies
- Breathing in the bacteria *F. tularensis*
- Contact with the blood of an infected animal, especially rabbits
- Eating or drinking contaminated food or water

INCIDENCE

- About 200 cases occur annually.
- This condition occurs more commonly in the south-central and western United States.

COMPLICATIONS

- Pneumonia
- Lung abscess
- Respiratory failure
- Rhabdomyolysis
- Meningitis
- Pericarditis
- Osteomyelitis

ASSESSMENT

HISTORY

- Tick bite
- Exposure to contaminated food or water
- Exposure to contaminated blood
- Abrupt onset of fever, chills, headache, and malaise

PHYSICAL FINDINGS

Ulceroglandular

- Ulcers at the site of inoculation
- Swollen regional lymph nodes

Glandular

- Swollen regional lymph nodes

Oculoglandular

- Painful
- Red eye
- Purulent exudates
- Swollen submandibular, preauricular, or cervical lymph nodes

Oropharyngeal

- Sore throat
- Abdominal pain
- Nausea
- Vomiting
- Diarrhea
- Occasionally, GI bleeding

Pneumonic

- Dry cough
- Dyspnea
- Pleuritic chest pain

Septicemic

- Fever, chills, myalgia, malaise, and weight loss
- Absence of ulcer

DIAGNOSTIC TEST RESULTS

LABORATORY

- A white blood cell count may be normal or elevated.
- Blood or sputum cultures are positive for *F. tularensis*.
- Serology may detect antibodies against *F. tularensis*.

IMAGING

- Chest X-ray may show pneumonia.

TREATMENT

GENERAL
◆ Proper skin care

DIET
◆ Increased fluid intake

MEDICATIONS
◆ I.V., I.M., or oral antibiotics
◆ Antipyretics

NURSING CONSIDERATIONS

NURSING DIAGNOSES
◆ Acute pain
◆ Diarrhea
◆ Hyperthermia
◆ Imbalanced nutrition: Less than body requirements
◆ Impaired gas exchange
◆ Impaired skin integrity
◆ Ineffective breathing pattern
◆ Risk for deficient fluid volume

EXPECTED OUTCOMES
The patient will:
◆ express feelings of comfort and relief from pain
◆ return to a normal elimination pattern
◆ remain afebrile
◆ maintain adequate nutritional intake
◆ express feelings of comfort in maintaining air exchange
◆ have warm, dry, and intact skin
◆ maintain adequate ventilation and oxygenation
◆ regain or maintain normal fluid balance.

NURSING INTERVENTIONS
◆ Give prescribed drugs.
◆ Replace lost fluids through diet or I.V. fluids.

MONITORING
◆ Intake and output
◆ Vital signs
◆ Signs of dehydration

PATIENT TEACHING

GENERAL
Be sure to cover:
◆ the disorder, diagnosis, and treatment
◆ drugs and potential adverse effects
◆ complications and when to notify the physician
◆ preventive measures, such as using insect repellent containing DEET on skin, or treating clothing with repellent containing permethrin.

RESOURCES
Organizations
National Center for Infectious Diseases — Division of Bacterial and Mycotic Diseases: *www.cdc.gov/ncidod/dbmd*
National Institute of Allergy and Infectious Diseases: *www.niaid.nih.gov*
U.S. Department of Labor Occupational Safety & Health Administration: *www.osha.gov*

Selected references
Buckingham, S.C. "Tick-borne Infections in Children: Epidemiology, Clinical Manifestations, and Optimal Management Strategies," *Paediatric Drugs* 7(3):163-76, 2005.
Daya, M., and Nakamura, Y. "Pulmonary Disease from Biological Agents: Anthrax, Plague, Q Fever, and Tularemia," *Critical Care Clinics* 21(4):747-63, vii, October 2005.
Farlow, J., et al. "Francisella Tularensis in the United States," *Emerging Infectious Diseases* 11(12):1835-841, December 2005.
Isherwood, K.E., et al. "Vaccination Strategies for Francisella Tularensis," *Advanced Drug Delivery Reviews* 57(9):1403-414, June 2005.
Schmitt, P., et al. "A Novel Screening ELISA and a Confirmatory Western Blot Useful for Diagnosis and Epidemiological Studies of Tularemia," *Epidemiology and Infection* 133(4):759-66, August 2005.

Ulcerative colitis

- Episodic inflammatory chronic disease that causes ulcerations of the mucosa in the colon
- Begins in the rectum and sigmoid colon and may extend upward into the entire colon
- Rarely affects the small intestine, except for the terminal ileum
- Produces congestion, edema (leading to mucosal friability), and ulcerations
- Range of severity from mild, localized disorder to fulminant disease that causes many complications

PATHOPHYSIOLOGY

- The disorder primarily involves the mucosa and the submucosa of the bowel.
- Crypt abscesses and mucosal ulceration may occur.
- The mucosa typically appears granular and friable.
- The colon becomes a rigid, foreshortened tube.
- In severe ulcerative colitis, areas of hyperplastic growth occur, with swollen mucosa surrounded by inflamed mucosa with shallow ulcers.
- Submucosa and the circular and longitudinal muscles may be involved.

CAUSES

- Exact cause unknown
- May be related to an abnormal immune response in the GI tract, possibly associated with genetic factors

RISK FACTORS

- Stress (may increase severity of an attack)
- Family history
- Jewish ancestry

INCIDENCE

- Ulcerative colitis occurs primarily in young adults, especially women.
- This disorder is more prevalent among Jews and higher socioeconomic groups.
- About 1 in 1,000 people are affected by this disorder.

- The onset of symptoms commonly peaks between ages 15 and 30 and again between ages 50 and 70.

COMPLICATIONS

- Nutritional deficiencies
- Perineal sepsis
- Anal fissure, anal fistula
- Perirectal abscess
- Perforation of the colon
- Hemorrhage, anemia
- Toxic megacolon
- Cancer
- Coagulation defects
- Erythema nodosum on the face and arms
- Pyoderma gangrenosum on the legs and ankles
- Uveitis
- Pericholangitis, sclerosing cholangitis
- Cirrhosis
- Cholangiocarcinoma
- Ankylosing spondylitis
- Strictures
- Pseudopolyps, stenosis, and perforated colon leading to peritonitis and toxemia
- Arthritis

HISTORY

- Remission and exacerbation of symptoms
- Mild cramping and lower abdominal pain
- Recurrent bloody diarrhea as often as 10 to 25 times daily
- Nocturnal diarrhea
- Fatigue and weakness
- Anorexia and weight loss
- Nausea and vomiting

PHYSICAL FINDINGS

- Liquid stools with visible pus, mucus, and blood
- Possible abdominal distention
- Abdominal tenderness
- Perianal irritation, hemorrhoids, and fissures
- Jaundice
- Joint pain

LABORATORY

- Stool specimen analysis reveals blood, pus, and mucus, but no pathogenic organisms.
- Other supportive laboratory tests show decreased serum levels of potassium, magnesium, hemoglobin, and albumin, as well as leukocytosis and increased prothrombin time; an elevated erythrocyte sedimentation rate correlates with the severity of the attack.

IMAGING

- Barium enema discloses the extent of disease and complications, such as strictures and carcinoma. This study isn't performed in a patient with active signs and symptoms.

DIAGNOSTIC PROCEDURES

- Sigmoidoscopy confirms rectal involvement in most cases by showing increased mucosal friability, decreased mucosal detail, and thick inflammatory exudates, edema, and erosions.
- Colonoscopy may be used to determine the extent of the disease and to evaluate the areas of stricture and pseudopolyps. This test isn't performed when the patient has active signs and symptoms.
- Biopsy, performed during colonoscopy, helps to confirm the diagnosis.

TREATMENT

GENERAL
- I.V. fluid replacement
- Blood transfusions, if needed

DIET
- Nothing by mouth (if severe)
- Parenteral nutrition (with severe disease)
- Supplemental feedings

ACTIVITY
- Rest periods during exacerbations

MEDICATIONS
- Corticotropin and adrenal cortico-steroids
- Sulfasalazine
- Mesalamine
- Antispasmodics and antidiarrheals
- Fiber supplements

SURGERY
- Treatment of last resort
- Proctocolectomy with ileostomy
- Pouch ileostomy
- Ileoanal reservoir with loop ileo-stomy
- Colectomy (after 10 years of active disease)

NURSING CONSIDERATIONS

NURSING DIAGNOSES
- Activity intolerance
- Acute pain
- Deficient fluid volume
- Diarrhea
- Disturbed body image
- Imbalanced nutrition: Less than body requirements
- Ineffective coping
- Risk for impaired skin integrity
- Risk for infection
- Risk for injury

EXPECTED OUTCOMES
The patient will:
- perform activities of daily living without excess fatigue or exhaustion
- express feelings of increased comfort and decreased pain
- maintain normal fluid volume
- regain normal bowel function
- express positive feelings about self
- maintain adequate caloric intake
- demonstrate effective coping skills
- maintain skin integrity
- remain free from signs and symptoms of infection
- avoid or minimize complications.

NURSING INTERVENTIONS
- Encourage verbalization and provide support.
- Provide diet therapy.
- Administer drug therapy.
- Give blood transfusions.
- Schedule care to allow for frequent rest periods.

MONITORING
- Response to treatment
- Fluid and electrolyte status
- Hemoglobin level and hematocrit
- Complications

After surgery
- Vital signs
- Wound site
- Pain level
- Bowel function
- Nasogastric tube function and drainage
- Skin integrity

PATIENT TEACHING

GENERAL
Be sure to cover:
- disorder, diagnosis, and treatment
- prescribed dietary changes
- importance of avoiding GI stimulants, such as caffeine, alcohol, and smoking
- medications administration, dosage, and possible adverse effects
- stoma care, after a proctocolectomy and ileostomy
- procedures to insert the catheter and care for the stoma, after a pouch ileostomy
- importance of regular physical examinations.

DISCHARGE PLANNING
- Refer the patient to a smoking-cessation program, if indicated.
- Refer the patient to an enterostomal therapist, if appropriate.

RESOURCES
Organizations
Crohn's & Colitis Foundation of America: *www.ccfa.org*
Digestive Disease National Coalition: *www.ddnc.org*
National Digestive Diseases Information Clearinghouse: *www.niddk.nih.gov/health/digest/nddic.htm*

Selected references
Handbook of Diseases, 3rd ed. Philadelphia: Lippincott Williams & Wilkins, 2004.
McNally, P. *GI/Liver Secrets*, 3rd ed. Philadelphia: Hanley & Belfus, Inc., 2006.
Sands, B.E. "Immunosuppressive Drugs in Ulcerative Colitis: Twisting Facts to Suit Theories?" *Gut* 55(4):437-41, April 2006.
Simmermacher, N.T. "Common Issues in Ostomy Care. Diarrhea and Excoriation in a Patient with an Ileoanal Reservoir," *Advance for Nurse Practitioners* 12(7):59-60, 62, July 2004.
Stein, P. "Ulcerative Colitis — Diagnosis and Surgical Treatment," *AORN Journal* 80(2):243-58, 261-62, August 2004.
Tanaka, M., and Kazuma, K. "Ulcerative Colitis: Factors Affecting Difficulties of Life and Psychological Well-Being of Patients in Remission," *Journal of Clinical Nursing* 14(1):65-73, January 2005.
Yamamoto, T., et al. "Safety and Clinical Efficacy of Granulocyte and Monocyte Adsorptive Apheresis Therapy for Ulcerative Colitis," *World Journal of Gastroenterology* 12(4):520-25, January 2006.

Urinary tract infection, lower

OVERVIEW

- Bacterial infection of the lower urinary tract system
- Two forms:
- Cystitis (infection of the bladder)
- Urethritis (infection of the urethra)
- Usually a ready response to treatment
- Possible recurring and resistant bacterial flare-ups during therapy
- Also known as *lower UTI*

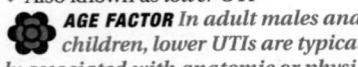 **AGE FACTOR** *In adult males and children, lower UTIs are typically associated with anatomic or physiologic abnormalities and require close evaluation.*

PATHOPHYSIOLOGY

- Local defense mechanisms in the bladder break down.
- Bacteria invade the bladder mucosa and multiply.
- Bacteria can't be readily eliminated by normal urination.
- The pathogen's resistance to prescribed antimicrobial therapy usually causes bacterial flare-up during treatment.
- Recurrent lower UTIs result from reinfection by the same organism or a new pathogen.

CAUSES

- Ascending infection by a single gram-negative, enteric bacterium, such as *Escherichia coli, Klebsiella, Proteus, Enterobacter, Pseudomonas,* and *Serratia*
- Simultaneous infection with multiple pathogens

RISK FACTORS

- Natural anatomic variations
- Inadequate fluid consumption
- Trauma or invasive procedures
- Urinary catheter
- Urinary tract obstructions
- Vesicourethral reflux
- Urinary stasis
- Diabetes
- Bowel incontinence
- Immobility

INCIDENCE

- Lower UTIs are nearly 10 times more common in females than in males (except elderly males), probably because natural anatomic features facilitate infection.
- Lower UTIs affect 10% to 20% of all females at least once.

COMPLICATIONS

- Damage to the urinary tract lining
- Infection of adjacent organs and structures

ASSESSMENT

HISTORY

- Urinary urgency and frequency
- Bladder cramps or spasms
- Pruritus
- Feeling of warmth during urination
- Nocturia or dysuria
- Urethral discharge (in men)
- Lower back or flank pain
- Malaise and chills
- Nausea and vomiting

PHYSICAL FINDINGS

- Pain or tenderness over the bladder
- Hematuria
- Fever
- Cloudy, foul-smelling urine

DIAGNOSTIC TEST RESULTS

LABORATORY

- Microscopic urinalysis may show red blood cell and white blood cell counts greater than 10 per high-power field, suggesting a lower UTI.
- Clean-catch urinalysis may show a bacterial count of more than 100,000/ml, confirming a lower UTI.
- Sensitivity testing determines the appropriate antimicrobial drug.
- If the patient history and physical examination warrant, a blood test or a stained smear of urethral discharge may rule out sexually transmitted diseases.

IMAGING

- Voiding cystourethrography or excretory urography may demonstrate congenital anomalies, predisposing the patient to recurrent UTIs.

TREATMENT

GENERAL
◆ Sitz baths or warm compresses

DIET
◆ Increased fruit juice intake, especially cranberry
◆ Increased fluid intake

MEDICATIONS
◆ Antimicrobials

SURGERY
◆ In case of recurrent infections from infected renal calculi, chronic prostatitis, or structural abnormalities

NURSING CONSIDERATIONS

NURSING DIAGNOSES
◆ Acute pain
◆ Disturbed sleep pattern
◆ Impaired urinary elimination
◆ Risk for infection
◆ Risk for injury
◆ Sexual dysfunction

EXPECTED OUTCOMES
The patient will:
◆ report increased comfort
◆ verbalize feeling well rested after undisturbed periods of sleep
◆ demonstrate skill in managing the urinary elimination problem
◆ remain free from further signs or symptoms of infection
◆ avoid or minimize complications
◆ reestablish sexual activity at the pre-illness level.

NURSING INTERVENTIONS
◆ Collect all urine specimens appropriately.
◆ Administer drug therapy.
◆ Encourage oral fluid intake unless contraindicated.
◆ Use sitz baths or warm compresses, as needed.

MONITORING
◆ Intake and output
◆ Urine characteristics
◆ Voiding patterns
◆ Vital signs
◆ Adverse effects of antimicrobial therapy

PATIENT TEACHING

GENERAL
Be sure to cover:
◆ disorder, diagnosis, and treatment
◆ completion of the prescribed course of antibiotics
◆ drug administration, dosage, and possible adverse effects
◆ warm sitz baths to relieve perineal discomfort
◆ proper cleaning after toileting.

RESOURCES
Organizations
American Association of Kidney Patients: *www.aakp.org*
National Institute of Diabetes & Digestive & Kidney Diseases: *www.niddk.nih.gov*

Selected references
Diseases, 4th ed. Philadelphia: Lippincott Williams & Wilkins, 2006.
Falagas, M.E., and Vergidis, P.I. "Urinary Tract Infections in Patients with Urinary Diversion," *American Journal of Kidney Diseases* 46(6):1030-1037, December 2005.
Schaeffer, A.J. "The Natural Course of Uncomplicated Lower Urinary Tract Infection in Women Illustrated by a Randomized Placebo-Controlled Study," *Journal of Urology* 173(2):467-68, February 2005.
Schroeder, A.R., et al. "Choice of Urine Collection Methods for the Diagnosis of Urinary Tract Infection in Young, Febrile Infants," *Archives of Pediatrics & Adolescent Medicine* 159(10):915-22, October 2005.
van Merode, T., et al. "Acute Uncomplicated Lower Urinary Tract Infections in General Practice: Clinical and Microbiological Cure Rates after Three- versus Five-Day Treatment with Trimethoprim," *European Journal of General Practice* 11(2):55-58, June 2005.

Urticaria and angioedema

OVERVIEW

- Common allergic reactions
- Occur separately or simultaneously
- Urticaria: may be acute (present for less than 6 weeks) or chronic (present for at least 6 weeks)
- Also known as *hives*

PATHOPHYSIOLOGY

- Urticaria is an episodic, rapidly occurring, usually self-limiting skin reaction. It involves only the superficial portion of the dermis, which erupts with local wheals surrounded by an erythematous flare.
- Angioedema involves additional skin layers and produces deeper, larger wheals, usually on the hands, feet, lips, genitalia, and eyelids. It causes diffuse swelling of loose subcutaneous tissue and may affect the upper respiratory and GI tracts.
- Several mechanisms and disorders may provoke urticaria and angioedema. They include immunoglobulin (Ig) E–induced release of mediators from cutaneous mast cells and binding of IgG or IgM to antigen, resulting in complement activation.

CAUSES

- Unknown
- Cholinergic trigger (heat, exercise, stress)
- Drug allergy
- Food allergy
- Hormones
- Inhalant allergens (animal dander, cosmetics)
- Insect bite
- Occupational skin exposure
- Rheumatological disease
- Thyroid abnormality
- Viral infection

INCIDENCE

- Urticaria and angioedema affect about 20% of people at some time in their lives.
- These disorders are more common after adolescence; the highest incidence is in people in their 30s.
- These disorders affect females more commonly than males.

COMPLICATIONS

- Skin abrasion and secondary infection
- Laryngeal edema
- Respiratory arrest
- Severe abdominal colic

ASSESSMENT

HISTORY

- Drug history, including nonprescription preparations such as vitamins, aspirin, and antacids
- Reported commonly troublesome foods and environmental factors
- Exposure to physical factors, such as cold, sunlight, exercise, and trauma
- Adverse reaction to iodinated contrast media used for diagnostic radiological studies

PHYSICAL FINDINGS

- Distinct, raised, evanescent dermal wheals surrounded by a reddened flare
- Nonpitting swelling of deep subcutaneous tissue on the eyelids, lips, genitalia, and mucous membranes that doesn't itch but may burn and tingle
- Respiratory stridor and hoarseness
- Anxiety, gasping for breath, and difficulty speaking
- Abdominal colic with or without nausea and vomiting
- Signs of anaphylaxis: hypotension, respiratory distress, stridor

DIAGNOSTIC TEST RESULTS

LABORATORY
◆ Decreased serum levels of C1, C2, and C4 inhibitors may confirm the diagnosis.

DIAGNOSTIC PROCEDURES
◆ Diagnosis may be confirmed through careful skin testing with the suspected offending substance to see if a local wheal and flare result.

TREATMENT

GENERAL
◆ Emergency measures if signs of anaphylaxis
◆ Limited contact with triggering factors
◆ Desensitization to the triggering antigen

DIET
◆ Avoidance of food allergens

MEDICATIONS
◆ Antihistamines
◆ Systemic glucocorticoids

NURSING CONSIDERATIONS

NURSING DIAGNOSES
◆ Acute pain
◆ Anxiety
◆ Disturbed body image
◆ Impaired oral mucous membrane
◆ Impaired skin integrity
◆ Ineffective airway clearance
◆ Ineffective breathing pattern
◆ Powerlessness
◆ Risk for infection
◆ Risk for injury

EXPECTED OUTCOMES
The patient will:
◆ express feelings of increased comfort and decreased pain
◆ express a reduced level of anxiety
◆ verbalize feelings about a changed body image
◆ maintain intact oral mucous membranes
◆ exhibit improved or healed lesions or wounds
◆ maintain a patent airway
◆ maintain respiratory rate within 5 breaths/minute of baseline
◆ express feelings of control over well-being
◆ remain free from signs or symptoms of infection
◆ avoid or minimize complications.

NURSING INTERVENTIONS
◆ Maintain a patent airway.
◆ Reduce or minimize environmental exposure to offending allergens and irritants, such as wool and harsh detergents.
◆ If food is a suspected cause, gradually eliminate foods from the diet, and watch for improvement.
◆ Administer drug therapy.

MONITORING
◆ Vital signs, with attention to respiratory status
◆ Skin, for signs of secondary infection caused by scratching
◆ Response to treatment

PATIENT TEACHING

GENERAL
Be sure to cover:
◆ disorder, diagnosis, and treatment
◆ how to identify the cause by recording exposure to suspected offending substances and the signs and symptoms that appear after exposure
◆ how to monitor nutritional status and nutrient replacement foods
◆ importance of keeping fingernails short to avoid abrading the skin when scratching
◆ signs and symptoms that indicate a skin infection
◆ how to use an epinephrine emergency kit if anaphylaxis occurs.

RESOURCES
Organizations
Allergic Diseases Resource Center: *www.worldallergy.org*
American Academy of Dermatology: *www.aad.org*
American College of Allergy, Asthma and Immunology: *www.acaai.org*

Selected references
Baxi, S., and Dinakar, C. "Urticaria and Angioedema," *Immunology and Allergy Clinics of North America* 25(2):353-67, vii, May 2005.

Bork, K., et al. "Hereditary Angioedema: New Findings Concerning Symptoms, Affected Organs, and Course," *American Journal of Medicine* 119(3):267-74, March 2006.

Kaplan, A.P., and Greaves, M.W. "Angioedema," *Journal of the American Academy of Dermatology* 53(3):373-88, September 2005.

Kasper, D.L., et al., eds. *Harrison's Principles of Internal Medicine*, 16th ed. New York: McGraw-Hill Book Co., 2005.

Mathelier-Fusade, P. "Drug-induced Urticarias," *Clinical Reviews in Allergy & Immunology* 30(1):19-24, February 2006.

The Merck Manual of Diagnosis & Therapy, 18th ed. Whitehouse Station, N.J.: Merck & Co., Inc., 2006.

Picado, C. "Non-steroidal Anti-Inflammatory Drugs-Induced Urticaria and Angioedema: More Research on Mechanisms Needed," *Clinical and Experimental Allergy* 35(6):698-99, June 2005.

Uterine cancer

- Proliferation of cancer cells in the endometrium
- Most common gynecologic cancer
- Also known as *endometrial cancer*

PATHOPHYSIOLOGY

- Uterine cancer is usually adenocarcinoma.
- Metastasis occurs late, usually from the endometrium to the cervix, ovaries, fallopian tubes, and other peritoneal structures. It may spread to distant organs, such as the lungs and the brain, by way of the blood or the lymphatic system; lymph node involvement can also occur.
- Less common uterine tumors include adenoacanthoma, endometrial stromal sarcoma, lymphosarcoma, mixed mesodermal tumors (including carcinosarcoma), and leiomyosarcoma.

CAUSES

- Exact cause unknown

RISK FACTORS

- Low fertility index and anovulation
- History of infertility or failure of ovulation
- Abnormal uterine bleeding
- Obesity
- Hypertension
- Diabetes
- Nulliparity
- Familial tendency
- History of uterine polyps or endometrial hyperplasia
- Prolonged estrogen therapy with exposure unopposed by progesterone
- Tamoxifen therapy
- Estrogren replacement therapy

INCIDENCE

- Uterine cancer is most common in postmenopausal women between ages 60 and 70. It's uncommon between ages 30 and 40 and rare before age 30.
- Most premenopausal patients have a history of anovulatory menstrual cycles or other hormonal imbalances.
- Annually about 33,000 new cases are reported; about 5,500 eventually are fatal.

COMPLICATIONS

- Anemia
- Intestinal obstruction
- Ascites
- Increasing pain
- Hemorrhage

HISTORY

- Presence of risk factors
- Spotting and protracted, heavy menses (in younger patient)
- In postmenopausal woman, possible bleeding beginning 12 or more months after menses stopped
- Vaginal discharge, initially watery, then increasingly blood streaked

PHYSICAL FINDINGS

- Palpable enlarged uterus (advanced disease)
- Abdominal tenderness

DIAGNOSTIC PROCEDURES

- Endometrial, cervical, or endocervical biopsy confirms the presence of cancer cells.
- Fractional dilatation and curettage are used to identify the problem when the disease is suspected but the endometrial biopsy result is negative.
- Multiple cervical biopsies and endocervical curettage pinpoint cervical involvement.
- A Papanicolaou test result may be normal or show abnormal cells.

OTHER

- Schiller's test involves staining the cervix and vagina with an iodine solution that turns healthy tissues brown. (Cancerous tissues resist the stain.)

TREATMENT

GENERAL
- Radiation therapy

DIET
- Well-balanced

MEDICATIONS
- Hormonal therapy
- Chemotherapy

SURGERY
- Total abdominal hysterectomy, bilateral salpingooophorectomy or, possibly, omentectomy with or without pelvic or para-aortic lymphadenectomy
- Total pelvic exenteration

NURSING CONSIDERATIONS

NURSING DIAGNOSES
- Acute pain
- Anxiety
- Disturbed body image
- Fear
- Impaired urinary elimination
- Ineffective coping
- Risk for infection
- Sexual dysfunction

EXPECTED OUTCOMES
The patient will:
- report feeling increased comfort and decreased pain
- express feelings of decreased anxiety
- express positive feelings about self
- discuss fears and concerns
- maintain adequate urine output
- demonstrate positive coping behaviors
- remain free from signs and symptoms of infection
- express feelings and perceptions about change in sexual performance with partner.

NURSING INTERVENTIONS
- Encourage verbalization and provide support.
- Administer drug therapy.
- Encourage the patient to breathe deeply and cough.

MONITORING
After surgery
- Wound site and drainage system
- Vital signs
- Postoperative complications
- Pain control

Internal radiation therapy
- Safety precautions (time, distance, and shielding)
- Movement (limited while source is in place)
- Vital signs
- Complications from radiation therapy, such as skin reaction, vaginal bleeding, abdominal discomfort, and dehydration

PATIENT TEACHING

GENERAL
Be sure to cover:
- disorder, diagnosis, and treatment
- preoperative and postoperative care
- (if the patient is premenopausal) that removal of her ovaries will induce menopause
- safety measures involved in internal radiation therapy
- dietary modifications
- drug administration, dosage, and possible adverse effects
- importance of follow-up examinations with a gynecologist.

DISCHARGE PLANNING
- Refer the patient to available resource and support services.

RESOURCES
Organizations
American Cancer Society:
www.cancer.org
Guide to Internet Resources for Cancer:
www.cancerindex.org
National Cancer Institute:
www.cancer.gov

Selected references
Ackermann, S., et al. "Awareness of General and Personal Risk Factors for Uterine Cancer Among Healthy Women," *European Journal of Cancer Prevention* 14(6):519-24, December 2005.

Ahlberg, K., et al. "Fatigue, Psychological Distress, Coping Resources, and Functional Status during Radiotherapy for Uterine Cancer," *Oncology Nursing Forum* 32(3):633-40, May 2005.

Atlas of Pathophysiology, 2nd ed. Philadelphia: Lippincott Williams & Wilkins, 2005.

Gold, M.A., et al. "Effects of Tubal Occlusion on Dissemination of Uterine Cancer," *International Journal of Gynecological Cancer* 14 (Suppl 1):6, September-October 2004.

Loizzi, V., et al. "Hormone Replacement Therapy on Ovarian and Uterine Cancer Risk and Cancer Survivors: How Shall We Do No Harm?" *International Journal of Gynecological Cancer* 15(3):420-25, May-June 2005.

Uterine leiomyomas

OVERVIEW

- Most common benign uterine tumors
- Tumors composed of smooth muscle that usually occur in the uterine corpus, although they may appear on the cervix or on the round or broad ligament
- Malignant in less than 0.1% of patients
- Also known as *myomas, fibromyomas,* or *fibroids*

PATHOPHYSIOLOGY

- Classified according to location, tumors may be located within the uterine wall (intramural) or protrude into the endometrial cavity (submucous) or from the serosal surface of the uterus (subserous).
- Size varies greatly.
- Tumors are usually firm and surrounded by a pseudocapsule composed of compressed but otherwise normal uterine myometrium.
- The uterine cavity may become larger, increasing the endometrial surface area. This can cause increased uterine bleeding.

CAUSES

- Unknown

RISK FACTORS

- Possible regulators of leiomyoma growth include:
- several growth factors including epidermal growth factor
- steroid hormones, including estrogen and progesterone (typically arise after menarche and regress after menopause, implicating estrogen as a promoter of leiomyoma growth).

INCIDENCE

- This disorder may affect three times as many Blacks as Whites; true incidence in either population is unknown.
- This disorder may occur at any age but is most common in women over age 30.

COMPLICATIONS

- Recurrent spontaneous abortion
- Preterm labor
- Malposition of the fetus
- Anemia secondary to excessive bleeding
- Bladder compression
- Infection
- Secondary infertility
- Bowel obstruction

ASSESSMENT

HISTORY

- Abnormal menstrual bleeding
- Urinary frequency, urgency, or incontinence
- Abdominal cramping during menstruation

PHYSICAL FINDINGS

- Pelvic pressure
- Abdominal distention

DIAGNOSTIC TEST RESULTS

LABORATORY

- Blood studies may show anemia from abnormal bleeding, which may support a diagnosis.

IMAGING

- An ultrasound allows an accurate assessment of the dimension, number, and location of tumors.
- A magnetic resonance imaging test may reveal calcified fibroids.

DIAGNOSTIC PROCEDURES

- Hysterosalpingography may detect myomas.

OTHER

- Patient history may reveal evidence.
- Bimanual examination may show an enlarged, firm, nontender, and irregularly contoured uterus (also seen with adenomyosis and other pelvic abnormalities).
- An endometrial biopsy may rule out endometrial cancer in patients who have abnormal uterine bleeding and are over age 35.
- Laparoscopy may corroborate other testing.

TREATMENT

GENERAL
◆ Blood transfusions

ACTIVITY
◆ As tolerated

MEDICATIONS
◆ Gonadotropin-releasing hormone agonists to rapidly suppress pituitary gonadotropin release
◆ Nonsteroidal anti-inflammatory drugs

SURGERY
◆ Abdominal, laparoscopic, or hysteroscopic myomectomy
◆ Myolysis
◆ Uterine artery embolization (radiologic procedure) to block uterine arteries using small pieces of polyvinyl chloride
◆ Hysterectomy

NURSING CONSIDERATIONS

NURSING DIAGNOSES
◆ Acute pain
◆ Anxiety
◆ Hopelessness
◆ Ineffective coping
◆ Ineffective sexuality patterns

EXPECTED OUTCOMES
The patient will:
◆ report increased comfort and decreased pain
◆ express feelings of decreased anxiety
◆ be involved in planning own care
◆ use available support systems, such as family and friends, to aid in coping
◆ express feelings about the condition and its effect on sexuality.

NURSING INTERVENTIONS
◆ Reassure the patient that she won't experience premature menopause if her ovaries are left intact.
◆ In a patient with severe anemia from excessive bleeding, give iron supplements and blood transfusions.
◆ Encourage the patient to verbalize her feelings and concerns related to the disease process and its effects on her lifestyle.

MONITORING
◆ Comfort level
◆ Amount of bleeding
◆ Response to treatment

PATIENT TEACHING

GENERAL
Be sure to cover:
◆ disorder, diagnosis, and treatment
◆ importance of reporting abnormal bleeding or pelvic pain immediately
◆ importance of regular gynecologic examinations.

RESOURCES
Organizations
American College of Obstetricians and Gynecologists: *www.acog.org*
Center for Uterine Fibroids: *www.fibroids.net*
National Uterine Fibroids Foundation: *www.nuff.org*
National Women's Health Information Center: *www.4woman.gov*

Selected references
Bachmann, G. "Expanding Treatment Option for Women with Symptomatic Uterine Leiomyomas: Timely Medical Breakthroughs," *Fertility and Sterility* 85(1):46-47, January 2006.
Baird, D.D., et al. "Luteinizing Hormone in Premenopausal Women May Stimulate Uterine Leiomyomata Development," *Journal for the Society of Gynecologic Investigation* 13(2):130-35, February 2006.
Hiller, J.Y., et al. "Uterine Artery Embolization: A Minimally Invasive Option to End Fibroid Symptoms," *Advance for Nurse Practitioners* 13(10):20-25, October 2005.
Ouyang, D.W., et al. "Obstetric Complications of Fibroids," *Obstetrics and Gynecology Clinics of North America* 33(1):153-69, March 2006.
Van Court, R.L. "Uterine Fibroids and Women's Right to Choose. Hysterectomies and Informed Consent," *Journal of Legal Medicine* 26(4):507-21, December 2005.

Vaginal cancer

- Proliferation of cancer cells in the vagina
- Rarest gynecologic cancer
- Usually appears as squamous cell carcinoma, but occasionally as melanoma, sarcoma, or adenocarcinoma

PATHOPHYSIOLOGY

- Because the vagina is a thin-walled structure with rich lymphatic drainage, vaginal cancer varies in severity, depending on its exact location and effect on lymphatic drainage.
- It may progress from an intraepithelial tumor to an invasive cancer.
- The upper third of the vagina is the most common site of vaginal cancer.

CAUSES

- Exact cause unknown

RISK FACTORS

- Advanced age (most likely risk factor) combined with:
- – trauma
- – chronic pessary use
- – use of chemical carcinogens (such as those in some sprays and douches)
- – use of diethylstilbestrol by the patient's mother during pregnancy
- – previous cancer of the endometrium, vulva, or cervix.

INCIDENCE

- Vaginal cancer usually occurs in women in their early to middle 50s.
- Rarely, rhabdomyosarcomas originate in the vagina in children.

COMPLICATIONS

- Metastasis may affect the cervix, uterus, and rectum.

HISTORY

- Presence of risk factors
- Bloody vaginal discharge
- Irregular or postmenopausal bleeding
- Urine retention or urinary frequency (if the lesion is close to the neck of the bladder)

PHYSICAL FINDINGS

- Ulcerated lesion in any area of the vagina

LABORATORY

- A Papanicolaou test may show abnormal cells.

DIAGNOSTIC PROCEDURES

- A biopsy may identify cancerous cells.
- A biopsy of the cervix and vulva may also be performed to rule out these areas as primary cancer sites.
- A colposcopy is used to locate lesions that may have been missed during the pelvic examination.

OTHER

- Lugol's solution painted on the suspected area may help to identify malignant areas by staining glycogen-containing normal tissue. (Abnormal tissue resists staining.)

TREATMENT

GENERAL
◆ Radiation therapy (preferred treatment for all stages of vaginal cancer)

DIET
◆ Well-balanced

ACTIVITY
◆ Limited (with internal radiation therapy)

MEDICATIONS
◆ Topical chemotherapy with fluorouracil and laser surgery

SURGERY
◆ May be recommended when tumor is so extensive that vagina's close proximity to the bladder and rectum allows only minimal tissue margins around resected vaginal tissue

NURSING CONSIDERATIONS

NURSING DIAGNOSES
◆ Acute pain
◆ Anxiety
◆ Disturbed body image
◆ Fear
◆ Impaired tissue integrity
◆ Ineffective coping
◆ Ineffective sexuality patterns
◆ Risk for infection

EXPECTED OUTCOMES
The patient will:
◆ experience feelings of increased comfort and decreased pain
◆ report that she feels less anxious
◆ express positive feelings about self
◆ voluntarily express fears and concerns
◆ experience an improvement in the condition of her ulcerated vaginal tissue, with decreased redness, swelling, and pain
◆ demonstrate positive coping behaviors
◆ express feelings and perceptions about change in sexual performance (with partner)
◆ exhibit no signs or symptoms of infection.

NURSING INTERVENTIONS
◆ Encourage verbalization and provide support.
◆ Administer drug therapy.

MONITORING
◆ Response to treatment
◆ Vaginal discharge

Internal radiation therapy
◆ Safety measures (time, distance, and shielding)
◆ Limited movement
◆ Complications from radiation therapy

PATIENT TEACHING

GENERAL
Be sure to cover:
◆ disorder, diagnosis, and treatment
◆ safety measures for radiation therapy
◆ importance of follow-up care
◆ importance of regular gynecologic check-ups
◆ adverse reactions to chemotherapy and ways to manage them
◆ signs and symptoms of infection and the need to report them to a practitioner immediately
◆ ways to avoid infection.

DISCHARGE PLANNING
◆ Refer the patient (and family) to American Cancer Society for resources and support services.

RESOURCES
Organizations
American Cancer Society:
www.cancer.org
Guide to Internet Resources for Cancer:
www.cancerindex.org
National Cancer Institute:
www.cancer.gov

Selected references
Atlas of Pathophysiology, 2nd ed. Philadelphia: Lippincott Williams & Wilkins, 2005.

Feng, Q., and Kiviat, N.B. "New and Surprising Insights into Pathogenesis of Multicentric Squamous Cancers in the Female Lower Genital Tract," *Journal of the National Cancer Institute* 97(24):1798-99, December 2005.

Gokaslan, H., et al. "Primary Malignant Melanoma of the Vagina: A Case Report and Review of the Current Treatment Options," *European Journal of Obstetrics, Gynecology, and Reproductive Biology* 121(2):243-48, August 2005.

Goker, B.O., et al. "A Case with Multiple Gynecological Malignancies," *International Journal of Gynecological Cancer* 15(2):372-76, March-April 2005.

Nomura, Y., et al. "Radiofrequency Ablation for the Treatment of Hemorrhagic Vaginal Cancer," *Journal of Vascular and Interventional Radiology* 16(11): 1557-58, November 2005.

Vancomycin intermediate-resistant *Staphylococcus*

- First discovered in mid-1996
- Staphylococci infection that has decreased susceptibility to vancomycin
- Common in chronically ill patients; most likely developing in health care setting
- Patient with methicillin-resistant *Staphylococcus aureus* (MRSA) normally most reliably and effectively treated with vancomycin; MRSA with decreased susceptibility to vancomycin possibly a sign that vancomycin-resistant strains are emerging
- Also called *VISA* and *glycopeptide intermediate-resistant* Staphylococcus aureus

PATHOPHYSIOLOGY

- Genes encode resistance and are carried on plasmids that transfer themselves from cell to cell.
- Resistance is mediated by enzymes that substitute a different molecule for the terminal amino acid so that vancomycin can't bind.

CAUSES

- Direct contact with infected or colonized patient or colonized health care worker or contact with a contaminated surface such as an overbed table

INCIDENCE

- Colonized patient is more than 10 times as likely to become infected with the organism as uncolonized patient, such as through a breach in the immune system.
- Four cases have been detected in the United States.
- This disorder has been noted in patients receiving multiple courses of vancomycin for MRSA infections.

COMPLICATIONS

- Sepsis
- Multisystem organ involvement
- Death in the immunocompromised patient

ASSESSMENT

HISTORY

- Possible breach in the immune system, surgery, or condition predisposing the patient to the infection
- Multiple antibiotic use

PHYSICAL FINDINGS

- The carrier patient is commonly asymptomatic but may exhibit signs and symptoms related to the primary diagnosis.
- The patient may exhibit cardiac, respiratory, or other major symptoms.

DIAGNOSTIC TEST RESULTS

LABORATORY

- Culture may show staphylococci with decreased susceptibility to vancomycin after 24-hour incubation.

aureus

TREATMENT

GENERAL
- With an infection, possibly no treatment
- Colonized patient in contact isolation until culture-negative or discharged
- Antimicrobial drugs

DIET
- No restrictions

ACTIVITY
- Rest periods when fatigued

MEDICATIONS
- Antimicrobials

NURSING CONSIDERATIONS

NURSING DIAGNOSES
- Acute pain
- Decreased cardiac output
- Deficient fluid volume
- Hyperthermia
- Impaired tissue integrity
- Ineffective tissue perfusion: Cardiopulmonary

EXPECTED OUTCOMES
The patient will:
- report decreased pain levels
- maintain adequate cardiac output
- have an adequate fluid volume
- remain afebrile
- maintain adequate circulation to impaired tissues
- attain and maintain hemodynamic stability.

NURSING INTERVENTIONS
- Consider grouping infected patients together and having the same nursing staff care for them.
- Institute contact isolation precautions.
- Ensure judicious and careful use of antibiotics. Encourage physicians to limit the use of antibiotics.
- Use infection-control practices, such as wearing gloves before and after contact with infectious body tissues and proper hand washing, to reduce the spread of VISA.

MONITORING
- Vital signs
- Response to treatment
- Complications

PATIENT TEACHING

GENERAL
Be sure to cover:
- disorder, diagnosis, and treatment
- importance of family and friends wearing personal protective equipment when they visit the patient
- how to dispose of protective equipment
- drug administration, dosage, and possible adverse effects.

RESOURCES
Organizations
National Center for Infectious Diseases: *www.cdc.gov/ncidod*
National Institute of Allergy and Infectious Diseases: *www.niaid.nih.gov*
National Library of Medicine: *www.nlm.nih.gov*

Selected references
Appelbaum, P.C. "The Emergence of Vancomycin-Intermediate and Vancomycin-Resistant *Staphylococcus Aureus*," *Clinical Microbiology and Infection* 12 Suppl 1:16-23, March 2006.

Bhateja, P., et al. "Characterisation of Laboratory-generated Vancomycin Intermediate Resistant *Staphylococcus Aureus* Strains," *International Journal of Antimicrobial Agents* 27(3):201-11, March 2006.

Cui, L., et al. "Correlation between Reduced Daptomycin Susceptibility and Vancomycin Resistance in Vancomycin-Intermediate *Staphylococcus Aureus*," *Antimicrobial Agents and Chemotherapy* 50(3): 1079-82, March 2006.

Howden, B.P. "Recognition and Management of Infections Caused by Vancomycin-Intermediate *Staphylococcus Aureus* (VISA) and Heterogenous VISA (hVISA)," *Internal Medicine Journal* 35 Suppl 2:S136-40, December 2005.

Kasper, D.L., et al., eds. *Harrison's Principles of Internal Medicine,* 16th ed. New York: McGraw-Hill Book Co., 2005.

Vancomycin-resistant enterococci

- Mutation of a common bacterium
- Easily spread by direct person-to-person contact
- Also called *VRE*

PATHOPHYSIOLOGY

- Genes encode resistance and are carried on plasmids that transfer themselves from cell to cell.
- Resistance is mediated by enzymes that substitute a different molecule for the terminal amino acid so that vancomycin can't bind.

CAUSES

- Direct contact with infected or colonized patient or colonized health care worker or contact with a contaminated surface such as an overbed table.

RISK FACTORS

- Immunocompromised condition
- Old age
- Indwelling catheter
- Major surgery
- Open wounds
- History of taking vancomycin or a third-generation cephalosporin
- History of enterococcal bacteremia, often linked to endocarditis
- Organ transplantation
- Prolonged or repeated hospital admissions
- Chronic renal failure
- Exposure to contaminated equipment or a VRE-positive patient

INCIDENCE

- This disorder has been reported in facilities in more than 40 states.
- Incidence rates have been as high as 14% in oncology units.

COMPLICATIONS

- Sepsis

HISTORY

- Possible breach in the immune system, surgery, or condition predisposing the patient to the infection
- Multiple antibiotic use

PHYSICAL FINDINGS

- Carrier commonly asymptomatic

LABORATORY

- VRE is isolated from stool or a rectal swab.

Taking precautions at home

Tell the patient's caregivers to:
- wash their hands with soap and water after physical contact with the patient and before leaving the home
- use towels only once when drying hands after contact
- wear disposable gloves if they expect to come in contact with the patient's body fluids and to wash hands after removing the gloves
- change linens routinely and whenever they become soiled
- clean the patient's environment routinely and when it becomes soiled with body fluids
- tell physicians and other health care personnel caring for the patient that the patient is infected with an organism resistant to multiple drugs.

GENERAL
- With an infection, possibly no treatment
- Colonized patient placed in contact isolation until culture-negative or discharged

ACTIVITY
- Rest periods when fatigued

MEDICATIONS
- Antimicrobials (VRE isolates not susceptible to vancomycin generally susceptible to other antimicrobial drugs)

NURSING DIAGNOSES
- Acute pain
- Decreased cardiac output
- Deficient fluid volume
- Hyperthermia
- Ineffective tissue perfusion: Cardiopulmonary

EXPECTED OUTCOMES
The patient will:
- report decreased pain levels
- maintain adequate cardiac output
- have an adequate fluid volume
- remain afebrile
- attain and maintain hemodynamic stability.

NURSING INTERVENTIONS
- Consider grouping infected patients together and having the same nursing staff care for them.
- Institute contact isolation precautions.
- Ensure judicious and careful use of antibiotics. Encourage physicians to limit the use of antibiotics.
- Use infection-control practices, such as wearing gloves and employing proper hand-washing techniques, to reduce the spread of VRE.

MONITORING
- Vital signs
- Response to treatment
- Complications

GENERAL
Be sure to cover:
- disorder, diagnosis, and treatment (see *Taking precautions at home*)
- importance of family and friends wearing personal protective equipment when visiting the patient
- how to dispose of protective equipment
- drug administration, dosage, and possible adverse effects.

RESOURCES
Organizations
National Center for Infectious Diseases: *www.cdc.gov/ncidod*
National Institute of Allergy and Infectious Diseases: *www.niaid.nih.gov*
National Library of Medicine: *www.nlm.nih.gov*

Selected references
Furuno, J.P., et al. "Methicillin-resistant Staphylococcus Aureus and Vancomycin-Resistant Enterococci Co-Colonization," *Emerging Infectious Diseases* 11(10):1539-44, October 2005.
Goldrick, B.A. "MRSA, VRE, and VRSA: How Do We Control Them in Nursing Homes?" *American Journal of Nursing* 104(8):50-51, August 2004.
Kolar, M., et al. "The Influence of Antibiotic Use on the Occurrence of Vancomycin-resistant Enterococci," *Journal of Clinical Pharmacy and Therapeutics* 31(1):67-72, February 2006.
Mascini, E.M., et al "Genotyping and Preemptive Isolation to Control an Outbreak of Vancomycin-resistant Enterococcus Faecium," *Clinical Infectious Diseases* 42(6):739-46, March 2006.

Varicella

- An acute, highly contagious viral infection
- The virus that causes chickenpox, thought to become latent until the sixth decade of life or later, causing herpes zoster (shingles)
- Transmission through direct contact and indirect contact
- Congenital varicella possible in infants whose mothers had acute infections in first or early second trimester
- Commonly known as *chickenpox*

PATHOPHYSIOLOGY

- Localized replication of the virus occurs (probably in the nasopharynx), leading to seeding of the reticuloendothelial system and development of viremia.
- Diffuse and scattered skin lesions result with vesicles involving the corium and dermis with degenerative changes (ballooning) and infection of localized blood vessels.
- Necrosis and epidermal hemorrhage result; vesicles eventually rupture and release fluid or are reabsorbed.
- Incubation period lasts 13 to 17 days.
- Infection is communicable from 48 hours before lesions erupt until after vesicles are crusted over.

CAUSES

- Varicella-zoster herpesvirus

INCIDENCE

- Chickenpox is most common in children ages 5 to 9 but can occur at any age.
- Neonatal infection is rare, probably because of transient maternal immunity.
- This disease occurs worldwide and is endemic in large cities with outbreaks occurring sporadically.
- Chickenpox equally affects all races and both sexes.
- Seasonal distribution varies; in temperate areas, incidence is higher during late winter and spring.

COMPLICATIONS

- With scratching due to severe pruritus: infection, scarring, impetigo, furuncles, and cellulitis
- Reye's syndrome
- Pneumonia
- Myocarditis
- Bleeding disorders
- Arthritis
- Nephritis
- Hepatitis
- Acute myositis
- Congenital varicella-caused hypoplastic deformity, limb scarring, retarded growth, and central nervous system and eye problems

HISTORY

- Recent exposure to someone with chickenpox
- Malaise
- Headache
- Anorexia

PHYSICAL FINDINGS

- Fever of 101° to 103° F (38.3° to 39.4° C)
- Crops of small, erythematous macules on the trunk or scalp
- Macules progressing to papules and then clear vesicles on an erythematous base (so-called "dewdrops on rose petals")
- Vesicles becoming cloudy and breaking easily; then scabs forming
- Rash that spreads to face and, rarely, to extremities
- Rash containing a combination of red papules, vesicles, and scabs in various stages
- Ulcers on mucous membranes of the mouth, conjunctivae, and genitalia

LABORATORY
- The virus can be isolated from vesicular fluid within the first 3 to 4 days of the rash.
- A Giemsa stain may distinguish the varicella zoster virus from the vaccinia variola virus.
- Serum samples contain antibodies 7 days after onset of symptoms.
- Serologic testing differentiates rickettsial pox from varicella.

TREATMENT

GENERAL
- Strict isolation until all vesicles have crusted over; for congenital chickenpox, no isolation

DIET
- Increased fluid intake

ACTIVITY
- Rest periods when fatigued

MEDICATIONS
- Antipruritics
- Antibiotics
- Analgesics and antipyretics
- Acyclovir (Zovirax)
- Varicella zoster immune globulin

NURSING CONSIDERATIONS

NURSING DIAGNOSES
- Disturbed body image
- Fatigue
- Hyperthermia
- Impaired skin integrity
- Readiness for enhanced management of therapeutic regimen
- Risk for imbalanced fluid volume
- Risk for infection
- Social isolation

EXPECTED OUTCOMES
The patient (or family) will:
- verbalize feelings about changed body image
- report or demonstrate an increased energy level
- remain afebrile
- exhibit improved or healed lesions or wounds
- demonstrate the skin care regimen
- maintain adequate fluid balance
- remain free from signs of secondary infection
- interact with family and peers to decrease feelings of isolation.

NURSING INTERVENTIONS
- Observe an immunocompromised patient for manifestations of complications, such as pneumonitis and meningitis, and report them immediately.
- Provide skin care comfort measures, such as calamine lotion, cornstarch, sponge baths, or showers.
- Administer varicella zoster immune globulin if ordered to lessen the severity of the disease.
- Institute strict isolation measures until all skin lesions have crusted.
- Prevent exposure to pregnant women.

MONITORING
- Response to treatment
- Complications
- Skin integrity
- Signs and symptoms of dehydration
- Signs and symptoms of infection
- Adverse drug reactions

PATIENT TEACHING

GENERAL
Be sure to cover:
- disorder, diagnosis, and treatment
- how to correctly apply topical antipruritics
- importance of good hygiene and keeping child's fingernails trimmed
- importance of the child avoiding scratching the lesions
- importance of the parents watching for and immediately reporting signs of complications (severe skin pain and burning possibly indicating a serious secondary infection)
- importance of refraining from giving the child aspirin because of its association with Reye's syndrome
- signs and symptoms of Reye's syndrome and the need to immediately report them to a practitioner.

RESOURCES
Organizations
Centers for Disease Control and Prevention — National Immunization Program: *www.cdc.gov/nip*
National Institute of Allergy and Infectious Diseases: *www.niaid.nih.gov*
World Health Organization: *www.who.int*

Selected references
Breuer, J. "Varicella Vaccination for Healthcare Workers," *British Medical Journal* 330(7489):433-34, February 2005.
Kasper, D.L., et al., eds. *Harrison's Principles of Internal Medicine*, 16th ed. New York: McGraw-Hill Book Co., 2005.
Neu, A.M. "Indications for Varicella Vaccination Post-Transplant," *Pediatric Transplantation* 9(2):141-44, April 2005.
Plourd, D.M., and Austin, K. "Correlation of a Reported History of Chickenpox with Seropositive Immunity in Pregnant Women," *Journal of Reproductive Medicine* 50(10):779-83, October 2005.
Sandy, M.C. "Herpes Zoster: Medical and Nursing Management," *Clinical Journal of Oncology Nursing* 9(4):443-46, August 2005.
Seward, J.F., and Orenstein, W.A. "Commentary: The Case for Universal Varicella Immunization," *Pediatric Infectious Disease Journal* 25(1):45-46, January 2006.

Varicocele

- A mass of dilated and tortuous varicose veins in the spermatic cord
- Commonly described as a "bag of worms" (see *Taking a close look at a varicocele*)

PATHOPHYSIOLOGY
- Because of a valvular disorder in the spermatic vein, blood pools in the pampiniform venous plexus.
- One function of the pampiniform plexus is to keep the testes slightly cooler than body temperature, which is the optimal temperature for sperm production.
- Incomplete blood flow through the testes thus interferes with spermatogenesis.
- Testicular atrophy may also occur because of the reduced blood flow.

CAUSES
- Incompetent or congenitally absent valves in the spermatic veins
- Tumor or thrombus obstructing the inferior vena cava (unilateral left-sided varicocele)

INCIDENCE
- This condition is present in 30% of all men diagnosed with infertility.
- This condition occurs in the left spermatic cord 95% of the time.
- This condition occurs in 10% to 15% of all males, usually between ages 13 and 18.

COMPLICATIONS
- Infertility
- Hydrocele

HISTORY
- Infertility
- Feeling of heaviness on affected side

PHYSICAL FINDINGS
- Palpation of "bag of worms" when the patient is upright
- Drained, can't be felt when patient is recumbent
- Testicular tenderness

GENERAL
- Physical examination confirms varicocele.

Taking a close look at a varicocele

Varicocele, an abnormal dilation of the veins of the spermatic cord, is asymptomatic, but it's important to identify and correct this condition in adolescent boys because it causes infertility.

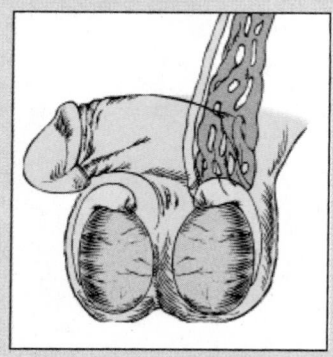

TREATMENT

GENERAL
◆ Scrotal support to relieve discomfort

SURGERY
◆ Surgical repair or removal involving ligation of the spermatic cord at the internal inguinal ring (if infertility is an issue)

NURSING CONSIDERATIONS

NURSING DIAGNOSES
◆ Acute pain
◆ Disturbed body image
◆ Fear
◆ Ineffective coping

EXPECTED OUTCOMES
The patient will:
◆ express feelings of increased comfort
◆ maintain positive outlook regarding body image
◆ express feelings regarding effect on fertility or other fears and concerns
◆ demonstrate adaptive coping behaviors.

NURSING INTERVENTIONS
◆ Promote the patient's comfort before and after surgery.
◆ After surgery, administer drug therapy.
◆ Apply an ice bag with a cover to reduce edema.
◆ Protect the wound from contamination.
◆ Allow the patient to perform as many normal daily activities as possible.

MONITORING
◆ Intake and output
◆ Comfort level
◆ Wound healing

PATIENT TEACHING

GENERAL
Be sure to cover:
◆ disorder, diagnosis, and treatment
◆ wound care.

RESOURCES
Organizations
American Urological Association: *www.auanet.org*
Cornell Institute for Reproductive Medicine – Center for Male Reproductive Medicine and Microsurgery: *www.maleinfertility.org*
Mayo Clinic: *www.mayoclinic.com*
The Merck Manuals Online Medical Library: *www.merck.com/mmhe*

Selected references
Al-Hunayan, A., et al. "Two-trocar Laparoscopic Varicocelectomy: Cost-Reduction Surgical Technique," *Urology* 67(3):461-65, March 2006.
Hassan, J.M., et al. "Hydrocele Formation Following Laparoscopic Varicocelectomy," *Journal of Urology* 175(3 Pt 1): 1076-1079, March 2006.
Nagler, H.M. "Is Antegrade Sclerotherapy a Valid Alternative for the Treatment of Varicocele?" *Nature Clinical Practice Urology* 2(9):424-25, September 2005.
Vasilios, S., et al. "Ultrasound Findings of an Intratesticular Varicocele. Report of a New Case and Review of the Literature," *International Urology and Nephrology* 38(1):115-18, 2006.
Williams, D.H., et al. "Varicocele: Surgical Techniques in 2005," *Canadian Journal of Urology* 13 Suppl 1:13-17, February 2006.

Varicose veins

- Dilated, tortuous veins, engorged with blood resulting from improper venous valve function
- Primary varicose veins originating in superficial veins (the saphenous veins and branches)
- Secondary varicose veins occurring in deep and perforating veins

PATHOPHYSIOLOGY

- A weakened valve allows backflow of blood to the previous valve in a vein.
- If the valve can't hold the pooling blood, it becomes incompetent, allowing even more blood to flow backward.
- As the volume of venous blood builds, pressure in the vein increases and the vein becomes distended.
- As the vein stretches, it loses elasticity, enlarges, and becomes tortuous.
- Hydrostatic pressure increases, plasma is forced out into surrounding tissue, and edema results.

CAUSES

- Congenital weakness of the valves or venous wall
- Deep vein thrombosis
- Occupations that necessitate standing for an extended period
- Pregnancy
- Tight clothing
- Trauma

INCIDENCE

- Varicose veins are common in middle adulthood.
- Primary varicose veins, which affect both legs, are found twice as often in women than in men.
- Secondary varicose veins are usually found in only one leg.

COMPLICATIONS

- Venous insufficiency
- Venous stasis ulcers

ASSESSMENT

HISTORY

- May be asymptomatic
- Feeling of heaviness in the legs that worsens in the evening and in warm weather
- Leg cramps at night
- Diffuse, dull, aching leg pain after prolonged standing or walking
- Aching legs during menses
- Fatigue
- Exercise possibly relieving symptoms because venous return improves

PHYSICAL FINDINGS

- Dilated, purplish, ropelike veins, especially in the calf
- Orthostatic edema and stasis of the calves and ankles
- Nodules along affected veins and valve incompetence
- In chronic condition, venous stasis ulcers, which must be differentiated from arterial and diabetic ulcerations

DIAGNOSTIC TEST RESULTS

IMAGING

- Ascending and descending venography may demonstrate venous occlusion and patterns of collateral flow.

IMAGING

- A photoplethysmography, a noninvasive test, may characterize venous blood flow by showing changes in the skin's circulation.
- Doppler ultrasonography quickly and accurately shows the presence or absence of venous backflow in deep or superficial veins.
- Venous outflow and reflux plethysmography may be used to detect deep venous occlusion.

Preventing varicose veins

Prevention of varicose veins involves identifying patients with increased risk factors, such as those in professions that require prolonged standing or time on the feet (such as nurses, surgeons, letter carriers, beauticians, teachers, and waiters). Other risk factors include obesity, heavy lifting, and pregnancy. People with these risk factors should be educated to rest their legs and elevate them periodically at work, wear supportive stockings, drink 2 to 3 qt (2 to 3 L) of fluid per day, and avoid crossing their legs.

TREATMENT

GENERAL
- Wearing elastic stockings
- Avoiding tight clothing
- For moderate varicose veins: wearing antiembolism stockings or elastic bandages
- For severe varicose veins: custom-fitted, surgical-weight stockings with graduated pressure

ACTIVITY
- Avoidance of prolonged standing
- Routine exercise
- Elevation of the legs

MEDICATIONS
- Sclerotherapy

SURGERY
- Stripping and ligation

NURSING CONSIDERATIONS

NURSING DIAGNOSES
- Activity intolerance
- Acute pain
- Disturbed body image
- Ineffective tissue perfusion: Peripheral

EXPECTED OUTCOMES
The patient will:
- carry out activities of daily living without excess fatigue or discomfort
- express feelings of increased comfort and decreased pain
- verbalize feelings about changed body image
- maintain adequate distal and collateral circulation.

NURSING INTERVENTIONS
- After stripping and ligation or after injection of a sclerosing agent, administer analgesics as ordered to relieve pain.
- Frequently check circulation in toes and observe elastic bandages for bleeding. When ordered, rewrap bandages at least once a shift, wrapping from toe to thigh, with the leg elevated. (See *Preventing varicose veins.*)

MONITORING
 WARNING *Watch for signs and symptoms of complications, such as sensory loss in the leg, calf pain, and fever.*
- Response to treatment
- Skin integrity
- Pain control

PATIENT TEACHING

GENERAL
Be sure to cover:
- importance of avoiding wearing constrictive clothing
- elevating the legs above heart level when possible and avoiding prolonged standing or sitting
- how to put on the elastic, antiembolism, or compression stockings before getting out of bed in the morning (or lying with the legs raised for 1 minute before putting on the stockings)
- how to avoid injury to the lower legs, ankles, and feet and the need to observe for altered skin integrity of those areas and to report any problems to the physician as soon as possible.

RESOURCES
Organizations
American Academy of Dermatology: *www.aad.org*
Mayo Clinic: *www.mayoclinic.com*
National Heart, Lung, and Blood Institute: *www.nhlbi.nih.gov*
Society for Vascular Surgery: *www.vascularweb.org*

Selected references
Foster, W., and Coghlan, G. "Medical Treatment of Varicose Veins," *Circulation* 112(19):e312, November 2005.
Goldman, M.P. "Intravascular Lasers in the Treatment of Varicose Veins," *Journal of Cosmetic Dermatology* 3(3):162-66, July 2004.
Kasper, D.L., et al., eds. *Harrison's Principles of Internal Medicine*, 16th ed. New York: McGraw-Hill Book Co., 2005.
Lin, S.D., et al. "Management of the Primary Varicose Veins with Venous Ulceration with Assistance of Endoscopic Surgery," *Annals of Plastic Surgery* 56(3):289-94, March 2006.
The Merck Manual of Diagnosis & Therapy, 18th ed., Whitehouse Station, N.J.: Merck & Co., Inc., 2006.
Palfreyman, S.J., et al. "Varicose Veins: A Qualitative Study to Explore Expectations and Reasons for Seeking Treatment," *Journal of Clinical Nursing* 13(3):332-40, March 2004.

Vasculitis

- Autoimmune condition that includes a broad spectrum of disorders characterized by blood vessel inflammation and necrosis
- Clinical effects dependent on the vessels involved and reflective of tissue ischemia caused by blood flow obstruction

PATHOPHYSIOLOGY

- The process is initiated by excessive circulating antigen, which triggers the formation of soluble antibody complexes. The reticuloendothelial system can't effectively clear these complexes, which are deposited in blood vessel walls.
- Increased vascular permeability (associated with the release of vasoactive amines by platelets and basophils) enhances this deposition. The deposited complexes activate the complement cascade and result in chemotaxis of neutrophils, which release lysosomal enzymes.
- Vessel damage and necrosis result.

CAUSES

- Several theories:
- Follows serious infectious disease and may be related to high doses of antibiotics
- Formation of autoantibodies directed at the body's own cellular and extracellular proteins, which can lead to the activation of inflammatory cells or cytotoxicity
- Cell-mediated (T-cell) immune response
- In atopic individuals, exposure to allergens

INCIDENCE

- Vasculitis can affect a person at any age (except for mucocutaneous lymph node syndrome, which affects only children).

COMPLICATIONS

- Renal failure, renal hypertension, glomerulitis
- Fibrous scarring of the lung tissue
- Stroke
- GI bleeding, intestinal obstruction
- Myocardial infarction and pericarditis
- Rupture of mesenteric aneurysms

ASSESSMENT

HISTORY

- Varied findings, depending on blood vessels involved
- Fever
- Weight loss
- Malaise
- Headache
- Abdominal pain
- Myalgias

PHYSICAL FINDINGS

- Polyarteritis nodosa (depends on body system)
- Hypertension (renal)
- Arthritic changes (musculoskeletal)
- Rash, purpura, nodules, and cutaneous infarcts (skin)
- Altered mental status and seizures (central nervous system)
- Respiratory distress, peripheral edema, hepatomegaly, peripheral vasoconstriction (cardiovascular)
- Blurred vision or sudden vision loss (eyes)

DIAGNOSTIC TEST RESULTS

DIAGNOSTIC PROCEDURES

- The results of biopsy of the affected vessel can help to confirm diagnosis.

TREATMENT

GENERAL

- Avoidance of antigenic drugs
- Avoidance of offending environmental substances

DIET

- Avoidance of antigenic foods

MEDICATIONS

- Corticosteroids
- Antihypertensives
- Analgesics
- Immunosuppressive agents
- Antineoplastics

NURSING CONSIDERATIONS

NURSING DIAGNOSES
- Activity intolerance
- Chronic pain
- Decreased cardiac output
- Disturbed body image
- Disturbed sensory perception (visual)
- Hyperthermia
- Imbalanced nutrition: Less than body requirements
- Impaired gas exchange
- Impaired oral mucous membrane
- Impaired physical mobility
- Impaired skin integrity
- Ineffective breathing pattern
- Ineffective tissue perfusion: Cardiopulmonary
- Risk for infection
- Risk for injury

EXPECTED OUTCOMES
The patient will:
- verbalize the importance of balancing activity, as tolerated, with rest
- express feelings of increased comfort and decreased pain
- maintain adequate cardiac output
- express positive feelings about self
- maintain optimal functioning within the confines of his visual impairment
- maintain a normal body temperature
- consume adequate daily caloric intake
- demonstrate adequate ventilation
- maintain intact oral mucous membranes
- maintain joint range of motion and muscle strength to the fullest extent possible
- experience healing of wounds and lesions without complications
- maintain a respiratory rate within 5 breaths/minute of baseline
- attain hemodynamic stability
- remain free from signs and symptoms of infection
- avoid complications.

NURSING INTERVENTIONS
- Assess for dry nasal mucosa. Instill nose drops to lubricate the mucosa and minimize crusting; irrigate nasal passages with warm normal saline solution.
- Keep the patient well hydrated (about 3 qt [3 L] of fluid daily).
- Make sure that a patient with decreased visual acuity has a safe environment.
- Regulate environmental temperature to prevent additional vasoconstriction caused by cold.
- Provide emotional support to the patient and family.

MONITORING
- Vital signs and neurologic status
- Signs and symptoms of organ involvement
- Laboratory values
- GI disturbances and renal function tests
- Intake and output
- Daily weight

PATIENT TEACHING

GENERAL
Be sure to cover:
- disorder, diagnosis, and treatment
- how to recognize adverse effects of drug therapy, watch for signs of bleeding, and report any of these findings to the physician
- importance of wearing warm clothes and gloves when going outside in cold weather.

DISCHARGE PLANNING
- Refer the patient to a smoking-cessation program, if appropriate.

RESOURCES
Organizations
Johns Hopkins Vasculitis Center: *www.vasculitis.med.jhu.edu*
Lupus Foundation of America: *www.lupus.org*
National Institute of Allergy and Infectious Diseases: *www.niaid.nih.gov*

Selected references
Kasper, D.L., et al., eds. *Harrison's Principles of Internal Medicine*, 16th ed. New York: McGraw-Hill Book Co., 2005.

Kim, S., and Dedeoglu, F. "Update on Pediatric Vasculitis," *Current Opinion in Pediatrics* 17(6):695-702, December 2005.

The Merck Manual of Diagnosis & Therapy, 18th ed., Whitehouse Station, N.J.: Merck & Co., Inc., 2006.

Rodriguez-Pla, A., and Stone, J.H. "Vasculitis and Systemic Infections," *Current Opinion in Rheumatology* 18(1):39-47, January 2006.

Russell, J.P., and Gibson, L.E. "Primary Cutaneous Small Vessel Vasculitis: Approach to Diagnosis and Treatment," *International Journal of Dermatology* 45(1):3-13, January 2006.

Ventricular septal defect

OVERVIEW

- Heart condition in which an opening in the septum between the ventricles allows blood to shunt between the left and right ventricles
- Most common congenital heart disorder
- Also known as *VSD*

PATHOPHYSIOLOGY

- The ventricular septum fails to close completely by the 8th week of gestation, as it would normally.
- VSDs are located in the membranous or muscular portion of the ventricular septum and vary in size.
- Some defects close spontaneously; in other defects, the entire septum is absent, creating a single ventricle.
- VSD isn't readily apparent at birth because right and left ventricular pressures are approximately equal, so blood doesn't shunt through the defect.
- As the pulmonary vasculature gradually relaxes, between 4 and 8 weeks after birth, right ventricular pressure decreases, allowing blood to shunt from the left to the right ventricle.

CAUSES

- Congenital

RISK FACTORS

- Fetal alcohol syndrome
- Coexists with additional birth defects, especially Down syndrome and other autosomal trisomies, renal anomalies, and cardiac defects, such as patent ductus arteriosus, tetralogy of Fallot, and coarctation of the aorta

INCIDENCE

- This disorder affects 2% to 7% of live births.
- This disorder is slightly more common in females.

COMPLICATIONS

- Heart failure
- Pneumonia

ASSESSMENT

HISTORY

- Dyspnea
- Cyanosis
- Slow weight gain
- Feeding difficulties
- Rapid grunting respirations

PHYSICAL FINDINGS

- Prominent anterior chest wall
- Clubbing
- Cyanosis
- With a large VSD, audible murmurs, loudest at the fourth intercostal space, usually with a thrill; pulmonic component of S_2 loud and widely split
- With fixed pulmonary hypertension, diastolic murmur possibly audible on auscultation, systolic murmur becoming quieter, and S_2 greatly accentuated
- Displacement of the point of maximal impulse to the left
- Typical murmur associated with a VSD, blowing or rumbling and varying in frequency
- In the neonate, moderately loud early systolic murmur along the lower left sternal border, possibly becoming louder and longer about the second or third day after birth
- In infants, murmur possibly loudest near the base of the heart, which may suggest pulmonary stenosis
- In small VSD, functional murmur or characteristic loud, harsh systolic murmur

DIAGNOSTIC TEST RESULTS

IMAGING

- Chest X-rays may be normal in small defects; in large VSDs, they may show cardiomegaly, left atrial and left ventricular enlargement, and prominent pulmonary vascular markings.
- Echocardiography may detect a large VSD and its location in the septum, estimate the size of a left-to-right shunt, suggest pulmonary hypertension, and identify associated lesions and complications.

DIAGNOSTIC PROCEDURES

- Electrocardiography is normal in children with small VSDs; in large VSDs, it shows left and right ventricular hypertrophy, suggesting pulmonary hypertension.
- Cardiac catheterization determines the size and exact location of the VSD, calculates the degree of shunting by comparing the blood oxygen saturation in each ventricle, determines the extent of pulmonary hypertension, and detects associated defects.

TREATMENT

GENERAL
- If the child has other defects and will benefit from delaying surgery, pulmonary artery banding to normalize pressures and flow distal to the band and prevent pulmonary vascular disease

DIET
- Low sodium
- Fluid restriction

ACTIVITY
- As tolerated

MEDICATIONS
- Digoxin (Lanoxin)
- Diuretics
- Antibiotics

After surgery
- Analgesics
- Antibiotics
- Vasopressors

SURGERY
- For small defects, simple suture closure
- For moderate to large defects, insertion of a patch graft using cardiopulmonary bypass

NURSING CONSIDERATIONS

NURSING DIAGNOSES
- Activity intolerance
- Decreased cardiac output
- Delayed growth and development
- Disabled family coping
- Imbalanced nutrition: Less than body requirements
- Impaired gas exchange
- Risk for infection

EXPECTED OUTCOMES
The patient (or family) will:
- carry out activities of daily living without weakness or fatigue
- maintain adequate cardiac output and hemodynamic stability, and have no arrhythmias
- demonstrate age-appropriate skills and behaviors to the extent possible
- agree to seek help from peer support groups or professional counselors to increase adaptive coping behaviors
- consume adequate daily caloric intake
- maintain adequate ventilation and oxygenation
- remain free from signs and symptoms of infection.

NURSING INTERVENTIONS
- Provide emotional support.
- Give prescribed drugs.

MONITORING
- Vital signs
- Signs of heart failure
- Intake and output
- Respiratory status

After surgery
- Hemodynamics
- Cardiac rhythm
- Oxygenation

PATIENT TEACHING

GENERAL
Be sure to cover:
- preventing complications until the child is scheduled for surgery or the defect closes
- watching for signs of heart failure, such as poor feeding, sweating, and heavy breathing
- drug administration, dosage, and possible adverse effects
- letting the child engage in normal activities
- importance of prophylactic antibiotics before and after surgery.

RESOURCES
Organizations
American Heart Association: *www.americanheart.org*
Cleveland Clinic Health Information Center: *www.clevelandclinic.org/health*
Mayo Clinic: *www.mayoclinic.com*

Selected references
Carminati, M., et al. "Transcatheter Closure of Congenital Ventricular Septal Defect with Amplatzer Septal Occluders," *American Journal of Cardiology* 96(12A):52L-58L, December 2005.

Diseases, 4th ed. Philadelphia: Lippincott Williams & Wilkins, 2006.

McCarthy, K.P., et al. "Perimembranous and Muscular Ventricular Septal Defects — Morphology Revisited in the Era of Device Closure," *Journal of Interventional Cardiology* 18(6):507-13, December 2005.

Walsh, M.A., et al. "Percutaneous Closure of Postoperative Ventricular Septal Defects with the Amplatzer Device," *Catheterizations and Cardiovascular Interventions* 67(3):445-51, March 2006.

Vesicoureteral reflux

OVERVIEW

- A genitourinary condition; urine flows from bladder back into ureters and eventually into renal pelvis or parenchyma
- Bladder empties poorly resulting in potential urinary tract infection (UTI); acute or chronic pyelonephritis with renal damage may result

PATHOPHYSIOLOGY

- Incompetence of the ureterovesical junction and shortening of intravesical ureteral musculature allow backflow of urine into the ureter when the bladder contracts during voiding.

CAUSES

- Acquired diverticulum (from outlet obstruction)
- Congenital anomalies of the ureters or bladder
- Cystitis
- Flaccid neurogenic bladder
- High intravesical pressure from outlet obstruction
- Inadequate detrusor muscle buttress in the bladder, stemming from congenital paraureteral bladder diverticulum
- Sometimes unknown

INCIDENCE

- **AGE FACTOR** *Most common during infancy in boys and during early childhood (ages 3 to 7) in girls.*
- Primary vesicoureteral reflux results from congenital anomalies that are most prevalent in females and rare in blacks.
- This disorder has also shown in up to 25% of asymptomatic siblings of children with diagnosed primary vesicoureteral reflux.
- **WARNING** *In children, fever, nonspecific abdominal pain, and diarrhea may be the only clinical effects. Rarely, children with minimal symptoms remain undiagnosed until puberty or later, when they begin to exhibit clear signs of renal impairment (anemia, hypertension, and lethargy).*

COMPLICATIONS

- Renal impairment
- UTIs

ASSESSMENT

HISTORY

- Urinary frequency and urgency
- Burning on urination

PHYSICAL FINDINGS

- In infants, hematuria or strong-smelling urine
- Hard, thickened bladder (hard mass deep in the pelvis) if posterior urethral valves are causing an obstruction in male infants

DIAGNOSTIC TEST RESULTS

LABORATORY

- A clean-catch urinalysis may show a bacterial count greater than 100,000/μl.
- A microscopic examination may reveal white blood cells, red blood cells, and an increased urine pH in the presence of infection. Specific gravity less than 1.010 demonstrates inability to concentrate urine.
- An elevated creatinine level (more than 1.2 mg/dl) and an elevated blood urea nitrogen level (more than 18 mg/dl) may indicate advanced renal dysfunction.

DIAGNOSTIC PROCEDURES

- Cystoscopy, with instillation of a solution containing methylene blue or indigo carmine dye, may confirm the diagnosis.
- Excretory urography may show dilated lower ureter, ureter visible for its entire length, hydronephrosis, calyceal distortion, and renal scarring.
- Voiding cystourethrography (either fluoroscopic or radionuclide) identifies and determines the degree of reflux and shows when reflux occurs. It may also pinpoint the causative anomaly.
- Nuclear cystography and renal ultrasound may detect reflux.

OTHER

- Catheterization of the bladder after the patient voids determines the amount of residual urine.

TREATMENT

DIET
◆ Increased fluid intake

MEDICATIONS
◆ Antibiotics

SURGERY
◆ UTI that recurs despite adequate prophylactic antibiotic therapy necessitates vesicoureteral reimplantation.
◆ Bladder outlet obstruction in neurogenic bladder requires surgery only if renal dysfunction is present.

NURSING CONSIDERATIONS

NURSING DIAGNOSES
◆ Acute pain
◆ Excess fluid volume
◆ Impaired urinary elimination
◆ Risk for infection
◆ Risk for injury

EXPECTED OUTCOMES
The patient (or family) will:
◆ report increased comfort
◆ maintain fluid balance
◆ demonstrate skill in managing the urinary elimination problem
◆ remain free from signs and symptoms of infection
◆ avoid or minimize complications.

NURSING INTERVENTIONS
◆ Encourage one of the parents to stay with the patient during all procedures.
◆ Explain the procedures to the parents and to the child, if he's old enough to understand.
◆ Give drug therapy.
◆ Make sure catheters are patent and draining well. Maintain sterile technique during catheter care.

MONITORING
◆ Intake and output
◆ Comfort level
◆ Vital signs

PATIENT TEACHING

GENERAL
Be sure to cover:
◆ utilizing the vesicoureteral reflux to double void (void once and then try to void again in a few minutes)
◆ voiding every 2 to 3 hours whether or not the urge exists
◆ recognizing and reporting recurring signs of UTI (painful, frequent, burning urination; foul-smelling urine)
◆ importance of completing the prescribed therapy or maintaining low-dose antibiotic prophylaxis.

DISCHARGE PLANNING
◆ After surgery, close medical follow-up is necessary even if symptoms haven't recurred.

RESOURCES
Organizations
American Urological Association: *www.auanet.org*
Mayo Clinic: *www.mayoclinic.com*
National Institute of Diabetes & Digestive & Kidney Diseases: *www.niddk.nih.gov*

Selected references
Afshar, K., et al. "Vesicoureteral Reflux and Complete Ureteral Duplication. Conservative or Surgical Management?" *Journal of Urology* 173(5):1725-727, May 2005.
Harrell, W.B., and Snow, B.W. "Endoscopic Treatment of Vesicoureteral Reflux," *Current Opinion in Pediatrics* 17(3): 409-11, June 2005.
Keating, M.A. "Role of Periureteral Injections in Children with Vesicoureteral Reflux," *Current Opinion in Urology* 15(6):369-73, November 2005.
Sole, K. "Endoscopic Treatment of Vesicoureteral Reflux Is Safe but Not Highly Effective," *Nature Clinical Practice Urology* 3(3):123, March 2006.
Wald, E.R. "Vesicoureteral Reflux: The Role of Antibiotic Prophylaxis," *Pediatrics* 117(3):919-22, March 2006.

Vitamin A deficiency

OVERVIEW

- Deficiency of vitamin A in the body possibly resulting in night blindness, decreased color adjustment, keratinization of epithelial tissue, and poor bone growth
- With therapy, excellent chance of reversing symptoms of night blindness and milder conjunctival changes; with corneal damage, emergency treatment necessary

PATHOPHYSIOLOGY

- A fat-soluble vitamin absorbed in the GI tract, vitamin A maintains epithelial tissue and retinal function.
- Healthy adults have adequate vitamin A reserves to last up to 1 year; children commonly don't.

CAUSES

- Decreased storage and transport of vitamin A from hepatic disease
- Inadequate dietary intake of foods high in vitamin A (liver, kidney, butter, milk, cream, cheese, and fortified margarine) or carotene, a precursor of vitamin A found in dark-green leafy vegetables, and yellow or orange fruits and vegetables
- Malabsorption caused by:
- Celiac disease
- Cystic fibrosis
- Giardiasis
- Habitual use of mineral oil as a laxative
- Obstructive jaundice
- Sprue
- Massive urinary excretion caused by:
- Cancer
- Tuberculosis
- Pneumonia
- Nephritis
- Urinary tract infection

INCIDENCE

- Vitamin A deficiency affects more than 80,000 people annually worldwide — mostly children in underdeveloped countries.
- Vitamin A deficiency is rare in the United States, although many disadvantaged children have substandard levels of vitamin A.

COMPLICATIONS

- Blindness
- Infections of the eyes and the respiratory or genitourinary tract

ASSESSMENT

HISTORY

- Night blindness (nyctalopia)
- Failure to thrive
- Apathy

PHYSICAL FINDINGS

- Dry, scaly skin
- Follicular hyperkeratosis
- Conjunctival changes
- Shrinking and hardening of the mucous membranes

DIAGNOSTIC TEST RESULTS

LABORATORY

- Carotene levels below 40 mcg/dl suggest vitamin A deficiency, but vary with seasonal ingestion of fruits and vegetables.
- Serum levels of vitamin A below 20 mcg/dl are diagnostic.

OTHER

- Dietary history and typical ocular lesions suggest vitamin A deficiency.

Foods that contain vitamin A

The following foods contain significant amounts of vitamin A:

- butternut squash
- cantaloupe
- carrots
- dandelion
- kale
- mangoes
- red peppers
- sweet potatoes.

GENERAL
- Cream-based or petroleum-based products for dry skin
- Control of underlying condition

DIET
- Increased intake of foods high in vitamin A

MEDICATIONS
- Vitamin A replacement
- Bile salts with biliary obstruction
- Pancreatin with pancreatic insufficiency

NURSING DIAGNOSES
- Delayed growth and development
- Disturbed sensory perception (visual)
- Imbalanced nutrition: Less than body requirements
- Impaired skin integrity
- Ineffective health maintenance
- Risk for infection
- Risk for injury

EXPECTED OUTCOMES
The patient will:
- achieve age-appropriate growth, behaviors, and skills to the fullest extent possible
- maintain optimal functioning within the confines of his visual impairment
- express understanding of diet high in vitamin A and improve vitamin levels
- maintain intact skin integrity and mucous membranes
- express understanding of dietary changes needed to improve nutritional status
- remain free from all signs and symptoms of infection
- avoid complications.

NURSING INTERVENTIONS
- Give prescribed oral vitamin A supplements with or after meals or parenterally.
- Provide information on foods high in vitamin A. (See *Foods that contain vitamin A.*)

MONITORING
- Signs of hypercarotenemia (orange coloration of the skin and eyes)
- Signs of hypervitaminosis A (children):
  – Rash
  – Hair loss
  – Anorexia
  – Transient hydrocephalus
  – Vomiting
- Signs of hypervitaminosis A (adults):
  – Bone pain
  – Hepatosplenomegaly
  – Diplopia
  – Irritability

GENERAL
Be sure to cover:
- signs of hypercarotenemia and hypervitaminosis
- dietary counseling on foods high in vitamin A.

DISCHARGE PLANNING
- Refer the patient for nutritional counseling and, if necessary, to an appropriate community agency.

RESOURCES
Organizations
American Dietetic Association: *www.eatright.org*
The Merck Manuals Online Medical Library: *www.merck.com/mmhe*
National Digestive Diseases Information Clearinghouse: *www.niddk.nih.gov/health/digest/nddic.htm*
World Health Organization: *www.who.int*

Selected references
Apushkin, M.A., and Fishman, G.A. "Improvement in Visual Function and Fundus Findings for a Patient with Vitamin A-Deficient Retinopathy," *Retina* 25(5):650-52, July-August 2005.

Bines, J.E., et al. "Vitamin A and E Deficiency and Lung Disease in Infants with Cystic Fibrosis," *Journal of Paediatrics and Child Health* 41(12):663-68, December 2005.

Diseases, 4th ed. Philadelphia: Lippincott Williams & Wilkins, 2006.

Kilic, S.S., et al. "Vitamin A Deficiency in Patients with Common Variable Immunodeficiency," *Journal of Clinical Immunology* 25(3):275-80, May 2005.

Penniston, K.L., and Tanumihardjo, S.A. "The Acute and Chronic Toxic Effects of Vitamin A," *American Journal of Clinical Nutrition* 83(2):191-201, February 2006.

Vitamin B deficiency

- ◆ Deficiency of vitamin B in the body
- ◆ Most common deficiencies: thiamine (B_1), riboflavin (B_2), niacin, pyridoxine (B_6), cobalamin (B_{12})

PATHOPHYSIOLOGY

- ◆ Vitamin B complex is a group of water-soluble vitamins essential to normal metabolism, cell growth, and blood formation. (See *Recommended daily allowance of B-complex vitamins.*)

CAUSES

Cobalamin deficiency

- ◆ Absence of intrinsic factor in gastric secretions
- ◆ Absence of receptor sites after ileal resection
- ◆ Diet low in animal protein
- ◆ Malabsorption syndromes associated with sprue, intestinal worm infestation, regional ileitis, and gluten enteropathy
- ◆ Medications
- ◆ Pernicious anemia

Niacin deficiency

- ◆ Carcinoid syndrome
- ◆ Corn as a dominant staple food
- ◆ Hartnup disease

Pyridoxine deficiency

- ◆ Destruction of pyridoxine in infant formulas by autoclaving
- ◆ Pyridoxine antagonists, such as isoniazid and penicillamine

Riboflavin deficiency

- ◆ Diet deficient in milk, meat, fish, green leafy vegetables, and legumes

Thiamine deficiency

- ◆ Inadequate dietary intake of vitamin B_1
- ◆ Malabsorption

RISK FACTORS

- ◆ Chronic alcoholism
- ◆ Prolonged diarrhea
- ◆ Exposure of milk to sunlight
- ◆ Treatment of legumes with baking soda

INCIDENCE

Cobalamin deficiency

- ◆ This condition is most common in those older than age 40.

Niacin deficiency

- ◆ This deficiency usually affects adults.

Pyridoxine deficiency

- ◆ This condition can occur at any age.
- ◆ This condition is rare.

Riboflavin deficiency

- ◆ This is the most common nutrient deficiency in the United States.

Thiamine deficiency

- ◆ This condition affects males and females equally.
- ◆ This condition can occur at any age.

COMPLICATIONS

- ◆ Cardiomegaly
- ◆ Circulatory collapse
- ◆ Beriberi
- ◆ Pellagra

⚡ **WARNING** *Because of a triad of symptoms, pellagra is sometimes called a "3-D" syndrome — dementia, dermatitis, and diarrhea. If not reversed by therapeutic doses of niacin, pellagra can be fatal.*

- ◆ Central nervous system disturbances

HISTORY

Cobalamin deficiency

- ◆ Pernicious anemia
- ◆ Anorexia
- ◆ Weight loss
- ◆ Constipation, diarrhea
- ◆ Glossitis
- ◆ Peripheral neuropathy

Niacin deficiency

- ◆ Backache
- ◆ Sore mouth, tongue, and lips
- ◆ Nausea, vomiting, and diarrhea
- ◆ Confusion, disorientation, and neuritis — if severe, may induce hallucinations and paranoia

Pyridoxine deficiency

- ◆ Presence of risk factors
- ◆ Fatigue
- ◆ Distal limb numbness
- ◆ Depression

Riboflavin deficiency

- ◆ Burning, itching, light sensitivity, and tearing of the eyes
- ◆ Neuropathy
- ◆ Signs of mild anemia
- ◆ Growth retardation

Thiamine deficiency

- ◆ Palpitations
- ◆ Dyspnea
- ◆ Constipation and indigestion

Recommended daily allowance of B-complex vitamins

VITAMIN	MEN (23 TO 50)	WOMEN (23 TO 50)	INFANTS	CHILDREN (1 TO 10)
B_1*	1.4 mg	1.4 mg	0.4 mg	0.7 to 12 mg
B_2*	1.6 mg	1.6 mg	0.5 mg	0.8 to 1.4 mg
Niacin*	18 mg	18 mg	5 to 8 mg	9 to 16 mg
B_6	2.2 mg	2.2 mg	0.4 mg	0.9 to 1.6 mg
B_{12}	3 mcg	3 mcg	0.3 mcg	2 to 3 mcg

*requirements per 1,000 kilocalories of dietary intake

PHYSICAL FINDINGS

Cobalamin deficiency
◆ Abdominal discomfort
◆ Peripheral neuropathy
◆ Ataxia, spasticity, and hyperreflexia

Niacin deficiency
◆ Dark, scaly dermatitis, especially on exposed parts of the body, that makes the patient appear to be severely sunburned
◆ Red mouth, tongue, and lips

Pyridoxine deficiency
◆ Weakness
◆ Confusion
◆ Glossitis
◆ Seborrheic dermatitis

Riboflavin deficiency
◆ Seborrheic dermatitis in the nasolabial folds, scrotum, and vulva and, possibly, generalized dermatitis involving the arms, legs, and trunk

Thiamine deficiency
◆ Tachycardia
◆ Ataxia, nystagmus, and ophthalmoplegia

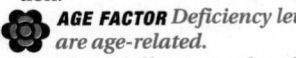

DIAGNOSTIC TEST RESULTS

LABORATORY

Cobalamin deficiency
◆ Cobalamin serum levels may measure less than 150 pg/ml.
◆ The Schilling test will measure absorption of radioactive cobalamin with and without an intrinsic factor.
◆ Gastric analysis and hemoglobin studies may uncover causation.

Niacin deficiency
◆ Niacin deficiency is measured by N-methyl nicotinamide in a 24-hour urine collection as micrograms per gram of creatinine.
◆ The adult deficiency level is less than 0.5 mcg/g.
◆ Pregnant women may measure less than 0.5 mcg/g in their first trimester; less than 0.6 mcg/g in their second trimester; and less than 0.8 mcg/g in their third trimester.

Pyridoxine deficiency
◆ Xanthurenic acid will measure more than 50 mg/day in a 24-hour urine collection after administration of 10 g of L-tryptophan.
◆ Decreased levels of serum and red blood cell transaminases may be seen.
◆ Reduced excretion of pyridoxic acid in urine may be seen.

Riboflavin deficiency
◆ Riboflavin deficiency is measured as micrograms per gram of creatinine in a 24-hour urine collection.
– Ages 1 to 3 will measure less than 150 mcg/g.
– Ages 4 to 6 will measure less than 100 mcg/g.
– Ages 7 to 9 will measure less than 85 mcg/g.
– Ages 10 to 15 will measure less than 70 mcg/g.
– Adults, less than 27 mcg/g.
◆ Pregnant women may measure less than 39 mcg/g in their second trimester, and less than 30 mcg/g in their third trimester.

Thiamine deficiency
◆ Thiamine deficiency is commonly measured as micrograms per deciliter in a 24-hour urine collection:

👁 **AGE FACTOR** *Deficiency levels are age-related.*
– *Ages 1 to 3 will measure less than 120 mcg/dl.*
– *Ages 4 to 6 will measure less than 85 mcg/dl.*
– *Ages 7 to 9 will measure less than 70 mcg/dl.*
– *Ages 10 to12 will measure less than 60 mcg/dl.*
– *Ages 13 to 15 will measure less than 50 mcg/dl.*
– *Adults will measure less than 27 mcg/dl.*
◆ Pregnant women may measure less than 23 mcg/dl in their second trimester, and less than 21 mcg/dl in their third trimester.

(continued)

GENERAL
Cobalamin deficiency
- Blood transfusion if severe

Pyridoxine deficiency
- Symptomatic

DIET
Cobalamin deficiency
- High in folate

Niacin deficiency
- Dietary enrichment (meats, fish, peanuts, brewer's yeast, enriched breads, and cereals rich in niacin; milk and eggs, in tryptophan)

Pyridoxine deficiency
- Dietary adjustments
- Increased carbohydrate intake before vigorous exercise

Riboflavin deficiency
- High in riboflavin foods (meats, enriched flour, milk and dairy products, green leafy vegetables, eggs, and cereal)

Thiamine deficiency
- High-protein, with adequate calorie intake and thiamine-rich foods (pork, peas, wheat bran, oatmeal, and liver)

MEDICATIONS
Cobalamin deficiency
- Parenteral cyanocobalamin in patients with reduced gastric secretion of hydrochloric acid, lack of intrinsic factor, some malabsorption syndromes, or ileum resections
- Folate

Niacin deficiency
- Supplemental B-complex vitamins
- Niacinamide

Pyridoxine deficiency
- Prophylactic pyridoxine therapy in infants and in children with seizure disorder
- Supplemental B-complex vitamins

Riboflavin deficiency
- Supplemental riboflavin

Thiamine deficiency
- B-complex vitamins
- Thiamine supplements or thiamine hydrochloride as part of a B-complex concentrate (with alcoholic beriberi)

NURSING DIAGNOSES
- Imbalanced nutrition: Less than body requirements
- Ineffective health maintenance

EXPECTED OUTCOMES
The patient will:
- express understanding of diet high in vitamin B and improve vitamin levels
- express understanding of dietary adjustments needed to improve nutritional status.

NURSING INTERVENTIONS
- Administer prescribed supplements.
- Explain all tests and procedures.

MONITORING
- Adverse effects from large doses of niacinamide, in patients with niacin deficiency
- Dietary intake
- Response to therapy

GENERAL

Be sure to cover:
◆ keeping an accurate dietary history
◆ that prognosis is good with treatment
◆ importance of adhering strictly to their prescribed treatment for the rest of their lives
◆ dietary adjustments.

DISCHARGE PLANNING

◆ Refer the patient to appropriate assistance agencies if his diet is inadequate due to adverse socioeconomic conditions.

RESOURCES

Organizations

American Dietetic Association: *www.eatright.org*
Mayo Clinic: *www.mayoclinic.com*
The Merck Manuals Online Medical Library: *www.merck.com/mmhe*
National Digestive Diseases Information Clearinghouse: *www.niddk.nih.gov/health/digest/nddic.htm*

Selected references

Diseases, 4th ed. Philadelphia: Lippincott Williams & Wilkins, 2006.

Flicker, L., et al. "Efficacy of B Vitamins in Lowering Homocysteine in Older Men: Maximal Effects for Those with B_{12} Deficiency and Hyperhomocysteinemia," *Stroke* 37(2):547-49, February 2006.

Henoun, L.N., et al. "Cobalamin Deficiency Due to Non-Immune Atrophic Gastritis in Elderly Patients. A Report of 25 Cases," *Journal of Nutrition, Health & Aging* 9(6):462, November-December 2005.

Kanbay, M., et al. "Portal Vein Thrombosis Due to Hyperhomocysteinemia Caused by Vitamin B-12 Deficiency," *Digestive Diseases and Sciences* 50(12):2362-63, December 2005.

Vitamin C deficiency

OVERVIEW

- Deficiency of vitamin C in the body
- Historically common among sailors and others deprived of fresh fruits and vegetables for long periods of time; uncommon today in the United States, except in alcoholics, people on restricted-residue diets, and infants weaned from breast milk to cow's milk without a vitamin C supplement
- Also known as *scurvy*

PATHOPHYSIOLOGY

- Deficiency of vitamin C can lead to scurvy or inadequate production of collagen, an extracellular substance that binds the cells of the teeth, bones, and capillaries.
- Because the body can't store this water-soluble vitamin in large amounts, the supply needs to be replenished daily.

CAUSES

- Diet lacking foods rich in vitamin C, such as citrus fruits, tomatoes, cabbage, broccoli, spinach, and berries
- Destruction of vitamin C in foods by overexposure to air or by overcooking
- Excessive ingestion of vitamin C during pregnancy, which causes the neonate to require large amounts of the vitamin after birth
- Marginal intake of vitamin C during periods of physiologic stress

INCIDENCE

- Vitamin C deficiency is rare in the United States.
- This condition can occur at any age.
- This condition affects males and females equally.

COMPLICATIONS

- Sudden death

ASSESSMENT

HISTORY

- Anorexia
- Limb and joint pain (especially in the knees)
- Insomnia
- Poor wound healing
- Irritability
- Depression
- Hysteria
- Hypochondriasis
- Fatigue

PHYSICAL FINDINGS

- Pallor
- Petechiae
- Ecchymoses
- Follicular hyperkeratosis (especially on the buttocks and legs)
- Swollen or bleeding gums (see *Scurvy's effect on gums and legs*)
- Loose teeth
- Ocular hemorrhages in the bulbar conjunctivae
- Beading, fractures of the costochondral junctions of the ribs or epiphysis

DIAGNOSTIC TEST RESULTS

LABORATORY

- Serum ascorbic acid levels are less than 0.2 mg/dl.
- White blood cell ascorbic acid levels are less than 30 mg/dl.

OTHER

- Dietary history may reveal an inadequate intake of ascorbic acid, which suggests vitamin C deficiency.

Scurvy's effect on gums and legs

In adults, scurvy causes swollen or bleeding gums and loose teeth.

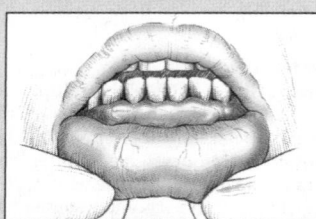

It also causes follicular hyperkeratosis, usually on the legs.

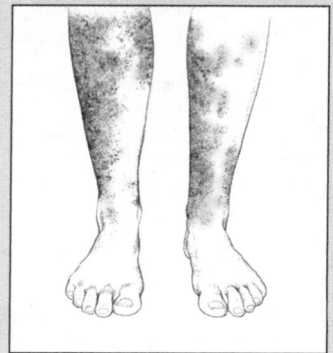

TREATMENT

DIET
◆ High in foods rich in vitamin C

MEDICATIONS
◆ Vitamin C supplements

Foods that contain vitamin C

The following foods contain significant amounts of vitamin C:
◆ blackberries
◆ broccoli
◆ brussels sprouts
◆ cantaloupe
◆ green and red peppers
◆ guava
◆ kale
◆ kiwi
◆ lemons
◆ oranges
◆ papaya
◆ peas
◆ strawberries
◆ tomatoes.

NURSING CONSIDERATIONS

NURSING DIAGNOSES
◆ Activity intolerance
◆ Acute pain
◆ Imbalanced nutrition: Less than body requirements
◆ Impaired oral mucous membrane
◆ Impaired skin integrity
◆ Ineffective health maintenance
◆ Risk for injury

EXPECTED OUTCOMES
The patient will:
◆ perform activities of daily living without excessive fatigue or exhaustion
◆ express feelings of increased comfort
◆ express understanding of diet high in vitamin C and improve vitamin levels
◆ maintain intact oral mucous membranes
◆ exhibit improved or healed wounds or lesions
◆ express understanding of dietary adjustments needed to improve nutritional status
◆ avoid or minimize complications.

NURSING INTERVENTIONS
◆ Give prescribed ascorbic acid orally or by slow I.V. infusion.
◆ Avoid moving the patient unnecessarily to avoid irritating painful joints and muscles.
◆ Encourage the patient to consume foods high in vitamin C. (See *Foods that contain vitamin C.*)

MONITORING
◆ Dietary intake

PATIENT TEACHING

GENERAL
Be sure to cover:
◆ importance of supplemental ascorbic acid
◆ good dietary sources of vitamin C
◆ not taking too much vitamin C because excessive doses of ascorbic acid may cause nausea, diarrhea, and renal calculi formation and may also interfere with anticoagulant therapy.

RESOURCES
Organizations
American Dietetic Association: *www.eatright.org*
The Merck Manuals Online Medical Library: *www.merck.com/mmhe*
National Digestive Diseases Information Clearinghouse: *www.niddk.nih.gov/health/digest/nddic.htm*

Selected references
Chaudhry, S.I., et al. "Scurvy: A Forgotten Disease," *Clinical & Experimental Dermatology* 30(6):735-36, November 2005.
Diseases, 4th ed. Philadelphia: Lippincott Williams & Wilkins, 2006.
Halligan, T.J., et al. "Identification and Treatment of Scurvy: A Case Report," *Oral Surgery, Oral Medicine, Oral Pathology, Oral Radiology, & Endodontics* 100(6):688-92, December 2005.
Lehmann, C., et al. "From Scurvy to Sepsis: Vitamin C – A Pill for All Seasons?" *Critical Care Medicine* 33(8):1881-882, August 2005.
Pimentel, L. "Scurvy: Historical Review and Current Diagnostic Approach," *American Journal of Emergency Medicine* 21(4):328-32, July 2003.

Vitamin D deficiency

OVERVIEW

- Deficiency of vitamin D in the body
- Also known as *rickets*

PATHOPHYSIOLOGY

- Deficiency of vitamin D causes failure of normal bone calcification, which results in rickets in infants and young children and osteomalacia in adults.
- With treatment, the prognosis is good; however, in rickets, bone deformities usually persist, while in osteomalacia, such deformities may disappear.

CAUSES

- Hepatic or renal disease
- Inadequate dietary intake of preformed vitamin D
- Malabsorption of vitamin D
- Malfunctioning parathyroid gland (decreased secretion of parathyroid hormone), which contributes to calcium deficiency (normally, absorption of calcium and phosphorus through the intestine controlled by vitamin D) and interferes with activation of vitamin D in the kidneys
- Too little exposure to sunlight
- Vitamin D-resistant rickets (refractory rickets, familial hypophosphatemia) from an inherited impairment of renal tubular reabsorption of phosphate (from vitamin D insensitivity)

INCIDENCE

- Vitamin D deficiency was once a common childhood disease, but now is rare in the United States.
- This condition occasionally appears in breast-fed infants who don't receive vitamin D supplementation and in infants receiving a formula with a nonfortified milk base.
- This condition may also occur in overcrowded, urban areas where smog limits sunlight penetration.
- The highest incidence of this deficiency occurs in black children who, because of their skin color, absorb less sunlight.

COMPLICATIONS

- Spontaneous fractures
- Abnormal gait
- Short stature

Recognizing bowlegs

This infant with rickets shows characteristic bowing of the legs.

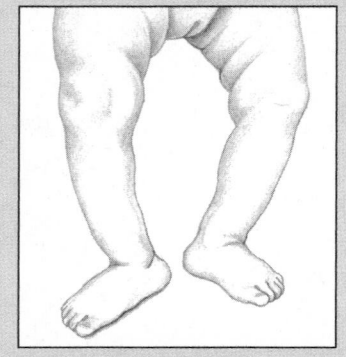

ASSESSMENT

HISTORY

- Spontaneous multiple fractures
- Pain in the legs and lower back

PHYSICAL FINDINGS

- Bowlegs (see *Recognizing bowlegs*)
- Knock-knees
- Rachitic rosary (beading of ends of ribs)
- Enlargement of wrists and ankles
- Pigeon breast
- Delayed closing of the fontanels
- Softening of the skull
- Bulging of the forehead

DIAGNOSTIC TEST RESULTS

LABORATORY
◆ Plasma calcium serum levels are less than 7.5 mg/dl.
◆ Serum inorganic phosphorus levels are less than 3 mg/dl.
◆ Serum citrate levels are less than 2.5 mg/dl.
◆ Alkaline phosphatase levels are less than 4 Bodansky units/dl.

IMAGING
◆ X-rays show characteristic bone deformities and abnormalities such as Looser's zones (pseudofractures).

TREATMENT

GENERAL
◆ Sunlight exposure

MEDICATIONS
◆ For osteomalacia and rickets (except when caused by malabsorption), massive oral doses of vitamin D or cod liver oil
◆ For rickets refractory to vitamin D or in rickets accompanied by hepatic or renal disease, 25-hydroxycholecalciferol, 1,25-dihydroxycholecalciferol, or a synthetic analogue of active vitamin D

NURSING CONSIDERATIONS

NURSING DIAGNOSES
◆ Acute pain
◆ Disturbed body image
◆ Imbalanced nutrition: Less than body requirements
◆ Impaired physical mobility
◆ Ineffective health maintenance
◆ Risk for injury

EXPECTED OUTCOMES
The patient will:
◆ express feelings of increased comfort
◆ express positive feelings about self
◆ express understanding of diet high in vitamin D and improve vitamin levels
◆ maintain optimal mobility within the confines of the disorder
◆ express understanding of dietary adjustments needed to improve nutritional status
◆ avoid injury and complications.

NURSING INTERVENTIONS
◆ Obtain a dietary history to assess the patient's current vitamin D intake.
◆ Administer supplementary aqueous preparations of vitamin D for chronic fat malabsorption, hydroxylated cholecalciferol for refractory rickets, and supplemental vitamin D for breast-fed infants.

MONITORING
◆ Dietary intake
◆ Comfort level

PATIENT TEACHING

GENERAL
Be sure to cover:
◆ watching for signs of vitamin D toxicity (headache, nausea, constipation and, after prolonged use, renal calculi).

DISCHARGE PLANNING
◆ If deficiency is due to socioeconomic conditions, refer the patient to an appropriate community agency.

RESOURCES
Organizations
American Dietetic Association: *www.eatright.org*
The Merck Manuals Online Medical Library: *www.merck.com/mmhe*
National Digestive Diseases Information Clearinghouse: *www.niddk.nih.gov/health/digest/nddic.htm*

Selected references
Diseases, 4th ed. Philadelphia: Lippincott Williams & Wilkins, 2006.
Francis, R.M. "Calcium, Vitamin D and Involutional Osteoporosis," *Current Opinion in Clinical Nutrition and Metabolic Care* 9(1):13-17, January 2006.
Grote, J. "Vitamin D Deficiency," *JAMA* 295(9):1002, March 2006.
Simonelli, C. "The Role of Vitamin D Deficiency in Osteoporosis and Fractures," *Minnesota Medicine* 88(11):34-36, November 2005.
Robinson, J.K. "Sun Exposure, Sun Protection, and Vitamin D," *JAMA* 294(12):1541-43, September 2005.
Wolpowitz, D., and Gilchrest, B.A. "The Vitamin D Questions: How Much Do You Need and How Should You Get It?" *Journal of the American Academy of Dermatology* 54(2):301-17, February 2006.

Vitamin E deficiency

◆ Deficiency of vitamin E in the body

PATHOPHYSIOLOGY
◆ Vitamin E (tocopherol) appears to act primarily as an antioxidant, preventing intracellular oxidation of polyunsaturated fatty acids and other lipids.
◆ Deficiency of vitamin E usually manifests as hemolytic anemia in low–birth-weight or premature neonates. With treatment, prognosis is good.

CAUSES
◆ Conditions associated with fat malabsorption
◆ In infants, usually results from consuming formulas high in polyunsaturated fatty acids fortified with iron but not vitamin E

INCIDENCE
◆ Vitamin E deficiency is uncommon in adults, but could possibly occur in people whose diets are high in polyunsaturated fatty acids, which increase vitamin E requirements, and in people with vitamin E malabsorption, which impairs red blood cell (RBC) survival.

COMPLICATIONS
◆ Disorders of reproduction
◆ Abnormalities of muscle, liver, bone marrow, and brain function
◆ Hemolysis of RBC
◆ Skeletal muscle dystrophy

HISTORY
◆ Intermittent claudication

PHYSICAL FINDINGS
◆ Edema
◆ Skin lesions

LABORATORY
◆ Serum alpha-tocopherol levels are below 0.5 mg/dl in adults and below 0.2 mg/dl in infants.
◆ Creatinuria, increased creatine kinase levels, hemolytic anemia, and an elevated platelet count support the diagnosis.

OTHER
◆ Dietary and medical histories suggest vitamin E deficiency.

Foods that contain vitamin E

The following foods contain significant amounts of vitamin E:
◆ almond oil
◆ almonds
◆ asparagus
◆ avocadoes
◆ canola oil
◆ corn
◆ corn oil
◆ cottonseed oil
◆ hazelnuts
◆ kiwi
◆ mangoes
◆ nuts
◆ olives
◆ safflower oil
◆ soybeans
◆ soybean oil
◆ sunflower seeds
◆ wheat germ
◆ wheat germ oil.

TREATMENT

DIET
◆ High in foods rich in vitamin E, such as vegetable oils, whole grains, dark green leafy vegetables, nuts, and legumes

MEDICATIONS
◆ Vitamin E supplementation

NURSING CONSIDERATIONS

NURSING DIAGNOSES
◆ Imbalanced nutrition: Less than body requirements
◆ Impaired skin integrity
◆ Ineffective health maintenance
◆ Ineffective tissue perfusion: Peripheral
◆ Risk for injury

EXPECTED OUTCOMES
The patient (or family) will:
◆ express understanding of diet high in vitamin E and improve vitamin levels
◆ maintain skin integrity
◆ express understanding of dietary adjustments needed to improve nutritional status
◆ exhibit signs of adequate peripheral perfusion
◆ avoid injury and complications.

NURSING INTERVENTIONS
◆ Encourage patient to consume foods high in vitamin E. (See *Foods that contain vitamin E.*)

MONITORING
◆ Dietary intake

PATIENT TEACHING

GENERAL
Be sure to cover:
◆ preventing deficiency by providing vitamin E supplements for low–birth-weight infants receiving formulas not fortified with vitamin E and for adults with vitamin E malabsorption
◆ dietary changes
◆ that food manufacturers fortify many products with vitamins and minerals
◆ that most adults in the United States get enough vitamin E in their normal diets to meet current recommendations. (Caution those on low-fat diets that low fat intake can decrease vitamin E intake if appropriate food choices aren't made.)

DISCHARGE PLANNING
◆ If deficiency is related to socioeconomic conditions, refer the patient to appropriate community agencies.

RESOURCES
Organizations
American Dietetic Association: *www.eatright.org*
National Digestive Diseases Information Clearinghouse: *www.niddk.nih.gov/health/digest/nddic.htm*

Selected references
Diseases, 4th ed. Philadelphia: Lippincott Williams & Wilkins, 2006.

Koscik, R.L., et al. "Preventing Early, Prolonged Vitamin E Deficiency: An Opportunity for Better Cognitive Outcomes Via Early Diagnosis Through Neonatal Screening," *Journal of Pediatrics* 147(3 Suppl):S51-56, September 2005.

Mas, E., et al. "Functional Vitamin E Deficiency in Apoe4 Patients with Alzheimer's Disease," *Dementia and Geriatric Cognitive Disorders* 21(3):198-204, 2006.

Puri, V., et al. "Isolated Vitamin E Deficiency with Demyelinating Neuropathy," *Muscle & Nerve* 32(2):230-35, August 2005.

Traber, M.G. "Vitamin E Regulation," *Current Opinion in Gastroenterology* 21(2):223-27, March 2005.

Vitamin K deficiency

- Deficiency of vitamin K in the body

PATHOPHYSIOLOGY

- Vitamin K is an element necessary for formation of prothrombin and other clotting factors in the liver; deficiency produces abnormal bleeding.
- If the deficiency is corrected, the prognosis is excellent.
- Vitamin K is found in specific foods and is also made by the bacteria that line the GI tract.

CAUSES

- Chronic hepatic disease
- Cystic fibrosis
- Malabsorption of vitamin K due to sprue, pellagra, bowel resection, ileitis, or ulcerative colitis
- Obstruction of the bile duct or bile fistula
- Prolonged use of drugs, such as the anticoagulant dicumarol and antibiotics that destroy normal intestinal bacteria

INCIDENCE

- Vitamin K deficiency is common among neonates in the first few days postpartum due to poor placental transfer of vitamin K and inadequate production of vitamin K-producing intestinal flora.

COMPLICATIONS

- Bleeding

HISTORY

- Prolonged or easy bleeding

PHYSICAL FINDINGS

- Ecchymosis
- Petechiae

LABORATORY

- A prothrombin time (PT) that's 25% longer than the normal range of 10 to 20 seconds confirms the diagnosis of vitamin K deficiency after other causes of prolonged PT (such as anticoagulant therapy or hepatic disease) have been ruled out.

Foods that contain vitamin K

The following foods contain significant amounts of vitamin K.

Breads, cereals, rice, and pasta
- Oats
- Wheat bran
- Whole wheat flour

Fruits
- Avocados

Vegetables
- Broccoli
- Cabbage
- Cauliflower
- Endive
- Kale
- Lentils (dry)
- Lettuce (iceberg)
- Soybeans
- Spinach
- Swiss chard
- Turnip greens
- Watercress

Organ meats
- Beef liver
- Chicken liver
- Pork liver

Fats, oils, sugars
- Corn oil
- Soybean oil

DIET
- Rich in foods high in vitamin K, such as green leafy vegetables, cereals, soybeans, and other vegetables

MEDICATIONS
- Vitamin K

NURSING DIAGNOSES
- Imbalanced nutrition: Less than body requirements
- Impaired skin integrity
- Ineffective health maintenance
- Risk for injury

EXPECTED OUTCOMES
The patient (or family) will:
- express understanding of diet high in vitamin K and show improved vitamin levels and laboratory values
- maintain skin integrity
- express understanding of dietary adjustments needed to improve nutritional status
- avoid injury and complications, and show decreased tendency to bleed easily.

NURSING INTERVENTIONS
- Encourage the patient to consume foods high in vitamin K. (See *Foods that contain vitamin K.*)
- Administer vitamin K to neonates and patients with fat malabsorption or with prolonged diarrhea caused by colitis, ileitis, or long-term antibiotic therapy.

MONITORING
- PT
- Signs of bleeding

GENERAL
Be sure to cover:
- warning against self-medication with or overuse of antibiotics, which destroy the intestinal bacteria necessary to generate significant amounts of vitamin K
- dietary counseling
- warning the patient to take safety precautions as vitamin K deficiency can cause increased risk of bruising and bleeding.

RESOURCES
Organizations
American Dietetic Association: *www.eatright.org*
The Merck Manuals Online Medical Library: *www.merck.com/mmhe*
National Digestive Diseases Information Clearinghouse: *www.niddk.nih.gov/health/digest/nddic.htm*

Selected references
Bhattacharyya, J., et al. "Congenital Vitamin K-Dependent Coagulation Factor Deficiency: A Case Report," *Blood Coagulation & Fibrinolysis* 16(7):525-27, October 2005.
Cashman, K.D. "Vitamin K Status May Be an Important Determinant of Childhood Bone Health," *Nutrition Reviews* 63(8):284-89, August 2005.
DeLoughery, T.G. "Critical Care Clotting Catastrophes," *Critical Care Clinics* 21(3):531-62, July 2005.
Diseases, 4th ed. Philadelphia: Lippincott Williams & Wilkins, 2006.

Vitiligo

OVERVIEW

- Hypopigmentation condition of the skin
- May cause a serious cosmetic problem
- Concurrent risk of other diseases, especially thyroid

PATHOPHYSIOLOGY

- Destruction of melanocytes and circulating antibodies results in hypopigmented areas.

CAUSES

- Apparently, both genetic and environmental components
- Associated concurrent diseases:
- – Addison's disease
- – Aseptic meningitis
- – Diabetes mellitus
- – Pernicious anemia
- – Thyroid dysfunction
- In about 30% of patients, first-degree relative with the same disorder
- Precipitating factors:
- – Stressful physical or psychological events
- – Chemical agents, such as phenols and catechols

INCIDENCE

- This disorder affects about 1% of U.S. population.
- This disorder can onset at any age.
- About 50% of all cases begin between ages 10 and 30.
- There is no racial predilection.
- Males and females are about equally affected. (Women tend to seek treatment more than men.)

COMPLICATIONS

- Extreme photosensitivity in depigmented areas
- Hypersensitivity reactions to therapeutic agents and to dyes or cosmetics used to camouflage lesions

ASSESSMENT

HISTORY

- Familial history of vitiligo

PHYSICAL FINDINGS

- Depigmented or stark white skin patches; almost imperceptible on fair-skinned whites
- Patches usually bilaterally symmetrical, with distinct borders that may be raised and hyperpigmented (see *Recognizing vitiligo*)
- Patches most likely over bony prominences, around orifices, within body folds, and at sites of traumatic injury
- Hair within lesions also possibly white
- Prematurely gray hair
- Ocular pigment changes

DIAGNOSTIC TEST RESULTS

DIAGNOSTIC PROCEDURES

- Wood's light examination in a darkened room may show vitiliginous patches in fair-skinned patients.
- A skin biopsy may confirm the diagnosis.

Recognizing vitiligo

This illustration shows characteristic depigmented skin patches in vitiligo. These patches are usually bilaterally symmetrical, with distinct borders.

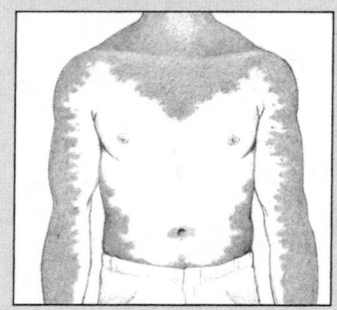

TREATMENT

GENERAL
- Sunscreens
- Cosmetics and skin dyes as cover-ups
- Rule out underlying thyroid disease

MEDICATIONS
- Repigmentation compounds
- Depigmentation creams

SURGERY
- Skin grafting

NURSING CONSIDERATIONS

NURSING DIAGNOSES
- Disturbed body image
- Risk for injury

EXPECTED OUTCOMES
The patient will:
- verbalize feelings about changed body image
- avoid complications.

NURSING INTERVENTIONS
- Encourage expression of feelings about appearance.
- Offer emotional support and reassurance.
- Reinforce treatment goals.

MONITORING
- Response to treatment
- Complications

PATIENT TEACHING

GENERAL
Be sure to cover:
- disorder, diagnosis, and treatment
- that exposure to sunlight also darkens normal skin in patients undergoing repigmentation therapy
- the use of sunscreen, sunglasses, and protective clothing
- that results of depigmentation are permanent
- adverse effects of sunlight.

DISCHARGE PLANNING
- Refer the patient to the National Vitiligo Foundation.

RESOURCES
Organizations
American Academy of Dermatology: *www.aad.org*
Dermatology Foundation: *www.dermfnd.org*
National Vitiligo Foundation: *www.nvfi.org*

Selected references
Don, P., et al. "Treatment of Vitiligo with Broadband Ultraviolet B and Vitamins," *International Journal of Dermatology* 45(1):63-65, January 2006.

Kostovic, K., and Pasic, A. "New Treatment Modalities for Vitiligo: Focus On Topical Immunomodulators," *Drugs* 65(4):447-59, 2005.

Leone, G., et al. "Tacalcitol and Narrow-Band Phototherapy in Patients with Vitiligo," *Clinical & Experimental Dermatology* 31(2):200-205, March 2006.

Ongenae, K., et al. "Psychosocial Effects of Vitiligo," *Journal of the European Academy of Dermatology and Venereology* 20(1):1-8, January 2006.

Tjioe, M., et al. "Topical Macrolide Immunomodulators: A Role in the Treatment of Vitiligo?" *American Journal of Clinical Dermatology* 7(1):7-12, 2006.

Volvulus

- Twisting of the intestine at least 180 degrees on itself
- Marked by sudden onset of severe abdominal pain
- Results in blood vessel compression
- Causes obstruction both proximal and distal to the twisted loop
- Occurs in a bowel segment long enough to twist, most commonly the sigmoid colon (small bowel a common site in children)
- Other common sites: the stomach and cecum

PATHOPHYSIOLOGY

- The colon twists on its mesentery.
- A closed loop obstruction occurs, affecting venous drainage and arterial inflow.
- Cecal volvulus is a congenital defect in the peritoneum with inadequate fixation of the cecum. (See *What happens in volvulus.*)

CAUSES

- Adhesions
- Anomaly of bowel rotation in utero
- Ingested foreign body
- Meconium ileus (in patients with cystic fibrosis)

RISK FACTORS

- Straining at stool
- Pregnancy
- Intestinal malignancy
- Hernia
- High-bulk diet
- History of previous attacks
- Use of chronic neuropsychotropic drugs
- Chronic constipation and laxative abuse

INCIDENCE

- The incidence of volvulus varies worldwide in cases involving the large bowel.
- This disorder accounts for 1% to 5% of all large-bowel obstructions in advanced Western populations.

- The most common sites for volvulus to occur include the sigmoid colon (80%), cecum (15%), transverse colon (3%), and splenic flexure (2%).
- This disorder is common in regions of Africa, Southern Asia, and South America.
- About 50% of large-bowel obstructions caused by volvulus occur in the "volvulus belt" of Africa and the Middle East.
- Volvulus affects men and women equally.

COMPLICATIONS

- Strangulation of the twisted bowel loop
- Bowel ischemia and infarction
- Bowel perforation

HISTORY

- Severe abdominal pain
- Bilious vomiting
- Constipation

PHYSICAL FINDINGS

- Abdominal distention
- Palpable abdominal mass

What happens in volvulus

Although volvulus may occur anywhere in a bowel segment long enough to twist, the most common site is the sigmoid colon, causing edema within the closed loop and obstruction at its proximal and distal ends.

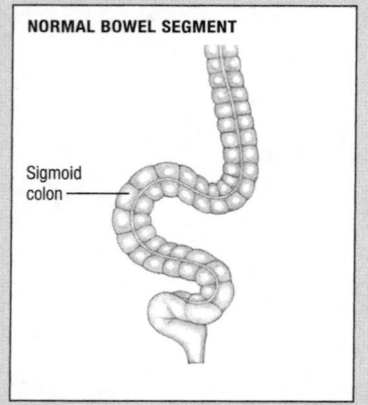

NORMAL BOWEL SEGMENT

Sigmoid colon

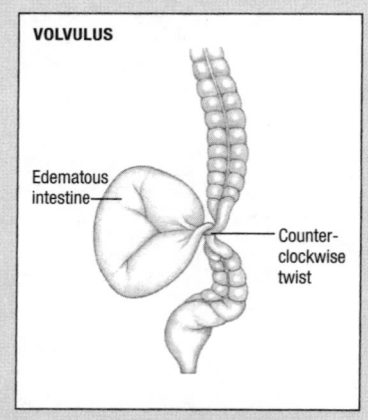

VOLVULUS

Edematous intestine

Counter-clockwise twist

DIAGNOSTIC TEST RESULTS

LABORATORY
- White blood cell count, in strangulation, is greater than 15,000/ml; in bowel infarction, it's greater than 20,000/ml.

IMAGING
- Abdominal X-rays may show multiple distended bowel loops and a large bowel without gas. In midgut volvulus, abdominal X-rays may be normal.
- Barium enema, in cecal volvulus, shows barium filling the colon distal to the affected section of cecum; in sigmoid volvulus, barium may twist to a point and, in adults, take on an "ace of spades" configuration.

TREATMENT

GENERAL
- For adults with sigmoid volvulus, nonsurgical treatment: proctoscopy to check for infarction and reduction by careful insertion of a flexible sigmoidoscope to deflate the bowel
- I.V. therapy

DIET
- Nothing by mouth until condition resolves

ACTIVITY
- Bed rest until condition resolves

MEDICATIONS
- Antibiotics
- Analgesics

SURGERY
- For children with midgut volvulus
- Detorsion (untwisting)
- Resection and anastomosis

NURSING CONSIDERATIONS

NURSING DIAGNOSES
- Acute pain
- Deficient fluid volume
- Imbalanced nutrition: Less than body requirements
- Ineffective tissue perfusion: GI
- Risk for infection

EXPECTED OUTCOMES
The patient will:
- express feelings of increased comfort and decreased pain
- maintain a normal fluid balance
- achieve adequate caloric and nutritional intake
- regain normal bowel function
- remain free from signs or symptoms of infection.

NURSING INTERVENTIONS
- Encourage verbalization and provide support.
- Give prescribed drugs.
- Give prescribed I.V. fluids.

MONITORING
- Pain control
- Bowel function
- Vital signs
- Fluid and electrolyte balance
- Nasogastric tube function and drainage
- Wound site

PATIENT TEACHING

GENERAL
Be sure to cover:
- disorder, diagnosis, and treatment
- preoperative teaching
- drug administration, dosage, and possible adverse effects
- signs and symptoms of infection
- importance of follow-up care.

RESOURCES
Organizations
Digestive Disease National Coalition: *www.ddnc.org*
National Digestive Diseases Information Clearinghouse: *www.niddk.nih.gov/health/digest/nddic.htm*

Selected references
Consorti, E.T., and Liu, T.H. "Diagnosis and Treatment of Caecal Volvulus," *Postgraduate Medical Journal* 81(962):772-76, December 2005.
McNally, P. *GI/Liver Secrets*, 3rd ed. Philadelphia: Hanley & Belfus, Inc., 2006.
Mourra, N., et al. "Chronic Schistosomiasis: An Incidental Finding in Sigmoid Volvulus," *Journal of Clinical Pathology* 59(1):111, January 2006.
Tiah, L, and Goh, S.H. "Sigmoid Volvulus: Diagnostic Twists and Turns," *European Journal of Emergency Medicine* 13(2):84-87, April 2006.
Tsang, T.K., et al. "Gastrointestinal: Sigmoid Volvulus," *Journal of Gastroenterology & Hepatology* 20(5):790, May 2005.

von Willebrand's disease

- Hereditary bleeding disorder characterized by prolonged bleeding time, moderate deficiency of clotting factor VIII (antihemophilic factor), and impaired platelet function
- Also known as *angiohemophilia*, *pseudohemophilia*, and *vascular hemophilia*

PATHOPHYSIOLOGY

- A mild to moderate deficiency of factor VIII and defective platelet adhesion prolongs coagulation time.
- Results from a deficiency of von Willebrand's factor (factor VIII_{VWF}), which appears to occupy the factor VIII molecule and may be necessary for the production of factor VIII and proper platelet function.
- Defective platelet function is characterized by decreased agglutination and adhesion at the bleeding site, reduced platelet retention when filtered through a column of packed glass beads, and diminished ristocetin-induced platelet aggregation.

CAUSES

- Acquired form identified in patients with cancer and immune disorders
- Inherited as an autosomal dominant trait

INCIDENCE

- This disorder affects males and females; tends to be more common in males.

COMPLICATIONS

- Hemorrhage

ASSESSMENT

HISTORY

- Possible familial history of the disease
- Easy bruising and frequent bleeding from the nose or gums (petechiae rare)
- Menorrhagia
- Hemorrhage after a laceration or surgery
- Possible episodes of GI bleeding

PHYSICAL FINDINGS

- Bruises
- Clinical bleeding

DIAGNOSTIC TEST RESULTS

LABORATORY

- Bleeding time is prolonged to more than 6 minutes.
- Partial thromboplastin time is slightly prolonged to more than 45 seconds.
- Factor VIII-related antigen levels are absent or reduced, and factor VIII activity level is low.
- In vitro platelet aggregation is defective using the ristocetin coagulation factor assay test.
- Platelet count and clot retraction are normal.

TREATMENT

GENERAL

- Depends on the symptoms and underlying type of disease
- Decreasing bleeding time by local measures and replacing factor VIII and, consequently, factor VIII_{VWF}
- Avoidance of aspirin

ACTIVITY

- Alternation of activities and rest periods if patient is fatigued after a bleeding episode

MEDICATIONS

- Cryoprecipitate (cryoprecipitated antihemophilic factor)
- Plasma products or vasopressin analogue
- Factor VIII concentrates

NURSING DIAGNOSES

- Activity intolerance
- Anxiety
- Disabled family coping
- Fatigue
- Ineffective coping
- Ineffective tissue perfusion: Cardiopulmonary
- Risk for deficient fluid volume
- Risk for injury

EXPECTED OUTCOMES

The patient (or family) will:
- verbalize the importance of balancing activity, as tolerated, with rest
- verbalize strategies to reduce anxiety level
- seek support systems and exhibit adequate coping behaviors
- express feelings of energy and decreased fatigue
- exhibit adequate coping skills
- show evidence of hemodynamic stability
- maintain normal fluid volume
- remain free from injury.

NURSING INTERVENTIONS

- Provide emotional support as necessary.
- During a bleeding episode, elevate the area if possible, and apply cold compresses and gentle pressure to the bleeding site. (Pressure is commonly the only treatment necessary.)
- Give prescribed drugs or transfusions.
- Prevent potential injury by using an electric razor, keeping the room free from clutter, and providing a cushioned sitting and sleeping surface (such as a convoluted foam mattress).

MONITORING

- Signs and symptoms of decreased tissue perfusion
- Vital signs
- Frequently, for bleeding from the skin, mucous membranes, and wounds
- After surgery, bleeding time or other clotting procedure for 24 to 48 hours and for signs of new bleeding
- Adverse reactions to blood products

PATIENT TEACHING

GENERAL

Be sure to cover:
- disorder, diagnosis, and treatment
- importance of notifying a physician after even minor trauma and before all surgery, including dental procedures, to determine whether replacement of blood components is necessary
- warnings against using aspirin and other drugs that impair platelet function (how to recognize over-the-counter medications that contain aspirin)
- special precautions to prevent bleeding episodes
- importance of wearing or carrying medical identification
- measures to control bleeding and how to prevent bleeding, unnecessary trauma, and complications.

DISCHARGE PLANNING

- Refer parents of an affected child for genetic counseling.

RESOURCES

Organizations

Centers for Disease Control and Prevention: *www.cdc.gov*
The Merck Manuals Online Medical Library: *www.merck.com/mmhe*
National Hemophilia Foundation: *www.hemophilia.org*

Selected references

Franchini, M. "Thrombotic Complications in von Willebrand Disease," *Hematology* 11(1):49-52, February 2006.

Handbook of Pathophysiology, 2nd ed. Philadelphia: Lippincott Williams & Wilkins, 2005.

James, A.H. "Von Willebrand Disease," *Obstetrical & Gynecological Survey* 61(2):136-45, February 2006.

Kasper, D.L., et al., eds. *Harrison's Principles of Internal Medicine*, 16th ed. New York: McGraw-Hill Book Co., 2005.

Michiels, J.J., et al. "Characterization, Classification, and Treatment of von Willebrand Diseases: A Critical Appraisal of the Literature and Personal Experiences," *Seminars in Thrombosis and Hemostasis* 31(5):577-601, November 2005.

Professional Guide to Diseases, 8th ed. Philadelphia: Lippincott Williams & Wilkins, 2005.

Tierney, L., et al. *Current Medical Diagnosis & Treatment* 2006. New York: McGraw-Hill Book Co., 2006.

Yoshida, K., et al. "Acquired von Willebrand Disease Type IIA in Patients with Aortic Valve Stenosis," *Annals of Thoracic Surgery* 81(3):1114-116, March 2006.

Vulvovaginitis

OVERVIEW

- Inflammation of the vulva (vulvitis) and vagina (vaginitis)
- Prognosis good with treatment

PATHOPHYSIOLOGY

- Because of the proximity of the vulva and vagina, inflammation of one usually precipitates inflammation of the other.

CAUSES

Vaginitis
- Bacterial infection (bacterial vaginosis)
- Fungal infection (*Candida albicans*)
- Protozoan infection (*Trichomonas vaginalis*)
- Venereal infection (*Neisseria gonorrhoeae*)
- Viral infection with venereal warts or herpes simplex virus Type 2

Vulvitis
- Allergic reactions, such as to douches or toilet paper
- Chemical irritations
- Parasitic infection (*Phthirus pubis*, crab louse)
- Poor personal hygiene
- Retention of a foreign body such as a tampon
- Traumatic injury

RISK FACTORS

- Pregnancy
- Hormonal contraceptives
- Diabetes mellitus
- Systemic broad-spectrum antibiotics
- Vaginal mucosa and vulval atrophy in menopausal women

INCIDENCE

- This disorder can occur at any age.
- This disorder affects most females at some time.

COMPLICATIONS

- Inflammation of the perineum
- Skin breakdown
- Secondary infection
- Dyspareunia
- Dysuria

ASSESSMENT

HISTORY

Trichomonal vaginitis
- Vaginal irritation and itching
- Urinary symptoms, such as burning and frequency

Candidal vaginitis
- Intense vaginal itching
- Thick, white, cottage cheese–like discharge

Bacterial vaginosis
- Fishy-smelling discharge
- May be asymptomatic

Gonorrhea
- Possibly no symptoms
- Dysuria

Acute vulvitis
- Vulvar burning, pruritus
- Severe dysuria
- Dyspareunia

PHYSICAL FINDINGS

Trichomonal vaginitis
- Thin, bubbly, green-tinged, and malodorous vaginal discharge

Candidal vaginitis
- Thick, white, cottage cheese–like discharge
- Red, edematous mucous membranes with white flecks on vaginal wall

Bacterial vaginosis
- Gray, foul, fishy-smelling discharge

Gonorrhea
- Profuse and purulent discharge

Acute vulvitis
- Vulvar edema and erythema

Herpesvirus infection
- Ulceration or vesicle formation on the perineum (active phase)
- Severe edema that may involve entire perineum (chronic infection)

DIAGNOSTIC TEST RESULTS

LABORATORY

- Wet slide preparation and microscopic examination of vaginal exudates are used in obtaining various test results:
- Vaginitis diagnosis requires identification of the infectious organism.
- In trichomonal infections, the presence of motile, flagellated trichomonads confirms the diagnosis.
- In monilial vaginitis, 10% potassium hydroxide is added to the slide; diagnosis requires identification of *C. albicans* fungus.
- In bacterial vaginosis, saline wet mount shows the presence of clue cells, giving it a stippled appearance.
- Gonorrhea requires a culture of vaginal exudate to confirm the diagnosis.
- Diagnosis of vulvitis or a suspected sexually transmitted disease (STD) may require a complete blood count, urinalysis, cytology screening, biopsy of chronic lesions to rule out cancer, and culture of exudate from acute lesions.

TREATMENT

GENERAL
- Cold compresses or cool sitz baths to relieve pruritus
- Warm compresses for severe inflammation
- Avoidance of drying soaps
- Loose clothing to promote air circulation
- For chronic vulvitis, changing problematic environmental factors

MEDICATIONS
- Antibacterials
- Antiprotozoal agents
- Topical corticosteroids
- Antipruritics
- Topical estrogen ointments
- Antivirals

NURSING CONSIDERATIONS

NURSING DIAGNOSES
- Acute pain
- Disturbed body image
- Ineffective coping
- Ineffective sexuality patterns
- Risk for impaired skin integrity
- Risk for infection

EXPECTED OUTCOMES
The patient will:
- express feelings of increased comfort
- express concerns about self-concept, self-esteem, and body image
- with her partner, use available counseling or support groups and develop effective coping mechanisms
- with her partner, verbalize feelings regarding the condition and how it affects their sexuality
- maintain intact skin integrity
- remain free from signs or symptoms of infection.

NURSING INTERVENTIONS
- Encourage expression of feelings.
- Help the patient to develop effective coping strategies.
- Provide comfort measures.
- Use meticulous hand-washing technique.
- Report cases of STDs to the local public health authorities.
- Administer drug therapy.

MONITORING
- Response to treatment
- Vaginal discharge
- Signs and symptoms of secondary infection

PATIENT TEACHING

GENERAL
Be sure to cover:
- disorder, diagnosis, and treatment
- correlation between sexual contact and spread of vaginal infections
- using condoms to prevent or decrease the spread of STDs
- notifying sexual partners of the need for treatment
- abstaining from sexual intercourse until the infection resolves
- completing prescribed drugs, even if symptoms subside
- proper application of vaginal ointments and suppositories
- importance of meticulous hand washing before and after drug administration
- preventing skin breakdown and secondary infections
- good hygiene practices
- wearing white cotton underpants and avoiding tight pants and panty hose
- abstaining from alcoholic beverages with metronidazole therapy
- that metronidazole therapy may turn the urine dark brown.

RESOURCES
Organizations
American College of Obstetricians and Gynecologists: *www.acog.org*
American Society for Reproductive Medicine: *www.asrm.org*

Selected references
Kokotos, F. "Vulvovaginitis," *Pediatrics in Review/American Academy of Pediatrics* 27(3):116-17, March 2006.

Merkley, K. "Vulvovaginitis and Vaginal Discharge in the Pediatric Patient," *Journal of Emergency Nursing* 31(4):400-402, August 2005.

Say, P.J., and Jacyntho, C. "Difficult-to-Manage Vaginitis," *Clinical Obstetrics and Gynecology* 48(4):753-68, December 2005.

Theroux, R. "Factors Influencing Women's Decisions to Self-treat Vaginal Symptoms," *Journal of the American Academy of Nurse Practitioners* 17(4):156-62, April 2005.

Warts

OVERVIEW

- Common, benign, skin growths
- Prognosis varies, some disappearing readily with treatment, others necessitating more vigorous and prolonged treatment
- Also known as *verrucae*

PATHOPHYSIOLOGY

- Warts are small harmless tumors of the skin caused by a virus.
- Most are well defined.
- Mode of transmission is probably through direct contact, but autoinoculation is possible.
- Warts are categorized by location and appearance.

CAUSES

- Infection with the human papillomavirus, a group of ether-resistant, deoxyribonucleic acid-containing papovaviruses

INCIDENCE

- The highest incidence occurs in children and young adults, but may occur at any age.

COMPLICATIONS

- Scarring
- Recurrence of wart
- Formation of keloid

ASSESSMENT

HISTORY

- Based on type and location
- Contact with someone who has warts

PHYSICAL FINDINGS

- Small, flat, usually painless lesion on forehead, cheeks, arms, or legs
- Rough, round, painful lesion on sole
- Rough growth around fingernails or toenails
- Small pink, moist lesions or cluster of lesions in the perineal area

DIAGNOSTIC TEST RESULTS

DIAGNOSTIC PROCEDURES

- Recurrent anal warts require sigmoidoscopy to rule out internal involvement, which may necessitate surgery.
- Skin biopsy may confirm diagnosis in some cases.

OTHER

- Visual examination usually confirms the diagnosis.

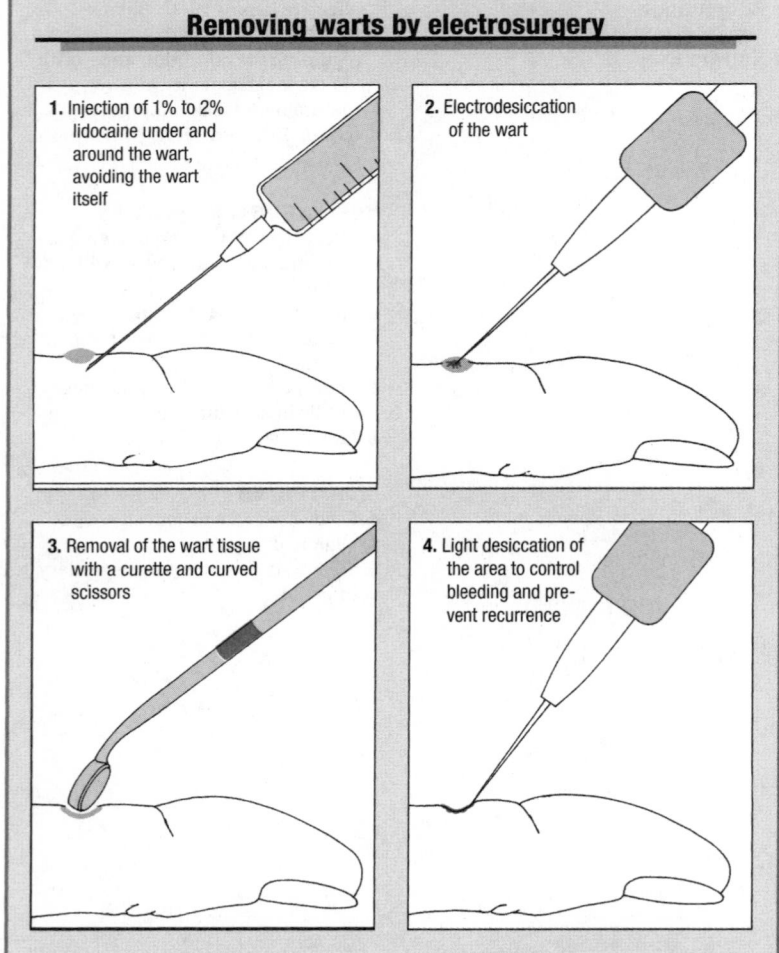

Removing warts by electrosurgery

1. Injection of 1% to 2% lidocaine under and around the wart, avoiding the wart itself

2. Electrodesiccation of the wart

3. Removal of the wart tissue with a curette and curved scissors

4. Light desiccation of the area to control bleeding and prevent recurrence

TREATMENT

GENERAL
- Cryotherapy

MEDICATIONS
- Acid therapy (primary or adjunctive)
- 25% podophyllin in compound with tincture of benzoin (for venereal warts)
- Carbon dioxide laser therapy

SURGERY
- Electrodesiccation and curettage (see *Removing warts by electrosurgery*)

NURSING CONSIDERATIONS

NURSING DIAGNOSES
- Acute pain
- Disturbed body image
- Impaired skin integrity
- Risk for infection

EXPECTED OUTCOMES
The patient will:
- report feelings of increased comfort and decreased pain
- express feelings about change in body image
- exhibit improved or healed lesions
- avoid or minimize the risk of secondary infection.

NURSING INTERVENTIONS
- During acid or podophyllin therapy, protect the surrounding area with petroleum jelly or sodium bicarbonate (baking soda).

MONITORING
- Response to treatment
- Bleeding
- Lesion healing

PATIENT TEACHING

GENERAL
Be sure to cover:
- that conscientious adherence to prescribed therapy is essential
- that the patient's sexual partner may also need treatment
- importance of avoiding direct contact with warts.

RESOURCES
Organizations
American Academy of Dermatology: *www.aad.org*
Dermatology Foundation: *www.dermfnd.org*
Mayo Clinic: *www.mayoclinic.com*
National Institute of Allergy and Infectious Diseases: *www.niaid.nih.gov*

Selected references
Davis, M., et al. "Response of Predominantly Recalcitrant Cutaneous Warts to Topical Chemotherapy," *Journal of the European Academy of Dermatology & Venereology* 20(2):232-34, February 2006.

Diseases, 4th ed. Philadelphia: Lippincott Williams & Wilkins, 2006.

Forbes, M.A., and Schmid, M.M. "Use of OTC Essential Oils to Clear Plantar Warts," *Nurse Practitioner* 31(3):53-57, March 2006.

Orchard, D. "The Treatment of Warts in Children," *Australasian Journal of Dermatology* 46(Suppl 2):A32, September 2005.

Professional Guide to Diseases, 8th ed. Philadelphia: Lippincott Williams & Wilkins, 2005.

West Nile encephalitis

OVERVIEW

- An infectious disease, part of a family of vector-borne diseases that also includes malaria, yellow fever, and Lyme disease
- Mortality rate from 3% to 15%; higher in elderly population
- Ticks infected with the virus found in Africa and Asia only; role of ticks in transmission and maintenance of the virus uncertain
- Also called *West Nile virus* or *airborne encephalitis*

PATHOPHYSIOLOGY

- Virus has an incubation period of 5 to 15 days after exposure.
- Mosquitoes become infected by feeding on birds contaminated with the virus. (See *Transmission routes of West Nile virus.*)
- The virus is transmitted to a human by the bite of an infected mosquito (mostly the *Culex* species).
- Disease primarily causes inflammation or encephalitis of the brain.

CAUSES

- A flavivirus commonly found in humans, birds, and other vertebrates in Africa, West Asia, and the Middle East

RISK FACTORS

- Recent chemotherapy
- Recent organ transplantation
- Immunocompromised state
- Pregnancy
- Advanced age
- Breast-feeding

INCIDENCE

- In temperate areas, this disease occurs mainly in late summer or early fall.
- In milder climates, it can occur year-round.
- The incidence is higher in areas with active cases.
- The highest incidence is in those older than age 50 and those with compromised immune systems.

COMPLICATIONS

- Neurologic impairment
- Seizures
- Bronchial pneumonia
- Death

ASSESSMENT

HISTORY

- Headache
- Myalgia
- Neck stiffness
- Possible recent exposure to bodies of water or dead birds, or recent mosquito bites
- Decreased appetite
- Nausea
- Vomiting
- Diarrhea

PHYSICAL FINDINGS

- Fever
- Rash
- Swollen lymph glands
- Stupor and disorientation
- Stiff neck
- Change in mental status

- Malaise
- Sore throat

DIAGNOSTIC TEST RESULTS

LABORATORY

- White blood cell (WBC) count is normal or increased.
- The enzyme-linked immunosorbent assay (ELISA) and the IgM Antibody Capture (MAC)-ELISA, allows a rapid and definitive diagnosis.
- Accurate diagnosis is possible only when serum or cerebrospinal fluid specimens are obtained while the patient is still hospitalized with acute illness and they show an elevated WBC count and protein levels.

IMAGING

- Magnetic resonance imaging may show inflammation.

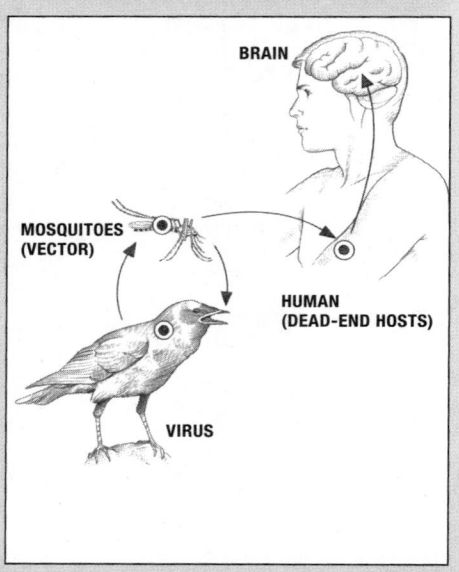

Transmission routes of West Nile virus

Birds are the reservoir of the West Nile virus, but they are unable to spread it. Mosquitoes serve as the vectors, spreading it from bird to bird and from birds to people. Humans are believed to be "dead-end hosts" because the virus can live and cause illness in humans, but it isn't believed that a feeding mosquito can acquire the virus from an infected person.

BRAIN

MOSQUITOES (VECTOR)

HUMAN (DEAD-END HOSTS)

VIRUS

GENERAL
◆ No specific treatment
◆ Respiratory support

DIET
◆ Increased fluid intake

ACTIVITY
◆ Rest periods when fatigued

MEDICATIONS
◆ Antipyretics

Preventing West Nile encephalitis

To reduce the risk of infection with West Nile encephalitis, advise patients to do the following:

◆ Stay indoors at dawn and dusk and in early evening when mosquitoes are biting.
◆ Wear long-sleeved shirts and long pants when outdoors.
◆ Apply insect repellent sparingly to exposed skin. Effective repellents contain 20% to 30% DEET (N,N-diethyltoluamide). DEET in high concentrations (greater than 30%) can cause adverse effects, particularly in children, and should be avoided; adults should apply repellent on children with no more than 10% DEET.
◆ Don't place repellent under clothing.
◆ Don't apply repellent over cuts, wounds, sunburn, or irritated skin.
◆ Wash repellent off daily and reapply as needed.

NURSING DIAGNOSES
◆ Acute pain
◆ Decreased cardiac output
◆ Deficient fluid volume
◆ Hyperthermia
◆ Impaired tissue integrity
◆ Ineffective tissue perfusion: Cardiopulmonary

EXPECTED OUTCOMES
The patient will:
◆ report decreased levels or absence of pain
◆ maintain adequate cardiac output
◆ maintain an adequate fluid volume
◆ remain afebrile
◆ maintain collateral circulation
◆ maintain hemodynamic stability.

NURSING INTERVENTIONS
◆ Maintain adequate hydration with I.V. fluids.
◆ Give prescribed medications.
◆ Provide respiratory support measures when needed.
◆ Follow standard precautions when handling blood or other body fluids.
◆ Report suspected cases of West Nile encephalitis to the state Department of Health.

MONITORING
◆ Fluid and electrolyte status
◆ Neurologic status
◆ Vital signs
◆ Intraventricular pressure

GENERAL
Be sure to cover:
◆ disorder, diagnosis, and treatment
◆ proper use of insect repellants, which can irritate the eyes and mouth, and to avoid applying repellant to the hands of children (shouldn't be applied to children younger than age 3) (see *Preventing West Nile encephalitis*)
◆ expected course and outcomes of the illness
◆ importance of drinking fluids to avoid dehydration
◆ how to stop mosquitoes from breeding by:
– cleaning out birdbaths and wading pools at least once per week
– cleaning roof gutters and downspout screens
– eliminating any standing water
– not allowing water to collect in trash cans
– turning over or removing containers in yards where rainwater collects, such as toys and old tires.

DISCHARGE PLANNING
◆ Refer the patient to an infectious disease specialist.

RESOURCES
Organizations
National Center for Infectious Diseases: *www.cdc.gov/ncidod*
National Institute of Allergy and Infectious Diseases: *www.niaid.nih.gov*
World Health Organization: *www.who.int*

Selected references
Abroug, F., et al. "A Cluster Study of Predictors of Severe West Nile Virus Infection," *Mayo Clinic Proceedings* 81(1):12-16, January 2006.
Avalos-Bock, S.A. "West Nile Virus and the U.S. Blood Supply: New Tests Substantially Reduce the Risk of Transmission via Donated Blood Products," *AJN* 105(12):34, 36-37, December 2005.
Civen, R., et al. "West Nile Virus Infection in the Pediatric Population," *Pediatric Infectious Disease Journal* 25(1):75-78, January 2006.

Zinc deficiency

OVERVIEW

- Insufficient amounts of zinc, an essential trace element that's a vital component of many enzymes and present in the bones, teeth, hair, skin, testes, liver, and muscles
- Good prognosis with correction of the deficiency

PATHOPHYSIOLOGY

- Zinc deficiency causes impairment of synthesis of deoxyribonucleic acid, ribonucleic acid and, ultimately, protein, and alters normal blood concentrations of vitamin A by mobilizing it from the liver.
- About 90% of zinc stores are in bone and skeletal muscle.

CAUSES

- Blood loss from parasitism
- Excessive intake of foods (containing iron, calcium, vitamin D, and the fiber and phytates in cereals) that bind zinc to form insoluble chelates that prevent its absorption
- Low dietary intake of foods containing zinc

RISK FACTORS

- Alcohol consumption
- Corticosteroids
- Celiac disease

INCIDENCE

- Zinc deficiency is most common in persons from underdeveloped countries, especially in the Middle East.
- Children are most susceptible to this deficiency during periods of rapid growth.

COMPLICATIONS

- Hypogonadism
- Dwarfism
- Hyperpigmentation

ASSESSMENT

HISTORY

- Weight loss
- Poor appetite
- Growth retardation
- Short stature
- Mental lethargy
- Diarrhea
- Intercurrent infections

PHYSICAL FINDINGS

- Sparse hair growth
- Rough skin
- Poor wound healing
- Striae
- White spots on fingernails
- Acne

DIAGNOSTIC TEST RESULTS

LABORATORY

- Fasting serum zinc levels may be less than 70 mcg/dl.

TREATMENT

GENERAL
◆ Correction of the underlying cause

DIET
◆ High in zinc

MEDICATIONS
◆ Zinc supplementation

NURSING CONSIDERATIONS

NURSING DIAGNOSES
◆ Delayed growth and development
◆ Disturbed body image
◆ Imbalanced nutrition: Less than body requirements
◆ Impaired skin integrity
◆ Ineffective health maintenance

EXPECTED OUTCOMES
The patient will:
◆ achieve age-appropriate growth and development to the fullest extent possible
◆ express positive feelings about self
◆ express understanding of diet high in zinc and improve zinc levels
◆ maintain skin integrity and exhibit improved or healed wounds or lesions
◆ express understanding of dietary adjustments needed to improve nutritional status.

NURSING INTERVENTIONS
◆ Administer drug therapy.
◆ Provide information about dietary sources of zinc. (See *Foods that contain zinc.*)

MONITORING
◆ Response to treatment

PATIENT TEACHING

GENERAL
Be sure to cover:
◆ taking zinc supplements with milk or meals to prevent gastric distress and vomiting
◆ following a balanced diet that includes foods high in zinc
◆ correct use of calcium and iron supplements.

RESOURCES
Organizations
American Dietetic Association: *www.eatright.org*
The Merck Manuals Online Medical Library: *www.merck.com/mmhe*
National Digestive Diseases Information Clearinghouse: *www.niddk.nih.gov/health/digest/nddic.htm*

Selected references
Beattie, J., and Kwun, I. "Is Zinc Deficiency a Risk Factor for Atherosclerosis?" *British Journal of Nutrition* 91(2):177-81, February 2004.
Gibson, R.S. "Zinc: The Missing Link in Combating Micronutrient Malnutrition in Developing Countries," *Proceedings of the Nutrition Society* 65(1):51-60, February 2006.
Shah, D., and Sachdev, H.P. "Zinc Deficiency in Pregnancy and Fetal Outcome," *Nutrition Reviews* 64(1):15-30, January 2006.
Shrimpton, R., et al. "Zinc Deficiency: What Are the Most Appropriate Interventions?" *British Medical Journal* 330(7487):347-49, February 2005.
Wilson, D., et al. "Apoptosis may Underlie the Pathology of Zinc-deficient Skin," *Immunology and Cell Biology* 84(1):28-37, February 2006.

Foods that contain zinc

The following foods contain significant amounts of zinc:
◆ beans
◆ dairy products
◆ fortified breakfast cereals
◆ nuts
◆ oysters
◆ poultry
◆ red meat
◆ seafood
◆ whole grains.

Index

---

i refers to an illustration; t refers to a table.

i refers to an illustration; t refers to a table.

i refers to an illustration; t refers to a table.

i refers to an illustration; t refers to a table.

i refers to an illustration; t refers to a table.

---

i refers to an illustration; t refers to a table.

i refers to an illustration; t refers to a table.